RUSH UNIVERSITY MEDICAL CENTER

# Review
*of*
# Surgery

## Fifth Edition

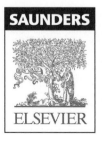

1600 John F. Kennedy Blvd.
Ste 1800
Philadelphia, PA 19103-2899

RUSH UNIVERSITY MEDICAL CENTER REVIEW OF SURGERY          ISBN: 978-1-4377-1791-4
**Copyright © 2011, 2007, 2000, 1994, 1988 by Saunders, an imprint of Elsevier Inc.**

---

**Notices**

Knowledge and best practice in this field are constantly changing. As new research and experience broaden our understanding, changes in research methods, professional practices, or medical treatment may become necessary.

Practitioners and researchers must always rely on their own experience and knowledge in evaluating and using any information, methods, compounds, or experiments described herein. In using such information or methods they should be mindful of their own safety and the safety of others, including parties for whom they have a professional responsibility.

With respect to any drug or pharmaceutical products identified, readers are advised to check the most current information provided (i) on procedures featured or (ii) by the manufacturer of each product to be administered, to verify the recommended dose or formula, the method and duration of administration, and contraindications. It is the responsibility of practitioners, relying on their own experience and knowledge of their patients, to make diagnoses, to determine dosages and the best treatment for each individual patient, and to take all appropriate safety precautions.

To the fullest extent of the law, neither the Publisher nor the authors, contributors, or editors assume any liability for any injury and/or damage to persons or property as a matter of products liability, negligence or otherwise, or from any use or operation of any methods, products, instructions, or ideas contained in the material herein.

---

**Library of Congress Cataloging-in-Publication Data**

Rush University Medical Center review of surgery.—5th ed. / [edited by] Jose M. Velasco ... [et al.].
        p. ; cm.
    Review of surgery
    Includes bibliographical references and index.
    ISBN 978-1-4377-1791-4 (pbk. : alk. paper)
1. Surgery—Examinations, questions, etc.   I. Velasco, Jose M.   II. Rush University Medical
Center.   III. Title: Review of surgery.
    [DNLM: 1. General Surgery—Examination Questions.   2. Surgical Procedures, Operative—Examination
Questions. WO 18.2]
    RD37.2.R88 2011
    617.0076—dc22

                                                                                    2011010539

*Acquisitions Editor:* Judith Fletcher
*Developmental Editor:* Lora Sickora
*Publishing Services Manager:* Anne Altepeter
*Project Manager:* Jessica L. Becher
*Design Direction:* Steve Stave
*Designer:* Lou Forgione

Printed in the United States of America

Last digit is the print number:   9   8   7   6   5   4   3   2   1

# Contributors

**Michael R. Abern, M.D.**
Chief Resident, Department of Urology, Rush University Medical Center, Chicago, Illinois
*Chapter 31, Gynecology, Neurosurgery, and Urology*

**Steven D. Bines, M.D.**
Associate Professor of Surgery, Rush Medical College, Chicago, Illinois
*Chapter 5, Surgical Infection and Transmissible Diseases and Surgeons*
*Chapter 11, Burns*
*Chapter 14, Breast*
*Chapter 33, Plastic and Reconstructive Surgery, Including Hand Surgery*

**Lisa N. Boggio, M.S., M.D.**
Assistant Professor of Medicine and Pediatrics, Division of Hematology, Rush University Medical Center, Chicago, Illinois
*Chapter 3, Hemostasis and Transfusion*

**John Butsch, B.A., M.S., M.D.**
Assistant Professor, Department of Surgery, SUNY at Buffalo; Assistant Professor, Department of Surgery, Buffalo General Hospital, Buffalo, New York
*Chapter 7, Perioperative Care and Anesthesia*

**Richard W. Byrne, M.D.**
Chairman, Professor, Department of Neurosurgery, Rush University Medical Center, Chicago, Illinois
*Chapter 31, Gynecology, Neurosurgery, and Urology*

**Edie Y. Chan, M.D.**
Assistant Professor of Surgery, Department of General Surgery, Division of Transplantation, Associate Program Director, Department of General Surgery, Rush University Medical Center, Chicago, Illinois
*Chapter 1, Physiologic Response to Injury*
*Chapter 6, Transplantation and Immunology*
*Chapter 10, Trauma*

**John D. Christein, M.D.**
Associate Professor, Department of Surgery, University of Alabama at Birmingham, Birmingham, Alabama
*Chapter 20, Stomach and Duodenum*

**Niki A. Christopoulos, M.D.**
Plastic and Reconstructive Surgeon, Department of Plastic and Reconstructive Surgery, Advocate Christ Medical Center, Oak Lawn, Illinois
*Chapter 33, Plastic and Reconstructive Surgery, Including Hand Surgery*

**Kyle G. Cologne, M.D.**
Resident Physician, Department of General Surgery, Rush University Medical Center, Chicago, Illinois
*Chapter 22, Colon, Rectum, and Anus*
*Chapter 26, Spleen and Lymphatic System*

**James A. Colombo, M.D.**
Partner, Park Ridge Anesthesia Associates, Department of Anesthesiology, Division of Critical Care Medicine, Advocate Lutheran General Hospital, Park Ridge, Illinois
*Chapter 7, Perioperative Care and Anesthesia*

**W. Christopher Croley, M.D., F.C.C.P.**
Assistant Professor of Anesthesiology, Medical Director, Surgical Intensive Care Unit, Co-Medical Director, Rush University Simulation Lab; Associate Director of Anesthesia Resident Education, Rush University Medical Center, Chicago, Illinois
*Chapter 7, Perioperative Care and Anesthesia*

**Shaun Daly, M.D.**
Resident, General Surgery, Rush University Medical Center, Chicago, Illinois
*Chapter 32, Pediatric*

**Gordon H. Derman, M.D.**
Assistant Professor of Plastic and Reconstructive Surgery, Senior Attending and Director of Hand Surgery, Department of Plastic and Reconstructive Surgery, Rush University Medical Center, Chicago, Illinois
*Chapter 33, Plastic and Reconstructive Surgery, Including Hand Surgery*

**Daniel J. Deziel, M.D.**
Professor of Surgery, Senior Attending Surgeon, Chairman, Department of General Surgery, Rush University Medical Center, Chicago, Illinois
*Chapter 23, Liver and Portal Venous System*
*Chapter 24, Gallbladder and Biliary Tract*
*Chapter 25, Pancreas*

**Joseph R. Durham, M.D., F.A.C.S., R.P.V.I.**
Chief, Division of Vascular Surgery, Medical Director, Vascular Laboratory, Department of Surgery, John H. Stroger, Jr. Hospital of Cook County, Chicago, Illinois
*Chapter 34, Principles of Ultrasound and Ablative Therapy*

**Nadine D. Floyd, M.D.**
Associate Clinical Professor, Department of Surgery, Indiana University School of Medicine-Fort Wayne, Surgeon, Center for Colon and Rectal Care, LLC, Fort Wayne, Indiana
*Chapter 8, Acute Abdomen*

**Crea Fusco, M.D.**
Resident, Department of General Surgery, Rush University Medical Center, Chicago, Illinois
*Chapter 9, Critical Care*

**Kiranjeet Gill, M.D.**
Resident, Department of General Surgery, Rush University Medical Center, Chicago, Illinois
*Chapter 23, Liver and Portal Venous System*

**Matthew J. Graczyk, M.D.**
Thoracic Surgery Resident, Department of Cardiovascular and Thoracic Surgery, Rush University Medical Center, Chicago, Illinois; Thoracic Surgeon, Abbott Northwestern Hospital and Virginia Piper Cancer Institute, Minneapolis, Minnesota
*Chapter 29, Thoracic Surgery*

**Alicia Growney, M.D.**
Assistant Professor of Surgery, Department of General Surgery, Rush University Medical Center, Chicago, Illinois
*Chapter 5, Surgical Infection and Transmissible Diseases and Surgeons*

**Alfred S. Guirguis, D.O., M.P.H.**
Assistant Professor in Gynecologic Oncology, Attending Professor in Gynecologic Oncology, Department of Obstetrics and Gynecology, Rush University Medical Center, Chicago, Illinois
*Chapter 31, Gynecology, Neurosurgery, and Urology*

**Tina J. Hieken, M.D.**
Associate Professor of Surgery, Rush Medical College, Attending, Department of Surgery, Rush University Medical Center, Chicago, Illinois; Attending, Department of Surgery, NorthShore University Health System, Skokie Hospital, Skokie, Illinois
*Chapter 12, Skin and Soft Tissue*
*Chapter 26, Spleen and Lymphatic System*
*Chapter 34, Principles of Ultrasound and Ablative Therapy*
*Chapter 37, Ethical Principles and Palliative Care*

**Robert S.D. Higgins, M.D., M.S.H.A**
John H. and Mildred C. Lumiey Medical Research Chair, Director, Ohio State University Comprehensive Transplant Center; Professor and Chief, Division of Cardiac Surgery, Ohio State University Cardiac Surgery, Columbus, Ohio
*Chapter 27, Cardiac Surgery*

**Edward F. Hollinger, M.D., Ph.D.**
Assistant Professor of Surgery, Assistant Attending, Department of General Surgery, Section of Abdominal Transplant, Rush University Medical Center, Chicago, Illinois
*Chapter 2, Wound Healing and Cell Biology*
*Chapter 6, Transplantation and Immunology*
*Chapter 36, Special Considerations in Surgery: Pregnant, Geriatric, and Immunocompromised Patients*
*Chapter 38, Evidence-Based Surgery and Applications of Biostatistics*

**Ai-Xuan L. Holterman, M.D.**
Professor of Surgery and Pediatrics, Department of Surgery and Pediatrics, Rush University Medical Center; Director of Pediatric Surgery, Rush Children's Hospital, Chicago, Illinois
*Chapter 32, Pediatric*

**Elizabeth A. Hooper, M.D.**
Resident, Department of General Surgery, Rush University Medical Center, Chicago, Illinois
*Chapter 6, Transplantation and Immunology*

**Kamran Idrees, M.D.**
Surgical Oncology Fellow and Clinical Instructor, Department of Surgery, Division of Surgical Oncology, University of Pittsburgh Medical Center, Pittsburgh, Pennsylvania
*Chapter 20, Stomach and Duodenum*

**Chad E. Jacobs, M.D.**
Assistant Professor of Surgery, Department of Cardiovascular Thoracic Surgery, Rush University Medical Center, Chicago, Illinois
*Chapter 3, Hemostasis and Transfusion*
*Chapter 4, Nutrition, Metabolism, and Fluid and Electrolytes*
*Chapter 7, Perioperative Care and Anesthesia*
*Chapter 28, Vascular Surgery*

**Jamie Elizabeth Jones, M.D.**
Fellow, Department of Surgery, Division of Trauma and Surgical Critical Care, Emory University, Atlanta, Georgia
*Chapter 10, Trauma*

**Muhammad Asad Khan, M.D.**
Assistant Professor, Division of Vascular and Endovascular Surgery, Upstate Medical University; Attending Vascular Surgeon, Department of Surgery, Syracuse VA Medical Center, Syracuse, New York
*Chapter 28, Vascular Surgery*

**Anthony W. Kim, M.D.**
Assistant Professor, Department of Surgery, Section of Thoracic Surgery, Yale University School of Medicine, New Haven, Connecticut
*Chapter 29, Thoracic Surgery*
*Chapter 39, Core Competencies and Quality Improvement*

**Michelle A. Kominiarek, M.D.**
Assistant Professor, Department of Obstetrics and Gynecology, Obstetrics and Gynecology, University of Illinois at Chicago, Chicago, Illinois
*Chapter 36, Special Considerations in Surgery: Pregnant, Geriatric, and Immunocompromised Patients*

**Katherine Kopkash, M.D.**
General Surgery Resident, Department of General Surgery, Rush University Medical Center, Chicago, Illinois
*Chapter 14, Breast*

**Vikram D. Krishnamurthy, M.D.**
Resident Physician, Department of General Surgery, Rush University Medical Center, Chicago, Illinois
*Chapter 34, Principles of Ultrasound and Ablative Therapy*

**Kalyan C. Latchamsetty, M.D.**
Assistant Professor, Department of Urology, Rush University Medical Center, Chicago, Illinois
*Chapter 31, Gynecology, Neurosurgery, and Urology*

**Benjamin Lind, M.D.**
Fellow, Section of Vascular Surgery, Department of Cardiovascular Thoracic Surgery, Rush University Medical Center, Chicago, Illinois
*Chapter 28, Vascular Surgery*

**Phillip S. LoSavio, M.D.**
Assistant Professor, Department of Otolaryngology, Rush University Medical Center, Chicago, Illinois
*Chapter 15, Head and Neck*

**Minh B. Luu, M.D., F.A.C.S.**
Assistant Professor of Surgery, Department of General Surgery, Rush University Medical Center, Chicago, Illinois
*Chapter 19, Esophagus*
*Chapter 30, Metabolic and Bariatric Surgery*

**Andrea Madrigrano, M.D.**
Assistant Professor of Surgery, Department of Surgery, Breast Surgeon, Department of General Surgery, Rush University Medical Center, Chicago, Illinois
*Chapter 14, Breast*

**Samuel M. Maurice, M.D.**
Craniofacial and Pediatric Plastic Surgery Fellow, Children's Healthcare of Atlanta at Scottish Rite, Atlanta, Georgia
*Chapter 33, Plastic and Reconstructive Surgery, Including Hand Surgery*

**Walter J. McCarthy, M.D.**
Professor of Surgery, Chief of Vascular Surgery, Department of Cardiovascular Thoracic Surgery, Rush University Medical Center, Chicago, Illinois
*Chapter 7, Perioperative Care and Anesthesia*
*Chapter 28, Vascular Surgery*

**Bruce C. McLeod, M.D.**
Professor, Department of Medicine and Pathology, Director, Blood Center, Rush University Medical Center, Chicago, Illinois
*Chapter 3, Hemostasis and Transfusion*

**Thomas A. Messer, M.D.**
Attending Surgeon, Director of Burn ICU, Division of Burns, Department of Trauma, John H. Stroger, Jr. Hospital of Cook County, Chicago, Illinois
*Chapter 11, Burns*

**Janet Deselich Millikan, M.S., R.D., L.D.N.**
Clinical Dietitian, Your Brainfood, Inc., Bloomingdale, Illinois
*Chapter 4, Nutrition, Metabolism, and Fluid and Electrolytes*

**Keith W. Millikan, M.D., F.A.C.S.**
Professor of Surgery, Department of General Surgery, Rush University Medical Center, Chicago, Illinois
*Chapter 19, Esophagus*

**Tricia Moo-Young, M.D.**
Fellow in Endocrine Surgery, Rush University Medical Center, Chicago, Illinois
*Chapter 16, Thyroid*
*Chapter 17, Parathyroid*
*Chapter 18, Adrenal*

**Jonathan A. Myers, M.D.**
Associate Professor of Surgery, Attending Surgeon, Department of General Surgery, Rush University Medical Center, Chicago, Illinois
*Chapter 30, Metabolic and Bariatric Surgery*
*Chapter 35, Principles of Minimally Invasive Surgery*

**Ferenc P. Nagy, M.D.**
Attending, Louisville Vascular Specialists, Jewish Hospital & St. Mary's HealthCare, Louisville, Kentucky
*Chapter 28, Vascular Surgery*

**Eric J. Okum, M.D.**
Voluntary Assistant Professor, University of Cincinnati, Cardiac, Vascular, and Thoracic Surgeons, Cincinnati, Ohio
*Chapter 27, Cardiac Surgery*

**R. Anthony Perez-Tamayo, M.D., Ph.D.**
Assistant Professor, Department of Cardiovascular and Thoracic Surgery, Rush University Medical Center; Chairman, Division of Cardiothoracic Surgery, John H. Stroger, Jr. Hospital of Cook County, Chicago, Illinois
*Chapter 27, Cardiac Surgery*

**Kyle A. Perry, M.D.**
Assistant Professor of Surgery, Division of General and Gastrointestinal Surgery, Ohio State University, Columbus, Ohio
*Chapter 35, Principles of Minimally Invasive Surgery*

**Troy Pittman, M.D.**
Fellow, Department of Plastic and Reconstructive Surgery, Rush University Medical Center, Chicago, Illinois
*Chapter 2, Wound Healing and Cell Biology*

**Anastasios C. Polimenakos, M.D., F.A.C.S., F.A.C.C.**
Assistant Professor of Surgery, Department of Pediatric Cardiovascular Surgery, Rush University Medical Center, Chicago, Illinois; Cardiovascular and Thoracic Surgeon, Department of Pediatric Cardiovascular and Thoracic Surgery, The Heart Institute for Children at Advocate Christ Medical Center, Oak Lawn, Illinois
*Chapter 27, Cardiac Surgery*

**Stathis J. Poulakidas, M.D., F.A.C.S.**
Assistant Professor, Department of Surgery, Rush University Medical Center; Director, Burn Services, Department of Trauma, John H. Stroger, Jr. Hospital of Cook County, Chicago, Illinois
*Chapter 11, Burns*

**Richard A. Prinz, M.D.**
Clinical Professor, Department of Surgery, University of Chicago Pritzker School of Medicine; Vice Chairman, Department of Surgery, NorthShore University Health System, Evanston, Illinois; Attending Surgeon, Department of Surgery, John H. Stroger, Jr. Hospital of Cook County, Chicago, Illinois
>    *Chapter 16, Thyroid*
>    *Chapter 17, Parathyroid*
>    *Chapter 18, Adrenal*

**Roderick M. Quiros, M.D., F.A.C.S.**
Surgical Oncologist, Cancer Care Associates, Department of Surgery, St. Luke's Hospital & Health Network, Bethlehem, Pennsylvania; Clinical Professor of Surgery, Temple University, Philadelphia, Pennsylvania
>    *Chapter 4, Nutrition, Metabolism, Fluid and Electrolytes*

**Lane A. Ritter, M.D.**
General Surgery Resident, Department of General Surgery, Rush University Medical Center, Chicago, Illinois
>    *Chapter 1, Physiologic Response to Injury*

**Theodore J. Saclarides, M.D.**
Professor of Surgery, Head, Section of Colon and Rectal Surgery, Department of General Surgery, Rush University Medical Center, Chicago, Illinois
>    *Chapter 8, Acute Abdomen*
>    *Chapter 21, Small Bowel and Appendix*
>    *Chapter 22, Colon, Rectum, and Anus*

**Edward B. Savage, M.D.**
Attending Surgeon, Department of Cardiothoracic Surgery, Cleveland Clinic Florida, Weston, Florida; Clinical Associate Professor, Florida International University—College of Medicine, Miami, Florida
>    *Chapter 27, Cardiac Surgery*

**David D. Shersher, M.D.**
Resident, Department of General Surgery, Rush University Medical Center, Chicago, Illinois
>    *Chapter 4, Nutrition, Metabolism, and Fluid and Electrolytes*

**Adam P. Smith, M.D.**
Resident, Neurological Surgery, Rush University Medical Center, Chicago, Illinois
>    *Chapter 31, Gynecology, Neurosurgery, and Urology*

**Mona Tareen, M.D.**
Assistant Professor, Director of Adult Palliative Care Service, Section of Geriatrics and Palliative Medicine, Rush University Medical Center, Chicago, Illinois; Associate Director, Midwest Hospice and Palliative Care Center, Glenview, Illinois
>    *Chapter 37, Ethical Principles and Palliative Care*

**Jacquelyn Turner, M.D.**
Resident, Department of General Surgery, Rush University Medical Center, Chicago, Illinois
>    *Chapter 21, Small Bowel and Appendix*
>    *Chapter 22, Colon, Rectum, and Anus*

**Martha L. Twaddle, M.D., F.A.C.P., F.A.A.H.P.M.**
Associate Professor of Medicine, Rush University Medical Center, Chicago, Illinois
>    *Chapter 37, Ethical Principles and Palliative Care*

**Leonard A. Valentino, M.D.**
Professor, Department of Pediatrics Senior Attending Physician, Department of Pediatrics, Internal Medicine, Biochemistry and Immunology/Microbiology, Rush University Medical Center, Chicago, Illinois
>    *Chapter 3, Hemostasis and Transfusion*

**José M. Velasco, M.D.**
Professor of Surgery, Rush Medical College; Associate Chair, Department of General Surgery, Rush University Medical Center, Chicago, Illinois; Vice Chair, Department of Surgery, NorthShore University Health System, Evanston, Illinois
>    *Chapter 4, Nutrition, Metabolism, and Fluid and Electrolytes*
>    *Chapter 7, Perioperative Care and Anesthesia*
>    *Chapter 9, Critical Care*
>    *Chapter 13, Hernia*
>    *Chapter 34, Principles of Ultrasound and Ablative Therapy*

**Thomas R. Witt, M.D., F.A.C.S.**
Associate Professor of Surgery, Senior Attending, Department of General Surgery, Rush University Medical Center, Chicago, Illinois
>    *Chapter 14, Breast*

**Norman Wool, M.D.**
Program Director, General Surgery Residency, Department of General Surgery, Rush University Medical Center, Chicago, Illinois
>    *Chapter 13, Hernia*

The fifth edition of the *Rush University Review of Surgery* is the first to be published without the participation of Dr. Steven G. Economou, the senior editor of the first two editions, who died in 2007. The remaining three editors of the first edition would like to honor his memory and pay tribute to his unique talent for the many students and surgeons who have benefited from his contributions.

The son of Greek immigrants, Dr. Economou lived modestly—early on of necessity; later by choice. As a surgeon, his exquisite technical skill and piercing intellect were legendary. He was accomplished at virtually every known general and oncologic operation. He was an ambidextrous artist who could create two separate illustrations, one with his right hand and one with his left, while simultaneously asking pointed questions of conference speakers. Above all, he was a teacher with a breadth of insight spanning the known arts and sciences. He taught by word, craft, and stunning example.

The *Rush University Medical Center Review of Surgery* is just one of Dr. Economou's many publications. With its inception, he harnessed a whirlwind of activity to produce an instant favorite on an international scale. In dedicating this fifth edition to his memory, we can only hope that it will elicit his slightly mischievous smile of affirmation, rather than a sharp wrap on the knuckles with a stout hemostat. We are accustomed to both.

**S.D. Bines, M.D.**
**D.J. Deziel, M.D.**
**T.R. Witt, M.D.**

*Try not to become a man of success but rather try to become a man of value.*

**—*Albert Einstein***

The editors of *Rush University Medical Center Review of Surgery* wish to dedicate this fifth edition to the memory of Steven G. Economou, the senior editor of the first two editions. His memory will stay with us forever, as will his legacy. Dr. Economou was relentless in the pursuit of excellence for his department. He was loved and respected by his patients and by those of us who were privileged to work with him.

To my wife, Aglae, for her unconditional love, her devotion, her tolerance, and her inveterate enthusiasm and perseverance. And to my children, Aglae and Jay Velasco, for helping me understand the joy of parenthood.

José M. Velasco, M.D.

I would be nothing without SAKER5. Thank you, guys. This book would not have happened without José Velasco. Thank you, José.

Steven D. Bines, M.D.

To Eileen Pehanich for her dedicated secretarial support.

Daniel J. Deziel, M.D.

To Mary, my wife.

Walter J. McCarthy, M.D.

To my parents, John and Joan, for making it all possible.
To my wife, Janet, for her never-ending understanding and support of my career.
To my children, Keith, Michael, Kyle, Kameron, Samantha, and John for inspiring my optimism for the future.

Keith W. Millikan, M.D.

To my family and for the endocrine surgery fellows.

Richard A. Prinz, M.D.

I thank my children, Kathryn, Stephanie, Deno, Alexandra (Zaz), and Dora for their love, support, and inspiration.

Theodore J. Saclarides, M.D.

# Preface

The editors of the *Rush University Medical Center Review of Surgery* are pleased to present the fifth edition of this book. It has been 23 years since one of the authors (S.B.) perceived a need to review the totality of surgery based on reading, examining, and discussing two major textbooks of surgery: *Textbook of Surgery, Thirteenth Edition*, by D.C. Sabiston and *Principles of Surgery, Fourth Edition*, by Seymour Schwartz. As questions were formulated and discussed, it became apparent that some of the issues were outside the purview of standard textbooks; consequently, consultants were invited to enrich the content of these sessions.

The first four editions provided an encompassing, yet concise and self-contained, review of surgery for a full spectrum of readers from students to residents, to surgeons preparing for general surgery certification or recertification, and to practitioners simply wishing to commit to lifelong learning. Surgery is more than an operating room activity. Once extensive knowledge is acquired, this base often needs to be modified, altered, and continuously updated. As this knowledge expands, it requires validation for alternatives of care to time-honored patterns of care, or for cementing more traditional methods. An adult may thus use various ways to acquire new knowledge—interaction with colleagues, written and online material, and interaction with a question/answer format. Testing of understanding of the material by comprehending the question, and by identifying the most correct answer, followed by a concise comment section, has always been the intent of this book.

The new edition of the *Rush University Medical Center Review of Surgery* seeks to integrate up-to-the-minute knowledge with rapidly evolving changes in surgical care, patient safety considerations, and the increasing adoption of multispecialty, disease-driven care. Minimal-access techniques, telementoring, and robotic technology have revolutionized delivery of care. Surgical practice is being transformed through an explosion of ground-breaking knowledge in basic science that is leading to incorporation of cellular and genetic concepts and rapid integration of innovative techniques in patient care. Furthermore, the American Board of Surgery has identified the need to structure the evaluation of surgeons' and residents' proficiency in practicing surgery based on core competencies. Surgeons and institutions are experiencing increased and close scrutiny regarding the quality, effectiveness, and efficiency of care rendered. In addition, simulation centers have been sprouting up throughout the country in an effort to meet some of these demands.

The entire book was examined fastidiously to make sure that the content and organization would reflect present concepts and paradigms of care. In addition, the editors have acknowledged the emerging role of online-based learning in the continuing education of surgeons and students. Furthermore, we solicited feedback from physicians preparing for the board examination throughout the country. As a result of our review, we have continued our emphasis on integration of basic science into clinical practice inasmuch as residents and surgeons need to be well versed in the fundamental scientific principles of clinical practice. Subspecialty residents reading this book before taking their board examination can expect an exposure to general surgery concepts that meet their needs. Conversely, general surgeons and residents in training should feel that they will become comfortable with a rich and encompassing content on basic sciences and clinical practice, as well as exposure to the fundamentals of various surgical subspecialties.

This fifth edition has been enhanced with changes in the book's editorial board, authorship, and electronic format, in addition to a comprehensive revision of its content and style. Chapters were completely reorganized and grouped into new sections. We elicited contributions from more than 60 authors, all chosen for their past or present affiliation to Rush University and their scientific sophistication. Each contributor is an active clinician in the field of medicine. Furthermore, some have presented articles, developed new concepts in their areas, and contributed to the education of their peers.

This comprehensive offering required the elimination of 7 chapters, incorporation of 4 new chapters, and extensive rewriting of the rest. This fifth edition includes 10 sections with 39 chapters, as opposed to 56 chapters in the fourth edition. The new chapters—Chapter 1: Physiologic Response to Injury; Chapter 36: Special Considerations in Surgery: Pregnant, Geriatric, and Immunocompromised Patients; Chapter 37: Ethical Principles and Palliative Care; and Chapter 39: Core Competencies and Quality Improvement—provide the reader with previously unexplored subjects in previous editions. The format of the questions was changed to select the best answer, breaking with the multiple-answer option of previous editions. The authors were asked to look at the questions as an integral component of the educational experience. Each subject was based on current practice and referenced to widely read textbooks of surgery. However, in this edition, we placed no restrictions on the reference base of suggested reading, except for the need to select evidence-based information, if available. We emphasized the use of vignettes or case studies, as opposed to scientific instruction, to give the reader a more realistic approach to learning.

In summary, we expect that the fifth edition of the *Rush University Medical Center Review of Surgery* will enable the reader to gain the knowledge needed in general surgery and associated specialties. This edition is integrated with a new electronic format and highlighted text. Access to supplemental content provided by Elsevier is an additional advantage of this integration. Placing this book on the web or on media should facilitate ease of access, and provide the user with immediate and interactive feedback.

**José M. Velasco, M.D.**

# Acknowledgments

*Large-scale success today is spelled "Teamwork." The successful teamworker doesn't wear a chip on his shoulder, doesn't look for slights, isn't constantly on alert lest his "dignity" be insulted. He puts the good of the house—the company or team—first. And if the whole prospers, he, as an active, effective, progressive part, will prosper with it.*

**—B.C. Forbes**

The editors of the fifth edition of the *Rush University Medical Center Review of Surgery* would like to recognize the contributions of an outstanding group of contributors who we believe upheld the high standard set by four previous editions. Of note, the editors invited junior faculty members to form an associate editor team to work closely with the contributors and the senior editors. They rapidly became an invaluable source of new approaches to learning, new concepts in patient care, and a limitless source of energy and knowledge. Foremost are the residents who, by desire and readiness, kept the writing and editing in constant motion.

We wish to thank all of those responsible for the publication of this edition, including Judith Fletcher, Lora Sickora, Jessica Becher, and the team at Elsevier, for their guidance and support throughout this process. Then there was Kathy Martin, who kept the organization and editing of this book in perpetual motion. She knew when and where to cajole, plead, and at times be firm, to get all the material ready. She organized the collective editing sessions every Saturday, and became the indispensable glue and liaison among all participants.

We are grateful to our patients, mentors, teachers, and members of our surgical team, without whom life would have less meaning.

# How to Use This Text

The topics in this fifth edition have been divided into 10 categories, which should facilitate review of the material for certification, or maintenance of certification, in general surgery. Special attention was given to input by residents from various programs throughout the country in regard to their needs concerning in-training examinations.

Each section contains a variable number of chapters, encompassing questions, and the corresponding comment and references attached to each question. Most questions are followed by one or more references that link them to a relevant textbook and to selected articles. Authors sought evidence-based material as appropriate. A *select best answer* format was chosen in accordance with the desire of those queried, and with the unanimous support of the associate editor group. At the end of each comment, a letter indicates the preferred answer. A list of references is included at the end of each chapter.

Words and phrases appearing in **boldface** type within the text indicate links to facilitate search of material to be reviewed.

# Contents

# SURGICAL PHYSIOLOGY

# CHAPTER 1

# Physiologic Response to Injury

*Lane A. Ritter, M.D., and Edie Y. Chan, M.D.*

1. Cytokines involved in the initial proinflammatory response include all of the following except:

   A. Interleukin-6

   B. Interleukin-10

   C. Tumor necrosis factor-$\alpha$

   D. Interleukin-1

   E. Interleukin-8

   *Ref.:* 1

**COMMENTS:** The complement cascade is the earliest humoral system activated in response to injury. C3a and C5a, the biologically active anaphylatoxins, induce the release of proinflammatory **cytokines**. Tumor necrosis factor-$\alpha$ (TNF-$\alpha$) and interleukin-1 (IL-1) are the key mediators of this cascade. IL-6 induces T and B cells, and IL-8 recruits and activates inflammatory cells at the site of injury. IL-10, in contrast, is one of the key mediators of the antiinflammatory response and acts to inhibit the aforementioned cytokines.

**ANSWER:** B

2. TNF-$\alpha$ release:

   A. Can be effectively blocked by anti–TNF-$\alpha$ antibodies to halt systemic inflammatory response syndrome (SIRS)

   B. Does not have any beneficial effects in the early phases of the inflammatory response

   C. Is primarily from leukocytes

   D. Promotes polymorphonuclear (PMN) cell adherence and further cytokine release

   E. Is always deleterious

   *Ref.:* 1

**COMMENTS:** **Tumor necrosis factor-$\alpha$** is a vital component of the early response, especially locally at the site of injury; it is released when the biologically active anaphylatoxins C3a and C5a are stimulated by the humoral system. Infusion of low doses of TNF-$\alpha$ in rats simulates the septic response with resulting fever, hypotension, fatigue, and anorexia. TNF-$\alpha$ promotes adherence of PMN cells to endothelium, production of prostaglandins by fibroblasts, and neutrophil activation and stimulates the release of multiple other cytokines from lymphocytes. TNF-$\alpha$ becomes deleterious when the proinflammatory stimuli become unchecked and leads to cellular damage and multi–organ system failure. TNF-$\alpha$ is released

by macrophages and natural killer cells, not leukocytes. Trials involving anti–TNF-$\alpha$ antibodies (NORASEPT, INTERSEPT) have not shown statistically significant improvement in patient outcomes.

**ANSWER:** D

3. Twenty-four hours after admission to the surgical intensive care unit (ICU), a postoperative patient is noted to have bright red blood through the nasogastric tube. All of the following have shown efficacy in preventing stress gastritis except:

   A. Sucralfate

   B. Proton pump inhibitors

   C. Enteral diet

   D. Histamine-2 (H$_2$) receptor antagonists

   E. Antacids

   *Ref.:* 2

**COMMENTS:** Stress-related gastritis can cause clinically significant bleeding in up to 5% to 10% of ICU patients; therefore, **stress ulcer** prophylaxis is now given routinely in most ICUs. These mucosal lesions are probably caused by gastric acid acting on poorly perfused or immunologically compromised mucosa. Mechanically ventilated, burn, head-injured, and coagulopathic patients are at increased risk, so aggressive preventive measures should be taken in these populations. Prophylaxis should be continued until patients are ingesting an enteral diet of more than 50% of their caloric goal because this is the best prevention of **stress gastritis**. Studies have supported the use of **sucralfate**, H$_2$ blockers, and **proton pump inhibitors** (PPIs) as effective pharmacologic prophylaxis. Sucralfate is activated in an acidic environment, where it binds exposed gastric mucosa and ulcers to form a protective barrier; a disadvantage is its interference with the absorption of other medications such as antibiotics, warfarin, and phenytoin. **Histamine$_2$ receptor antagonists** seem to be superior to sucralfate in preventing clinically important bleeding. There is currently no superiority of PPIs over H$_2$ blockers for stress ulcer prophylaxis. Previously, it was thought that H$_2$ blocker use had a greater association with nosocomial pneumonia (compared with sucralfate) because of gastric bacterial colonization and subsequent aspiration. However, more recent trials have not demonstrated any difference between sucralfate and H$_2$ receptor antagonists in the rate of ventilator-associated pneumonia. Antacids have not shown efficacy in preventing stress-related mucosal lesions in ICU patients and are not considered appropriate prophylactic agents.

**ANSWER:** E

4. Acute respiratory distress syndrome (ARDS) develops in an acutely injured patient. If an alveolar biopsy specimen were taken within the first 24 hours, the histologic examination would demonstrate:

   A. Influx of protein-rich fluid and leukocytes

   B. Preservation of type II pneumocytes

   C. Bacterial colonization

   D. Alveolar hemorrhage

   E. High levels of collagen and fibronectin

   *Ref.:* 2

**COMMENTS: Acute respiratory distress syndrome** involves three distinct phases: the early, exudative, phase is characterized by disruption of the alveolar epithelium with an influx of protein-rich fluid and leukocytes. Type II pneumocytes are damaged and therefore surfactant production is halted. The second, fibroproliferative, phase includes the arrival of mesenchymal cells that produce collagen and fibronectin. The third, or resolution, phase involves gradual remodeling and clearance of edema. Typically, ARDS is not associated with either hemorrhage or bacterial colonization.

**ANSWER: A**

5. A 35-year-old man is admitted to the surgical ICU with a diagnosis of acute alcoholic pancreatitis. **Systemic inflammatory response syndrome** (SIRS) develops and the patient requires 8 L of fluid resuscitation to keep his central venous pressure higher than 10 mm Hg. You have a high index of suspicion for the development of abdominal compartment syndrome (ACS). This clinical entity:

   A. Requires immediate decompressive laparotomy for intraabdominal pressures greater than 20 mm Hg

   B. Results in hypocapnia

   C. Is associated with decreased systemic vascular resistance

   D. Will not affect cerebral perfusion

   E. Should be suspected in any patient taking vasopressors who requires more than 6 L of resuscitative fluid over a short period

   *Ref.:* 2

**COMMENTS:** The diagnosis of **abdominal compartment syndrome** requires a high level of clinical suspicion. Any patient requiring vasopressors and receiving more than 6 L crystalloid or 6 units of blood over a 6-hour period should be monitored closely for signs of ACS. It is generally accepted that most patients with intraabdominal pressure greater than 25 mm Hg will have clinically significant sequelae that will ultimately require decompression. One of the hallmarks of ACS is the development of hypercapnia secondary to decreased pulmonary compliance and hypoventilation as a result of increased pressure on the diaphragm. ACS is associated with markedly increased systemic vascular resistance and does indeed result in secondary cerebral hypoperfusion because of decreased venous outflow.

**ANSWER: E**

6. A patient is brought to the surgical ICU after emergency exploratory laparotomy for fecal peritonitis. The operation was prolonged and required 10 L of fluid resuscitation. All of the following measurements and tests can be used to monitor for ACS except:

   A. Bladder pressure

   B. Central venous pressure

   C. Urine output

   D. Airway pressure

   E. Abdominal examination

   *Ref.:* 2

**COMMENTS: Bladder pressure** is accepted as the most accurate objective measure that directly correlates to **intraabdominal pressure**. It is easily obtained by transducing a needle inserted into the port of a standard urinary drainage catheter after instilling 25 mL of saline into the bladder; the transducer should be zeroed at the level of the pubic symphysis. Serial measurements should be performed every 2 to 4 hours to delineate the pressure trend. Normal intraabdominal pressure is 5 to 10 mm Hg. Pressure greater than 12 mm Hg suggests an element of intraabdominal hypertension as mentioned previously; pressure greater than 25 mm Hg is generally accepted as an indication for decompressive laparotomy. It is also important to consider abdominal perfusion pressure, that is the difference between the mean arterial pressure and the intraabdominal pressure. Other screening considerations include decreasing urine output, increasing airway pressure, and increasing abdominal distension, although these observations are less specific. Central venous pressure has not been used as a standard screening tool for ACS.

**ANSWER: B**

7. A patient is brought to the emergency department after being found unresponsive. Electroencephalography (EEG) indicates status epilepticus. A potential secondary clinical consequence is:

   A. Meningitis

   B. Hypothermia

   C. Myoglobinuria

   D. Cerebrovascular accident

   E. Hypoglycemia

   *Ref.:* 2

**COMMENTS:** Status epilepticus is an entity that should be considered in any patient with recurrent or persistent seizure activity or in those who do not wake up after seizure activity. One of the potential systemic complications is **rhabdomyolysis**, which would result in myoglobinuria, elevated serum creatine kinase, and pigmented granular urinary casts. The other options are potential primary causes of seizure activity. Rhabdomyolysis is a direct result of muscle injury and can be caused by prolonged seizure activity, major trauma, drug overdose, vascular embolism, extremity compartment syndrome, malignant hyperthermia, neuroleptic malignant syndrome, myositis, severe exertion, alcoholism, and medications such as statins, macrolide antibiotics, and cyclosporine.

**ANSWER: C**

8. An obese patient with a body mass index (BMI) of 50 just underwent a laparoscopic gastric bypass. Because of the technical difficulty of the case, the procedure lasted 8 hours. The

patient was doing well postoperatively until 4 hours later, when the nurse noted a change in urine color from yellow to dark brown. She also says that the patient's output has decreased and his creatinine has risen from 1.0 to 1.5. Which test would confirm the cause of these findings?

A. Renal ultrasound

B. Haptoglobin

C. Serum creatine kinase

D. Complete blood count

E. Urine electrolytes

*Ref.:* 3

**COMMENTS: Rhabdomyolysis** can occur postoperatively in obese patients whose back and buttock muscles were compressed against the operating table for a prolonged procedure. Preventive measures include the use of larger tables to better distribute body weight, effective padding at all pressure points, intraoperative changing of patient position, and limitation of operative times. Physicians should have a high index suspicion for rhabdomyolysis in this patient population so that early recognition and treatment can prevent the potentially devastating consequence of acute renal failure (ARF) in this already high-risk group. Creatine kinase should be measured in any patient complaining of muscle pain or in whom dark urine, oliguria, or rising plasma creatinine develops.

**ANSWER:** C

9. The primary algorithm to treat the patient in Question 8 includes all of the following except:

A. Loop diuretics

B. Mannitol

C. Aggressive intravenous fluid resuscitation

D. Sodium bicarbonate

E. Serial basic metabolic panels

*Ref.:* 3

**COMMENTS:** The goal of the treatment algorithm for **rhabdomyolysis** is to prevent **acute renal failure**. The cause of rhabdomyolysis-induced ARF is multifactorial and includes hypovolemia, ischemia, direct tubule toxicity caused by the heme pigment in **myoglobin**, and intratubular obstruction by casts. Treatment of rhabdomyolysis is to induce prompt polyuria with sufficient intravenous fluid resuscitation to produce 1.5 to 2 mL/kg/hr of urine. Concurrently, urine alkalinization with a goal urine pH of greater than 6.5 should be instituted with sodium bicarbonate to prevent precipitation of casts and obstruction of nephrons. Mannitol may also act as a free radical scavenger in addition to a diuretic, although this is somewhat controversial. Loop diuretics can be used as an alternative if brisk urine output cannot be achieved with the aforementioned measures, but it has the disadvantage of acidifying the urine.

**ANSWER:** A

10. You suspect that a patient has ARF secondary to hypovolemia. All of the following are appropriate initial treatments except:

A. Check the hemoglobin level.

B. Give intravenous fluid boluses.

C. Start a vasopressor infusion to keep mean arterial pressure (MAP) greater than 65 mm Hg.

D. Calculate the fractional excretion of sodium ($FE_{Na}$).

E. Rule out causes of outflow obstruction.

*Ref.:* 3

**COMMENTS:** Nephrogenic injury in patients with **hypovolemia** occurs when the renal arteries constrict in response to increased levels of epinephrine, angiotensin II, and vasopressin and the nephrons receive inadequate delivery of oxygen. The goal of treatment is to quickly reverse shock and restore renal blood flow. The primary treatment is always intravenous fluid resuscitation. Active bleeding and obstruction should be ruled out. **Fractional excretion of sodium** should be calculated to confirm your cause. Vasopressors should be avoided whenever possible because the resultant vasoconstriction will actually exacerbate the ischemic insult to the kidneys.

**ANSWER:** C

11. Which of the following is true concerning intravenous contrast–induced renal toxicity?

A. The highest prevalence is caused by the intravenous contrast material used for computed tomography (CT).

B. Most patients with a rise in creatinine eventually require renal replacement therapy.

C. The cause of renal injury is precipitation of iodinated contrast material within the tubules.

D. Use of contrast agents with a lower osmolarity can significantly reduce the risk for renal injury.

E. N-Acetylcysteine has been shown to be highly effective in preventing renal failure.

*Ref.:* 3

**COMMENTS:** It is true that contrast agents with lower osmolarity have a lower risk for toxicity in high-risk patients. Most patients with **contrast-induced nephropathy** experience a transient rise in creatinine that peaks in 2 to 6 days and then returns to normal; only a small percentage eventually require dialysis. The highest prevalence is found in patients who have undergone angiography. Experimental evidence suggests that the renal toxicity is secondary to the production of oxygen radicals. N-Acetylcysteine is an antioxidant that has been theorized to counteract the effect of oxygen radicals at the renal tubule level, although the results of studies have thus far been equivocal. If there is no contraindication to volume expansion, this has generally been accepted as the best prophylaxis against contrast-induced renal toxicity in high-risk patients. Volume expansion can be achieved with either isotonic saline or isotonic bicarbonate solution given for several hours before and after infusion of the contrast agent; the effectiveness of one regimen over the other has not been proved definitively.

**ANSWER:** D

12. A liver transplant candidate has worsening encephalopathy and decreased urine output. Laboratory and physiologic abnormalities that are present in patients with hepatorenal syndrome (HRS) include all of the following except:

A. High urinary sodium

B. High urinary osmolality

C. Azotemia

D. Vasodilation

E. Oliguria

*Ref.: 2*

COMMENTS: **Hepatorenal syndrome** is characterized by azotemia, oliguria, low urinary sodium (<10 mEq/L), and high urinary osmolality. It is theorized to be caused by a combination of systemic vasodilation, hypovolemia, and increased activity of the renin-angiotensin-aldosterone system associated with chronic liver failure. Although this syndrome does occur spontaneously in patients with advanced cirrhosis, specific precipitants are more common. Such precipitants include sepsis (especially spontaneous bacterial peritonitis), increased intraabdominal pressure secondary to tense ascites, gastrointestinal bleeding, and hypovolemia. It is important to prevent excessive diuresis with diuretics or lactulose or aggressive paracentesis without intravascular repletion to avoid precipitating HRS. Treatment of HRS should be aimed at reversing these causative factors. Transjugular intrahepatic portosystemic shunt (TIPS) placement has shown modest improvement in renal function in patients who are not candidates for or are awaiting liver transplantation. The best treatment to reverse renal failure is treatment of the underlying primary liver disease or successful orthotopic liver transplantation.

ANSWER: A

13. Which one of the following may suggest an acute adrenal crisis:

A. Random cortisol level of 34 mcg/dL

B. Hypothermia

C. Hyperglycemia

D. Hypokalemia

E. Increase in cortisol of 5 mcg/dL after stimulation with cosyntropin

*Ref.: 2*

COMMENTS: Impairment of the normal stress response of the hypothalamic-pituitary-adrenal axis can result in **acute adrenal insufficiency** in postoperative or critically ill patients. Clinical suspicion should be raised in any patient with persistent hypotension or sepsislike symptoms. Supporting laboratory findings may include hyponatremia, hyperkalemia, hypoglycemia, and azotemia. The diagnosis can be made with a random cortisol level of less than 15 mcg/dL. A patient with a cortisol level of 15 to 34 mcg/dL should undergo a cosyntropin stimulation test. An increase of less than 9 mcg/dL is suggestive of adrenal insufficiency.

ANSWER: E

14. A patient with type 2 diabetes has a blood glucose level of 700 mg/dL and mental status changes. Although no ketones are evident on urinalysis, the patient has severe serum electrolyte abnormalities, including hypernatremia. Treatment of this condition differs from that of diabetic ketoacidosis (DKA) in that:

A. Insulin infusion should be initiated immediately

B. More aggressive fluid replacement should be instituted after calculating the free water deficit

C. The potassium level should be monitored closely

D. Glucose infusion should begin once the blood glucose level is less than 250 mg/dL

E. The patient should be evaluated for an inciting infection

*Ref.: 2*

COMMENTS: This patient has **hyperosmolar hyperglycemic nonketotic syndrome** (HHNS). The key to differentiating this condition from the other hyperglycemic emergency, **diabetic ketoacidosis**, is lack of ketone formation. This phenomenon occurs because intrinsic pancreatic insulin secretion remains more intact, although significantly impaired, enough to prevent fatty acid lipolysis and ketoacidosis. The changes in mental status and degree of hyperglycemia tend to be more severe, and there is no anion gap acidosis. Consequently, the time from onset to diagnosis and treatment tends to be longer in patients with HHNS than in those with DKA. Patients with HHNS can have a total body water deficit of up to 100 to 200 mL/kg. Aggressive intravascular repletion is the mainstay of therapy and needs be more dramatic than in DKA, although care must be taken to avoid decreasing serum osmolality greater than 3 mOsm/kg/hr to prevent the development of acute cerebral edema. As for DKA, insulin infusion, close monitoring and correction of electrolytes, and treatment of precipitating conditions are the other goals of treatment. Both entities can quickly progress to severe shock with cardiovascular collapse, severe metabolic acidosis, and death if not recognized and treated immediately.

ANSWER: B

15. Stress-related hyperglycemia is thought to be due to increased release of all of the following except:

A. Glucocorticoids

B. Growth hormone

C. Thyroid-stimulating hormone (TSH)

D. Glucagon

E. Epinephrine

*Ref.: 2*

COMMENTS: Stress-related **hyperglycemia** is present in critically ill or injured patients who have increased blood glucose levels without a background diagnosis of diabetes. It is thought to be due to insulin resistance secondary to increased release of counterregulatory hormones. Increased catecholamine and cortisol levels suppress pancreatic insulin release. Glucagon stimulates glycogenolysis and gluconeogenesis. Because hyperglycemia in the perioperative period has been associated with increased morbidity and mortality, tight glucose control in surgical ICU patients has become an important quality control measure.

ANSWER: C

16. The physiologic parameters used in the definition of SIRS include all of the following except:

A. Temperature lower than 36° C

B. Respiratory rate greater than 20 breaths/min

C. $Paco_2$ less than 32 mm Hg

D. Systolic blood pressure lower than 90 mm Hg

E. Heart rate greater than 90 beats/min

*Ref.: 2, 4*

---

**BOX 1-1  Criteria for Four Categories of Systemic Inflammatory Response Syndrome**

**Systemic Inflammatory Response Syndrome (SIRS) (2 or more of the following):**
- Temperature (core) >38° C or <36° C
- Heart rate >90 beats/min
- Respiratory rate of >20 breaths/min for patients spontaneously ventilating or a $Paco_2$ of <32 mm Hg
- White blood cell count >12,000 cells/mm³ or <4000 cells/mm³ or >10% immature (band) cells in the peripheral blood smear

**Sepsis**

Same criteria as for SIRS but with a clearly established focus of infection

**Severe Sepsis**

Sepsis associated with organ dysfunction and hypoperfusion
Indicators of hypoperfusion:
- Systolic blood pressure <90 mm Hg
- >40–mm Hg fall from normal systolic blood pressure
- Lactic acidemia
- Oliguria
- Acute mental status changes

**Septic Shock**

Patients with severe sepsis who:
- Are not responsive to intravenous fluid infusion for resuscitation
- Require inotropic or vasopressor agents to maintain systolic blood pressure

---

**COMMENTS:** Coined by Bone and colleagues in 1992 at the American College of Chest Physicians/Society of Critical Medicine (ACCP/SCCM) Consensus Conference, the definition of **systemic inflammatory response syndrome** includes abnormalities in temperature, heart rate, respiratory rate, $Paco_2$, and white blood cell count (Box 1-1). Blood pressure is not included in the consensus definition of SIRS.

**ANSWER:**  D

17. The syndrome of multi–organ system failure (MOF):

 A. Involves sequential insults that lead to systemic hyperinflammation

 B. Requires the documentation of active infection

 C. Has decreased in incidence over the past decade

 D. Requires diagnosis within 3 days of the systemic insult

 E. Demonstrates consistent improvement after blood transfusion

*Ref.: 2*

**COMMENTS:** The "two-event" model of **multi-organ system failure** involves an initial insult that results in a primed inflammatory response; sequential events during this vulnerable period then lead to a dysfunctional state of hyperinflammation. MOF can develop without overt infection. It has been shown to occur in a bimodal distribution: early, within 3 days of the initial insult, and late, 6 to 8 days after the insult. Blood transfusion has been shown to have immunomodulatory effects and may be detrimental in patients with MOF. MOF has actually increased in incidence, probably because of the improved initial survival of critically ill patients.

**ANSWER:**  A

18. Critically ill patients who undergo a major abdominal operation enter a stressed state of starvation. This condition differs from nonstressed starvation in that:

 A. The primary substrates for metabolism are generated by lipolysis

 B. The glucose-using tissue requires 300 kcal/day

 C. It can be maintained for up to 90 days

 D. There is an expected ebb and flow phase of starvation

 E. Its hallmark is an anabolic state

*Ref.: 5*

**COMMENTS:** Metabolism in the stressed, starved state is very different from that in the nonstressed, starved state. In nonstressed starvation (hypometabolic), the primary substrates for metabolism are free fatty acids generated by lipolysis, with only a small amount of proteolysis occurring to provide the 300 kcal/day needed for glucose-dependent tissues; this condition can be maintained in the nonstressed state for up to 90 days. In the stressed **starvation** state, there is a brief hypometabolic "ebb" phase followed by a pronounced hypermetabolic "flow" phase. The hallmarks are catabolism, proteolysis, and gluconeogenesis.

**ANSWER:**  D

19. A patient in the surgical ICU has severe nutritional deficiencies secondary to dysphagia and resulting anorexia. An echocardiogram demonstrates an ejection fraction of just 25%, and the patient complains of diffuse muscle soreness. You should consider a deficiency of which mineral as the cause of these clinical sequelae?

 A. Copper

 B. Selenium

 C. Chromium

 D. Zinc

 E. Manganese

*Ref.: 5, 6*

**COMMENTS: Selenium** deficiency is a rare condition that has received attention because of the reversible nature of its effects. It produces cardiomyopathy, diffuse skeletal myalgia, loss of pigmentation, and erythrocyte macrocytosis. Selenium is a trace mineral that is found in seafood and meat; it is also ingested in grains and seeds, but in this form the content depends on the concentration of selenium in the soil. Garlic, asparagus, Brazil nuts, and mushrooms are all good sources of dietary selenium. The dose appropriate for daily supplementation is very small; beneficial and toxic effects occur within a very narrow range for this trace mineral. Parenteral nutrition will typically include 100 micrograms of selenium daily, with normal dietary intake being approximately 70 to 150 micrograms/day.

**ANSWER:**  B

20. Preservation of normothermia in surgical patients is important and has become one of the goals of the Surgical Care Improvement Project (SCIP). All of the following are negative outcomes that have been directly associated with perioperative hypothermia except:

 A. Coagulopathy

 B. Wound infections

C. Nosocomial pneumonia

D. Myocardial ischemia

E. Delayed wound healing

*Ref.:* 7

**COMMENTS: Hypothermia** results in peripheral vasoconstriction, which leads to decreased subcutaneous oxygen tension and antibiotic delivery. Both neutrophil activity and leukocyte chemotaxis are impaired. All of these sequelae give rise to an increased incidence of wound infections. Globally reduced enzyme function leads to coagulopathy. Collagen cross-linking and therefore wound healing are affected by hypothermia. An increased risk for myocardial ischemia in patients with known coronary artery disease has been associated with hypothermic states. There has not been a direct correlation between the development of nosocomial pneumonia and hypothermia. SCIP Inf-10 aims to achieve a target temperature of 36.0°C in perioperative patients by using active warming methods.

**ANSWER:** C

21. Perioperative β-adrenergic blockade has been shown to reduce morbidity and mortality in which scenario?

A. 42-year-old man undergoing inguinal hernia repair with hypertension treated with hydrochlorothiazide

B. 28-year-old woman with acute postoperative hypertension after emergency appendectomy

C. 55-year-old man taking metoprolol at home for hypertension now in septic shock after exploratory laparotomy

D. 45-year-old woman taking metoprolol at home for congestive heart failure after laparoscopic cholecystectomy

E. 70-year-old man undergoing colon resection with no known cardiac risk factors

*Ref.:* 7, 8

**TABLE 1-1  Cardiac Risk Indices**

| Variables | Points | Comments |
|---|---|---|
| Goldman Cardiac Risk Index, 1977 | | |
| 1. Third heart sound or jugular venous distention | 11 | 0-5 points = 1%* 6-12 points = 7% |
| 2. Recent myocardial infarction | 10 | 13-25 points = 14% |
| 3. Non–sinus rhythm or premature atrial contraction on ECG | 7 | >26 points = 78% |
| 4. >5 premature ventricular contractions | 7 | |
| 5. Age >70 years | 5 | |
| 6. Emergency operation | 4 | |
| 7. Poor general medical condition | 3 | |
| 8. Intrathoracic, intraperitoneal, or aortic surgery | 3 | |
| 9. Important valvular aortic stenosis | 3 | |
| Revised Cardiac Risk Index | | |
| 1. Ischemic heart disease | 1 | Each increment in |
| 2. Congestive heart failure | 1 | points increases the |
| 3. Cerebral vascular disease | 1 | risk for postoperative |
| 4. High-risk surgery | 1 | myocardial morbidity |
| 5. Preoperative treatment of diabetes with insulin | 1 | |
| 6. Preoperative creatinine >2 mg/dL | 1 | |

ECG, Electrocardiography.
*Cardiac complication rate.

**COMMENTS:** Perioperative β-**blockers** have been shown to reduce morbidity and mortality in select patient groups, including patients undergoing high-risk surgical procedures (vascular, cardiac, thoracic) and those with a Revised Goldman Cardiac Risk Index of greater than 2 (Table 1-1). Now emphasized as a quality measure by the SCIP, β-blockers should not be discontinued in the perioperative period in patients who were taking them preoperatively. Several studies have demonstrated that β-blocker withdrawal is associated with increased 1-year mortality in surgical patients.

**ANSWER:** D

22. Strategies that have been suggested to decrease the risk for postoperative pulmonary complications include all of the following except:

A. Routine nasogastric tube decompression

B. Lung expansion maneuvers

C. Preoperative smoking cessation

D. Postoperative epidural anesthesia

E. Use of intraoperative short-acting neuromuscular blocking agents

*Ref.:* 9

**COMMENTS: Postoperative pulmonary complications** include atelectasis, pneumonia, prolonged mechanical ventilation, bronchospasm, and exacerbation of underlying lung disease. Aggressive pulmonary toilet, smoking cessation, epidural analgesia, and minimal neuromuscular blockade have indeed been shown to be effective means of reducing postoperative respiratory complications. In contrast, because systemic reviews have found that routine use of nasogastric decompression increases pulmonary complications, **nasogastric tubes** should be used postoperatively only when specifically indicated for the operative procedure. An early **postoperative fever** is most likely due to **atelectasis** causing a respiratory shunt secondary to alveolar collapse. This results in varying degrees of hypoxemia. Persistent collapse leaves alveoli prone to bacterial colonization. Aggressive pulmonary toilet with incentive spirometry, forced coughing, and frequent turning is the best prevention.

**ANSWER:** A

23. All of the following are true concerning the sympathetic nervous system except:

A. Circulating epinephrine is produced mainly in the adrenal gland and secreted as a hormone.

B. Most circulating norepinephrine is derived from synaptic nerve clefts.

C. Activation of the sympathetic nervous system results in vasoconstriction, tachycardia, and tachypnea.

D. Norepinephrine acts primarily as a neurotransmitter.

E. Up to 5% of norepinephrine and 15% of dopamine are produced by the enteric nervous system.

*Ref.:* 10

**COMMENTS:** Secretion of **catecholamines** by the **sympathetic nervous system** is classically known as the "fight or flight" response. The first four choices represent the classic pathways of the sympathetic response. The enteric organs have actually been found to produce up to 37% of norepinephrine and greater than 50% of the dopamine found in the body.

**ANSWER:** E

24. Which of the following is true concerning the state of circulating cortisol in a patient with severe sepsis?

   A. Cortisol binds to steroid receptors on the cell membrane.

   B. Cortisol induces an increase in α- and β-adrenergic receptors on cells.

   C. Cortisol exacerbates the inflammatory response.

   D. Cortisol decreases the sensitivity of adrenergic receptors to catecholamines.

   E. The increase in cortisol level is not proportional to the degree of stress.

*Ref.:* 10

**COMMENTS:** There is up to a sixfold increase in free **cortisol** levels in response to the stress of critical illness. Cortisol does indeed induce an increase in adrenergic receptors on cell membranes in an effort to improve hemodynamic stability. It also sensitizes the receptors to catecholamines and suppresses the inflammatory response. Cortisol binds to intracellular steroid receptors, and its increase is proportional to the degree of stress.

**ANSWER:** B

25. Euthyroid sick syndrome is diagnosed in a patient in the surgical ICU. All of the following are part of this clinical phenomenon except:

   A. The patient behaves as though clinically hypothyroid

   B. Normal or decreased total serum thyroxine ($T_4$) level

   C. Increased serum reversed triiodothyronine ($rT_3$) level

   D. Decreased TSH level

   E. Decreased total serum $T_3$ level

*Ref.:* 10, 11

**COMMENTS:** The hallmark of this diagnosis is that the patient behaves neither clinically **hypothyroid** nor hyperthyroid. The other choices are the expected laboratory findings in patients with this syndrome. Referred to alternatively as **euthyroid sick syndrome**, low $T_3$ syndrome, low $T_4$ syndrome, and nonthyroidal illness, considerable debate exists regarding whether this syndrome represents a pathologic process or an adaptive response to systemic illness that allows the body to lower its tissue energy requirements. In light of this controversy, no consensus has been reached on how to treat this entity or whether any treatment at all is necessary. Because interpretation of thyroid function tests in critically ill patients is complex, they should therefore not be done in the ICU setting unless a thyroid disorder is strongly suspected.

**ANSWER:** A

**REFERENCES**

1. O'Leary PJ, Tabuenca A, editors: *The physiologic basis of surgery*, Philadelphia, 2008, Lippincott Williams & Wilkins.
2. Adams CA, Biffl WL, Cioffi WG: Surgical critical care. In Townsend CM, Beauchamp RD, Evers BM, et al, editors: *Sabiston textbook of surgery: the biological basis of modern surgical practice*, ed 18, Philadelphia, 2008, WB Saunders.
3. Mullins RJ: Acute renal failure. In Cameron JL, editor: *Current surgical therapy*, ed 9, Philadelphia, 2008, CV Mosby.
4. Jan BU, Lowry SF: The septic response. In Cameron JL, editor: *Current surgical therapy*, ed 9, Philadelphia, 2008, CV Mosby.
5. Keating KP, Marshall W: Nutritional support in the critically ill. In Cameron JL, editor: *Current surgical therapy*, ed 9, Philadelphia, 2008, CV Mosby.
6. Tawa NE, Fischer JE: Metabolism in surgical patients. In Townsend CM, Beauchamp RD, Evers BM, et al, editors: *Sabiston textbook of surgery*, ed 18, Philadelphia, 2008, WB Saunders.
7. Thomsen RW, Martinez EA, Simon BA: Perioperative care and monitoring of the surgical patient: evidence-based performance practices. In Cameron JL, editor: *Current surgical therapy*, ed 9, Philadelphia, 2008, CV Mosby.
8. Crisostomo PR, Meldrum DR, Harken AH: Cardiovascular pharmacology. In Cameron JL, editor: *Current surgical therapy*, ed 9, Philadelphia, 2008, CV Mosby.
9. Mendez-Tellez PA, Dorman T: Postoperative respiratory failure. In Cameron JL, editor: *Current surgical therapy*, ed 9, Philadelphia, 2008, CV Mosby.
10. Rosemeier F, Berenholtz S: Endocrine changes with critical illness. In Cameron JL, editor: *Current surgical therapy*, ed 9, Philadelphia, 2008, CV Mosby.
11. Sipos JA, Cance WG: Thyroid disease in the intensive care unit. In Gabrielli A, Layon AJ, Yu M, editors: *Civetta, Taylor & Kirby's critical care*, ed 4, Philadelphia, 2009, Lippincott Williams & Wilkins.

# CHAPTER 2

# Wound Healing and Cell Biology

*Edward F. Hollinger, M.D., Ph.D., and Troy Pittman, M.D.*

1. A 41-year-old woman undergoes complex repair of a deep laceration in her hand. When removing the dressing on postoperative day 2, a large clot with mild surrounding erythema is encountered. Which of the following statements regarding the inflammatory phase of wound healing is true?

   A. It lasts up to 24 hours after the injury is incurred.

   B. Initial vasodilation is followed by subsequent vasoconstriction.

   C. Bradykinin causes vasoconstriction, which inhibits migration of neutrophils to the healing wound.

   D. The complement component C5a and platelet factor attract neutrophils to the wound.

   E. The presence of neutrophils in the wound is essential for normal wound healing.

   *Ref.:* 1-5

**COMMENTS:** The **inflammatory phase** starts immediately after the injury occurs and lasts up to 72 hours. After the injury, there is a transient period (about 10 minutes) of vasoconstriction followed by active vasodilation. These events are mediated by substances released secondary to the local tissue injury. Vasoactive components such as **histamine** cause brief periods of vasodilation and increased vascular permeability. The **kinins** (bradykinin and kallidin) are released by the enzymatic action of kallikrein, which is formed after activation of the coagulation cascade. These components, in addition to those of the complement system, stimulate the release of **prostaglandins** (particularly PGE$_1$ and PGE$_2$), which work in concert to maintain more prolonged vessel permeability, not only of capillaries but also of larger vessels. In addition, these substances, particularly the complement component C5a and platelet-derived factors such as platelet-derived growth factor (PDGF), act as chemotactic stimuli for **neutrophils** to enter the wound. Although neutrophils can phagocytize bacteria from a wound, the results of studies involving clean wound healing show that healing can proceed normally without them. **Monocytes**, however, must be present for normal wound healing because in addition to their role in phagocytosis, they are required to trigger a normal fibroblast response. The later phases of wound healing include the proliferative or regenerative phase and the remodeling phase. The **proliferative phase** is marked by the appearance of fibroblasts in the wound, which leads to the formation of granulation tissue. The **remodeling phase** involves an increase in wound strength secondary to collagen remodeling and lasts up to 1 year after the initial injury. The three main phases of wound healing may occur sequentially or simultaneously.

**ANSWER:** D

2. A 55-year-old woman with a history of venous stasis ulcers is evaluated for a nonhealing ulcer on the medial aspect of the lower part of her leg. Application of topical ointment to the ulcer and compression stockings have allowed partial healing. However, she states that regardless of the various interventions, the ulcer never completely heals. Which of the following statements regarding wound epithelialization is true?

   A. Integrins act as a key modulator of the interaction between epithelial cells and the surrounding environment.

   B. Structural support and attachment between the epidermis and dermis are provided by tight cell junctions.

   C. Early tensile strength of the wound is a direct result of collagen deposition.

   D. A reepithelialized wound develops hair follicles and sweat glands like those seen in normal skin.

   E. Contact inhibition can prevent collagen deposition and result in a chronic (nonhealing) wound.

   *Ref.:* 2, 4-6

**COMMENTS:** Migration of **epithelial cells** is one of the earliest events in wound healing. Shortly after injury and during the inflammatory phase, basal epithelial cells begin to multiply and migrate across the defect, with fibrin strands being used as the support structure. **Integrins** are the main cellular receptors involved in epithelial migration; they act as sensors and integrators between the extracellular matrix and the epithelial cell cytoskeleton. Tight junctions within the epithelium contribute to its impermeability, whereas the basement membrane contributes to structural support and attachment of the epidermis to the dermis. Surgical incisions seal rather promptly and after 24 hours are protected from the external environment. Early **tensile strength** is a result of blood vessel ingrowth, epithelialization, and protein aggregation. After covering the wound, the epithelial cells keratinize. The reepithelialized wound has no sweat glands or hair follicles, which distinguishes it from normal skin. Control of the cellular process during wound epithelialization is not completely understood, but it appears to be regulated in part by **contact inhibition**, with growth being arrested when two or more similar cells come into surface contact. Derangements in the control of this process can result in epidermoid malignancy. **Malignancy** is more frequently observed in wounds resulting from ionizing radiation or chemical injury, but it can occur in any wound when the healing process has been chronically disrupted. For example, squamous cell carcinoma may develop in patients with chronic burn wounds or osteomyelitis (Marjolin ulcer).

**ANSWER:** A

**3.** A 31-year-old man undergoes his second exploratory laparotomy for bowel obstruction secondary to Crohn's disease. The patient expresses concern regarding the long-term complications related to his midline incision since he has taken steroids for the last year. Which of the following statements regarding the role of collagen in wound healing is true?

A. Collagen synthesis in the initial phase of injury is the sole responsibility of endothelial cells.

B. Net collagen content increases for up to 2 years after injury.

C. At 3 weeks after injury, more than 50% of the tensile strength of the wound has been restored.

D. Tensile strength of the wound increases gradually for up to 2 years after injury; however, it generally reaches a level of only about 80% of that of uninjured tissue.

E. Tensile strength is the force necessary to reopen a wound.

*Ref.:* 2, 3, 6

**COMMENTS: Synthesis of collagen** by **fibroblasts** begins as early as 10 hours after injury and increases rapidly; it peaks by day 6 or 7 and then continues more slowly until day 42. Collagen continues to mature and remodel for years. Its solubility in saline solution and the thermal shrinkage temperature of collagen reflect the intermolecular cross-links, which are directly proportional to collagen age. After 6 weeks, there is no measurable increase in net collagen content. However, synthesis and turnover are ongoing for life. Historical accounts of sailors with scurvy (with impaired collagen production) who experienced reopening of previously healed wounds illustrate this fact. **Tensile strength** correlates with total collagen content for approximately the first 3 weeks of wound healing. At 3 weeks, the tensile strength of skin is 30% of normal. After this time, there is a much slower increase in the content of collagen until it plateaus at about 6 weeks. Nevertheless, tensile strength continues to increase as a result of intermolecular bonding of collagen and changes in the physical arrangement of collagen fibers. Although the most rapid increase in tensile strength occurs during the first 6 weeks of healing, there is slow gain for at least 2 years. Its ultimate strength, however, never equals that of unwounded tissue, with a level of just 80% of original skin strength being reached. **Tensile strength** is measured as the load capacity per unit area. It may be differentiated from **burst strength**, which is the force required to break a wound (independent of its area). For example, in wounds of the face and back, burst strength is different because of differences in skin thickness, even though tensile strength may be similar. Corticosteroids affect wound healing by inhibiting fibroblast proliferation and epithelialization. The latter effect can be reversed by the administration of vitamin A.

**ANSWER:** D

**4.** Which of the following is correct regarding cell signaling?

A. Cytokines are exclusively peptide mediators.

B. Autocrine mediators are secreted by a cell and act on adjacent cells of a different type.

C. Cytokines are usually produced by cells specialized for only that purpose.

D. The effects of hormones are generally local rather than global.

E. Growth factors are frequently mediated by second messenger systems such as diacylglycerol (DAG) and cyclic adenosine monophosphate (cAMP).

*Ref.:* 7-9

**COMMENTS: Cytokines** are proteins, glycoproteins, or peptides that bind to target cell surface receptors to stimulate a cellular response. They are important mediators of wound healing. Cytokines can reach target cells by paracrine, autocrine, or intracrine routes. **Paracrine** mediators are produced by one cell and act on an adjacent target cell. **Autocrine** mediators are secreted by a cell and act on cell surface receptors on the same cell. **Intracrine** mediators act within a single cell. Hormones are released by cells and act on a distant target (endocrine route). Although the distinction between cytokines and hormones has blurred, in general, hormones are secreted from specialized glands (e.g., insulin, parathyroid hormone), and cytokines are secreted by a wide variety of cell types. Hormones typically induce body-wide effects, whereas the effects of cytokines may be more localized (e.g., wound healing at the site of an injury). Generally, **growth factors** are named according to their tissue of origin or their originally discovered action. Growth factors interact with specific membrane receptors to initiate a series of events that ultimately lead to stimulation of cell growth, proliferation, or differentiation. The intermediate events activate a variety of second messenger systems mediated by agents such as inositol 1,4,5-triphosphate ($IP_3$), DAG, and cAMP.

**ANSWER:** E

**5.** A 25-year-old man is seen in the office with complaints of contracture of his left index finger after a burn injury. Which of the following statements is true about growth factors?

A. Epidermal growth factor (EGF) stimulates the production of collagen.

B. Vascular endothelial growth factor (VEGF) and PDGF both stimulate angiogenesis by binding to a common receptor.

C. Fibroblast growth factor (FGF) stimulates wound contraction.

D. Transforming growth factor-β (TGF-β) is stored in endothelial cells.

E. Tumor necrosis factor-α (TNF-α) inhibits angiogenesis.

*Ref.:* 3, 6, 10, 11

**COMMENTS: Epidermal growth factor** was the first cytokine described. It is a potent mitogen for epithelial cells, endothelial cells, and fibroblasts. EGF stimulates synthesis of fibronectin, angiogenesis, and collagenase activity. **Platelet-derived growth factor** is released from the alpha granules of platelets and is responsible for the stimulation of neutrophils and macrophages and for increasing production of TGF-β. PDGF is a mitogen and chemotactic agent for fibroblasts and smooth muscle cells and stimulates angiogenesis, collagen synthesis, and collagenase activity. **Vascular endothelial growth factor** is similar to PDGF but does not bind to the same receptors. VEGF is mitogenic for endothelial cells. Its role in promoting angiogenesis has led to interest in anti-VEGF therapies for cancer. **Fibroblast growth factor** has acidic and basic forms whose actions are identical but whose strengths differ (basic FGF is 10 times stronger than acidic FGF). FGF is mitogenic for endothelial cells, fibroblasts, keratinocytes, and myoblasts; stimulates wound contraction and epithelialization; and induces the production of collagen, fibronectin, and proteoglycans. It is an important mediator of angiogenesis. **Transforming growth**

factor-β is released from the alpha granules of platelets and has been shown to regulate its own production in an autocrine manner. TGF-β stimulates fibroblast proliferation and the production of proteoglycans, collagen, and fibrin. It is an important mediator of fibrosis. Administration of TGF-β has been suggested as an approach to reduce scarring and reverse the inhibition of wound healing by glucocorticoids. **Tumor necrosis factor-α** is a mitogen for fibroblasts and is produced by macrophages. It stimulates angiogenesis and the synthesis of collagen and collagenase.

**ANSWER: C**

6. A 34-year-old man sustained a gunshot wound to his abdomen that necessitated exploratory laparotomy and small bowel resection. Two weeks after the initial operation, he was reexplored for a large intraabdominal abscess. Which of the following will result in the most rapid gain in strength of the new incision?

   A. A separate transverse incision is made.

   B. The midline scar is excised with a 1-cm margin.

   C. The midline incision is reopened without excision of the scar.

   D. The midline incision is left to heal by secondary intention.

   E. The rate of gain in strength is not affected by the incision technique.

   *Ref.: 2, 3, 6*

**COMMENTS:** When a normally-healing wound is disrupted after approximately the fifth day and then reclosed, return of wound strength is more rapid than with primary healing. This is termed the **secondary healing effect** and appears to be caused by elimination of the lag phase present in normal primary healing. If the skin edges more than about 7 mm around the initial wound are excised, the resulting incision is through essentially uninjured tissue, so accelerated secondary healing does not occur.

**ANSWER: C**

7. A 29-year-old black woman is scheduled for incision and drainage of a breast abscess that has recurred three times despite ultrasound-guided needle drainage. The patient has a history of keloid formation and is concerned about an unsightly scar on her breast. Which of the following statements concerning wound healing is true?

   A. Keloids contain an overabundance of fibroblasts.

   B. A hypertrophic scar extends beyond the boundaries of the original wound.

   C. Improvement is usually seen with keloid excision followed by intralesional steroid injection.

   D. An incision placed perpendicular to the lines of natural skin tension will result in the least obvious scar.

   E. Hypertrophic scars occur most commonly on the lower extremities.

   *Ref.: 2, 3, 6*

**COMMENTS:** **Keloids** are caused by an imbalance between collagen production and degradation. The result is a scar that extends beyond the boundaries of the original wound. The absolute number of fibroblasts is not increased. Treatment of keloids is difficult. There is often some improvement with excision and intralesional

steroid injection. If this technique is not successful, excision and radiation treatment can be used. **Hypertrophic scars** contain an overabundance of collagen, but the dimensions of the scar are confined to the boundaries of the original wound. Hypertrophic scars are often seen in the upper part of the torso and across flexor surfaces. Scar formation is affected by multiple factors, including the patient's genetic makeup, wound location, age, nutritional status, infection, tension, and surgical technique. In planning surgical incisions, an effort to parallel natural tension lines will promote improved wound healing.

**ANSWER: C**

8. An 85-year-old nursing home patient is found to have a worsening stage III sacral pressure ulcer. The ulcer is débrided and tissue for culture obtained. Tissue cultures reveal $10^8$ organisms per gram of tissue after operative débridement. What is the next most appropriate step in management of the patient's wound?

   A. Muscle flap coverage

   B. Wound vacuum-assisted closure (VAC)

   C. Intravenous antibiotics

   D. Repeat débridement

   E. Débridement with immediate application of a split-thickness skin graft

   *Ref.: 2, 3, 6, 12*

**COMMENTS:** The National Pressure Ulcer Advisory Panel has recommended a **staging system for pressure sores** that is useful in planning treatment. Stage I is represented by the presence of nonblanching erythema of intact skin. Stage II is characterized by partial-thickness skin loss involving the epidermis or dermis. Clinically, the ulcer is manifested as a blister, abrasion, or a shallow crater. Stage III is full-thickness skin loss with involvement of the underlying subcutaneous tissue. Stage III wounds may extend down to but not through the underlying fascia. Stage IV represents full-thickness skin loss with extensive destruction or tissue necrosis of underlying structures, which may include muscle and bone. Studies have shown that wounds with quantitative cultures revealing more than $10^6$ organisms per gram of tissue that undergo reconstruction with skin or even muscle flaps have a significantly greater risk for complications, including infection, accumulation of fluid, and wound dehiscence. Similarly, a skin graft is unlikely to survive in an environment with such a high bacterial inoculate. **Negative pressure wound therapy**, such as with the **wound vacuum-assisted closure system**, involves the use of a sponge and an occlusive dressing connected to a suction apparatus in a closed system. In patients with large wounds, a wound VAC may serve as a bridge to reduce wound size for definitive reconstruction. It has been shown to be effective in reducing wound edema, controlling wound drainage, encouraging diminution of wound size, and facilitating the formation of granulation tissue. Although studies show that wound VAC therapy may reduce bacterial counts over time, the most appropriate management of this patient is repeat débridement of the wound. Intravenous antibiotics may be indicated to treat underlying osteomyelitis.

**ANSWER: D**

9. A 30-year-old man is scheduled for definitive management of his open wounds after undergoing embolectomy and fasciotomies on his left lower extremity. Which of the following statements is true regarding the use of split- and full-thickness skin grafts?

A. A split-thickness skin graft undergoes approximately 40% shrinkage of its surface area immediately after harvesting.

B. A full-thickness skin graft undergoes approximately 10% shrinkage of its surface area immediately after harvesting.

C. Secondary contraction is more likely to occur after adequate healing of a full-thickness skin graft than after adequate healing of a split-thickness skin graft.

D. Sensation usually returns to areas that have undergone skin grafting.

E. Skin grafts may be exposed to moderate amounts of sunlight without changing pigmentation.

*Ref.:* 2, 3, 6

**COMMENTS: Skin grafts** are considered to be **full thickness** when they are harvested at the dermal-subcutaneous junction. **Split-thickness** skin grafts are those that contain epidermis and variable partial thicknesses of underlying dermis. They are usually 0.018 to 0.060 inch in thickness. Cells from epidermal appendages deep to the plane of graft harvest resurface the donor site of a split-thickness skin graft in approximately 1 to 3 weeks, depending on the depth. The donor site requires a moist environment to promote epithelialization, and such an environment is maintained by using polyurethane or hydrocolloid dressings. Because a full-thickness graft removes all epidermal appendages, the defects must be closed primarily. When a skin graft is harvested, there is immediate shrinkage of the surface area of the graft. This process, known as **primary contraction**, is due to recoil of the elastic fibers of the dermis. The thicker the skin graft, the greater the immediate shrinkage, with full-thickness grafts shrinking by approximately 40% of their initial surface area and split-thickness grafts shrinking by approximately 10% of their initial surface area. Shrinkage must be considered when planning the amount of skin to harvest for covering a given size wound. **Secondary contraction** occurs when contractile myofibroblasts in the bed of a granulating wound interact with collagen fibers to cause a decrease in the wound's surface area. Secondary contraction is greater in wounds covered with split-thickness grafts than in those covered with full-thickness grafts. The amount of secondary contracture is inversely proportional to the amount of dermis included in the graft rather than the absolute thickness of the graft. Dermal elements hasten the displacement of myofibroblasts from the wound bed.

Sensation may return to areas that have been grafted as long as the bed is suitable and not significantly scarred. Although sensation is not completely normal, it is usually adequate for protection. This process begins at about 10 weeks and is maximal at 2 years. Skin grafts appear to be more sensitive than normal surrounding skin to melanocyte stimulation during exposure to ultraviolet sunlight. Early exposure to sunlight after grafting may lead to permanently increased pigmentation of the graft and should be avoided. Dermabrasion or the application of hydroquinones may be of benefit in reducing this pigmentation.

**ANSWER:  D**

10. A 45-year-old woman undergoes bilateral transverse rectus abdominis muscle (TRAM) breast reconstruction after modified radical mastectomy. The patient is scheduled for postoperative radiation therapy and is concerned that this will affect her ability to heal her wounds. Which of the following statements regarding wound healing in this patient is true?

A. Denervation has a profound effect on wound contraction and epithelialization.

B. A bacterial count of 1000 organisms per square centimeter retards wound healing.

C. Chemotherapy beginning 10 to 14 days after primary wound closure has little effect on the final status of a wound.

D. Tissue ischemia is the main component of tissue damage after irradiation.

E. Postoperative radiation therapy should be delayed at least 4 to 6 months after surgery to decrease the incidence of wound complications.

*Ref.:* 2-4, 6, 13

**COMMENTS:** Denervation has no effect on **wound contraction** or **epithelialization**. Flap wounds in paraplegics heal satisfactorily when other factors, such as nutrition and temperature, are controlled. Subinfectious bacterial levels appear to accelerate wound healing and the formation of granulation tissue. However, when the level reaches $10^6$ organisms per square centimeter of wound, healing is delayed because of decreased tissue oxygen pressure, increased collagenolysis, and a prolonged inflammatory phase. Various chemotherapeutic agents affect wound healing. Most **antimetabolic agents** (e.g., 5-fluorouracil) do not delay wound healing, although agents such as doxorubicin have been shown to delay wound healing. When chemotherapy begins 10 to 14 days after wound closure, little effect is noted on its final status despite a demonstrable early retardation in wound strength. Tissue ischemia may not be the primary factor involved in chronic wound-healing problems associated with **irradiation**. Such problems are most likely related to changes within the nuclei and concomitant cytoplasmic malformation. To decrease wound complications, it is usual to delay surgery until at least 3 to 4 weeks after full-dose irradiation and to avoid radiation therapy for at least 3 to 4 weeks after surgery.

**ANSWER:  C**

11. A 21-year-old graduate student has a large hypertrophic scar on the lower part of her face. The patient had sustained a laceration on her face 2 years previously after hitting her face on the side of a swimming pool. Which of the following statements regarding scar revision is true?

A. Scar maturation refers to the change in size of the wound in the first 1 to 2 months.

B. Scar revision should have been performed in the first 3 months after injury to minimize fibrosis.

C. Revision should be performed earlier in children than in adults.

D. It corrects undesirable pigmentation.

E. Scar revision should be delayed approximately 1 year to allow maturation.

*Ref.:* 2, 3, 6

**COMMENTS:** Changes in pliability, pigmentation, and configuration of a scar are known as **scar maturation**. This process continues for many months after an incision, so it is generally recommended that revision not be carried out for approximately 12 to 18 months because natural improvement can be anticipated within this period. In general, scar maturation occurs more rapidly in adults than in children. Most erythematous scars show little improvement after revision, therefore scar revision should not be undertaken for correction of undesirable scar color alone.

**ANSWER:  E**

**12.** A 68-year-old diabetic man undergoes a below-knee amputation. The patient's postoperative course is complicated by severe depression and anorexia. Before discharge the patient is started on a multivitamin regimen. Which of the following statements regarding wound healing is true?

A. Vitamin A is needed for hydroxylation of lysine and proline in collagen synthesis.

B. High doses of vitamin C improve wound healing.

C. Vitamin E is involved in the stimulation of fibroplasia, collagen cross-linking, and epithelialization.

D. Zinc deficiency results in delayed early wound healing.

E. Iron deficiency had been linked to defects in long-term wound remodeling.

*Ref.:* 2, 3, 6

**COMMENTS: Vitamin A** is involved in the stimulation of fibroplasia and epithelialization. Although there has been no conclusive evidence of efficacy in humans, in animal studies vitamin A has been shown to reverse the inhibitory effects of glucocorticoids on the inflammatory phase of wound healing and epithelialization. **Vitamin C** is a necessary cofactor in the hydroxylation and cross-linking of lysine and proline in collagen synthesis. Deficiencies in vitamin C (scurvy) can lead to the production of inadequately hydroxylated collagen, which either degrades rapidly or never forms proper cross-links. Doses higher than physiologic doses do not improve wound healing. **Vitamin E** is applied to wounds and incisions by many patients, but there is no evidence to support the use of vitamin E in wound healing. Large doses of vitamin E have been found to inhibit wound healing. **Zinc** is a necessary cofactor of RNA and DNA polymerase, and deficiencies have been linked to poor early wound healing. **Iron** (specifically, the ferrous iron) is necessary for converting hydroxyproline to proline. However, chronic anemia and iron deficiency have not been linked to delayed or impaired wound healing.

**ANSWER:** D

**13.** A 46-year-old man is evaluated shortly after undergoing radiation therapy and chemotherapy for primary laryngeal cancer. He also gives a history of long-term steroid use for rheumatoid arthritis. The patient complains of a chronic, nonhealing wound on his neck, just over his right clavicular head. Which statement regarding the treatment of this wound is true?

A. The wound should be treated with compression dressings.

B. The wound should be treated with injected steroids.

C. The patient should start taking vitamin A, and the wound should be covered with antimicrobial dressings.

D. The patient should start taking vitamin C, and the wound should be kept open to air.

E. The wound should be excised and a skin graft applied.

*Ref.:* 11, 14

**COMMENTS: Radiation** results in progressive endarteritis obliterans and microvascular damage to the skin, which leads to skin ischemia and fibrotic interstitial changes. This leaves wounds in the skin particularly prone to infection. The use of antimicrobial dressings capable of maintaining a moist environment is ideal for these wounds. Research also supports the use of **hyperbaric oxygen** and growth factors to promote wound healing. Patients taking steroids should receive daily **vitamin A** supplements. Wounds in these patients show decreased rates of angiogenesis, collagen deposition, and cellular proliferation. Wounds should be kept free of bacterial contamination.

**ANSWER:** C

**14.** A 25-year-old ballet dancer with a history of anorexia nervosa arrives at the emergency department with right lower quadrant pain. After an appendectomy, a wound infection at the surgical site requires débridement. The patient is placed on an antibiotic regimen, and the wound is packed with wet-to-dry dressings. Regarding wound healing and malnutrition, which of the following statements is true?

A. Hypoproteinemia leads to decreased levels of arginine and glutamine, which are essential in wound healing.

B. Cell membranes rapidly become dehydrated in the absence of vitamin E, resulting in delayed wound healing.

C. Zinc is essential to the fibroblast's ability to cross-link collagen.

D. Vitamin D serves an immunomodulatory role in wound healing.

E. The patient should be treated with high-dose vitamin C, vitamin A, and zinc.

*Ref.:* 2, 15

**COMMENTS:** Adequate amounts of protein, carbohydrates, fatty acids, and vitamins are essential for wound healing. **Hypoproteinemia** results in decreased delivery of the essential amino acids used in the synthesis of collagen. **Carbohydrates** and **fats** provide energy for wound healing, and in their absence, proteins are rapidly broken down. **Fatty acids** are vital components of cell membranes. **Vitamin C** is a cofactor for hydroxylation of lysine and proline during collagen synthesis, and deficiency leads to decreased collagen cross-linking by fibroblasts. Vitamin C is also effective in providing resistance to infection. **Vitamin A** is essential for normal epithelialization, proteoglycan synthesis, and enhanced immune function. **Vitamin D** is required for normal calcium metabolism, but it is also involved in promoting immune function in the skin. **Vitamin E** has not been shown to play a role in wound healing. **Zinc** deficiency leads to deficient formation of granulation tissue and inhibition of cellular proliferation. Increased administration of vitamins and minerals does not accelerate wound healing and often has a deleterious effect.

**ANSWER:** D

**15.** A 56-year-old man underwent total thyroidectomy for papillary cancer. On the first postoperative day, the patient complains of circumoral tingling and muscle weakness. Which of the following statements regarding the electrical properties of cell membranes is not true?

A. Ions flow through hydrophilic channels formed by specific transmembrane proteins.

B. Lipids provide the ability to store electric charge (capacitance).

C. Active pumps maintain the ionic gradients necessary for a resting membrane potential.

D. Initiation of an action potential depends on voltage-gated channels.

E. Large numbers of sodium ions rush in during the initial phase of a nerve action potential.

*Ref.:* 16, 17

**COMMENTS:** This patient has clinical findings associated with hypocalcemia. Specific transmembrane proteins provide hydrophilic paths for the ions (primarily $Na^+$, $K^+$, $Ca^{2+}$, and $Cl^-$) involved in electrical signaling. The amino acid sequence in specific regions of these proteins determines the selectivity for ions. The lipid component of the plasma membrane provides the capability of storing electric charge (**capacitance**), and the protein component provides the capability of resisting electric charge (**resistance**). Establishment and maintenance of a **resting cell membrane potential** requires the separation of charge maintained by membrane capacitance, selective permeability of the plasma membrane, concentration gradients (intracellular versus extracellular) of the permeant ions, and impermeant intracellular anions. Active pumping by the sodium (sodium-potassium adenosine triphosphatase [$Na^+,K^+$-ATPase]) or calcium pumps generally maintains the ionic concentration gradients. **Action potentials** are regenerative (self-sustaining) transient depolarizations caused by the activation of voltage-sensitive sodium and potassium channels. Only a small volume of sodium ions is necessary to initiate an action potential. In fact, the amount of sodium ions that flow into a typical nerve cell during an action potential would change the intracellular $Na^+$ concentration by only a few parts per million.

**ANSWER:** E

16. An 84-year-old woman with colon cancer undergoes a right hemicolectomy. Her estimated blood loss is 700 mL. Shortly after surgery, her urine output falls to 10 mL/h. She is administered several liters of normal saline. On the second postoperative day, the patient complains of severe swelling of her hands and feet. Which cell junction acts as a transmembrane linkage without an intracellular communication function?

   A. Tight junction

   B. Gap junction

   C. Desmosome

   D. Connexon

   E. All of these junctions have an intracellular communication function

*Ref.:* 16, 18

**COMMENTS:** Any patient undergoing abdominal surgery will sustain a certain amount of capillary leakage. A proposed mechanism involves increased release of nitric oxide, which causes vasodilation in precapillary cells, vasoconstriction in postcapillary cells, and ultimately results in increased third-spacing of fluids. There are three major types of cell junctions: gap junctions, desmosomes, and tight junctions. **Gap junctions** are the most common and function primarily in intercellular communication but also in cellular adhesion. The connection between cells maintained by a gap junction is not particularly stable; it depends on a variety of complexes on each cell but not on connecting proteins (hence the term *gap*). Gap junctions serve as a pathway of permeability between cells for many different molecules up to weights of 1000 daltons. **Connexons** are protein assemblies formed by six identical protein subunits. They span the intercellular gap of the lipid bilayer to form an aqueous channel connecting the bilayers. **Desmosomes** function as cellular adhesion points but do not provide a pathway of communication. They are linked by filaments that function as transmembrane linkers, but desmosomes are not points of true cell fusion. **Tight junctions**, in contrast, are true points of cell fusion and are impermeable barriers. They prevent leakage of molecules across the epithelium in either direction. They also limit the movement of membrane proteins within the lipid bilayer of the plasma membrane and therefore maintain cells in a differentiated polar state.

**ANSWER:** C

17. A 42-year-old woman with a history of end-stage renal disease is being evaluated for cadaveric renal transplantation. Which of the following statements regarding cell surface antigens is true?

   A. Cell surface antigens are generally glycoproteins or glycolipids.

   B. Histocompatibility antigens are not cell surface antigens.

   C. ABO antigens are glycoproteins.

   D. ABO antibodies are present at birth.

   E. HLA antigens have an extracellular hydrophobic region and an intracellular hydrophilic region.

*Ref.:* 19

**COMMENTS:** **Cell surface antigens** are generally glycoproteins or glycolipids that are anchored to either a protein or a lipid. Common examples include the ABO blood group antigens and the histocompatibility antigens. Antigens of the **ABO system** are glycolipids whose oligosaccharide portions are responsible for the antigenic properties. The structures of the blood group oligosaccharides occur commonly in nature and lead to the stimulation needed to produce anti-A or anti-B antibodies after a few months of life. **HLA antigens** are two-chain glycoproteins that are anchored in the cell membrane at the carboxyl terminal. These antigens contain an extracellular hydrophilic region, a transmembrane hydrophobic region, and an intracellular hydrophilic region. This transmembrane structure allows extracellular signals to be transmitted to the interior of the cell.

**ANSWER:** A

18. A 36-year-old man is evaluated at the office because of complaints of fatigue, weight gain, and irritability. Routine laboratory tests are performed and his thyroid-stimulating hormone (TSH) level is found to be 11.0. The patient is concerned about his condition and inquires about the relationship between hypothyroidism and his symptoms. Which of the following statements regarding second messenger systems is true?

   A. Most receptor proteins (such as G proteins) are completely extracellular.

   B. Both the "first messenger" and "second messenger" mediators of cell signaling function within the cell cytoplasm.

   C. Adenylate cyclase stimulates the conversion of cAMP to adenosine triphosphate (ATP).

   D. $IP_3$ generally increases cytoplasmic calcium concentrations.

   E. $IP_3$ and DAG together lead to inactivation of protein kinase C.

*Ref.:* 7, 8, 16

**COMMENTS:** The **thyrotropin** (TSH) receptor is a $G_{\alpha s}$ receptor found mainly on the surface of thyroid follicular cells. When activated, it stimulates increased production of thyroxine ($T_4$) and triiodothyronine ($T_3$).

Several families of receptor proteins have been identified. The most common is the **G protein** (guanine nucleotide–binding protein) family, a subset of guanosine triphosphatase (GTPase) enzymes. All G protein–coupled receptors have a characteristic seven transmembrane domains. Binding of an extracellular ligand causes a conformational change in the receptor that allows it to exchange guanosine diphosphate (GDP) for guanosine triphosphate (GTP) on the intracellular portion of the G protein. The intracellular portion of the "large" (heterotrimeric) G protein–coupled receptor consists of three subunits, $G_\alpha$, $G_\beta$, and $G_\gamma$. Other "small" (monomeric) G protein receptors have only a homologue of the $G_\alpha$ portion. There are several important subsets of the "large" G protein receptors, and they are classified according to the specific intracellular pathway that is activated.

$G_{\alpha s}$ stimulates membrane-associated **adenylate cyclase** to produce **cyclic adenosine monophosphate** from ATP. cAMP is a second messenger that activates **protein kinase A**, which results in the phosphorylation of downstream targets. $G_{\alpha s}$ ligands include adrenocorticotropic hormone (ACTH), calcitonin, glucagon, histamine ($H_2$), TSH, and many others. $G_{\alpha i}$ inhibits the production of cAMP from ATP. $G_{\alpha i}$ ligands include acetylcholine ($M_2$ and $M_4$), dopamine ($D_2$, $D_3$, and $D_4$), and histamine ($H_3$ and $H_4$). $G_{\alpha q}$ activates **phospholipase C**, which cleaves phosphatidylinositol 4,5-bisphosphate ($PIP_2$) into inositol **1,4,5-triphosphate** and **diacylglycerol**. $IP_3$ mediates the release of calcium from intracellular reservoirs, such as the endoplasmic reticulum (ER), sarcoplasmic reticulum (SR) in muscle, and mitochondria. $IP_3$ and DAG together work to activate **protein kinase C**, which can modulate membrane permeability and activate gene transcription. $G_{\alpha q}$ ligands include histamine ($H_1$), serotonin (5-$HT_2$), and muscarinic receptors.

The most well known "small" G protein receptors are the **Ras family** GTPases. The Ras receptors influence a wide variety of processes in the cell, including growth, cellular differentiation, and cell movement.

Chemical messengers can influence intracellular physiology via several mechanisms. Some **ligands**, such as acetylcholine (binding to the nicotinic cholinergic receptor) or norepinephrine (binding to the potassium channel in cardiac muscle), directly bind to ion channels in the cell membrane to alter their conductance. Some lipid-soluble messengers, such as steroid and thyroid hormones, enter the cell and bind to nuclear or cytoplasmic receptors, which then bind to DNA to increase transcription of selected mRNA. Many other extracellular messengers bind to the extracellular portion of transmembrane receptor proteins to trigger the release of intracellular mediators. The extracellular ligands are termed the "**first messenger**," whereas the intracellular mediators are "**second messengers**." Examples of second messengers include $IP_3$, DAG, calcium, and cAMP.

**ANSWER:** D

19. A 67-year-old man undergoes revascularization of his right lower extremity after sustaining thrombosis secondary to a popliteal artery aneurysm. Shortly after surgery, a compartment syndrome of the affected limb develops and is attributed to reperfusion injury. Research suggests that ER stress may be responsible for apoptosis after ischemia. Which of the following statements regarding the ER is not true?

A. Rough ER is a primary site of lipid synthesis.

B. Smooth ER plays an important role in the metabolism of drugs.

C. Ribosomes attached to the rough ER manufacture proteins for use within the cell.

D. The SR is found mainly in epithelial cells.

E. The SR plays an important role in gluconeogenesis.

*Ref.:* 18, 20

**COMMENTS:** The **endoplasmic reticulum** is part of a network that includes **mitochondria**, **lysosomes**, microbodies, the **Golgi complex**, and the **nuclear envelope**. This network forms an intracellular circulatory system that allows vital substrates to reach the interior of the cell for transportation and assembly. There are two types of ER. **Rough endoplasmic reticulum** is coated with **ribosomes** and functions as the site of synthesis of membrane and secreted proteins. Other ribosomes that circulate freely in the cytoplasm synthesize proteins destined to remain within the cell. **Smooth endoplasmic reticulum** plays a major role in metabolic processes, including the synthesis of lipids and steroids, metabolism of carbohydrates (especially gluconeogenesis), drug detoxification, and molecular conjugation. Smooth ER contains the enzyme **glucose-6-phosphatase**, which converts glucose-6-phosphate to glucose during gluconeogenesis. Cells that synthesize large amounts of protein for export have abundant rough ER, whereas cells that make steroids (e.g., those in the adrenal cortex) generally have smoother ER. The smooth ER is continuous with the nuclear envelope. The **sarcoplasmic reticulum** is a distinct type of smooth ER found in striated and smooth muscle. The SR contains large stores of calcium, which it sequesters and then releases when the cell is stimulated. Release of calcium from the SR plays a major role in **excitation-contraction coupling**, which allows muscle cells to convert an electric stimulus to a mechanical response.

**ANSWER:** B

20. A 43-year-old woman is undergoing external beam radiation therapy for invasive breast cancer. Biopsy of the tumor shows a relatively high mitotic index, indicative of active growth. Which portion of the cell cycle in actively dividing cells is most sensitive to ionizing radiation?

A. S phase

B. M phase

C. $G_1$ phase

D. $G_2$ phase

E. All phases are equally radiosensitive

*Ref.:* 21

**COMMENTS:** The primary mechanism by which **ionizing radiation** induces cell death is direct and indirect injury to **deoxyribonucleic acid** (DNA). Ionizing radiation can cause lethal damage (damage that cannot be repaired; for example, most double-strand DNA breaks) or sublethal damage (damage that can be repaired if conditions are correct; for example, most single-strand DNA breaks). Factors that increase the cell's ability to repair damage make it less sensitive to ionizing radiation. The cell division cycle is divided into four distinct phases. Replication of DNA occurs in the synthesis (S) phase, whereas nuclear division and cell fission occur in the mitotic (M) phase. The intervals between these two phases are called the gap (G) phases. Cells in **M phase** (mitosis) have the least capability to repair sublethal damage and hence are the most radiation sensitive. Cells in **S phase** have the most capability of repairing damage and consequently are the most radiation resistant. Resting cells ($G_0$) are less sensitive to radiation injury than cells that are actively dividing (and proceeding through the cell cycle). Cancer cells are generally less differentiated (with less ability to repair DNA damage) and more rapidly dividing than normal tissue. The fact that tumor cells are usually more sensitive to radiation than surrounding normal tissue is an important determinant of the utility of radiation therapy.

**ANSWER: B**

21. A 56-year-old man is transferred from the county jail with complaints of hemoptysis, fever, and chills. The patient had undergone left lower lobectomy 6 years ago for an isolated lung nodule. Chest radiography on admission shows a lesion in the left upper lobe that is concerning for tuberculosis. The cell wall of *Mycobacterium tuberculosis* prevents lysosomes from fusing with phagosomes, which contributes to its tendency to lead to granuloma formation. Which of the following statements regarding endocytosis is not true?

   A. Phagocytosis refers to engulfment of particulate matter.

   B. Pinocytosis refers to the engulfment of soluble material.

   C. Only specialized cells of the immune system are capable of endocytosis.

   D. Opsonins increase the likelihood of phagocytosis by binding to the antigen.

   E. Antibodies and complement fragments can serve as opsonins.

*Ref.:* 7, 20

**COMMENTS:** All cells are capable of **endocytosis**, which is the process of internalizing extracellular molecules by engulfing the molecule within the cell membrane. **Pinocytosis** (cell drinking) is the engulfment of soluble material. **Phagocytosis** (cell eating) is the process by which cells ingest solids. For cells of the immune system, such as macrophages, dendritic cells, and polymorphonuclear leukocytes, phagocytosis is particularly important in recognizing and combating pathogens. In phagocytosis the cell membrane surrounding the engulfed material pinches off and forms a vesicle called a **phagosome**. The phagosome maintains the material separate from the cytosol of the cell. The phagosome fuses with a **lysosome**, which leads to degradation of the engulfed material. Degradation can be oxygen dependent (by the production of reactive oxygen species) or okygen independent (generally by proteolytic enzymes and cationic proteins).

   Typically, both the target (antigen) and the phagocyte are negatively charged. This limits their ability to come into close proximity. **Opsonins** are molecules that act to enhance phagocytosis. **Opsonization** occurs when antigens are bound by antibody or complement molecules (or both). Phagocytic cells express receptors (Fc, CR1) that bind opsonin molecules (antibody, C3b), which greatly increases the affinity of the phagocyte for the antigen. Phagocytosis is an unlikely event if the antigen is not opsonized.

**ANSWER: C**

22. Which of the following statements regarding lysosomes is true?

   A. Primary lysosomes usually contain extracellular material targeted for digestion.

   B. Lysosomal enzymes work effectively in the acidic pH of the cytoplasm.

   C. Serum levels of lysosomal acid phosphatases may have prognostic value in diseases such as prostate cancer.

   D. Lysosomal storage diseases such as Tay-Sachs result from unregulated activity of lysosomal enzymes.

   E. To better isolate their hydrolytic enzymes, lysosomes are resistant to fusion with other cell membranes.

*Ref.:* 18, 20

**COMMENTS: Lysosomes** are membrane-bound organelles that contain acid hydrolases. Heterolysosomes are involved in the endocytosis and digestion of extracellular material, whereas autolysosomes are involved in digestion of the cell's own intracellular material. **Primary lysosomes** are formed by the addition of hydrolytic enzymes (from the rough ER) to endosomes from the Golgi complex. Combining a primary lysosome with a phagosome creates a **phagolysosome**. Lysosomal enzymes are hydrolases that are resistant to autolysis. They function best in the acidic milieu of the lysosome; the slightly alkaline pH of the surrounding cytosol helps protect the cell from injury if the lysosome leaks. **Acid phosphatase** is a marker enzyme for lysosomes. Different forms of acid phosphatase are found in lysosomes from various organs, and serum levels may be indicative of disease (for example, prostatic acid phosphatase may have prognostic significance in prostate cancer).

   One of the distinguishing characteristics of lysosomal membranes is their ability to fuse with other cell membranes. Lysosomal membranes have a high proportion of lipids in a micellar configuration, primarily because of the presence of the phospholipid **lysolecithin**. This increased micellar configuration facilitates fusion of the lysosome membrane with the phagosome membrane for digestion and with the plasma membrane for secretion. Steroids are thought to work partially by stabilizing lysosomal membranes, thereby inhibiting membrane fusion and enzyme release. Lysosomes may engage in **autophagocytosis**, which is thought to be important for cell turnover, cell remodeling, and tissue changes. Several **lysosomal storage diseases**, such as Tay-Sachs, Gaucher, and Pompe disease, are caused by inactive or missing lysosomal digestive proteins. These genetic diseases lead to the accumulation of normally degraded substrates within the cell.

**ANSWER: C**

23. An 81-year-old woman undergoes a Hartman procedure for perforated diverticulitis. Postoperatively, the patient remains hypotensive and norepinephrine is administered. On day 2, parenteral nutrition is initiated. Which of the following statements regarding oxidative phosphorylation and mitochondria is true?

   A. Glycoproteins are transported into the mitochondrial matrix to facilitate oxidative phosphorylation.

   B. The citric acid cycle takes place within the inner mitochondrial membrane.

   C. Oxidative phosphorylation via ATP synthase converts adenosine diphosphate (ADP) to ATP.

   D. Electrochemical (proton) gradients provide the energy to power chemosmotic production of ATP.

   E. Mitochondrial DNA is almost exclusively paternally derived.

*Ref.:* 22

**COMMENTS:** Metabolic substrates such as fats, proteins, and glycoproteins are converted to **fatty acids and pyruvate** and transported into mitochondria. Within the mitochondrial matrix they are metabolized by the **citric acid (Krebs) cycle** to produce the reduced forms of **nicotinamide adenine dinucleotide** (NADH) and **flavin adenine dinucleotide** ($FADH_2$). The reducing power of these substrates fuels transfer of electrons from electron donors to receptors as **oxidative phosphorylation**. The resultant high-energy electrons pass along the electron transport chain and release the energy used to move protons across the inner mitochondrial membrane to generate potential energy in the form of electrical and pH gradients. **ATP synthase** uses the energy obtained from allowing protons to flow down this gradient to synthesize **adenosine triphosphate** from **adenosine diphosphate**. This process is called **chemosmosis**. Three ATP molecules are generated for each mole of oxygen consumed. **Mitochondrial DNA** is transmitted only from the mother because sperm contains few mitochondria. During **sepsis**, inhibited mitochondrial function as a result of hypoxia or other mediators of sepsis has been postulated to contribute to organ injury through accelerated oxidant production and by promoting cell death.

**A N S W E R :**   D

24. Inflammatory breast cancer is diagnosed in a 36-year-old woman. A decision is made to treat the patient with radiation, along with paclitaxel and doxorubicin. Which of the following statements regarding cellular motility and contractility is true?

   A. Actin fibers are found mainly in muscle cells.

   B. The interactions between actin and myosin that underlie the contraction of skeletal muscle require calcium but not ATP.

   C. Intermediate filaments extend from the centrosome to the nucleus.

   D. The proteins kinesin and dynein are required for directional transport of cellular components along the microtubules.

   E. The microtubules used to form the spindle apparatus are synthesized de novo before each mitosis.

*Ref.:* 8, 16

**COMMENTS:** The **cytoskeleton** provides the structural framework for the cell. It is composed of three main types of protein polymers: actin filaments, intermediate filaments, and microtubules. **Actin filaments** are found in nearly all types of cells. They form a cortical layer beneath the plasma membrane of most cells, the stress fibers of fibroblasts, and the cytoskeleton of microvilli of intestinal epithelial cells. In muscle cells, the interaction between the heads of myosin (thick filaments) and actin (thin filaments) requires hydrolysis of ATP to separate the filaments at the end of the power stroke. Calcium and troponin C (an actin-associated protein) are also required to expose the binding site for myosin on the actin filament. **Intermediate filaments** are a heterogeneous group of proteins that extend from the nucleus to the cell surface. They interact with other cytoskeletal filaments and binding proteins to produce their effects.

   **Microtubules** arise from the **centrosome**, with the cell's microtubule-organizing center being located near the nucleus. Microtubules are in a constant dynamic equilibrium between assembly and disassembly. Movement of cellular components, such as vacuoles, along the microtubules requires ATP and either of two associated proteins: **kinesin** for movement away from the centrosome and **dynein** for movement toward it. Cilia and flagella contain columns of doublet microtubules in a 9-2 arrangement (nine doublets in a circle surrounding two central doublets). Movement is accomplished when the doublets slide along each other in a process mediated by dynein and fueled by hydrolysis of ATP. Microtubules also play an important role in cell division. Assembly of the **mitotic spindle** involves replication and splitting of the microtubule-organizing center into the two spindle poles and

reorganization of the cytoskeletal microtubules to form the spindle apparatus. **Taxanes** function as mitotic inhibitors by inhibiting depolymerization of the mitotic spindle, which results in a "frozen" mitosis. Paclitaxel is a natural taxane that prevents depolymerization of cellular microtubules. The **vinca alkaloids** (e.g., vinblastine, vincristine) also inhibit cell division, but by disrupting the mitotic spindle. Doxorubicin (Adriamycin) intercalates between DNA base pairs and impairs the progression of topoisomerase II, which unwinds DNA for transcription.

**A N S W E R :**   D

25. A 26-year-old with a history of type 2 neurofibromatosis is scheduled to undergo resection of an acoustic neuroma. The *NF2* gene is located on the long arm of chromosome 22. Which of the following statements regarding chromosomes is not true?

   A. The nucleus contains the entire cellular DNA.

   B. Histones compact and organize the DNA strands.

   C. Interactions between DNA and proteins expose specific genes and control their expression.

   D. During mitosis, the spindle apparatus attaches to the chromosome at the centromere.

   E. Telomeres maintain chromosomal length through the replication cycles.

*Ref.:* 23

**COMMENTS:** **Chromosomes** are formed by the combination of double-stranded helical DNA with **histones** and other proteins. The interactions between DNA and proteins stabilize the chromosomal structure. Most cellular DNA is located in the **nucleus**, although a small portion is found in the **mitochondria**. Each chromosomal double helix contains approximately 108 base pairs. There are several levels of organizational restructuring, from DNA and histones binding to form **chromatin** all the way to the complex folded structure of the chromosome itself. To express a gene, that portion of the chromosome must be unfolded and unwrapped to expose the DNA double helix. **Gene expression** is regulated by the binding of nonchromosomal proteins, called **transcription factors**, to specific regions of the DNA (enhancer and promoter sequences). Several distinct regions of chromosomes are identifiable: the **origins of replication** (sites of initiation of DNA synthesis), the **centromere** (site of spindle attachment during mitosis), and **telomeres** (specialized end structures that maintain the length of the chromosome through replication cycles).

**A N S W E R :**   A

26. A 25-year-old man is admitted to the trauma intensive care unit after sustaining multiple gunshot wounds to the abdomen that necessitated several small bowel resections. On postoperative day 12 the patient begins to have spiking fevers. Blood cultures grow *Serratia*, and the patient is started on an antibiotic regimen that includes gentamicin. Aminoglycosides bind the ribosomal 30S subunit, thereby inhibiting bacterial protein production. Which of the following statements regarding protein synthesis is not true?

   A. Transcription of messenger RNA occurs in the nucleus.

   B. Messenger RNA moves from the nucleus to the cytoplasm and attaches to free ribosomes in the cytoplasm.

   C. The enzyme RNA polymerase catalyzes the transcription of messenger RNA from DNA.

D.  Introns are placed into the DNA transcript by splicing.

E.  Posttranslational processing includes glycosylation and enzymatic cleavage.

*Ref.:* 24

**COMMENTS:** The sequence of nucleotides in DNA determines the amino acid sequence of the protein. Protein synthesis involves (1) **transcription** of messenger RNA from the gene that codes for the protein, (2) **translation** of the messenger RNA into a protein, and (3) **posttranslational processing** of the protein, which may involve enzymatic cleavage or glycosylation of the protein. Transcription takes place in the nucleus, whereas translation and posttranslational processing occur in the rough ER, Golgi complex, or free ribosomes in the cytoplasm. Transcription of messenger RNA from DNA occurs by assembly of complementary base pairs on the DNA template one nucleotide at a time. This step is catalyzed by the enzyme **RNA polymerase**. Eukaryotic genes are interrupted by noncoding regions called **introns**. Introns are removed from the RNA transcript by splicing. The resulting messenger RNA is moved to the cytoplasm, in which it binds to **ribosomes** to begin translation. The initial step in protein synthesis is attachment of the messenger RNA to a ribosome that is preloaded with transfer RNA that recognizes the start codon (three bases) AUG and thus sets the reading frame for the translation. Subsequent binding of aminoacyl-transfer RNA to the ribosomes that match the three nucleotide codons specifying each amino acid results in peptide synthesis as the ribosome moves along the messenger RNA molecule. The first portion of the protein that is synthesized is an amino terminal leader called the **signal peptide**. At this stage, the ribosome becomes attached to the rough ER. As translation continues, the signal peptide is inserted into the rough ER membrane by another transmembrane protein and later cleaved as the peptide elongates.

**ANSWER:** D

27. A 27-year-old woman sustains an incomplete T10 spinal cord injury after falling off a horse. The patient is given 30 mg/kg of methylprednisolone. Which of the following is true regarding steroid hormones and their receptors?

A.  Steroid hormones are synthesized from proteins.

B.  In the bloodstream, steroid hormones often dimerize to facilitate transport.

C.  Steroid hormone receptors are found only in the cytoplasm.

D.  Heat shock proteins (HSPs) are usually associated with cytosolic steroid hormone receptors.

E.  Binding of the steroid hormone to a receptor induces a second messenger cascade to alter cellular metabolism.

*Ref.:* 16

**COMMENTS:** Steroid hormones are synthesized from **cholesterol**. Their lipophilic nature allows them to cross cell membranes easily. Steroid hormones can be divided into five groups based on their receptors: **glucocorticoids**, **mineralocorticoids**, **androgens**, **estrogens**, and **progestogens**. In the bloodstream, steroid hormones are generally bound to specific **carrier proteins** such as sex hormone–binding globulin or corticosteroid-binding globulin. Receptors for steroid hormones are most commonly located in the **cytosol**, although they are also found in the nucleus and on the cell membrane. After binding to the steroid hormone, steroid receptors often dimerize. For many cytosolic steroid receptors, binding of the ligand induces a conformational change and releases **heat shock proteins**. Nuclear steroid receptors are not generally associated with HSPs. HSPs themselves have several roles, including functioning as intracellular chaperones for other proteins, serving as **transcription factors**, and facilitating antigen binding. They may also serve as targets for therapeutics. Ultimately, the activated steroid receptor must enter the nucleus to serve as a transcription factor for augmentation or suppression of the expression of particular genes. The resulting messenger RNA leaves the nucleus for the ribosomes, where it is translated to produce specific proteins.

**ANSWER:** D

28. A 55-year-old man with a history of hepatitis C cirrhosis has complaints of nausea, fever, and progressive lethargy. Part of his evaluation includes an assessment of his hepatitis C viral load. Which of the following tests would be most useful in assessing his hepatitis C viral load?

A.  Western blot

B.  Gel electrophoresis

C.  Fluorescence microscopy

D.  Polymerase chain reaction (PCR)

E.  Expression cloning

*Ref.:* 16

**COMMENTS:** **Western blot** is a technique used to detect specific proteins in a sample. An antibody to the protein of interest is used as a probe. **Gel electrophoresis** is a method for separating proteins or nucleic acids according to size, mass, or composition. It is based on the differential rate of movement of the molecules of interest through a gel when an electric field is applied. **Polymerase chain reaction** is a technique by which DNA may be massively amplified. Primers or oligonucleotides are synthesized to complement one strand of the DNA to be amplified. Amplification involves three temperature-cycled steps: (1) heating for separation (denaturation) of the double-helix structure into two single strands, (2) cooling for hybridization of each single strand with its primer (annealing), and (3) heating for DNA synthesis (elongation). The steps are repeated with exponential amplification of the DNA of interest. When RNA is used, reverse transcriptase is employed initially to transcribe the RNA to DNA before amplification. **Quantitative polymerase chain reaction** can be used in real time to measure the starting concentration of DNA or RNA in a sample, for example, the amount of hepatitis C RNA in a blood sample. With **expression cloning**, DNA coding for a protein of interest is cloned into a **plasmid** (extrachromosomal DNA molecule) that can be inserted into a bacterial or animal cell. The cell expresses the protein, which allows the production of sufficient amounts for study. **Fluorescence microscopy** is performed by labeling a component of interest in a sample with a molecule that absorbs light at one wavelength and emits light at another (fluorescence).

**ANSWER:** D

29. Which of the following methods is most useful for determining the RNA content of a sample?

A.  Southern blotting

B.  Northern blotting

C.  Western blotting

D. PCR

E. None of the above

*Ref.:* 24

**COMMENTS: Blotting** is a method used to study macromolecules (DNA, RNA, or proteins) separated by **gel electrophoresis** (usually by size) and transferred onto a carrier (technically, the transfer is the "blot"). The macromolecules can then be visualized by specific probes or staining methods. A **Southern blot** is used for detection of specific DNA sequences. A **Northern blot** performs the same function but for RNA or mRNA samples. A **Western blot** is used to detect specific proteins in a sample, with an antibody to the protein of interest being used as a probe. An **Eastern blot** is a modification of the Western blot technique that is used to detect posttranslational modification of proteins. There are several other modifications of the technique; for example, Southwestern blotting is used to detect DNA-binding proteins. The origin of the nomenclature is derived from the Southern blot, which is named for its inventor biologist Edwin Southern.

**A N S W E R :**   B

30. What enzyme is responsible for the catalysis of deoxynucleoside triphosphates into DNA?

    A. DNA helicase

    B. DNA ligase

    C. DNA polymerase

    D. DNA primase

    E. All of the above

*Ref.:* 23

**COMMENTS: DNA polymerases** are enzymes that catalyze the assembly of deoxynucleoside triphosphates into DNA. There are several types of DNA polymerases. DNA polymerase III promotes DNA elongation by nucleotide linkage, whereas DNA polymerase I functions to fill gaps and repair DNA. **DNA helicase** is the enzyme involved in unwinding the double-stranded DNA into individual strands before replication, transcription, or repair. **DNA primase** catalyzes the formation of RNA primers used to initiate DNA synthesis. **DNA ligase** joins the DNA fragments generated by the degradation of RNA primers.

**A N S W E R :**   C

31. In DNA replication, what type of mutation is specifically associated with the generation of a stop codon?

    A. Point mutation

    B. Missense mutation

    C. Nonsense mutation

    D. Frameshift mutation

    E. Neutral mutation

*Ref.:* 7

**COMMENTS:** A change in a single base pair is known as a **point mutation**. A single amino acid change resulting from a point mutation is known as a **missense mutation**. A missense mutation may cause changes in the structure of the protein that lead to altered biologic activity. **Nonsense mutations** occur if a point mutation results in the replacement of an amino acid codon with a stop codon. Nonsense mutations lead to premature termination of translation and often result in the loss of encoded protein. **Frameshift mutations** occur when a few base pairs are added or deleted and lead to the introduction of unrelated amino acids or stop codons. A neutral mutation occurs when the change results in the substitution of a different but chemically similar amino acid. Frequently, the amino acids are similar enough that little or no change occurs in the resultant protein.

**A N S W E R :**   C

**R E F E R E N C E S**

1. Alarcon LH, Fink MP: Mediators of the inflammatory response. In Townsend CM, Beauchamp RD, Evers BM, et al, editors: *Sabiston textbook of surgery: the biological basis of modern surgical practice*, ed 18, Philadelphia, 2008, WB Saunders.

2. Ethridge RT, Leong M, Phillips LG: Wound healing. In Townsend CM, Beauchamp RD, Evers BM, et al, editors: *Sabiston textbook of surgery: the biological basis of modern surgical practice*, ed 18, Philadelphia, 2008, WB Saunders.

3. Fine NA, Mustoe TA: Wound Healing. In Mulholland MW, Lillemoe KD, Doherty GM, et al, editors: *Greenfield's surgery: scientific principles and practice*, ed 4, Philadelphia, 2006, Lippincott Williams & Wilkins.

4. Simmons RL, Steel DL: *Basic science review for surgeons*, Philadelphia, 1992, WB Saunders.

5. Gupta S, Lawrence WT: Wound healing normal and abnormal mechanisms and closure techniques. In O'Leary JP, Tabuenca A, editors: *The physiologic basis of surgery*, ed 4, Philadelphia, 2008, Lippincott Williams & Wilkins.

6. Barbul A, Efron DT: Wound healing. In Brunicardi FC, Andersen DK, Billiar TR, et al, editors: *Schwartz's principles of surgery*, ed 9, New York, 2010, McGraw-Hill.

7. Ko TC, Evers BM: Molecular and cell biology. In Townsend CM, Beauchamp RD, Evers BM, et al, editors: *Sabiston textbook of surgery: the biological basis of modern surgical practice*, ed 18, Philadelphia, 2008, WB Saunders.

8. Williams JA, Dawson DC: Cell structure and function. In Mulholland MW, Lillemoe KD, Doherty GM, et al, editors: *Greenfield's surgery: scientific principles and practice*, ed 4, Philadelphia, 2006, Lippincott Williams & Wilkins.

9. Rosengart MR, Billiar TR: Inflammation. In Mulholland MW, Lillemoe KD, Doherty GM, et al, editors: *Greenfield's surgery: scientific principles and practice*, ed 4, Philadelphia, 2006, Lippincott Williams & Wilkins.

10. Peacock EE Jr.: Symposium on biological control of scar tissue, *Plast reconstr surg* 41:8–12, 1968.

11. Barbul A: Immune aspects of wound repair, *Clin Plast Surg* 17:433–442, 1990.

12. Galiano RD, Mustoe TA: Wound care. In Aston S, Seasley R, Thorne C, editors: *Grabb and Smith's plastic surgery*, ed 6, Philadelphia, 2007, Lippincott-Raven.

13. Basson MD, Burney RE: Defective wound healing in patients with paraplegia and quadriplegia, *Surg Gynecol Obstet* 155:9–12, 1982.

14. Gurtner GC: Wound Healing: Normal and Abnormal. In Aston S, Seasley R, Thorne C, editors: *Grabb and Smith's plastic surgery*, ed 6, Philadelphia, 2007, Lippincott-Raven.

15. Martindale RG, Zhou M: Nutrition and metabolism. In O'Leary JP, Tabuenca A, editors: *The physiologic basis of surgery*, ed 4, Philadelphia, 2008, Lippincott Williams & Wilkins.

16. Reeves ME: Cell biology. In O'Leary JP, Tabuenca A, editors: *The physiologic basis of surgery*, ed 4, Philadelphia, 2008, Lippincott Williams & Wilkins.

17. Transport across cell membranes. In Lodish H, Berk A, Zipursky SL, et al, editors: *Molecular cell biology*, New York, 1999, Scientific American Books.

18. Biomembranes and the subcellular organization of eukaryotic cells. In Lodish H, Berk A, Zipursky SL, et al, editors: *Molecular cell biology*, New York, 1999, Scientific American Books.

19. Protein sorting, organelle biogenesis and protein secretion. In Lodish H, Berk A, Zipursky SL, et al, editors: *Molecular cell biology*, New York, 1999, Scientific American Books.
20. The dynamic cell. In Lodish H, Berk A, Zipursky SL, et al, editors: *Molecular cell biology*, New York, 1999, Scientific American Books.
21. Radiosensitivity and cell age in the mitotic cycle. In Hall EJ, Amato JG, editors: *Radiobiology for the radiologist*, ed 6, Philadelphia, 2005, Lippincott Williams & Wilkins.
22. Cellular energetics, glycolysis, aerobic oxidation and photosynthesis. In Lodish H, Berk A, Zipursky SL, et al, editors: *Molecular cell biology*, New York, 1999, Scientific American Books.
23. DNA replication, repair and recombination. In Lodish H, Berk A, Zipursky SL, et al, editors: *Molecular cell biology*, New York, 1999, Scientific American Books.
24. Recombinant DNA and genomics. In Lodish H, Berk A, Zipursky SL, et al, editors: *Molecular cell biology*, New York, 1999, Scientific American Books.

# CHAPTER 3

# Hemostasis and Transfusion

*Chad E. Jacobs, M.D.; Leonard A. Valentino, M.D.;*
*Lisa N. Boggio, M.S., M.D.; and Bruce C. McLeod, M.D.*

1. With regard to normal hemostasis, which of the following statements is true?

   A. Vascular disruption is followed by vasoconstriction mediated by vasoactive substances released by activated platelets.

   B. Platelet adhesion is mediated by fibrin monomers.

   C. The endothelial surface supports platelet adhesion and thrombus formation.

   D. Heparin inhibits adenosine diphosphate (ADP)-stimulated platelet aggregation.

   E. A prolonged bleeding time may be due to thrombocytopenia, a qualitative platelet defect, or reduced amounts of von Willebrand factor.

   *Ref.:* 1-3

**COMMENTS:** Blood fluidity is maintained by the action of inhibitors of blood coagulation and by the nonthrombogenic vascular surface. Three physiologic reactions mediate initial **hemostasis** following vascular injury: (1) the vascular response (vasoconstriction) to injury; (2) platelet activation, adherence, and aggregation; and (3) generation of thrombin with subsequent conversion of fibrinogen to fibrin. Injury exposes subendothelial components and induces vasoconstriction independent of platelet participation, which results in decreased blood flow but an increase in local shear force. Within seconds, platelets are activated by the increase in shear force and adhere to exposed subendothelial collagen by a mechanism dependent on the participation of von Willebrand factor. Adhesion stimulates the release of platelet ADP, thereby mediating the recruitment of additional platelets. Fibrinogen binds to activated platelet receptors, and platelet aggregation follows to create a primary hemostatic plug. Formation of the plug requires calcium and magnesium and is not affected by heparin. Bleeding time measurements reflect the time that it takes to form this platelet plug. A reduction in platelet number or function, loss of vascular integrity, or a reduction in the amount or function of von Willebrand factor may prolong the bleeding time.

**ANSWER:** E

2. With regard to drug effects and platelet function, which of the following statements is true?

   A. Vasoconstricting agents such as epinephrine, prostaglandin $G_2$ and $H_2$ ($PGG_2$ and $PGH_2$), and thromboxane $A_2$ reduce levels of cyclic adenosine monophosphate (cAMP) and induce platelet aggregation.

   B. Vasodilators such as prostaglandin $E_1$ ($PGE_1$), prostacyclin ($PGI_2$), theophylline, and dipyridamole elevate cAMP levels and block platelet aggregation.

   C. Aspirin and indomethacin interfere with platelet release of ADP and inhibit aggregation.

   D. Furosemide competitively inhibits $PGE_2$.

   E. The effect of aspirin is reversible in 2 to 3 days.

   *Ref.:* 1-4

**COMMENTS:** Aspirin, indomethacin, and most other nonsteroidal antiinflammatory drugs (NSAIDs) are inhibitors of prostaglandin synthesis. They block the formation of $PGG_2$ and $PGH_2$ from platelet arachidonic acid and, as a result, inhibit **platelet aggregation**. $PGI_2$, $PGE_1$, and thromboxane $A_2$ stimulate cAMP production, whereas dipyridamole and theophylline derivatives block its degradation. Aspirin inhibits thromboxane production, acetylates fibrinogen, interferes with fibrin formation, and makes fibrin susceptible to accelerated fibrinolysis. The effect of aspirin begins within 2 hours, is irreversible, and lasts the 7- to 9-day life span of affected platelets. The clinical result is increased bruising and bleeding and increased risk for surgical bleeding. Platelet counts are normal, but the bleeding time is prolonged. Furosemide competitively inhibits ADP-induced platelet aggregation and reduces the response of platelets to $PGG_2$. Furosemide may also cause thrombocytopenia. A wide variety of drugs inhibit platelet function.

**ANSWER:** B

3. With regard to blood coagulation, which of the following statements is true?

   A. The principal complex initiating blood coagulation is the tissue factor (TF)–factor VIIa complex.

   B. Coagulation is initiated in the fluid phase of blood.

   C. Only endothelial cells express TF.

   D. The factor Xa-Va complex converts fibrinogen to fibrin in quantities sufficient to activate platelets.

   E. Antithrombin is the main regulator of blood coagulation.

   *Ref.:* 1, 2

**COMMENTS: Coagulation** is initiated on a phospholipid surface, such as the monocyte or fibroblast membrane, following expression of TF. TF binds factor VII, which is then activated by minor proteolysis through an autocatalytic mechanism or by the action of thrombin or other serine proteases. The TF–factor VIIa complex is a potent serine protease that activates factors X and IX. Factor Xa combines with factor Va on the phospholipid surface to convert prothrombin to thrombin. The amount of thrombin generated by this reaction is insufficient for the formation of a stable fibrin clot. It is sufficient, however, to activate platelets, dissociate factor VIII from von Willebrand factor, and activate factors V, VIII, and XI. Factor IXa, formed by the action of the TF–factor VIIa complex, binds to activated platelets and associates with factor VIIIa, which then recruits circulating factor X to the platelet surface and converts it to factor Xa. Platelet-bound factor Xa and its cofactor, factor Va, generate sufficient quantities of thrombin to form a stable fibrin clot. The catalytic activity of the TF–factor VIIa–factor Xa complex is regulated by tissue factor pathway inhibitor (TFPI). TFPI binds to factor Xa, thereby limiting the activity of the complex.

**A N S W E R :**   A

4. With regard to fibrinolysis, which of the following statements is true?

   A. Plasmin is not a significant factor in fibrinolysis.

   B. Plasminogen deficiency results in a clinical bleeding disorder.

   C. Plasmin acts only on cross-linked fibrin polymers.

   D. Ischemia is a potent activator of the fibrinolytic system.

   E. Physiologic fibrinolysis does not occur.

*Ref.:* 1-3

**COMMENTS:** Plasminogen is converted to plasmin by a number of enzymes, including blood-borne activators and tissue activators such as thrombin, streptokinase, urokinase, and kallikrein. Ischemia is also a potent stimulator of activation of the fibrinolytic system. Plasmin acts on fibrin, fibrinogen, factor V, and factor VIII. Physiologic **fibrinolysis** is the result of the natural affinity of plasminogen for fibrin. Plasminogen is incorporated into the clot, and fibrinolysis is locally controlled. Pathologic fibrinolysis occurs when plasminogen that is free in plasma is activated, which leads to the proteolysis of fibrinogen, fibrin, and other coagulation factors. Unrestrained fibrinolysis can result in bleeding for several reasons: small fibrin fragments are capable of interfering with normal platelet aggregation, large fibrin fragments join the clot instead of the normal monomers and produce an unstable clot, fibrin fragments interfere with cleavage of fibrinogen by thrombin, and destruction of clotting factors other than fibrin results in a consumptive coagulopathy. Blood and platelets contain antifibrinolytic substances capable of inhibition of plasminogen. Physiologic fibrinolysis plays an important role in tissue repair, cancer metastasis, ovulation, and embryo implantation. Disorders of fibrinolysis can result from excessive activity (bleeding) or insufficient activity (thrombosis).

**A N S W E R :**   D

5. With regard to measurement of bleeding times, which of the following statements is true?

   A. Spontaneous bleeding may occur with platelet counts higher than 15,000/µL.

   B. Platelet counts higher than 150,000/µL exclude the possibility of a primary hemostatic disorder.

   C. Bleeding time is a predictor of surgical bleeding.

   D. Platelet counts higher than 50,000/µl are usually associated with a normal bleeding time and adequate surgical hemostasis.

   E. Normal bleeding time excludes von Willebrand disease as a potential factor affecting surgical hemostasis.

*Ref.:* 1, 3

**COMMENTS:** The **bleeding time** is a crude measure of platelet function, the number of platelets, or both. The normal value is 3 to 9 minutes and implies normal platelet function and counts greater than 50,000/µl. Spontaneous bleeding rarely occurs when the platelet count is greater than 30,000/µl. The bleeding time is prolonged in patients with normal platelet counts in whom qualitative abnormalities are present as a primary platelet disorder or one secondary to drugs, uremia, or liver disease or in those who have thrombasthenia or a variety of other defects in platelet function. Patients with defective platelets or capillaries, those with von Willebrand disease, and those with a history of recent ingestion of aspirin, NSAIDs, antibiotics (penicillins and cephalosporins), and a wide variety of miscellaneous drugs also have prolonged bleeding times. False-negative (normal) bleeding times are frequently due to the technical difficulty of performing the test and its lack of sensitivity. For example, only 60% of patients with von Willebrand disease have a prolonged bleeding time. Other tests of **platelet function** include assessment of platelet aggregation in response to a variety of agonists.

**A N S W E R :**   D

6. Which of the following conditions is associated with an isolated prothrombin time (PT) prolongation?

   A. von Willebrand disease

   B. Factor VIII deficiency (hemophilia A)

   C. Common pathway factor deficiencies (factors II, V, and X and fibrinogen)

   D. Therapeutic anticoagulation with warfarin (Coumadin)

   E. Therapeutic anticoagulation with heparin

*Ref.:* 1, 2

**COMMENTS:** The one-stage **prothrombin time** is used to measure the function of fibrinogen and factors II, V, X, and VII. The **partial thromboplastin time** (PTT) reflects the function of fibrinogen and factors II, V, X, VIII, IX, XI, and XII. Fibrinogen and factors II, V, and X are common to both tests. Both tests require comparison with normal control values obtained daily in the laboratory. Because of the antithrombin effect of heparin, even trace amounts prolong the PTT and thrombin time. At least 5 hours must elapse after the last dose of intravenous heparin before the PTT can be reliably interpreted. The thrombin time is a measure of the ability to generate fibrin and is prolonged by deficiencies and abnormalities of fibrinogen or the presence of heparin or fibrinogen degradation products. The thrombin time, together with the PT and PTT, can distinguish whether factors are deficient in the first or second stage of coagulation. A normal PT and thrombin time with an abnormal PTT in the absence of clinical bleeding suggest deficiencies of factor XII, high-molecular-weight kininogen, or prekallikrein or the presence of a lupus anticoagulant. The same laboratory values obtained for a bleeding patient suggest deficiency of factor VIII, IX, or XI. A normal PTT and thrombin time with an abnormal PT suggest factor VII deficiency. A prolonged thrombin time with an abnormal PTT and PT suggests the presence of hepatocellular liver disease or a consumptive coagulopathy if the platelet count is decreased or an abnormality of fibrinogen if the platelet count is normal. Factor VIII is synthesized in the endothelial cells of the liver and is therefore not affected by hepatocellular disease. A decrease in factor VIII can be used to differentiate consumptive coagulopathy (reduced levels of all factors) from hepatocellular liver disease (reduced levels of all factors except factor VIII). The PTT is also prolonged by heparin administration and can be used to monitor its efficacy. Calculation of the **international normalized ratio** (INR) from the PT is the preferred method of controlling anticoagulation with warfarin (Coumadin). Vitamin K is necessary for the full function of factors II, VII, IX, and X, and therefore its deficiency is reflected by prolongation of both the PT and PTT.

**ANSWER:** D

7. All of the following statements regarding complications of transfusion are false except:

A. Febrile reactions are rare.

B. Gram-positive organisms are the most common contaminants of stored blood.

C. Screening for minor antigens should be repeated every week when multiple transfusions are given.

D. A small amount (more than 0.1 cc) of intravenous air is well tolerated.

E. Malaria, Chagas disease, human T-cell leukemia virus I (HTLV-I), acquired immunodeficiency syndrome (AIDS), and hepatitis can be transmitted by blood transfusions.

*Ref.:* 1, 4

**COMMENTS:** Febrile reactions are the most common **complications** of red blood cell and platelet transfusions and occur once per 100 units given. Fever and chills are the usual symptoms. If mild, these symptoms respond to antipyretics. In severe cases, they are treated with opiates. Urticarial reactions are the most common reaction to plasma transfusions. They usually respond to antihistamines. Anaphylactic reactions are rare and are treated with epinephrine and steroids. Although unusual, gram-negative organisms capable of surviving at 4° C are the most common cause of bacterial contamination of banked blood. Platelets, which are optimally stored at room temperature and are being used increasingly, are a more frequent source of sepsis, usually with gram-positive organisms. Air embolism has become rare since bottles have been replaced by collapsible plastic containers. Even small volumes of air have the potential to cause fatal complications and should be avoided whenever possible. Hepatitis viruses B and C (HBV and HCV), human immunodeficiency virus (HIV), HTLV-I and HTLV-II, malaria, Chagas disease, and other infections can be transmitted by transfusion. Specific testing of donors is available for HBV, HCV, HIV, and HTLV. Health, immigration, and travel histories are used to exclude donors who may harbor malaria or Chagas disease and are being used to control a perceived "theoretical risk" for variant Creutzfeldt-Jakob disease. Recipient alloimmunization to "minor" antigens may occur after multiple transfusions, in which case red blood cells lacking the relevant antigen must be transfused. To detect or exclude such alloimmunization, recipient serum samples should be screened for antibodies. This screening should be repeated every 48 to 72 hours if multiple transfusions are given. It can take several hours to identify the blood's antibody specificity (e.g., anti-C and anti-K antibodies) and find donor red blood cells that lack the relevant antigen or antigens. This unavoidable delay

can be problematic for same-day surgery patients who have not had a blood bank sample drawn in advance.

**ANSWER:** E

8. With regard to evaluating bleeding in surgical patients, which of the following statements is true?

A. Bleeding from a resected prostatic bed indicates poor local hemostasis.

B. The most common cause of surgical bleeding is incomplete mechanical hemostasis.

C. ε-Aminocaproic acid is an excellent topical hemostatic agent for nonmucosal wounds.

D. Bleeding from a surgical wound along with bleeding from other sites implies poor local hemostasis.

E. The bleeding time is an excellent predictor of surgical bleeding.

*Ref.:* 1, 2, 4

**COMMENTS: Bleeding from the surgical wound** suggests ineffective local hemostasis, particularly if associated wounds (e.g., drain sites, tracheostomy wounds, or intravenous infusion sites) are not bleeding. An exception is isolated bleeding from a resected prostatic bed, in which prostate-borne plasminogen activators can be activated by urokinase. Activation is inhibited by ε-aminocaproic acid. Blood transfusions can lead to bleeding via a number of mechanisms. Transfusion of more than one blood volume produces thrombocytopenia by dilution. Patients bleeding after a large number of blood transfusions should be considered thrombocytopenic and be treated as such. Nonetheless, additional evaluation is indicated because an alternative explanation for transfusion-associated bleeding is a hemolytic transfusion reaction. In such an instance, disseminated intravascular coagulopathy (DIC) is caused by thromboplastic activity of factors liberated from the stroma of lysed red blood cells. Extracorporeal circulation may induce hemostatic failure as a result of thrombocytopenia, inadequate reversal of heparinization, or overadministration of protamine. Septic surgical patients may bleed because of endotoxin-induced thrombocytopenia. Defibrination and bleeding may occur in patients with meningococcemia, *Clostridium perfringens* sepsis, or staphylococcal sepsis. Uncommonly, an operation on tissues rich in fibrinolytic activity, such as those of the pancreas, liver, or lungs, may lead to pathologic fibrinolysis and bleeding.

**ANSWER:** B

9. When evaluating a patient who bleeds unexpectedly, which of the following statements is true?

A. The most reliable test for detecting patients at risk for bleeding is a platelet count.

B. Infants who do not bleed during circumcision have normal hemostatic function.

C. An isolated episode of gastrointestinal bleeding is often associated with generalized hemostatic disorders.

D. Jaundice is a sign of an underlying congenital bleeding disorder.

E. The presence of healthy parents and siblings does not exclude the possibility of a primary hemostatic disorder.

*Ref.:* 2, 3

**COMMENTS:** No single test for detecting patients at **risk for bleeding** exists. The best protocol is a complete history and physical examination. Many normal individuals consider themselves to have a positive bleeding history. Because aspirin is contained in a wide variety of over-the-counter medications, its use is easily overlooked in the patient's medical history. Circumcision typically involves significant trauma to tissues and activation of the TF–factor VIIa pathway. Just 30% of affected males bleed following circumcision. Only rarely do patients with a bleeding disorder undergo tooth extraction or tonsillectomy without encountering a bleeding problem. Some patients with a severe bleeding disorder experience bleeding with tooth eruption. Isolated gastrointestinal bleeding is unusual in patients with congenital bleeding disorders. Epistaxis is one of the most common symptoms of von Willebrand disease and platelet disorders. Excessive menstrual flow (menorrhagia), but not intermenstrual bleeding, is common in patients with hemostatic disorders. Because inherited bleeding defects may be autosomal dominant, autosomal recessive, or sex-linked recessive, an inquiry into the family history should account for bleeding problems in grandparents, aunts, uncles, and cousins. Since patients' assessment of severity is subjective, objective indicators should be sought, such as need for a prolonged hospital stay for minor surgery, transfusion, and anemia. A search for ecchymosis or petechiae, particularly near pressure points, is essential. The lesions of hereditary hemorrhagic telangiectasia are found on the lips, underneath the fingernails, and around the anus. Signs of liver disease suggest the presence of an acquired deficiency of the prothrombin complex, not a predisposition to primary hemostatic disorders.

**ANSWER:** E

10. With regard to classic hemophilia, which of the following statements is true?

   A. The incidence in the general population is 1 in 5000.

   B. A given patient's baseline factor VIII or IX level may fluctuate with stress.

   C. Muscle compartment bleeding is the most common orthopedic problem.

   D. Factor VIII replacement therapy is required before any elective surgery.

   E. Therapy with cryoprecipitated plasma is free of risk for hepatitis.

*Ref.:* 1-3

**COMMENTS:** Bleeding in patients with **hemophilia** usually appears during early childhood. Hemarthrosis is the most common orthopedic problem. Epistaxis, hematuria, and intracranial bleeding may occur. Equinus contracture, Volkmann contracture of the forearm, and flexion contracture of the elbows or knees are sequelae of these bleeding episodes. Retroperitoneal or intramural intestinal bleeding may produce abdominal symptoms. The level of factor VIII or IX in plasma (which tends to remain stable throughout life) determines the tendency to bleed. Spontaneous bleeding is frequent in patients with severe disease, defined as less than 1% factor VIII or IX activity. Bleeding typically occurs with trauma in patients with moderately severe disease, defined as 1% to 5% factor activity. In patients with mild hemophilia A or B, defined as 6% to 25% factor activity, bleeding typically occurs only with major trauma or surgery. The factor VIII or IX level must be raised to at least 30% to achieve hemostasis and control minor hemorrhage. A level of approximately 50% is required to control joint and muscle bleeding, whereas a level of 80% to 100% is necessary to treat life-threatening hemorrhage (central nervous system, retroperitoneal,

or retropharyngeal bleeding) and to prepare patients for elective surgery. After elective surgery, levels of 25% should be maintained for at least 2 weeks. Transmission of hepatitis or HIV, the development of neutralizing antibodies, and qualitative platelet dysfunction are possible complications of factor replacement therapy. Appropriate replacement includes infusions of factor VIII and factor IX. These products are available in both recombinant and highly purified concentrates that are virally inactivated. Cryoprecipitate is not optimal replacement therapy for factor VIII and von Willebrand factor, does not contain factor IX, and is associated with a risk of viral transmission.

**ANSWER:** D

11. A 12-year-old boy with known factor VIII deficiency has a painful, swollen, immobile right knee. The clinician suspects hemarthrosis. Therapeutic options include which of the following?

   A. Immediate aspiration and compression dressings to prevent cartilage necrosis

   B. Compression dressings and immobilization to prevent further bleeding

   C. Immediate aspiration after appropriate factor VIII replacement therapy

   D. Initial trial of factor VIII therapy, compression dressings, cold packs, and rest followed by active range-of-motion exercises

   E. None of the above is an appropriate option

*Ref.:* 1, 2

**COMMENTS:** Treatment of **hemarthrosis** is aimed at preventing chronic synovitis and degenerative arthritis. Early, intensive factor VIII therapy is critical for limiting the extent of hemorrhage. Factor VIII replacement therapy is most effective when initiated before swelling of the joint capsule. Frequently, replacement therapy is initiated before the onset of any objective physical findings, when the patient perceives only subtle signs of joint hemorrhage. Factor VIII therapy, joint rest, compression dressing, and cold packs constitute the usual initial therapy. Aspiration is to be avoided. The goal of treatment of hemarthrosis is maintenance of range of motion. Active range-of-motion exercises should begin 24 hours after factor VIII therapy. Compression and cold packs should be continued for 3 to 5 days.

**ANSWER:** D

12. With regard to von Willebrand disease, which of the following statements is true?

   A. It is more common than hemophilia.

   B. It is best treated with cryoprecipitated plasma.

   C. Factor VIII levels are constant over time in a given patient.

   D. There is an associated platelet abnormality in 30% of patients.

   E. Bleeding after elective surgery is rare.

*Ref.:* 1, 2

**COMMENTS: von Willebrand disease** is the most common congenital bleeding disorder, with 1% of the population being affected. The prevalence of patients with symptomatic bleeding is approximately 1 in 1000. Most patients have mild disease unless challenged by trauma or surgery. von Willebrand disease is associated with a variable deficiency of both von Willebrand factor and factor VIII. A platelet defect is also present in most patients. The severity of coagulation abnormalities varies from patient to patient and from time to time for a given patient. In all but 1% to 2% of patients, the bleeding manifestations are milder than those of classic hemophilia. In the same group of patients with type 3 von Willebrand disease, bleeding is more severe than in hemophilia. Bleeding is treated with desmopressin (DDAVP), which induces the release of von Willebrand factor from storage sites in endothelial cells and platelets. The effect of DDAVP is rapid, with maximal procoagulant effects being reached in 1 to 2 hours. The effects dissipate quickly (within 12 to 24 hours), thus necessitating repeated dosing. When more than two or three doses of DDAVP are given, the effects may diminish or are absent. DDAVP is most effective for type 1 disease and is not effective for type 3 disease. Because of a risk for thrombocytopenia, DDAVP is specifically contraindicated for type 2B disease but may be effective for other forms of type 2 disease. In type 3 and most type 2 von Willebrand disease, specific von Willebrand factor replacement product should be administered.

**A N S W E R :**  A

13. With regard to hereditary hemostatic disorders, which of the following statements is not true?

   A. Deficiencies of any of the four vitamin K–dependent factors (II, V, VII, and X) may be treated with stored plasma.

   B. Factor VII has the shortest intravascular half-life of any clotting factor.

   C. Factor IX deficiency is clinically indistinguishable from factor VIII deficiency.

   D. Factor V is known as a labile factor.

   E. Factor XI deficiency is treated with plasma.

*Ref.:* 2, 4

**COMMENTS:** Factor V is not vitamin K dependent. Factor VIII and IX deficiencies are clinically indistinguishable. Bleeding in patients with factor IX deficiency (Christmas disease) is treated with factor IX concentrate. Prothrombin complex concentrate (PCC) contains mainly the **vitamin K–dependent clotting factors**. Use of PCC may be complicated by thrombosis or DIC. In older patients, administration of PCC should be accompanied by prophylactic administration of low-dose heparin. Deficiency of factor XI (Rosenthal syndrome) or factor V is treated with plasma. Because factor V is labile and activity is lost with storage, fresh plasma is necessary. Deficiency of factor VII is treated with recombinant activated factor VII (rFVIIa), and deficiency of factor X (Stuart-Prower deficiency) or II is treated with plasma or PCC. The duration and frequency of treatment with plasma-derived products are inversely proportional to the intravascular half-life.

**A N S W E R :**  A

14. True statements regarding acquired hypofibrinogenemia include which of the following?

   A. The thrombin time aids in differentiating primary fibrinolysis from DIC.

   B. Release of excessive plasminogen activators causes pathologic fibrinolysis.

   C. Primary fibrinolysis can be differentiated from DIC on the basis of the PT, PTT, and thrombin time.

   D. The most important aspect of the treatment of DIC is adequate heparinization.

   E. Thrombocytopenia is common with pure fibrinolysis.

*Ref.:* 1-3

**COMMENTS:** DIC results from the introduction of thromboplastic material into the circulation, which leads to activation of the coagulation system and secondary "protective" **fibrinolysis** (Box 3-1). Transfusion reactions, crush injuries, hemorrhagic perinatal complications, disseminated cancer, and bacterial sepsis have been implicated as causes. The release of excessive plasminogen-activating substances leads to primary pathologic fibrinolysis. Shock, hypoxia, sepsis, disseminated prostate cancer, cirrhosis, portal hypertension, and peritoneovenous shunts are possible causes. The thrombin time is a measurement of the clotting time of plasma. In the absence of heparin or the by-products of fibrinolysis, fibrinogen abnormalities or deficiencies may be detected. Pathologic fibrinolysis causes a prolonged thrombin time, as well as rapid whole blood clot dissolution. Whole blood clot lysis, which normally takes as long as 48 hours, may occur in as few as 2 hours in patients with increased fibrinolysis. The presence of a paraprotein may cause false-positive results for the thrombin time and other tests based on whole blood clotting measurements. Differentiation between DIC and "protective" fibrinolysis on laboratory grounds alone is difficult, although thrombocytopenia is rarely seen with pure fibrinolysis. For both entities, treating the underlying medical or surgical problem is the most important single step. With **disseminated intravascular coagulopathy**, maintenance of a patent microcirculation is important. Adequate fluid volumes and heparinization may be necessary. Active bleeding should be appropriately treated with factor replacement and does not accelerate DIC. Clotting factors can be replenished with fresh frozen plasma and cryoprecipitate. Heparin alone is rarely useful for the treatment of acute DIC. Activated protein C concentrates may be beneficial. Administration of heparin to patients with primary pathologic fibrinolysis can be dangerous, as is administering ε-aminocaproic acid to patients with secondary fibrinolysis. Correction of the underlying cause is the most important component in the treatment of DIC.

**A N S W E R :**  B

---

**BOX 3-1  Examples of Disseminated Intravascular Coagulation Syndromes**

**"Fast" DIC**

Amniotic fluid embolism
Abruptio placentae
Septic abortion
Septicemia
Massive tissue injury
Incompatible blood transfusion
Purpura fulminans

**"Slow" DIC**

Acute promyelocytic leukemia
Dead fetus syndrome
Transfusion of activated prothrombin complex concentrates
Carcinomas
Kasabach-Merritt syndrome
Liver disease

---

15. With regard to polycythemia vera, which of the following statements is not true?

   A. Spontaneous thrombosis is a complication of polycythemia vera.

B. Spontaneous hemorrhage is a possible complication of polycythemia vera.

C. The reason for bleeding is a deficit in platelet function.

D. A hematocrit of less than 48% and a platelet count of less than 400,000/µl are desirable before an elective operation is performed on a patient with polycythemia vera.

E. Postoperative complication rates may be as high as 60%.

*Ref.:* 2, 3

**COMMENTS:** Patients with untreated **polycythemia** vera are at high risk for postoperative bleeding or thrombosis. The complication rate is highest with uncontrolled erythrocytosis. Increased viscosity and platelet count, along with a tendency toward stasis, may explain the spontaneous thrombosis seen in patients with polycythemia vera. Patients most likely to bleed are those with platelet counts greater than 1.5 million/µl. Polycythemia vera may cause a qualitative defect in platelet function. When possible, surgery should be delayed until the hematocrit and platelet count can be medically reduced. Phlebotomy may help in acute situations. Complication rates as high as 46% have been reported in patients with polycythemia vera undergoing surgery. Spontaneous hemorrhage, thrombosis, a combination of hemorrhage and thrombosis, and infection are the major complications.

**ANSWER:** E

16. With regard to anticoagulation, which of the following statements is not true?

A. Warfarin (Coumadin) inhibits the generation of vitamin K–dependent factors (II, VII, IX, and X).

B. Heparin enhances the effect of antithrombin on thrombin-mediated conversion of fibrinogen to fibrin.

C. Theoretically, 1.28 mg of protamine neutralizes 1 mg of heparin.

D. The effects of vitamin K reversal take 48 hours.

E. An INR of 1.5 or less is considered safe for surgery.

*Ref.:* 2, 5

**COMMENTS:** With meticulous hemostatic technique, many operations can be performed on patients with an **international normalized ratio** of 1.5 or less. Exceptions include operations on the eye or the prostate, neurosurgical procedures, or blind needle aspiration. In these cases, an INR of less than 1.2 is required. Patients who are undergoing anticoagulant treatment with warfarin and require emergency surgery may be given plasma to immediately reverse the warfarin effect. Alternatively, vitamin K may be given orally or subcutaneously at least 6 hours preoperatively to reverse the effect of warfarin on vitamin K–dependent factors. The INR should be determined again before surgery, and if it is not below 1.5, plasma should be administered. The efficacy of rFVIIa and PCC in reversing the INR has been demonstrated in several clinical scenarios. These agents have the advantage of directly activating the hemostatic mechanism and generating high concentrations of thrombin. Use of rFVIIa should be reserved for patients with life-threatening hemorrhage and a significantly elevated INR (>6) in whom emergency surgery is anticipated. An INR greater than 1.5 is a contraindication to intramuscular medications.

**ANSWER:** D

17. With regard to the storage of banked blood, which of the following statements is true?

A. Packed red blood cells stored in additive solution (AS-3) and kept at 4° C are suitable for transfusion for 3 months.

B. Platelets in banked blood retain their function for 3 days.

C. Factors II, VII, IX, and XI are stable at 4° C.

D. A decrease in red blood cell oxygen affinity occurs during storage as a result of a decrease in 2,3-diphosphoglycerate (2,3-DPG) levels.

E. There is a significant rate of hemolysis in stored blood.

*Ref.:* 4

**COMMENTS: Packed red blood cells** properly collected and stored at 4° C in AS-3 additive solution are "good" for 42 days. The proportion of cells removed from the circulation within 24 hours of transfusion increases with time that the blood is in storage, with about 25% being depleted at 42 days. This percentage defines satisfactory shelf life. Any blood component that has been stored in an "open" system (e.g., frozen red blood cells after thawing and deglycerolization) has a useful life of just 24 hours because of concerns about contamination. Cells that survive the first 24 hours live out their remaining life span, and some transfused cells can be detected for up to 120 days—the life span of a normal red blood cell. **Platelets in packed red blood cells** become nonfunctional during the first 6 hours of storage. Red blood cell adenosine triphosphate (ATP) and 2,3-DPG levels fall during storage. Oxygen affinity is increased until 2,3-DPG levels rise again after transfusion. Factors II, VII, IX, and XI are stable at 4° C, whereas factors V and VIII are not. To maintain factor V and VIII activity, plasma must be frozen shortly after the blood is drawn (fresh frozen plasma). Lactic acid concentrations increase and the pH falls in packed red blood cells during storage, whereas potassium and ammonia concentrations rise steadily. The citrate used for preservation may reduce plasma ionized calcium if large volumes are transfused. These metabolites are especially significant in pediatric patients and in those with impaired liver or renal function (or both).

**ANSWER:** C

18. In cirrhotic patients who are actively bleeding, the coagulopathy of end-stage liver disease can be differentiated from DIC most readily by estimation of which of the following factors?

A. Factor II

B. Factor V

C. Factor VII

D. Factor VIII:C

E. Factor X

*Ref.:* 3

**COMMENTS:** Of all of the coagulation factors, only factor VIII:C is not produced by hepatocytes. It is manufactured by reticuloendothelial cells, and levels are typically increased in the presence of **cirrhosis**. Reductions in factor VIII:C are observed in patients with DIC because it is consumed along with the other coagulation factors.

**ANSWER:** D

**19.** With regard to leukocytes in cellular blood components (red blood cells and platelets), which of the following statements is true?

    A. Febrile reactions occur in 10% of all transfusions.

    B. Washing red blood cells with saline solution is the best way to remove leukocytes.

    C. Leukocyte reduction lowers the rate of febrile reactions to cellular components from 10% to 1%.

    D. Leukocyte reduction of cellular components lowers the risk of alloimmunization to HLA antigens in transfusion recipients.

    E. Leukocyte reduction of cellular components lowers the risk of wound infection in transfused surgical patients.

*Ref.:* 4

**COMMENTS: Transfused leukocytes** may interact with preexisting recipient HLA antibodies. In addition, leukocytes in platelets that are stored at room temperature may elaborate pyrogenic cytokines during storage, such as interleukin-6. Either mechanism may cause a febrile reaction in a susceptible recipient. Leukocyte reduction filters are 100 to 1000 times more effective than washing for removing leukocytes from packed red blood cells. Thus, filtration is the preferred method. (Washed red blood cells are virtually free of plasma proteins and can be given safely to patients who have had severe allergic or anaphylactic reactions to plasma.) Less than 1% of transfusions cause a (usually mild) febrile reaction. Fifty percent to 70% of these reactions may be prevented by leukocyte reduction. Use of leukocyte-reduced components to avoid febrile reactions is justified only in patients who have repeated reactions despite premedication with antipyretics. A more important indication for leukocyte-reduced components is to prevent the formation of HLA antibodies in candidates for kidney, heart, or lung transplantation and in patients expected to need long-term platelet support. Despite a long-standing suspicion that transfusions may be immunosuppressive, large prospective controlled studies have not shown lower mortality rates, shorter hospital stays, or lower rates of postoperative infection in transfused surgical patients who received only leukocyte-reduced cellular components.

**ANSWER: D**

**20.** With regard to hemolytic transfusion reactions, which of the following statements is true?

    A. They are generally caused by ABO incompatibility.

    B. Urticaria and pruritus are the most common symptoms.

    C. Acidification of the urine prevents precipitation of hemoglobin.

    D. Intravenous diphenhydramine (Benadryl) should be given immediately.

    E. Laboratory findings include a negative direct hemoglobin test result and no free hemoglobin in a posttransfusion blood sample.

*Ref.:* 4

**COMMENTS:** The most common cause of a fatal **hemolytic transfusion reaction** is a clerical error that results in the transfusion of red blood cells of the wrong ABO type of blood. Because the severity is proportional to the antigen dose, constant awareness, early recognition, and immediate intervention are important. Hemolytic reactions lead to complement-mediated intravascular red blood cell destruction, hemoglobinemia, and hemoglobinuria. They also lead to the release of vasoactive amines through the activation of complement. This in turn results in shock, renal ischemia, tubular necrosis, and renal failure proportional to the depth and duration of hypotension. Red blood cell lipids initiate DIC in 8% to 30% of patients in whom a full unit of mismatched blood has been transfused. However, as little as 10 mL can produce serious hypotension and DIC. Typical signs and symptoms include chills, fever, lumbar and chest pain, pain at the infusion site, and hypotension. In anesthetized patients, diffuse bleeding and continued hypotension suggest the diagnosis. Laboratory criteria are positive direct antiglobulin test results, hemoglobinemia with free hemoglobin concentrations higher than 5 mg/dL, and serologic confirmation of incompatibility. Because hemoglobin is a highly chromogenic molecule, small amounts (as little as 30 mg/dL) can be detected visually. The hemoglobin from as little as 5 mL of red blood cells makes the plasma pink and produces hemoglobinuria. Treatment includes stopping the transfusion, inserting a bladder catheter, and administering mannitol and bicarbonate to encourage excretion of alkaline urine. This helps prevent precipitation of hemoglobin in the renal tubules, which could contribute to tubular necrosis. If oliguria develops, appropriate fluid management and possibly dialysis are begun. The most important treatment is restoration of blood pressure and renal perfusion. Vasopressors may be necessary. A sample of the recipient's blood is compared with pretransfusion samples to confirm incompatibility. Results of the direct antiglobulin test remain positive for as long as incompatible red blood cells continue to circulate. The serum bilirubin level can be monitored to chart the increase in indirect bilirubin caused by hemolysis.

**ANSWER: A**

## REFERENCES

1. Rutherford EJ, Brecher ME, Fakhry SM, et al: Hematologic principles in surgery. In Townsend CM, Beauchamp RD, Evers BM, et al, editors: *Sabiston textbook of surgery: the biological basis of modern surgical practice,* ed 18, Philadelphia, 2008, Elsevier.
2. Gonzalez EA, Jastrow KM, Holcomb JB, et al: Hemostasis, surgical bleeding and transfusion. In Brunicardi FC, Andersen DK, Billiar TR, et al, editors: *Schwartz's principles of surgery,* ed 9, New York, 2010, McGraw-Hill.
3. Colman RW, Hirsh J, Marder VJ, et al, editors: *Hemostasis and thrombosis: basic principles and practice,* ed 5, Philadelphia, 2006, JB Lippincott.
4. Simon TL, Snyder EL, et al, editors: *Rossi's principles of transfusion medicine,* ed 4, Oxford, 2009, Wiley-Blackwell.
5. Sorensen B, Johansen P, Nielsen GL, et al: Reversal of the international normalized ratio with recombinant activated factor VII in central nervous system bleeding during warfarin thromboprophylaxis: clinical and biochemical aspects, *Blood Coagul Fibrinolysis* 14:469–477, 2003.

# CHAPTER 4

# Nutrition, Metabolism, and Fluid and Electrolytes

*José M. Velasco, M.D., and Chad E. Jacobs, M.D.*

## A. Fluid and Electrolytes
*David D. Shersher, M.D.*

1. Which of the following statements regarding total body water is false?

    A. In males, approximately 60% of total body weight is water

    B. The percentage of total body weight that is water is higher in males than in females

    C. Lean individuals have a greater proportion of water (relative to body weight) than do obese individuals

    D. The percentage of total body water decreases with age

    E. The majority of body water is contained within the interstitial fluid compartment

*Ref.:* 1-3

**COMMENTS:** Approximately 50% to 75% of body weight is water. In males, 60% (±15%) of body weight is water, and in females, 50% (±15%) of body weight is water. Age and lean body mass also contribute to differences in the percentage of total body weight that is water. Since fat contains little water, lean individuals have a greater proportion of **body water** than do obese individuals of the same weight. Because females have more subcutaneous fat in relation to lean mass than do males, they have less body water. Total body water decreases with age as a result of decreasing lean muscle mass. Infants have an unusually high ratio of total body water to body weight: up to 75% to 80%. By 1 year of age, however, the percentage of body water approaches that of adults.

Body water is divided into three functional compartments: the **intracellular fluid (ICF) compartment** (40% of body weight) and the **extracellular fluid (ECF) compartment** (20% of body weight), which is further subdivided into the interstitial (15% of body weight) and intravascular (5% of body weight) fluid compartments.

**ANSWER:** E

2. Which of the following statements regarding the distribution, composition, and osmolarity of body fluid compartments is not true?

    A. Most intracellular water resides in skeletal muscle.

    B. The principal extracellular cation is sodium.

    C. Nonpermeable proteins determine the effective osmotic pressure between the interstitial and intravascular (plasma) fluid compartments.

    D. Calcium greatly determines the effective osmotic pressure between the ICF and ECF compartments

    E. The principal extracellular anions are chloride and bicarbonate.

*Ref.:* 1

**COMMENTS:** The ICF compartment (accounting for 40% of total body weight) is contained mostly within skeletal muscle. The principal **intracellular cations** are potassium and magnesium, whereas the principal intracellular anions are proteins and phosphates. In the ECF compartment (20% of total body weight), which is subdivided into the interstitial (extravascular) and the intravascular (plasma) fluid compartments, the principal cation is sodium, whereas the principal anions are chloride and bicarbonate. The interstitial compartment has a rapidly equilibrating functional component and a slowly equilibrating, relatively nonfunctional component consisting of fluid within connective tissue and cerebrospinal and joint fluid (termed **transcellular water**). Intravascular fluid (plasma) has a higher concentration of nondiffusible organic proteins than do interstitial fluids. These plasma proteins act as multivalent anions. As a result, the concentration of inorganic anions is lower but the total concentration of cations is higher in intravascular fluid than in interstitial fluid. This relationship is explained in the **Gibbs-Donnan equilibrium equation**: the product of the concentrations of any pair of diffusible cations and anions on one side of a semipermeable membrane equals the product of the same pair on the other side.

In each body compartment the concentration of osmotically active particles is 290 to 310 mOsm. Although total osmotic pressure represents the sum of osmotically active particles in the fluid compartment, the effective osmotic pressure depends on osmotically active particles that do not freely pass through the semipermeable membranes of the body. The nonpermeable proteins in plasma are responsible for the effective osmotic pressure between plasma and the interstitial fluid compartment (the colloid osmotic pressure). The effective osmotic pressure between the ECF and ICF compartments is due mainly to sodium, the major extracellular cation, which does not freely cross the cell membrane. Because water moves freely between the compartments, the **effective oncotic pressure** within the various body fluid compartments is considered to be equal after fluid equilibration. An increase in the effective oncotic pressure of the ECF compartment (such as an increase in sodium concentration) causes movement of water from the intracellular space to the extracellular space until the osmotic pressure equalizes. Conversely, loss of sodium (hyponatremia) from the extracellular space results in movement of water into the intracellular space. Thus, the ICF contributes to correcting the changes in concentration and composition in the ECF. Isotonic ECF losses (losses in volume without change in concentration) generally do not cause transfer of water from the intracellular space as long as the osmolarity remains unchanged. Isotonic volume losses result in changes in ECF volume.

**A N S W E R :  D**

3. Which of the following statements regarding changes in volume status of the ECF compartment is true?

   A. Hyponatremia is diagnostic of excess ECF volume.

   B. Hypernatremia is diagnostic of depletion of ECF volume

   C. Excess extracellular volume is usually iatrogenic or due to renal or cardiac failure.

   D. Central nervous system symptoms appear after tissue signs with acute volume loss.

   E. The concentration of serum sodium is directly related to extracellular volume.

   *Ref.:* 1, 2

**COMMENTS:** The serum concentration of sodium is not necessarily related to the volume status of the ECF compartment. **Volume deficit** or excess can exist with high, low, or normal serum sodium concentrations. Volume deficit is the most frequent volume disorder encountered during surgery. Its most common cause is loss of isotonic fluid (i.e., fluid having the same composition as ECF), for example, through hemorrhage, vomiting, diarrhea, fistulas, or third-spacing. With acute volume loss, central nervous symptoms (e.g., sleepiness and apathy progressing to coma) and cardiovascular signs (e.g., orthostasis, hypotension, tachycardia, and coolness in the extremities) appear first, along with decreasing urine output. Tissue signs (e.g., decreased turgor, softness of the tongue with longitudinal wrinkling, and atonicity of muscles) usually do not appear during the first 24 hours. In response to hypovolemia, body temperature may be slightly decreased. It is therefore important to also monitor the body temperature of hypovolemic patients. Signs and symptoms of sepsis may be depressed in volume-depleted patients. The abdominal pain, fever, and leukocytosis associated with peritonitis may be absent until ECF volume is restored.

   **Volume overload** is generally either iatrogenic or the result of renal insufficiency or heart failure. Both plasma and the interstitial fluid spaces are involved. The signs are those of circulatory overload and include distended veins, bounding pulses, functional murmurs, edema, and basilar rales. These signs may be present in young, healthy patients, but these patients can compensate for moderate to severe volume excess without overt failure or pulmonary edema developing. In elderly patients, however, congestive

heart failure (CHF) with pulmonary edema may develop quite rapidly.

**A N S W E R :  C**

4. Which one of the following is not a stimulus for ECF expansion?

   A. Hemorrhage leading to a reduction in blood volume

   B. Increased capillary permeability after major surgery

   C. Peripheral arterial vasoconstriction

   D. Negative interstitial fluid hydrostatic pressure

   E. Colloid oncotic pressure

   *Ref.:* 3

**COMMENTS:** Approximately 85% of the ECF that is within the vascular compartment resides in the venous circulation. Therefore, the remaining 15% resides within the arterial system. The vascular compartment, otherwise known as **plasma fluid**, constitutes approximately a third of the ECF. **Interstitial fluid** (i.e., fluid between the cells) makes up approximately two thirds of the ECF. The **extracellular fluid** constitutes a third of total body water, whereas the ICF represents two thirds. Expansion of ECF is primarily driven by three mechanisms, all of which have the final common stimuli of reduction of intravascular volume. The first mechanism, hemorrhage, is directly responsible for the reduction in blood volume. Through various pathways, this drop in volume signals the retention and sequestration of fluid in the intravascular space. Increased capillary permeability, the second mechanism, occurs following major surgery and is due to the loss of endothelial integrity. This loss of integrity is mediated by several humoral factors that act on the endothelium. The end result of loss of endothelial integrity is extravasation of protein-rich fluid into the interstitium, with a consequent increase in the interstitial fluid space. This constitutes the third mechanism of ECF expansion. Serum albumin is a major determinant of **colloid oncotic pressure**, and hypoalbuminemia could lead to transudation of fluid from the vascular to the interstitial compartment. This concept is expressed mathematically by the **Starling equation**: $Qf = Kf \times (Pv - Pt) - \delta \times (COP - TOP)$, where $Qf$ is fluid flux, $Kf$ is the capillary filtration coefficient, $Pv$ is vascular hydrostatic pressure, $Pt$ is interstitial hydrostatic pressure, $\delta$ is a reflection coefficient (which defines the effectiveness of the membrane in preventing flow of solutes), $COP$ is colloid osmotic pressure, and $TOP$ is tissue osmotic pressure.

**A N S W E R :  C**

5. Which of the following humoral factors increases arterial vasodilation while not decreasing protein permeability in the capillary membranes?

   A. Bradykinin

   B. Nitric oxide (NO)

   C. Atrial natriuretic factor

   D. Histamine

   E. Platelet-activating factor

   *Ref.:* 1

**COMMENTS:** The **protein permeability** characteristics of capillary membranes are quantified by a numeric value termed the **reflection coefficient**. This value ranges from 0 to 1 and is conceptualized as the fraction of plasma protein that "reflects" back from the capillary wall when water crosses. The higher the coefficient, the more impermeable the capillary is to protein. Therefore, the oncotic pressure of the plasma volume declines as the reflection coefficient decreases. Certain intravascular factors can reduce the reflection coefficient and increase arterial vasodilation. Bradykinin, atrial natriuretic factor, histamine, and platelet-activating factor increase microvascular membrane permeability while causing arterial vasodilation. NO, although it causes arterial vasodilation, does not increase microvascular membrane permeability. Membrane permeability causes a shift of fluid and plasma proteins into the interstitium and thereby decreases the intravascular compartment. The protein-rich edema in the interstitium can adversely affect the ability to combat infection.

**ANSWER:** B

---

6. Which of the following statements regarding hypervolemia in postoperative patients is not true?

   A. Hypervolemia can be produced by the administration of isotonic salt solutions in amounts that exceed the loss of volume.

   B. Acute overexpansion of the ECF space is usually well tolerated in healthy individuals.

   C. Avoidance of volume excess requires daily monitoring of intake and output and determinations of serum sodium concentrations to guide accurate fluid administration.

   D. The most reliable sign of volume excess is peripheral edema.

   E. The earliest sign of volume excess is weight gain

   *Ref.:* 1, 2

**COMMENTS:** The earliest sign of **volume excess** during the postoperative period is weight gain. Normally, during this period the patient is in a catabolic state and is expected to lose weight ($\frac{1}{4}$ to $\frac{1}{2}$ lb/day). Circulatory and pulmonary signs of overload appear late and usually represent massive overload. Peripheral edema does not necessarily indicate excess volume. In a patient with edema but without additional evidence of volume overload, other causes of peripheral edema should be considered. The most common cause of excess volume in a surgical patient is the administration of isotonic salt solutions in amounts that exceed the loss of volume. In a healthy individual, such overload is usually well tolerated. However, if excess fluid is administered for several days, the ability of the kidneys to secrete sodium may be exceeded, thus resulting in hypernatremia.

**ANSWER:** D

---

7. Which of the following statements regarding loop diuretics is not true?

   A. Loop diuretics act on the thick ascending limb of the loop of Henle in the nephron.

   B. Loop diuretics increase blood flow to the kidney.

   C. Magnesium and calcium are unaffected during diuresis.

   D. Loop diuretics increase venous capacitance.

   E. Loop diuretics inhibit the sodium-potassium-chloride cotransporter.

   *Ref.:* 1, 3

**COMMENTS: Loop diuretics**, most commonly furosemide, are potent inhibitors of the sodium-potassium-chloride cotransporter. They act by competing for the chloride-binding site at the thick ascending limb of the loop of Henle. The effect is inhibition of sodium reabsorption resulting in diuresis. Magnesium, potassium, and calcium will likewise be excreted with the net increase in urine output. Therefore, it is important to monitor their serum levels to prevent depletion while a patient is being treated with a loop diuretic.

Loop diuretics are commonly used for pulmonary edema because of their potency. In addition to inhibition of sodium absorption, they increase blood flow to the kidneys by stimulating vasodilatory prostaglandins and increase venous capacitance, which can quickly relieve pulmonary edema, even before diuresis and natriuresis have occurred. These three mechanisms help decrease ECF volume. Loop diuretics, such as furosemide or bumetanide, are extensively protein bound and must reach their intratubular site of action through active proximal tubular secretion.

**ANSWER:** C

---

8. Which of the following pairing statements regarding daily fluid balance is incorrect?

   A. Daily water intake, 2000 to 2500 mL

   B. Average stool loss, 1000 mL

   C. Average insensible loss, 600 mL

   D. Average urine volume, 800 to 1500 mL

   E. Average increase in insensible loss in a febrile patient, 250 mL/day for each degree of fever

   *Ref.:* 2

**COMMENTS:** The average individual has an intake of 2000 to 2500 mL of water per day—1500 mL is ingested orally and the remainder is acquired in solid food. Daily losses include 250 mL in stool, 800 to 1500 mL in urine, and approximately 600 mL as insensible loss. To excrete the products of normal daily catabolism, an individual must produce at least 500 to 800 mL of urine. In healthy individuals, 75% of insensible loss occurs through the skin and 25% through the lungs. Insensible loss from the skin occurs as loss of water vapor through the skin and not by evaporation of water secreted by the sweat glands. In febrile patients, insensible loss through the skin may increase to 250 mL/day for each degree of fever. Losses from sweating can be as high as 4 L/h. In a patient with a tracheostomy who is being ventilated with unhumidified air, insensible loss from the lungs may increase to 1500 mL/day.

**ANSWER:** B

---

9. Which of the following statements concerning the sodium concentration of various fluids is incorrect?

   A. Pancreatic secretions, 140 mEq/L

   B. Sweat, 40 mEq/L

   C. Gastric secretions, 50 mEq/L

   D. Saliva, 100 mEq/L

   E. Ileostomy output, 125 mEq/L

   *Ref.:* 3

**COMMENTS:** Average **daily salt intake** ranges from 50 to 90 mEq sodium chloride. Usually, the kidneys excrete excess salt as it is encountered. Under conditions of reduced intake or increased extrarenal fluid loss, renal sodium excretion can be reduced to less than 1 mEq/day. Conversely, in patients with malfunctioning kidneys, sodium loss may be as high as 200 mEq/L of urine. The electrolyte composition of sweat and gastrointestinal secretions varies. Sweat represents a hypotonic loss of fluids. The average sodium concentration in sweat is 15 to 60 mEq/L. Insensible loss from the skin and lungs consists of pure water. Although the various gastrointestinal secretions vary in composition, gastrointestinal losses are usually isotonic or slightly hypotonic. Pancreatic secretions have high bicarbonate concentrations (75 mEq/dL), in contrast to that of bile. Stomach, small intestine, and biliary fluids have relatively high chloride concentrations. Duodenal, ileal, pancreatic, and biliary fluids contain levels of sodium that approximate those seen in plasma. Saliva is relatively high in potassium, a fact that is important to remember when managing a patient with a salivary fistula (Table 4-1). The concentration of sodium varies with gland stimulation and circadian rhythm; it ranges from 3 mmol/L to 70 mmol/L.

**TABLE 4-1 Electrolyte Composition**

| Fluid | $Na^+$ | $K^+$ | $H^+$ | $Cl^-$ | $HCO_3^-$ |
|---|---|---|---|---|---|
| Sweat | 30-50 | 5 | 45-55 | — | — |
| Gastric | 40-65 | — | 90 | 100-140 | — |
| Biliary | 135-155 | 5 | — | 80-110 | 70-90 |
| Pancreatic | 135-155 | 5 | — | 55-75 | 70-90 |
| Ileostomy | 120-130 | 10 | — | 50-60 | 50-70 |
| Diarrhea | 25-50 | 35-60 | — | 20-40 | 30-45 |

Management of fluid losses should take into account the electrolyte composition of the fluid, as well as that of the solution being used to replace these fluids. Lactated Ringer solution contains 130 mEq/L of sodium and 109 mEq/L of chloride. It also contains 4 mEq/L of potassium, 3 mEq/L of calcium, and 28 mEq/L of lactate. This is in contrast to 0.9% normal saline solution, which contains 154 mEq/L of both sodium and chloride. On the other hand, hypertonic 3% saline solution contains 513 mEq/L of both sodium and chloride.

**A N S W E R :** D

10. With regard to distributional shifts during an operation, which of the following statements is true?

A. The surface area of the peritoneum is not large enough to account for significant third-space loss.

B. Approximately 1 to 1.5 L/h of fluid is needed during an operation.

C. Blood is replaced as it is lost, without modification of the basal operative fluid replacement rate.

D. Sequestered ECF is predominantly hypotonic.

E. A major stimulus to ECF expansion is peripheral vasoconstriction.

*Ref.:* 1-3

**COMMENTS:** The **functional ECF volume** decreases during major abdominal operations largely because of sequestration of fluid in the operative site as a consequence of (1) extensive dissection, (2) fluid collection within the lumen and wall of the small bowel, and (3) accumulation of fluid in the peritoneal cavity. The surface area of the peritoneum is 1.8 m². When irritated, it can account for a functional loss of several liters of fluid that is not readily apparent. It is generally agreed that this lost volume should be replaced during the course of an operation with isotonic saline solution as a "mimic" of sequestered ECF. Although there is no set formula for intraoperative fluid therapy, useful guidelines for

replacement include the following. (1) Blood is replaced as it is lost, regardless of additional fluid therapy, provided that the patient meets the criteria for transfusion: hemoglobin concentration less than 7 g/dL. (2) Lost ECF should be replaced during the operative procedure; delay in replacement until after the operation is complicated by adrenal and hypophyseal compensatory mechanisms that respond to operative trauma during the immediate postoperative period. (3) Approximately 0.5 to 1.0 L/h of fluid is needed during the course of an operation, to a maximum of 2 to 3 L during a 4-hour procedure, unless there are measurable losses.

**A N S W E R :** C

11. With regard to intraoperative management of fluids, which of the following statements is true?

A. In a healthy person, up to 500 mL of blood loss may be well tolerated without the need for blood replacement.

B. During an operation, functional ECF volume is directly related to the volume lost to suction.

C. Functional ECF losses should be replaced with plasma.

D. Administration of albumin plays an important role in the replacement of functional ECF volume loss.

E. Operative blood loss is usually overestimated by the surgeon.

*Ref.:* 1, 2

**COMMENTS:** It is now believed that the routine use of albumin to replace blood and **ECF losses** intraoperatively is not indicated and may be potentially harmful. Maintenance of cardiac and pulmonary function by replacing blood with blood products and ECF with "mimic" solutions can be achieved without the addition of albumin. In general, it is believed that blood should be replaced as it is lost. However, it is usually unnecessary to replace blood loss of less than 500 mL. Operative blood loss is usually underestimated by the surgeon by 15% to 40% in comparison to the isotopically measured loss, a factor that may contribute to the detection of anemia during the immediate postoperative period.

**A N S W E R :** A

12. With regard to postoperative fluid management, which of the following statements is not true?

A. Insensible loss is approximately 600 mL/day.

B. Insensible loss may increase to 1500 mL/day.

C. About 800 to 1000 mL of fluid is needed to excrete the catabolic end products of metabolism.

D. Lost urine should be replaced milliliter for milliliter.

E. Lost gastrointestinal fluids should be replaced milliliter for milliliter.

*Ref.:* 1-3

**COMMENTS: Postoperative fluid management** requires assessment of the patient's volume status and evaluation for possible disorders in concentration or composition. All measured and insensible losses should be treated by replacement with appropriate fluids. In patients with normal renal function, the amount of potassium given is 40 mEq/day for replacement of renal excretion. An additional 20 mEq should be given for each liter of gastrointestinal loss. Insensible water loss is usually constant in the range of

600 mL/day. It can be increased to 1500 mL/day by hypermetabolism, hyperventilation, or fever. Insensible loss is replaced with 5% dextrose in water. Insensible loss may be offset by an insensible gain of water from excessive catabolism in postoperative patients who require prolonged intravenous fluid therapy. Approximately 800 to 1000 mL/day of fluid is needed to excrete the catabolic end products of metabolism. Because the kidneys are able to conserve sodium in a healthy individual, this amount can be replaced with 5% dextrose in water. A small amount of salt is usually added, however, to relieve the kidneys of the stress of sodium resorption. If there is a question regarding urinary sodium loss, measurement of urinary sodium levels helps determine the type of fluid that can best be used. Urine volume should not be replaced milliliter for milliliter because high output may represent diuresis of the fluids given during surgery or the diuresis that takes place to eliminate excessive fluid administration. Sensible or measurable losses such as those from the gastrointestinal tract are usually isotonic and should therefore be treated by replacement in equal volumes with isotonic salt solutions. The type of salt solution selected depends on determination of the patient's serum sodium, potassium, and chloride levels. In general, replacement fluids are administered at a steady rate over a period of 18 to 24 hours as losses are incurred (Table 4-2).

**ANSWER: D**

**TABLE 4-2  Composition and Osmolality of Intravenous Solutions**

| | Na+ (mEq/L) | Cl− (mEq/L) | Glucose (g/L) | Osmolality (mOsm/kg) |
|---|---|---|---|---|
| Lactated Ringer solution* | 130 | 109 | — | 272 |
| 0.9% NaCl (normal saline) | 154 | 154 | — | 308 |
| 0.45% NaCl (½ normal saline) | 77 | 77 | — | 154 |
| D₅W | — | — | 50 | 252 |
| D₁₀W | — | — | 100 | 505 |
| D₅₀W | — | — | 500 | 2520 |
| 3% NaCl (hypertonic saline) | 513 | 513 | — | 1026 |

D₅W, 5% dextrose in water.
*Also contains K+ (4 mEq/L), CaH (3 mEq/L), and lactate (28 mEq/L).

13. With regard to abnormalities in serum sodium concentration, which of the following statements is true?

    A. Changes in serum sodium concentration usually produce changes in the status of ECF volume.

    B. The chloride ion is the main determinant of the osmolarity of the ECF space.

    C. Extracellular hyponatremia leads to depletion of intracellular water.

    D. Dry, sticky mucous membranes are characteristic of hyponatremia.

    E. Preservation of normal ECF has higher precedence than does maintenance of normal osmolality.

*Ref.:* 1, 2

**COMMENTS:** Although extracellular volume may change without a change in serum sodium concentration (as occurs after isotonic volume losses), changes in serum sodium concentration usually produce changes in ECF volume because the serum sodium concentration is the main determinant of the osmolarity of the ECF space. Alterations in its concentration produce concomitant shifts in water volume. Signs and symptoms of hypernatremia and hyponatremia are not generally present unless the changes are severe or the alteration in sodium concentration occurs rapidly.

**Hyponatremia** is caused by excessive intake of hypotonic fluids or salt loss that exceeds water loss. With hyponatremia, decreased extracellular osmolarity causes a shift of water into the intracellular compartment. When such a shift occurs, central nervous system symptoms caused by increased intracranial pressure develop, and tissue signs of excess water are noted. Central nervous system symptoms include muscle twitching, hyperactive tendon reflexes, and when the hyponatremia is severe, convulsions and hypertension. Tissue signs include salivation, lacrimation, watery diarrhea, and "fingerprinting" of the skin. When hyponatremia develops rapidly, signs and symptoms may appear at sodium concentrations of less than 130 mEq/L. Acute dilution of osmolality can occur if patients with an ECF deficit are given sodium-free water. The hyponatremia is exacerbated in hypovolemic patients because of secretion of antidiuretic hormone (ADH) as a result of the hypothalamic-pituitary response to both elevated ECF osmolality and a reduction in ECF volume. The normal response of the hypothalamic-pituitary axis to hyponatremia is suppression of ADH release, and as the dilute urine is excreted, there is a corrective increase in serum [Na+]. A moderate or severely hyponatremic patient should have undetectable blood levels of ADH. Preservation of normal ECF has higher precedence than does maintenance of normal osmolality. In symptomatic patients, administration of hypertonic (3%) solutions of sodium may be indicated to correct the problem in those with severe hyponatremia who are at risk for seizures. In less severe cases, restriction of free water and judicious infusion of normal saline solution are usually sufficient. In patients with acute hyponatremia and [Na+] less than 120 mEq/L, the rate of infusion of sodium-containing solutions should not increase serum [Na+] more rapidly than 0.25 mEq/L/h.

**Chronic hyponatremia** develops slowly, and patients may have sodium levels as low as 120 mEq/L before becoming symptomatic. Severe hyponatremia may be associated with the onset of irreversible oliguric renal failure. Patients with a closed head injury are sensitive to even mild hyponatremia because of increased intracellular water, which exacerbates the increased intracranial pressure associated with the head injury. The **syndrome of inappropriate release of antidiuretic hormone** (SIADH) and chronic renal failure are frequent causes of hyponatremia. The diagnosis of SIADH can be made only in euvolemic patients who have a serum osmolality of less than 270 mmol/kg H₂O along with inappropriately concentrated urine.

**Hypernatremia** is the result of excessive free water loss or salt intake. Central nervous system signs and symptoms associated with hypernatremia include restlessness, weakness, delirium, and maniacal behavior. The tissue signs are characteristic and include dryness and stickiness of mucous membranes, decreased salivation and tear production, and redness and swelling of the tongue. Body temperature is usually elevated, occasionally to a lethal level. An acute onset of hypernatremia increases ECF osmolality and contracts the size of the ICF compartment. Patients have moderate hypernatremia if their serum [Na+] is 146 to 159 mEq/L. Water loss is the most common explanation for acute hypernatremia. Neurologic damage as a result of contraction of brain cell volume is the primary risk associated with hypernatremia. Patients with **diabetes insipidus** or **nephrogenic diabetes insipidus** have a failure to synthesize and release ADH or a failure of the renal tubular cells to respond to ADH, respectively, thus leading to hypernatremia. Treatment of patients with hypernatremia secondary to dehydration involves the administration of water. Hypernatremic patients are frequently hypovolemic, and these patients are treated by the intravenous infusion of isotonic saline solution until the volume deficit has been restored. A rapid decline in ECF osmolality in a severely hypernatremic patient can lead to cerebral injury as a result of cellular swelling. [Na⁺] should be lowered at a rate not to exceed 8 mEq/day (Table 4-3). Patients with central diabetes insipidus are treated with desmopressin (1-desamino-8-D-arginine vasopressin [DDAVP]). **Desmopressin** is a synthetic analogue of ADH.

**A N S W E R :   A**

---

**TABLE 4-3   Given a Patient with Hypernatremia (Serum [Na⁺] = 160 mEq/L), the Estimated Change in [Na⁺] after Infusion of 1 L**

$$\frac{\text{Change in}\left[Na^+\right]}{L} = \frac{\text{Infusate}\left[Na^+\right] - \text{Serum}\left[Na^+\right]}{TBW + 1}$$

| Infusate | Woman Aged 70 Years 50 kg × 0.45 = 22.5 L TBW | Man Aged 20 Years 80 kg × 0.60 = 48.0 L TBW |
|---|---|---|
| D₅W | $\frac{0-160}{22.5+1} = -6.8$ | $\frac{0-160}{48+1} = -3.3$ |
| D₅ 0.2% NaCl | $\frac{34-160}{22.5+1} = -5.4$ | $\frac{34-160}{48+1} = -2.6$ |
| D₅ 0.45% NaCl | $\frac{77-160}{22.5+1} = -3.5$ | $\frac{77-160}{48+1} = -1.7$ |

D₅W, 5% dextrose in water; TBW, total body water.

---

**14.** Which of the following does not contribute to the development of hypernatremia?

A. Excessive sweating

B. Hyperlipidemia

C. Lactulose

D. Glycosuria

E. Inadequate maintenance fluids

*Ref.: 3*

**COMMENTS:** **Hypernatremia** is less common than hyponatremia in postoperative patients and is a reflection of elevated serum osmolality and hypertonicity. It is indicative of a deficiency of free water relative to the sodium concentration. Decreased intake of water, increased loss of water, and increased intake of sodium are the main mechanisms responsible for the development of hypernatremia. Loss of the thirst mechanism and an inability to access free water are mechanisms by which hypernatremia secondary to decreased intake of water can develop. Excessive sweating and large evaporative losses are mechanisms of loss of free water. Agents such as lactulose, sorbitol, and carbohydrate malabsorption can cause osmotic diarrhea and result in relative losses of hypotonic fluid. Similarly, hyperglycemia causing glycosuria or diuresis in a catabolic patient excreting excess urea can also cause an osmotic diuresis. Both hyperlipidemia and hyperproteinemia are responsible for an entity known as pseudohyponatremia, which occurs when excess lipids or proteins displace water and create a falsely measured hyponatremia.

**A N S W E R :   B**

**15.** Which of the following conditions is not associated with hypernatremia?

A. Diabetes insipidus

B. Tumor lysis syndrome

C. Steven-Johnson syndrome

D. Primary hypodipsia

E. Enterocutaneous fistula

*Ref.: 1*

**COMMENTS:** **Diabetes insipidus** is characterized by the excretion of large volumes of dilute urine, which can lead to **hypernatremia**. Patients with primary hypodipsia, a rare neurologic deficit of the thirst center, have an impaired or absent thirst response to an increase in extracellular tonicity. Tumor or infection may be responsible for this defect. Dermatologic conditions such as second-degree burns and exfoliative dermatitis can substantially increase transcutaneous water loss and thereby result in the rapid onset of dehydration and hypernatremia. Dehydration from vomiting, diarrhea, or uncompensated loss of hypotonic gastrointestinal fluid, such as occurs with fistulas or endoluminal tubes, may cause hypernatremia. Tumor lysis syndrome, a condition involving cell breakdown and release of their intracellular contents after some chemotherapies, typically develops in patients treated with vinca alkaloid chemotherapy; it causes hyperkalemia, hyperphosphatemia, hyperuricemia, and ultimately, renal failure. Tumor lysis syndrome does not cause hypernatremia.

**A N S W E R :   B**

**16.** Which of the following clinical situations can be associated with hypovolemic hyponatremia?

A. CHF

B. SIADH

C. Cirrhosis

D. Hyperglycemia

E. Gastrointestinal losses

*Ref.: 1, 2*

**COMMENTS:** **Hyponatremia** in a surgical patient can be classified into hypervolemic, euvolemic, and hypovolemic categories, which can then be further subclassified according to tonicity (hypertonic, >290 mOsm; isotonic, 280 to 290 mOsm; and hypotonic, <280 mOsm). For simplicity and rapid clinical evaluation, volume status can be used to direct treatment. **Hypervolemic hyponatremia** may be caused by increased intake of water, postoperative secretion of ADH, and high ECF volume states such as cirrhosis and CHF. Hyponatremia can develop in patients with edema and ascites secondary to CHF, nephrotic syndrome, or cirrhosis despite having an expanded overall volume of extracellular water. These patients have an excess of sodium but an even greater proportional increase in water volume. Their pathophysiologic condition entails an overall contracted intravascular volume, which stimulates the release of vasopressin from the hypothalamus centrally. Peripherally, renal hypoperfusion contributes to water retention. Fluid restriction is crucial to the treatment of this type of hyponatremia. In patients with severe hyponatremia, small volumes of hypertonic saline solution may be administered. Diuresis may be used but is generally unsuccessful. Hemodialysis may be performed in extreme circumstances of fluid excess. **Euvolemic hyponatremia** may be caused by hyperglycemia, hyperlipidemia or hyperproteinemia (termed *pseudohyponatremia* because of relative hyperosmolar protein, lipid, or glucose-rich plasma drawing fluid from the interstitial space and diluting plasma sodium), SIADH, water intoxication, and diuretics. SIADH is characterized by functional reabsorption of free water and subsequent dilution of plasma sodium. **Hypovolemic hyponatremia** may be caused by decreased overall sodium intake, gastrointestinal losses, renal losses associated with the use of diuretics (especially thiazide diuretics), and primary renal disease.

Conversely, hypernatremia can also be subdivided into volume states. Hypervolemic hypernatremia may be caused by iatrogenic sodium administration or mineralocorticoid excess (e.g., aldosteronism, Cushing disease, congenital adrenal hyperplasia). Euvolemic hypernatremia may be associated with renal (renal disease, diuretics, or diabetes insipidus) or nonrenal free water loss through the skin or gastrointestinal tract. Hypovolemic hypernatremia can likewise be subdivided into nonrenal and renal water loss.

**ANSWER: E**

17. With regard to diabetes insipidus, which of the following statements is true?

    A. Diabetes insipidus causes hypervolemic hyponatremia.

    B. Central diabetes insipidus cannot be corrected by the administration of desmopressin.

    C. Treatment of diabetes insipidus requires correction of hypernatremia at a rate faster than 12 mEq/day.

    D. Alcohol intoxication can mimic diabetes insipidus.

    E. Lithium administration could induce central diabetes insipidus.

*Ref.:* 1, 3

**COMMENTS: Diabetes insipidus** is one of the causes of hypovolemic hypernatremia and is marked by continual production of dilute urine of less than 200 mOsm/kg $H_2O$ in the context of serum osmolarity of extracellular fluid greater than 300 Osm/L. Patients can have either central (lack of production of ADH by the hypothalamus) or nephrogenic diabetes insipidus (lack of response of the distal tubule of the nephron to ADH). Alcohol causes suppression of vasopressin release and can mimic central diabetes insipidus. Treatment of hypernatremia consists of slow correction of sodium by the administration of free water. Whenever hypernatremia develops, a relative free water deficit exists and must be replaced. The water deficit can be approximated by using the following formula: water deficit = total body water $\times$ [(1 − 140 ÷ serum sodium)]. Usually, the rate of correction of hypernatremia should not exceed 12 mEq/L/day. The aim should be to correct approximately half the deficit over the first 24 hours. Too rapid correction of hypernatremia may lead to cerebral edema and seizures.

Desmopressin is a synthetic analogue of ADH that can be used to mimic arginine vasopressin (AVP) and to differentiate between central and nephrogenic diabetes insipidus. It is the agent of choice for treating patients with central diabetes insipidus because the drug increases water movement out of the collecting duct but does not have the vasoconstrictive effects of ADH. **Central diabetes insipidus** will respond to desmopressin, whereas nephrogenic diabetes insipidus will not. Unlike vasopressin, desmopressin is only renally active and does not have the vasoactive side effects. Lithium and amphotericin B can induce nephrogenic, not central diabetes insipidus.

**ANSWER: D**

18. A 30-year-old, 70-kg woman has symptomatic hyponatremia. Her serum sodium level is 120 mEq/L (normal level, 140 mEq/L). Her sodium deficit is:

    A. 500 mEq/L

    B. 600 mEq/L

    C. 700 mEq/L

    D. 800 mEq/L

    E. 400 mEq/L

*Ref.:* 1

**COMMENTS:** Correction of changes in concentration depends in part on whether the patient is symptomatic. If symptomatic **hypernatremia** or **hyponatremia** is present, attention is focused on prompt correction of the abnormal concentration to the point that the symptoms are relieved. Attention is then shifted to correction of the associated abnormality in volume. The sodium deficiency in this patient is estimated by multiplying the sodium deficit (normal sodium concentration minus observed sodium concentration) by total body water in liters (60% of body weight in males and 50% of body weight in females). For the patient in question, the calculation is as follows: total body water = 70 kg $\times$ 0.5 = 35 L. Sodium deficit = (140 − 120 mEq/L) $\times$ 35 L = 700 mEq sodium chloride.

Initially, half the calculated amount of sodium is infused as 3% sodium chloride. The infusion is given slowly because rapid infusion can cause symptomatic hypovolemia. Rapid correction of hyponatremia can be associated with irreversible central nervous system injury (central pontine and extrapontine myelinolysis). Once the symptoms are alleviated, the patient should be reassessed before additional infusion of sodium is begun. In patients with profound hyponatremia, a correction of no more than 12 mEq/L/24 h should be achieved. If the original problem was associated with a volume deficit, the remainder of the resuscitation can be accomplished with isotonic fluids (sodium chloride in the presence of alkalosis, and sodium lactate in the presence of acidosis). Care must be taken when treating hyponatremia associated with volume excess. In this setting, after the symptoms are alleviated with a small volume of hypertonic saline solution, water restriction is the treatment of choice. Infusion of hypertonic saline solution in this setting has the potential to further expand the extracellular intravascular volume and is contraindicated in patients with severely compromised cardiac reserve. In such a case, peritoneal dialysis or hemodialysis may be preferred for removing excess water.

**ANSWER: C**

19. A postoperative patient has a serum sodium concentration of 125 mEq/L and a blood glucose level of 500 mg/dL (normal level, 100 mg/dL). What would the patient's serum sodium concentration be (assuming normal renal function and appropriate intraoperative fluid therapy) if the blood glucose level were normal?

    A. 120 mEq/L

    B. 122 mEq/L

    C. 137 mEq/L

    D. 142 mEq/L

    E. 147 mEq/L

*Ref.:* 1-3

**COMMENTS: Serum osmolality** is described as the amount of solutes per unit of water. It can be measured with an osmometer or it can be calculated. It is reported as milliosmoles per liter. Calculation of serum osmolality is performed with the following equation:

$$P_{osm} = 2 \times Na\,(mEq/L) + \frac{Glucose\,(mg\%)}{18}$$
$$+ \frac{Blood\ urea\ nitrogen\,(mg\%)}{2.8}$$

The serum concentrations of sodium, urea, and glucose are required, whereas that of chloride is not required for the calculation. Simply doubling the serum sodium concentration provides an adequate estimate of serum osmolality.

As a general rule, each 100-mg/dL rise in the blood glucose level above normal is equivalent to a 1.6- to 3.0-mEq/L fall in the apparent serum sodium concentration. For example, if the patient has a blood glucose level of 500 mg/dL, or 400 mg/dL above normal, this is equivalent to a 12-mEq/L change in the serum sodium level. If this patient has a measured sodium concentration of 125 mEq/L, the sodium concentration is actually 137 mEq/L once the excess extracellular water has been eliminated.

**ANSWER: C**

20. With regard to postoperative hyponatremia, which of the following statements is not true?

A. It may easily occur when water is used to replace sodium-containing fluids or when the water given exceeds the water lost.

B. In patients with head injury, hyponatremia despite adequate salt administration is usually caused by occult renal dysfunction.

C. In oliguric patients, cellular catabolism with resultant metabolic acidosis increases cellular release of water and can contribute to hyponatremia.

D. Hyperglycemia may be a cause of hyponatremia.

E. Patients with salt-wasting nephropathy could have normal blood urea nitrogen and creatinine values.

*Ref.:* 1, 2

**COMMENTS:** Abnormalities in sodium concentration do not usually occur during the postoperative period if the functional ECF volume has been adequately replaced during the operation. The sodium concentration generally remains normal because the kidneys retain the ability to excrete moderate excesses of water and solute administered during the early postoperative period. Hyponatremia does occur when water is given to replace lost sodium-containing fluids or when the amount of water given consistently exceeds the amount of water lost. In patients with head injury, hyponatremia may develop despite adequate salt administration because of excessive secretion of ADH with resultant increased water retention.

Patients with preexisting renal disease and loss of concentrating ability may elaborate urine with a high salt concentration. This **salt-wasting** phenomenon is commonly encountered in elderly patients and is often not anticipated because the blood urea nitrogen and creatinine levels are within normal limits. When there is doubt, determination of the urine sodium concentration can help clarify the diagnosis. Oliguria reduces the daily water requirement and can lead to hyponatremia if not anticipated. Cellular catabolism in patients without adequate caloric intake can lead to gain of significant quantities of water released from the tissues. Hyperglycemia may produce a depressed serum sodium level by exerting an osmotic force in the extracellular compartment, thus diluting serum sodium levels.

**ANSWER: B**

21. An elderly patient with adult-onset diabetes mellitus is admitted to the hospital with severe pneumonia. All of the following conditions can be associated with this patient condition except:

A. Hypokalemia

B. Hyperkalemia

C. Nonketotic hyperosmolar coma

D. Hypophosphatemia

E. Hyponatremia

*Ref.:* 1

**COMMENTS:** Elderly patients with adult-onset diabetes mellitus are at risk for the development of **nonketotic hyperosmolar coma** during sepsis. As a result of the development of a nonketotic hyperglycemic hyperosmolar state, hypokalemia and hyperglycemia may also occur. Treatment of these patients should include a reduction in the glucose load provided and the administration of isotonic fluid. Patients may also benefit from the administration of insulin. Systemic bacterial sepsis is also often accompanied by a drop in the serum sodium concentration, possibly because of interstitial or intracellular sequestration. It is treated by withholding free water, restoring ECF volume, and treating the source of sepsis.

**ANSWER: B**

22. Which one of the following clinical signs or symptoms is not associated with serum sodium concentrations below 125 mEq/L?

A. Headache

B. Hallucinations

C. Bradycardia

D. Hypoventilation

E. Hyperthermia

*Ref.:* 2, 3

**COMMENTS:** In most patients with **symptomatic hyponatremia**, the serum sodium concentration decreases below 125 mEq/L. When the concentration falls below 125 mEq/L, clinical signs and symptoms may occur, including headache, nausea, lethargy, hallucinations, seizures, bradycardia, hypoventilation, and occasionally coma. Hypothermia, not hyperthermia, occurs.

**ANSWER: E**

23. With regard to potassium, which of the following statements is not true?

A. Normal dietary intake of potassium is 50 to 100 mEq/day.

B. In patients with normal renal function, most ingested potassium is excreted in urine.

C. More than 90% of the potassium in the body is located in the extracellular compartment.

D. Critical hyperkalemia (>6 mEq/L) is rarely encountered if renal function is normal.

E. Administration of sodium bicarbonate shifts potassium from the extracellular space (ECF) to the intracellular space (ICF).

*Ref.:* 1, 2

**COMMENTS:** The average daily dietary intake of potassium is 50 to 100 mEq. In patients with normal renal function and normal serum potassium levels, most ingested potassium is excreted in urine. More than 90% of the body's potassium stores is within the intracellular compartment at a concentration of 150 mEq/L. Although the total extracellular potassium concentration is just 50 to 70 mEq (4.5 mEq/L), this concentration is critical for cardiac and neuromuscular function. Significant quantities of intracellular potassium are released in response to severe injury, surgical stress, acidosis, and a catabolic state. However, dangerous hyperkalemia (>6 mEq/L) is rarely encountered if renal function is normal. The administration of bicarbonate shifts potassium from the ECF across the cell membrane into the ICF.

**ANSWER:** C

24. Which of the following electrocardiographic (ECG) findings is not associated with hyperkalemia?

A. Peaked T waves

B. Prolonged PR interval

C. Loss of the P wave

D. Narrowing of the QRS complex

E. T waves higher than R waves in more than one lead

*Ref.:* 1, 2

**COMMENTS:** **Hyperkalemia** occurs when the serum potassium level exceeds 5 mmol/L. As potassium increases, changes in the resting membrane potential of cells impair depolarization and repolarization and lead to cardiac arrhythmias. The signs of hyperkalemia are generally limited to cardiovascular and gastrointestinal symptoms. Gastrointestinal symptoms include nausea, vomiting, intermittent intestinal colic, and diarrhea. ECG changes could be the first manifestation of hyperkalemia (Figure 4-1) and include

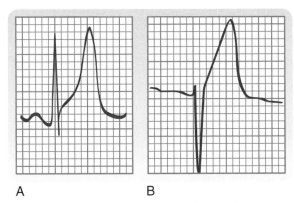

**Figure 4-1.  A,** Electrocardiographic (ECG) changes indicating hyperkalemia. The T wave is tall, narrow, and symmetrical. **B,** ECG changes indicating acute myocardial infarction. The T wave is tall but broad based and asymmetrical. *(From Somers MP, Brady WJ, Perron AD, et al: The prominent T wave: Electrocardiographic differential diagnosis, Am J Emerg Med 20:243–251, 2002.)*

peaked T waves and a prolonged PR interval, which are characteristic early findings. These ECG changes may be seen with potassium concentrations greater than 6 mEq/L. Symmetrically peaked T waves indicate dangerous hyperkalemia, particularly if the T waves are higher than the R wave in more than one lead. At higher potassium concentrations (7 mmol/L), loss of P waves, slurring, or widening of the QRS complexes occurs. As [K$^+$] exceeds 8 mmol/L, sudden lethal arrhythmias ensue, such as asystole, ventricular fibrillation, or a wide pulseless idioventricular rhythm.

**ANSWER:** D

25. Which one of the following is least useful in the immediate treatment of hyperkalemia?

A. Calcium salts

B. Sodium bicarbonate

C. Potassium-binding resins

D. Glucose and insulin

E. Hemodialysis

*Ref.:* 1-3

**COMMENTS:** The most dreaded complication of **hyperkalemia** is the development of a lethal arrhythmia. Immediate management includes ECG monitoring and cessation of all potassium supplementation and potassium-sparing drugs. **Calcium** is administered intravenously to stabilize the membrane potential and decrease myocardial excitability. It acts in less than 5 minutes and the effects last for 30 to 60 minutes. **Sodium bicarbonate** drives potassium into cells, thereby transiently reducing serum potassium levels. Its actions last 15 to 30 minutes. **Insulin and glucose** also facilitate entry of potassium into cells, with an almost immediate onset of action. In cases of severe hyperkalemia, **hemodialysis** is the definitive and most rapid method of decreasing extracellular potassium. **Potassium-binding resins**, such as sodium polystyrene sulfonate (Kayexalate), begin lowering serum potassium within 1 to 2 hours and last 4 to 6 hours. Rectal administration of these binding resins is more effective than oral formulations. However, enemas with sodium polystyrene sulfonate combined with sorbitol have been associated with colon necrosis and perforation. Kaliuresis through the administration of diuretics such as acetazolamide is also effective in reducing serum potassium levels.

**ANSWER:** C

26. With regard to hypokalemia, which of the following statements is not true?

A. Potassium and hydrogen ions are exchanged for sodium in the renal tubule.

B. Respiratory acidosis is associated with increased renal potassium loss.

C. Hypokalemia can cause decreased deep tendon reflexes.

D. Flattened T waves and a prolonged QT interval are associated with hypokalemia.

E. Intravenous potassium administration should not exceed 40 to 60 mEq/h.

*Ref.:* 1, 2

**COMMENTS:** Hypokalemia is more common than hyperkalemia in surgical patients. Hypokalemia can result from increased renal excretion, prolonged administration of potassium-free fluids, hyperalimentation with inadequate potassium replacement, or gastrointestinal losses. Respiratory and metabolic **alkaloses** result in increased renal potassium loss because potassium is preferentially excreted in an attempt to preserve hydrogen ions. Loss of gastrointestinal **secretions** can also be a significant cause of potassium depletion. This problem is compounded if potassium-free fluids are used for volume replacement. Signs of hypokalemia, including **paralytic ileus**, diminished or absent **tendon reflexes**, weakness, and even flaccid **paralysis**, are related to decreased muscle contractility. ECG changes include **flattened or inverted T waves**, U waves, and **prolongation of the QT interval**. The best treatment of hypokalemia is prevention. Gastrointestinal losses should be treated by the administration of fluids containing enough potassium to replace daily obligatory loss (20 mEq/day), as well as the additional losses in gastrointestinal drainage. As a rule, no more than 40 to 60 mEq of potassium should be added to each liter of intravenous fluid, and the rate of potassium administration should never exceed 40 to 60 mEq/h.

**ANSWER:　B**

---

27. Which one of the following is not associated with hypocalcemia?

    A. Shortening of the QT interval

    B. Painful muscle spasms

    C. Perioral or fingertip tingling

    D. Seizures in children

    E. Prolongation of the QT interval

*Ref.: 1-3*

**COMMENTS:** The symptoms of **hypocalcemia** are generally seen at serum levels of less than 8 mg/dL. Symptoms include numbness and tingling in the circumoral area and in the tips of the fingers and toes. Signs include hyperactive deep tendon reflexes, positive **Chvostek sign**, positive **Trousseau sign**, muscle and abdominal cramps, tetany with carpal pedal spasm, or convulsions. The electrocardiogram may show prolongation of the QT interval. Calcium is found in three forms in the body: **protein bound** (≈50%, mostly to albumin); diffusible calcium combined with anions such as bicarbonate, phosphate, and acetate (5%); and **ionized** (≈45%). Patients with severe alkalosis may have symptoms of hypocalcemia despite normal serum calcium levels because the ionized calcium is markedly decreased. Conversely, hypocalcemia without signs or symptoms may be present in patients with hypoproteinemia and a normal ionized fraction. Acute symptoms can be relieved by the intravenous administration of calcium gluconate or calcium chloride. Patients requiring prolonged replacement can be treated with oral calcium, often given with vitamin D.

**ANSWER:　A**

---

28. Which one of the following clinical scenarios is not associated with acute hypocalcemia?

    A. Fluid resuscitation from shock

    B. Rapid infusion of blood products

    C. Improper administration of phosphates

    D. Vitamin D–deficient diets

    E. Acute pancreatitis

*Ref.: 1*

**COMMENTS:** Infusion of large volumes of **isotonic fluid** can cause a modest reduction in serum calcium levels. The concomitant decrease in magnesium also impairs vitamin D activity and makes correction of the hypocalcemia more difficult. Administration of a **citrate load** during rapid transfusion of blood products can lead to severe hypocalcemia, hypotension, and cardiac failure. In this setting, calcium should be replaced at a dose of 0.2 g/500 mL of blood transfused. Most patients receiving slow, elective blood transfusions do not require calcium supplementation. **Acute pancreatitis** causes precipitation of calcium salts in the abdomen and may contribute to hypocalcemia. Other common causes include necrotizing fasciitis, renal failure, gastrointestinal fistula, and hypoparathyroidism. In general, calcium replacement should be monitored by measuring the concentration of ionized calcium.

**ANSWER:　D**

---

29. Which of the following disturbances is not associated with tumor lysis syndrome?

    A. Hypocalcemia

    B. Hyperuricemia

    C. Hyperkalemia

    D. Hypermagnesemia

    E. Hyperphosphatemia

*Ref.: 1*

**COMMENTS:** **Tumor lysis syndrome** is a constellation of electrolyte abnormalities that results from massive tumor cell necrosis secondary to antineoplastic therapy. **Hypocalcemia, hyperphosphatemia, hyperuricemia**, and **hyperkalemia** may occur. Hypocalcemia results from the release of intracellular stores of phosphate, which binds with ionized serum calcium to form calcium phosphate salts. Chemotherapy directed against solid tumors, especially **lymphomas**, is most commonly associated with tumor lysis syndrome. **Acute renal failure** can occur and prevent spontaneous correction of the electrolyte abnormalities. Hypermagnesemia is not associated with tumor lysis syndrome.

**ANSWER:　D**

---

30. An asymptomatic patient is found to have a serum calcium level of 13.5 mg/dL. Which of the following medications should be avoided?

    A. Bisphosphonates

    B. Thiazide diuretics

    C. Mithramycin

    D. Calcitonin

    E. Corticosteroids

*Ref.: 1*

**COMMENTS: Hypercalcemia** can affect the gastrointestinal, renal, musculoskeletal, and central nervous systems. Early symptoms include fatigability, lassitude, weakness, anorexia, nausea, and vomiting. Central nervous symptoms can progress to stupor and coma. Other symptoms include headaches and the three P's: pain, polydipsia, and polyuria. The critical serum calcium level for hypercalcemia is 16 to 20 mg/mL. Prompt treatment must be instituted at this level, or the symptoms may progress to death. Two major causes of hypercalcemia are **hyperparathyroidism** and **metastatic disease**. Metastatic breast cancer in patients receiving estrogen therapy is the most common cause of hypercalcemia associated with metastases.

Oral or intravenous **phosphates** are useful for reducing hypercalcemia by inhibiting bone resorption and forming calcium phosphate complexes that are deposited in the soft tissues. Intravenous phosphorus, however, has been associated with the acute development of hypocalcemia, hypotension, and renal failure. For this reason, it should be given slowly over a period of 8 to 12 hours once daily for no more than 2 to 3 days. Intravenous **sodium sulfate** is effective, but no more so than saline diuresis. **Bisphosphonates** reduce serum calcium levels by suppressing the function of osteoclasts and thus reducing the bone resorption of calcium. With some malignant conditions such as breast cancer, bisphosphonates may be administered prophylactically to prevent hypercalcemia. **Mithramycin** lowers serum calcium levels in 24 to 48 hours by inhibiting bone resorption. A single dose may normalize serum calcium levels for several weeks.

**Calcitonin** is produced by the parafollicular cells of the thyroid gland and functions by inducing renal excretion of calcium and suppressing osteoclast bone resorption. Calcitonin can produce a moderate decrease in serum sodium levels, but the effect is lost with repeated administration. Because **corticosteroids** decrease resorption of calcium from bone and reduce intestinal absorption, they are useful for treating hypercalcemic patients with sarcoidosis, myeloma, lymphoma, or leukemia. Their effects, however, may not be apparent for 1 to 2 weeks. **Chelating agents**, such as ethylenediaminetetraacetic acid (EDTA), are not indicated since they can result in metastatic calcification, acute renal failure, and hypocalcemia. **Thiazide diuretics** are contraindicated because they are calcium sparing (and are often implicated as a cause of iatrogenic hypercalcemia). Acute hypercalcemic crisis from hyperparathyroidism is treated by stabilizing the patient and performing a parathyroidectomy.

**A N S W E R :** B

---

31. A 45-year-old alcoholic man is found to have hypomagnesemia. Which of the following statements about magnesium is true?

A. The distribution of nonosseous magnesium is similar to that of sodium.

B. Calcium deficiency cannot be adequately corrected until the hypomagnesemia is addressed.

C. Magnesium depletion is characterized by depression of the neuromuscular and central nervous systems.

D. Magnesium supplementation should be stopped as soon as the serum level has normalized.

E. The treatment of choice for magnesium deficiency is oral magnesium phosphate.

*Ref.:* 1, 2

**COMMENTS:** The body contains 2000 mEq of **magnesium**, half of which is contained in bone. Most of the remaining magnesium is **intracellular** (a distribution similar to that of potassium). Plasma levels range between 1.5 and 2.5 mEq/L. Normal dietary intake is 240 mg/day, most of which is excreted in feces. The kidneys excrete some magnesium but can help conserve magnesium when a deficiency is present. **Hypomagnesemia** (like calcium deficiency) is characterized by **neuromuscular** and **central nervous system hyperactivity**. Hypomagnesemia can occur with

starvation, malabsorption, protracted loss of gastrointestinal fluid, and prolonged parenteral therapy without proper magnesium supplementation. When there is an accompanying **calcium deficiency**, the latter cannot be successfully treated until the hypomagnesemia is corrected.

**Magnesium deficiency** is treated with parenteral administration of magnesium sulfate or magnesium chloride. The extracellular magnesium concentration can be restored rapidly, but therapy must be continued for 1 to 2 weeks to replenish the intracellular component. To avoid magnesium deficiency, patients managed with hyperalimentation should receive 12 to 24 mEq of magnesium daily. Oral supplementation and intramuscular injection are alternative routes for replacement but are not preferred. **Magnesium toxicity** is rare except in the setting of renal insufficiency. Immediate treatment is infusion of **calcium chloride** or **calcium gluconate**; if the symptoms persist, dialysis may be required.

**A N S W E R :** B

---

32. Apnea develops in a postoperative patient from narcotics. His Pco₂ is 60. With regard to acid-base buffering, which of the following is false?

A. The major extracellular buffer is bicarbonate.

B. Intracellular pH and extracellular pH are usually the same.

C. The major intracellular buffer consists of proteins and phosphate salts.

D. Hydrogen ions cannot directly pass through the cell membrane.

E. Treating acidosis with bicarbonate infusion can cause cell death.

*Ref.:* 1

**COMMENTS:** Two separate physiologic buffering systems exist. **Intracellular buffering** is mediated mainly by proteins and phosphate, whereas **extracellular buffering** is mediated by the bicarbonate–carbonic acid system. When serum hydrogen ion concentrations are high (decreased pH), hydrogen ions and sodium bicarbonate form carbonic acid and sodium chloride. Eventually, this reaction yields **water** and **carbon dioxide**. The carbon dioxide is expired through alveolar ventilation or crosses cell membranes to contribute to intracellular hydrogen stores. The opposite occurs with an increase in serum pH. This equilibrium can be represented as

$$HCl + NaHCO_3 \rightleftharpoons NaCl + H_2CO_3 \rightleftharpoons H_2O + CO_2$$

Hydrogen ions cannot pass through the cell membrane because of their polarity, so a nonpolar buffering shuttle such as carbon dioxide is needed. **Intracellular pH** is maintained at 7.1, whereas **extracellular pH** is normally 7.4 (Table 4-4). The major intracellular buffering system is composed of **proteins** (which have binding sites for intracellular hydrogen ions) and **phosphate salts.** When serum pH is low, a **bicarbonate infusion** can prevent intracellular accumulation of hydrogen ion. However, with excess infusion of bicarbonate, the bicarbonate–carbonic acid equation is pushed to the right to generate more carbon dioxide, which must be expired. If ventilation is inadequate, excess carbon dioxide can pass into cells, oversaturate the intracellular buffering system, and lead to cell death.

**A N S W E R :** B

**TABLE 4-4  Six-Step Sequential Approach to Interpretation of Arterial Blood Gases with Supplemental Information from Serum Sodium, Potassium, and Chloride Concentrations***

| Observation | Interpretation | Intervention |
|---|---|---|
| Is pH other than 7.40? | Acidosis if <7.35 Alkalosis if >7.45 | Clinical evaluation for causal disease |
| Is pH <7.20 or >7.55? | Severe disorder | Prompt correction required |
| Is $Paco_2$ other than 40 mm Hg? | Ventilation compensates or contributes to the disorder | Change ventilation so that $Paco_2$ compensates |
| Is base deficit other than zero? | Bicarbonate loss/gain compensates or contributes to the disorder | Infuse $NaCO_3$ or HCl to correct proton concentration |
| Does urine pH reflect acidosis/ alkalosis? | Acid/alkaline urine indicates that renal function compensates or contributes | Renally active drugs or electrolyte replacement so that nephrons contribute |
| Is anion gap† <12 mmol/L? | Values above 12 mmol/L suggest lactic acidosis or ketoacidosis | Correct primary metabolic problem |

*The goal is to achieve a normal pH of 7.40.
†Anion gap = $[Na^+] + [K^+] - [Cl^-]$.

33. A 70-year-old man with sepsis has a pH of 7.18. Which of the following statements is true regarding his metabolic acidosis?

    A. Tissue hypoxia leads to increased oxidative metabolism.

    B. Acute compensation for metabolic acidosis is primarily renal.

    C. Metabolic acidosis results from the loss of bicarbonate or the gain of fixed acids.

    D. The most common cause of excess acid is prolonged nasogastric suction.

    E. Restoration of blood pressure with vasopressors corrects the metabolic acidosis associated with circulatory failure.

*Ref.: 1, 4*

**COMMENTS:** **Metabolic acidosis** results from the retention or gain of fixed acids (e.g., through diabetic acidosis or lactic acidosis) or the loss of bicarbonate (e.g., through diarrhea, small bowel fistula, or renal tubular dysfunction). Initial compensation is **respiratory** (by hyperventilation). **Renal compensation** is slower and occurs through the same means as the renal compensation for respiratory acidosis: excretion of acid salts and retention of bicarbonate. This compensation depends on normal renal function. When kidney damage interferes with the ability to excrete acid and resorb bicarbonate, metabolic acidosis may rapidly progress to profound levels. The most common cause of metabolic acidosis in surgical patients is **circulatory failure**, with tissue hypoxia and anaerobic metabolism leading to the accumulation of lactic acid. Resuscitation with vasopressors or infusion of bicarbonate does not correct the underlying problem. Replacement of volume with a balanced electrolyte solution, blood, or both results in restoration of the circulation, hepatic clearance of lactate, consumption of the formed bicarbonate, and clearance of carbonic acid by the lung. Excessive use of **bicarbonate** can cause metabolic alkalosis, which in combination with other sequelae such as hypothermia and low levels of 2,3-diphosphoglycerate (from banked blood), shifts the oxygen-hemoglobin distribution curve to the left and thereby compromises oxygen delivery.

**ANSWER:  C**

34. A 70-kg man with pyloric obstruction secondary to ulcer disease is admitted to the hospital for resuscitation after 1 week of prolonged vomiting. What metabolic disturbance is expected?

    A. Hypokalemic, hyperchloremic metabolic acidosis

    B. Hyperkalemic, hypochloremic metabolic alkalosis

    C. Hyperkalemic, hyperchloremic metabolic acidosis

    D. Hypokalemic, hypochloremic metabolic alkalosis

    E. None of the above

*Ref.: 1, 4*

**COMMENTS:** A common problem seen in patients with persistent emesis is **hypokalemic, hypochloremic metabolic alkalosis**. To compensate for the alkalosis associated with the loss of chloride- and hydrogen ion–rich fluid from the stomach, bicarbonate excretion in urine is increased. The bicarbonate is usually excreted as a sodium salt. However, in an attempt to conserve intravascular volume, aldosterone-mediated sodium absorption occurs and leads to potassium and hydrogen excretion. This compounds the alkalosis and results in a paradoxical aciduria. Management includes resuscitation with isotonic saline solutions and aggressive replacement of lost potassium.

**ANSWER:  D**

**REFERENCES**

1. Mullins RJ: Schock, electrolytes, and fluid. In Townsend CM, Beauchamp RD, Evers BM, et al, editors: *Sabiston textbook of surgery: the biological basis of modern surgical practice*, ed 18, Philadelphia, 2008, WB Saunders.
2. Shires GT: Fluid and electrolyte management of the surgical patient. In Brunicardi FC, Andersen DK, Billiar TR, et al, editors: *Schwartz's principles of surgery*, ed 9, New York, 2010, McGraw-Hill.
3. Fenves AZ, Rao A, Emmett M: Fluids and electrolytes. In O'Leary JP, editor: *The physiologic basis of surgery*, ed 4, Philadelphia, 2008, Lippincott Williams & Wilkins.
4. Jan BV, Lowry SF: Systemic response to injury and metabolic support. In Brunicardi FC, Andersen DK, Billiar TR, et al, editors: *Schwartz's principles of surgery*, ed 9, New York, 2010, McGraw-Hill.

# B. The Endocrine and Metabolic Response to Stress

*Roderick M. Quiros, M.D., F.A.C.S.*

1. Which of the following is true with regard to the metabolic response to stress as described by Cuthbertson:

   A. The flow phase of Cuthbertson's two-phase model of the metabolic response to injury is characterized by physiologic responses designed to restore tissue perfusion and circulating volume.

   B. The ebb phase begins once the patient is successfully resuscitated.

   C. The ebb phase entails both a catabolic and an anabolic period.

   D. The flow phase occurs initially after traumatic injury.

   E. The anabolic phase starts after wounds have closed and is characterized by the return of normal homeostasis.

   *Ref.: 1*

COMMENTS: The **metabolic response to injury** is traditionally broken down into two phases outlined by Cuthbertson. The first part of the response is known as the ***ebb phase***, which is composed of physiologic responses designed to restore tissue perfusion and maintain circulating volume immediately after injury. The ***flow phase*** follows once the patient is resuscitated. It can be further broken down into catabolic and anabolic phases. The catabolic phase is characterized by a hyperdynamic response that includes hypermetabolism, hyperglycemia, and water retention. The anabolic phase begins after injuries have started to heal and is characterized by return to normal homeostasis.

ANSWER: E

2. All of the following activate the sympathoadrenal and hypothalamic-pituitary axes during stress or injury except:

   A. Pain

   B. Hypovolemia

   C. Acidosis

   D. Hypercapnia

   E. Acetylcholine

   *Ref.: 1*

COMMENTS: In response to **stress** or injury, neural afferent signals converge on the brain to activate the sympathetic nervous system and hypothalamic stimulation. Catecholamines are released from the sympathetic nervous system and result in increases in blood pressure, heart rate, cardiac output, and minute ventilation. Hypothalamic release of corticotropin-releasing hormone leads to release of corticotropin from the pituitary gland, which in turn induces the adrenal cortex to synthesize and release cortisol. These responses are designed to compensate for lost circulatory volume, maintain organ perfusion, and provide the energy substrates needed for organ function. Pain is a potent activator of these pathways. Hypovolemia simulates baroreceptors in the aorta and carotid bodies, which stimulates these pathways. Chemoreceptors in the carotid bodies and aorta are activated by hypoxemia, acidosis, and hypercapnia. These receptors also trigger the hypothalamic-pituitary-adrenal axis. Cytokines can likewise affect these pathways, though in a less direct manner since they do not have direct neural input into these axes. Acetylcholine has antiinflammatory effects and is not part of the afferent response to injury.

ANSWER: E

3. All of the following are a part of the systemic inflammatory response syndrome (SIRS) except:

   A. Temperature of 36° C or lower

   B. Pulse lower than 56 beats/min

   C. Respiratory rate of 20 breaths/min or higher

   D. White blood cell count of 12,000/μl or greater

   E. 10% or greater band forms on complete blood count (CBC) with differential

   *Ref.: 2*

COMMENTS: The clinical spectrum of **SIRS** includes two or more of the following criteria:

- Temperature of 38° C or higher or 36° C or lower
- Pulse of 90 beats/min or greater
- Respiratory rate of 20 breaths/min or greater or a $Paco_2$ of 32 mm Hg or lower
- White blood cell count of 12,000/μl or greater or 4000/μl or lower or 10% or more band forms on the CBC with differential

   SIRS is a sterile response. Sepsis includes an identifiable source of infection in addition to SIRS.

ANSWER: B

4. Which of the amino acids is critical to the synthesis of catecholamines?

   A. Tyrosine

   B. Phenylalanine

   C. Glutamate

   D. Aspartic acid

   E. Methionine

   *Ref.: 1*

**COMMENTS:** Tyrosine from the diet or from conversion of phen-ylalanine is the prime substrate for the synthesis of cate-cholamines. Tyrosine is hydroxylated to form dihydroxyphenylala-nine (dopa), which undergoes decarboxylation to form dopamine. Dopamine is then hydroxylated to form norepinephrine. Norepi-nephrine is subsequently methylated in the adrenal medulla to form epinephrine.

**A N S W E R :**   A

5. All of the following are secreted as part of the endocrine response to stress except:

   A. Corticotropin

   B. ADH

   C. Growth hormone

   D. Thyroid hormone

   E. None of the above

*Ref.:* 1

**COMMENTS: Trauma** induces the release of **hormones,** which directly affect the metabolism of carbohydrate, fat, and protein. Corticotropin is released from the pituitary gland and stimulates the release of cortisol, which stimulates hepatic gluconeogenesis and increases release of amino acids from skeletal muscles. Release of ADH from the posterior pituitary gland in response to decreases in effective circulating plasma volume leads to increased peripheral vasoconstriction, increased water reabsorption, increased hepatic gluconeogenesis, and glycogenolysis. Growth hormone is released from the anterior pituitary and increases amino acid uptake and hepatic protein synthesis. Release of thyroid hormone increases after injury in response to release of thyroid-stimulating hormone (TSH) from the anterior pituitary after injury. It induces glycolysis and gluconeogenesis and increases the metabolic rate and heat production.

**A N S W E R :**   E

6. Which of the following is true with regard to the renin-angiotensin system?

   A. It is activated by an increase in the renal tubular sodium concentration.

   B. Angiotensinogen is found in the renal medulla.

   C. Angiotensin-converting enzyme in the liver converts angiotensin I to angiotensin II.

   D. Angiotensin II stimulates the release of aldosterone.

   E. Angiotensin II decreases splanchnic vasoconstriction.

*Ref.:* 1

**COMMENTS:** The **renin-angiotensin system** is activated by decreases in renal arterial blood flow and renal tubular sodium concentration, as well as increased β-adrenergic stimulation. Renin is secreted from the juxtaglomerular cells of the renal afferent arteriole. Renin converts angiotensinogen in the liver to angioten-sin I. Angiotensin-converting enzyme produced by the lung con-verts angiotensin I to angiotensin II. Angiotensin II simulates the release of aldosterone, increases peripheral and splanchnic vaso-constriction, and decreases the renal excretion of salt and water.

**A N S W E R :**   D

7. Which of the following is not an action of cortisol in a meta-bolically stressed patient?

   A. It stimulates release of insulin by the pancreas.

   B. It induces insulin resistance in muscles and adipose tissue.

   C. It stimulates release of lactate from skeletal muscle.

   D. It induces release of glycerol from adipose tissue.

   E. It leads to immunosuppression.

*Ref.:* 2

**COMMENTS: Cortisol** is the major glucocorticoid released during **physiologic stress**. After injury, levels are elevated in pro-portion to the degree of stress to the patient. Metabolically, cortisol potentiates the actions of glucagon and epinephrine, which is mani-fested as hyperglycemia. It also stimulates enzymatic activities favoring hepatic gluconeogenesis. In skeletal muscle, cortisol induces protein degradation and release of lactate, which serves as a substrate for hepatic gluconeogenesis. It also potentiates the release of free fatty acids, triglycerides, and glycerol from adipose tissue to provide additional energy sources. In a stressed patient, cortisol induces insulin resistance in muscles and adipose tissue. All these actions are directed at increasing blood glucose levels in the stressed system. Answer A is therefore incorrect because insulin causes a decrease in blood glucose levels. Additionally, glucocor-ticoids cause depressed cell-mediated immune responses (decreased killer T-cell and natural killer cell function, as well as T-cell genera-tion) and delayed hypersensitivity responses.

**A N S W E R :**   A

8. Which of the following are effects of epinephrine in response to injury?

   A. It enhances the adherence of leukocytes to vascular endo-thelial membranes.

   B. It stimulates the release of aldosterone.

   C. It inhibits the secretion of thyroid hormones.

   D. It increases glucagon secretion.

   E. It decreases lipolysis in adipose tissue.

*Ref.:* 2

**COMMENTS:** The **catecholamines** norepinephrine and epi-nephrine are increased up to fourfold in plasma immediately after injury. In the liver, epinephrine promotes glycogenolysis, gluco-neogenesis, lipolysis, and ketogenesis. It decreases insulin release and increases glucagon secretion. Epinephrine increases lipolysis in adipose tissue and induces insulin resistance in skeletal muscle. The overall effect of these actions is stress-induced hyperglycemia. Catecholamines also increase the secretion of thyroid and parathy-roid hormones as part of the stress response. Epinephrine induces leukocyte demargination from vascular endothelial membranes, which is manifested as leukocytosis.

**A N S W E R :**   D

9. Which of the following substances has been shown to be useful as a measurable marker of the response to injury?

   A. Tumor necrosis factor-α (TNF-α)

   B. Interleukin-2 (IL-2)

   C. IL-6

D. IL-10

E. C-reactive protein (CRP)

Ref.: 2

COMMENTS: **Cytokines** released as part of the **stress response** have a myriad of effects that both drive and inhibit the inflammatory process. TNF-α is among the earliest detectable cytokines after injury. It is secreted by macrophages, Kupffer cells, neutrophils, natural killer cells, T lymphocytes, mast cells, and endothelial cells, among others. It has a half-life of less than 20 minutes. TNF-α induces significant shock and catabolism. IL-2 is secreted by T lymphocytes and has a half-life of less than 10 minutes. It promotes lymphocyte proliferation, immunoglobulin production, and gut barrier integrity. It also regulates lymphocyte apoptosis. IL-6 is released by macrophages, B lymphocytes, neutrophils, basophils, mast cells, and endothelial cells. It has a long half-life and prolongs the survival of activated neutrophils. It is a potent inducer of acute phase proteins in the liver. IL-10 is secreted by B and T lymphocytes, macrophages, basophils, and mast cells. It is an antiinflammatory cytokine and has been shown to reduce mortality in animal models of sepsis and acute respiratory distress syndrome (ARDS). CRP is useful as a marker of the response to injury because it reflects the degree of inflammation fairly accurately. CRP levels are not subject to diurnal variations and do not change with feeding. Consequently, it is used as a biomarker of inflammation and response to treatment.

ANSWER:  E

10. Which of the following is true regarding reactive oxygen metabolites:

A. Reactive oxygen metabolites are synthesized and stored within leukocytes before being released in response to injury.

B. Reactive oxygen metabolites cause injury by oxidation of unsaturated fatty acids within cell membranes.

C. Cells secreting reactive oxygen metabolites are immune to damage after release of these metabolites.

D. In ischemic tissue, the mechanisms for production of reactive oxygen metabolites are downregulated.

E. Reactive oxygen metabolites are quenched by inhibitory cytokines.

Ref.: 2

COMMENTS: **Reactive oxygen metabolites** are short-lived, highly reactive molecules that cause tissue injury by oxidation of fatty acids within cell membranes. They are produced during anaerobic glucose oxidation, with resulting production of superoxide anion from the reduction of oxygen. Superoxide anion is further metabolized to hydrogen peroxide and hydroxyl radicals. Cells are not immune to injury from the reactive oxygen metabolites that they release, but they are usually protected from damage by oxygen scavengers such as glutathione and catalases, not inhibitory cytokines. In ischemic tissues, the mechanisms for production of oxygen metabolites are actually activated, but because of the lack of oxygen supply, production of reactive oxygen metabolites is kept to a minimum. Once blood flow is restored, oxygen is redelivered, thereby allowing large quantities of reactive oxygen metabolites to be produced, which in turn leads to reperfusion injury.

ANSWER:  B

11. Which of the following statements about eicosanoids is true?

A. Their synthesis is dependent on enzymatic activation of phospholipase A₂.

B. They originate from lymphocytes around the site of injury.

C. They are stored within inflammatory cells and released on tissue injury.

D. The production of leukotrienes is dependent on enzymatic activation of cyclooxygenase.

E. The production of prostaglandins is dependent on enzymatic activation of lipoxygenase.

Ref.: 2

COMMENTS: **Eicosanoids** are a class of mediators that includes **prostaglandins**, thromboxanes, leukotrienes, hydroxyeicosatetraenoic acids, and lipoxins. They are secreted by all nucleated cells except for lymphocytes. Phospholipids are converted by phospholipase A₂ into arachidonic acid. Arachidonic acid is then metabolized by cyclooxygenase to yield cyclic endoperoxides and eventually prostaglandins and thromboxanes. Alternatively, arachidonic acid is metabolized by lipoxygenase to yield hydroperoxyeicosatetraenoic acid and, eventually, hydroxyeicosatetraenoic acid and leukotrienes. Eicosanoids are not stored within cells but are synthesized and released in response to hypoxia or direct tissue injury. Other substances such as endotoxin, norepinephrine, vasopressin, angiotensin II, bradykinin, serotonin, acetylcholine, cytokines, and histamine can also induce the production and release of eicosanoids. Eicosanoids have a variety of deleterious effects, including acute lung injury, pancreatitis, and renal failure. They are extremely potent in promoting capillary leakage, leukocyte adherence, neutrophil activation, bronchoconstriction, and vasoconstriction.

ANSWER:  A

12. Which of the following is true regarding the kallikrein-kinin system?

A. Bradykinins are potent vasoconstrictors produced in ischemic tissues.

B. Bradykinins are stored in macrophages and released in response to tissue injury.

C. Bradykinin release and elevation are proportional to the magnitude of injury.

D. Bradykinin antagonists have been shown to improved survival in septic trauma patients.

E. Release of bradykinin is actually decreased in sepsis.

Ref.: 2

COMMENTS: **Bradykinins** are vasodilators produced by kininogen degradation by the protease kallikrein. **Kallikrein** circulates in blood and tissues in inactive form until is activated by Hageman factor, trypsin, plasmin, factor XI, kaolin, and collagen. Bradykinins increase capillary permeability, which leads to tissue edema. They also increase renal vasodilation, thereby leading to a reduction in renal perfusion pressure, which in turn activates the renin-angiotensin system and culminates in retention of sodium and water. Bradykinins are released during hypoxia and ischemia and after hemorrhage, sepsis, and endotoxemia. Elevations in bradykinins are proportional to the magnitude of the injury present. Studies in which bradykinin antagonists have been used to reduce the effects of sepsis show no improvement in survival.

**ANSWER: C**

13. Which of the following is true with regard to the complement cascade in the setting of injury?

    A. Complement deactivates granulocyte activation.

    B. Complement induces the release of TNF-α and IL-1.

    C. Complement induces the relaxation of endothelial smooth muscle.

    D. The complement components C3b and C5b are strong anaphylotoxins.

    E. The complement cascade is inhibited by hemorrhage.

*Ref.: 3*

**COMMENTS:** Ischemia and endothelial injuries lead to the activation of **complement**, a series of plasma proteins involved in the inflammatory response. Complement is activated with release of the biologically active anaphylotoxins C3a and C5a during hemorrhage. These components cause granulocyte activation and aggregation, increased vascular permeability, smooth muscle contraction, and release of histamine and arachidonic acid metabolites. They also promote the release of TNF-α and IL-1, both major cytokines in the inflammatory response. Although activation of complement can lead to the destruction and lysis of invading organisms, overactivation may result in tissue destruction and damage, as seen in ARDS.

**ANSWER: B**

14. Which of the following is true with regard to the inflammatory response?

    A. Clot at the site of injury is the primary chemoattractant for neutrophils and monocytes.

    B. Migration of neutrophils to the site of injury is inhibited by the release of serotonin.

    C. Mast cells appear at the site of injury after migrating to the injury via chemoattractants such as cytokines.

    D. Surgical or traumatic injury is associated with upregulation of cell-mediated immunity via type 1 helper T (T$_H$1) cells and downregulation of antibody-mediated immunity via type 2 helper T (T$_H$2) cells.

    E. Eosinophils involved in the inflammatory response are inactivated by the complement anaphylatoxins C3a and C5a.

*Ref.: 2*

**COMMENTS:** Formation of clot at the site of injury serves at the primary **chemoattractant** for **neutrophils** and monocytes during the **inflammatory** response of the body to injury. Migration of neutrophils along with platelets through the vascular endothelium occurs within hours of injury and is facilitated by serotonin, platelet-activating factor, and prostaglandin E$_2$. **Mast cells** are preexistent in tissues and are therefore the first to be involved in the inflammatory response. They release histamine, cytokines, eicosanoids, proteases, and TNF-α, which results in local vasodilation, capillary leakage, and recruitment of other inflammatory cells to the area. In severe injuries, there is a reduction in cell-mediated

immunity and T$_H$1 cytokine production and a shift toward antibody-mediated immunity through the action of T$_H$2 cells. A T$_H$1 response is favored in lesser injuries; with intact cell-mediated opsonizing capability and antibody immunity against microbial infections; and with activation of monocytes, B lymphocytes, and cytotoxic T lymphocytes. A shift to the T$_H$2 response is associated with more severe injuries and includes activation of eosinophil, mast cell, and B-lymphocyte antibody production. Eosinophils involved in the inflammatory response are activated by IL-3, granulocyte-macrophage colony-stimulating factor (GM-CSF), IL-5, platelet-activating factor, and the complement anaphylatoxins C3a and C5a.

**ANSWER: A**

15. The initial recruitment of neutrophils to endothelial surfaces is mediated primarily by:

    A. Immunoglobulins

    B. Integrins

    C. Selectins

    D. All of the above

    E. None of the above

*Ref.: 2*

**COMMENTS:** In endothelial injury, the initial recruitment of inflammatory leukocytes, specifically **neutrophils**, to the endothelial surfaces is mediated by adhesion molecules known as **selectins**, which are found on cell surfaces. Neutrophil rolling in the first 20 minutes after injury is mediated by P-selectin, which is stored within endothelial cells. After 20 minutes, P-selectin is degraded and L-selectin becomes the primary mediator of leukocyte rolling. Firm adhesion and transmigration of neutrophils through the endothelium and into the site of injury are mediated by integrins and the immunoglobulin family of **adhesion molecules**, including intercellular adhesion molecule (ICAM), vascular cell adhesion molecule (VCAM), and platelet–endothelial cell adhesion molecule (PECAM).

**ANSWER: C**

16. Which of the following regarding macrophages/monocytes is true?

    A. Macrophages and monocytes become hyperresponsive to *continued* injury/insult after trauma.

    B. Functional impairment in macrophage/monocyte capability may persist for a week and is overcome with the development and growth of newer, more immature monocytes.

    C. Macrophages present peptides in association with major histocompatibility complex (MHC) class II molecules to prime CD8$^+$ cytotoxic T lymphocytes.

    D. Human leukocyte antigen/MHC II expression on monocytes increases after major injury.

    E. Macrophages present peptides in association with MHC class I molecules to prime CD4$^+$ helper T lymphocytes.

*Ref.: 4*

**COMMENTS:** After the initial short-lived hyperactivation involving release of TNF and IL-1, **macrophages** and **monocytes** actually become hyporesponsive. Deactivation of these cells results in a type of immunologic paralysis. With stress, these cells release prostaglandin $E_2$, which has immunosuppressive effects. It inhibits T-cell mitogenesis, along with IL-1 and TNF-α production. This functional impairment in the patient's innate cellular immunity lasts for up to 7 days, until newly recruited monocytes are produced to bolster the immune response. Additional mediators such as transforming growth factor-β (TGF-β), IL-10, and IL-4 are also secreted after stress or trauma and inhibit the capability of macrophages and monocytes to present antigen to T cells, thereby contributing to impairment in antigen-specific immunity as well. The overall decrease in the adaptive immune response has been found to be associated with decreased resistance to infection. The functional impairment in macrophage/monocyte capability may persist for up to 7 days and is overcome with the development and growth of newer, more immature monocytes, which may lack the abilities of their predecessor monocytes. HLA-DR/MHC II expression on monocytes decreases after major injury, with prolonged depression being associated with an increased infection rate. Macrophages present peptides in association with MHC class I molecules to prime $CD8^+$ cytotoxic T lymphocytes and peptides in association with MHC class II to prime $CD4^+$ helper T lymphocytes.

**ANSWER: B**

17. Which of the following is true regarding NO?

    A. NO is inhibited by acetylcholine stimulation.

    B. NO is expressed constitutively.

    C. NO can induce platelet adhesion and thus lead to microthrombosis.

    D. NO has a half-life of 5 minutes.

    E. NO is formed from the oxidation of L-alanine.

*Ref.:* 2

**COMMENTS: Nitric oxide** is derived from the endothelial surfaces in response to acetylcholine stimulation, hypoxia, endotoxins, and cellular injury. It is expressed constitutively at low levels and helps maintain normal vascular smooth muscle relaxation. It reduces platelet adhesion and aggregation, thus making thrombosis of small vessels less likely. It is diffusible, with a half-life measured in seconds. NO is formed from the oxidation of L-arginine via the enzyme NO synthase.

**ANSWER: B**

18. Which of the following regarding TNF-α is true?

    A. Predominantly a local mediator that induces the classic inflammatory febrile response to injury by stimulating local prostaglandin activity in the anterior hypothalamus.

    B. Effective in promoting the maturation/recruitment of functional leukocytes needed for a normal cytokine response. Delays apoptosis of macrophages and neutrophils, which may contribute to organ injury.

    C. Has both a proinflammatory and antiinflammatory role. Is a mediator of the hepatic acute phase response to injury. Induces neutrophil activation, but also delays disposal of neutrophils. Can attenuate TNF-α and IL-1 activity, thereby curbing the inflammatory response.

    D. An inducer of muscle catabolism and cachexia during stress by shunting available amino acids to the hepatic circulation as fuel substrates. Also activates coagulation

and promotes the expression/release of adhesion molecules, prostaglandin $E_2$, platelet-activating factor, glucocorticoids, and eicosanoids.

    E. Promotes T-cell proliferation, production of immunoglobulins, and gut barrier integrity.

*Ref.:* 2

**COMMENTS: Cytokines** are the most potent mediators of the inflammatory response. On a local level, they promote wound healing and proliferation of microorganisms. In excess levels, as sometimes occurs during the response to injury, they may induce hemodynamic instability, which can lead to organ failure or death. There is considerable overlap regarding the effects of cytokines with regard to promoting or attenuating the inflammatory response. Choice A describes IL-1. Choice B describes GM-CSF. Choice C describes IL-6. Choice D describes TNF-α. Choice E describes IL-2.

**ANSWER: D**

19. Which of the following is considered an antiinflammatory cytokine?

    A. IL-1

    B. IL-4

    C. IL-6

    D. IL-8

    E. Interferon-γ (IFN-γ)

*Ref.:* 4

**COMMENTS:** The alterations in the hemodynamic, metabolic, and immune responses evident in stressed patients are orchestrated by endogenous polypeptides known as **cytokines**. They are produced by immune cells in direct response to injury, with levels correlating with the degree of tissue damage. Despite considerable overlap in bioactivity among cytokines, they are commonly classified by their predominant effect as proinflammatory or antiinflammatory. Those commonly considered proinflammatory include IL-1, IL-6, IL-8, and IFN-γ. Those usually considered antiinflammatory include IL-4, IL-10, IL-13, and TGF-β.

**ANSWER: B**

20. Which of the following is true with regard to TNF-α and IL-1?

    A. Levels of soluble molecules that antagonize the effects of TNF-α and IL-1 have been shown to be predictive of organ failure.

    B. Secretion of TNF-α and IL-1 is conducive to a hypocoagulable state during acute injury.

    C. Secretion of TNF-α and IL-1 in response to injury leads to downregulation of the synthesis of NO and subsequent vasoconstriction.

    D. TNF-α and IL-1 have a long half-life, which makes them effective markers for determining the magnitude and severity of the inflammatory response.

    E. TNF-α and IL-1 have no natural antagonists; rather, their systemic effects diminish because of natural cytokine degradation.

*Ref.:* 4

**COMMENTS: Tumor necrosis factor-α** and **Interleukin-1** are overproduced in patients after posttraumatic inflammation. They induce increased synthesis of NO; activation of the **cyclooxygenase** and **lipoxygenase** pathways, which leads to the formation of thromboxanes and prostaglandins; and production of platelet-activating factor, intracellular adhesion molecules, and selectins, which is conducive to hypercoagulability. TNF-α and IL-1 have a short half-life, thus making them unreliable predictors of the severity of injury in the clinical setting. Soluble molecules that antagonize their effects are more stable and have been found to be predictive of lethal outcome and end-organ failure. IL-1 receptor antagonist (IL-1Ra) binds to the IL-1 receptor and blocks IL-1 activity. Soluble TNF receptor I and II (sTNF-RI and sTNF-RII) bind biologically active TNF and antagonize its effects.

**ANSWER: A**

21. All of the following with regard to IL-6 are true except:

    A. IL-6 is a sensitive marker for the degree of tissue injury.

    B. IL-6 induces the synthesis of CRP.

    C. IL-6 secretion is inhibited by TNF-α and IL-1.

    D. IL-6 levels peak early after injury.

    E. IL-6 has antiinflammatory effects.

    *Ref.: 4*

**COMMENTS: Interleukin-6** is a very sensitive marker for the degree of tissue injury. It is secreted by monocytes, macrophages, neutrophils, T and B cells, endothelial cells, smooth muscle cells, and fibroblasts. IL-6 expression is induced by bradykinin, TGF-β, platelet-derived growth factor, TNF-α, and IL-1, among others. IL-6 levels peak early after injury, with levels found to be predictive of risk for and mortality from organ failure after trauma. IL-6 induces the synthesis of acute phase proteins such as fibrinogen, complement factors, $\alpha_1$-antitrypsin, and CRP. CRP itself is a marker for states with increased inflammation and in addition is predictive of adverse outcomes following secondary surgery. IL-6 also has some antiinflammatory effects, including inhibition of proteases and reduction of TNF-α and IL-1 synthesis; furthermore, it can cause the release of immunosuppressive glucocorticoids.

**ANSWER: C**

22. All of the following with regard to IL-8 are true except:

    A. IL-8 levels after injury have been shown to correlate with the onset of multiorgan failure.

    B. IL-8 exerts important inhibitory effects on polymorphonuclear cells.

    C. IL-8 is associated with ARDS.

    D. Local hypoxia induces production of IL-8 from macrophage.

    E. IL-8 does not produce the hemodynamic instability characteristic of TNF-α and IL-1.

    *Ref.: 4*

**COMMENTS:** Like IL-6, **Interleukin-8** levels peak within the first 24 hours after injury. Prolonged elevation of IL-8 is predictive of the onset of multiorgan failure and even mortality. IL-8 is secreted by monocytes, macrophages, neutrophils, and endothelial cells. It is a potent chemoattractant for polymorphonuclear cells,

particularly in the lung, where it is thought to have a role in initiating ARDS. Local hypoxia is thought to play a role in stimulating IL-8 production by pulmonary macrophages. Circulating polymorphonuclear cells migrate in response to IL-8 production, thereby leading to massive infiltration into the lungs, which in turn can progress to full-blown ARDS. Interestingly, IL-8 does not produce the hemodynamic instability characteristic of TNF-α and IL-1.

**ANSWER: B**

23. Which of the following with regard to IL-10 is true?

    A. IL-10 is a strong proinflammatory cytokine.

    B. IL-10 is secreted primarily by platelets in response to injury.

    C. IL-10 inhibits some proinflammatory cytokines such as IL-1.

    D. IL-10 has a short half-life and is therefore not a useful marker for assessing the severity of injury.

    E. IL-10 secretion is inhibited by the stress of surgical procedures.

    *Ref.: 4*

**COMMENTS: Interleukin-10** originates from T cells and monocytes. It has strong antiinflammatory properties and is capable of inhibiting the synthesis of proinflammatory cytokines such as IL-1 and TNF-α. IL-10 also induces a reduction in class II MHC molecules on monocytes, thereby leading to downregulation of the immune response. IL-10 levels in trauma patients have been shown to reflect the severity of injury and are predictive of patients in whom sepsis or multiorgan dysfunction syndrome will develop. Release of IL-10 is increased in direct proportion to tissue damage, thus suggesting that more invasive surgical procedures augment release of IL-10.

**ANSWER: C**

24. Which of the following with regard to metabolism during fasting is true?

    A. The main source of fuel in short-term fasting (<5 days) is derived from hepatic glycogen stores.

    B. Norepinephrine, vasopressin, and angiotensin II promote the assembly of glycogen chains during fasting.

    C. In prolonged starvation, ketone bodies become the primary fuel source for the brain.

    D. Lipid stores in adipose tissue provide 80% of the caloric expenditure during starvation.

    E. Release of free fatty acids is stimulated by an increase in serum insulin levels.

    *Ref.: 2*

**COMMENTS:** The normal adult contains up to 400 g of carbohydrates in the form of glycogen. Of this, approximately 100 g is stored in the liver and up to 250 g is stored in skeletal, cardiac, and smooth muscle cells. **Glycogen stores** within muscle are not readily available for systemic use but are available for the energy needs of muscle cells. In the **fasting state**, hepatic glycogen stores are therefore depleted rapidly, with a fall in serum glucose concentration in less than 16 hours. Glucagon, norepinephrine, vasopressin, and angiotensin II promote the utilization of glycogen stores.

After that time, glucose must come from gluconeogenesis in the liver, with lactate from skeletal muscle serving as a substrate. The result, in simple starvation and fasting, is protein degradation in skeletal muscle. In prolonged starvation, systemic proteolysis is reduced as vital organs (myocardium, brain, renal cortex, skeletal muscle) start to use ketone bodies as a primary fuel source. In continued fasting, lipid stores provide an additional source of glucose and supply up to 40% of the caloric expenditure during starvation. Up to 160 g of free fatty acids and glycerol can be mobilized from adipose tissue in a fasting 70-kg patient. Release of free fatty acids is stimulated in part by a reduction in serum insulin levels and in part by an increase in circulating glucagon and catecholamine levels.

**ANSWER:** C

**25.** All of the following regarding insulin therapy are true except:

A. Hyperglycemia increases the morbidity of critically ill patients in the surgical intensive care unit (ICU) setting without significantly affecting mortality rates.

B. Maintaining blood glucose levels of 80 to 110 mg/dL is beneficial in surgical ICU patients.

C. Hyperglycemia impairs macrophage ability.

D. Insulin has antiinflammatory effects.

E. Hyperglycemia promotes coagulation.

*Ref.:* 4

**COMMENTS:** Prospective, randomized data from Van den Berge and colleagues show that hyperglycemia increases mortality rates in critically ill surgical ICU patients. Hyperglycemia promotes oxidative stress, coagulation, and phagocyte dysfunction. Advanced glycation end products resulting from hyperglycemia are themselves proinflammatory. Insulin has anabolic, antiinflammatory, and antiapoptotic effects. For all these reasons, **insulin therapy** for **tight blood glucose control** has been shown to improve outcomes in ICU patients.

**ANSWER:** A

**26.** Which of the following provides the main energy source during critical illness/injury?

A. Skeletal muscle

B. Liver

C. Adipose tissue

D. Kidney

E. Gut

*Ref.:* 2

**COMMENTS:** Lipids are nonprotein, noncarbohydrate fuel sources that minimize **protein breakdown** in injured patients. In response to catecholamines released during stress, triglyceride lipase induces fat mobilization/lipolysis from adipose stores. Glycerol is released and provides a substrate for hepatic gluconeogenesis. Fatty acids are released and processed into ketone bodies by the liver to provide an additional fuel source. Free fatty acids can also serve as a direct source of energy for such tissues as cardiac, kidney, liver, and muscle cells.

**ANSWER:** C

**27.** Which of the following is correct with respect to the respiratory quotient (RQ)?

A. RQ = 1: greater oxidation of protein for fuel

B. RQ > 1: overfeeding/greater carbohydrate oxidation

C. RQ = 0.7: greater oxidation of carbohydrate for fuel

D. RQ = 0.85: greater oxidation of fatty acid for fuel

E. RQ < 1: excess breakdown of proteins for fuel

*Ref.:* 2

**COMMENTS:** The **respiratory quotient** is a unitless number used for the calculation of basal metabolic rate when estimated from carbon dioxide production. It is calculated from the ratio of $CO_2$ produced and $O_2$ consumed. The RQ in patients in metabolic balance usually ranges from 1.0, the value expected for pure carbohydrate oxidation, to 0.7, the value expected for pure fat oxidation. A mixed diet of fat and carbohydrate results in an average value between these numbers. The RQ may rise above 1.0 in an organism oxidizing carbohydrate to produce fat, as in overfeeding. In summary,

RQ = 1: greater oxidation of carbohydrate for fuel
RQ > 1: overfeeding/greater carbohydrate oxidation
RQ = 0.7: greater oxidation of fatty acid for fuel
RQ = 0.85: oxidation of equal amounts of fatty acids and glucose

**ANSWER:** B

## REFERENCES

1. Zukerbraun BS, Harbrecht BG: The physiologic response to injury. In Peitzman AB, Rhoes M, Schwab CW, et al, editors: *The trauma manual: trauma & acute care surgery*, ed 3, New York, 2008, Lippincott Williams & Wilkins.
2. Jan BV, Lowry SF: Systemic response to injury and metabolic support. In Brunicardi FC, Andersen DK, Billiar TR, et al, editors: *Schwartz's principles of surgery*, ed 9, New York, 2010, McGraw-Hill.
3. Phelan HA, Esatman AL, Frotan A, Gonzales RP: Shock and hypoperfusion states. In O'Leary JP, Tabuenca A, Capote LR, editors: *The physiologic basis of surgery*, ed 4, New York, 2008, Lippincott Williams & Wilkins.
4. Faist E, Trentzsch H: The Immune Response. In Feliciano DV, Mattox KL, Moore EE, editors: *Trauma*, ed 6, New York, 2007, McGraw-Hill Medical.

# C. Nutrition

*Janet Deselich Millikan, M.S., R.D., L.D.N.*

1. For an adult patient consuming a normal diet, which of the following is the most calorically dense energy source?

   A. Fat

   B. Alcohol

   C. Protein

   D. Carbohydrate

   E. Water

   *Ref.:* 1

**COMMENTS:** See Question 2.

**ANSWER:** A

2. The gastrointestinal tract can secrete and reabsorb how much water in the form of gastric juices per day (in a 70-kg adult male)?

   A. 1 to 2 L/day

   B. 4 to 5 L/day

   C. 6 to 7 L/day

   D. 8 to 10 L/day

   E. 50 L/day

   *Ref.:* 2

**COMMENTS:** Understanding **body composition** is important for comprehending the metabolic changes that occur in various clinical settings. The science of nutrition is primarily the study of nutrient metabolism at the cellular level. The digestive tract allows the utilization of nutrients via various mechanisms of digestion, including ingestion of food, separation of nutrients from food (digestion), movement of nutrients into the body for use (absorption), and release of by-products. Interruption of any of these stages of intake, digestion, and absorption creates a deviation from normal nutrition and can lead to unfavorable nutritional status. For a 70-kg man, body composition can be generalized as follows in terms of percentage of body weight: 40% ICF; 20% ECF, composed of 13% interstitial fluid, 2% transcellular fluid, and 5% plasma; 7% minerals; 18% protein; and 15% lipid. Fat stores can equal 160,000 kcal, with higher stores present in obese individuals. Lean body mass proteins can supply 30,000 kcal of the body's energy stores. Although energy in the diet is provided entirely by carbohydrates (4 kcal/g), fats (9 kcal/g), proteins (4 kcal/g), and alcohol (7 kcal/g), maintenance of fluid status is essential for nutrient use and nutritional equilibrium. The end products of protein, carbohydrate, and fat oxidation include water, with 1 g of carbohydrate yielding 0.6 mL of water, 1 g of protein yielding 0.42 mL; and 1 g of fat yielding 1.07 mL. In addition, the gastrointestinal tract may secrete and reabsorb as much as 8 to 10 L/day of water as digestive juices in the following estimated amounts: saliva, 1500 mL; gastric

juice, 2500 mL; bile, 500 mL; pancreatic juices, 700 mL; intestinal juices, 3000 mL; and water intake, 2000 mL. Regulation of fluid via the thirst mechanism and ADH allows stable fluid status.

**ANSWER:** D

3. Glucagon mobilizes which of the following:

   A. Glycogen from muscle tissue

   B. Liver glycogen

   C. Insulin to improve cellular uptake of glucose

   D. Glucose to the liver for storage

   E. None of the above

   *Ref.:* 3

**COMMENTS:** See Question 4.

**ANSWER:** A

4. The protein-sparing effect of glucose administration begins to be manifested after the administration of how much glucose?

   A. 1 L of 5% dextrose in water ($D_5W$)

   B. 2 L of $D_5W$

   C. 3 L of $D_5W$

   D. 4 L of $D_5W$

   E. 5 L of $D_5W$

   *Ref.:* 1

**COMMENTS:** **Dietary carbohydrates** provide 4 kcal/g and can be classified as complex (polymeric) or simple (monomeric or dimeric). The major role of carbohydrates in the body is to provide energy for body tissues to use for metabolic processes. Approximately 30% to 60% of the calories consumed are in the form of carbohydrates. Digestion of starches begins orally via salivary amylase, followed by pancreatic and intestinal enzymes (amylase and disaccharidases) to reduce complex carbohydrates to disaccharides (maltose, sucrose, and lactose), which can then be hydrolyzed to primary derivatives of carbohydrates—the monosaccharides or hexoses (glucose, fructose, and galactose)—via specific disaccharidases. Glucose is the preferred fuel in humans, with all metabolism beginning or ending with this hexose. The monosaccharides are transported to the liver via the portal circulation. They form pyruvate or glycogen, or they are used by red blood cells or the brain or in the formation of fat in adipose tissue.

   In a 70-kg man, the liver can store as much as 70 g of **glycogen** (10% of the liver's wet weight), thereby allowing a 12- to 24-hour nutritional reservoir during fasting, and 120 g (1% to 2%) of the wet weight of the muscle mass can be attributed to glycogen. Release of muscle glycogen to the bloodstream, as seen with liver glycogen, cannot occur because muscle tissue lacks glucose-6-phosphatase. Thus, liver glycogen is the glucose reserve used to maintain blood glucose levels as needed.

Blood glucose levels are regulated by hormones in response to carbohydrate intake. Insulin secretion increases with intake of glucose, and glucagon secretion declines, thus allowing increased uptake of glucose by liver, muscle, and adipose tissue. Conversely, glucagon mobilizes liver glycogen via the cyclic adenosine monophosphate (cAMP) protein kinase system when blood glucose levels decrease because of decreased intake. Glucose tolerance is determined by the rate at which mechanisms of glucose removal can operate. Administration of 100 g of glucose (or 1 mg/kg/min) has a protein-sparing effect that suppresses the use of nitrogen (from amino acids) for gluconeogenesis.

All major pathways of carbohydrate metabolism start or end with glucose. The three major types of glucose metabolism are (1) glycolysis, a process by which all cells can oxidize glucose to pyruvate (aerobic conditions), lactate (anaerobic conditions), and adenosine triphosphate (ATP); (2) oxidation of acetyl coenzyme A (CoA) from carbohydrates, fat, or protein for use by the tricarboxylic acid cycle; and (3) the hexose monophosphate shunt (pentose phosphate shunt), which produces reduced nicotinamide adenine dinucleotide phosphate (NADPH), a reducing agent, and enables the degradation of sugars other than hexoses. In addition to glucose from outside sources, gluconeogenesis (formation of glucose from a large variety of noncarbohydrate substrates, including amino acids, lactate, pyruvate, propionate, and glycerol) and glycogenolysis (formation of glucose from glycogen) allow glucose production endogenously when exogenous sources are not available. Endogenous glucose production allows maintenance of plasma glucose levels in the fasting state at a rate of approximately 2 to 3 mg/kg/min. Dietary fiber is a complex carbohydrate that is enzymatically digested and not considered a source of nourishment. Fiber includes cellulose (insoluble) and noncellulose (soluble) forms (including pectins, gums, mucilages, and hemicelluloses), which are broken down by bacterial flora in the gut and degraded primarily in the colon. **Soluble fiber** is thought to have numerous benefits, including (1) hypocholesterolemic effects; (2) production of short-chain fatty acids, which have trophic effects throughout the intestinal tract; (3) improvement of blood glucose levels by decreasing the rate of glucose absorption; and (4) protection from bacterial translocation.

**ANSWER:** B

5. Glutamine is an amino acid that:

   A. Is categorized as an essential amino acid

   B. Is found only in muscle tissue

   C. Has been shown to be conditionally essential during stress

   D. Maintains stable levels in plasma during stress

   E. Can be eliminated from the diet during times of stress

*Ref.: 4*

**COMMENTS:** See Question 7.

**ANSWER:** C

6. Which amino acids can be metabolized outside the liver and are a local source of energy for muscle?

   A. Leucine, isoleucine, valine

   B. Alanine, arginine, lysine

   C. Ethionine, glutamine, lysine

   D. Phenylalanine, tyrosine, histidine

   E. None of the above

*Ref.: 5*

**COMMENTS:** See Question 7.

**ANSWER:** A

7. What are the dietary protein recommendations for a 60-kg woman with intact protein stores?

   A. 0.7 to 0.8 g/kg/day (30 to 45 g/day)

   B. 0.8 to 1.0 g/kg/day (48 to 60 g/day)

   C. 1.2 to 1.5 g/kg/day (72 to 90 g/day)

   D. 2 to 4 g/kg/day (120 to 240 g/day)

   E. 5 to 6 g/kg/day (300 to 360 g/day)

*Ref.: 6*

**COMMENTS: Body proteins** are made up of 20 different amino acids, each of which has a different metabolic fate and function in the body. There are three categories of amino acids: (1) essential amino acids, which cannot be synthesized by the body; (2) nonessential amino acids, which can be synthesized de novo in the body; and (3) conditionally essential amino acids, which consist of nonessential amino acids that are considered essential during stress or trauma if their use exceeds the body's capacity for synthesis and an outside source is required. The dietary protein requirement for adults is 0.8 g/kg/day; that is, approximately 20% of the calories consumed should be in the form of protein. One gram of nitrogen equals 6.24 g of protein.

Protein digestion is a result of the sequential hydrolysis of peptide bonds of the protein to form amino acids and peptides by the action of pepsin and pancreatic enzymes (trypsin, chymotrypsin, and carboxypolypeptidase). Protein metabolism depends on numerous endogenous mediators, including endocrine hormones (insulin and glucagon), prostaglandins, cytokines, and lymphokines, with health status and intake determining which substance takes precedence. Endogenous protein production is estimated to be 70 g/day, and approximately 250 g of protein is mobilized daily within the body. Protein breakdown is thought to match protein input, with 60% of protein intake being converted to urea, 25% used to form new amino acids, and 15% used for the synthesis of new protein. Urine contains 90% of all nitrogen lost, with small amounts lost via the skin and stool. Cellular protein and amino acids are thought to be in constant equilibrium in terms of degradation and synthesis. Continuous turnover of protein and amino acids (the amount of synthesis or degradation taking place over time) occurs at the following rates: 30% in muscle, 50% in viscera, and 20% in plasma, without which daily protein requirements would be higher. The liver is the site of urea production, biosynthesis of nonessential amino acids, and degradation of all amino acids. Excess amino acids can be oxidized for energy, stored as fat or glycogen, or excreted. Glutamate dehydrogenase, present in both the cytoplasm and mitochondria of the liver, is the primary enzyme responsible for transamination of amino acids to the end products α-ketoglutarate and ammonia. The **branched-chain amino acids**, which include leucine, isoleucine, and valine, are the only amino acids metabolized outside the liver. Branched-chain amino acids are extensively oxidized by muscle and adipose tissue and are a local source of energy for muscle.

Preservation of lean body mass is essential during times of stress because synthesis and catabolism are elevated. Providing adequate calorie and protein can help minimize losses to preserve lean body mass, but beneficial amounts vary depending on patient weight and the severity of the illness or trauma. **Glutamine**, the most abundant amino acid in the body, accounts for 50% of the amino acids in muscle, and concentrations can fall during times of stress because of the body's inability to meet increases in body requirements for the amino acid. A decrease in muscle and plasma concentrations of glutamine in severe illness has been associated with a worse prognosis.

**ANSWER: A**

8. Which of the following forms of fat constitute 95% to 98% of fat in the body?

   A. Glycerides

   B. Phospholipids

   C. Sterols

   D. Cholesterol

   E. Linoleic acid

   *Ref.:* 7

**COMMENTS:** See Question 10.

**ANSWER: A**

9. What is the primary substrate for the formation of bile acids?

   A. Cholesterol

   B. Triglycerol

   C. Triglycerides

   D. Phospholipids

   E. Insulin

   *Ref.:* 7

**COMMENTS:** See Question 10.

**ANSWER: A**

10. In diabetic patients or those in a fasting state, lipolysis can exceed carbohydrate breakdown and:

    A. Elevate insulin utilization

    B. Increase the production of fatty acids, which are then converted to ketones

    C. Decrease lipase utilization

    D. Decrease acetoacetate production

    E. Improve a patient's response to medical therapies

    *Ref.:* 3

**COMMENTS: Fat** is considered the most calorie-dense macronutrient in the diet and provides 9 kcal/g. The structure of fat is characterized by its relative lack of oxygen, which necessitates longer oxidative processes than do the less calorie-yielding carbohydrates. Three main forms of fat are found in the body: glycerides, phospholipids, and sterols. **Glycerides**, principally triglycerides and triglycerol (fatty acid and glycerol), are the storage forms of fat and are the most abundant forms in food; they account for

approximately 95% to 98% of ingested fat and the fat in tissues. **Essential fatty acids** (linoleic, linolenic, and arachidonic acids) cannot be synthesized by humans. Phospholipids are ingested in small amounts and are mainly constituents of cell membranes and myelin sheaths. Sterols consist primarily of cholesterol. Triglycerides store calories, protect organs, and act as insulators. Cholesterol and phospholipids make up cell membranes and are substrates for other essential substances. **Cholesterol** is the substrate for the formation of bile acids (the primary bile acids are cholate and chenodeoxycholate) and steroid hormones (aldosterone, progesterone, estrogen, and androgens). **Phospholipids** are substrates for prostaglandins, leukotrienes, and thromboxanes.

Dietary fat is digested in the small intestine. The end products of triglyceride digestion are free fatty acids and monoglycerides. Cholesterol (esters) and phospholipids are hydrolyzed by pancreatic cholesterol ester hydrolase and phospholipase $A_2$, respectively. Once absorbed, the triglycerides, cholesterol esters, and phospholipids are formed and combined with small amounts of protein to generate lipoproteins. **Lipoproteins** (very low density, low density, and high density) act as transporters for various forms of fat to their ultimate destination (i.e., liver and adipose tissue). It should be noted that only medium-chain fatty acids, which are made up of fewer than 12 carbons, can be directly absorbed via the portal circulation and bypass the lymphatic system. Various hormonal and substrate factors influence rates of **lipolysis** of adipose tissue. Utilization of fat energy relies on adipose cell lipase, which is regulated by epinephrine, norepinephrine, glucagon, and adrenocorticotropic hormone. Insulin inhibits lipolysis. Lipolysis results in the formation of glycerol and eventually glucose or pyruvate in the liver. If fat breakdown exceeds carbohydrate degradation for energy, which is common in diabetic patients and in the fasting state, fatty acids are converted to **ketones** (acetoacetate and β-hydroxybutyrate), and oxidation by the tricarboxylic acid cycle is decreased. The ketones are released into the circulation from the liver and converted back to acetyl CoA for use in the citric acid cycle in peripheral tissues. In the heart, muscle, and renal cortex, ketone **acetoacetate** is the predominant fuel, whereas in the brain and red blood cells, glucose is the predominant fuel. Omega-3 fatty acid (linolenic) is the focus of much research because of its potential benefits in curbing cardiovascular disease. During periods of stress, enteral and parenteral supplementation of omega-3 fatty acid may improve clinical outcomes by curbing the production of highly inflammatory eicosanoids. Sources of omega-3 fatty acids include canola oil, flax seed, and leafy vegetables.

**ANSWER: B**

11. Which of the following vitamins is water soluble?

    A. Vitamin A

    B. Vitamin D

    C. Vitamin E

    D. Vitamin C

    E. Vitamin K

    *Ref.:* 8

**COMMENTS: Vitamins**, trace elements, and ultratrace elements are necessary for the release of energy from carbohydrate, fat, and protein; for transfer and delivery of oxygen; and for tissue repair. Vitamins can be either water soluble (vitamin C and B vitamins—thiamin, niacin, riboflavin, folate, vitamin $B_6$, vitamin $B_{12}$, biotin, and pantothenic acid) or fat soluble (vitamins A, D, E, and K, which dissolve in organic solvents). **Trace elements** exist as organic ions and include calcium, phosphorus, potassium, sodium, chloride, magnesium, iron, and sulfur. **Ultratrace elements** are elements that normally constitute less than 1 mcg/g of an organism and include aluminum, arsenic, boron, bromine, cadmium, chromium, fluorine, germanium, iodine, lead, lithium, molybdenum, nickel, rubidium, selenium, silicon, tin, and vanadium. Because early detection of deficiencies may be difficult, patients with malnutrition should be assumed to have inadequate vitamin and mineral intake. Various factors can affect a patient's micronutrient status, including nutritional intake, medications, availability, and losses via wounds, stool, urine, and metabolic needs.

**ANSWER:** D

12. Which of the following equations is thought to be the best predictor of the resting metabolic rate in critically ill, nonobese patients?

   A. Harris-Benedict equation

   B. ASPEN equation

   C. Fick equation

   D. Penn State 2003 equation

   E. Arizona State equation

*Ref.:* 9

**COMMENTS:** See Question 14.

**ANSWER:** D

13. Which of the following visceral proteins has the shortest half-life?

   A. Retinol-binding prealbumin

   B. Albumin

   C. Transferrin

   D. Thyroxine-binding prealbumin

   E. Serum globulin

*Ref.:* 10

**COMMENTS:** See Question 14.

**ANSWER:** A

14. Which of the following information would not be a typical component of the Subjective Global Assessment tool?

   A. Weight changes

   B. Serum albumin level

   C. Changes in muscle mass

   D. Dietary changes

   E. Evaluation of gastrointestinal symptoms

*Ref.:* 11

**COMMENTS:** **Malnutrition** is common in hospitalized patients, with as many as 50% having moderate malnutrition, which significantly increases morbidity and mortality, particularly in surgical or highly stressed patients. **Nutrition assessment** is done through a review of the patient's medical history, physical examination, anthropometric characteristics, and laboratory data related to

ingestion, digestion, absorption, and excretion. See the American Society for Parenteral and Enteral Nutrition (ASPEN) Chart Reference—Screening and Assessment. **Subjective Global Assessment** is a tool that uses the patient's history and physical examination and is less reliant on objective laboratory data and anthropometrics. Additionally, appetite and weight loss, though simple, seem to be as good a predictor of nutritional risk when correlated with global assessment scores. Anthropometric data—height and weight—help relate body size to nutritional needs. A drastic change in weight within a short time (days) is an indication of fluid shifts and should be evaluated appropriately. Adjustments in weight expectations and macronutrient needs should be made for obese patients and those with amputations. Estimates of fat and muscle mass via midarm circumference and **triceps skinfold thickness** are not widely used for the assessment of hospitalized patients, but they have shown merit in patients monitored long-term.

**Visceral protein** stores include **albumin** (half-life, 18 to 21 days), **transferrin** (half-life, 8 to 10 days), thyroxine-binding **prealbumin** (half-life, 1 to 2 days), and **retinol-binding protein** (half-life, 10 hours). Evaluation of proteins with a shorter half-life is most useful in acute care settings. **Nitrogen balance** is the state when protein intake (nitrogen input) and nitrogen output are equal. **Nitrogen output** is monitored through 24-hour urine collection and determination of urinary urea nitrogen (UUN) levels. One gram of protein equals 6.24 g of nitrogen. Therefore, protein input (24-hour UUN + 4 for insensible losses) equals the nitrogen balance. The total **lymphocyte count** and the results of **delayed hypersensitivity testing** to measure compromised immune function resulting from malnutrition may be affected by many nonnutritional factors. Therefore, the validity of these tests as a measure of malnutrition is debated.

The most common type of malnutrition seen in hospitalized patients is **protein-calorie malnutrition** as a result of partial or total starvation. Seven days is the absolute maximum period for which a patient should have severely limited nutritional intake. Consequently, early determination of the patient's daily nutritional requirements is important. Many equations and formulas have been developed and studied to determine energy expenditure, including the **Harris-Benedict** equation to determine energy needs in hospitalized patients. The **Penn State 2003**, **Swinamer**, and **Ireton-Jones equations** are thought to be the most accurate predictors of the resting metabolic rate in nonobese, critically ill patients. Clinicians have found that a range of 20 to 35 kcal/kg when determining calorie needs tends to work during the initial assessment of patients. The most accurate means of measuring energy expenditure in the hospital setting is to use **indirect calorimetric measurements** (via a metabolic cart) to measure the resting metabolic rate.

The recommended daily allowance for protein is 0.8 g/kg in healthy adults. An increased need for protein is seen with the catabolic response to injury, with 1.2 to 1.5 g of protein per kilogram or higher necessary for protein synthesis in stressed patients (i.e., postsurgical or sepsis patients). A **nonprotein calorie–nitrogen ratio** of 150 : 1 in a nonstressed individual or 80 : 1 to 100 : 1 in a stressed individual is typically recommended. Given the availability of endogenous glucose, excessive infusion of parenteral glucose can lead to unwanted side effects, including (1) elevated blood glucose levels; (2) increased rate of fat synthesis leading to fatty liver disease; and (3) increased water and carbon dioxide production, which can result in respiratory compromise and possibly water overload. Glucose administration should be kept below 5 mg/kg/min to prevent these complications. For patients with hepatic disease, protein requirements are based on the stress level. A patient with encephalopathic episodes requires branched-chain amino acids since they do not require metabolism by the liver and can be converted to energy locally in the muscle. Patients with renal disease and acute failure, without dialysis, are typically permitted only 0.4 to 0.6 g/kg of protein. Protein needs increase with dialysis, and such needs should be determined on an individual basis.

**A N S W E R :   B**

15. The decreased insulin-glucagon ratio seen during simple starvation allows:

    A. Increased lipogenesis

    B. Increased lipolysis

    C. Increased protein synthesis

    D. Increased glycogen production

    E. Decreased lipolysis

    *Ref.:* 3

**COMMENTS:** See Question 17.

**A N S W E R :   B**

16. Which amino acid is released in large amounts to be used by the liver during simple starvation?

    A. Valine

    B. Serine

    C. Glutamine

    D. Cysteine

    E. Homocysteine

    *Ref.:* 3

**COMMENTS:** See Question 17.

**A N S W E R :   C**

17. During simple starvation, gluconeogenesis is important for:

    A. Glycogen storage

    B. Lipogenesis to continue to allow adequate fat storage

    C. Protein synthesis to progress to allow muscle health

    D. Tissues that use only glucose for fuel, such as the brain and blood, which depend on this process for fuel

    E. None of the above

    *Ref.:* 3

**COMMENTS:** Surgical patients may be at risk for both simple **starvation** and **stress hypermetabolism**, depending on the severity of disease, length of recovery, and the surgical procedure performed and its consequences. Simple starvation results when nutrient intake does not meet energy requirements. Energy expenditure characteristically decreases to help match energy intake, and metabolic responses occur to preserve muscle mass. Initially, during early fasting, the glycogen derived from glycogenolysis supplies glucose for obligatory glucose-using tissues (i.e., red blood cells and brain). Lipogenesis is curtailed since lactate, pyruvate, and amino acids are not diverted to glucose production. The Cori cycle is then activated, which allows the glucose produced by gluconeogenesis in the liver to be converted back to lactate through glycolysis in the peripheral tissues. Skeletal muscle releases amino acids via the alanine cycle, which provides carbon for gluconeogenesis in the liver. The Cori and alanine cycles are important

because tissues that use only glucose (i.e., brain, blood, renal medulla, and bone marrow) depend on hepatic gluconeogenesis, primarily from lactate, glycerol, and alanine, during starvation. Glycerol and protein are important substrates for net glucose synthesis. **Protein metabolism** adapts to starvation as follows: (1) the synthesis of protein decreases because energy sources to generate production are not available, (2) protein catabolism is reduced as other fuels become the primary sources of energy for many tissues, and (3) decreased ureagenesis and urinary nitrogen loss reflect protein sparing (in the initial stages of starvation, the rate of urea nitrogen loss is greater than 10 g/day, with a decline to less than 7 g/day after weeks of starvation). Alanine, glutamine, and glycine are released in large amounts to be used by the liver and kidney for net glucose formation. **Glucose synthesis** in the liver during simple starvation is linked to the synthesis of urea because of the increased transamination.

During **starvation**, the insulin-glucagon ratio is decreased, which allows activation of lipolysis and suppression of lipogenesis. Levels of fatty acids are increased during starvation and they are used as alternative fuels by many tissues that prefer fat as a fuel source (i.e., kidney, cardiac muscle, and skeletal muscle). The liver uses fatty acids to meet the energy needs for gluconeogenesis. The acetyl CoA generated by the oxidation of fatty acids in the liver is converted to ketones. As **ketone** (acetoacetate and β-hydroxybutyrate) levels rise, they can cross the blood-brain barrier to supply fuel, but some glucose is still required. The use of fatty acids as a primary fuel source allows the sparing of body proteins for gluconeogenesis. This sparing effect is important for maintenance of immune functions and liver and respiratory muscle function. An RQ of 0.6 to 0.7 during simple starvation reflects the fact that fat is the body's primary fuel source during simple starvation.

**A N S W E R :   D**

18. Hyperglycemia during stress hypermetabolism can be attributed to:

    A. Increased insulin resistance

    B. Increased glycogen storage

    C. Decreased lipolysis

    D. Increased glycogenesis

    E. Increased insulin uptake

    *Ref.:* 12

**COMMENTS:** See Question 19.

**A N S W E R :   A**

19. Stress hypermetabolism is characterized by:

    A. Decreased body temperature

    B. Hypoglycemia and glycogenesis

    C. Fluid imbalance and increased resting metabolic rate

    D. Decreased gluconeogenesis and proteolysis

    E. Decreased urinary protein retention

    *Ref.:* 12

**COMMENTS:** In contrast to simple starvation, activation of **stress hypermetabolism** occurs following surgery, trauma, or sepsis to provide energy and substrates for tissue repair and to activate immune function and the inflammatory response. In the initial period, known as the **ebb phase**, a decline in oxygen consumption is seen, along with poor circulation, fluid imbalance, and cellular shock lasting 24 to 36 hours. As the body adapts (**flow phase**), enhanced cellular activity and increased hormonal stimulation take place and lead to an elevated metabolic rate, body temperature, and nitrogen loss. This phase can last days, weeks, or months.

Nutrients are used during hypermetabolism in response to the stress and during the hormonal and inflammatory mediator response to the injury. The earliest stages of response are characterized by increases in gluconeogenesis, resting energy expenditure (REE), proteolysis, ureagenesis, and urinary nitrogen loss. Clinical signs include tachypnea, increased body temperature, and tachycardia, with laboratory results showing increased leukocytosis, hyperlactatemia, azotemia, and hyperglycemia. Liver production of glucose during stress is increased through gluconeogenesis and glycogenolysis (Cori cycle), which are stimulated by endocrine (hormonal) changes: increased cortisol, increased glucagon, increased catecholamines, and decreased insulin. Overall use of protein as an oxidative fuel source by the liver is increased, and typically there is increased turnover of branched-chain amino acids.

**Hyperglycemia** is characteristic during stress, with (1) increased glycogenolysis occurring initially to elevate the blood glucose level, followed by (2) increased glucose production and (3) reduced peripheral utilization later in response to the stress. Gluconeogenesis in the liver continues despite hyperglycemia. Typically, neither glucose nor insulin infusion can control blood glucose levels (or gluconeogenesis) during times of extreme stress. As a result, protein stores are depleted and insulin resistance continues. Unsuppressed glucose production leads to low rates of glycogen storage, lipolysis, and oxidation of fat. Continuous circulation of insulin, resulting from high plasma glucose levels, prevents extended use of the body's vast fat stores for energy. Increased fatty acid oxidation occurs with hypermetabolism and results in decreased plasma linoleic and arachidonic acid levels, which can lead to essential fatty acid deficiency in 10 days if exogenous sources are not supplied. Low visceral blood flow rates lead to complications in nutrient utilization and cellular responses. Supplying nutrients intraluminally may help with ischemic injury. Hemodynamic stability must be considered when deciding where feeding tubes should be placed, how quickly feedings should be advanced, and how well the bowel is functioning to achieve the goal of preventing/decreasing gastrointestinal ischemia.

**ANSWER:** C

20. Which of the following can lead to errors in information obtained from indirect calorimetry when using the metabolic cart?

A. The patient ate breakfast at 7:45 AM and walked to the bathroom before the 8 AM test.

B. The patient is ventilator dependent.

C. The patient is losing weight after 2 weeks of a nutrition support regimen.

D. The patient underwent hemodialysis 2 days before being tested.

E. The experience of the personnel administering the test is limited.

*Ref.:* 13

**COMMENTS: Energy expenditure** and the resulting caloric needs can be estimated for stressed patients through various equations that have been developed. **Indirect calorimetric** studies measure a hospitalized patient's energy released and gas exchange via a portable metabolic cart at the patient's bedside. In both ventilator-dependent and non–ventilator-dependent patients, energy expenditure can be accurately determined to allow the provision of optimal macronutrient prescription. The use of indirect calorimetry to determine a patient's nutritional needs has proved useful because certain diagnoses or clinical conditions, such as amputation and sepsis, can alter REE. Indirect calorimetry can also be used to determine whether the nutrition prescription is contributing to metabolic or respiratory problems or whether the nutritional support is accurate. The indirect calorimeter measures $O_2$ consumption ($\dot{V}_{O_2}$) and $CO_2$ production ($\dot{V}_{CO_2}$), which enables the calculation of **resting energy expenditure** and **respiratory quotient**. The abbreviated Weir equation is **REE = 1.44 [3.9($\dot{V}_{O_2}$) + 1.1($\dot{V}_{CO_2}$)]**, where $\dot{V}_{O_2}$ is $O_2$ consumption in milliliters per minute, $\dot{V}_{CO_2}$ is $CO_2$ production in milliliters per minute, and REE is expressed in kilocalories per day.

REE is typically 10% greater than **basal energy expenditure** (BEE). REE is generally obtained via the metabolic cart for an alert person in a postabsorptive state, and the value reflects 75% to 90% of **total energy expenditure** (TEE). An additional factor of 1.1 to 1.3 is required to account for the thermodynamic effects of food, shivering, physical activity, illness, and injury in estimations of TEE. When the REE value obtained through indirect calorimetric studies is compared with results predicted with the **Harris-Benedict equation**, the following assessments can be made regarding a patient's metabolic state: (1) 110% greater than predicted REE = hypermetabolism, (2) 90% to 100% of predicted REE = normometabolism, and (3) REE measured at 90% less than predicted REE = hypometabolism. Calculation of the RQ allows the clinician to alter the nutrient content of feedings to optimize macronutrient intake. The RQ is the ratio of $CO_2$ expired ($\dot{V}_{CO_2}$) to the amount of $O_2$ inspired ($\dot{V}_{O_2}$): RQ = $\dot{V}_{CO_2}/\dot{V}_{O_2}$.

In general, the following nutritional changes can be suggested for the RQ values obtained. An RQ greater than 1 indicates excessive calorie load and necessitates decreased caloric intake. An RQ of 1 indicates a need to decrease carbohydrates, increase lipids, or both. An RQ of less than 0.82 requires an increase in total energy intake. Mixed substrate oxidation with an RQ of 0.85 to 0.95 is considered ideal. Normal deviations in RQ can be seen after eating (RQ = 1.0), in diabetes (RQ = 0.71), and in starvation (RQ = 0.83). Numerous factors can affect the accuracy of indirect calorimetry, including but not limited to positive end-expiratory pressure (PEEP) greater than 12 cm $H_2O$, hyperventilation, leaking chest tube, bronchopleural fistula, errors in calibration or leaking tubes of the indirect calorimeter, and hemodialysis.

**ANSWER:** C

21. A 35-year-old man is admitted to the ICU following a diagnosis of acute pancreatitis. After initial resuscitation, the patient's condition improves and enteral tube feedings are started through a postpyloric tube. Initial intolerance to a tube feeding regimen requires the clinician to:

A. Immediately discontinue the tube feeding regimen and start total parenteral nutrition (TPN)

B. Add water to feeding regimen to dilute the feedings for better tolerance

C. Consider slowing the tube feeding regimen and progress to the goal rate less aggressively

D. Immediately change the tube feeding formula

E. Increase the tube feeding rate per hour

*Ref.:* 14

**COMMENTS:** See Question 22.

**ANSWER:** C

22. A 67-year-old woman with a history of atrial fibrillation is admitted to the emergency department with complaints of abdominal pain out of proportion to the physical findings. The patient undergoes diagnostic mesenteric angiography, followed by revascularization of the superior mesenteric artery. At a second-look operation, small bowel resection and right hemicolectomy are performed. The remaining proximal jejunum measures 100 cm. What is the minimum amount of small intestine required for absorption of nutrients before considering the use of enteral feedings?

   A. 20 cm of small intestine

   B. 50 cm of small intestine

   C. 100 cm of small intestine

   D. 120 cm of small intestine

   E. 250 cm of small intestine

*Ref.:* 14

**COMMENTS: Enteral nutrition** is the provision of a liquid formula diet by mouth or tube into some area of the gastrointestinal tract to maintain or improve nutritional status and to preserve gut integrity. The decision to use enteral nutrition is based on the premise that patients receiving enteral feedings have been found to have fewer septic complications than those receiving TPN, probably because of less bacterial translocation in the gut in the former. Good evidence supports the concept that delivery of early enteral nutrition in critically ill patients improves clinical outcomes even if the initial amounts are suboptimal. The functional capacity of the gut must be considered before prescribing enteral nutrition therapy. There must be (1) at least 100 cm of small intestine for absorption of nutrients, (2) an intact ileocecal valve, and (3) adequate airway protection. Conditions contraindicating use of the gastrointestinal tract include gastroparesis, intestinal obstruction, paralytic ileus, high-output enteric fistula, short bowel syndrome, severe gastrointestinal bleeding, no access to the gastrointestinal tract, aggressive nutrition not wanted by the patient, short-term need for enteral nutrition (<5 to 7 days), severe malabsorption, and hemodynamic instability. Previously contraindicated conditions for enteral feedings have been reviewed extensively, and certain conditions now seem more plausible when considering enteral support with careful clinical review, specific tube placement, and very diligent monitoring of feedings for intolerance. Such conditions include diarrhea/vomiting, gastrointestinal fistula, gastrointestinal bleeding, mechanical obstruction, and situations involving poor digestion and absorption.

Once it has been established that the patient cannot consume adequate nutrition by mouth and that the enteral route can be used, various tubes can be used to deliver the feedings. Nasogastric tubes are preferred for short-term feedings (<4 weeks) and can be inserted in the stomach, duodenum, or jejunum. Long-term feedings (>4 to 6 weeks) require the placement of a more permanent gastrointestinal access device: (1) a percutaneous enteral device (gastric, gastric jejunal, or direct jejunal), (2) a laparoscopically placed tube (gastrostomy or jejunostomy), or (3) a surgically placed tube (gastrostomy or jejunostomy). There are three methods for administering enteral feedings: (1) bolus or gravity, in which 250 to 500 mL of formula is administered quickly several times per day to patients with relatively normal digestion and absorption; (2) intermittent feeding, administered several times per day over a period of at least a half-hour to allow gastric emptying similar to that seen with

normal eating; and (3) continuous feeding. In continuous feeding, the formula is typically full strength, initiated at a slow rate (20 to 40 mL/h), and advanced as tolerated until the goal rate is reached.

Most complications associated with tube feeding can be prevented with proper monitoring. Complications can be metabolic (e.g., overhydration or underhydration), gastrointestinal (e.g., diarrhea, nausea, vomiting, delayed gastric emptying, constipation, or abdominal distention), or mechanical (e.g., the wrong tube size or a cracked tube). Note that the typical tube feeding regimen requires additional water to ensure adequate hydration. **Diarrhea** has been estimated to occur in 2.3% of the enteral population and in 34% to 41% of critically ill patients. Diarrhea may be related to (1) factors not associated with the feeding formula, including medications or antibiotics, fecal impaction, hypoalbuminemia, enteric pathogens, preexisting medical conditions, inflammatory syndromes, or sepsis, or (2) factors related to the tube feeding formula, including too rapid an infusion rate, too rapid initiation or progression, lactose intolerance, microbe contamination, lack of fiber, the osmolality of the formula, or a high fat content in the formula. The diarrhea may be controlled by (1) medications such as diphenoxylate and atropine or Loperamide once *Clostridium difficile* has been ruled out as a cause of the diarrhea, (2) changing to continuous feeding, or (3) slowing the rate of tube feeding until tolerance is established, before initiation of medication to control the problem.

**ANSWER:** C

23. Which type of formula might be appropriate for a patient who has had nothing per mouth for more than a week and has a partially functioning gastrointestinal tract?

   A. Elemental formula

   B. Concentrated formula

   C. Specialty formula

   D. Modular formula

   E. Superconcentrated formula

*Ref.:* 15

**COMMENTS:** See Question 24.

**ANSWER:** A

24. Which of the following is one of the most common food allergies that must be considered when deciding on a tube feeding formula?

   A. Rice allergy

   B. Soy allergy

   C. Nut allergy

   D. Corn syrup allergy

   E. Citrus fruit allergy

*Ref.:* 16

**COMMENTS:** Many formulas exist for use in tube-fed patients. Carbohydrate is usually provided from intact macronutrient sources, including maltodextrin, hydrolyzed cornstarch, corn syrup solids, and sucrose. Protein sources are casein, soy, whey, lactalbumin, or free amino acids. Fat content may consist of long-chain triglycerides derived from vegetable oil or medium-chain triglycerides derived from coconut or palm kernel oil. Enteral formulas are divided into six product categories. **Standard formulas** mimic the American diet, with 50% to 60% of calories being derived from carbohydrates, 10% to 15% from protein, and 25% to 40% from fat (e.g., Isocal, Osmolite). These formulas are isosmolar to blood (300 mOsm/kg) and are used for patients with functioning gastrointestinal tracts who have been receiving nothing by mouth for less than 7 days. **Concentrated formulas** are similar to the standard formula in terms of content to meet the patient's nutritional requirements, but the density per milliliter is greater than that of standard formulas because of the decreased water content (e.g., TwoCal HN, Isosource 1.5). They are typically used in patients with fluid restrictions or those receiving bolus or nighttime feedings. **High–nitrogen-protein formulas** contain more than 15% of calories supplied by nitrogen and protein (e.g., Isosource HN, Osmolite HN, and Replete). These formulas are used for patients with higher than normal protein needs (e.g., malnourished, catabolic, or elderly patients with increased protein requirements). **Elemental formulas** are advocated for patients who have been receiving nothing by mouth for more than 7 days and those with partially functioning gastrointestinal tracts (e.g., Alitraq and Peptamen). They contain hydrolyzed macronutrients, which require less digestion and are potentially better tolerated until the patient is able to transition back to intact nutrients. Generally, the formulas are low in fat or contain fewer long-chain triglycerides and are hyperosmolar (>450 mOsm/kg). **Fiber-containing** or blenderized formulas contain fiber supplied from added soy polysaccharides or natural food sources, respectively. Fiber formulas are intended to regulate bowel function by eliminating diarrhea and constipation (e.g., Jevity, FiberSource, Replete with Fiber). Fructooligosaccharides are short-chain oligosaccharides that are similar to other dietary fibers but can be digested quickly by colonic bacteria to produce short-chain fatty acids. Short-chain fatty acids help promote intestinal growth and water and sodium absorption and provide an energy source for colonocytes. **Blenderized formulas** differ from fiber formulas in that they are regular foods and therefore contain all the components of nutrients naturally occurring in foods (e.g., Compleat). **Specialty formulas** are available for patients with liver, renal, and pulmonary disease and diabetes (e.g., for ARDS/chronic obstructive pulmonary disease (COPD), Oxepa; for pulmonary disease, **Nutren Pulmonary**; for liver disease, Hepatic-Aid II; and for renal failure, Nepro). Their composition varies, depending on the disease state, but they generally have high osmolality and are nutritionally inadequate. The benefit of such formulas remains controversial. **Food allergy** considerations are important when selecting an enteral formula. Nuts, fruits, and milk are the most common food allergy triggers for 20% of the population of allergy sufferers. Gluten tolerance should also be a consideration. Some enteral products contain lactose, which causes bloating, cramping, and diarrhea in some patients. Because of electrolyte imbalances or the need for varied macronutrient content, some patients have needs that cannot be met by the available commercial products. Enteral feeding modules can be used to create a patient-specific formula (**modular formula**) that addresses the carbohydrate, protein, and fat requirements. Vitamins and mineral products are available as well.

**ANSWER:** C

25. A 65-year-old man is admitted to the hospital because of profuse diarrhea after small bowel resection for an ischemic bowel that resulted in short bowel syndrome. The patient is resuscitated and TPN started. What is the maximum infusion rate for lipids when using TPN?

   A. 0.5 g/kg/day

   B. 1.5 g/kg/day

   C. 2.5 g/kg/day

   D. 3.0 g/kg/day

   E. 4.0 g/kg/day

*Ref.:* 17, 18

**COMMENTS:** See Question 26.

**ANSWER:** C

26. How many calories are provided in one 500-mL bottle of 20% intravenous fat solution?

   A. 150 kcal

   B. 550 kcal

   C. 800 kcal

   D. 1000 kcal

   E. 4000 kcal

*Ref.:* 17

**COMMENTS:** A patient whose nutritional needs cannot be met via the oral or enteral route requires **total parenteral nutrition**, the basic goal of which is to meet nutritional needs and maintain or improve metabolic balance safely. Indications for TPN include a nonfunctioning gastrointestinal tract (i.e., short bowel syndrome, intractable vomiting, or diarrhea), the need for bowel rest (e.g., as in severe pancreatitis), and severe malnutrition when the patient has been unable to eat for 5 to 7 days or longer. Two types of solution are available: (1) traditional dextrose and amino acid solutions, in which lipids are piggybacked into the solution, and (2) total nutrient admixture (TNA), which contains all three macronutrients dispensed from a single container. An automated compounding device is needed for accurate mixing, and as with all TPN, mixing should be done under laminar airflow to control bacterial contamination. Crystalline protein and synthetic amino acids are the **protein** sources for TPN solutions, with standard base solutions ranging from 8.5% to 10.0% amino acids (0.5 L of a 8.5% solution contains 42.5 g of protein). HepatAmine 8% is an amino acid solution sometimes used for patients with encephalopathy since it contains an increased percentage of branched-chain amino acids. Commercially available **dextrose** solutions contain 5% to 70% glucose (50 to 700 g/L). The final solution (i.e., after all solutions are added) typically contains 15% to 35% dextrose. The monohydrate form of dextrose is used for TPN and provides 3.4 kcal/g on oxidation. Carbohydrates should be administered at a rate no greater than 5 mg/kg/min via TPN, which is the maximum oxidation rate of glucose. **Peripheral venous nutrition**, at concentrations of less than 10% dextrose and 3% protein (<100 g/day), should be administered only short-term (no less than 5 days and no longer than 2 weeks) since higher concentrations may promote thrombosis because of low peripheral blood flow, thereby preventing the provision of adequate calories or protein (or both) via this method. Fat solutions are considered isotonic and can be administered peripherally or centrally without concern about thrombosis. **Fat solutions** are available in 10%, 20%, and 30% solutions, which provide 1.1, 2.0, and 3.0 kcal/mL, respectively. Fats can be administered intermittently, continuously, or via TNA. Monitoring clearance by checking triglyceride levels is key to ensuring tolerance to lipid infusions. Patients should also be observed for signs of chills, fever, headaches, or back pain with initiation of fat solutions to rule out intolerance. Fat should be administered at no faster a rate than 2.5 g/kg/day. Lipid solutions should be administered cautiously to patients with ARDS, severe liver disease, or increased metabolic stress because fat may exacerbate these conditions. Patients with hypertriglyceridemia (>250 mg/dL), lipid nephrosis, egg allergy, or acute pancreatitis associated with hyperlipidemia should not be given fat emulsions. **Vitamins and minerals** should be supplied to meet the recommended daily allowance. Vitamin K must be ordered separately based on coagulation status. Electrolytes are added to TPN to maintain or achieve electrolyte homeostasis, with individual electrolyte needs depending on the patient's disease state, renal function, drug therapy, hepatic function, and nutritional status.

**ANSWER:** D

27. Refeeding syndrome is characterized by which of the following electrolyte abnormalities?

    A. Hyponatremia, hypokalemia, and hypercalcemia

    B. Hyperphosphatemia, hypokalemia, and hypocalcemia

    C. Hypokalemia, hypomagnesemia, and hypophosphatemia

    D. Hypocalcemia, hyponatremia, and hypomagnesemia

    E. Hyperkalemia, hypernatremia, and hypercalcemia

*Ref.:* 18

**COMMENTS:** See Question 28.

**ANSWER:** C

28. Hyperglycemia in a surgical patient receiving TPN may best be managed by:

    A. Oral hypoglycemics

    B. Decreasing the dextrose load and doubling the amount of fat

    C. Adding regular insulin to the TPN

    D. Discontinuing TPN for 2 weeks and then trying to start TPN again

    E. Increasing the concentration of protein and carbohydrate calories and decreasing that of lipids

*Ref.:* 18

**COMMENTS:** Complication with use of TPN include (1) **mechanical**, (2) metabolic, and (3) nutritional complications. The incidence of pneumothorax is usually higher in emergency situations and in nutritionally depleted patients. Arterial injury, air embolism, brachial plexus injury, thoracic duct injury, lymphatic injury, catheter embolus, venous thrombosis, and poor catheter position, among other problems, are possible mechanically related complications. Catheter-related sepsis can be expected at a rate of 2% to 5%. The rate of line sepsis is 20% to 30%. Important steps to help prevent line infections include appropriate skin preparation before an operative procedure, ultrasound guidance, appropriate maintenance of the central line, frequent catheter changes, careful use of multiple-lumen catheters, and appropriate antibiotic and thrombolytic treatment if sepsis develops.

A number of **metabolic complications** may result from TPN. Standard use of vitamins and solutions with trace element has eliminated the problem of deficiency states seen with extended TPN during the early stages of its use. Excess glucose can (1) increase blood glucose levels and induce hyperosmolar nonketotic coma; (2) lead to dehydration; (3) lead to lipogenesis with subsequent hepatic abnormalities (e.g., fatty liver); and (4) increase $CO_2$ production, which may compromise respiratory function. Because rebound hypoglycemia can occur with discontinuation of TPN, weaning to 50 mL/h before complete discontinuation is

important. Treatment of **hyperglycemia** in TPN patients typically consists of the addition of regular (not long-acting) insulin to the parenteral solution along with stringent monitoring of glucose levels. **Fat deficiency** can occur if fat is not provided at least twice weekly to meet essential fatty acid requirements. Clinical signs of essential fatty acid deficiency include dry skin, poor wound healing, and hair loss. Hepatic toxicity and benign transient abnormalities on liver function tests can occur. Gut atrophy and bacterial translocation can occur with gut disuse. Depletion or an excess of vitamins and minerals can cause unwanted deficiencies or elevated levels of nutrients (e.g., hyperkalemia or hypokalemia and hyperphosphatemia or hypophosphatemia). **Refeeding syndrome** results when glucose is administered quickly to an individual with poor nutrient intake before TPN. Subsequent rapid serum depletion of magnesium, phosphorus, or potassium develops. **Immunologic impairment** as a result of large doses or rapid lipid administration has been shown to occur. It is thought that once the lipoprotein lipase system becomes overloaded, the reticuloendothelial system helps rid the body of excessive amounts of lipids, which cause neutrophils to become lipid saturated and affects their ability to function. Therefore, careful monitoring of lipid levels by determination of triglyceride concentrations is important.

**Nutritional complications** of TPN include overfeeding and underfeeding. Careful assessment and monitoring of the patient's nutritional status help ensure appropriate feeding regimens. Conditions such as acalculous cholecystitis, steatosis, and gut atrophy could occur and lead to significant morbidity.

**ANSWER:** C

29. Which of the following is not true regarding nutritional support of hospitalized obese patients?

    A. Enteral feedings are not a choice for this patient population because of the inability to meet calorie and protein requirements.

    B. Vascular and enteral access may be difficult in obese patients.

    C. Critically ill obese patients have an inability to mobilize fat stores to use as an energy source.

    D. Underfeeding may be advantageous in obese patients to limit metabolic complications.

    E. Fat sources in feedings should be eliminated.

*Ref.:* 19

**COMMENTS:** See Question 30.

**ANSWER:** A

30. A 40-year-old man undergoes gastric bypass surgery for morbid obesity. This patient should:

    A. Eat only high-protein foods

    B. Begin feeding regimen with small amounts of regular foods

    C. Begin with small amounts of water

    D. Eat high-calorie foods six times a day

    E. Eat only small amounts of high-fat foods

*Ref.:* 20

**COMMENTS:** The incidence of overweight or obesity in adults in the United States is on the rise, with 65% of adults being overweight or obese according to the 1999-2002 National Health and

Nutrition Examination Survey (NHANES). **Obesity** can affect or complicate conditions involving the cardiac, respiratory, gastrointestinal, endocrine, and musculoskeletal systems; psychosocial relationships; and immunity and cancer risk. Other care issues that can affect nutrition management include problems with enteral and vascular access and weight limits for the equipment used for various procedures. Nutrition support regimens for critically ill obese patients must be able to provide appropriate nutrition without giving rise to complications. Challenges in providing nutritional support for critically ill obese patients include altered metabolism and determination of the most appropriate energy requirements. A critically ill overweight/obese patient has an inability to mobilize fat stores during critical illness, which results in accelerated use of lean body mass and endogenous protein stores with increased insulin production. Determining the appropriate energy requirements is most important in the obese population to curb the loss of lean body mass and allow healing and improved patient status. Indirect calorimetry remains the best tool for determining energy needs. The most reliable predictive nutrition equation for this population is debatable and dependent on the primary goal of nutrition intervention: weight maintenance, modest weight reduction, keeping nutritional support complications at bay, or a combination of these goals. Current research seems to support hypocaloric, high-protein feedings to help minimize metabolic abnormalities and decrease the loss of lean body mass. For critically ill obese patients being mechanically ventilated, use of the Ireton-Jones 1992 or Penn State 1998 equations may be the best predictive equations to use for developing feeding regimens.

**Bariatric surgery** has emerged as a viable weight loss method for patients with medically significant obesity and morbidly obese patients who are unable to achieve or sustain weight loss. Nutritional issues are complex in this population. Patients are expected to lose 50% to 60% of their presurgery weight. Therefore, numerous postoperative nutritional complications are possible. Malnutrition, vitamin and mineral deficiencies, failure of weight loss, dehydration, anemia, and dumping syndrome may occur. Gastrointestinal problems may include nausea, constipation, abdominal pain, marginal ulcers, incisional hernias, vomiting, diarrhea, gallstones, gastritis, and intestinal obstruction. Oral feeding resumes on postoperative day 1 with small volumes of water. A 3-day progression from clear liquids to pureed foods is recommended, with small-volume feedings of 30 to 60 mL at each feeding. The diet eventually returns to regular foods given in small, frequent meals, along with the following general instructions: (1) stop eating when full; (2) chew food well, to a pulplike consistency; (3) avoid high-calorie liquids, especially those with ice cream; and (4) make mealtimes last 30 minutes. Because of bypass of 90% of the stomach, entire duodenum, and a small portion of the jejunum, supplemental nutrient recommendations are necessary. A multivitamin, vitamin B$_{12}$, calcium, and in some instances iron are typically prescribed.

**ANSWER:  C**

31. Which of the following is true when considering the nutritional status of a geriatric patient?

    A. Muscle wasting can be a pathologic process that is mistaken for normal aging.

    B. Liver function does not affect the selection of nutrition regimens.

    C. Enteral nutrition is not an option because of slowed gut function.

    D. Body mass index (BMI) is the best anthropometric measurement for determining nutritional status in an elderly patient.

    E. Laboratory tests cannot be used to evaluate nutritional status.

*Ref.:* 21

**COMMENTS:** Determining the most appropriate nutrition support interventions in **elderly** surgical patients can be difficult because of the aging process. Use of the BMI and anthropometrics often results in inaccurate measurements because of age-related changes. Many pathologic processes mistaken for normal aging are related to nutrition or affect nutritional status (anthropometrics and biochemical and hematologic aspects) and can include muscle wasting, weight loss, undernutrition, problems with balance and endurance, declining cognition, and depression. Multiple age-related changes in the renal, liver, cardiovascular, and muscular systems can affect overall health and nutrition regimens for surgical patients. Enteral nutrition may be an option for an elderly patient with poor nutritional intake before surgery. Commonly, enteral nutrition has been used in patients with dementia, cancer, dysphagia secondary to stroke, and other neurologic problems. Conditions for which the benefits of enteral support have been demonstrated in the elderly include short-term use in those with stroke and cancer when significant decreases in body mass can probably be prevented, the patient is a candidate for physical therapy, or recovery is probable. Semistarvation, decreased appetite, and decreases in the metabolic rate are seen with changes in cortisol and thyroid metabolism. The use of TPN is indicated in elderly patients with no functional gastrointestinal tract, prolonged ileus, obstruction of the gastrointestinal tract, severe diarrhea/malabsorption, mesenteric ischemia, and peritonitis. Prolonged use of nutrition therapy may have limitations because of financial constraints, lack of home care support systems, and inadequate patient capabilities.

**ANSWER:  A**

## REFERENCES

1. Blundell JE, Stubbs J: Diet composition and control of food intake in humans. In Bray GA, Bouchard C, editors: *Handbook of obesity: etiology and pathophysiology,* New York, 2004, Marcel Dekker.
2. Regulation of gastrointestinal function: In Ganong WF, editor: *Review of medical physiology,* ed 22, New York, 2005, McGraw Hill Lange Medical.
3. Berg JM, Tymoczko JL, Stryer L, editors: *Biochemistry,* New York, 2002, WH Freeman.
4. Saito H, Furukawa S, Matsuda T: Glutamine as an immunoenhancing nutrient, *JPEN J Parenter Enteral Nutr* 23(Suppl 5):S59–S61, 1999.
5. Reeds PJ: Dispensable and indispensable amino acids for humans, *J Nutr* 130:S1835–S1840, 2000.
6. Ettinger S: Macronutrients: carbohydrates, protein, and lipids. In Mahan JK, Escott-Stumps S, editors. *Krause's food, nutrition, and diet therapy,* ed 10, Philadelphia, 2000, WB Saunders.
7. Digestion and absorption. In Ganaong WF: *Review of medical physiology,* ed 22, New York, 2005, McGraw Hill Lange Medical.
8. Food and Nutrition Board, Institute of Medicine: *Dietary reference intakes for vitamin C, vitamin E, selenium, and carotenoids,* Washington, DC, 2004, National Academy Press.
9. Frankenfield DC, Rowe WA, Smith JS, et al: Validation of several established equations for resting metabolic rate in obese and nonobese people, *J Am Diet Assoc* 103:1152–1159, 2003.
10. Fuhrman MP, Charney P, Mueller CM: Hepatic proteins and nutritional assessment, *J Am Diet Assoc* 104:1258–1264, 2004.
11. Makhija S, Baker J: The Subjective Global Assessment: a review of its use in clinical practice, *Nutr Clin Pract* 23:405–409, 2008.
12. Chioléro R, Revelly J, Tappy L: Energy metabolism in sepsis and injury, *Nutrition* 13(Suppl 9):S45–S51, 1997.
13. Holdy KE: Monitoring energy metabolism with indirect calorimetry: Instruments, interpretation, and clinical application, *Nutr Clin Pract* 19:447–454, 2004.

14. ASPEN Board of Directors and the Clinical Guideline Task Force: Guidelines for the use of parenteral and enteral nutrition in adult and pediatric patients, *JPEN J Parenter Enteral Nutr* 26(Suppl 1):SA1–SA138, 2002.

15. Parrish CR: Enteral formula selection: a review of selected product categories, *Pract Gastroenterol* 29:44, 2005.

16. Malone A: Enteral formula selection. In Charney P, Malone A, editors: ADA pocket guide to enteral nutrition, vol 63, Chicago, 2006, American Dietetic Association.

17. Sacks GS, Mayhew S, Johnson D: Parenteral nutrition implementation and management. In Merritt R, De Legge M, Holcombe B, et al: *The A.S.P.E.N. Nutrition support practice manual*, ed 2, Silver Spring, Md, 2005, American Society for Parenteral and Enteral Nutrition.

18. Matarese LE: Metabolic complications of parenteral nutrition therapy. In Gottschlich MM, Furhman MP, Hammond KA, et al, editors: *The science and practice of nutrition support: a case-based care curriculum*. Dubuque, Iowa, 2001, Kendall/Hunt.

19. Levi D, Goodman ER, Patel M, et al: Critical care of the obese and bariatric surgical patient, *Crit Care Clin* 19:11–32, 2003.

20. Shikovra S: Techniques and procedures: surgical treatment for severe obesity: the state of the art for the new millennium, *Nutr Clin Pract* 15:13–22, 2000.

21. Mitchell-Eady C: Nutritional assessment of the elderly. In Chernoff R, editor: *Geriatric nutrition: the health professional's handbook.* Sudbury, Mass, 2006, Jones & Barllett.

# CHAPTER 5

# Surgical Infection and Transmissible Diseases and Surgeons

*Alicia Growney, M.D., and Steven D. Bines, M.D.*

## A. Surgical Infection

1. A patient is seen at the hospital after a trip to Texas with a 2-week history of fever, chills, cough, and right-sided pleuritic chest pain. The patient has otherwise been healthy and does not take any medication. He does not have any allergies. Physical examination showed an icteric young man with a temperature of 102° F (38.9° C) and tender hepatomegaly. Breath sounds are decreased in the right lower lobe. A computerized axial tomographic (CT) scan of the chest and abdomen shows a mass in the right lobe of the liver compatible with an abscess. Which of the following empirical antibiotic therapies should be started?

   A. Ampicillin, gentamicin, and clindamycin

   B. Levofloxacin and gentamicin

   C. Piperacillin/tazobactam, clindamycin, and amikacin

   D. Cefoxitin, gentamicin, and metronidazole

   E. Imipenem and clindamycin

   *Ref.:* 1, 2

**COMMENTS:** This patient has a **liver abscess**, the two possible causes being bacterial or amebic in origin. The symptoms of both may be similar, and clinical differentiation between them is not usually possible. The diagnosis can be made by requesting serologic studies for ameba or by obtaining an aspirate of the fluid collection. Before identifying the etiologic agent, the empirical antimicrobial treatment must cover polymicrobial bacterial infection (including aerobic gram-negative rods and anaerobes), as well as *Entamoeba histolytica*.

   Gentamicin and levofloxacin provide good coverage for gram-negative organisms. Cefoxitin covers both gram-positive and gram-negative organisms. Clindamycin and metronidazole are effective against anaerobes. In addition, metronidazole is the antimicrobial of choice for *E. histolytica*. Imipenem and piperacillin/tazobactam cover both gram-negative organisms and anaerobes. Because of the emergence of multidrug resistant bacteria, the best initial combination for empirical broad antibiotic coverage is a second-generation cephalosporin and an aminoglycoside with metronidazole.

**ANSWER:** D

2. A patient with recurrent duodenal ulcer is referred for surgical consultation. He has been having recurrent abdominal pain for the last 2 years. Fifteen months ago, upper endoscopy showed a duodenal ulcer. The patient was treated with ranitidine and his condition improved, but the symptoms recurred. Upper endoscopy confirmed a recurrent ulcer, and the result of a *Campylobacter*-like organism (CLO) test was positive. The patient was treated with a combination of two antibiotics and a proton pump inhibitor for 2 weeks. Which of the following tests best assesses eradication of *Helicobacter pylori* after completion of treatment?

   A. Urea breath test

   B. CLO test

   C. Biopsy and culture

   D. Serum antibody (by enzyme-linked immunosorbent assay [ELISA])

   E. Stool antibody test

   *Ref.:* 3

**COMMENTS:** Surgery for the treatment of peptic ulcers is indicated only in the following circumstances: intractable hemorrhage, perforation, and obstruction. The patient does not have any of these conditions. Furthermore *Helicobacter pylori*, the most important pathophysiologic factor in the development of duodenal ulcer, was never adequately treated. Treatment options for *H. pylori* are numerous, but they must always include an $H_2$ blocker or a proton pump inhibitor plus at least two antibiotics. The antibiotics most commonly used are amoxicillin, clarithromycin, and metronidazole. Bismuth-containing regimens have also been used. Depending on the combination used, the length of treatment varies from 2 to 4 weeks.

   Methods of diagnosing *H. pylori* can be divided into two categories: invasive and noninvasive. Biopsy and the **campylobacter pylori** test require endoscopy, but all the other tests do not. Like the CLO test, the urea breath test takes advantage of the ability of *H. pylori* to split urea. However, the urea breath test only requires the patient to "blow," whereas the CLO test is conducted on a piece of tissue. The serologic test for *H. pylori* antibody is useful but of limited value in determining the success of therapy. There is no stool "antibody" test for *H. pylori*, but a stool antigen test is available and is as sensitive as the urea breath test.

Since there is no need for repeated endoscopy in this patient, the clinician must consider the relative merits of the noninvasive methods. Because antibody test results may remain positive after treatment, the best choice is the urea breath test, which determines the presence of live *H. pylori*.

**ANSWER:** A

3. A woman is recovering well after surgery for appendicitis complicated by secondary peritonitis. A second-generation cephalosporin (cephamycin) was administered perioperatively. On her third day of hospitalization, urine culture reveals *Candida* spp. and *Enterococcus faecalis*. The patient has remained afebrile since surgery, and her vital signs are stable. Physical examination reveals an intubated young woman who is awake and calm. Her abdomen is soft and nontender, and she has a urinary catheter in place. Her white blood cell count is 5.4 thou/cu mm with a normal differential count. Urinalysis revealed many white blood cells, many epithelial cells, and many bacteria. Which of the following is the best treatment for this woman?

A. Resume cephamycin.

B. Start fluconazole and vancomycin.

C. Start amphotericin B and linezolid.

D. Start amphotericin B bladder washes and vancomycin.

E. There is no need for antimicrobials.

*Ref.:* 1

**COMMENTS:** A **positive culture** result does not always indicate infection or the need for treatment. Urinary catheters predispose to urinary tract infections. However, infections generally produce symptoms such as fever, abdominal pain, dysuria, frequency, and leukocytosis. This patient has contaminated urine (many epithelial cells) with colonization by several microorganisms. There is no need to treat her. It may be advisable to change or remove her catheter and repeat a urinalysis and urine culture. When more than one organism is seen in the urine, it is most likely a contaminated sample.

**ANSWER:** E

4. A 10-year-old boy who recently emigrated from Mexico has had a 2-day illness characterized by fever, odynophagia, dysphagia, and drooling at the mouth. Physical examination reveals a child in a toxic condition with a temperature of 102° F (38.9° C), tachycardia, and tachypnea. There is mild tenderness in the submandibular area and few palpable lymph nodes. The suspected diagnosis is epiglottitis, which is confirmed with a CT scan of the neck. Blood culture results are positive. What kind of organism will probably be seen on Gram stain?

A. Gram-positive cocci in pairs and chains

B. Gram-positive cocci in clusters

C. Slender gram-negative rods

D. Gram-negative coccobacilli

E. Spirochetes

*Ref.:* 1

**COMMENTS:** The patient has acute **epiglottitis**, most likely attributable to *Haemophilus influenzae* type B, which is recovered from the blood in up to 100% of cases. Classically, the patient is a 2- to 4-year-old boy with a short history of fever, irritability,

dysphonia, and dysphagia, which can occur at any time of the year. However, the widespread use of *H. influenzae* type B vaccine in developed countries has led to a marked decline in invasive disease with this organism. The disease is still common in developing countries, however. *Haemophilus* species are gram-negative coccobacilli. Treatment includes early intubation, with plans for cricothyroidotomy or tracheotomy if intubation fails, and antibiotic such as ceftriaxone or ampicillin/sulbactam.

**ANSWER:** D

5. A diabetic patient has recently been discharged from the hospital after intracranial bleeding. He is readmitted for aspiration pneumonia. His condition deteriorates rapidly, with hypotension and multiorgan dysfunction. Which of the following treatments is contraindicated?

A. Volume resuscitation

B. Antibiotics

C. Activated protein C

D. Intensive insulin therapy for hyperglycemia

E. Low-dose hydrocortisone

*Ref.:* 4

**COMMENTS:** **Severe sepsis** is characterized by multiorgan dysfunction with or without shock and is due to a generalized inflammatory and procoagulant response to infection. Efforts to improve the outcome with anticytokine therapy along with antibiotics and supportive care have until recently not been associated with improved survival. Recently, a randomized, double-blind, placebo-controlled multicenter trial evaluating recombinant **activated protein C** has demonstrated a survival benefit in patients with severe sepsis. However, activated protein C treatment was associated with an increased risk for bleeding and is contraindicated in patients with recent hemorrhagic stroke. Fluid resuscitation and antibiotics are mainstays in the treatment of sepsis. Intensive insulin therapy that maintains serum glucose levels at 80 to 110 mg/dL reduces morbidity and mortality in critically ill patients. The mechanism is unknown, but it is possible that correcting hyperglycemia may improve neutrophil function. The use of **corticosteroids** for sepsis remains controversial. High doses of corticosteroids may in fact worsen outcomes by increasing the frequency of secondary infections. However, low doses of corticosteroids may be beneficial in septic patients, who may have "relative" adrenal insufficiency despite elevated levels of circulating cortisol. Although the issue is controversial, the use of low-dose hydrocortisone is not contraindicated in this patient.

**ANSWER:** C

6. A patient in whom angioedema develops after the administration of penicillin is scheduled for a craniotomy to ablate a seizure focus. Which of the following choices is appropriate for antibiotic prophylaxis?

A. Cefazolin from the time of surgery and then for 7 days

B. No antibiotic prophylaxis

C. Vancomycin at the time of induction and then for 3 to 5 days

D. Vancomycin at the time of induction

E. Vancomycin and gentamicin at the time of induction

*Ref.:* 5, 6

**COMMENTS:** The degree of wound contamination (clean versus contaminated procedure) combined with host factors (e.g., diabetes, advanced age, obesity, immunodeficiency, and nutritional status) and procedure-related factors (e.g., presence of foreign material and the degree of trauma to host tissues) determines the overall risk for the development of a **surgical site infection** (SSI). Despite state-of-the-art aseptic technique, bacterial contamination of the surgical wound is inevitable. Microorganisms that colonize the skin, such as *Staphylococcus aureus*, coagulase-negative staphylococci, and streptococci, are the most common wound pathogens, particularly during clean procedures. SSIs associated with contaminated procedures are frequently polymicrobial and are due to the normal flora of the entered viscus (i.e., coliforms and anaerobic bacteria associated with colonic procedures). **Prophylactic antibiotics** are clearly indicated for most clean-contaminated and contaminated procedures and effectively decrease the rate of SSI. Antibiotic prophylaxis for clean surgery remains controversial in certain cases. However, when bone is incised, as in craniotomy, sternotomy, and placement of orthopedic hardware, antibiotic prophylaxis has proven efficacy in decreasing the incidence of SSIs. Antibiotics selected for clean procedures must have excellent activity against skin microorganisms. Cefazolin is the usual choice. However, as in this case, severe penicillin allergy prevents the use of other β-lactams, including cephalosporins and the carbapenems. Vancomycin is the usual alternative. In addition, clindamycin and trimethoprim/sulfamethoxazole may also be effective prophylactic agents for neurosurgical procedures. The timing of antibiotic administration is critical, and for best results they should be given within 30 minutes of the surgical incision. Redosing during a prolonged procedure is recommended to maintain serum concentrations. The duration of antibiotic prophylaxis following surgery remains a source of disagreement, although administration of antibiotics beyond 24 hours is rarely indicated.

**ANSWER:** D

7. Endocarditis prophylaxis is recommended for which of the following patients?

A. A patient with mitral valve prolapse but without murmur who is undergoing lithotripsy for renal calculi

B. A patient with a history of rheumatic fever and normal cardiac valves who is undergoing prostatic biopsy

C. A patient with a prosthetic aortic valve who is undergoing pulmonary resection

D. A patient with severe hypertrophic cardiomyopathy who is undergoing endoscopic retrograde cholangiography for biliary obstruction

E. A patient previously treated for streptococcal endocarditis who is undergoing colonoscopy

*Ref.:* 7

**COMMENTS: Antibiotic prophylaxis for endocarditis** is recommended for patients with certain cardiac conditions who are undergoing any dental procedure that involves the gingival tissues or periapical region of a tooth and for any procedure involving perforation of the oral mucosa. In addition, patients undergoing procedures on the respiratory tract or those with skin or soft tissue infections should also receive prophylaxis. The cardiac conditions associated with the highest risk for adverse outcomes from infective endocarditis for which prophylaxis is indicated before the previously listed procedures include prosthetic heart valves, history of infective endocarditis, congenital heart disease (CHD) limited to unrepaired cyanotic CHD, repaired CHD with prosthetic

material or devices during the first 6 months after the procedure, repaired CHD with residual defects at the site or adjacent to the site of a prosthesis, and cardiac transplantation recipients with cardiac valvulopathy. Prophylaxis against viridans group streptococci with a penicillin, cephalosporin, or clindamycin is recommended. Routine prophylaxis in patients undergoing gastrointestinal or genitourinary procedures is no longer recommended.

**ANSWER:** C

8. A patient is infected with human immunodeficiency virus (HIV). His last CD4+ T-lymphocyte count was 50 cells/mm³, and his viral load was 100,000 copies/mL. He comes to the hospital with the sudden onset of right hemiparesis. He has been afebrile. A CT scan and magnetic resonance imaging (MRI) of the brain show multiple ring-enhancing lesions in the left cerebral hemisphere. The *Toxoplasma* IgG antibody test result is positive. He has received pyrimethamine and sulfadiazine for 12 days. Neurologically, the patient is stable. Which of the following is the next best step?

A. Repeat MRI of the brain.

B. Continue the same antibiotic therapy for an additional 10 days and reassess.

C. Switch treatment to pyrimethamine with the addition of clindamycin and reassess whether the patient improves clinically in 10 to 14 days.

D. Add corticosteroids to the treatment regimen.

E. Perform a positron emission tomographic (PET) or single-photon emission computed tomographic (SPECT) scan.

*Ref.:* 8

**COMMENTS:** Up to 90% of **human immunodeficiency virus**-infected patients with advanced disease (<100 CD4+ cells/mm³), multiple ring-enhancing lesions, and a positive *Toxoplasma* IgG antibody test result have cerebral **toxoplasmosis**. Empirical treatment with pyrimethamine, sulfadiazine, and folinic acid is recommended. Most patients with central nervous system (CNS) toxoplasmosis respond rapidly to this therapy, with nearly 90% of patients demonstrating neurologic improvement at 2 weeks. Radiographic improvement occurs at a slower pace, with approximately 50% improvement on repeated MRI of the brain occurring within 3 weeks of initiating treatment. For patients who do not improve by 2 weeks, a brain biopsy is indicated. Although **lymphoma** is the most likely alternative diagnosis in patients with acquired immunodeficiency syndrome (AIDS) and CNS lesions, up to 25% of brain biopsy specimens reveal toxoplasmosis. Thallium-201 (SPECT) or PET scans may provide useful information in that a "cold" lesion revealed by SPECT or hypometabolic lesions seen on PET scanning are consistent with infection. However, false-positive and false-negative results can occur with these functional imaging studies. Pyrimethamine plus sulfadiazine or clindamycin is considered first-line therapy for toxoplasmosis. The addition of corticosteroids may be useful in the treatment of increased intracranial pressure. However, this antiinflammatory effect may make interpretation of clinical and radiographic responses difficult.

**ANSWER:** A

9. Which of the following statements regarding the collection of blood for culture is false?

A. The optimal timing for drawing blood for culture is approximately 1 hour before the onset of fever.

B. Blood collected via intravascular devices for culture should be paired with blood obtained by peripheral venipuncture.

C. At least two sets of blood cultures should be obtained for any patient with suspected bacteremia.

D. A minimum of 10 mL of blood should be collected for each set of cultures.

E. Blood collected via intravascular devices for culture does not need to be paired with blood obtained by peripheral venipuncture.

*Ref.:* 9

**COMMENTS:** Early studies demonstrated that rigors and fever often follow bacteremia by 30 to 90 minutes. Since circulatory phagocytes are generally effective in removing bacteria from the bloodstream, collection of blood for culture should occur as early as possible in the course of a febrile episode. Good data document that two or three sets of **blood cultures** containing at least 10 mL of blood per set are sufficient for demonstrating most episodes of bacteremia or fungemia. After adequate skin antisepsis, peripheral venipuncture sites are preferred for blood collection for culture. Central venous catheters are frequently used for blood collection but should be paired with a peripheral blood draw to aid in the interpretation of a positive test result. A positive blood culture result obtained from intravenous catheters combined with a negative result from a blood culture obtained from a peripheral site may represent only colonization of the line and not true bacteremia.

**ANSWER:** E

10. Which of the following statements regarding anaerobic bacterial infections is true?

A. Anaerobic bacteria are common inhabitants of the skin and mucous membranes.

B. *Bacteroides* spp. are the most common isolates in intraabdominal anaerobic infections.

C. If appropriate cultures are obtained, anaerobes are found in more than 75% of intraabdominal abscesses.

D. Proper treatment of anaerobic infections consists of surgical drainage, débridement of necrotic tissue, and appropriate antibiotic therapy.

E. All of the above.

*Ref.:* 1

**COMMENTS: Anaerobic bacteria** are normal inhabitants of the skin, mucous membranes, and gastrointestinal tract. In fact, anaerobic bacteria outnumber aerobic organisms by more than 10:1 in the oral cavity and by more than 1000:1 in the colon. Therefore, it is not surprising that anaerobes are cultured from up to 90% of intraabdominal abscesses. The most common pathogens in this group are *Bacteroides* spp. *Bacteroides fragilis* is an important co-pathogen in the pathogenesis of intraabdominal abscesses. As with most serious infections, proper treatment involves appropriate drainage of abscesses and débridement of devitalized tissue when present, as well as appropriate antibiotic therapy. Antibiotics with excellent broad-spectrum anaerobic activity include the carbapenems (imipenem, meropenem, and ertapenem), β-lactam/β-lactamase combinations (ampicillin/sulbactam, ticarcillin/clavulanate, and piperacillin/tazobactam), and metronidazole. Although the second-generation cephalosporins (i.e., cefoxitin and cefotetan) and clindamycin also provide anaerobic coverage, over the past decade an

increase in resistance of *Bacteroides* organisms to these agents has been observed. For example, as many as 30% of *B. fragilis* isolates are resistant to clindamycin.

**ANSWER:** E

11. The use of tigecycline is not indicated for which of the following?

A. Methicillin-resistant *S. aureus* (MRSA) bacteremia

B. Community-acquired pneumonia

C. Ventilator-associated pneumonia caused by vancomycin-resistant enterococci (VRE)

D. *Enterobacter* cultured from an intraabdominal abscess

E. *Klebsiella pneumonia* soft tissue infection

*Ref.:* 10

**COMMENTS: Tigecycline** is part of a new class of antibiotics called the glycylcyclines and has a broad spectrum of activity against gram-positives, gram-negatives, aerobes, and anaerobes, including MRSA. It has no activity against *Pseudomonas* or *Proteus*. It is indicated in the treatment of complicated skin and soft tissue infections, complicated intraabdominal infections, and community-acquired pneumonia. Treatment of infections caused by VRE with tigecycline has not been well studied in clinical trials.

**ANSWER:** C

12. Which of the following statements regarding tetanus prophylaxis is false?

A. A patient has a minor, clean wound. His second tetanus shot was 4 years ago. He requires a dose of tetanus toxoid. Antitetanus immunoglobulin is not required.

B. A patient has a minor, clean wound. His third tetanus shot was 5 years ago. He does not require any additional prophylaxis.

C. A patient has a dirty wound. He completed three tetanus shots when he was a child but has not had a tetanus booster in 20 years. He is immune and does not require additional toxoid or antitetanus immunoglobulin.

D. A patient has a dirty wound. He does not remember when and how many tetanus shots he received in the past. He requires a toxoid dose. Antitetanus immunoglobulin is also required.

E. A hematopoietic stem cell transplant (HSCT) recipient should begin reimmunization with tetanus toxoid 12 months after transplantation.

*Ref.:* 11

**COMMENTS:** Approximately 100 cases of tetanus occur in the United States annually. **Tetanus** develops in nonimmune individuals after a penetrating injury is inoculated with spores of *Clostridium tetani*. With appropriate local anaerobic conditions, these spores germinate and produce a neurotoxin, tetanospasmin, that is responsible for the signs and symptoms of tetanus. The majority of cases of tetanus occur in older adults (>60 years) who have waning immunity. The need for active immunization with tetanus toxoid or passive immunization with human tetanus immunoglobulin (or both) depends on the nature of the wound and the immune status of the patient. Tetanus toxoid and immunoglobulin are indicated for patients with dirty (tetanus-prone) wounds who have received fewer than three doses of tetanus toxoid in the past or whose immunization status is unknown. Dirty wounds include those contaminated with feces, saliva, or soil and wounds related to punctures, gunshots, crush injury, burns, or frostbite. Tetanus toxoid is indicated only for patients with dirty wounds who have received three doses of toxoid more than 10 years ago and have not received a booster within 5 years of the injury. Patients with clean, minor wounds require tetanus toxoid if they have received fewer than three doses of toxoid less than 10 years ago and have not received a booster or the patient's immune status is unknown. Immunocompromised patients undergoing chemotherapy and HSCT recipients may be at increased risk for tetanus. HSCT recipients should begin reimmunization with tetanus toxoid 12 months after transplantation.

**ANSWER:**   C

---

13. Match each agent in the left-hand column with one or more mechanisms of antimicrobial action in the right-hand column.

| | |
|---|---|
| A. Carbapenems | a. Impairment of bacterial DNA synthesis |
| B. Aminoglycosides | b. Inhibition of cell wall synthesis |
| C. Quinolones | c. Disruption of ribosomal protein synthesis |
| D. Cephalosporins | d. Disruption of cell wall cation homeostasis |
| E. Vancomycin | e. Disruption of the cytoplasmic membrane |

*Ref.:* 12

**COMMENTS:** All the antimicrobial agents listed are **bactericidal agents** (i.e., their associated mechanisms of action result in bacterial death). **Bacteriostatic agents** (e.g., tetracyclines, chloramphenicol, erythromycin, clindamycin, and linezolid) act by preventing bacterial growth but do not result in bacterial death. They work primarily through inhibition of ribosomal protein synthesis. Both carbapenems and cephalosporins are β-lactam antibiotics and hence have a similar mode of activity. Enzymes located within the bacterial cytoplasmic membrane are responsible for peptide cross-linkage. These enzymes are called penicillin-binding proteins (PBPs) and are the site at which β-lactam drugs bind. Such binding interferes with bacterial cell wall synthesis and eventually results in cell lysis. Gram-negative bacteria contain a variable number of various PBPs. Each β-lactam antibiotic has various affinities for the various PBPs. Vancomycin is a glycopeptide that also inhibits bacterial cell wall synthesis and assembly. Vancomycin complexes to cell wall precursors and prevents elongation and cross-linkage, thereby making the cell susceptible to lysis. This antibacterial activity is limited to gram-positive organisms. Aminoglycosides bind irreversibly to the 30S bacterial ribosome and interfere with protein synthesis. For this activity to take place, they must penetrate the cell wall, which occurs optimally under aerobic conditions. Unlike other antibiotics that inhibit protein synthesis, aminoglycosides are bactericidal. This feature is due to their disruptive effect on calcium and magnesium homeostasis within the cell wall. Quinolones inhibit topoisomerase II (DNA gyrase) and topoisomerase IV, which impairs DNA synthesis in bacteria. Appreciation of the mechanism of action of antimicrobials may have a bearing on the selection of alternative therapies when bacterial resistance to the drug of choice develops.

**ANSWER:**   A-b; B-c,d; C-a; D-b; E-b

---

14. Which of the following statements concerning cephalosporins is not correct?

A. Cefazolin is a reasonable choice for nosocomial urinary tract infection.

B. Cefoxitin monotherapy is effective for the treatment of hospital-acquired intraabdominal sepsis.

C. Ceftriaxone is effective against *Pseudomonas aeruginosa.*

D. Cefepime is effective against enterococci.

E. Cefepime is effective against Enterobacteriaceae and *S. aureus.*

*Ref.:* 1

**COMMENTS: Cephalosporins** are chemically similar to penicillins and have similar mechanisms of action and toxicities. Because cephalosporins are more stable in the presence of bacterial β-lactamases, they have a broader spectrum of antibacterial activity than do penicillins. Cephalosporins are loosely classified into four major groups, or generations, based mainly on the spectrum of antimicrobial activity. In general, first-generation cephalosporins have better coverage for gram-positive organisms, and later generations exhibit improved activity against gram-negative bacteria. Cefazolin is a first-generation cephalosporin that has good coverage of gram-positive cocci. It is also effective against some community-acquired gram-negative bacteria, such as *Escherichia coli,* but its gram-negative coverage is not adequate, and resistance to it is common. Cefazolin is not appropriate treatment of nosocomial urinary tract infection. Cefoxitin is a second-generation cephalosporin that has demonstrated efficacy in the treatment of intraabdominal, pelvic, and gynecologic infections. These infections are generally due to facultative gram-negative bacilli and anaerobic organisms, especially *B. fragilis.* However, approximately 15% of *B. fragilis* isolates may be resistant. Nosocomially acquired organisms, such as Enterobacteriaceae and *S. aureus,* may be resistant to cefoxitin, thus making cefoxitin monotherapy a poor choice for nosocomial intraabdominal infections. Ceftriaxone is a third-generation cephalosporin that is widely used for community-acquired pneumonia and meningitis. It has excellent coverage against *Streptococcus pneumoniae.* This cephalosporin does not cover *P. aeruginosa,* but other third-generation cephalosporins such as ceftazidime do. Cefepime is a fourth-generation cephalosporin that combines the spectra of first- and third-generation cephalosporins. This agent has broad activity against Enterobacteriaceae, *P. aeruginosa,* and methicillin-susceptible *S. aureus.* However, cefepime has poor activity against enterococci and *B. fragilis.*

**ANSWER:**   D

---

15. Adverse events associated with the use of quinolones include all of the following except:

A. Tendinitis and possible tendon rupture

B. Seizures

C. Arthropathy in children

D. *Clostridium difficile* colitis

E. Narrowing of the QT interval

*Ref.:* 1

**COMMENTS:** The **quinolones** are antibiotics that exert their bactericidal effect by inhibiting topoisomerase II (DNA gyrase) and topoisomerase IV, thereby impairing DNA synthesis. These antibiotics have a broad spectrum of activity that covers many gram-positive cocci, but they are not active against MRSA, and some of them, such as ciprofloxacin, may not adequately treat infections with *S. pneumoniae*, gram-positive bacilli (anthrax), and many gram-negative species. Gatifloxacin and moxifloxacin have anaerobic activity. Most quinolones also have activity against *Mycobacterium tuberculosis* and atypical respiratory pathogens such as *Mycoplasma pneumoniae*, *Chlamydia pneumoniae*, and *Legionella* spp. Adverse effects of quinolones include gastrointestinal intolerance, antibiotic-associated colitis, cutaneous reactions, hepatotoxicity (trovafloxacin was withdrawn from the market for this reason), prolongation of the QT interval (leading to ventricular arrhythmias), and Achilles tendon rupture. Quinolone use is generally avoided in children because animal studies suggest that these drugs cause cartilage erosion. However, children receiving quinolones have rarely experienced joint symptoms, and they appear to be reversible. Results of MRI studies performed to identify subclinical cartilage damage have been negative.

**ANSWER:** E

16. Which of the following is not characteristic of aminoglycosides?

A. Active against a broad spectrum of gram-negative aerobes and useful for synergy against some gram-positive cocci

B. Emergence of resistant bacterial strains

C. Narrow margin between therapeutic and toxic blood levels

D. Nephrotoxicity, ototoxicity, and neuromuscular paralysis

E. Excellent activity in abscesses in which gram-negative organisms are involved

*Ref.:* 1

**COMMENTS:** Until the mid-1980s, **aminoglycosides** were the only reliable empirical treatment of serious gram-negative infections. However, the introduction of third-generation cephalosporins, extended-spectrum penicillins, carbapenems, and quinolones has reduced the frequency of aminoglycoside use. The mechanism of action of aminoglycosides involves irreversible binding to the 30S bacterial ribosome. However, aminoglycosides must first penetrate the cell wall, and since this step is oxygen dependent, it does not occur under anaerobic conditions. For this reason, aminoglycosides have no activity against anaerobic bacteria or facultative bacteria in an anaerobic environment (e.g., an abscess). Aminoglycosides are useful against gram-negative aerobes, including *P. aeruginosa*, and they are effective as synergistic agents (usually in combination with a β-lactam or vancomycin) against *Staphylococcus epidermidis*, *S. aureus*, and enterococci. Resistance to aminoglycosides does occur. Selection of an aminoglycoside should be based on local patterns of resistance. Aminoglycosides are difficult to use clinically because of their low therapeutic-to-toxic level ratio. Monitoring of serum concentrations of aminoglycosides is usually required to achieve safe and therapeutic blood levels. The two major toxic side effects are nephrotoxicity and ototoxicity. The ototoxicity, both auditory and vestibular, is potentially more significant because it is nonreversible and cumulative. The auditory toxicity affects the response to higher frequencies, which makes early detection difficult. The nephrotoxicity is usually a dose-dependent, reversible, acute tubular necrosis that produces nonoliguric renal failure. Paralysis can occur after the administration of aminoglycosides and is due to inhibition of presynaptic release of acetylcholine and postsynaptic blockade of acetylcholine receptors at the neuromuscular junction. Neuromuscular blockade is a rare but potentially lethal event. This risk is increased in patients receiving tubocurarine, succinylcholine, or similar agents and in patients with myasthenia gravis. This effect is reversible with the intravenous administration of calcium carbonate.

**ANSWER:** E

17. For which of the following conditions are perioperative antibiotics not indicated?

A. Perforated appendix

B. Open fracture of the humerus

C. Mastectomy

D. Traumatic colonic perforation

E. Cholecystectomy for acute cholecystitis

*Ref.:* 13

**COMMENTS:** Surgical wounds can be classified according to their risk for infection. Clean wounds are defined as nontraumatic in origin. No evidence of inflammation is encountered during surgery, and no breaks in surgical technique occur. There must also not be a breach of the respiratory, alimentary, or genitourinary tract. A good example of a clean surgical wound is a mastectomy wound. Generally, **antibiotic prophylaxis** is not needed for such procedures. However, in cases of clean-contaminated or contaminated wounds, the use of perioperative antibiotics is indicated. A clean-contaminated wound is a nontraumatic wound in which a minor break in surgical technique occurs or in which the respiratory, gastrointestinal, or genitourinary tract has been entered without significant spillage. Examples include transection of the appendix or cystic duct in the absence of acute inflammation or entrance into the biliary or genitourinary tract without evidence of infected bile or urine. Some debate exists regarding antibiotic prophylaxis for elective open and laparoscopic cholecystectomy. Several studies suggest that wound infection rates are similar in patients regardless of whether they receive prophylactic antibiotics. However, patients considered to be at high risk for infectious complications, including those 60 years or older and those undergoing procedures with evidence of acute inflammation, common bile duct stones, or jaundice, probably benefit from perioperative antibiotics. Patients who have previously undergone biliary tract operations or endoscopic retrograde cholangiopancreatography should also receive perioperative antibiotics. Contaminated wounds include traumatic wounds (e.g., open fractures) and wounds from operations involving a major break in surgical technique, such as gross spillage from the gastrointestinal tract or entrance into the genitourinary or biliary tract in the presence of acute infection. This category also includes dirty wounds, defined as old traumatic wounds with devitalized tissue and those involving existing clinical infections, such as perforated appendix.

**ANSWER:** C

18. Which of the following statements regarding clostridial infections is true?

A. The presence of clostridial organisms in a surgical or traumatic wound does not warrant immediate antibiotic administration and surgical intervention.

B. The oxidation-reduction potential in contaminated tissues is a significant factor in the development of a clostridial infection.

C. Despite the potentially fulminant course of clostridial infections, the skin overlying clostridial cellulitis may not be discolored or edematous.

D. Clostridial myonecrosis (gas gangrene) should be treated with immediate surgical débridement, antibiotics, and hyperbaric oxygenation.

E. A frozen section of soft tissue without polymorphonuclear infiltrates rules out the diagnosis of clostridial myonecrosis.

*Ref.:* 1

**COMMENTS: Clostridial organisms** are ubiquitous and are a common contaminant of traumatic wounds. In most wounds, however, the high oxidation-reduction potential of the surrounding healthy tissues prevents colonization and invasion of these tissues. In such cases, the presence of clostridia is clinically insignificant. When colonization with clostridia occurs in the presence of necrotic tissue, proliferation and invasion of other tissue can occur and lead to clostridial cellulitis. This form of clostridial infection is confined to the superficial fascial planes, and although it may spread rapidly, systemic effects may be mild and the skin of normal color. Clostridial myonecrosis occurs when the deeper muscular compartments are invaded, usually by *Clostridium perfringens*. The inaccessibility of systemic antibiotics to this ischemic, necrotic tissue, coupled with the low oxidation-reduction potential of such wounds, permits rapid dissemination of clostridia through the muscular compartments. Symptoms of clostridial myonecrosis are variable: pain out of proportion to the findings on physical examination; systemic toxicity; a rapidly spreading zone of cellulitis; bronzing of the skin; and a thin, watery, brown discharge. Gram staining reveals large numbers of gram-positive rods and an absence of neutrophils. In the appropriate clinical setting, an innocuous appearance of the postoperative wound does not exclude the possibility of clostridial sepsis. Therapy should include immediate surgical débridement and antibiotic therapy (penicillin G plus clindamycin). Adjuvant hyperbaric oxygen treatment may be helpful, but it has not been evaluated in a randomized, controlled trial.

**A N S W E R :** E

**19.** Which of the following statements regarding diabetic foot infections is false?

A. Acute diabetic foot infections are often caused by gram-positive organisms.

B. Chronic diabetic foot infections are polymicrobial.

C. To diagnose an infection in a patient with a chronic wound, a foul odor and redness must be present.

D. MRSA infections are associated with a worse outcome.

E. Impaired host defenses allow low-virulence colonizers such as coagulase-negative staphylococci and *Corynebacterium* spp. to become pathogens.

*Ref.:* 1

**COMMENTS:** See Question 20.

**A N S W E R :** C

**20.** Which of the following regarding the treatment of diabetic foot infections is true?

A. Acute diabetic foot infections are caused by monomicrobial gram-negative aerobes.

B. The use of antibiotics for an uninfected chronic wound facilitates wound closure and prevents future infection.

C. Sharp débridement of necrotic or unhealthy tissue facilitates wound healing and removes a potential reservoir for bacteria.

D. Avoiding direct pressure on the wound facilitates healing.

E. The administration of granulocyte-stimulating factors (GSFs) results in faster resolution of the infection.

*Ref.:* 14

**COMMENTS:** Diabetic patients have a higher risk for foot infections because of factors such as vascular insufficiency, decreased sensation, hyperglycemia, and impairment of the immune system, particularly neutrophil dysfunction. Deep tissue biopsy of the infected foot is the preferred method of culture. Acute **diabetic foot infections** are often caused by monomicrobial aerobic gram-positive cocci (*S. aureus* and β-hemolytic streptococci, especially group B), whereas patients with chronic wounds and those who have recently received antibiotic therapy generally have polymicrobial gram-positive and gram-negative aerobes and anaerobes within their wound, including enterococci, *Enterobacter*, obligate anaerobes, and *P. aeruginosa*. Initial therapy is usually empirical and based on the severity of infection and available microbiology data (culture results or Gram stain). A majority of mild infections can be treated with orally dosed antimicrobials directed against aerobic gram-positive cocci. In patients with more severe infections or extensive chronic infections, parenteral broad-spectrum antibiotics with activity against gram-positive cocci (including MRSA) and gram-negative and obligate anaerobic organisms is warranted. The diagnosis of infection in patients with chronic wounds includes the presence of purulent secretions (pus) and two or more of the following: redness, warmth, swelling or induration, and pain or tenderness. MRSA infections are associated with worse outcomes, and impaired host defenses allow low-virulence colonizers such as coagulase-negative staphylococci and *Corynebacterium* spp. to become pathogens. In addition to antibiotics, early incision and drainage of abscesses with débridement of devitalized tissue, immobilization, and supportive care are important in the total management of a diabetic foot. In the presence of significant vascular insufficiency, revascularization of the distal end of the lower extremity may improve healing and prevent amputation. Radioactive studies using technetium-99 (bone scan) or gallium citrate or indium-labeled leukocyte scans have poor specificity and should not be performed routinely. MRI has become the imaging study of choice for diagnosing osteomyelitis (OM).

Continued used of antimicrobials is not warranted for the entire time that the wound is open or for the management of clinically uninfected ulceration either to enhance wound healing or as prophylaxis against infection. Local wound care with sharp débridement of necrotic or unhealthy tissue promotes wound healing and removes a potential reservoir of pathogens. Avoiding direct pressure on the wound and providing off-loading devices facilitate wound healing. Administration of granulocyte colony-stimulating factors (G-CSFs) does not accelerate the resolution of infection but may significantly reduce the need for operative procedures.

**A N S W E R :** D

**21.** Which of the following clinical situations or laboratory results require systemic antifungal therapy?

A. A single positive blood culture result obtained from an indwelling intravascular catheter

B. *Candida* identified from a drain

C. Oral candidiasis

D. *Candida* isolated from a drain culture in a patient who recently underwent surgery for colonic perforation

E. Mucocutaneous candidiasis

*Ref.:* 1

**COMMENTS: Candidemia** is associated with significant morbidity (e.g., endocarditis, septic arthritis, and ophthalmitis) and mortality (approximately 40%). Management of candidemia, particularly in patients with intravascular devices, remains controversial. Although some patients—usually immunocompetent patients—spontaneously clear the bloodstream after removal of the intravascular device, other patients—particularly those who are immunosuppressed—have disseminated disease and require systemic antifungal therapy. There are no accurate diagnostic tests or methods for selecting high-risk patients to determine those who require systemic antifungal therapy. Therefore, all patients with at least one positive blood culture result for *Candida* should be treated with an antifungal agent. All nonsurgically implanted lines should be removed, and if continued central venous access is required, a new line should be placed at a new site (not exchanged over a guidewire). Some would attempt to sterilize the bloodstream without the removal of tunneled catheters or subcutaneous ports. However, in patients with persistent candidemia or septic shock, these devices should also be removed. **Amphotericin B** and **fluconazole** appear to have similar efficacy in the treatment of candidemia. **Voriconazole** and **caspofungin** are new antifungal agents that are also effective against *Candida*. These agents may be particularly useful for non-*albicans* species such as *Candida krusei* or *Candida glabrata*, which are less susceptible to fluconazole. All patients with candidemia should be evaluated for manifestations of disseminated disease, such as ocular involvement or OM. *Candida* identified from a surgical drain most likely represents colonization and does not require systemic antifungal therapy. Mucocutaneous candidiasis can be treated with local nystatin or clotrimazole.

**ANSWER: A**

**22.** Which of the following statements regarding antifungal agents is false?

A. Voriconazole is at least as effective as amphotericin B against invasive aspergillosis.

B. Intravenous voriconazole is relatively contraindicated in patients with renal failure.

C. Voriconazole causes irreversible changes in vision.

D. Caspofungin is at least as effective as amphotericin B for the treatment of invasive candidiasis and, more specifically, candidemia.

E. Caspofungin is not effective in the treatment of cryptococcal meningitis.

*Ref.:* 15, 16

**COMMENTS: Voriconazole** is a broad-spectrum triazole that is active against *Aspergillus* spp. It is a selective inhibitor of the fungal cytochrome P-450 system used in the production of ergosterol for synthesis of the cell membrane. A randomized trial comparing voriconazole with amphotericin B for primary treatment of invasive **aspergillosis** showed that initial therapy with voriconazole led to better responses and improved survival. The survival rate at 12 weeks was 70.8% in the voriconazole group and 57.9% in the amphotericin B group, and voriconazole resulted in fewer severe side effects than did amphotericin B. In patients with a creatinine clearance rate of less than 50 mL/min, voriconazole should be given orally (not intravenously) since the intravenous vehicle (cyclodextrin) may accumulate and cause liver failure. Patients receiving voriconazole may experience episodes of visual changes, which are reversible.

**Caspofungin** is an echinocandin with an antifungal spectrum that includes *Candida* and *Aspergillus* spp., but not *Cryptococcus neoformans*. Caspofungin inhibits the synthesis of β-(1-3)-D-glycan, an essential component of the cell wall that is present in susceptible organisms. A recent study showed that the clinical outcome with caspofungin was similar to that with amphotericin B for the primary treatment of invasive candidiasis and candidemia.

**ANSWER: C**

**23.** Match each clinical characteristic or agent in the left-hand column with the correct infecting organism or organisms in the right-hand column.

| | |
|---|---|
| A. Fibrosing mediastinitis | a. *Candida albicans* |
| B. Amphotericin | b. *Nocardia asteroides* |
| C. Intertrigo | c. *Actinomyces israelii* |
| D. Brain abscess | d. *C. neoformans* |
| E. Pelvic mass | e. *Histoplasma capsulatum* |

*Ref.:* 1, 17

**COMMENTS: Amphotericin B** remains an important agent for the treatment of **systemic mycotic infections**, including candidiasis, mucormycosis, cryptococcosis, histoplasmosis, coccidioidomycosis, sporotrichosis, and aspergillosis. Amphotericin B is a fungicidal agent. Binding of amphotericin B to ergosterol in the fungal cell membrane alters permeability, with leakage of intracellular ions and macromolecules leading to cell death. Adverse events such as infusion reactions and nephrotoxicity are common with the conventional (deoxycholate) form of the drug. New lipid formulations of amphotericin B have been developed and are associated with a reduction in toxicity without sacrificing efficacy. Newer triazoles (voriconazole and posaconazole) and echinocandins (caspofungin, micafungin, and anidulafungin) are emerging as alternative broad-spectrum antifungal agents. Histoplasmosis is predominantly a pulmonary infection caused by *H. capsulatum*, a dimorphic fungus endemic to the Mississippi and Ohio River valleys and along the Appalachian Mountains. Histoplasmosis has been associated with massive enlargement of the mediastinal lymph nodes secondary to granulomatous inflammation. During the healing process, fibrotic tissue can cause postobstructive pneumonia or constriction of the esophagus or superior vena cava and result in dysphagia or superior vena cava syndrome (or both). **Actinomycosis** is caused by a group of gram-positive higher-order bacteria that are part of the normal flora found in the oral cavity, gastrointestinal tract, and female genital tract. Typically, infections with *Actinomyces* spp. often occur after disruption of mucosal surfaces and lead to oral and cervical disease, pneumonia with empyema, and intraabdominal or pelvic abscesses. Placement of intrauterine devices has been associated with pelvic abscess secondary to this organism. Sinus tract formation is common as these organisms extend, unrestricted, through tissue planes. High-dose penicillin and surgical drainage are generally required for cure. *Nocardia* spp., other higher-order bacteria, are found in soil, organic matter, and water. Human infection occurs after inhalation or skin inoculation. Chronic pneumonia can occur, usually in immunocompromised patients. Skin lesions and brain abscesses are common with disseminated infection.

Prolonged treatment with sulfonamides in combination with other antibiotics is required for cure. *C. neoformans* causes meningitis and pulmonary disease. Infection is common in the setting of immunodeficiency, such as organ transplantation and AIDS, but it may also occur in immunocompetent hosts. *C. albicans* is a common inhabitant of the mucous membranes and gastrointestinal tract. Intertrigo is one form of cutaneous candidiasis that occurs in skinfolds where a warm moist environment exists. Vesiculopustules develop, enlarge, rupture, and cause maceration and fissuring. Obese and diabetic patients are at risk for the development of candidal intertrigo. Local care, including nystatin powder, is usually effective.

**A N S W E R :**    A-e; B-a,d,e; C-a; D-b; E-c

24. Which of the following statements is correct regarding spontaneous bacterial peritonitis (SBP; primary peritonitis) in a cirrhotic patient?

    A. Infection is usually polymicrobial.

    B. Ascitic fluid culture results are always positive.

    C. The most likely pathogenic mechanism is translocation from the gut.

    D. Twenty-one days of antibiotic treatment may be adequate.

    E. Infection-related mortality has declined to less than 10%.

    *Ref.:* 18, 19

**COMMENTS: Spontaneous bacterial peritontis** is a monomicrobial infection, with enteric gram-negative rods accounting for 60% to 70% of episodes of SBP. *E. coli* is the most frequently recovered pathogen, followed by *K. pneumoniae*. Streptococcal species, including pneumococci and enterococci, are also important pathogens. Ascitic fluid culture results are negative in many cases, but inoculation of blood culture bottles at the bedside yields bacterial growth in approximately 80% of cases. SBP most likely develops from the combination of prolonged bacteremia secondary to abnormal host defense, intrahepatic shunting, and impaired bactericidal activity of ascetic fluid. Transmural migration of gut flora and transfallopian spread of vaginal bacteria to the peritoneal space may also occur. Initial antimicrobial treatment should include coverage against aerobic gram-negative organisms. A third-generation cephalosporin, such as cefotaxime or ceftriaxone, is a reasonable choice. The duration of antibiotic treatment is unclear. Two weeks has been suggested, but shorter courses (5 days) may have similar efficacy. Although the in-hospital mortality rate approaches 40%, infection-related mortality has declined significantly (10%). Unfortunately, the probability of recurrence is 70% at 1 year, with 1- and 2-year survival rates being 30% and 20%, respectively.

**A N S W E R :**    E

25. Which of the following patients with cirrhosis benefit from prophylactic antibiotic therapy to decrease the risk for SBP?

    A. Patients awaiting liver transplantation

    B. Patients hospitalized with acute gastrointestinal bleeding

    C. Patients with ascitic fluid protein levels of greater than 1 g/100 mL

    D. Patients who have recovered from a previous episode of SBP

    E. Patients with ascitic fluid protein levels of less than 1 g/100 mL

    *Ref.:* 19

**COMMENTS:** Randomized trials have demonstrated that **secondary prophylaxis** with oral norfloxacin, 400 mg/day, or trimethoprim/sulfamethoxazole, one double strength tablet five times per week decreases the risk for **recurrent spontaneous bacterial peritontis** from 68% to 20%. However, overall mortality in these patients is unchanged in comparison to those not receiving secondary prophylaxis. Another observation is that long-term quinolone use has been associated with the development of infection with quinolone-resistant bacteria. In approximately 30% to 40% of patients with cirrhosis hospitalized for acute gastrointestinal bleeding, infection develops during the hospitalization. Norfloxacin (400 mg a day for 7 days) decreased the incidence of infective episodes involving gram-negative bacteria. The risk for SBP increases tenfold in patients with an ascitic fluid protein concentration of less than 1 g/100 mL fluid. Norfloxacin, 400 mg/day, during hospitalization decreases the incidence of SBP in these patients as well. Patients hospitalized while awaiting liver transplantation are probably at risk for SBP and may therefore benefit from antibiotic prophylaxis. Active infection is a contraindication to liver transplantation.

**A N S W E R :**    C

26. Which of the following statements regarding secondary peritonitis is false?

    A. It usually occurs as a result of perforation of an intraabdominal viscus.

    B. Carbapenems, aminoglycosides, and fourth-generation cephalosporins have equal efficacy in treatment studies.

    C. Increased age, cancer, cirrhosis, and systemic illness are factors that increase the mortality rate.

    D. Sequestration of bacteria within fibrin clots leads to intraabdominal abscess formation.

    E. The most common organism cultured from the abdomen is *E. coli*.

    *Ref.:* 1, 13

**COMMENTS: Secondary peritonitis** usually occurs as a result of perforation of an intraabdominal viscus: perforated peptic ulcer, appendix, or diverticulum or penetrating gastrointestinal trauma. The infection is polymicrobial, with facultative aerobes and anaerobes acting synergistically. One study revealed an average of 2.5 anaerobes and 2 facultative aerobes identified per case of secondary peritonitis. *E. coli* is the most common isolate in culture. *Bacteroides* spp. are the most frequent anaerobes cultured from abdominal infections. About $10^{12}$ bacteria reside in the colon per gram of feces, with 90% of these bacteria being anaerobic organisms. Any process that impairs immunologic function or is associated with general debilitation increases mortality. Age, cancer, hepatic cirrhosis, and the presence of a systemic illness have been shown to increase mortality. One of the defense mechanisms of the peritoneal cavity is the production of fibrin to sequester bacteria for limiting systemic spread. Such sequestration leads to the formation of intraabdominal abscesses, which generally require drainage for cure. Treatment of secondary peritonitis requires surgical intervention for removal of the source of infection and systemic antibiotics for eradication of residual bacteria. Antibiotics selected should include agents with broad-spectrum coverage for facultative aerobes, gram-negative bacilli, and anaerobes. Carbapenems are a good empirical choice for treatment. Aminoglycosides and fourth-generation cephalosporins lack anaerobic activity.

**A N S W E R :**    B

**27.** A 32-year-old HIV-positive intravenous drug user is admitted to the hospital following a seizure. Examination reveals a right pronator drift. MRI of the brain reveals two ring-enhancing lesions. All of the following diagnoses should be considered except:

A. Progressive multifocal leukoencephalopathy (PML)

B. Glioblastoma multiforme

C. Toxoplasmosis

D. Lymphoma

E. Bacterial endocarditis

*Ref.:* 8

**COMMENTS:** With the widespread use of highly active antiretroviral therapy, the incidence of neurologic disease in HIV-infected individuals has declined. Major **human immunodeficiency virus–related central nervous system** diseases include the AIDS-dementia complex, meningitis, myelopathy, opportunistic infections (e.g., cryptococcosis, PML secondary to JCpoly omavirus, cytomegalovirus [CMV], herpes, and toxoplasmosis), and neoplasms (primary CNS lymphoma). For patients with advanced HIV disease (CD4+ T-cell count <100 cells/mm$^3$) who have focal neurologic disease and ring-enhancing lesions on brain imaging, the two major diagnostic considerations are toxoplasmosis and primary CNS lymphoma. PML is also a possibility in AIDS patients, but CNS lesions are not usually associated with cerebral edema. In addition, one should consider non–HIV-associated conditions, including primary brain tumors such as glioma and bacterial brain abscesses, which may occur in the setting of bacterial endocarditis and intravenous drug abuse. Current management recommendations for HIV-infected patients with focal brain lesions include approximately 2 weeks of empirical therapy for toxoplasmosis, followed by brain biopsy if radiographic or clinical deterioration occurs.

**ANSWER:** A

**28.** Persistent *Salmonella* bacteremia has been diagnosed in a 68-year-old man with a history of diabetes, hypertension, and peripheral vascular disease. The patient's only complaints are fever and back pain. Transesophageal echocardiography showed normal findings. Which of the following tests should be recommended to confirm the clinical suspicion?

A. CT scan of the chest and abdomen

B. Duplex ultrasound of the lower extremities

C. Explorative laparotomy

D. Bone marrow culture and stool culture

E. No further tests warranted

*Ref.:* 1

**COMMENTS:** The patient has persistent bacteremia without evidence of cardiac involvement. However, an **endovascular infection**, such as an infected aortic atherosclerotic aneurysm, is a probable diagnosis in this patient. *S. aureus* and *Salmonella* spp. are common pathogens infecting preexisting atherosclerotic vessels. MRI, CT scanning, and sonographic studies may reveal the presence of an aneurysm but often do not provide adequate preoperative detail. Nuclear studies, such as gallium- or indium-labeled leukocyte scans, may help localize intraarterial infection, but they have low sensitivity (<30%). Although antibiotic therapy is needed for this disease, the vascular lesion is rarely sterilized, and aneurysmal enlargement with rupture is the rule. A high index of suspicion is required for early diagnosis since mortality rates

exceed 80% if rupture recurs. If possible, perioperative angiography is usually performed to better delineate the extent of the aneurysm and operative approach.

**ANSWER:** A

**29.** Which of the following regarding complicated intraabdominal infections is true?

A. They can be treated with intravenous antibiotics to eliminate the need for more invasive interventions.

B. Isolated bacteria from colonic perforations are often aerobic gram-negative organisms.

C. The infectious isolates from acute necrotizing pancreatitis and colonic perforation are similar.

D. Bowel injuries secondary to penetrating, blunt, or iatrogenic trauma repaired within 12 hours of injury require no more than 72 hours of antibiotics.

E. Single-agent therapy is often inadequate.

*Ref.:* 20

**COMMENTS:** Complicated **intraabdominal infections** are defined as infections that extend beyond the hollow viscus of origin into the peritoneal space and result in either peritonitis or abscess formation. These infections require either operative or percutaneous intervention in addition to the administration of antibiotics for resolution. For community-acquired infections, the pathogen isolated varies according to the location of the perforation along the gastrointestinal tract. More proximal infections are due to facultative and aerobic gram-positive and gram-negative organisms. Terminal ileum/colonic perforations result from facultative and obligate anaerobes such as *E. coli*, enterococci, and streptococci. Infections resulting from necrotizing pancreatitis are due to pathogens similar to those found in colonic perforation infections. Bowel injuries caused by penetrating, blunt, or iatrogenic trauma and repaired within 12 hours of injury are adequately treated with 24 hours or less of antibiotics. Randomized prospective trials have demonstrated that single-agent therapies with β-lactam/β-lactamase inhibitor combinations, carbapenems, or cephalosporins are adequate in the treatment of complicated intraabdominal infections.

**ANSWER:** C

**30.** A patient with AIDS who has never been treated with antiretroviral therapy is admitted to the hospital after 2 weeks of fever with postprandial right upper quadrant pain. His serum alkaline phosphatase level is elevated, and a sonographic study of the gallbladder reveals a thickened gallbladder wall with pericholecystic fluid but no evidence of gallstones. Which of the following organisms is not commonly responsible for this clinical syndrome?

A. CMV

B. *Cryptosporidium*

C. *Campylobacter* spp.

D. *Mycobacterium avium*

E. *Rhodococcus equi*

*Ref.:* 8

**COMMENTS:** AIDS-associated cholangiopathy is a condition characterized by pain and cholestasis along with bile duct stenosis, similar to the clinical picture seen with sclerosing cholangitis. The condition may be idiopathic or associated with opportunistic biliary infection, most commonly with cryptosporidia. Other infectious causes include CMV, Microsporida, and *Cyclospora*. Treatment consists of antimicrobial drugs and relief of mechanical obstruction, usually by endoscopic methods (sphincterotomy, dilation, and stenting). Hepatic disease and elevated levels of liver enzymes are common in patients with HIV infection, particularly those with late-stage disease. Patients often have coexisting chronic infection with hepatitis B virus (HBV) or hepatitis C virus (HCV). A multitude of opportunistic infections may affect the liver, including *Mycobacterium avium-intracellulare*, CMV, and *Candida albicans*. These patients may have clinical findings similar to those with cholangiopathy but do not have the ductal changes detected on ultrasound or endoscopic retrograde cholangiographic studies.

**ANSWER:** E

31. A 45-year-old man infected with HIV is evaluated for a persistently symptomatic posterior anal fissure with associated edematous tags. His CD4$^+$ T-cell count is 100 cells/mm$^3$. Which of the following statements regarding surgical treatment are true?

A. Wound healing is unaffected by the stage of HIV disease.

B. Internal anal sphincterotomy is unlikely to cause incontinence.

C. Internal anal sphincterotomy is contraindicated in HIV-positive patients.

D. Operative morbidity is correlated with the CD4$^+$ T-cell count.

E. Unlike the general population, anal fissures in HIV-positive patients tend to be anterior rather than posterior.

*Ref.:* 21

**COMMENTS:** Anorectal surgery in HIV-positive patients should be approached with caution and concern regarding wound healing during the postoperative period. A distinction should be made among HIV-negative patients, asymptomatic HIV-positive patients, and patients with AIDS. In the first two categories, wound healing can be expected to occur within the usual 6 weeks following the operation. A patient with symptomatic HIV disease, particularly those with CD4$^+$ T-cell counts of less than 200 cells/mm$^3$, may have very poor healing. Only 12% are healed within the first month, and a third may take longer than 6 months to heal. Furthermore, if a sphincterotomy is performed, most patients will have some impairment of continence postoperatively. In light of these factors, a thorough evaluation of potential risk factors and, if possible, determination of HIV status are advised before proceeding with anorectal surgery in groups at high risk of becoming infected. CD4$^+$ counts have been shown to be correlated with morbidity. Sixty-five percent morbidity rates have been seen in patients with CD4$^+$ counts of less than 200 cells/mm$^3$, as opposed to 7% morbidity rates in patients with counts greater than 200 cells/mm$^3$. In summary, cautiously performed anorectal surgery in an asymptomatic HIV-positive patient is appropriate. Anorectal surgery in a patient with AIDS, however, may be followed by prolonged wound healing and functional impairment.

**ANSWER:** D

32. Which of the following previously healthy patients scheduled for an operation should undergo HIV antibody testing?

A. A 35-year-old man seen for removal of a lipoma in the anterior triangle of the neck. A routine preoperative complete blood count reveals a white cell count of

4500 cells/mL with a normal differential, hemoglobin level of 13 g/dL, and platelet count of 81,000/mL.

B. A 40-year-old man seen for repair of an inguinal hernia. Physical examination reveals white, adherent, nonremovable plaques on the lateral aspect of his tongue.

C. A 28-year-old woman seen for removal of a breast lump in whom a painful vesicular rash along the T8-10 dermatomes develops on the right side.

D. A 20-year-old man undergoing nephrectomy for living related donor transplantation.

E. All of the above.

*Ref.:* 1

**COMMENTS:** Several risk groups have been identified in whom **human immunodeficiency virus testing** is indicated, including persons with sexually transmitted diseases and persons in high-risk categories, such as injected drug users, homosexual and bisexual men, hemophiliacs, patients with active tuberculosis (TB), and pregnant women. Donors of blood or organs should be tested. Certain clinical or laboratory findings should also prompt HIV testing. Such findings include idiopathic thrombocytopenia, oral hairy leukoplakia, reactivation varicella-zoster virus infection involving more than one dermatome, unexplained oral candidiasis, persistent vulvovaginal candidiasis, and herpes simplex virus infection resistant to treatment.

**ANSWER:** E

33. Which of the following statements about HIV-positive patients with gastrointestinal bleeding is incorrect?

A. The most common cause of lower gastrointestinal bleeding is CMV colitis.

B. Ganciclovir therapy prevents rebleeding in patients with documented CMV disease.

C. Kaposi sarcoma is the most frequent AIDS-associated cause of upper gastrointestinal bleeding.

D. Upper gastrointestinal bleeding is usually secondary to infection.

E. Lower gastrointestinal bleeding is less common than upper gastrointestinal bleeding.

*Ref.:* 22

**COMMENTS: Gastrointestinal bleeding** is a relatively infrequent complication in **human immunodeficiency virus-**infected individuals. Upper gastrointestinal bleeding is more frequent than lower gastrointestinal hemorrhage and is usually unrelated to HIV infection (e.g., caused by peptic ulcer disease, esophageal varices secondary to portal hypertension, or a Mallory-Weiss tear). However, in patients with advanced HIV infection, AIDS-associated causes such as Kaposi sarcoma become more common. **Cytomegalovirus infection** can produce disease at all levels of the gastrointestinal tract and is the most common cause of colitis and lower gastrointestinal hemorrhage in AIDS patients. Ganciclovir is effective therapy for CMV disease of the gastrointestinal tract and prevents recurrent hemorrhage. Significant bone marrow suppression with neutropenia is a frequent side effect of ganciclovir therapy. In stable patients, endoscopy with biopsy is the initial diagnostic procedure of choice for HIV-infected patients with gastrointestinal bleeding.

**ANSWER:** D

**34.** Patient factors that have been shown to increase the risk for postoperative infection include all of the following except:

A. Diabetes mellitus

B. Nicotine use

C. Prolonged hospitalization before surgery

D. Obesity

E. *S. aureus* carrier status

*Ref.:* 23, 24

**COMMENTS:** Patients with elevated hemoglobin $A_{1c}$ levels have an increased incidence of **surgical site infections** after cardiac surgery. Nicotine impedes wound healing, which is thought to increase the risk for SSIs. Current smoking is an independent risk factor for mediastinal or sternal wound infections following cardiac surgery. Postoperative infections are at least twice as likely to develop in carriers of *S. aureus* as in noncarriers. Other important factors are advanced age, ischemia secondary to vascular disease, previous radiation exposure, and obesity. The length of the preoperative hospital stay is a much less significant problem than in previous years.

**A N S W E R :  C**

**35.** Which of the following statements regarding CMV infection and solid organ transplantation is false?

A. Symptomatic infection occurs 2 to 6 months after transplantation.

B. Patients being treated for acute rejection are at increased risk for the development of symptomatic CMV infection.

C. Transmission can occur through the donor organ.

D. Reactivation of latent infection is associated with the greatest risk for the development of severe disease.

E. CMV infection may be associated with premature atherosclerosis in cardiac transplant patients.

*Ref.:* 25, 26

**COMMENTS:** **Cytomegalovirus** is the most important pathogen affecting recipients of **solid organ transplants**. Symptomatic CMV disease may develop in as many as 50% of allograft recipients, usually 2 to 6 months after transplantation. CMV-seronegative recipients who are primarily infected are at greatest risk for the development of severe CMV disease. Primary infection can occur through the donor organ, unscreened blood products, or intimate contact with a viral shedder. Reactivation of latent infection is less likely to cause severe disease. Patients receiving Muromonab CD-3 (OKT3)/antilymphocyte globulin (ALG) therapy for acute rejection also appear to be at risk for the development of CMV disease. In addition to clinical disease directly attributable to CMV infection, CMV has indirect immunomodulatory activity. Symptomatic CMV infections are associated with an increased incidence of bacterial infections and opportunistic infections such as aspergillosis and *Pneumocystis carinii* pneumonia. In heart transplant patients, acute rejection and accelerated atherosclerosis are associated with CMV infection. Ganciclovir is the most commonly used agent for the prevention of CMV infection and disease; however, there is growing concern regarding the emergence of ganciclovir resistance.

**A N S W E R :  D**

**36.** A 28-year-old man who sustained closed head trauma in a motor vehicle accident a month earlier comes to the emergency department with a 3-day history of progressive headache, fever, and confusion. His wife reports the recent onset of clear drainage from his left naris. Physical examination reveals a temperature of 102° F (38.9° C), a stiff neck, and no rash. Which of the following statements concerning the patient is true?

A. He most likely has bacterial meningitis secondary to *S. aureus.*

B. Antiretroviral prophylaxis has been beneficial in preventing bacterial meningitis after head trauma.

C. Empirical antibiotics should include an extended-spectrum cephalosporin and vancomycin.

D. Corticosteroid administration with antibiotics is not indicated.

E. He requires immediate surgical intervention for repair of cerebrospinal fluid leakage.

*Ref.:* 27, 28

**COMMENTS:** The patient probably sustained a basilar skull fracture and a dural rent, with subsequent development of a dural fistula from the subarachnoid space and nasal cavity or paranasal sinuses. **Cerebrospinal fluid rhinorrhea** may occur and can easily be diagnosed by detecting the presence of $\beta_2$-transferrin in nasal secretions. In patients with known basilar skull fracture, cerebrospinal fluid rhinorrhea develops in approximately 10%. Of these patients, bacterial meningitis develops in up to 30%. *S. pneumoniae* is the most common pathogen (65% of cases). Other organisms, such as *H. influenzae, Neisseria meningitidis,* and *S. aureus,* account for the remaining cases. Empirical treatment should include an extended-spectrum cephalosporin (ceftriaxone, cefotaxime, or cefepime) and vancomycin since the incidence of $\beta$-lactam–resistant pneumococci is increasing. Prophylactic antibiotics have no proven benefit and may predispose to meningitis from antibiotic-resistant gram-negative bacteria. A recent prospective study demonstrated a survival advantage in patients with pneumococcal meningitis who received corticosteroids before or at the time of antibiotic administration. Spontaneous closure of the dural fistula is less likely in patients with a delayed manifestation of cerebrospinal fluid leakage with meningitis, and surgical repair is indicated. Diagnostic studies to identify the site of the fistula and treatment of any CNS infection should be completed before surgical intervention.

**A N S W E R :  C**

**37.** A large painful swelling in the right inguinal area has developed in a 25-year-old man who recently returned from Southeast Asia. He admits to having unprotected sex during his visit, and a small painless ulcer had developed on his penis and healed without a scar 2 weeks earlier. Physical examination reveals a temperature of 102° F (38.9° C) and firm right inguinal adenopathy with areas of fluctuance. Which of the following is appropriate in the management of this patient?

A. Obtain an incisional biopsy specimen of the inguinal nodes.

B. Perform serologic tests for *Chlamydia trachomatis,* syphilis, and HIV.

C. Start oral penicillin.

D. Perform a CT scan of the chest and abdomen for staging of the disease.

E. Perform a PET scan to rule out lymphoma.

*Ref.:* 1

**COMMENTS:** Few **sexually transmitted diseases** are characterized by **inguinal lymphadenopathy** with or without associated ulcers involving the genitalia. These diseases include lymphogranuloma venereum (LGV), syphilis, granuloma inguinale, chancroid, and sometimes herpes simplex. The findings in this patient are classic for LGV, which is caused by *C. trachomatis* serovars L1 to L3. LGV has three stages. Initially, there is a small, painless ulcer that heals without scarring, followed (in days to weeks) by discrete inguinal lymphadenopathy that is generally unilateral (in two thirds of cases). The swollen lymph nodes may coalesce to form abscesses and sinus tracts if untreated. Incisional biopsy is contraindicated in these patients because of the potential for sinus tract formation. Healing can occur without treatment as hardened inguinal masses develop and slowly involute. Relapse occurs in approximately 20% of untreated patients. The disease, which is endemic in Southeast Asia, Africa, India, South America, and the Caribbean Islands, is diagnosed by serologic testing and resolves with doxycycline, 100 mg twice daily for 21 days. The differential diagnosis of inguinal lymphadenopathy in this age group includes the sexually transmitted diseases mentioned earlier and sometimes lymphoma, but a CT scan is clearly not warranted at this stage.

**ANSWER:** B

38. Which of the following statements regarding HCV infection is false?

A. The prevalence of HCV infection in health care workers (HCWs) is similar that in the general population.

B. Chronic HCV infection occurs in 75% to 85% of patients after acute infection.

C. Hepatic failure as a result of chronic HCV infection is the most common indication for liver transplantation.

D. Pegylated interferon plus ribavirin is effective therapy for the majority of patients with chronic HCV infection.

E. Factors associated with the development of cirrhosis include male gender, alcohol use, and coinfection with HIV.

*Ref.:* 1, 29

**COMMENTS:** Persons with **acute hepatitis C virus infection** are typically asymptomatic (60% to 70%) or have mild clinical illness. Fulminant hepatitis is rare. Chronic HCV infection develops in approximately 75% to 80% of persons with acute HCV infection. Cirrhosis develops in 10% to 20% of chronically infected individuals, usually after more than 20 years of infection. Liver failure from chronic HCV infection has become the leading indication for liver transplantation. Increased alcohol use, male gender, HIV coinfection, and HCV genotype 1 are associated with more severe liver disease. Hepatocellular carcinoma can be a late complication in 1% to 2% of patients with cirrhosis. Antiviral therapy is recommended for individuals at increased risk for progressive liver disease, as demonstrated by persistently elevated serum transaminase levels, detectable HCV RNA levels, and moderate inflammation in liver biopsy specimens. The combination of pegylated interferon and ribavirin is the most effective regimen to date.

However, up to 60% of patients receiving this treatment fail to achieve a sustained virologic response. Predictors of a poor response include HCV genotype 1 (most frequent genotype in the United States), more extensive fibrosis in liver biopsy specimens, and high baseline HCV RNA levels. Adverse events (e.g., bone marrow suppression and fatigue) are common and significant and lead to discontinuation of combination therapy in 20% of patients. The prevalence of HCV infection is highest in injected drug users and patients undergoing hemodialysis. Overall, nearly 2% of the U.S. population has persistent HCV infection. Although transmission of HCV to HCWs occurs after approximately 3% of needle-stick exposures involving HCV-infected patients, the prevalence of HCV infection in HCWs, including surgeons, is similar to that in the general population.

**ANSWER:** D

39. Which of the following markers is clinically useful for predicting progression to AIDS in persons infected with HIV-1?

A. $CD4^+$ T-cell count greater than 600 cells/mm$^3$

B. p24 antigen level

C. HIV-1 RNA plasma viral load

D. Serum neopterin level

E. Serum $\beta_2$-microglobulin level

*Ref.:* 1

**COMMENTS:** The **human immunodeficiency virus plasma viral load** strongly predicts the rate of decrease in $CD4^+$ T lymphocytes and progression to AIDS and death. Progression to AIDS within 6 years occurs in 80% of HIV-infected individuals with viral loads greater than 30,000 copies/mL, as compared with 55.2%, 31.7%, 16.6%, and 5.4% of individuals with viral loads of 10,000 to 30,000, 3001 to 10,000, 501 to 3000, and less than 500 copies/mL, respectively. The baseline viral load is a stronger predictor of progression of disease and outcome than is the $CD4^+$ T-cell count. However, the combination of HIV load and $CD4^+$ T-cell count gives the best prognostic estimate for HIV-infected individuals. The $CD4^+$ T-cell count reflects the degree of immunocompromise and is most useful for determining the risk for opportunistic infection. The normal $CD4^+$ T-cell count is greater than 600 cells/mm$^3$. Symptomatic HIV infection usually begins when $CD4^+$ T-cell counts fall below 350 cells/mm$^3$. Opportunistic infections, such as *P. carinii* pneumonia, occur when $CD4^+$ T-cell counts fall below 200 cells/mm$^3$. Without antiretroviral treatment, the median time from infection to the development of AIDS is approximately 11 years. p24 antigen is one of the major core proteins of HIV. It can be detected during the acute phase of HIV infection and during late symptomatic disease. Serum neopterin produced by macrophages stimulated by interferon and $\beta_2$-microglobulin levels reflect lymphocytic turnover. Although both may be found in HIV-infected individuals, neither is specific for HIV infection.

**ANSWER:** C

40. Which statement about *M. tuberculosis* treatment and prophylaxis is true?

A. Two-drug treatment with isoniazid (INH) and rifampin (RIF) for 9 months is standard therapy for active pulmonary TB.

B. Treatment failure can be due to drug resistance or nonadherence.

C. HIV-infected individuals require prolonged therapy for active TB.

D. INH prophylaxis for latent TB is given for at least 12 months.

E. INH prophylaxis should not be given to individuals with recent conversion from purified protein derivative (PPD)-negative to PPD-positive status.

*Ref.:* 30

**COMMENTS:** Recent Centers for Disease Control and Prevention (CDC) guidelines recommend that all patients with **active pulmonary tuberculosis** receive four-drug therapy consisting of INH, RIF, pyrazinamide, and ethambutol for the initial 2 months of treatment. For patients with drug-susceptible TB and negative sputum test results after 2 months of therapy, treatment can be completed with 4 months of INH and RIF. Extrapulmonary disease requires 6 to 9 months of treatment, except for meningitis, which is treated for 1 year. HIV-infected individuals are treated similar to non–HIV-infected patients with TB. However, significant drug-drug interactions may occur with antiretroviral agents and TB drugs and may alter therapeutic decisions. Treatment failures are generally due to nonadherence by patients to multidrug regimens. Currently, local health departments have directly observed therapy programs to improve compliance with and completion of anti-TB medication regimens. Another cause of treatment failure is infection with **multidrug-resistant strains of *Mycobacterium tuberculosis***. Conditions associated with a higher rate of resistance include TB in those known to have a higher prevalence of drug resistance, such as Asians or Hispanics and previously treated individuals; persistence of culture-positive sputum after 2 months of therapy; and known exposure to drug-resistant TB.

Certain individuals are at considerable risk for the development of active TB once infected (latent TB). TB skin testing (Mantoux/PPD) is useful for identifying latent TB in high-risk individuals. Three cut points have been recommended for defining a positive tuberculin reaction: greater than 5 mm, greater than 10 mm, and greater than 15 mm of induration. Persons considered at highest risk (>5 mm of induration) include individuals with HIV infection, recent contacts with TB patients, and organ transplant patients. Individuals also at risk (>10-mm induration) include injected drug users, residents of nursing homes and prisons, hospital employees, and recent immigrants from countries with a high prevalence of TB. These individuals, who are at considerable risk for the development of active TB once infected, should receive 9 months of INH therapy.

**ANSWER:** B

41. A 50-year-old woman with a history of severe dilated cardiomyopathy and placement of a left ventricular assist device (LVAD) is admitted to the hospital with fever and *S. aureus* bacteremia. Which of the following statements regarding LVAD-associated infection is not true?

A. LVAD-associated infection is a common event that occurs in up to 50% of LVAD recipients.

B. LVAD-associated bacteremia is a contraindication to cardiac transplantation.

C. The majority of LVAD-associated infections occur within 1 month of implantation.

D. Gram-positive bacteria are responsible for most LVAD-associated bacteremias.

E. The optimal duration of antibiotic therapy for LVAD-associated bacteria is poorly defined.

*Ref.:* 31

**COMMENTS: Left ventricular assist device** implantation has become an effective means of treating severe heart failure in patients awaiting cardiac transplantation. Unfortunately, device-related infection is common and occurs in nearly 50% of LVAD recipients. Localized infections involving the drive line exit site or LVAD pocket occur but are frequently associated with bacteremia. The majority (60%) of LVAD-associated infections occur within 30 days of implantation. Gram-positive bacteremia accounts for more than 75% of infections, with staphylococci being the most frequent blood isolate. Although short courses of systemic antibiotics for localized infections may be curative, the optimal duration of antibiotic therapy for LVAD-associated bacteremia is unclear. Relapse is common, and systemic antibiotics should generally be continued through transplantation.

Transplantation is not contraindicated in patients with recent LVAD-associated bacteremia. Posttransplant outcomes, such as length of hospitalization and 1-year survival rates, are not different in infected and noninfected LVAD patients.

**ANSWER:** C

42. Suspicion of OM in a diabetic foot ulcer should be raised in all of the following except:

A. Deep ulcer that overlies a bony prominence

B. An ulcer that does not heal after 2 weeks of appropriate therapy

C. A patient with a swollen foot and a history of foot ulceration

D. Unexplained high white blood cell count or inflammatory markers in a patient with a diabetic foot ulcer

E. Evidence of cortical erosion and periosteal reaction on plain radiography

*Ref.:* 14

**COMMENTS:** See Question 43.

**ANSWER:** B

43. Which of the following is true regarding OM in a diabetic foot?

A. A nuclear medicine tagged white blood cell scan is the best way to diagnose OM.

B. The only reported successful treatment of OM includes resection of the infected bone.

C. A presumptive diagnosis of OM cannot be made even if bone destruction is seen on plain film underneath an ulcer.

D. Bone biopsy is often difficult to perform and invasive and should be avoided.

E. Selected patients may benefit from implanted antibiotics, hyperbaric oxygen therapy, or revascularization.

*Ref.:* 14

**COMMENTS: Osteomyelitis** impairs healing of the wound and acts as a nidus for recurrent infection. It should be suspected in any deep or extensive ulcer, in one that overlies a bony prominence, and in an ulcer that does not heal after 6 weeks of appropriate therapy. In addition, concern for OM is raised in a patient with a swollen foot and a history of foot ulceration, the presence of a "sausage toe" (red, swollen digit), unexplained high white blood cell count, or inflammatory markers. Bone destruction underneath an ulcer seen on radiographs or probing of an ulcer down to bone is OM until proved otherwise. MRI is the most useful available imaging modality to diagnose OM, as well as to characterize any underlying soft tissue infection. The "gold standard" for diagnosis of OM remains isolation of bacteria from a bone sample with concomitant histologic findings of inflammatory cells and osteonecrosis.

When treating a **diabetic foot infection**, if there are no hard signs to indicate the presence of OM and plain radiographs do not demonstrate any evidence of bone pathology, the patient should be treated for about 2 weeks for the soft tissue infection. If there is persistent concern for OM, plain films should be repeated in 2 to 4 weeks to look for evidence of cortical erosion, periosteal reaction, or mixed radiolucency and sclerosis. Radioisotope scans are more sensitive than plain radiographs for diagnosis but are expensive and can be time consuming. If findings on plain films are only consistent with but not characteristic of OM, the clinician should consider the following: (1) additional **imaging studies**—MRI is preferred but nuclear medicine scans with leukocyte or immunoglobulin techniques would be the second choice; (2) empirical treatment for an additional 2 to 4 weeks with repeated radiographs to look for progression of bone changes; and (3) bone biopsy (operative or percutaneous fluoroscopic or CT guidance), especially if the etiologic pathogen or susceptibilities need to be established. Some physicians would perform biopsies for midfoot or hindfoot lesions because these are more difficult to treat and lead to higher-level amputations.

Traditionally, resection of a bone with chronic OM was necessary for cure; however, some nonrandomized case series report clinical success in 65% to 80% of patients treated nonoperatively with prolonged (3 to 6 months) antibiotic therapy. When treatment of OM fails, the clinician should consider whether the original diagnosis was correct, whether there is any remaining necrotic or infected bone or surgical hardware that needs to be removed, and whether the antimicrobials selected were appropriate, achieved an effective concentration within the bone, and were used for a sufficient duration. Selected patients may benefit from implanted antibiotics, hyperbaric oxygen therapy, revascularization, long-term or intermittent antibiotic administration, or amputation.

**ANSWER:** E

44. Which of the following regarding hospital-acquired pneumonia (HAP), ventilator-associated pneumonia (VAP), and health care–associated pneumonia (HCAP) is false?

A. They are the most common nosocomial infection.

B. They are usually caused by aerobic gram-negative bacilli.

C. They are rarely due to viral or fungal pathogens in immunocompetent patients.

D. Infection resulting from aspiration is usually due to anaerobes.

E. Gram-positive coccal isolates are more common patients with head trauma.

*Ref.:* 32

**COMMENTS:** See Question 45.

**ANSWER:** A

45. Which of the following are risk factors for HAP, VAP, or HCAP caused by multidrug-resistant pathogens?

A. Hospitalization for 5 or more days

B. Antimicrobial therapy or hospitalization in the preceding 90 days

C. Home wound care

D. Immunosuppressive disease or therapy

E. All of the above

*Ref.:* 32

**COMMENTS:** HAP, HCAP, and VAP are the second most common **nosocomial infections** after urinary tract infection. They result in significant morbidity and mortality. They are due to a wide spectrum of bacterial pathogens and are often polymicrobial, especially in patients with acute respiratory distress syndrome. They are rarely due to viral or fungal agents in immunocompetent patients. Isolation of *Candida* from endotracheal aspirates of immunocompetent patients usually represents colonization.

Common pathogens include aerobic gram-negative bacilli, including *P. aeruginosa, E. coli, K. pneumoniae,* and *Acinetobacter* spp. There has been an emergence of pneumonia associated with gram-positive cocci (*S. aureus,* particularly MRSA) , and it is more commonly seen in diabetics, patients with head trauma, and those hospitalized in the intensive care unit. Infection with anaerobic organisms may follow aspiration in nonintubated patients but is rare in VAP.

Early-onset HAP or VAP occurring within the first 4 days of hospitalization carries a better prognosis than does late-onset infections (5 days or more), which are more likely to be due to multidrug-resistant bacterial pathogens and result in increased morbidity and mortality. Additional risk factors for multidrug-resistant bacterial pathogens such as *Pseudomonas, Acinetobacter* spp., MRSA, and *K. pneumoniae* include antimicrobial therapy or hospitalization in the preceding 90 days, a high frequency of antibiotic resistance in the community or in the specific hospital unit, and immunosuppressive disease or therapy. Risk factors for multidrug-resistant pathogens in patients with HCAP include residence in a nursing home or long-term care facility, home infusion therapy, chronic dialysis within 30 days, home wound care, and a family member with a multidrug-resistant pathogen.

*P. aeruginosa* is the most common gram-negative bacterial pathogen that causes multidrug-resistant HAP/VAP, with some isolates being susceptible only to polymyxin B. Most MRSA infections are treated successfully with linezolid, although MRSA isolates resistant to linezolid are emerging.

Early administration of a broad-spectrum antibiotic in adequate doses and deescalation of the initial antibiotic therapy on the basis of cultures and clinical response are essential. Failure to adequately treat the infection because of delayed initiation of appropriate therapy has been associated with increased mortality. Guidelines have been established by the American Thoracic Society and the Infectious Disease Society of America for empirical therapy in immunocompetent adults with bacterial causes of HAP, VAP or HCAP; treatment should include either ceftriaxone, a fluoroquinolone, ampicillin/sulbactam, or ertapenem if there is no suspicion of a multidrug-resistant pathogen.

**ANSWER:** E

**REFERENCES**

1. Mandell GL, Bennett JE, Dolin R: *Principles and practice of infectious diseases,* ed 5, Philadelphia, 2000, Churchill Livingstone.
2. Chen SC, Wu WY, Yeh CH, et al: Comparison of *Escherichia coli* and *Klebsiella pneumonia* liver abscesses, *Am J Med Sci* 334:97–105, 2007.
3. Suerbaum S, Michetti P: *Helicobacter pylori* infection, *N Engl J Med* 347:1175–1186, 2002.
4. Bernard GR, Vincent JL, Laterre PF, et al: Efficacy and safety of recombinant human activated protein C for severe sepsis, *N Engl J Med* 344:699–709, 2001.

5. ASHP therapeutic guidelines on antimicrobial prophylaxis in surgery: American Society of Health-System Pharmacists, *Am J Health Syst Pharm* 56:1839–1888, 1999.

6. Barie PS: Surgical site infections: epidemiology and prevention, *Surg Infect (Larchmt)* 3(Suppl 1):9–21, 2002.

7. Wilson W, Taubert KA, Gewitz M, et al: Prevention of infective endocarditis: guidelines from the American Heart Association, *J Am Dent Assoc* 138:739–745, 2007.

8. Dolin R, Masur H, Saag MS: *AIDS therapy*, ed 2, Philadelphia, 2003, Churchill Livingstone.

9. Magadia RR, Weinstein MP: Laboratory diagnosis of bacteremia and fungemia, *Infect Dis Clin North Am* 15:1009–1024, 2001.

10. Karageorgopoulos DE, Falagas ME: New antibiotics: optimal use in current clinical practice, *Int J Antimicrob Agents* 34(Suppl 4):S55–S62, 2009.

11. Kretsinger K, Broder KR, Cortese MM, et al: Preventing tetanus, diphtheria, and pertussis among adults: use of tetanus toxoid, reduced diphtheria toxoid and acellular pertussis vaccine, *MMWR Recomm Rep* 55(RR-17):1–37, 2006.

12. Katzung BG: *Basic and clinical pharmacology*, ed 8, New York, 2001, McGraw-Hill.

13. Anaya DA, Dellinger EP: Surgical infections and choice antibiotics. In Townsend CM, Beauchamp RD, Evers BM, et al, editors: *Sabiston textbook of surgery: the biological basis of modern surgical practice*, ed 18, Philadelphia, 2008, WB Saunders.

14. Lipsky BA, Berendt AR, Deery HG, et al: Diagnosis and treatment of diabetic foot infections, *Clin Infect Dis* 39:885–910, 2004.

15. Mora-Duarte J, Betts R, Rotstein C, et al: Comparison of caspofungin and amphotericin B for invasive candidiasis, *N Engl J Med* 347:2020–2029, 2002.

16. Herbrecht R, Denning DW, Patterson TF, et al: Voriconazole versus amphotericin B for primary therapy of invasive aspergillosis, *N Engl J Med* 347:408–415, 2002.

17. Garrett HE Jr, Roper CL: Surgical intervention in histoplasmosis, *Ann Thorac Surg* 42:711–722, 1986.

18. Bhuva M, Ganger D, Jenssen D: Spontaneous bacterial peritonitis: an update on evaluation, management, and prevention, *Am J Med* 97:169–175, 1994.

19. Such J, Runyon BA: Spontaneous bacterial peritonitis, *Clin Infect Dis* 27:669–674, 1998.

20. Solomkin JS, Mazuski JE, Baron EJ, et al: Guidelines for the selection of anti-infective agents for complicated intra-abdominal infections, *Clin Infect Dis* 37:997–1005, 2003.

21. Beck DE, Wexner SD: *Fundamentals of anorectal surgery*. New York, 1992, McGraw-Hill.

22. Chalasani N, Wilcox CM: Gastrointestinal hemorrhage in patients with AIDS, *AIDS Patient Care STDs* 13:343–346, 1999.

23. Arnold MA, Barbul A: Surgical site infections. In Cameron JL, editor: *Current surgical therapy*, ed 9, Philadelphia, 2008, CV Mosby.

24. Cheadle, WG: Risk factors for surgical site infection, *Surg Infect* (Larchmt) 7:S7–S11, 2006.

25. Simon DM, Levin S: Infectious complications of solid organ transplantations, *Infect Dis Clin North Am* 15:521–549, 2001.

26. Razonable RR: Infections in solid organ transplant recipients. Conference report: highlights from the 40th annual meeting of Infectious Diseases Society of America, October 24–27, 2002.

27. de Gans J, van de Beek D, et al: Dexamethasone in adults with bacterial meningitis, *N Engl J Med* 347:1549–1556, 2002.

28. Chawdhury MH, Tunkel AR: Antibacterial agents in infections of the central nervous system, *Infect Dis Clin North Am* 14:391–408, 2000.

29. Centers for Disease Control and Prevention: Recommendations for prevention and control of hepatitis C virus infection and HCV-related chronic disease, *MMWR Recomm Rep* 47(RR-19):1–39, 1998.

30. American Thoracic Society; CDC; Infectious Diseases Society of America: Treatment of tuberculosis, *MMWR Recomm Rep* 52(RR-11):1–77, 2003.

31. Argenziano M, Catenese KA, Moazami N, et al: The influence of infection on survival and successful transplantation in patients with left ventricular assist devices, *J Heart Lung Transplant* 16:822–831, 1997.

32. Guidelines for the management of adults with hospital-acquired, ventilator-associated, and healthcare-associated pneumonia, *Am J Respir Crit Care Med* 171:388–416, 2005.

# B. Transmissible Diseases and Surgeons

1. Which of the following is not considered standard precautions for reducing the spread of transmissible diseases?

   A. Hand washing before contact with a patient

   B. Hand washing after glove removal

   C. Wearing gloves during contact with a patient

   D. Negative pressure airflow

   E. Eye protection

   *Ref.:* 1

**COMMENTS: Standard, or universal, precautions** are designed to prevent the spread of transmissible disease by contact with blood, body fluids, or any other potentially infected material. These precautions apply to *all* patients *all* of the time. Hand washing is fundamental and should be performed before and between each contact with a patient and after glove removal. Gloves are worn when contacting a potentially contaminated area. Surgical masks and eye protection are required if mucous membrane or eye exposure is possible. Gowns are part of standard precautions when more extensive blood or fluid exposure may occur. Specific engineering controls for airflow and processing of air are integral to preventing spread of certain airborne pathogens and as such are not a component of basic standard precautions. Specific procedures for infection control are mandated by federal regulatory agencies. Surgeons and all health care workers (HCWs) must be familiar with the specific infection control policies and procedures established at their places of work.

**ANSWER:** D

2. A 68-year-old woman is admitted to the hospital for neurosurgery after being found comatose at home. The patient lives alone, but her neighbor states that she has been "acting strangely" for the last several weeks. No additional history is available. MRI of the brain reveals evidence of focal cerebritis and enlarged ventricles along with enhancement of the basilar meninges. A chest radiograph shows upper lobe consolidation. Results of a rapid HIV test are positive. The patient is taken to the operating room for placement of a ventricular drain. Which type of isolation would be needed for this patient in the postoperative period?

   A. Standard and airborne precautions

   B. Airborne precautions

   C. Droplet precautions

   D. Contact precautions

   E. Reverse isolation

   *Ref.:* 2

**COMMENTS:** This **human immunodeficiency virus**-infected patient has evidence of meningitis, cerebritis, and upper lobe pneumonia. The unifying diagnosis is pulmonary and cerebral **tuberculosis**. This patient requires airborne precautions.

A variety of infection control measures are implemented to decrease the risk for transmission of microorganisms in hospitals. Standard precautions are used for the care of all patients. Hand washing between patient contact and the use of barrier protection, such as gloves, gowns, and masks, to minimize exposure to potentially infectious body fluids (e.g., blood, feces, wound drainage) are important components of standard precautions and all infection control programs.

In addition to standard precautions, **airborne precautions** are used for patients with known or suspected illness transmitted via small airborne droplets ($\leq 5\ \mu m$). TB, measles, smallpox, and varicella (chickenpox) are examples of diseases requiring airborne precautions. Because these organisms can be dispersed widely by air currents and may remain suspended in the air for long periods, special air handling and ventilation are necessary. Patients requiring airborne precautions are placed in "negative pressure" rooms, and all persons entering the room require an N95 mask.

In addition to standard precautions, **droplet precautions** are used for patients with suspected or proven invasive disease caused by *H. influenzae* or *N. meningitidis* (e.g., pneumonia, meningitis, or sepsis) or other respiratory illnesses such as diphtheria, pertussis, pneumonic plague, influenza, mumps, and rubella. The droplets produced by these illnesses are usually generated by coughing but are larger than the droplets described earlier ($>5\ \mu m$), travel only short distances (<3 feet), and do not remain suspended in air. Patients require a private room, and persons entering the room require a surgical mask.

In addition to standard precautions, contact precautions apply to specific patients infected or colonized with epidemiologically important organisms spread by direct contact with a patient or contact with items in the patient's environment. These organisms may demonstrate antibiotic resistance and include MRSA, vancomycin-resistant *S. aureus*, VRE, and multidrug-resistant gram-negative bacilli. Enteric pathogens such as *C. difficile* and skin infections such as impetigo (group A streptococci), herpes simplex, and scabies also require contact precautions.

**ANSWER:** A

3. Which of the following statements regarding MRSA is false?

   A. MRSA is a common nosocomial pathogen, but it can also be detected in the community.

   B. The treatment of choice is vancomycin.

   C. Treatment of surgical patients with intranasal mupirocin decreases wound infection rates with MRSA.

   D. Hospitalized patients colonized with MRSA require contact isolation.

E. MRSA is less virulent than methicillin-sensitive *S. aureus*.

*Ref.:* 3-5

**COMMENTS:** Staphylococci are the most common cause of nosocomial infections in surgical patients. Recent reports suggest that carriage of **methicillin-resistant S. aureus** ™in the community has increased, and more infections with this organism are being seen in persons without health care–associated risks (nosocomial risks).

At the beginning of the antibiotic era, *S. aureus* was susceptible to penicillins. Resistance developed to penicillin via β-lactamase production, and new antibiotics were discovered, including the penicillinase-resistant penicillins (methicillin, oxacillin, nafcillin, etc). MRSA is by definition resistant to methicillin. Methicillin is not used in clinical practice because it induces interstitial nephritis, but it is still used in the laboratory to differentiate methicillin-susceptible *S. aureus* (MSSA) from MRSA. Vancomycin or linezolid can be used to treat MRSA. *S. aureus* strains with intermediate susceptibility to vancomycin and vancomycin-resistant *S. aureus* have been reported in the United States.

Although some studies suggest that mortality after MRSA infection is higher that that after **methicillin-susceptible S. aureus** infection, the increased death rate is most likely due to comorbid conditions and not to differences in virulence between MSSA and MRSA. Hospitalized patients colonized with MRSA require contact isolation to avoid spread of the bacteria to other patients. A recent prospective, randomized, placebo-controlled study showed that intranasal mupirocin did not significantly reduce *S. aureus* SSIs. However, it did significantly reduce the rate of all nosocomial *S. aureus* infections in the patients who were *S. aureus* carriers.

**ANSWER:** C

4. Which of the following statements regarding hand hygiene is false?

A. HCWs should clean their hands with an antiseptic-containing agent before and after each contact with a patient.

B. The use of soap and water for hand washing is required when hands are visibly soiled with blood or body fluids.

C. Adherence to hand hygiene guidelines by HCWs is generally poor.

D. Alcohol-based hand rubs are inferior to antimicrobial soaps for hand decontamination.

E. VRE and MRSA are frequently isolated from the hands of HCWs.

*Ref.:* 6

**COMMENTS: Hand washing** by HCWs may be the single most effective measure for preventing nosocomial infection. The spread of bacteria, particularly antibiotic-resistant organisms such as MRSA and VRE, from contaminated HCWs to patients is well documented. Despite recommendations to wash hands before and after all contact with patients, adherence to such policies by HCWs has been poor. Although hand washing with soap and water is required when hands are visibly soiled with blood, the widespread use of alcohol-based hand rubs by HCWs between patient contacts may decrease the spread of resistant bacteria to patients. Alcohol-based products are superior to antimicrobial soaps for standard hand decontamination. Alcohol-based hand rubs have the broadest spectrum of antimicrobial activity among the available hand hygiene products, and their use results in a rapid reduction in microbial skin counts. The ability to make these rubs available at the entrance to patients' rooms, at the bedside, or in pocket-sized containers to be carried by HCWs may improve compliance with hand hygiene policies. The CDC has recently published guidelines for hand hygiene in heath care settings that include recommendations for hand-washing antisepsis, hand hygiene techniques, and surgical hand antisepsis.

**ANSWER:** D

5. Current CDC recommendations concerning HCWs and H1N1 virus include all of the following except:

A. All HCWs should be vaccinated for H1N1 virus.

B. If H1N1 develops, the HCW must stay out of work for a total of 9 days.

C. If H1N1 develops, the HCW must stay out of the hospital for at least 24 hours after fever is no longer present (without fever-reducing medication).

D. If in contact with a patient suspected of having H1N1, the HCW should follow standard precautions and wear an N95 respirator.

E. All persons coming in and out of the hospital should be screened for flulike symptoms unless they have been vaccinated.

*Ref.:* 7

**COMMENTS:** All HCWs should be vaccinated for **H1N1**. If symptoms of the virus develop, the CDC recommends that the HCW should stay out of work for 7 days from the onset of symptoms *or* for 24 hours after becoming afebrile without any fever-reducing medication, whichever is shortest. All persons coming in contact with a person suspected or proved to have H1N1 should wear an N95 respiratory mask in addition to following standard precautions. Moreover, it is now recommended that everyone coming in and out of the hospital, including visitors, be screened for flulike symptoms unless they have been vaccinated for H1N1.

**ANSWER:** B

6. Contraindication to receiving the attenuated live nasal vaccine for H1N1 virus include all of the following except:

A. Age younger than 2 years

B. Age 50 years or older

C. Pregnancy

D. Age younger than 3 years

E. Children/adolescents who take aspirin

*Ref.:* 7

**COMMENTS:** Currently, the CDC states that the attenuated live **H1N1 nasal vaccine** is safe for all healthy individuals aged 2 to 49. Contraindications include children 2 years or younger, adults 50 years or older, pregnant patients, and patients with a preexisting medical condition that places them at high risk for complications from influenza (chronic heart or lung disease, diabetes, or kidney failure; illnesses that weaken the immune system; or patients who take medications that can weaken the immune system). The nasal vaccine is also contraindicated in children younger than 5 years with a history of recurrent wheezing, in children or adolescents who take aspirin, in anyone with a history of Guillain-Barré syndrome occurring after receiving influenza vaccine, and in anyone with a severe allergy to eggs.

**ANSWER:** D

---

7. A nonvaccinated surgical resident is exposed to a patient with H1N1, and fevers and upper respiratory symptoms subsequently develop. Which is the correct treatment?

A. Amantadine

B. Rimantadine

C. Fever-reducing medications and supportive care

D. Oseltamivir

E. None of the above

*Ref.:* 7

**COMMENTS: H1N1** has been shown to be resistant to the adamantane class of drugs (including amantadine and rimantadine) and susceptible to oseltamivir (oral) and zanamivir (nasal). It is recommended that in addition to treating the symptoms and supportive care, persons suspected of having H1N1 should start either oseltamivir or zanamivir therapy. If the symptoms worsen, patients may require hospitalization and more invasive support.

**ANSWER:** D

---

8. Which type of hepatitis virus has a DNA genome?

A. Hepatitis A

B. Hepatitis B

C. Hepatitis C

D. All of the above

E. None of the above

*Ref.:* 8

**COMMENTS:** Five viruses (hepatitis A, B, C, D, and E) are recognized as causes of **acute hepatitis.** They have some similar and some dissimilar features in how they are transmitted and in the potential consequences of infection. HBV contains partially double-stranded DNA. All the other types are RNA viruses. Hepatitis D (delta hepatitis) is an incomplete virus or virus particle with small, circular RNA. It must coexist with HBV to replicate and produce infection. The diagnosis of hepatic viral infection and determination of disease status depend on the detection of viral proteins encoded by these genomes or the presence of antibodies to them.

**ANSWER:** B

---

9. Worldwide, which of the following is the most common mode of transmission of HCV?

A. Fecal-oral

B. Sexual

C. Parenteral

D. Vertical (childbirth)

E. Contaminated water

*Ref.:* 8, 9

**COMMENTS:** HCV is primarily spread by parenteral routes. Sexual transmission can also occur but is less common than with HBV. Injected drug use currently accounts for most HCV transmission in the United States. Injected drug use leads to transmission of HCV by direct transfer of infected blood on shared needles or syringes and by contamination of drug preparation equipment. Blood transfusions were an important method of spread before the availability of screening. Routine testing of donors for evidence of HCV infection was initiated in 1990, and multiantigen testing was implemented in 1992 and has reduced the risk for infection to 0.001% per unit transfused.

**ANSWER:** C

---

10. What is the prevalence of HCV infection in the United States?

A. 0.2%

B. 2%

C. 5%

D. 10%

E. 20%

*Ref.:* 9, 10

**COMMENTS:** The prevalence of HCV infection in the United States is approximately four times greater than the prevalence of HIV infection. The rate in HCWs, including general, orthopedic, and oral surgeons, is no higher. As would be expected, some populations have a much higher prevalence, including hemophiliacs (60% to 90%), injected drug users (60% to 90%), and chronic hemodialysis patients (up to 60%).

**ANSWER:** B

---

11. The clinical course of the majority of patients with HCV infection is characterized by which one of the following?

A. Acute constitutional symptoms and jaundice

B. Acute fulminant hepatic failure

C. Development of chronic hepatitis

D. Progression to cirrhosis

E. Development of hepatocellular carcinoma

*Ref.:* 8, 9

**COMMENTS:** The incubation period for HCV infection is about 5 to 10 weeks. Most acute infections are asymptomatic, but about 25% of patients may have constitutional symptoms and elevated aminotransferase levels. Fulminant, acute hepatic failure is rare. Infection with HCV is particularly serious, however, because patients with chronic HCV infection can progress to cirrhosis (20%), liver failure (10%), and hepatocellular carcinoma (1% to 5%). Chronic HCV infection may be associated with more severe or progressive liver disease in patients with concurrent hepatopathy, especially alcoholics. Chronic HCV infection is now the leading indication for liver transplantation. In comparison, chronic infection develops in only about 10% of individuals infected with HBV.

**ANSWER:** C

---

12. A surgical resident is stuck with an HCV-contaminated hollow-bore needle. Which of the following tests should be done initially?

A. Detection of HCV RNA

B. Detection of HCV surface antigen

C. Detection of HCV antibodies by enzyme immunoassay

D. Measurement of viral load

E. Detection of HCV core antigen

*Ref.:* 9

**COMMENTS:** The initial screening test for HCV is an antibody immunoassay. The person stuck with the contaminated needle should have baseline testing performed. Since it can take up to 6 months for a person to seroconvert, called the window period, people who have been stuck with a contaminated needle not only require baseline testing but will also need follow-up testing in 6 months.

**ANSWER:** C

13. Which of the following blood tests confirm HCV infection?

A. Detection of HCV RNA

B. Detection of HCV surface antigen

C. Detection of HCV antibodies by enzyme immunoassay

D. Detection of HCV antibodies and alanine aminotransferase levels of 500 to 1000

E. Measurement of HCV viral load

*Ref.:* 9

**COMMENTS:** The **screening test for HCV** is an immunoassay for anti-HCV antibodies. Although the results are positive in 90% of patients infected with HCV, the predictive value of the test is limited when the prevalence of infection is low. In addition, anti-HCV antibodies may not be detectable for up to 18 weeks following exposure. Their presence does not differentiate the state of infection. Qualitative reverse transcriptase polymerase chain reaction (RT-PCR) for detection of HCV RNA is confirmatory. Infection may also be confirmed by recombinant immunoblot assay for HCV antibody.

**ANSWER:** A

14. Which of the following is an important risk factor for transmission of HIV to the surgeon after a percutaneous injury?

A. The source patient has advanced HIV infection with a CD4+ T-cell count of less than 50 cells/mm$^3$.

B. The surgeon sustains a deep puncture injury.

C. Blood was visible on the sharp object causing the injury.

D. The injury was caused by a device that had entered a blood vessel of the source patient before injury.

E. All of the above.

*Ref.:* 11

**ANSWER:** E

**COMMENTS:** See Question 15.

15. What is the approximate probability of transmission of HCV to an HCW through a needlestick injury from an infected source?

A. 0.3%

B. 3%

C. 5%

D. 30%

E. 50%

*Ref.:* 8, 9

**COMMENTS:** The risk for **transmission of HIV** after percutaneous exposure to HIV-infected blood is about 0.3%. This risk is influenced by several factors, including depth of the injury and the presence of undiluted blood on the device causing the injury. Exposure to blood from patients in the terminal stages of AIDS, which probably reflects high titers of circulating virus, also increases the risk to HCWs. Although no prospective study demonstrating benefit from postexposure prophylaxis with antiretroviral agents has been completed, a retrospective case-control study suggests that in those who receive zidovudine prophylaxis after exposure, the odds of HIV infection were reduced significantly (by approximately 80%). Postexposure prophylaxis, which now includes at least two antiretroviral agents, should be started immediately (within 72 hours) in HCWs with high-risk injuries.

HCWs are at risk for contracting transmissible viral disease when stuck by needles with contaminated blood or by exposure of mucosal membranes to blood or other body fluids. The risk for documented seroconversion is approximately 3% to 10% for HCV. The risk for HBV infection after needlestick injury is 5% to 30%. The risk of for HCV infection following mucous membrane or other cutaneous exposure has not been defined. The risk for HIV infection with mucous membrane exposure is about 0.1%. When exposure occurs, the infected area should be washed thoroughly with soup and water. The source should be tested for infection with HBV, HCV, and HIV. The risk of contracting HIV infection is greatest with hollow needles, with deep intramuscular injury, or when the exposure involves a greater amount of virus (i.e., from a larger amount of blood or a source with late-stage HIV infection).

**ANSWER:** C

16. The operating surgeon is stuck with a needle while performing elective repair of an inguinal hernia. The patient is known to be HIV negative, but his HCV status is unknown. The patient has a known history of intravenous drug abuse. In addition, the operating surgeon is hepatitis B immune because of previous vaccination. Which one of the following measures is appropriate?

A. Prophylactic antiviral treatment

B. Administration of HCV vaccine and immunoglobulin if the surgeon is HCV antibody negative

C. Baseline testing of the surgeon and patient for HCV and follow-up testing of the surgeon at 4 to 6 months

D. No testing for the surgeon indicated if the patient tests negative for HCV

E. Prophylactic administration of HCV immunoglobulin in addition to baseline testing of both the surgeon and patient and follow-up testing of the surgeon in 4 to 6 months

*Ref.:* 7, 9

**COMMENTS:** Anytime that someone is inadvertently stuck with a needle from a patient with unknown **HCV status,** both the patient and the person stuck should undergo baseline testing for HCV. In addition, the person stuck should have follow-up testing at 4 to 6 months. There is no treatment that has proven efficacy in reducing the risk for seroconversion with HCV; therefore, no prophylaxis for HCV infection is currently indicated.

**ANSWER:** C

17. During an emergency appendectomy, a surgical resident sustains an injury from a contaminated hollow-bore needle with spontaneous bleeding. Which one of the following blood-borne organisms is most likely to be transmitted, assuming that the patient was infected with all of them?

A. HIV

B. HBV

C. HCV

D. *Plasmodium* spp. (malaria)

E. *Treponema pallidum* (syphilis)

*Ref.:* 12

**COMMENTS:** All the organisms mentioned are potentially transmissible through the exposure described. After significant exposure to **blood-borne pathogens**, the risk is about 30% for acquiring hepatitis B, 3% for hepatitis C, and 0.3% for HIV disease. Malaria and syphilis may be acquired through blood transfusion, and acquisition through a needlestick is theoretically possible. Because of the high risk associated with hepatitis B exposure, it is recommended that all HCWs be vaccinated against HBV. In the event that a nonimmune HCW is exposed to HBV, it is recommended that the HCW receive hepatitis B immune globulin (HBIG) within 7 days of the exposure and also start a vaccination series. Postexposure prophylaxis with antiretroviral drugs may be indicated after exposure to HIV-infected blood. There is no postexposure prophylaxis available against HCV.

**ANSWER:** B

18. A surgical resident sustains a needlestick with a hollow-bore needle contaminated with the blood of a patient who is hepatitis B antigen positive. The resident completed a series of three hepatitis B vaccines 1 year ago, but his antibody response was not checked. Which of the following statements best describes management of this case?

A. Observation only is indicated since the source does not have active HBV infection.

B. The resident needs a booster of hepatitis B vaccine.

C. The resident should receive HBIG immediately.

D. The resident should receive HBIG and a hepatitis B vaccine booster immediately.

E. The resident needs to be tested for anti–hepatitis B antibody immediately. If the test result is negative, proceed as in alternative D.

*Ref.:* 13

**COMMENTS:** HCWs who sustain injuries from needles contaminated with blood containing **hepatitis B virus** have a risk for the development of serologic evidence of HBV infection as high as 62%. The source patient is hepatitis B antigen positive, which is an indication of active HBV infection. The resident has been vaccinated against HBV, but his immune status is unknown and

should be determined. If the resident is anti–hepatitis B antibody positive, no intervention is necessary. However, if anti–hepatitis B antibody negative, HBIG (which can be given up to 7 days after the exposure) and a hepatitis B vaccine booster should be administered. If the resident was never vaccinated, HBIG should be administered immediately and the hepatitis B vaccination series begun.

**ANSWER:** E

19. Which of the following clinical conditions is identified by the presence of antibodies in the serum against hepatitis B surface antigen (anti-HBs) in the absence of hepatitis B core antigen (anti-HBc) and hepatitis B surface antigen (HBsAg)?

A. The patient is susceptible to HBV infection.

B. The patient is immune because of HBV vaccination.

C. The patient has an active acute infection with HBV.

D. The patient has chronic active hepatitis with HBV.

E. The patient has recovered from an HBV infection with subsequent natural immunity.

*Ref.:* 8, 14

**COMMENTS: Testing for hepatitis B surface antigens** will be positive in both patients who have been immunized against HBV and those who were previously infected. To distinguish the two clinical situations, one must use other testing. HBsAg positivity indicates an active infection, either acute or chronic. Anti-HBc–positive results indicates that a person either currently has an active infection or has been infected with HBV in the past. If both are negative in the setting of positive anti-HBs, the person has been vaccinated but never infected with HBV.

**ANSWER:** B

20. A nonimmune surgical resident is stuck by a contaminated needle from an HBsAg-positive source. Which of the following is the correct initial treatment?

A. None because the patient does not have active HBV infection and is immune to HBV

B. Interferon

C. Vaccination against HBV

D. HBIG

E. Vaccination against HBV and administration of HBIG

*Ref.:* 8

**COMMENTS:** The best method of preventing **occupational hepatitis B virus infection** is to vaccinate all HVWs at risk if they do not have natural immunity from previous infection. When exposure occurs, the affected area should be immediately and thoroughly washed with soap and water. The source is tested for HBV, HCV, and HIV. If the source tests positive for HBV, nonimmune individuals are given HBIG for passive prophylaxis and are vaccinated. If a previously vaccinated individual incurs a needle injury, titers should be checked and a dose of vaccine given if titers are not detected. Interferon is not used for prophylaxis following acute exposure but may be useful for some patients with chronic HBV or HCV infection.

**ANSWER:** E

21. A surgical resident is placing a central venous catheter in a patient who is HIV positive and is stuck with the needle. Which of the following regarding postexposure prophylaxis is true?

  A. No prophylaxis necessary; however, the surgical resident should have a baseline HIV test performed and follow-up tests in 3 and 6 months.

  B. The resident should have a baseline HIV test performed and follow-up testing in 3 and 6 months and, in addition, begin combined triple antiretroviral therapy.

  C. The resident should have a baseline HIV test performed and follow-up testing in 3 and 6 months and, in addition, begin single antiretroviral therapy.

  D. The resident should have a baseline HIV test performed and follow-up testing in 3 and 6 months and, in addition, begin therapy with two antiretroviral drugs.

  E. The resident should begin combined triple antiretroviral therapy and have an HIV test performed in 6 months.

*Ref.: 7, 9*

COMMENTS: Most occupationally **acquired human immuno-deficiency virus infection** has been documented in nurses or laboratory technicians. Postexposure drug prophylaxis should be initiated as soon as possible, ideally within 2 hours. In cases in which the status of the source is unknown, standard **serologic testing** (enzyme immunoassay and Western blot) is indicated, but the results may take several days. A rapid HIV test can now give results within 1 hour. However, serologic test results may be negative in infected individuals for 3 to 12 weeks following acquisition of the virus. The decision to start postexposure drug prophylaxis must therefore consider any known risk factors that the source may have, regardless of the serologic results. **Postexposure prophylaxis** consists of multidrug therapy with a combination of nucleoside and protease inhibitors. Adverse side effects are frequent and sometimes severe. Recommendations for postexposure prophylaxis continue to evolve. The most effective method of reducing the risk for transmission of HIV in a person stuck with a needle from a known HIV-positive patient is to begin combined triple antiretroviral therapy. The first dose should be given as soon after exposure as possible. Besides a baseline HIV test, this person should undergo additional follow-up testing at both 3 and 6 months.

ANSWER: B

22. Which of the following markers is the most clinically useful for monitoring the course of a person infected with HIV?

  A. Viral load

  B. CD4$^+$ T-cell count

  C. Serum neopterin

  D. Serum oligoclonal immunoglobulins

  E. Serum p24 antigen level

*Ref.: 7, 15*

COMMENTS: The **CD4+ T-cell count**, although somewhat imperfect, is the most useful determination for monitoring the course of an HIV infection. The normal CD4$^+$ count is greater than 600 cells/mm$^3$ with most counts ranging from 800 to 1200 cells/mm$^3$. Symptomatic disease usually begins when the CD4$^+$ count falls below 300 to 400 cells/mm$^3$. Opportunistic infections begin to occur when the CD4$^+$ cell count is less than 200 cells/mm$^3$. The time course of this decline in CD4$^+$ T-cell count is prolonged and may take more than 10 years. Direct quantification of viral load with plasma viremia shows increasing viral titers as the disease progresses. $\beta_2$-Microglobulin is shed into the serum in HIV-infected patients and reflects increased lymphocyte turnover. **Neopterin** is produced by macrophages stimulated by interferon. Although both are found in increasing amounts as HIV infection progresses, neither of these two determinations is specific for HIV infection, and they are generally used in a research setting. Determination of p24 antigen is specific for HIV but not very sensitive.

ANSWER: B

23. The chance of an HIV-infected individual transmitting infection best correlates with which of the following?

  A. CD4$^+$ T-cell count

  B. Viral load

  C. Absolute lymphocyte count less than 1000 cells/mm$^3$

  D. Active opportunistic infection

  E. Whether the patient is currently receiving antiretroviral therapy

*Ref.: 7, 9, 16*

COMMENTS: Blood measurements of **viral load** reflect the risk for transmission of HIV by any route: parenteral, sexual, or perinatal. The risk of acquiring HIV infection through occupational exposure also correlates with the viral load in the source. Both viral load and the CD4$^+$ count reflect the stage of the disease in that patients with late viral infection have low CD4$^+$ levels and high viral counts. Opportunistic infections are also more prevalent as CD4$^+$ counts fall and immunodeficiency worsens. **Clinical acquired immunodeficiency syndrome** is defined in patients with positive HIV serologic findings when CD4$^+$ counts are less than 200 cells/mm$^3$ or when one of a number of defined associated conditions exists. The list of these AIDS-defining conditions includes specific opportunistic infections, neoplasms, and degenerative conditions.

ANSWER: B

24. A 36-year-old man with HIV infection and a CD4$^+$ count of less than 500 cells/mm$^3$ has an incarcerated ventral hernia. In addition to standard precautions, which one of the following is recommended?

  A. Avoidance of prosthetic mesh

  B. Broader preoperative prophylactic antibiotic coverage than for a patient who is HIV negative

  C. Prophylactic trimethoprim/sulfamethoxazole in addition to standard preoperative antibiotics

  D. Disposable surgical instruments

  E. None of the above

*Ref.: 9*

COMMENTS: Beyond the universal precautions that are used for all patients, there are no specific recommendations regarding the preoperative or **intraoperative management of patients with human immunodeficiency virus** infection. Operative treatment should be performed according to the surgical condition and antiretroviral drug therapy administered according to the status of the HIV disease. Prophylactic antibiotics or prosthetic materials are used for the same indications as for non–HIV-infected individuals. Trimethoprim/sulfamethoxazole is used for the prophylaxis of *P. carinii* pneumonia in patients with clinical AIDS but has nothing to do with surgical prophylaxis. Standard surgical instruments and sterilization techniques are appropriate. The use of disposable instruments is often convenient and simple when performing minor procedure outside the main operating room.

**ANSWER:** E

25. A 28-year-old woman with AIDS has right upper quadrant pain and on ultrasound examination is found to have acute cholecystitis. Which of the following is the appropriate therapy?

   A. The patient should begin antibiotic therapy but should undergo no surgical intervention because of her immune status.

   B. The patient should begin antibiotic therapy and have a percutaneous cholecystostomy tube placed.

   C. The patient should begin antibiotic therapy and undergo open cholecystectomy.

   D. The patient should begin antibiotic therapy and undergo laparoscopic cholecystectomy.

   E. None of the above.

*Ref.: 17*

**COMMENTS:** AIDS and **human immunodeficiency virus** infection are not contraindications to **laparoscopy.** These patients should be managed according to routine general surgery principles. A patient with AIDS and acute cholecystitis should be treated with appropriate antibiotics and laparoscopic cholecystectomy unless the patient is not stable enough or has other comorbid conditions that make surgery too dangerous.

**ANSWER:** D

26. The operative mortality rate after laparotomy in patients with AIDS has most closely been associated with which of the following?

   A. Total lymphocyte count less than 1000 cells/mm$^2$

   B. CD4$^+$ T-cell count less than 500/mm$^3$

   C. Active opportunistic infection

   D. Duration of HIV infection

   E. Emergency surgery

*Ref.: 18*

**COMMENTS: Prognostic factors in acquired immunodeficiency syndrome patients** undergoing abdominal operations have not been extensively analyzed. The cumulative operative mortality rate after major abdominal procedures is approximately 20%. Most deaths are related to the patient's underlying disease and not to specific operative complications. Emergency operations have been associated with higher mortality rates than have elective procedures, particularly in patients with intestinal perforations because of opportunistic infections such as CMV. However, there is no convincing evidence that patients with HIV infection without AIDS-defining criteria have an inordinate risk for death or complications after abdominal surgery.

**ANSWER:** E

27. Laparotomy is performed on a 26-year-old, HIV-positive man who has been hospitalized with abdominal pain, intractable diarrhea, and a perforated viscus. He has a 2-cm cecal perforation, and the colon is dilated throughout. Select the most appropriate therapy.

   A. Primary repair of the perforation with placement of a drain

   B. Primary repair of the perforation with a diverting ileostomy

   C. Ileocecal resection with primary anastomosis

   D. Ileocecal resection with primary anastomosis and a diverting ileostomy

   E. Abdominal colectomy with ileostomy and a Hartmann procedure

*Ref.: 14, 19*

**COMMENTS:** Infection of the gastrointestinal tract with CMV is one of the most common causes of **intestinal perforation in human immunodeficiency virus-infected patients** and is an AIDS-defining condition. The diagnosis is based on demonstration of intranuclear inclusion bodies on a biopsy specimen. Initial treatment consists of antiviral agents and support. Surgery is indicated for perforation, bleeding, or obstruction as a result of stricture formation. CMV perforations are most frequently ileocolic in location. They can involve the small intestines, stomach, or duodenum. Operative management of colon perforations is resection without anastomosis. Determination of the extent of resection has various considerations, but since the entire colon is typically involved, total abdominal colectomy is often advisable. Such patients are often desperately ill, and appropriate and timely surgical intervention and aggressive support are necessary for survival.

**ANSWER:** E

28. A 30-year-old HIV-positive man undergoes repair of an incarcerated inguinal hernia. His CD4$^+$ T-cell count is 300 cells/mm$^2$. Postoperatively, a wound infection develops at his incision site. Which of the following organisms is most likely responsible?

   A. CMV

   B. *Staphylococcus*

   C. *Candida* spp.

   D. *E. coli*

   E. None of the above

*Ref.: 9*

**COMMENTS:** Even in a patient with a low CD4$^+$ T-cell count, the most likely source of a **wound infection** will be from the same flora that affects patients with normal immune systems. In patients undergoing inguinal hernia repair, the most likely cause of a wound infection is *Staphylococcus*.

**ANSWER:** B

29. A 32-year-old, HIV-positive injected drug user is admitted following a seizure. Examination reveals a pronator drift. A CT scan of the head with intravenous contrast material shows two ring-enhancing lesions. Which of the following statements is true?

A. Primary CNS lymphoma is the most likely diagnosis.

B. Biopsy should be performed on all enhancing lesions in HIV-infected patients.

C. Toxoplasmosis is the most likely diagnosis.

D. Pyrimethamine is an effective agent for primary prophylaxis of this condition, but it is not very effective for its treatment.

E. The neurologic symptoms are unrelated to AIDS.

*Ref.:* 7, 15, 20

**COMMENTS:** Ten percent of AIDS patients experience a neurologic symptom as the first sign of their illness, and one or more neurologic deficits eventually develop in 40% of AIDS patients. Major **human immunodeficiency virus-related central nervous system** diseases include HIV encephalopathy, meningitis, myelopathy, opportunistic infections (PML caused by papovavirus, CMV, herpes, *Toxoplasma gondii*, and *C. neoformans*), neoplasms (primary CNS lymphoma), and cerebrovascular complications. *T. gondii*, the protozoan that causes toxoplasmosis, accounts for 50% to 70% of focal brain lesions in these patients and is the most common cause of focal enhancing lesions on CT. Ten percent to 25% of focal lesions are **central nervous system lymphomas**. Primary CNS lymphoma is a rare intracranial tumor in the general population, in whom it accounts for only 1.5% of primary brain tumors. However, it is significantly more common in HIV-infected patients, even when compared with other immunosuppressed populations. Current management recommendations for HIV-infected patients with focal brain lesions include 2 to 3 weeks of empirical treatment of toxoplasmosis, followed by biopsy if the radiologic or clinical condition deteriorates.

**ANSWER:** B

30. Select the true statement regarding splenectomy in HIV-infected patients.

A. The laparoscopic approach is contraindicated.

B. HIV-associated thrombocytopenia is the primary indication.

C. It is associated with a 30% risk for overwhelming postsplenectomy infection.

D. Splenectomy may accelerate progression to AIDS.

E. All of the above.

*Ref.:* 9, 14, 21

**COMMENTS: Thrombocytopenia** similar to but immunologically distinct from classic idiopathic thrombocytopenic purpura develops in approximately 10% to 20% of patients with asymptomatic **human immunodeficiency virus disease**. Initial treatment with corticosteroids produces a response in most (80%) patients. Those who fail to respond or who relapse when steroid use is tapered are appropriate candidates for splenectomy. Splenectomy yields a favorable result in 80% of patients. Neither the morbidity of splenectomy nor the risk for overwhelming postsplenectomy infection appears to be increased in HIV-infected patients. Likewise, there is no evidence that absence of the spleen worsens HIV disease. In fact, it has been suggested that splenectomy may actually slow disease progression in some patients. Other occasional indications for splenectomy in HIV-related conditions include opportunistic infections, abscesses, and malignancies.

**ANSWER:** B

31. A 60-year-old immigrant from China is admitted to the hospital with fevers and a cough productive of bloody sputum. A chest radiograph demonstrates a right upper lobe infiltrate. The patient's TB exposure is unknown. Which of the following precautions is appropriate?

A. No precautions are necessary.

B. The patient should be admitted to a shared room but be required to wear a mask.

C. The patient should be admitted to a private room but does not need a mask during transport.

D. The patient should be admitted to a private room and should wear a mask during transport.

E. The patient should be admitted to a negative pressure private room and wear a mask during transport.

*Ref.:* 7

**COMMENTS: Airborne precautions** are necessary to reduce the exposure of staff and other patients to individuals with suspected pulmonary or laryngeal **tuberculosis**. Early recognition of patients at risk for TB is critical, including patients with possible symptoms of TB and those at higher risk for active disease. Typical symptoms include persistent cough, bloody sputum, fever, night sweats, and weight loss. A chest radiograph may show a cavitary lesion or upper lobe infiltrate. Individuals at higher risk include the homeless, elderly, known contacts of TB cases, injected drug users, foreign-born individuals, and patients with HIV infection, renal failure, malignancy, or immunosuppression. The largest growing proportion of new TB cases is in the HIV-infected and immunosuppressed population. Persons with suspected TB must have their face covered with a surgical mask during transport and should be admitted to a private negative airflow room equipped with engineering controls specifically designed to reduce airborne exposure. Precautions must be implemented promptly for any suspected case and should not be delayed to wait for confirmation by acid-fast bacillus (AFB) culture results, which may take weeks. Staff entering the patient's room must wear special particulate filter respirators (fit testing required) or equivalent respirator systems. Use of appropriate respiratory equipment for protection of HCWs is mandated by the Occupational Safety and Health Administration (OSHA) and the National Institute of Occupational Safety and Health (NIOSH).

**ANSWER:** E

32. The patient described in Question 31 is scheduled for bronchoscopy. Which of the following statements is correct?

A. The endoscopy staff should wear a powered air-purifying respirator (PAPR) during bronchoscopy.

B. The endoscopy staff should take prophylactic INH for 3 days after the procedure.

C. Bronchoscopy should be performed with the patient under general anesthesia and the use of endotracheal intubation.

D. Bronchoscopy should be deferred if the patient's tuberculin skin test result is positive.

E. Bronchoscopy is contraindicated until the result of the PPD test is available.

*Ref.:* 1

**COMMENTS:** Health care providers are at increased risk for exposure to **tuberculosis** during cough-inducing or aerosolizing procedures, such as bronchoscopy, endotracheal intubation, or suctioning. Respiratory protection requires use of a particulate filter respirator or a PAPR. The latter device provides filtered air to a hood that is worn. Use of a PAPR may be recommended when prolonged exposure is possible, such as during bronchoscopy. The risk for infection depends on the concentration of droplet nuclei and the duration of exposure. The diagnosis of pulmonary TB is made presumptively on the basis of the tuberculin skin test and chest radiograph results and confirmed by AFB smear and culture results. Bronchoscopy is indicated for the diagnosis of patients with undiagnosed pulmonary infection and for the exclusion of cancer, regardless of the skin test results.

**ANSWER:** A

33. A surgical resident performs endotracheal intubation of a patient. The patient is unknown to the resident, and the resident had not worn a mask during intubation. Subsequently, the resident is informed that the patient has active TB. The resident has had previous negative PPD tests. The appropriate measure for the resident is:

A. No intervention is necessary.

B. The resident should have a PPD test performed and prophylactic INH started regardless of the result.

C. The resident should have a PPD test performed and prophylactic INH started only if the result is positive and the resident does not have symptoms of active infection.

D. The resident should have a PPD test performed and INH started only if the result is positive and symptoms develop in the resident.

E. The resident does not need a PPD test but should have chest radiography performed.

*Ref.:* 7

**COMMENTS:** Exposure to ***M. tuberculosis*** is determined by skin testing. If there is any concern for exposure to active disease, especially in a high-risk situation such as intubation in which the resident is directly exposed to respiratory secretions, the patient should have a PPD test performed. If the PPD results are positive, the resident should begin treatment with INH. A chest radiograph should not be performed in place of the PPD test. If symptoms develop, a chest radiograph is warranted. Infection develop in less than 10% of exposed individuals. Skin testing is performed at least annually in HCWs. The majority of PPD-positive individuals have old exposures. When PPD test results are positive, however, a chest radiograph and sputum for AFB smear and culture are obtained. **Isoniazid prophylaxis** is indicated for persons younger than 35 years with positive skin test results and those older than 35 years with high-risk conditions (i.e., HIV infection, injected drug use, contact with a known TB source, from a medically underserved population, foreign born, or those with abnormal chest radiograph results). The duration of prophylaxis is 6 to 12 months. Active pulmonary TB is diagnosed by sputum AFB smear or culture analysis (or both). The standard treatment of active disease involves a multidrug regimen with INH, RIF, and other drugs (pyrazinamide, ethambutol, or streptomycin) for months. Surgical therapy (usually resection) is occasionally necessary for patients who fail medical therapy or for those in whom persistent problems develop, such as a residual lung cavity or destruction, bronchiectasis, or hemoptysis.

**ANSWER:** C

34. A 60-year-old woman with a history of multiple soft tissue abscesses has a recurrent abscess on her right thigh. This patient had a recent hospitalization for exacerbation of congestive heart failure, during which she was in the hospital for 5 days. Because of her history of previous MRSA abscesses, vancomycin therapy is started. On morning rounds all of the following precautions should be taken except:

A. Washing hands before examining the patient

B. Wearing gloves while examining the patient

C. Wearing a mask while examining the patient

D. Wearing a gown while examining the patient

E. Washing hands after examining the patient

*Ref.:* 1

**COMMENTS: Contact precautions** are indicated in this patient and include washing one's hands both before and after leaving the patient's room and donning both a gown and gloves while in the patient's room. Wearing a mask is not indicated for patients who are on contact precautions.

**ANSWER:** C

35. An 80-year-old woman who lives in a nursing home and who had just finished a 10-day course of antibiotics has abdominal pain and profuse diarrhea. Her stool is tested and comes back positive for *C. difficile*. What is the most appropriate initial management?

A. Oral vancomycin

B. Intravenous vancomycin

C. Metronidazole

D. Vancomycin enemas

E. Supportive treatment only

*Ref.:* 14

**COMMENTS:** The most appropriate initial treatment of *C. difficile colitis* is metronidazole. If the patient is not improving, it is appropriate to try *oral* vancomycin. In refractory severe cases it is also appropriate to use vancomycin enemas.

**ANSWER:** C

36. All of the following precautions are appropriate for the patient in Question 35 except:

A. The physician should wear both gloves and a gown when examining the patient.

B. If possible, there should be a disposable stethoscope dedicated to that patient in the room.

C. The patient should be placed in a private room.

D. All visitors should wear gloves, a gown, and a mask.

E. Hands should be washed before entering and after leaving the patient's room.

*Ref.:* 1, 14

**COMMENTS:** This patient is on contact precautions because of *C. difficile* **colitis** since it is spread by direct contact. Appropriate precautions include donning a gown and gloves and washing hands both before entering and after leaving the patient's room. There is no indication for anyone to wear a mask in this patient's room. In addition, the patient should be placed in a private room. It is also ideal to have a disposable stethoscope dedicated to that patient to avoid spreading *C. difficile*. If not available, the stethoscope must be cleaned after use.

## ANSWER: D

## REFERENCES

1. Centers for Disease Control and Prevention (CDC): Healthcare-associated infections (HAIs). Available at www.cdc.gov/hai.
2. Garner JS: Guidelines for isolation precautions in hospitals. The Hospital Infection Control Practices Advisory Committee, *Infect Control Hosp Epidemiol* 17:53–80, 1996.
3. Perl TM, Cullen JJ, Wenzel RP, et al: Intranasal mupirocin to prevent postoperative *Staphylococcus aureus* infections, *N Engl J Med* 346:1871–1877, 2002.
4. Salgado CD, Farr BM, Calfee DP: Community-acquired methicillin-resistant *Staphylococcus aureus*: a meta-analysis of prevalence and risk factors, *Clin Infect Dis* 36:131–139, 2003.
5. Centers for Disease Control and Prevention (CDC): Vancomycin-resistant *Staphylococcus aureus*—Pennsylvania, 2002, *MMWR Morb Mortal Wkly Rep* 51:902, 2002.
6. Boyce JM, Pittet D, et al: Guidelines for hand hygiene in healthcare settings: recommendations of the Healthcare Infection Control Practices Advisory Committee and the HICPAC/SHEA/APIC/IDSA Hand Task Force. Society for Healthcare Epidemiology of America Association for Professionals in Infection Control/Infectious Diseases Society of America, *MMWR Recomm Rep* 51(RR-16):1–45, 2002.
7. Centers for Disease Control and Prevention website: www.cdc.gov.
8. Dellinger EP: Surgical infections. In Mulholland MW, Lillemoe KD, Doherty GM, editors: *Greenfield's surgery: scientific principles and practice*, ed 4, Philadelphia, 2006, Lippincott Williams & Wilkins.
9. Bartlett JG: Occupational exposure to HIV and other blood-borne pathogens. In Cameron JL, editor: *Current surgical therapy*, ed 9, Philadelphia, 2008, CV Mosby.
10. Recommendations for prevention and control of hepatitis C (HCV) virus and HCV-related chronic disease. Centers for Disease Control and Prevention, *MMWR Recomm Rep* 47(RR-19):1–39, 1998.
11. Dolin R, Masur H, Saag MS: *AIDS therapy*, ed 2, Philadelphia, 2003, Churchill Livingstone.
12. Mandell GL, Bennett JE, Dolin R: *Principles and practice of infectious diseases*, ed 5, Philadelphia, 2000, Churchill Livingstone.
13. U.S. Public Health Service: Updated U.S. Public Health Service guidelines for the management of occupational exposures to HBV, HCV, and HIV and recommendations for postexposure prophylaxis, *MMWR Recomm Rep* 50(RR-11):1–52, 2001.
14. Anaya DA, Dellinger EP: Surgical infections and choice antibiotics. In Townsend CM, Beauchamp RD, Evers BM, et al, editors: *Sabiston textbook of surgery: the biological basis of modern surgical practice*, ed 18, Philadelphia, 2008, WB Saunders.
15. Public Health Service guidelines for the management of health care worker exposures to HIV and recommendations for postexposure prophylaxis. Centers for Disease Control and Prevention, *MMWR Recomm Rep* 47(RR-7):1–33, 1998.
16. 1993 Revised classification system for HIV infection and expanded surveillance case definition for AIDS among adolescents and adults, *MMWR Recomm Rep* 41(RR-17):1–19, 1992.
17. HIV InSite website by the University of California San Francisco, Section of Surgery in Patients with HIV: http://hivinsite.ucsf.edu
18. Deziel DJ, Hyser MJ, Doolas A, et al: Major abdominal operations in acquired immunodeficiency syndrome, *Am Surg* 56:445–450, 1990.
19. Beck DE, Wexner SD: *Fundamentals of anorectal surgery*, New York, 1992, McGraw-Hill.
20. HIV InSite website by the University of California San Francisco, Section of Toxoplasmosis and HIV. Available at http://hivinsite.ucsf.edu
21. Tsoukas CM, Bernard NF, Abrahamowicz M, et al: Effect of splenectomy on slowing human immunodeficiency virus disease progression, *Arch Surg* 133:25–31, 1998.

# CHAPTER 6

# Transplantation and Immunology

*Elizabeth A. Hooper, M.D.; Edie Y. Chan, M.D.; and Edward F. Hollinger, M.D., Ph.D.*

1. A 53-year-old African-American man with diabetic nephropathy receives a cadaveric renal transplant from a 30-year-old healthy donor. Which of the following statements is false.

A. The 1-year graft survival rate is 90%.

B. The patient's life expectancy following transplantation more than doubles in diabetic patients.

C. The primary cause of graft loss after 5 years is chronic rejection.

D. Treatment of chronic rejection has improved significantly over the past 10 years.

E. Treatment of renal failure with transplantation becomes cost-effective at the end of the second transplant year.

*Ref.:* 1-3

**COMMENTS:** The graft survival rate is 89% for all deceased donor transplants. Grafts from extended-criteria donors have a decreased 1-year survival rate of 81%, whereas grafts from traditional-criteria donors have a 90% survival rate at 1 year. Recipients of living donor grafts have a 95% 1-year graft survival rate. For patients with diabetes, the average life expectancy is 8 years if no transplantation occurs. In contrast, patients receiving a transplant have an increase in average life expectancy of 19 years. **Graft loss as a result of acute rejection** has continued to follow a declining trend since the introduction of cyclosporine in the 1980s and tacrolimus in the 1990s. However, the incidence of graft loss because of **chronic rejection** has not changed significantly over the past 10 years. Despite improvements in immunosuppression and monitoring of opportunistic diseases, the 5-year survival rate after kidney transplantation is 70% for non–extended-criteria grafts, with most grafts being lost to chronic rejection. Transplantation becomes cost-effective when compared with dialysis at the end of the second year.

**ANSWER: D**

2. A 60-year-old woman has renal failure secondary to hypertension; she is undergoing hemodialysis and waiting for a cadaveric renal transplant. Which of the following statements regarding kidney transplantation is true?

A. Crossmatching is performed before kidney transplantation to prevent graft loss from chronic cellular rejection.

B. A positive crossmatch is an absolute contraindication to cadaveric renal transplantation.

C. Hyperacute rejection is responsive to additional immunotherapy.

D. Routine screening of potential recipients with the panel-reactive antibody (PRA) test can predict the presence of donor-specific antibodies.

E. ABO incompatibility is an absolute contraindication to kidney transplantation.

*Ref.:* 4, 5

**COMMENTS: Hyperacute rejection** of a transplanted kidney generally occurs within minutes of reperfusion and is due to the presence of preformed immunoglobulin G (IgG) antibodies in the recipient's serum. These antibodies attach to major histocompatibility antigens (HLA-A, HLA-B, and HLA-DR) on the donor vascular endothelium. The test for donor-specific antibodies is called a **crossmatch** and is performed on all potential donors just before transplantation.

A positive crossmatch result is a relative contraindication to cadaveric renal transplantation. With cadaveric kidneys, there is insufficient time for preoperative plasmapheresis and intravenous immunoglobulin until a negative crossmatch is obtained. This increases the risk of immunologic graft loss. Patients undergoing living related renal transplantation with a positive crossmatch result can be treated to remove the antibody (through plasmapheresis, the administration of gamma globulin, or both) and agents such as Rituxamab (anti-CD-20) can be used to decrease antibody production. If a subsequent crossmatch result is negative following treatment, living related or unrelated renal transplantation can be performed with an acceptable success rate. Potential recipients of ABO-compatible renal allografts develop donor-specific HLA antibodies of the IgG class from antigen exposure because of transfusions, pregnancy, or previous transplants. The presence of donor-specific antibodies can be predicted by periodically testing the reactivity of the recipient's serum to a panel of common A, B, and DR antigens and expressing the result as a percentage. This test is referred to as the **panel-reactive antibody**. The higher the PRA result at the time of transplantation, the more likely a patient is to have an episode of antibody mediated rejection. Previous recipients of ABO-incompatible allografts have had a high incidence of hyperacute rejection from preformed isoagglutinins, also of the IgG type, which attach to A and B antigens expressed by the vascular endothelium. However, success in Japan with **ABO-incompatible donors** and an increasing shortage of donors have resulted in recent evaluation of the use of ABO-incompatible renal allografts. The combination of modern immunosuppression and the use of plasmapheresis to remove isoagglutinins has resulted in acceptable graft survival rates. Recent studies have shown success with type A2 kidneys transplanted into type O recipients.

**ANSWER: D**

**3.** A 43-year-old woman undergoing dialysis for end-stage renal disease secondary to hypertension is placed on the transplantation waiting list. Allocation of cadaveric renal allografts is not dependent on which of the following?

A. Number of prior kidney transplants

B. HLA compatibility

C. Previous living kidney donor status

D. PRA test results

E. Time spent on the waiting list

*Ref.:* 4

**COMMENTS:** Allocation of cadaveric renal allografts is dependent on the length of time that the recipient has been maintained on hemodialysis, HLA compatibility, PRA results, and any previous history of kidney donation by the waiting recipient. Age is not a factor. HLA antigens are inherited on chromosome 6, and although multiple HLA antigens have been identified, kidney recipients and donors undergo tissue typing for only three antigens: HLA-A, HLA-B, and HLA-DR. Since these antigens are inherited from each parent, usually as a codominant allele, offspring have two HLA-A antigens, two HLA-B antigens, and two HLA-DR antigens. Siblings have a 25% chance of being HLA identical, a 50% chance of sharing one haplotype, and a 25% chance of being HLA dissimilar. **HLA matching** for all six antigens has resulted in improved long-term outcome in patients undergoing both living related and cadaveric renal transplantation. As a result, cadaveric organs that match for all six antigens are **allocated nationwide**. If no six-antigen matches can be found for a cadaveric renal allograft, the organ is placed locally, with points given for the number of HLA matches, PRA results, and time spent on the waiting list.

**ANSWER:** A

**4.** Which of the following best describes the preservation process for kidneys procured for transplantation?

A. Continuous pulsatile perfusion with solutions that mimic intracellular electrolytes has proved to be superior to simple cold storage.

B. Continuous pulsatile perfusion uses lactated Ringer solution for preservation.

C. Simple cold storage allows longer preservation time because of its simplicity.

D. University of Wisconsin (UW) solution contains lactobionate, which suppresses hypothermia-induced cell swelling.

E. Simple cold storage is equivalent to continuous pulsatile perfusion when storage times are longer than 24 hours.

*Ref.:* 1

**COMMENTS:** In 1987, **University of Wisconsin solution** was introduced at the University of Wisconsin by Belzer and Southard. This solution contains **lactobionate**, an osmotic agent that serves to inhibit calcium-dependent enzymes. This reduces hypothermia-related changes, including swelling of cells. **Pulsatile perfusion** is expensive and has been shown only to reduce delayed graft function. There is no difference in graft survival rates when comparing simple storage with pulsatile perfusion. For kidneys undergoing pulsatile perfusion, cryoprecipitated homologous plasma or other preservation solution is used, not crystalloid such as lactated Ringer solution.

**ANSWER:** D

**5.** A 30-year-old woman with lupus receives a kidney transplant. Two hours later she is anuric. Vital statistics about the kidney include a cold ischemia time of 10 hours, a 60-year-old donor, a negative crossmatch, and PRA of 80%. Select the best next step of management:

A. Immediate angiogram to rule out arterial occlusion

B. Immediate sonographic studies to verify vessel patency

C. Immediate reexploration

D. Immediate administration of high-dose steroids to treat rejection

E. Magnetic resonance angiography to determine vessel patency

*Ref.:* 6

**COMMENTS:** The most common cause of delayed graft function following kidney transplantation is **acute tubular necrosis** (ATN). However, ATN is usually characterized by urine production in the range of 10 to 30 mL/h, which generally declines to 0 to 5 mL/h over the first 24 hours. Although surgical complications such as vascular thrombosis and ureteral obstruction are rare, they must be excluded in patients who have anuria immediately after kidney transplantation. The initial test of choice is a **Doppler ultrasound** to verify vessel patency, exclude the presence of a fluid collection secondary to a hematoma or a urinoma that may be impinging on the graft, and rule out arterial or venous obstruction from kinking of one or both vessels. If no flow is seen in either the renal artery or vein, reexploration is indicated. Ultrasound is a quick, reliable, and noninvasive test to evaluate vessels and detect hydronephrosis and fluid collections; it should be performed before returning to the operating room.

**ANSWER:** B

**6.** A 30-year-old type 1 brittle diabetic patient with diabetic nephropathy receives a simultaneous pancreas and kidney (SPK) transplant. Which of the following statements is true?

A. Elevation of plasma glucose levels in the early postoperative period is indicative of pancreas rejection.

B. Bladder drainage is preferred because it is associated with fewer complications.

C. Most surgeons prefer enteric drainage because the incidence of complications attributed to bladder drainage, such as acidosis and urinary tract infections, is decreased.

D. Most surgeons prefer bladder drainage because the incidence of infections is reduced by avoiding contamination with enteric contents.

E. The preferred enteric drainage of the pancreatic allograft is the cecum.

*Ref.:* 7

**COMMENTS:** The first sign of **renal rejection** in an SPK transplant recipient may be elevated serum creatinine levels. Elevation of glucose in the immediate postoperative period can be a sign of vascular compromise. In long-term patients, elevated glucose is a late sign of rejection. Enteric drained pancreas transplants have a lower leak rate than those drained to the bladder, however a leak in an enteric anastomosis is more likely to result in graft loss. Long-term complications of bladder drainage include acidosis, infection, and cystitis from the loss of bicarbonate into the bladder. Bladder drainage is commonly converted to enteric drainage because of acidosis and recurrent urinary tract infections. **Enteric drainage** of the pancreas does not have a higher infection rate than bladder drainage. The preferred enteric drainage site is the small bowel.

**ANSWER:** C

7. Which of the following would exclude a patient from whole-organ pancreatic transplantation?

   A. History of hypoglycemic unawareness without end-organ damage

   B. History of coronary artery bypass grafting

   C. History of diabetic neuropathy

   D. History of lower extremity peripheral vascular disease

   E. None of the above

   *Ref.:* 1

**COMMENTS:** When considering pancreas transplantation, the benefits must be weighed against the risks of surgery and lifelong immunosuppression. **Brittle diabetic patients** are candidates for pancreatic transplantation regardless of the presence of end-organ damage. Pancreas transplantation may be lifesaving in patients with severe hypoglycemic unawareness. In patients with good glycemic control and no evidence of end-organ damage, the risks associated with lifelong immunosuppression may outweigh the benefits of insulin independence. There is good evidence that optimal glycemic control decreases the progression of microvascular complications of diabetes. This is significant for patients with diabetic nephropathy, neuropathy, and retinopathy. Vascular disease of the coronary arteries and peripheral vasculature is also common in diabetics and is a significant factor in the preoperative evaluation process. The **cardiac** status of a potential recipient must be fully evaluated. In those with significant coronary disease, cardiac revascularization may be required before transplantation. **Peripheral vascular disease** does not exclude a patient from transplantation but may change the operative planning regarding placement of.

**ANSWER:** E

8. In a uremic diabetic patient who undergoes SPK transplantation, which of the following statements regarding the secondary complications of diabetes and pancreatic transplantation is false?

   A. Diabetic retinopathy generally improves after pancreatic transplantation.

   B. Recurrence of diabetic nephropathy in renal allografts can be avoided.

   C. Diabetic neuropathy can improve after pancreatic transplantation.

   D. Patients with advanced diabetic neuropathy have an improved survival rate after pancreatic transplantation.

   E. Diabetic gastropathy may stabilize.

   *Ref.:* 7

**COMMENTS: Retinopathy** has not been shown to reverse with successful transplantation, but by 3 years after transplantation, there is often no further progression. In control groups including those with failed pancreatic transplantation, retinopathy usually progresses. With normoglycemia, **nephropathy** may not only be

halted but also actually reversed. Comparisons of diabetics who have undergone kidney transplantation alone versus pancreas recipients have shown remodeling of the basement membrane in normoglycemic patients. This reversal is seen in patients with normoglycemia for at least 5 years. Patients with **neuropathy** have improvement in both motor and sensory indices following successful pancreatic transplantation. The combination of diabetes and severe neuropathy leads to a lower survival rate. Improvement in long-term glucose control results in improved neural function and subsequent improved survival rates. Like other neuropathies, **diabetic gastropathy** stabilizes.

**ANSWER:** A

9. Regarding liver transplantation for patients chronically infected with hepatitis C virus (HCV), which of the following statements is true?

   A. Posttransplant reinfection with HCV occurs in only 50% of patients.

   B. Combination interferon and ribavirin therapy is effective in treating recurrent hepatitis C.

   C. Posttransplant reinfection with HCV causes cirrhosis in approximately 80% of patients at 5 years after liver transplantation.

   D. The clinical course of hepatitis C after reinfection is less virulent than that of the original infection.

   E. Allograft failure secondary to recurrence of HCV infection is the most common cause of death and retransplantation in recipients with HCV infection.

   *Ref.:* 8-10

**COMMENTS:** The most common indication for liver transplantation worldwide is HCV infection. Most patients with chronic **hepatitis C virus infection** who develop cirrhosis have had the infection for more than 20 years. Patients chronically infected with HCV who undergo liver transplantation uniformly become reinfected within a matter of days. No therapy is effective in preventing reinfection. Cirrhosis develops much earlier in the transplanted allograft, with approximately 5% to 20% of patients exhibiting cirrhosis on biopsy at 5 years following transplantation. **Combination therapy** with interferon and ribavirin eradicates the recurrent infection in a small percentage of patients (approximately 25% to 36%) after transplantation. The most common cause of death and retransplantation in recipients with HCV infection is recurrence of hepatitis C.

**ANSWER:** E

10. Mr. Smith is a 58-year-old gentleman with hepatitis B–associated cirrhosis. Regarding liver transplantation in patients chronically infected with hepatitis B virus (HBV), which of the following statements is true?

    A. The frequency of de novo infection in patients with grafts from donors who are hepatitis B core antibody positive is 5%.

    B. The presence of HBV DNA or hepatitis Be antigen (HBeAg) in the serum of recipients before transplantation increases the risk for posttransplant recurrence.

    C. The frequency of recurrence is higher in patients with fulminant HBV infection.

D. The risk for posttransplant HBV infection is 50% in patients who have detectable surface antigen.

E. The risk for transmission through blood products is 1 in 500,000.

*Ref.:* 11

COMMENTS: Before availability of the reverse transcriptase inhibitors lamivudine and adefovir, liver transplantation in patients chronically infected with HBV had an unacceptably high rate of recurrence. However, patients now undergoing transplantation for liver failure secondary to **hepatitis B virus infection** have excellent outcomes, with a negligible rate of recurrence of the native infection. Patients who test positive for e antigen or for HBV DNA have an increased risk for recurrent infection. Patients with fulminant hepatic failure secondary to HBV infection have the lowest risk for the development of recurrent infection. The frequency of de novo infection in patients who receive a hepatitis B core antibody–positive liver is approximately 50%. The risk for transmission of HBV from blood products is 1 in 200,000 per unit of screened packed red blood cells.

ANSWER:  B

11. A 58-year-old man undergoes orthotopic liver transplantation (OLT) for cirrhosis secondary to HCV infection. At the time of transplantation he receives induction immunosuppression therapy. All of the following may be used as induction agents except:

A. Alemtuzumab (Campath)

B. Sirolimus (Rapamune)

C. Basiliximab (Simulect)

D. Rabbit antithymocyte globulin (Thymoglobulin)

E. Steroids

*Ref.:* 12

COMMENTS: **Rabbit antithymocyte globulin** is an antilymphocyte globulin commonly used for induction therapy. It has antibodies against CD2, CD3, CD4, CD8, CD11a, CD18, CD25, HLA-DR, and HLA class I. Clinical trials have shown it to be an effective drug for preventing acute rejection after transplantation. **Basiliximab** is a chimeric anti-CD25 monoclonal antibody that blocks IL-2 stimulation of T-cells by competitively binds to the interleukin-2 (IL-2) receptor without activating it. **Alemtuzumab** is a humanized monoclonal antibody against CD52 that is expressed on B cells, T cells, monocytes, and macrophages. Use of this drug leads to depletion of lymphocytes for approximately 2 to 6 months. Though rarely used alone, high-dose **steroids** may be used as an induction agent. **Rapamycin** is used only for maintenance immunosuppression.

ANSWER:  B

12. Which of the following is the most commonly used primary maintenance immunosuppressive agent?

A. Tacrolimus (Prograf)

B. Azathioprine (Imuran)

C. Mycophenolate (CellCept)

D. Rapamycin (Sirolimus)

E. Prednisone

*Ref.:* 12, 13

COMMENTS: **Tacrolimus** was first isolated from *Streptomyces tsukubaensis*. It is approximately 100 times more potent than cyclosporine. A U.S. multicenter trial in 1994 randomized 478 liver transplant recipients to either tacrolimus- or cyclosporine-based immunosuppression. This trial demonstrated that tacrolimus was associated with significantly fewer episodes of acute steroid-resistant or refractory rejection. Mycophenolate mofetil, azathioprine, and sirolimus are not as potent as tacrolimus and are rarely used alone. **Prednisone** administered as monotherapy is not the standard of care. Steroids are used for their unique immunosuppressive qualities, such as reduction in the synthesis of IL-2 and interferon-$\gamma$ (INF-$\gamma$). They also inhibit the secretion of IL-1 from macrophages.

ANSWER:  A

13. After OLT 2 years earlier for autoimmune hepatitis, a 30-year-old woman is seen in the clinic for routine follow-up and complains of diarrhea. Which of the following statements is true regarding the toxicity of immunosuppressive agents?

A. The calcineurin inhibitors cyclosporine, tacrolimus, and rapamycin are nephrotoxic.

B. Mycophenolate and rapamycin are toxic to the gastrointestinal system.

C. Tacrolimus has been associated with an increased incidence of posttransplant diabetes.

D. Cyclosporine and tacrolimus can cause hirsutism and gingival hyperplasia.

E. Cyclosporine and tacrolimus can cause thrombocytopenia.

*Ref.:* 12-14

COMMENTS: All immunosuppressive agents have toxicities, but they can be minimized by using various combinations of the agents at lower dosages. Both **tacrolimus** and **cyclosporine** cause renal vasoconstriction, which leads to nephrotoxicity by reducing renal blood flow. **Rapamycin** is not nephrotoxic, but causes thrombocytopenia and hypercholesterolemia. After binding with the receptor, cyclosporine and tacrolimus each bind to calcineurin and form a larger complex. **Calcineurin** is a calcium-dependent protein that plays a crucial role in activation of transcription of the IL-2 gene. This signaling takes place in T cells. Inhibition prevents further phosphorylation and stops the second messenger cycle, thereby halting propagation of the immune response. **Mycophenolate** inhibits purine synthesis, which is essential for the proliferative responses of T and B cells to mitogens. However, it can also cause gastrointestinal side effects, such as diarrhea, flatulence, and bloating. Mycophenolate is the only immunosuppressive agent that frequently causes toxicity in the gastrointestinal system. **Tacrolimus** has been associated with an increase in posttransplant diabetes. Only cyclosporine is also associated with hirsutism, gingival hyperplasia, and thrombocytopenia.

ANSWER:  C

14. A 35-year-old man with a body mass index of 22 underwent kidney transplantation 6 weeks earlier for focal segmental

glomerular sclerosis. He has a sense of fullness in his pelvis and increased urinary frequency. On physical examination the ipsilateral lower extremity is painless but noticeably swollen. Ultrasound of the lower extremities is negative for deep venous thrombosis. An ultrasound of the transplanted kidney shows normal flow and a heterogenous a fluid collection adjacent to the bladder. A diagnosis of lymphocele is made. Treatment of a lymphocele after kidney transplantation may include all except which of the following?

A. Percutaneous drainage regardless of symptoms

B. Percutaneous drainage with sclerosis

C. Prolonged external percutaneous drainage

D. Observation if asymptomatic

E. Laparoscopic internal marsupialization

*Ref.:* 6

**COMMENTS: Lymphoceles** develop after kidney transplantation in up to 50% of recipients, usually as a result of inadequate ligation of the iliac lymphatics. They do not require intervention if asymptomatic. However, if they compress the kidney or obstruct the ureter intervention is necessary. Initial treatment usually involves percutaneous drainage. If the lymphocele recurs, most surgeons would place an external drain percutaneously under ultrasound or computed tomographic (CT) guidance. **Percutaneous drainage with sclerosing agents** such as povidone-iodine can be used, but such treatment can have a directly toxic effect on the transplanted kidney limiting there. If the lymphocele reaccumulates and becomes symptomatic after removal of the external drain, **internal drainage** by marsupialization is indicated. The marsupialization involves fenestrating the peritoneum to drain the lymphocele into the peritoneal cavity. This can be done as an open procedure or laparoscopically with ultrasound guidance.

**ANSWER:** A

15. Liver transplantation may be contraindicated for which of the following?

A. Cirrhosis from prior alcohol use

B. Stage II hepatocellular carcinoma (HCC) with cirrhosis

C. A 30-year-old patient with liver failure and uncorrected pulmonary hypertension

D. A 30-year-old patient with liver failure and hepatopulmonary syndrome

E. A 30-year-old patient with liver failure and portal vein thrombosis

*Ref.:* 15-18

**COMMENTS:** Patients with **alcoholic liver disease** who are abstinent for more than 6 months and have good psychosocial support are considered good candidates for liver transplantation because of the low risk for alcohol recidivism. As a group their long-term survival rate may be one of the highest because they are often not subject to viral hepatitis and other progressive diseases that may recur in the transplanted liver. Alcohol use is frequently encountered in patients who are evaluated for other diseases, and they too should be abstinent for a certain defined period. Patients awaiting liver transplantation are currently classified by the Model for End-Stage Liver Disease (MELD) system. The MELD system is based on points (0 to 40) calculated from a logarithmic formula that uses a patient's bilirubin and creatinine levels and the prothrombin time. Patients also receive additional points for HCC and hepatopulmonary syndrome.

Hypoxemia from **severe pulmonary hypertension** is an absolute contraindication to transplantation. Pulmonary hypertension is defined as a mean pulmonary artery pressure greater than 25 mmHg with normal pulmonary capillary wedge pressure. The overall right heart dysfunction in these patients will not withstand reperfusion. The overall prevalence of pulmonary hypertension in the general population is 0.13%, although in patients with portal hypertension it is significantly higher, 0.73%. For patients with liver failure, pulmonary hypertension can be classified as mild (mean pulmonary pressure of 25 to 35), moderate (mean pulmonary pressure of 35 to 45), or severe (mean pulmonary pressure >45). Pulmonary artery pressure higher than 50 mm Hg despite therapy correlates with a nearly 100% mortality rate. Patients with untreated severe pulmonary hypertension who undergo liver transplantation are at very high risk for cardiac death from right ventricular failure immediately following reperfusion. Fortunately, for moderate and severe pulmonary hypertension, treatment with epoprostenol or prostacyclin by constant infusion can reduce pulmonary pressure to a range at which liver transplantation can be successful. Liver transplantation may be contraindicated in patients with **severe pulmonary hypertension** unresponsive to prostacyclin. For patients who do respond, prostacyclin can be gradually weaned after transplantation and pulmonary pressure will remain normal.

**Hepatopulmonary syndrome** is essentially the opposite of pulmonary hypertension. Pulmonary capillaries serving unoxygenated areas of the lung respond to the liver disease by dialating, which causes a significant reduction in pulmonary systolic pressure and increases the shunt fraction to as high as 10% to 20% (normal shunt fraction is 7%). As a result, patients require increasing amounts of supplemental oxygen. However, transplantation is curative, and the shunt fraction is reduced to normal often within a few days, although complete resolution may take up to 15 months. **Portal venous thrombosis** can be corrected by thrombectomy at the time of transplantation or by superior mesenteric vein grafting.

**ANSWER:** C

16. A 62-year-old woman comes to the emergency department because of nausea and vomiting. She underwent OLT for alcoholic cirrhosis 5 weeks earlier. Her white blood cell count is 1.0 cell/mL. Which of the following is the most likely cause of her clinical symptoms.

A. Wound infection

B. Cytomegalovirus (CMV)

C. Pneumonia

D. Bowel obstruction

E. Rejection

*Ref.:* 19

**COMMENTS: Cytomegalovirus** has the highest incidence of infection in seronegative recipients who receive seropositive organs. Early CMV disease occurs most commonly between 3 and 8 weeks after transplantation. Late disease can also occur. Treatments for rejection such as antilymphocytic or antithymocyte globulin increase the incidence of CMV infection. The most common symptoms of CMV are malaise, anorexia, myalgia, and arthralgia. Laboratory abnormalities include thrombocytopenia, neutropenia, and elevated liver enzymes. CMV infection can have clinical manifestations that include gastrointestinal tract inflammation, hepatitis, and in severe cases, pneumonia. The mainstay of therapy is **ganciclovir**.

**ANSWER:** B

17. Which of the following statements regarding CMV infection is true?

   A. Infection with CMV following kidney transplantation is the strongest predictor of poor long-term survival.

   B. The incidence of symptomatic CMV infection is declining secondary to the use of screening tests.

   C. Patients at highest risk for the development of CMV infection are those who test seropositive for CMV IgG.

   D. CMV infection is more likely than infection with polyomavirus (BK) virus to cause chronic allograft nephropathy.

   E. CMV infection can be indistinguishable from acute Epstein-Barr virus (EBV) infection.

*Ref.: 20*

**COMMENTS:** With development of the effective antiviral agent ganciclovir, acute rejection, not CMV infection, is now the strongest predictor of poor allograft survival. The incidence of **CMV** infection is declining, probably because of very effective tests for viral load in the serum, such as CMV pp65 antigen and CMV DNA testing and early prophylaxis. Patients who are at the highest risk for CMV are those who test seronegative for CMV IgG and receive an allograft from a donor seropositive for CMV IgG. CMV infection is usually an acute, systemic infection that can result in gastritis, hepatitis, pneumonitis, retinitis, and bone marrow suppression. CMV infection rarely involves only one *organ* and seldom causes chronic nephropathy. Infection with **polyomavirus** is usually isolated to the kidney and the urinary system. BK infection can cause nephropathy in the transplanted kidney. Active infection is associated with progressive loss of graft function, a condition also known as polyomavirus-associated nephropathy. Acute infection with **Epstein-Barr virus** generally causes inflammation of the gastrointestinal tract in the form of gastritis, enteritis, or colitis and is thus clinically similar to CMV infection. The two can easily be distinguished by checking serum viral loads with quantitative CMV DNA and EBV DNA testing. In addition, biopsy specimens from inflamed gastrointestinal mucosa can be specifically stained for each virus.

**ANSWER:** B

18. A 40-year-old man is seen in the office with an enlarged groin lymph node. He underwent kidney transplantation 3 years ago. An excisional biopsy specimen is consistent with posttransplant lymphoproliferative disorder (PTLD). Which of the following statements is true?

   A. The use of antilymphocyte globulin is a risk factor for PTLD.

   B. The incidence of PTLD is elevated in patients with pretransplant seronegative EBV titers.

   C. PTLD is more common in recipients who seroconvert their CMV status.

   D. PTLD develops more commonly in children than in adults.

   E. All of the above.

*Ref.: 20, 21*

**COMMENTS: Posttransplant lymphoproliferative disorder** represents a spectrum of diseases related to **Epstein-Barr virus** infection, including infectious mononucleosis, benign proliferation of B cells, and lymphoma. In a transplant recipient, clones of EBV-transformed B cells are generated as a result of infection with EBV from the donor or personal contact. Because of impaired immunity, transplant recipients are unable to control the clonal expansion of EBV-infected B cells, and may develop hyperplasia (an EBV-induced tumor) or neoplasia (lymphoma). Risk factors for the development of PTLD include the use of antilymphocytic globulin or polyclonal antibodies as induction agents. The risk for PTLD can be increased up to 75 times the standard risk in a previously seronegative EBV patient in whom a primary EBV infection develops after transplantation. Asymptomatic transplant recipients at risk or symptomatic recipients are surveyed for EBV infection by quantitative polymerase chain reaction analysis of peripheral blood. CMV infection in a negative recipient with a positive donor serum titer (CMV IgG) and CMV infection in a CMV-mismatched patient (donor positive for CMV IgG and recipient negative for CMV IgG) can also increase the risk for PTLD. The disease is more common in children than in adults. Patients with elevated serum levels of EBV are usually treated by decreasing the dosage of immunosuppressive agents and administering either acyclovir or ganciclovir. Patients with hyperplastic tumors are generally treated by terminating the administration of immunosuppressive agents and initiating treatment with acyclovir or ganciclovir. Patients with unresponsive hyperplastic tumors can be treated with the anti–B-cell (anti-CD20) antibody rituximab (Rituxan). CHOP (cyclophosphamide, hydroxydaunorubicin, Oncovin [vincristine], and prednisone) therapy is usually reserved for patients with lymphoma.

**ANSWER:** E

19. Which of the following does not predict a patient's long-term survival rate following liver transplantation?

   A. Pretransplant MELD score

   B. Age of the recipient

   C. Prolonged warm ischemia time

   D. Use of antilymphocytic globulin

   E. Pretransplant intensive care unit admission

*Ref.: 13, 22*

**COMMENTS:** The **Model for End-Stage Liver Disease** score can predict pretransplant mortality, but it does not predict posttransplant survival. MELD scores are derived from the continuous disease severity scale designed for patients after transjugular intrahepatic portosystemic shunting. **Pretransplant functionality** of the patient can relate to posttransplant outcomes. The survival rate for patients immediately after liver transplantation is related to the severity of the illness before transplantation. Statistics show that patients who are well enough to reside at home with liver disease at the time of transplantation have a 91.4% 1-year survival rate. In contrast, patients who had been hospitalized have an 84.5% survival rate. Those in an **intensive care unit** before transplantation have a 79.9% survival rate, and those on life support have a 69.7%

survival rate. Increasing **recipient age** correlates with decreased long-term survival. The deleterious effects of increased warm ischemia time have been well established by analysis of the United Network for Organ Sharing (UNOS) database. In retrospective reviews, **Rabbit antithymocyte globulin** has been associated with decreased rates of acute rejection. It also may be given to limit the use of nephrotoxic agents (tacrolimus, cyclosporine) in patients with renal dysfunction after transplantation.

**ANSWER:** A

20. A 4-year-old child with hepatoblastoma requires a liver transplant. Which of the following would constitute an appropriate liver graft?

A. Graft from a donor of similar size and habitus

B. Split liver graft from an adult cadaveric donor and transplantation of the appropriate segment

C. Left lobe or left lateral segment of a liver from an living adult donor

D. All of the above

E. None of the above

*Ref.:* 23-25

**COMMENTS:** Over the past 10 years there has been a substantial expansion in the availability of donor grafts for pediatric liver transplantation. Previously, many children died while waiting for an appropriately sized donor to become available. Now, with the application of **segmental liver resection** techniques, full-size cadaveric liver grafts can be reduced to the appropriate volume for pediatric recipients. In addition, resection of the left lobe or the left lateral segment from a living adult donor can be performed, with comparable survival of the recipient and minimal risk to the donor.

**ANSWER:** D

21. Six months after renal transplantation, a 56-year-old woman is admitted to the hospital with high fever, an elevated serum creatinine level, disseminated varicella skin lesions, and bilateral pulmonary infiltrates. Which of the following statements is true?

A. The treatment of choice is intravenous acyclovir with or without hyperimmunoglobulin.

B. Bronchoscopic examination is unnecessary.

C. The patient does not need to be placed in isolation.

D. The immunosuppressive drug regimen should maintained to decrease the risk of rejection.

E. The peak incidence of this disease is 3 years after transplantation.

*Ref.:* 26, 19

**COMMENTS:** The incidence of **herpes zoster** (**shingles**) is 7.9% in renal transplant recipients, and it usually occurs during the first 9 months after transplantation. Intravenous, followed by oral acyclovir usually prevents systemic dissemination and leads to rapid healing of the skin lesions. The levels of immunosuppressive agents should be drastically reduced to prevent death. **Respiratory isolation** is necessary to prevent spread of infection to other patients. **Bronchoscopic examination** is advisable to rule out superinfection with bacterial, fungal, or other opportunistic organisms. **Intravenous acyclovir** with or without

hyperimmunoglobulin (varicella-zoster immune globulin) is the therapy of choice. The peak incidence of herpes zoster occurs within the first posttransplant year as a result of high levels of immunosuppression.

**ANSWER:** A

22. With respect to de novo post–renal transplant diabetes mellitus, which of the following statements is false?

A. It is more common in African-American recipients.

B. Most patients do not require long-term insulin therapy.

C. Risk factors include weight, age, and family history.

D. It has become less common since the introduction of tacrolimus.

E. Diabetes is more common with higher steroid doses.

*Ref.:* 27

**COMMENTS:** New-onset diabetes after transplantation (NODAT) occurs at rates of 9.1%, 16%, and 24% at 12, 24, and 36 months after transplantation, respectively. Steroids, cyclosporine, and tacrolimus are diabetogenic. There is a direct relationship between steroid dosage and the incidence of NODAT. **Tacrolimus**-based immunosuppressive therapy was associated with a 15% incidence of NODAT. Rates are dose dependent and fall with decreased levels of tacrolimus. **Cyclosporine**-based immunosuppressive therapy resulted in only a 9% incidence of NODAT. Risk factors include age, obesity, family history of diabetes, and African-American race. The potential mechanisms include decreased insulin secretion, increased insulin resistance, and a toxic effect of tacrolimus and cyclosporine on pancreatic beta cells. In only 25% of patients with NODAT does persistent hyperglycemia develop, and 50% of patients in this group ultimately require insulin replacement therapy.

**ANSWER:** D

23. A 55-year-old is being evaluated for renal transplantation. His creatinine clearance is less than 10 mL/min. His past medical history is significant for hepatitis C following intravenous drug use 20 years ago. With respect to hepatitis and renal transplantation, which of the following statements is true?

A. Hepatitis C is an absolute contraindication to organ donation.

B. All hepatitis B surface antigen–positive patients are poor renal transplant candidates.

C. The presence of HCV antibody is an independent risk factor for graft failure after transplantation.

D. HCV-positive recipients have a poor prognosis.

E. HCV-positive individuals should never be used as a donor.

*Ref.:* 26

**COMMENTS:** Patients with **preexisting hepatitis C** who have a low viral load, normal liver function, and minimal chronic active hepatitis on liver biopsy are acceptable recipients for a renal transplant. Donors with a similar profile may be acceptable for such a patient but not for a recipient who does not have hepatitis C. Meta-analyses have shown hepatitis C has been shown to be an independent risk factor for death and graft failure after renal transplantation based on meta-analyses. Twenty-year survival rates are 88% for non-HCV patients versus 64% for HCV-positive recipients. **Hepatitis B** surface antigen–positive patients who have stable liver function and test negative for e antigen do fairly well after renal transplantation with low-dose immunosuppressive therapy. However, recipients who are HBV DNA positive and HBeAg positive have a much higher risk for mortality.

**ANSWER: C**

24. The incidence of primary nonfunction of a liver allograft following transplantation ranges from 2% to 10%. Immediately after the liver transplantation procedure, which of the following is not associated with this clinical syndrome?

A. Metabolic alkalosis

B. Hyperkalemia

C. Reduced mental status

D. Marked elevation in liver enzyme levels

E. Minimal bile output (if a T-tube biliary drainage catheter is in place)

*Ref.:* 28

**COMMENTS: Primary nonfunction** of a liver allograft is a poorly understood clinical syndrome associated with markedly abnormal function of the allograft (i.e., severe coagulopathy, acidosis, hyperkalemia, poor mental status, continued hyperdynamic cardiac function with high cardiac output, low systemic vascular resistance with liver failure, poor bile output, and usually renal failure). Recipients with normally functioning grafts have marked metabolic alkalosis secondary to metabolism of the citrate component of bicarbonate (from banked blood given during the transplant procedure) by the liver graft during the immediate posttransplant period. Within the first 24 hours after liver transplantation, patients with normally functioning grafts return to normal cardiac hemodynamics. The most specific pretransplant predictor of primary nonfunction is the amount of **macrosteatosis** (extracellular fat globules) in the liver allograft. Studies have shown that when greater than 30% of the cross-sectional area of a liver biopsy specimen exhibits macrosteatosis, the incidence of primary dysfunction may reach 13%. Other possible predictors of primary nonfunction include high levels of vasopressor support in the donor and cold ischemia time. Although a variety of strategies have been used in attempts to ameliorate this syndrome, the only treatment is prompt retransplantation.

**ANSWER: A**

25. Which of the following would exclude a patient with HCC from becoming a transplant candidate?

A. A single 1-cm lesion in the liver with microvascular invasion

B. Two lesions each less than 2 cm

C. A solitary 1-cm HCC lesion in the lung

D. A single 4.8-cm HCC lesion in segment VIII

E. Portal vein thrombus

*Ref.:* 15, 29

**COMMENTS: Orthotopic liver transplantation** is an excellent option for stage I and stage II HCC. It has an advantage over resection because of the multifactorial nature of **Hepatocellular carcinoma**. Approximately 80% to 90% of patients with HCC also have cirrhosis. OLT allows excision of the tumor and removal of the underlying disease, which should decrease the likelihood of recurrence. OLT can be considered for any stage I or stage II tumor. This limits OLT to patients without distant metastases, those with negative lymph nodes and either $T_1$ or $T_2$ disease. $T_1$ disease is a solitary tumor without vascular invasion (regardless of size). $T_2$ disease is a solitary tumor with vascular invasion or a combination of tumors all less than 5 cm in size. These groupings were developed on the basis of the way in which these tumors behave. Conventionally, OLT is an option for solitary tumors less than 5 cm in size or multiple tumors of up to three in number, all smaller than 3 cm. Distant metastasis is an absolute contraindication to transplantation. Portal vein thrombosis is a relative contraindication to transplantation.

**ANSWER: C**

26. A 32-year-old woman is seen in the emergency department with an acute onset of confusion. Her laboratory work reveals markedly elevated transaminase levels, hyperbilirubinemia, and coagulopathy. Which of the following is not a potential indication for transplantation in a patient with fulminant hepatic failure?

A. A history of progressive jaundice over the past month

B. Acute overdose of acetaminophen

C. Acute infection with hepatitis A virus

D. Prothrombin time greater than 100 seconds

E. CMV affecting multiple organs

*Ref.:* 30, 31

**COMMENTS: Fulminant hepatic failure** can be caused by a multitude of injuries to the liver, including but not limited to acetaminophen toxicity and infection with hepatitis A virus, HBV, EBV, parvovirus, CMV, varicella-zoster virus, and herpes simplex virus. Other causes include *Bacillus cereus* infection, other illicit drugs such as ecstasy, antiretroviral drugs, and pregnancy-related disorders (the syndrome of hemolysis, elevated liver enzymes, and low platelet count [HELLP] and acute fatty liver of pregnancy). Though not standardized, most centers follow the criteria established by the **King's College Hospital** in London. Patients with acetaminophen overdose have a persistent acidosis (pH <7.30) or prothrombin time longer than 100 seconds plus serum creatinine levels greater than 300 μmol/L (>3.4 mg/dL) and grade 3 or 4 encephalopathy. In non–acetaminophen-caused fulminant hepatic failure the criteria are a prothrombin time longer than 100 seconds irrespective of encephalopathy or any three of the following: cryptogenic hepatitis or other drug toxicity, age younger than 10 years or older than 40 years, jaundice, duration of encephalopathy of less than 7 days, prothrombin time longer than 50 seconds, or serum bilirubin level greater than 300 μmol/L (17.5 mg/dL). By definition, jaundice progressing over more than a 7-day period would exclude a diagnosis of fulminant hepatic failure even though the encephalopathy may be acute in onset.

**ANSWER: A**

27. A 26-year-old man is found to be brain-dead after a gunshot wound to the head. His family consents to organ donation. Which of the following is a contraindication to organ donation?

A. Positive hepatitis B core antibody

B. Active hepatitis C

C. History of basal cell carcinoma 5 years previously

D. Donor liver biopsy with 10% steatosis

E. Creutzfeldt-Jakob disease

*Ref.:* 32

**COMMENTS:** There are both absolute and relative contraindications to **organ donation**. **Absolute contraindications** include transmissible agents that may cause death or severe disease in the recipient. These include Creutzfeldt-Jakob disease and other prion diseases such as kuru. Other contraindications include human immunodeficiency virus (HIV), disseminated or invasive viral infections, mycobacterial infections, fungal infections, or systemic bacterial infections such as methicillin-resistant *Staphylococcus aureus* (MRSA). **Active malignancy** is an absolute contraindication to donation. Low-grade skin cancers such as basal cell carcinoma do not exclude a donor. Five-year disease-free survival in the donor from any cancer is considered cure by UNOS. However, the type and the biologic behavior of the tumor should be considered. Late recurrence is seen with breast and lung cancer, and therefore additional caution is warranted even beyond the 5-year disease-free interval. **Relative contraindications** include age of the donor, hepatic steatosis, damaged organs, infection, and viral infection. Age older than 60 years places a donated organ in the extended-criteria category. Steatosis greater than 60% has a unacceptably high risk for primary nonfunction and is contraindicated; however, livers with steatosis of less than 30% have not been shown to have higher rates of nonfunction or lower graft survival rates than non-fatty livers. Liver transplantation from hepatitis B core antibody–positive donors results in a 22% to 100% seroconversion rate in hepatitis B core antibody–negative recipients. HBV-positive livers can be transplanted with concurrent postoperative treatment with hepatitis B immune globulin (HBIG) and lamivudine. The ideal recipient for a hepatitis B core antibody–positive donor is a patient who already has hepatitis B and would undergo treatment after transplantation regardless of donor status. Donors with hepatitis C should donate to only hepatitis C–positive recipients. The disease is transmitted universally. Recipients with hepatitis C will reinfect the new liver even if it is hepatitis C negative. Studies have shown no difference between patient survival, graft survival, or severity of recurrent hepatitis C disease.

**ANSWER:** E

28. Which of the following statements regarding the immune response is true?

A. The primary immune response is more intense and rapid than the secondary immune response.

B. A cell-mediated immune response consists primarily of T lymphocytes.

C. T lymphocytes are the precursors of plasma cells, which produce antibodies.

D. The immune response has three phases, the first being the establishment of memory.

E. Immunoglobulins (IgG versus IgE versus IgM) are all identical except at the variable region.

*Ref.:* 12, 33

**COMMENTS:** The **immune response** is characterized by a series of reactions triggered by an immunogen. Immunogens include substances recognized as foreign, or "nonself" (e.g., virus, bacteria, and histoincompatible tissues), as well as substances that are "altered self" or "modified self" (e.g., most tumor antigens). All immune responses, whether primary or secondary, are characterized by three phases: (1) **cognitive phase** (recognition of nonself antigen), (2) **activation phase** (proliferation of immunocompetent cells or lymphocytes), and (3) **effector phase** (development of immunologic memory). The primary immune response is the result of the first (or primary) exposure to a specific antigen. The secondary response results from a second (or subsequent) exposure to the same antigen. It is more rapid and more intense than the primary response and is a result of the phenomenon of immunologic memory.

There are two basic types of immune response: cell-mediated immune response (cellular immunity), mediated primarily by T lymphocytes, and humoral immune response, mediated primarily by B lymphocytes. **B lymphocytes**, or **B cells**, differentiate into antibody-producing plasma cells after activation. They develop in the fetal liver and the bone marrow. B lymphocytes are precursors of plasma cells and can be identified by specific antigen-binding sites on their surface. Plasma cells ultimately produce the antibodies that are found in serum and that may be transferred passively in serum. **T lymphocytes**, or **T cells**, mature in the thymus from multipotential cells derived from the bone marrow. Plasma cells produce immunoglobulins. Within a subgroup of **immunoglobulins**, IgG versus another IgG, the variable portions consist of both the light and heavy chains. The number of chains is constant. IgG has two heavy chains and two light chains joined by disulfide bonds that create a dimeric structure, whereas the IgM structure is made of multiple chains that create a pentamer.

**ANSWER:** B

29. Which of the following statements regarding T cells is true?

A. T cells finish development in the thymus and then migrate to the bone marrow.

B. The various types of T cells can be identified by the binding of specific monoclonal antibodies to antigens on the cell surface.

C. Helper T cells can be activated to produce antibodies.

D. Cytotoxic T cells can destroy target cells by recognizing foreign antigens at the target cell nucleus.

E. Cell-mediated immunity can be transferred passively in serum.

*Ref.:* 12, 33

**COMMENTS:** T lymphocytes (T cells) mature in the thymus, whereas B lymphocytes mature in the fetal liver and the bone marrow. The thymus, liver, and bone marrow are referred to as the primary lymphoid organs. The **T lymphocytes** subsequently migrate to the secondary lymphoid organs: the spleen, lymph nodes, and dispersed lymphoid tissues found in the bronchus, urogenital tract, and gut (i.e., Peyer patches). The T lymphocytes cycle through the bloodstream from these points in search of nonself antigens. Lymphocytes that differentiate into T cells and B cells express various clusters of antigens on their membranes. All T cells express the cell surface antigen–specific receptor designated CD3, whereas B cells express the cell surface antigen–specific receptors CD19 and CD20. **CD3⁺ T cells** can be distinguished and subdivided further by the expression of additional differentiation antigens on the T-cell surface (T-cell receptors): cytotoxic T cells (CD3/CD8), suppressor T cells (CD3/CD8), helper/inducer T cells (CD3/CD4), and delayed-type hypersensitivity T cells (CD3/CD4).

**Cytotoxic T cells** are capable of destroying a target cell by recognizing a foreign or "modified-self" antigen and class I major histocompatibility complex (MHC) molecules on the target cell surface. **Helper T cells** consist of $T_H1$ and $T_H2$ cells. They appear to work together in a regulatory circuit with each having a negative effect on the other. $T_H1$ cells are proinflammatory and release IFN-γ. $T_H2$ cells release interleukins to promote B-cell differentiation and maturation. **Delayed-type hypersensitivity T cells** bring macrophages and other inflammatory cells to areas in which delayed-type hypersensitivity reactions occur through the production of various chemoattractant molecules known collectively as chemokines.

**ANSWER:** B

30. Which of the following statements regarding T-cell activation is true?

   A. Antigen recognition is not specific, which allows clonal expansion and differentiation.

   B. Antigen expression requires the T cell to be MHC compatible with the antigen-presenting cell.

   C. T cells produce IL-1 in response to antigen presentation.

   D. Plasma cells are responsible for the synthesis of IL-2.

   E. T cells recognize soluble antigen.

*Ref.:* 12, 33

**COMMENTS:** When antigen enters a lymph node or the spleen, it may first be phagocytized by a macrophage, which processes the antigen and expresses it on the cell surface for presentation to B and T cells. Macrophages that do this are called antigen-presenting cells. **Other antigen-presenting cells** include dendritic cells (a macrophage-like cell found in the skin, lymph nodes, and other tissues) and a subset of B lymphocytes. Recognition of the antigen is highly specific and accomplished only by T-lymphocyte clones that have a receptor specific to that antigen. When antigen is presented to the T cell, **macrophages** produce IL-1, T cells produce IL-2, and T cells increase the expression of IL-2 receptor on the surface. This activation by IL-2 causes T cells to proliferate. Helper T cells interact with B cells to stimulate their differentiation into plasma cells that produce antibodies. **Activated T cells**, not plasma cells, produce IL-2. T cells require interaction with the MHC, and they do not directly recognize unbound circulating antigen.

**ANSWER:** B

31. Which of the following statements regarding interleukins is true?

   A. All interleukins will only upregulate the immune system.

   B. IL-8 is a neutrophil chemotactic factor.

   C. Interleukins are produced only by leukocytes.

   D. IL-10 produces fever and inflammation.

   E. Prednisone upregulates the effect of IL-1.

*Ref.:* 12, 33, 34

**COMMENTS: Interleukins** are a group of cytokines that function in many various ways to upregulate and downregulate the immune system. IL-3 functions as a hematopoietic growth factor. IL-4, IL-6, and IL-10 are the interleukins that have

known inhibitory functions. **Interleukin-4** inhibits the secretion of cytokines by macrophages. IL-6 inhibits tumor necrosis factor (TNF). **Interleukin-10** inhibits monocyte/macrophage function and counteracts the inflammatory cytokines. IL-4, IL-6, and IL-10 also have other stimulatory functions. IL-8 attracts neutrophils to the site of inflammation by movement through the vascular endothelium. **Interleukin-1** is responsible for fever and inflammation and also leads to the proliferation of T and B cells. Interleukins are produced by a variety of cells, including macrophages and monocytes, T and B lymphocytes, mast cells, stromal cells of the thymus and bone marrow, fibroblasts, epithelial cells, and endothelial cells. Most of the interleukins stimulate a particular or just a few varieties of leukocytes. **Glucocorticoid administration** inhibits the synthesis of IL-1 (among others), thus downregulating the inflammatory and immune response.

**ANSWER:** B

32. Which of the following statements regarding the cytokine IL-1 is false?

   A. The major cells that produce IL-1 are monocytes and macrophages.

   B. IL-1 may induce fever.

   C. T-lymphocyte production of IL-2 is inhibited by IL-1.

   D. IL-1 may augment wound healing by increasing fibroblast proliferation and collagen synthesis.

   E. IL-1 binds to CD121.

*Ref.:* 33, 34

**COMMENTS:** Cells of the immune system cells are regulated by a variety of cytokines that are, in general, categorized according to their cell of origin. One of these cytokines, **interleukin-1**, is a key regulator of inflammation, wound healing, and the immune response. It is produced primarily by macrophages but is also produced by neutrophils, fibroblasts, natural killer (NK) cells, keratinocytes, endothelial cells, and vascular smooth muscle cells. IL-1 can induce endothelial cells to produce prostaglandins, platelet-activating factor, and plasminogen activator, which can lead to vasodilation and hypotension by promoting endothelial leakage and intravascular thrombosis. IL-1 binds to CD121 receptors. It directly stimulates the thermoregulatory center of the hypothalamus, thereby inducing fever. IL-1 stimulates the liver to produce several acute phase proteins. It plays a key role in joint inflammation by inducing synovial cells to produce prostaglandin $E_2$, collagenase, and phospholipase. IL-1 mediates wound healing by activating basophils and eosinophils, stimulating neutrophil and macrophage activity, and locally increasing fibroblast proliferation and collagen synthesis. **Interleukin-1 induces the proliferation** of T and B lymphocytes, IL-2 production, and expression of the IL-2 receptor. IL-1 stimulates the release of other cytokines, including interferon, IL-3, IL-6, and colony-stimulating factors. The effects of IL-1 on immunity are greatly amplified through the stimulation of other cytokines. IL-1 and TNF-α are currently being studied as therapeutic agents for autoimmune disease, such as inflammatory bowel disease, psoriasis, and rheumatoid arthritis.

**ANSWER:** C

33. Which of the following statements regarding TNF is true?

   A. TNF is produced only by monocytes and macrophages.

   B. Release of TNF is stimulated by exotoxins.

C. TNF is an anabolic stimulant to the host that results in the deposition of fat.

D. TNF is responsible for the cachexia associated with metastatic disease.

E. TNF-α expression increases in response to glucocorticoid exposure.

*Ref.:* 33, 34

**COMMENTS: Tumor necrosis factor** is so named because of its ability to cause hemorrhagic necrosis in methylcholanthrene-induced sarcomas in mice. **Tumor necrosis factor-α** is produced primarily by monocytes and macrophages but also by neutrophils and NK cells. It stimulates the activity of neutrophils and induces endothelial cells to produce IL-1 and synovial cells and fibroblasts to produce prostaglandin $E_2$ and collagenase. TNF-α enhances the procoagulant activity of endothelial surfaces, increases vascular permeability, degranulates neutrophils, and stimulates the release of superoxides and arachidonic acid metabolites. In gram-negative shock, endotoxin stimulates the release of TNF-α, which leads to hypotension, disseminated intravascular coagulation, and even death. TNF stimulates catabolism in muscle and fat cells, thereby leading to an increase in anaerobic glycolysis, protein breakdown, and lipolysis. It is largely responsible for the cachexia associated with metastatic disease. TNF-α also has a role in stimulating and mediating apoptosis. TNF-α is produced in lesser quantities when glucocorticoids are present. **Glucocorticoids** downregulate the signaling pathway that transcribes the TNF gene.

**ANSWER:** D

34. Which of the following statements regarding interferons is true?

A. INF-γ is produced by macrophages.

B. Interferon production is inhibited by infection.

C. Interferons have a direct antiproliferative effect on $T_H2$ cells.

D. Cytokine production by macrophages is inhibited by interferons.

E. Interferons have a direct antiproliferative effect on $T_H1$ cells.

*Ref.:* 33, 34

**COMMENTS: Interferons** are glycoproteins produced by a variety of cells in response to viral infection or other stimulants. Interferons block viruses in two ways: through signaling pathways and by inhibition of the translation machinery (protein synthesis). The three major classifications of interferons are based on their cells of origin: **Interferon-α**, produced mainly by macrophages; **interferon-β**, produced by epithelial cells, fibroblasts, and macrophages; and **interferon-γ**, produced by T lymphocytes and NK cells. Interferons have a direct antiproliferative effect on cells but can also induce differentiation. Interferons decrease the activity of $T_H2$ cells but promote the differentiation of immature $CD4^+$ cells into committed $T_H1$ cells. This explains their usefulness as anticancer agents, although some anticancer effects may also result from stimulation of the cytotoxic activity of macrophages, NK cells, and cytotoxic T cells. Interferons stimulate a variety of cells to release other mediators and cytokines.

**ANSWER:** C

35. Which of the following statements regarding rejection of solid organ transplants is true?

A. Hyperacute rejection begins in the operating room with reperfusion of the transplanted organ.

B. Liver transplants are especially susceptible to hyperacute rejection.

C. Most immunosuppressive medications are used to prevent chronic rejection.

D. The major cause of graft failure is acute rejection.

E. Chronic rejection is characterized histologically by lymphocyte infiltration.

*Ref.:* 1

**COMMENTS:** There are three types of **solid organ rejection** that are based on the timing of the rejection: hyperacute rejection, acute rejection, and chronic rejection. The immunologic mechanism varies among these types of rejection. **Hyperacute rejection** occurs immediately and is the result of preformed antibody binding to the allograft on reperfusion of the organ. Hyperacute rejection is due to ABO incompatibility or a high titer of antidonor HLA-I antibodies in the recipient. For kidney, heart, pancreas, and lung transplants, current protocols include preoperative testing for ABO incompatibility or HLA antibodies (or both). For reasons not completely elucidated, liver transplants are resistant to this process. Liver transplants are performed without HLA matching and can be performed without ABO typing, although the ABO type is usually matched. **Acute rejection** occurs days to weeks following transplantation. Since acute rejection is initiated by T-cell immunity, most medications for preventing and treating it are directed toward T-cell suppression. Microscopically, acute rejection is characterized by a lymphocytic infiltrate, with plasma cells and eosinophils being seen on tissue biopsy specimens. **Chronic rejection** occurs months to years after transplantation and is the major cause of graft failure and mortality with all organ transplants. There is loss of normal histologic structure, fibrosis, and atherosclerosis, with intergraft expression of certain cytokines. Chronic rejection is the final common pathway of various insults, including repeated bouts of acute rejection, drug toxicity, chronic mechanical obstruction, recurrent infections, noncompliance with immunosuppressive medications, and pretransplant organ issues such as ischemia time and older organ donors. There is no defined therapy for chronic rejection, but it is believed that a better understanding of cytokine-mediated atherosclerosis would help in the development of treatments and prevention of chronic rejection.

**ANSWER:** A

## REFERENCES

1. Markmann JF, Yeh HA, Naji A, et al: Transplantation of abdominal organs. In Townsend CM Jr, et al, editors: *Sabiston textbook of surgery: the biological basis of modern surgical practice,* ed 18, Philadelphia, 2008, WB Saunders.
2. Chapman JR: The recipient of a renal transplant. In Morris PJ, Knechtle SJ, editors: *Kidney transplantation: principles and practice,* ed 6, Philadelphia, 2008, WB Saunders.
3. Knectle SJ, Morris PJ: Results of renal transplantation. In Morris PJ, Knechtle SJ, editors: *Kidney transplantation: principles and practice,* ed 6, Philadelphia, 2008, WB Saunders.
4. Fuggle SV, Taylor CJ: Histocompatability in renal transplantation. In Morris PJ, Knechtle SJ, editors: *Kidney transplantation: principles and practice,* ed 6, Philadelphia, 2008, WB Saunders.
5. Stegall MD, Gloor JM: Transplantation in the sensitized recipient and across ABO blood Groups. In Morris PJ, Knechtle SJ, editors: *Kidney*

*transplantation: principles and practice*, ed 6, Philadelphia, 2008, WB Saunders.

6. Allen RD: Vascular Complication after kidney transplantation. In Morris PJ, Knechtle SJ, editors: *Kidney transplantation: principles and practice*, ed 6, Philadelphia, 2008, WB Saunders.

7. Kobayashi TA, Sutherland DE, et al: Pancreas and kidney transplantation for diabetic nephropathy. In Morris PJ, Knechtle SJ, editors: *Kidney transplantation: principles and practice*, ed 6, Philadelphia, 2008, WB Saunders.

8. Sears D, Davis GL: Natural history of hepatitis C. In Busuttil RW, Klintmalm GK, editors: *Transplantation of the liver*, ed 2, Philadelphia, 2005, WB Saunders.

9. Charlton MR, Narayanan Menon KV: Late complications of liver transplantation and recurrence of disease. In Busuttil RW, Klintmalm GK, editors: *Transplantation of the liver*, ed 2, Philadelphia, 2005, WB Saunders.

10. Demetris AJ, Nalesnik M, Randhawa P, et al: Histological patterns of rejection and other causes of liver dysfunction. In Busuttil RW, Klintmalm GK, editors: *Transplantation of the liver*, ed 2, Philadelphia, 2005, WB Saunders.

11. Roche B, Samuel D: Transplantation for viral hepatitis A and B. In Busuttil RW, Klintmalm GK, editors: *Transplantation of the liver*, ed 2, Philadelphia, 2005, WB Saunders.

12. Grainger DK, Ildstad ST: Transplantation immunology and immunosuppression. In Townsend CM Jr, Beauchamp RD, Evers BM, et al, editors: *Sabiston textbook of surgery: the biological basis of modern surgical practice*, ed 18, Philadelphia, 2008, WB Saunders.

13. Chinnakotla S, Klintmalm GB: Induction and maintenance of immunosuppression. In Busuttil RW, Klintmalm GK, editors: *Transplantation of the liver*, ed 2, Philadelphia, 2005, WB Saunders.

14. Russell NK, Knight, SR, Morris PJ: Cyclosporine. In Morris PJ, Knechtle SJ, editors: *Kidney transplantation: principles and practice*, ed 6, Philadelphia, 2008, WB Saunders.

15. Fink SA, Brown RS Jr: Current indications, contraindications, delisting criteria, and timing for liver transplantation. In Busuttil RW, Klintmalm GK, editors: *Transplantation of the liver*, ed 2, Philadelphia, 2005, WB Saunders.

16. Ramsay MA: Anesthesia for liver transplantation. In Busuttil RW, Klintmalm GK, editors: *Transplantation of the liver*, ed 2, Philadelphia, 2005, WB Saunders.

17. Mai ML, Yip DS, Keller CA, et al: Pretransplantation evaluation: pulmonary, cardiac, and renal. In Busuttil RW, Klintmalm GK, editors: *Transplantation of the liver*, ed 2, Philadelphia, 2005, WB Saunders.

18. Desai NM, Olthoff KM: Portal vein thrombosis and other venous anomalies in liver transplantation. In Busuttil RW, Klintmalm GK, editors: *Transplantation of the liver*, ed 2, Philadelphia, 2005, WB Saunders.

19. Holt CD, Winston DJ: Infections after liver transplantation. In Busuttil RW, Klintmalm GK, editors: *Transplantation of the liver*, ed 2, Philadelphia, 2005, WB Saunders.

20. Fishman JA, Davis JO: Infection in renal transplant recipients. In Morris PJ, Knechtle SJ, editors: *Kidney transplantation: principles and practice*, ed 6, Philadelphia, 2008, WB Saunders.

21. Kirk AL: Antibodies and fusion proteins. In Morris PJ, Knechtle SJ, editors: *Kidney transplantation: principles and practice*, ed 6, Philadelphia, 2008, WB Saunders.

22. Ghobrial RM, Klintmalm GB: Outcome predictors in liver transplantation. In Busuttil RW, Klintmalm GK, editors: *Transplantation of the liver*, ed 2, Philadelphia, 2005, WB Saunders.

23. Alonso EM, Besedovsky A, et al: General criteria for pediatric transplantation. In Busuttil RW, Klintmalm GK, editors: *Transplantation of the liver*, ed 2, Philadelphia, 2005, WB Saunders.

24. De Ville de Goyet J, Rogiers X, Otte JB: Split-liver transplantation for the pediatric and adult recipient. In Busuttil RW, Klintmalm GK, editors: *Transplantation of the liver*, ed 2, Philadelphia, 2005, WB Saunders.

25. Tanaka K, Inomata Y: Living related liver transplantation in pediatric recipients. In Busuttil RW, Klintmalm GK, editors: *Transplantation of the liver*, ed 2, Philadelphia, 2005, WB Saunders.

26. Said AD, Safar NA, Wells J, et al: Liver disease in renal transplant recipients. In Morris PJ, Knechtle SJ, editors: *Kidney transplantation: principles and practice*, ed 6, Philadelphia, 2008, WB Saunders.

27. Kasiske BE, Israni AJ: Cardiovascular complications after renal transplantation. In Morris PJ, Knechtle SJ, editors: *Kidney transplantation: principles and practice*, ed 6, Philadelphia, 2008, WB Saunders.

28. Nissen NN, Colquhoun SD: Graft failure: etiology, recognition, and treatment. In Busuttil RW, Klintmalm GK, editors: *Transplantation of the liver*, ed 2, Philadelphia, 2005, WB Saunders.

29. Stone MJ, Fulmer JM, Klintman GB: Transplantation for primary hepatic malignancy. In Busuttil RW, Klintmalm GK, editors: *Transplantation of the liver*, ed 2, Philadelphia, 2005, WB Saunders.

30. Riordan SM, Williams R: Transplantation for fulminant hepatic failure. In Busuttil RW, Klintmalm GK, editors: *Transplantation of the liver*, ed 2, Philadelphia, 2005, WB Saunders.

31. VanThiel DH, Mindikoglu AL, et al: Unusual indications for liver transplantation. In Busuttil RW, Klintmalm GK, editors: *Transplantation of the liver*, ed 2, Philadelphia, 2005, Elsevier.

32. Fondevila C, Ghobrial RM: Donor selection and management. In Busuttil RW, Klintmalm GK, editors: *Transplantation of the liver*, ed 2, Philadelphia, 2005, WB Saunders.

33. Bromberg JS, Magee JC: Transplant immunology. In Mulholland MW, Lillemoe KD, Doherty GM, et al, editors: *Greenfield's surgery: scientific principles and practice*, ed 4, Philadelphia, 2006, Lippincott Williams & Wilkins.

34. Alarcon LH, Fink MP: Mediators of the inflammatory response. In Townsend CM Jr, Beauchamp RD, Evers BM, et al, editors: *Sabiston textbook of surgery: the biological basis of modern surgical practice*, ed 18, Philadelphia, 2008, WB Saunders.

# CHAPTER 7

# Perioperative Care and Anesthesia

*Chad E. Jacobs, M.D., and Walter J. McCarthy, M.D.*

## A. Perioperative Care

*José M. Velasco, M.D., and John Butsch, B.A., M.S., M.D.*

1. Regarding tight control of serum glucose levels in diabetic patients undergoing cardiac surgery, which of the following statements is true?

   A. It has no effect on postoperative complications.

   B. It significantly reduces the incidence of deep sternal wound infections.

   C. It enhances phagocytosis.

   D. It increases urine production.

   E. Tighter glucose control decreases in-hospital mortality.

   *Ref.: 1-6*

COMMENTS: Diabetes mellitus impairs wound healing. In addition, tissue perfusion is decreased because of both macrovascular and microvascular disease. **Hyperglycemia** may also result in osmotic diuresis, which may lead to a decrease in effective hypovolemia. Hyperglycemia is a known risk factor for postoperative deep sternal wound infection because it alters the normal physiologic response to infection. It is associated with impaired phagocytosis, lymphocyte dysfunction, immunoglobulin inactivation, activation of the complement component C3, and impaired deposition of collagen in wounds. Tight control of blood glucose levels in diabetic patients during the postoperative period via a continuous insulin infusion pump improves wound healing and reduces the incidence of postoperative sternal wound infections. When blood glucose levels are maintained between 80 and 120 mg/dL, the postoperative sternal wound infection rate approaches that found in nondiabetic patients. Correction of the blood glucose level to normal limits restores both neutrophil chemotaxis and phagocytosis. Moreover, it reverses the reduced $CD4^+$ cell counts found in patients with poorly controlled diabetes. Although there are many studies attributing postoperative benefit with tight glucose control, it is difficult to discern the beneficial effects of glucose versus insulin and the adverse effects of hypoglycemia. Insulin plays a role as an antiinflammatory and antioxidant hormone, which might contribute to the benefits seen in these studies. In a recent meta-analysis including 29 studies, **tight glucose control** was not associated with a significant reduction in hospital mortality, but there was a markedly increased risk for hypoglycemia in 21% of the studies—which may negate the beneficial effects of normoglycemia.

ANSWER: B

2. The perioperative management of a patient whose diabetes has been controlled by diet alone consists of determination of the blood glucose level and which of the following?

   A. Continuation of diet and determination of the serum glucose level before surgery

   B. Subcutaneous administration of regular insulin

   C. Oral hypoglycemic agents initiated 3 days before surgery

   D. Insulin infusion beginning 1 hour before surgery

   E. Increased oral carbohydrate intake to prevent ketosis

   *Ref.: 7*

COMMENTS: Patients whose diabetes is controlled by diet alone do not require any special preoperative measures other than **monitoring serum glucose**. Insulin and oral hypoglycemic agents are not necessary and may cause hypoglycemia. Oral hypoglycemic agents stimulate insulin secretion (sulfonylurea) or decrease intestinal absorption (metformin). Patients being treated with oral hypoglycemic agents should stop taking them before any major operation, and their blood glucose level should be controlled with insulin as needed. Increasing carbohydrate consumption will cause hyperglycemia and place the patient at risk for infection.

ANSWER: A

3. Regarding diabetic patients, which of the following statements is false?

   A. Glycosylated hemoglobin ($HbA_{1c}$) accounts for 4% to 7% of the total hemoglobin.

   B. High levels of $HbA_{1c}$ result in a higher complication rate.

   C. Long-acting insulin should be replaced with intermediate-acting insulin preoperatively.

   D. Operations commonly result in elevated blood glucose levels and higher ketone body levels.

   E. Short-acting insulin and 5% to 10% glucose should be administered in separate bags to optimize blood glucose control.

   *Ref.: 4*

**COMMENTS: Management of diabetic patients** is complex because of the metabolic effects of the disease and the possible presence of complications such as cardiovascular, renal, and neurologic diseases. Tight control of the blood glucose level is imperative. Ideally, blood glucose levels should be 80 to 110 mg/dL during fasting and below 180 mg/dL postprandially. Normally, **HbA$_{1c}$** accounts for 4% to 7% of the total hemoglobin. Poor control of glycemia will result in higher HbA$_{1c}$ levels. However, there is no evidence that high levels of HbA$_{1c}$ are associated with a higher risk for complications, provided that the blood glucose level is carefully monitored and controlled. Diabetic and nondiabetic patients experience higher blood glucose levels because of suppression of endogenous insulin secretion, the action of counterregulatory hormones, and infusion of glucose solutions. In preparing diabetic patients for major operations, all use of long-acting insulins and oral hypoglycemic agents should be suspended. When renal function is impaired, metformin may lead to lactic acidosis.

**ANSWER: B**

4. When evaluating a patient with known or suspected adrenal insufficiency, which of the following statements is false.

A. When indicated, the dose of glucocorticoid (generally hydrocortisone) should be adjusted in response to the anticipated surgical stress.

B. The signs and symptoms of acute adrenal insufficiency may mimic those of septic shock.

C. Hyponatremia, hyperkalemia, and hypoglycemia are frequently present.

D. The sudden development of hypotension in these patients should be treated immediately with 100 mg of hydrocortisone intravenously.

E. Appropriate laboratory studies, including determinations of serum cortisol and electrolyte levels, should be conducted and interpreted before initiation of therapy.

*Ref.: 1, 2*

**COMMENTS: Adrenal insufficiency** can be classified as primary or secondary. The three main causes of secondary insufficiency include exogenous glucocorticoids, operative correction of endogenous hypercortisolism, and abnormalities of the hypothalamus or pituitary gland. The hypothalamus secretes corticotropin-releasing factor, which stimulates the **anterior pituitary to release adrenocorticotropic hormone** (ACTH). ACTH stimulates the adrenal production of cortisol. Cortisol activates a negative feedback mechanism that affects both the hypothalamus and the anterior pituitary. Acute, or relative, adrenal insufficiency is a rare condition that may be manifested clinically as septic shock. It is associated with electrolyte abnormalities (hyponatremia and hyperkalemia), hypotension, nausea, vomiting, abdominal pain, weakness, and dizziness. The diagnosis should be considered in any patient with a history of tuberculosis or any patient undergoing long-term glucocorticoid therapy. While laboratory studies are being conducted, suspected adrenal insufficiency should be treated with a 100-mg loading dose of hydrocortisone or its equivalent. The laboratory studies should include determinations of cortisol, electrolyte, blood urea nitrogen, and creatinine levels, as well as a complete blood count. If blood pressure fails to return to normal within 1 to 2 hours after administration of the hydrocortisone bolus, an adrenal crisis is unlikely. If adrenal insufficiency is supported by the patient's response to hydrocortisone and a serum cortisol level of less than 20 mg/dL, an ACTH stimulation test can be used to confirm the diagnosis.

**ANSWER: E**

5. Regarding the ACTH stimulation test in patients with suspected adrenal insufficiency, which of the following statements is true?

A. The ACTH stimulation test is useful in determining the functional status of the hypothalamic-pituitary-adrenal (HPA) axis.

B. This test is based on the blood glucose response to a standard dose of ACTH.

C. If the ACTH test result is abnormal, 6-week perioperative steroid coverage is indicated.

D. This test is not indicated for a patient taking chronic topical steroid preparations.

E. All of the above.

*Ref.: 1, 2, 4*

**COMMENTS:** In patients with **adrenal gland suppression** or adrenal insufficiency, it is important to determine whether the HPA axis is intact. Basically, the ACTH test determines the response of a patient's adrenal gland (cortisol) to ACTH stimulation. A normal response includes a baseline cortisol level greater than 20 mg/dL and an elevation of the cortisol level of at least 7 mg/dL following an ACTH bolus. A patient who demonstrates a normal response to ACTH stimulation (i.e., a cortisol level >600 mg/L at 30 minutes) does not need additional glucocorticoid therapy. An abnormal response to ACTH stimulation indicates that either the HPA axis is not intact, the adrenal gland is insufficient, or both. In patients for whom surgical intervention results in the need for perioperative glucocorticoid therapy, the **ACTH stimulation test** can be used to determine when the function of the HPA axis normalizes. In addition, this test should be used to assess the integrity of the HPA axis in patients being managed with chronic inhaled or topical steroid preparations.

**ANSWER: A**

6. A patient with a long-term history of rheumatoid arthritis is scheduled for emergency colon resection. Which of the following statements is true?

A. Sudden hypotension and tachycardia should be treated with a 100-mg bolus of hydrocortisone and perioperative glucocorticoid treatment.

B. The patient is at increased risk for infection.

C. The patient might benefit from an epidural catheter.

D. Before elective reversal of the colostomy, the patient needs an ACTH stimulation test.

E. All of the above.

*Ref.: 4, 8*

**COMMENTS:** This patient suffers from a medical condition that is often treated with long-term steroid therapy, which may lead to **acute adrenal insufficiency**, particularly during periods of stress. Acute adrenal crisis can be manifested as a shocklike syndrome. Treatment should be instituted while investigating possible causes. If acute adrenal insufficiency is present, the patient will improve following the hydrocortisone injection, and perioperative administration of glucocorticoid should be continued. Patients maintained on long-term steroid therapy are at increased risk for postoperative infection, impaired wound healing, increased skin friability, and gastrointestinal bleeding. Epidural anesthesia reduces the perioperative stress response in patients at risk for adrenal insufficiency.

**The ACTH stimulation test** assesses the integrity of the HPA axis. Although a negative test result indicates that perioperative glucocorticoids are not necessary, a positive result indicates that steroid replacement therapy may be helpful but does not predict the clinical response to surgical stress. There is considerable variation in cortisol secretion among individuals undergoing operations. However, cortisol secretion rates greater than 200 mg/day in the first postoperative day are rare. Patients who have received more than 80 mg/day of hydrocortisone or its equivalent for longer than 3 weeks can be considered to have suppression of the HPA axis. They require **perioperative stress therapy** with 100 mg of hydrocortisone, followed by 100 to 150 mg in three divided doses. Tapering to preoperative maintenance doses can be accomplished in 2 to 3 days. In general, patients who have taken any dose of corticosteroid for less than 3 weeks or who are being managed chronically with alternative therapy should take the same dose perioperatively. In high-risk patients, one should also consider the anesthetic since etomidate inhibits the 11β-hydroxylase enzyme that converts 11β-deoxycortisol into cortisol and predictably reduces cortisol synthesis for up to 48 hours after a single intubating dose of this hypnotic agent.

**ANSWER:** E

7. Which of the following statements concerning preoperative management of patients with pheochromocytoma is true?

A. α-Adrenergic blockade with phenoxybenzamine requires a minimum of 4 to 6 weeks.

B. A β-blocker is indicated in patients with tachycardia.

C. Determination of 24-hour urine metanephrine levels confirms adequate α-adrenergic blockade.

D. Intraoperative hypotension following resection of the tumor is best treated with vasopressors and glucocorticoids.

E. Morphine and phenothiazines should be avoided preoperatively.

*Ref.:* 1, 9, 10

**COMMENTS:** Preoperative management of patients with **pheochromocytoma** requires control of hypertension and volume contraction. **α-Adrenergic blockade** prevents intraoperative hypertensive crises and allows fluid replacement to prevent hypovolemia after removal of the tumor. Several classes of medications have been investigated, including α-adrenergic and **β-adrenergic blockers**, calcium channel blockers, and **α-methylparatyrosine**. Calcium channel blockers are effective in patients with coronary vasospasm, and there is some evidence that metyrosine decreases intraoperative complications. Phenoxybenzamine is the drug of choice for α-adrenergic blockade. Initial doses begin around 10 mg/day in two divided dose, with ranges of 10 to 240 mg/day being required. The average dose is about 45 mg/day, and therapy may require 2 weeks to become effective. Therapy is considered effective when a patient's symptoms have disappeared and blood pressure control is adequate (blood pressure <160/90); orthostatic hypotension may be present. The absence of ST-segment depression on the electrocardiogram (ECG) and the presence of no more than one premature ventricular contraction per 5-minute period are indicators of adequate treatment and predictors of relatively few perioperative complications. If a patient's symptoms have not resolved or if the pulse is higher than 100 beats per minute, β-adrenergic blockade therapy is added. β-Adrenergic blockers should not be used for tachycardia until α-blockade has been established or a hypertensive crisis can occur. Once the catecholamine-secreting tumor is removed, persistent vasodilation may result in

hypovolemia, thereby increasing the need for intravenous fluids. All patients should have an arterial line inserted, and a central venous pressure monitor or a pulmonary catheter may prove useful in perioperative management. In addition, patients may seem somnolent or sedated for long as 24 hours postoperatively as a result of α-adrenergic blockade therapy. Morphine and phenothiazines may precipitate a hypertensive crisis and should be avoided preoperatively. Anesthetic agents may trigger catecholamine secretion. Enflurane and isoflurane have been used successfully. Intraoperative hypertension is treated with sodium nitroprusside, and cardiac arrhythmias are best treated with short-acting β-blockers.

**ANSWER:** E

8. A 33-year-old woman is scheduled for elective cholecystectomy. Preoperative evaluation shows the presence of mild to moderate hypothyroidism. Select the next most appropriate action:

A. Proceed with surgery with the knowledge that minor perioperative complications could develop.

B. Postpone surgery until a euthyroid state is achieved.

C. Proceed with surgery while beginning treatment with levothyroxine.

D. Proceed with surgery while beginning treatment with thionamides.

E. Proceed with surgery if severe clinical symptoms are not present.

*Ref.:* 8-20

**COMMENTS:** Mild to moderate **hypothyroidism** is a diagnosis that applies to patients who are not in myxedema coma and do not exhibit severe clinical symptoms. Systolic and diastolic myocardial function is impaired in patients with chronic hypothyroidism, with congestive heart failure occasionally occurring in hypothyroid patients in the absence of underlying heart disease. Hypothyroidism causes a decrease in cardiac output by reducing the heart rate and contractility. Patients with hypothyroidism are predisposed to pericardial effusion and may have a higher incidence of atherosclerotic heart disease. Hypoventilation may be present because of respiratory muscle weakness and impaired pulmonary response to hypoxia and hypercapnia. These patients have decreased gut motility, constipation, and hyponatremia because of a reduction in clearance of free water. Hypothyroidism is also associated with a decrease in red blood cell mass, which causes normochromic normocytic anemia. Although elective procedures may be performed on these patients safely, they are at increased risk for hypotension and congestive heart failure, along with postoperative gastrointestinal and neuropsychiatric complications. Elective operations should be postponed in these patients, but urgent or emergency ones can proceed, provided that thyroid replacement is begun with levothyroxine. Thionamides are used for the treatment of hyperthyroidism.

**ANSWER:** B

9. Regarding thyroid dysfunction in surgical patients, which of the following statements is true?

A. An operation can precipitate myxedema coma in patients with severe hypothyroidism.

B. Iodine administration is more likely to trigger an exacerbation of hyperthyroidism in patients with Graves disease than in those with toxic multinodular goiter.

C. Hypothyroidism is unlikely to result in postoperative complications.

D. All of the above.

E. None of the above.

*Ref.:* 14-17, 20-25

**COMMENTS: Severe hypothyroidism** is a medical emergency with a high mortality rate (50%). Symptoms and signs include decreased mental status, hypoventilation, and hypothermia. In both Graves disease and toxic multinodular goiter, iodine may worsen the hyperthyroidism. Antithyroid medication (thionamide) should be given at least 1 hour before the administration of iodine. Postoperative hypothyroidism can occur in any patient with chronic hypothyroidism when replacement therapy is not resumed within 10 days. Treatment of severe hypothyroidism consists of the administration of hydrocortisone followed by levothyroxine. Fluid restriction may be necessary if hyponatremia exists.

**ANSWER:** A

10. Which of the following agents is not a recommended treatment for the management of thyroid storm crisis?

A. β-Blockers

B. Thionamide

C. Iodine solution

D. Aspirin

E. Acetaminophen

*Ref.:* 22, 26, 27

**COMMENTS:** Patients with hyperthyroidism should not undergo a surgical procedure until clinical euthyroidism has been achieved. **β-Blockers** will control the symptoms of increased adrenergic tone, whereas thionamides will block the synthesis of new hormone. Iodine solution has been used both to decrease vascularity of the gland and to block the release of thyroid hormone. Acetaminophen is preferred over aspirin to treat hyperpyrexia because aspirin can cause increased serum levels of free thyroxine ($T_4$) and triiodothyronine ($T_3$) by interfering with protein binding. In emergency situations, hydration, cooling blankets, and a combination of glucocorticosteroids, β-blockers, and iopanoic acid therapy can restore patients with thyrotoxicosis to an acceptable state of clinical euthyroidism within 5 days, even if this treatment does not normalize thyroid-stimulating hormone levels. It can be difficult to diagnose thyroid storm. A medical history, clinical symptoms, and routine laboratory tests are necessary. Burch and Wartofsky developed a score to assess the likelihood of **thyroid storm** that involves the use of seven clinical variables: body temperature, heart rate, central nervous system (CNS) symptoms, gastrointestinal symptoms, congestive heart failure, atrial fibrillation, and jaundice. Total scores exceeding 45 were "highly suggestive" of thyroid storm.

**ANSWER:** D

11. Regarding the use of epidural anesthesia in patients with severe chronic obstructive pulmonary disease (COPD) who are undergoing upper abdominal operations, which of the following statements is true?

A. Epidural anesthesia is preferred to avoid the respiratory depressant effects of general anesthetics.

B. The use of epidural anesthesia has consistently led to a decreased incidence of postoperative pulmonary complications.

C. Postoperative epidural analgesia leads to a higher incidence of postoperative respiratory depression than does patient-controlled analgesia with morphine.

D. None of the above.

E. All of the above.

*Ref.:* 28, 29

**COMMENTS:** In general, **epidural or spinal anesthesia** is preferred for patients with severe COPD who are scheduled to undergo operations outside the abdominal cavity, particularly lower extremity operations. Although procedures involving the lower part of the abdomen can frequently be performed with epidural or spinal anesthesia, upper abdominal operations usually require supraumbilical incisions, which would necessitate higher levels of epidural anesthesia. Patients with severe COPD may not tolerate such high levels because they may result in decreased expiratory reserve volume, ineffective cough, and inability to clear secretions. General anesthesia allows better control of ventilation in these patients, thus optimizing ventilation and oxygenation. Studies have been inconclusive regarding whether epidural anesthesia results in a decreased incidence of postoperative pulmonary complications. Generally, it is believed that the risk for postoperative pulmonary complications is independent of the choice of intraoperative anesthesia. However, postoperative epidural analgesia may decrease the risk for complications after upper abdominal and thoracic surgery. The ideal anesthesia for patients with severe COPD would include an epidural catheter for postoperative pain control and general anesthesia for intraoperative management. Intravenous narcotics are associated with higher postoperative respiratory depression, and they may not be as effective in treating pain in these patients.

**ANSWER:** D

12. Regarding preoperative pulmonary function tests (PFTs), which of the following statements is false?

A. PFTs help predict postoperative pulmonary complications in patients undergoing abdominal operations.

B. PFTs conducted before and after bronchodilator therapy are useful in determining optimal management.

C. The history and physical examination are more useful than PFTs in predicting postoperative pulmonary complications.

D. Patients with a functional residual capacity of less than 50% of forced vital capacity should undergo ventilation-perfusion testing before pneumonectomy.

E. All of the above.

*Ref.:* 28, 29

**COMMENTS:** Routine use of preoperative PFTs in all patients with **preexisting pulmonary disease** is controversial. **Pulmonary function tests** have a positive predictive value for postoperative pulmonary complications in patients undergoing lung resection. However, the routine use of PFTs for abdominal operations often does not predict postoperative pulmonary complications. Instead, PFTs can be used as tools to provide optimal preoperative management and assist in the postoperative care of patients (i.e., patients with bronchospastic disease whose PFT results improve after bronchodilator therapy). Clinical factors such as smoking, wheezing, and increased sputum production on the preoperative work-up are more predictive of potential postoperative complications. Patients with a functional residual capacity of less than 50% of forced vital capacity who are scheduled for lung resection should undergo ventilation-perfusion studies to determine their predicted postoperative pulmonary function.

**ANSWER:** A

13. A 25-year-old asthmatic patient is scheduled for elective inguinal hernia repair. In the holding area, he exhibits severe wheezing bilaterally. Which of the following would be the best initial approach?

   A. Administer local anesthesia with sedation and avoid unnecessary airway manipulation.

   B. Administer albuterol nebulizer treatment in the holding area and proceed with the operation if the patient is not wheezing.

   C. Postpone surgery until the patient's asthma is under control.

   D. Administer spinal anesthesia and intravenous corticosteroids.

   E. Provide supplemental steroids intraoperatively if the patient states that he uses steroid inhalers.

*Ref.: 28, 29*

**COMMENTS:** This patient may have uncontrolled or poorly controlled **asthma**. Although inguinal hernia repair is considered a low-stress operations, unexpected complications can occur with both the surgical procedure and anesthesia. Since this is an elective procedure, the patient's asthmatic attack should be managed preoperatively. A single treatment may not be sufficient for adequate therapy. The use of spinal or local anesthesia with sedation does not ensure that the patient will not require a general anesthetic, particularly if the spinal block or sedation is inadequate. Patients using inhaled steroids as part of their asthma management do not require supplemental steroids.

**ANSWER:** C

14. An 85-year-old with severe COPD is scheduled for elective cholecystectomy. Preoperatively, which one of the following steps will not help reduce the risk for postoperative pulmonary complications?

   A. Cessation of smoking for at least 8 weeks

   B. Prophylactic antibiotics for patients with productive yellowish sputum

   C. Preoperative incentive spirometry

   D. Laparoscopic technique

   E. Inspiratory-to-expiratory ratio of 1 : 1 while intubated

*Ref.: 28, 29*

**COMMENTS:** Patients with **chronic obstructive pulmonary disease** are at increased risk for postoperative pulmonary complications. The risk can be reduced if effective measures are taken in the perioperative period. Patients should be instructed to stop smoking. Frequently, however, there is insufficient time to achieve the beneficial effects of this maneuver. It takes at least 8 weeks of cessation before any decrease in postoperative pulmonary complications can be realized. Cessation for 2 weeks will improve carbon monoxide levels, but secretions still can be a problem, and ciliary function

may take longer to return. Patients with COPD should be free of any acute exacerbations of bronchospasm or infection. Increased sputum production or a change in the color of sputum is an indication that an underlying infection could exist. If pulmonary infection is present, antibiotic therapy should be instituted and the patient treated for the appropriate amount of time before undergoing surgery. Incentive spirometry may help prevent postoperative pulmonary complications, along with deep breathing, coughing, and chest physical therapy. In patients with COPD, if at all possible the cholecystectomy should be done via laparoscopy to avoid a painful upper abdominal incision and to preserve better diaphragmatic function. COPD patients need a prolonged expiratory phase while on the respirator.

**ANSWER:** E

15. In morbidly obese patients, obstructive sleep apnea often results in all but which of the following conditions?

   A. Right ventricular failure

   B. Hypoxemia

   C. Hypercapnia

   D. Polycythemia

   E. Left ventricular failure

*Ref.: 28*

**COMMENTS: Morbidly obese patients** (body mass index >40) have an increased incidence of obstructive sleep apnea (25%). Right ventricular failure can occur secondary to the effects of obstructive sleep apnea. Chronic arterial hypoxemia and hypercapnia often lead to polycythemia, pulmonary hypertension, and right heart failure. These patients are at increased risk for the development of left ventricular failure, but not as a direct result of sleep apnea. Increased stroke volume may lead to enlargement of the left ventricle. In addition, systemic hypertension causes left ventricular hypertrophy, which added to the effects of increased stroke volume, ultimately results in systolic and diastolic dysfunction. The higher incidence of ischemic heart disease found in these patients also increases the risk for left ventricular failure.

**ANSWER:** E

16. Obese patients have an increased risk for deep venous thrombosis for all but which of the following reasons?

   A. Increased abdominal weight and venous stasis

   B. Polycythemia

   C. Infrequent ambulation

   D. Increased incidence of ischemic heart disease

   E. Lengthy operations because of difficult exposure

*Ref.: 28*

**COMMENTS: Obese patients** are at much higher risk than nonobese patients for **deep venous thrombosis**. Venous stasis increases the risk for deep venous thrombosis. Increased abdominal weight leads to decreased venous return secondary to compression of the inferior vena cava. Polycythemia leads to decreased vascular flow. If an obese patient has difficulty walking preoperatively, it is likely that postoperative mobilization will be unsatisfactory and lead to increased risk. Prolonged operations result in longer periods of venous stasis during the intraoperative course, thereby increasing the risk. Preventive therapy should be instituted before induction of anesthesia by administering regular **heparin or low-molecular-weight heparin** along with **intermittent sequential venous compression boots**. It is important to encourage early ambulation in this patient population.

**ANSWER: D**

17. Regarding tracheal intubation in morbidly obese patients, which of the following statements is true?

 A. The body habitus of these patients (i.e., short, thick necks) makes intubation difficult. However, it does not compromise ventilation.

 B. The diagnosis of obstructive sleep apnea should not alter management of the airway.

 C. Hypoxemia following induction of anesthesia and during intubation is the result of diminished functional residual capacity.

 D. Awake intubation is contraindicated.

 E. All of the above.

*Ref.:* 28

**COMMENTS:** Management of a **morbidly obese patient's airway** can be difficult. The approach to intubation must take into consideration a number of factors. Such patients often have short thick necks, large tongues, limited mouth and neck mobility, and increased thoracic and abdominal pressure. For these reasons, both ventilation and intubation can be difficult. Patients with obstructive sleep apnea frequently have redundant soft tissue in the airway, which makes visualization of the vocal cords extremely difficult. In fact, obese patients with sleep apnea and abnormalities on airway examination should be considered for awake intubation. In experienced hands, awake fiberoptic intubation with prior topical application of local anesthetic and small amounts of sedation is ideal. If general anesthesia is induced and difficulty with intubation and ventilation ensues, obese patients can rapidly become desaturated and hypoxemic. This is due to both an increased rate of oxygen consumption and decreased functional residual capacity. Oxygenation with 100% oxygen before induction of anesthesia helps decrease the rate of desaturation but does not eliminate this risk.

**ANSWER: C**

18. A 65-year-old patient with no significant past medical history and normal laboratory values is scheduled for laparoscopic inguinal hernia repair. While waiting in the preoperative holding area, his ECG shows an irregularly irregular rhythm without P waves. His heart rate varies between 70 and 85 beats per minute. Which of the following constitutes appropriate management of this patient?

 A. Cancel the operation and order a stress test.

 B. Cancel the operation and immediately start treatment with digoxin.

 C. Perform transthoracic echocardiography and proceed with the operation if the result is normal and the heart rate is controlled.

 D. Proceed with the operation and place the patient on an aspirin regimen postoperatively.

 E. Administer cardioversion.

*Ref.:* 30

**COMMENTS:** This patient has **atrial fibrillation**. Arrhythmias in this setting typically appear in elderly patients and are frequently associated with pain or severe anxiety. The possibility of a new arrhythmia in association with these diseases is less than 1% in the absence of signs suggesting cardiac disease or thyrotoxicosis. Therefore, immediate stress testing is unnecessary. This patient's heart rate is within normal limits, thus making the administration of digoxin unwarranted. Proceeding with surgery is an acceptable course of management, provided that the ventricular rate is controlled and there are no signs of acute illness. A transthoracic echocardiogram should rule out structural heart disease and atrial clot. Anticoagulation is recommended only if the risk for thromboembolism is higher than the risk for postoperative bleeding. Intravenous heparin with the initiation of oral warfarin, not aspirin, is the anticoagulation therapy of choice.

 **Cardioversion** is not indicated as the initial management step in this patient since there is no hemodynamic instability. Moreover, 85% of the patients in whom atrial fibrillation develops revert to sinus rhythm with medication. Of those who are discharged from the hospital with atrial fibrillation, 98% revert to sinus rhythm within 2 months of the operation. Perioperative atrial fibrillation may be related to autonomic nervous system changes associated with an inflammatory response. Although it may seem logical that rhythm conversion would be more advantageous than rate control, this is not true. Controlling the ventricular response rate either pharmacologically or by ablation of the atrioventricular node and implantation of a pacemaker allows the use of less toxic medications, which results in fewer adverse drug reactions and hospitalizations.

**ANSWER: C**

19. A patient in the postanesthesia care unit is in no apparent distress. The vital signs are stable except for a heart rate of 128 beats per minute that is irregular with no P waves. Which of the following treatment options would not be appropriate initial therapy?

 A. Metoprolol

 B. Diltiazem

 C. Digoxin

 D. Adenosine

 E. All are appropriate options

*Ref.:* 31

**COMMENTS:** This patient has **atrial fibrillation** with a rapid ventricular response. Treating this patient with β-blockers such as metoprolol or calcium channel blockers such as diltiazem would be appropriate. Calcium channel blockers are especially advantageous in patients who cannot tolerate β-blockade, such as those with bronchospastic disease or congestive heart failure. Digoxin may also be used, although recent studies suggest that it may be ineffective in high adrenergic states such as those that are present postoperatively. Supraventricular tachycardia, not atrial fibrillation, responds to adenosine. Direct current cardioversion is not an appropriate first-line therapy in a hemodynamically stable patient. Had the aforementioned patient been hypotensive, complaining of angina, or in pulmonary edema, cardioversion would have been appropriate.

**ANSWER: D**

20. Atrial fibrillation develops in a 65-year-old patient 4 days after a coronary arterial bypass graft operation. The vital signs are

stable, and the laboratory test values are normal. Which of the following statements pertains to this patient?

A. The patient is not at increased risk for stroke.

B. The duration and cost of the patient's hospital stay will be increased.

C. The duration of atrial fibrillation is inconsequential.

D. Anticoagulation therapy with heparin should be started immediately.

E. All of the above.

*Ref.: 30-32*

**COMMENTS:** The risk for **stroke** in postoperative cardiac patients in whom atrial fibrillation develops doubles in comparison to those without atrial fibrillation. The duration of the hospital stay will increase by an average of 1 to 2 days, and the median cost will increase significantly. The duration of atrial fibrillation is crucial to determining therapy. The risk for thromboembolism in patients without sinus rhythm is markedly increased after 48 hours. Therefore, anticoagulation should be strongly considered in patients with an indeterminate duration of atrial fibrillation, even in the immediate postoperative period. A reasonable treatment plan consists of intravenous heparin, titrated to maintain a partial thromboplastin time of two to three times normal, and subsequent administration of warfarin to maintain an international normalized ratio between 2.0 and 3.0. In general, atrial fibrillation is associated with a five-fold to sixfold increased risk for stroke in comparison to normal individuals. The addition of anticoagulation therapy decreases the risk by 68%.

**ANSWER:** B

21. Indicate which of the following statements in regard to delaying elective noncardiac surgery is not true.

A. Elective noncardiac surgery should be delayed for at least 2 weeks and optimally for 4 to 6 weeks after coronary artery stenting.

B. Elective noncardiac surgery should be delayed at least 3 months after myocardial infarction (MI).

C. Elective noncardiac surgery should be delayed at least 1 week after coronary artery angioplasty without stent placement.

D. Elective noncardiac surgery should be delayed in patients with stage 3 hypertension.

E. All of the above.

*Ref.: 30, 33*

**COMMENTS:** The "6-month rule" formerly observed for delaying **elective noncardiac surgery** after **acute myocardial infarction** was based on the results of perioperative management of patients with recent MI reported nearly 3 decades ago. Current management and risk stratification do not use the 3- and 6-month intervals traditionally discussed in the past. Rather, current management of MI provides for risk stratification during convalescence, and the risk for adverse perioperative complications depends more on the amount of residual myocardium at risk for severe ischemia and infarction than on the age of the previous MI. Although no specific current studies have evaluated the timing of elective noncardiac surgery after MI, it appears reasonable to delay elective surgery for 4 to 6 weeks after uncomplicated MI, assuming that noninvasive testing does not indicate residual myocardium at risk.

The timing of elective surgery after percutaneous coronary intervention (PCI) involving **angioplasty** with or without stenting depends on the temporally related risks for vessel thrombosis, restenosis, and bleeding related to the antiplatelet therapy used in the acute phase after PCI. Delaying surgery for at least 1 week after balloon angioplasty has the theoretical benefits of allowing healing of the vessel injury and reducing the risk for vessel thrombosis. Delaying elective surgery for 2 weeks and ideally for 4 to 6 weeks will allow partial endothelialization of a coronary stent, as well as decrease the risk for bleeding related to antiplatelet therapy (typically used for 4 to 6 weeks after stenting). Stage 3 hypertension (systolic blood pressure ≥180 mm Hg and diastolic blood pressure ≥110 mm Hg) should be controlled before elective surgery. Effective control of blood pressure can often be achieved by the administration of oral antihypertensive medication for several days to weeks. If an operation is urgent, more aggressive therapy can reduce blood pressure preoperatively, but there is a significantly greater risk for intraoperative blood pressure lability, with the potential development of hypotension and severe hypertension.

**ANSWER:** B

22. A 65-year-old man with a long-standing history of hypertension and a 25-pack-per-year history of smoking is scheduled for elective laparoscopic hernia repair. On examination, his blood pressure is 150/90. The ECG shows nonspecific ST-segment changes. Appropriate interventions would include which of the following?

A. Cancelling the procedure

B. Obtaining a more detailed history regarding the level of exercise and daily activity

C. Requesting a cardiac consultation

D. Perioperative administration of a β-blocker and changing the operation to open hernia repair with local anesthesia

E. None of the above

*Ref.: 30, 33*

**COMMENTS:** Current recommendations regarding **preoperative cardiac evaluation for noncardiac surgery** are based on the theory that random testing and screening for cardiac disease in the absence of clinical findings or changes in a patient's history are not cost-effective and do not appear to reduce perioperative cardiovascular morbidity and mortality. The approach to the patient needs to consider both the surgical risk factors for a cardiac complication and the patient's cardiac risk factors.

High-risk **predictors of cardiac complications** include known coronary artery disease, unstable angina, severe stenotic valvular disease, essential hypertension, and recent documented MI. Intermediate predictors of coronary disease include advanced age, poor exercise tolerance, congestive heart failure, rhythm other than sinus rhythm, and insulin-dependent diabetes. High-risk surgical procedures include any emergency procedure, procedures involving the aorta or other major vasculature, and long procedures entailing large blood loss and fluid shifts. Intermediate procedures include major orthopedic procedures and prostate, carotid artery, and head or neck operations.

For a patient undergoing a low- to intermediate-risk procedure who has more than two intermediate to high predictors of cardiac risk, the history and physical findings will guide the necessity for further work-up. If the history and exercise tolerance have been stable and routine laboratory studies such as ECGs are unchanged, elective procedures of low to intermediate risk can proceed without additional intervention. When additional history or records cannot be obtained, the urgency of surgery must be considered in situations in which the history and physical findings suggest progression of coronary artery disease.

Cardiac consultation should be used to answer specific questions regarding disease status and not simply to request "clearance." Appropriate use of consultation services may include further testing when indicated by changes in a patient's history or findings on physical examination. As a general rule, if nothing in the history or physical examination indicates a need for intervention, an intervention is not required simply because the patient is undergoing an operation.

Although available data indicate that appropriate **β-blockade therapy** may reduce the incidence of preoperative morbidity and mortality, there is no evidence that one type of anesthetic technique is superior to another. The approach should involve optimizing the patient's condition and making reasonable predictions of risk rather than attempting alternative measures in the hope of reducing the likelihood of complications.

**A N S W E R :** B

---

**23.** A patient is scheduled for colon resection secondary to diverticulitis. The patient's history is significant for coronary artery disease, hypertension, and insulin-dependent diabetes. The patient underwent two-vessel angioplasty 6 months previously, is symptom free, and exercises three times per week. Appropriate preoperative testing would include which of the following?

A. ECG

B. Treadmill stress test

C. Dobutamine echocardiographic stress test

D. Angiogram

E. None of the above

*Ref.:* 30, 33

**COMMENTS:** In the absence of a change in a patient's clinical history or physical findings, only routine testing appropriate for age and gender needs to be conducted. In a patient who has undergone coronary artery bypass grafting within 5 years or had normal findings during an interventional **cardiac work-up** within 2 years, no further testing is warranted unless dictated by changes in the history or findings on physical examination. When indicated, exercise stress testing is the preferred test. Routine treadmill testing provides much useful information, including the patient's functional capacity, areas of myocardium in which ischemia may occur, and a heart rate at which ischemia may occur. For patients who cannot exercise on a treadmill, chemical stress testing is the next preferred method of assessing ventricular function. **Angiography** is generally reserved for patients with known cardiac disease, recent MI or unstable angina, or severe stenotic valvular disease. In such patients, an acute intervention such as angioplasty (stenting) or balloon valvuloplasty may be indicated before noncardiac surgery. In addition, although coronary artery bypass grafting is not generally indicated to improve the outcome after noncardiac surgery, angioplasty may identify patients who do require coronary artery bypass grafting or valve replacement before elective noncardiac surgery. When surgery is needed on an urgent or emergency basis, the patient's condition should be medically optimized and interventional studies reserved for the postoperative period.

**A N S W E R :** A

---

**24.** In patients with intermediate predictors of cardiac risk who are scheduled for intermediate- or high-risk surgical procedures, which of the following interventions can reduce perioperative morbidity and mortality?

A. Continuous intraoperative ST-segment monitoring

B. Regional anesthesia when indicated

C. Transesophageal echocardiography

D. Routine use of intravenous nitroglycerin

E. β-Blockade therapy

*Ref.:* 30, 34, 35

**COMMENTS:** It is unclear whether certain anesthetic techniques or intraoperative monitors can reliably reduce **perioperative morbidity and mortality**. Continuous ST-segment monitoring is a noninvasive, safe, readily available, inexpensive component of routine intraoperative monitoring. Even though it has proved useful in the early detection of myocardial ischemia, it has not been shown to favorably affect the overall incidence of perioperative MI or death. Although regional anesthesia seems safer than general anesthesia, no studies have corroborated such a claim. **Transesophageal echocardiography** is very safe and provides pertinent information regarding volume status, contractility, and regional wall motion abnormalities. However, it requires an experienced operator since adequate views may not always be obtainable, particularly during procedures involving the thorax and upper part of the abdomen.

**Perioperative nitroglycerin administration** has been used to optimize cardiac perfusion in high-risk patients because it causes dilation of epicardial vessels and is an effective therapy for angina. Topical nitrates are not recommended in the operating room since absorption may be adversely affected by changes in body temperature and cutaneous blood flow. Although intravenous nitroglycerin is commonly used, no studies have clearly demonstrated its efficacy in reducing perioperative cardiac morbidity and mortality. β-Blockade therapy reduces perioperative and long-term complications related to myocardial morbidity and death from MI. It is thought to decrease the incidence of myocardial complications via several mechanisms, including reduction of myocardial oxygen demand and stabilization of intravascular plaques and thrombi. Although there is controversy regarding how soon the medications can be given to see the best benefit, cardiac complications can be reduced in patients with the **administration of β-blockers** 3 to 4 hours before surgery, and these effects can last for 2 years postoperatively, but such patients may have a higher incidence of stroke and other mortality according to the **POISE (PeriOperative Ischemia Evaluation) trial**. Other drugs, such as calcium channel blockers and $α_2$-agonists, have not been shown to have the same effect as β-blockade.

**A N S W E R :** E

---

**25.** Which of the following statements regarding perioperative β-blocker use is true?

A. Perioperative β-blockade can reduce intraoperative myocardial ischemia in at-risk patients.

B. Perioperative β-blockade can reduce postoperative myocardial ischemia in at-risk patients.

C. Perioperative β-blockade can reduce postoperative cardiac death and nonfatal MI after major vascular surgery.

D. Perioperative β-blockade should be initiated preoperatively and continued for several days postoperatively in patients at risk for cardiac events.

E. All of the above.

*Ref.:* 33, 35

**COMMENTS:** In 2001, the Agency for Healthcare Research and Quality found sufficient clinical evidence to justify the widespread implementation of **perioperative β-blockade**. Patients with known coronary disease, positive preoperative stress evaluation results, or known risk factors for cardiac complications and those undergoing intermediate- to high-risk procedures will probably benefit from perioperative β-blockade. This observation has best been documented in vascular surgery patients, in whom reductions in intraoperative and postoperative ischemia, perioperative MI, and cardiac mortality have been demonstrated. The greatest benefit appears to accrue in patients with more than one of the following risk factors: high-risk surgery, known coronary artery disease, cerebrovascular disease, diabetes mellitus, or chronic renal insufficiency. Even though specific guidelines have not yet been developed, continuation of β-blockade for up to a month postoperatively appears logical. Despite widespread use of this protocol, recent trials have begun to question the universality of their use. In the POISE trial, patients who were randomized to the treatment group received a starting dose of 100 mg metoprolol given orally 2 to 4 hours before surgery and 100 mg given 0 to 6 hours after surgery, followed by 200 mg every day for 30 days. They concluded that although major postoperative cardiac events were reduced in the metoprolol group, overall mortality and the incidence of stroke were higher. There are some inherent problems with this study, and the final recommendation may be to dose and titrate high-risk patients 1 to 2 weeks before surgery to achieve the best benefit. The risk for perioperative MI is greatest in the first 24 to 96 hours after surgery, but it persists for up to 1 week postoperatively.

**ANSWER:** E

26. Regarding the scenarios listed below, which one of the operations should proceed as scheduled?

A. An 80-year-old scheduled for cataract surgery who has a pulse of 60 and blood pressure of 180/110 and is completely asymptomatic

B. A 67-year-old scheduled for left total hip arthroplasty who has a pulse of 80 and blood pressure of 180/110, is asymptomatic, and takes β-blockers

C. A 65-year-old hypertensive scheduled for bilateral total knee arthroplasty who has a pulse of 90 and blood pressure of 130/70 and who takes angiotensin-converting enzyme (ACE) inhibitors

D. An 80-year-old scheduled for bilateral laparoscopic hernia repair who has a pulse of 42 and blood pressure of 100/60 and who has a pacemaker and is taking β-blockers

E. None of the above operations should proceed

*Ref.:* 30, 32

**COMMENTS:** Management of hypertension in the perioperative period remains controversial. Nonetheless, several studies have consistently shown that a preoperative diastolic blood pressure higher than 110 mm Hg confers an increased risk for major morbidity. Aggressive perioperative normalization may not reduce the risk. However, the patient in scenario A is scheduled for a low-risk operation, unlike the patient in scenario B. Therefore, the operation in scenario A can be performed safely as long as the patient has adequate follow-up. ACE inhibitors have been associated with severe perioperative hypotension during major surgery, especially in patients who receive an epidural catheter as part of their management. The patient in scenario D may have a pacemaker malfunction that needs to be evaluated. β-Blockers have been shown to decrease

intraoperative ischemia and should be continued. Calcium channel blockers and diuretics may also be continued.

**ANSWER:** A

27. Evidence-based strategies for perioperative renal protection include which of the following?

A. Fenoldopam, 0.01 mcg/kg/min intravenously

B. Mannitol, 0.5 to 1 g/kg intravenously

C. Furosemide, 20 to 40 mg intravenously

D. *N*-Acetylcysteine

E. None of the above

*Ref.:* 36-41

**COMMENTS:** None of these drugs have been approved as a renoprotective agent by the U.S. Food and Drug Administration, and none has consistently shown clear benefit, although all have theoretical benefits. **Fenoldopam** preserves medullary blood flow without significant systemic effects. **Mannitol** promotes diuresis, which should minimize sludging of tubular fluid, and seems to be a free radical scavenger. However, it increases osmolarity and may lead to hypovolemia. **Loop diuretics**, such as furosemide (Lasix), reduce the metabolism of tubular cells and should enable patients to better tolerate ischemia. Therapeutic measures with proven efficacy are hydration before and after the administration of contrast material and use of the minimal dose required (not exceeding a volume of contrast medium of 5 mL/kg of body weight divided by the serum creatinine level in milligrams per deciliter). Other modalities that have not shown clear evidence of prevention are the use of *N*-acetylcysteine, isosmolar contrast media, bicarbonate infusion, or purine antagonists (theophylline, aminophylline). The use of continuous venovenous hemofiltration in high-risk patients has been shown to be effective.

**ANSWER:** E

28. Regarding urinary retention after ambulatory surgery, which of the following statements is not true?

A. Urinary retention is most frequently associated with herniorrhaphy and anorectal procedures.

B. Spinal anesthesia, but not general anesthesia, is a predisposing factor for postoperative urinary retention.

C. Postoperative urinary retention can frequently be asymptomatic.

D. Ambulatory surgery patients must void as a criterion for discharge.

E. Overzealous administration of intravenous fluids (>1200 mL) can cause urinary retention.

*Ref.:* 1, 2, 35, 42

**COMMENTS:** Patients at risk for **postoperative urinary retention** include those with a previous history of retention and those undergoing procedures such as herniorrhaphy and anorectal operations. Both spinal anesthesia and general anesthesia are predisposing factors, especially when the latter is associated with the use of anticholinergic drugs. Although bladder overdistention is a significant factor contributing to postoperative urinary retention, many patients are asymptomatic with bladder volumes exceeding 600 mL. Even though low-risk patients may be discharged safely without the requirement to void, consideration should be given to catheterization of high-risk patients before discharge. Patients at high risk for postoperative urinary retention should have ready access to a medical facility and be instructed to return to a medical facility if still unable to void 8 to 12 hours after discharge from an ambulatory surgical facility. Judicious use of intravenous fluids may reduce the incidence of postoperative urinary retention in patients at high risk.

**ANSWER: B**

29. Initial treatment of a postoperative headache 24 hours after spinal anesthesia for outpatient knee arthroplasty includes all but which of the following?

    A. Oral fluids

    B. Bed rest

    C. Oral analgesics

    D. Caffeine

    E. Epidural blood patch

    *Ref.: 29*

**COMMENTS: Post–dural puncture headache** (PDPH) results from decreased intracranial pressure (ICP) secondary to leakage of cerebrospinal fluid from the dural defect created by the spinal needle. The incidence of PDPH can be decreased primarily by reducing the needle size and, to a lesser extent, by using needles of improved design. Increased oral fluid intake, remaining recumbent, and the use of oral analgesics can reduce cephalgia, as well as other symptoms, such as visual disturbances, auditory disturbances, and nausea. Caffeine may also be helpful in reducing symptoms. An epidural blood patch is a more aggressive approach that is typically reserved for severe, persistent symptoms. Epidural injection of 10 to 20 mL of autologous blood collected from a fresh venipuncture is associated with successful relief of severe, persistent PDPH symptoms in 90% of patients.

**ANSWER: E**

30. Which statement about postoperative nausea and vomiting (PONV) after ambulatory surgery is false.

    A. PONV is associated with opioid use.

    B. PONV occurs less frequently following anesthetic induction with propofol than with thiopental.

    C. PONV prophylaxis should be administered to all patients before ambulatory surgery.

    D. PONV is increased in adults who are not required to ingest oral fluids before discharge.

    E. PONV is one of the most prevalent factors leading to delay in discharge after outpatient procedures.

    *Ref.: 29, 43, 44*

**COMMENTS:** PONV is one of the most prevalent factors leading to delay in discharge from ambulatory surgical centers or unanticipated hospitalization after outpatient procedures. Both pain and the treatment of pain with opioids are associated with increased risk for PONV. "**Balanced analgesia**" with use of nonopioid medications such as ketorolac (a nonsteroidal anti-inflammatory drug) and adjuvant methods of analgesia such as wound infiltration with local anesthetic and local or regional nerve blocks can substantially

reduce the use of **opioids** and associated PONV. Use of propofol as an induction drug is known to reduce the incidence of PONV, although the effect is lessened after long surgical procedures unless it is infused during the procedure or another dose of propofol is administered toward the conclusion of a long procedure. Because of the cost and side effects of antiemetic drugs, prophylaxis for all patients undergoing ambulatory surgery is not recommended. However, prophylaxis for patients at high risk for PONV can be cost-effective by reducing the length of the postoperative stay and improving patients' satisfaction. Although in a comparison between ondansetron, 8 mg, and metoclopramide, 10 mg, significant improvement in reducing PONV was noted with ondansetron, a new class of antiemetics, substance P or NK1 receptor antagonists, have shown improvement over ondansetron in terms of vomiting. In a simplified risk score developed by Apfel, when none, one, two, three, or four of the risk factors (being female, history of PONV or motion sickness, nonsmoking status, postoperative opioids) are present, the patient's risk for PONV is about 10%, 20%, 40%, 60%, or 80% respectively. Although oral fluid intake before discharge does not increase the risk for PONV in adult patients, eliminating oral fluid intake as a discharge criterion does not reduce the risk for PONV. Therefore, patients should be allowed to decide to accept or decline oral fluids as they desire before discharge.

**ANSWER: C**

31. Regarding skin preparation in a 35-year-old man scheduled for inguinal hernia repair, which of the following is an effective measure?

    A. Clip the hair from the operative site.

    B. Paint the operative site with chlorhexidine gluconate/alcohol.

    C. Allow the povidone-iodine solution to dry.

    D. All of the above.

    E. None of the above.

    *Ref.: 1*

**COMMENTS:** The sole reason for preparing the patient's skin before an operation is to reduce the risk for wound infection. A preoperative antiseptic bath is not necessary for most surgical patients. Hair should not be removed from the operative site unless it physically interferes with accurate anatomic approximation of the wound edges. If hair must be removed, it should be clipped in the operating room. Shaving hair from the operative site, particularly on the evening before surgery or immediately before the wound incision, increases the risk for wound infection. The necessary reduction in microorganisms can be achieved by using povidone-iodine or chlorhexidine gluconate both for mechanical cleansing of the intertriginous folds and the umbilicus and for painting the operative site. Simply applying the agents (painting or spraying) is an effective means of disinfection of the skin. Povidone-iodine and chlorhexidine/alcohol should be allowed to dry.

**ANSWER: D**

32. Regarding the risk associated with surgery in patients with liver disease, which of the following is not true?

    A. Halothane and enflurane reduce hepatic arterial blood flow.

    B. Hypercapnia increases portal blood flow.

C. Fentanyl, not morphine or meperidine, is the preferred narcotic agent.

D. Patients with Child class B cirrhosis undergoing cardiac operations have a high mortality rate.

E. Laparoscopic cholecystectomy can be performed safely in patients with compensated Child class A cirrhosis.

*Ref.:* 36, 37

**COMMENTS:** Routine laboratory screening of otherwise healthy surgical candidates for unsuspected liver disease is controversial. However, a carefully taken history to identify risk factors for liver disease permits adequate initial evaluation. Isoflurane is preferred over halothane because it increases hepatic arterial blood flow. Hypercapnia should be avoided since it triggers sympathetic splanchnic stimulation and leads to decreased portal flow. Fentanyl or sufentanil are the narcotic agents of choice. The metabolism of morphine and diazepam can be prolonged in patients with liver disease. Lorazepam is preferred since it is eliminated by glucuronidation. Cardiac operations are associated with a high mortality rate in patients with Child class B cirrhosis because of the higher risk for infection and bleeding. Celiotomy leads to a greater reduction in hepatic arterial blood flow than do extraabdominal or laparoscopic operations. In patients with cirrhosis, the Child-Pugh and Model for End-Stage Liver Disease (MELD) classifications are the most useful predictors of mortality and morbidity. A MELD score of less than 10, 10 to 14, and higher than 14 correspond to classes A, B, and C. Postoperatively, bilirubin levels and the prothrombin time should be monitored closely. Preoperative correction of coagulopathic states is mandatory.

**ANSWER:** B

**REFERENCES**

1. Neumayer L, Vargo D: Principles of preoperative and operative surgery. In Townsend CM, Beauchamp RD, Evers BM, et al, editors: *Sabiston textbook of surgery: the biological basis of modern surgical practice*, ed 18, Philadelphia, 2008, WB Saunders.
2. Alarcon LH: Physiologic monitoring of the surgical patient. In Brunicardi FC, Andersen DK, Billiar TR, et al, editors: *Schwartz's principles of surgery*, ed 9, New York, 2010, McGraw-Hill.
3. Furnary AP, Zerr KJ, Grunkemeier GL, et al: Continuous intravenous insulin infusion reduces the incidence of deep sternal wound infection in diabetic patients after cardiac surgical procedures, *Ann Thorac Surg* 67:352–362, 1999.
4. Bartlett RH, Rich PB: Endocrine problems. American College of Surgeons ACS Surgery Principles and Practice. Retrieved May 2003 from www.acssurgery.com.
5. Dandona P, Thusu K, Hafeez R, et al: Effect of hydrocortisone on oxygen free radical generation by mononuclear cells, *Metabolism* 47:788–791, 1998.
6. Wiener RS, Wiener DC, Larson RJ. Benefits and risks of tight glucose control in critically ill adults: a meta-analysis, *JAMA.* 2008;300:933–944
7. Ansara MF, Gryer PE, Scharp DN: Diabetes mellitus. American College of Surgeons ACS Surgery Principles and Practice. Retrieved May 2003 from www.acssurgery.com.
8. Vinclair M, Broux C, Faure P, et al: Duration of adrenal inhibition following a single dose of etomidate in critically ill patients, *Intensive Care Med* 34:714–719, 2008.
9. Kinney MA, Narr BJ, Warner MA: Perioperative management of pheochromocytoma, *J Cardiothorac Vasc Anesth* 16:359–369, 2002.
10. Steinsapir J, Carr AA, Prisant LM, et al: Metyrosine and pheochromocytoma, *Arch Intern Med* 157:901–906, 1997.
11. Braverman LE, Utiger RD, editors: *The thyroid*, ed 6, Philadelphia, 1991, JP Lippincott, pp 1002–1004.
12. Steinberg AD: Myxedema and coronary artery disease: a comparative autopsy study, *Ann Intern Med* 68:338–344, 1968.
13. Abbott TR: Anaesthesia in untreated myxoedema: report of two cases, *Br J Anaesth* 39:510–514, 1967.
14. Kim JM, Hackman L: Anesthesia for untreated hypothyroidism: report of three cases, *Anesth Analg* 56:299–302, 1977.
15. Weinberg AD, Brennan MD, Gorman CA, et al: Outcome of anesthesia and surgery in hypothyroid patients, *Arch Intern Med* 143:893–897, 1983.
16. Ladenson PW, Levin AA, Ridgway EC, et al: Complications of surgery in hypothyroid patients, *Am J Med* 77:261–266, 1984.
17. Appoo JJ, Morin JF: Severe cerebral and cardiac dysfunction associated with thyroid decompensation after cardiac operations, *J Thorac Cardiovasc Surg* 114:496, 1997.
18. Catz B, Russell S. Myxedema, shock and coma: seven survival cases, *Arch Intern Med* 108:407–417, 1961.
19. Holvey DN, Goodner CJ, Nicoloff JT, et al: Treatment of myxedema coma with intravenous thyroxine, *Arch Intern Med* 113:89–96, 1964.
20. Ragaller M, Quintel M, Bender HJ, et al: Myxedema coma as a rare postoperative complication, *Anaesthesist* 42:179–183, 1993.
21. Bennett-Guerrero E, Kramer DC, Schwinn DA: Effect of chronic and acute thyroid hormone reduction on perioperative outcome, *Anesth Analg* 85:30–36, 1997.
22. Roti E, Robuschi G, Gardini E, et al: Comparison of methimazole, methimazole and sodium ipodate, and methimazole and saturated solution of potassium iodide in the early treatment of hyperthyroidoid Graves' disease, *Clin Endocrinol (OXF)* 28:305–314, 1988.
23. Baeza A, Aguayo J, Barria M, et al: Rapid preoperative preparation in hyperthyroidism, *Clin Endocrinol (OXF)* 35:439–442, 1991.
24. Nabil N, Miner DJ, Amatruda JM: Methimazole: an alternative route of administration, *J Clin Endocrinol Metab* 54:180–181, 1982.
25. Walter RM Jr., Bartle WR: Rectal administration of propylthiouracil in the treatment of Graves' disease, *Am J Med* 88:69–70, 1990.
26. Burch HB, Wartofsky L: Hyperthyroidism, *Curr Ther Endocrinol Metab* 5:64–70, 1994.
27. Burch HB, Wartofsky L: Life-threatening thyrotoxicosis. Thyroid storm, *Endocrinol Metab Clin North Am* 22:263–277, 1993.
28. Stoelting RK, Dierdorf SF: *Anesthesia and Co-Existing Disease*, ed 4, Philadelphia, 2000, Churchill Livingstone.
29. Barash PG, Cullen BF, Stoelting RK: *Clinical Anesthesia*, ed 4, Philadelphia, 2001, Lippincott Williams & Wilkins.
30. Eagle KA, Berger PB, Calkin H, et al: ACC/AHA guideline update for perioperative cardiovascular evaluation of non-cardiac surgery: a report of the American College of Cardiology/American Heart Association Task Force on Practice Guidelines 2002. Retrieved June 2003 from www.acc.org/clinical/guidelines/perio/update/periupdate_index.htm.
31. Amar D, Zhang H, Leung DH, et al: Older age is the strongest predictor of postoperative atrial fibrillation, *Anesthesiology* 96:352–356, 2002.
32. Bharucha D, Marinchak R, Kowey P. Arrhythmias after cardiac surgery: atrial fibrillation and atrial flutter. *Up to Date* 2003. Available at www.uptodate.com.
33. Miller RS: *Anesthesia*, vol. 2, ed 5, Philadelphia, 2000, Churchill Livingstone.
34. Mangano DT, Layug EI, Wallace A, et al: Effect of atenolol on mortality and cardiovascular morbidity after noncardiac surgery. Multicenter Study of Perioperative Ischemia Research Group, *N Engl J Med* 335:1713–1720, 1996.
35. POISE study group: Effects of extended-release metoprolol succinate in patients undergoing non-cardiac surgery (POISE trial): a randomized controlled trial, *Lancet* 371:1839–1847, 2008.
36. Newman MF, editor: *Perioperative Organ Protection*, Philadelphia, 2003, Lippincott Williams & Wilkins.
37. Friedman LS: The risk of surgery in patients with liver disease, *Hepatology* 29:1617–1623, 1999.
38. Solomon R, Werner C, Mann D, et al: Effects of saline, mannitol, and furosemide to prevent acute decreases in renal function induced by radiocontrast agents, *N Engl J Med* 331:1416–1420, 1994.
39. Cox CD, Tsikouris JP: Preventing contrast nephropathy: what is the best strategy? A review of the literature, *J Clin Pharmacol* 44:327–337, 2004.
40. Barrett BJ, Parfrey PS: Clinical practice: preventing nephropathy induced by contrast medium, *N Engl J Med* 2006; 354:379–386.

41. Guastoni C, De Servi S, D'Amicoc M: The role of dialysis in contrast-induced nephropathy: doubts and certainties, *J Cardiovasc Med (Hagerstown)* 8:549–557, 2007.
42. Pavlin DJ, Pavlin EG, Fitzgibbon DR, et al: Management of bladder function after outpatient surgery, *Anesthesiology* 91:42–50, 1999.
43. Apfel CC, Malhotra A, Leslie JB: The role of neurokinin-1 receptor antagonists for the management of postoperative nausea and vomiting, *Curr Opin Anaesthesiol* 21:427–432, 2008.
44. Apfel CC, Korttila K, Abdalla M, et al: A factorial trial of six interventions for the prevention of postoperative nausea and vomiting, *N Engl Med* 350:2441–2451, 2004.

# B. Anesthesia

*W. Christopher Croley, M.D., F.C.C.P., and James A. Colombo, M.D.*

1. During a tracheostomy, a flash is noted in the surgical field while using electrocautery. Which of the following is the correct sequence of steps in management of the patient?

   A. Extinguish the flames with saline solution or water; turn off all anesthetic gases, including $O_2$; and then hyperventilate with 21% $O_2$ through the endotracheal tube (ETT).

   B. Extinguish the flames with saline solution or water, turn off all anesthetic gases except $O_2$, and then hyperventilate with 100% $O_2$ through the ETT.

   C. Stop the ventilation; disconnect all anesthetic gas supply, including $O_2$; extinguish the flames with saline solution or water; remove the ETT; ventilate the patient with a mask; and then reintubate.

   D. Extinguish the flames with saline solution or water; remove all draping immediately; stop the ventilation; disconnect all anesthetic gas supply, including $O_2$; allow the patient to awaken; and then extubate.

   E. Stop the ventilation; disconnect all anesthetic gas supply, including $O_2$; extinguish the flames with saline solution or water; and resume ventilation.

   *Ref.:* 1

COMMENTS: **Airway fires** occur most often during laser airway surgery but can take place in any $O_2$-rich environment where igniting stimuli may exist. Any combustible material, including polyvinyl chloride tubing, surgical drapes, and human tissue, can ignite. Both the surgeon and the anesthesiologist should take the following steps simultaneously: stop all gas flow, including $O_2$; extinguish the fire with water or saline solution; and remove the ETT or any foreign body present in the airway (e.g., bronchoscope or gauze). Mask ventilation is performed until the trachea is reintubated. Bronchoscopy is then performed to determine the extent of the airway damage and to remove any foreign bodies that may be present. The trachea should be left intubated for at least 24 hours after an airway fire, and humidified gases should be administered through the ETT or tracheostomy tube. The use of steroids is controversial and probably of no benefit.

**ANSWER: C**

2. Effective management of gastric acid aspiration includes which of the following?

   A. Tracheal intubation and saline lavage of the lungs

   B. Prophylactic antibiotic therapy

   C. Prophylactic steroid therapy

   D. Suctioning and controlled ventilation with positive end-expiratory pressure (PEEP)

   E. Diuresis

   *Ref.:* 1-4

COMMENTS: **Gastric aspiration** can be a fatal complication. The severity of the injury is determined by the volume and pH of the gastric fluid aspirated. Fluid with a pH of less than 2.5 and a volume greater than 0.4 mL/kg (approximately 30 mL for an adult) is associated with a greater degree of pulmonary damage.

Initial treatment should begin with intubation, suctioning of aspirated fluid, testing the pH of the fluid (if readily available), and positive pressure ventilation with PEEP. The level of PEEP is determined by the ability to adequately oxygenate ($Pao_2$ >60 mm Hg) the patient, ideally with the fractional concentration of oxygen in inspired gas ($Fio_2$) below 60%. Saline lavage is not indicated because it has been shown to aggravate injury. Prophylactic antibiotic and steroid therapy is not indicated. With the initiation of positive pressure ventilation and loss of fluid into the damaged lung parenchyma, patients are often intravascularly depleted. Thus, empirical diuretic therapy is not appropriate.

Antibiotic therapy may be indicated in cases of aspiration in patients receiving enteral feeding but is not indicated as a general prophylactic maneuver. Steroid medications are not indicated in the initial stages of aspiration.

**ANSWER: D**

3. A 30 year old man undergoes hernia repair with spinal anesthesia. He calls the next day complaining of a headache that worsens with moving from a supine to a sitting position. He also has complaints of tinnitus. Initial treatment should include which of the following?

   A. Bed rest, increased fluid intake, and analgesics

   B. Urgent computed tomographic scan of brain to check for increased ICP

   C. Intravenous caffeine administration

   D. Placement of an epidural blood patch

   E. Remaining in the sitting position

   *Ref.:* 1

COMMENTS: **Post spinal anesthesia headache** is typically characterized by frontal or occipital cephalgia that worsens with sitting or standing and is usually relieved by assuming a supine position. Initial treatment is conservative and consists of bed rest, fluids, and analgesics. Caffeine administration may be of benefit if conservative measures fail. PDPH may be associated with neurologic findings. Common complaints are tinnitus, diplopia, and decreased hearing acuity. An epidural blood patch usually provides immediate relief of symptoms and is administered if conservative measures are ineffective in relieving severe symptoms after 24 hours. Factors associated with an increased incidence of PDPH include young age, female gender, large (cutting) spinal needles, and the direction of needle insertion. Insertion of spinal needle with a cutting bevel (Quincke design) in a direction nonparallel to the dural fibers (which are aligned in a vertical plane running cephalad to caudad) is associated with a higher incidence of PDPH. Informing the anesthesiologist that PDPH has occurred is helpful in guiding further treatment if required.

**ANSWER: A**

4. For a trauma patient with suspected intracranial hypertension, which intravenous anesthetic agent is contraindicated, even when mechanical ventilation is controlled?

   A. Midazolam

   B. Methohexital

   C. Thiopental

   D. Ketamine

   E. Morphine

*Ref.:* 1, 2

**COMMENTS:** Benzodiazepines (midazolam), opioids (morphine), and barbiturates (methohexital and thiopental) decrease cerebral blood flow and the cerebral metabolic rate, which in turn decrease ICP. **Ketamine** is an arylcyclohexylamine structurally related to phencyclidine. Ketamine increases the cerebral metabolic rate and cerebral blood flow and therefore ICP. Hence, ketamine is contraindicated when **intracranial hypertension** is suspected.

**ANSWER: D**

5. Intubation of a spontaneously breathing but obtunded patient with a closed head injury is best accomplished by which of the following?

   A. Application of topical lidocaine to the nares, spontaneous ventilation, and "blind" nasal intubation

   B. Induction with thiopental, muscle relaxation with succinylcholine, and oral tracheal intubation

   C. Awake fiberoptic intubation

   D. Awake tracheostomy with local anesthesia

   E. Awake rigid laryngoscopy

*Ref.:* 1, 3, 4

**COMMENTS:** Securing an airway in a trauma patient can be difficult. Concurrent cervical injury should be suspected in a patient with a head injury. All **airway management** should be done while maintaining in-line axial cervical stabilization. All the methods listed are acceptable for intubating this patient, but the ideal method would attenuate increases in ICP via thiopental induction, which can decrease cerebral blood flow and the cerebral metabolic rate by 40% to 60%. Succinylcholine causes small, transient increases in ICP (approximately 4 mm Hg), but these increases are offset by the ICP-reducing effect of thiopental. In addition, the muscle paralysis induced by succinylcholine prevents coughing, which can increase ICP by 50 to 70 mm Hg. Nasal intubation carries the risk of damage to the cribriform plate when preexisting fractures are present, and epistaxis can cause airway compromise in an obtunded patient. Blind intubation under these circumstances is therefore less desirable than other methods of securing an artificial airway. Tracheostomy should be performed whenever airway distortion prevents prompt intubation by other methods. In some situations, tracheostomy is the appropriate initial approach to securing the airway.

**ANSWER: B**

6. Use of succinylcholine should be avoided for which of the following patients?

   A. Patients with burns to 40% of their body surface area in need of emergency intubation 2 hours after injury

   B. Patients with burns to 40% of their body surface area in need of emergency intubation 5 days after injury

   C. Patients arriving at the emergency room immediately after sustaining an acute spinal cord injury (complete T4 injury)

   D. Children younger than 2 years

   E. Patients with end-stage renal disease and normal serum electrolyte levels

*Ref.:* 1, 2, 5

**COMMENTS:** Succinylcholine is a depolarizing **muscle relaxant**. It causes paralysis by depolarizing the motor end plate via repeated generation of action potentials. This results in an efflux of potassium ions and a transient rise in extracellular potassium levels. This increase is approximately 0.5 mEq/L in patients without neurologic deficits or severe muscular injury. Since the number of motor end plates is markedly increased (i.e., sensitization) 3 to 5 days after neurologic or muscular injury, administration of depolarizing muscle relaxants, such as succinylcholine, at this time can cause large increases in extracellular potassium and cardiac arrest. Therefore, succinylcholine should be used only in an acute setting (immediately after injury) for patients with burns or spinal cord injury in whom such sensitization is not observed within the first 1 to 2 days of injury. There are no contraindications to the use of succinylcholine in healthy children. The presence of renal failure does not preclude the use of succinylcholine if serum potassium levels are within a normal range.

**ANSWER: B**

7. Which of the following determines the spread of local anesthetics in cerebrospinal fluid?

   A. Addition of a narcotic to the local anesthetic

   B. Baricity of the local anesthetic

   C. Patient's body surface area

   D. Anesthetic volume

   E. Dose of the agent administered

*Ref.:* 1, 2

**COMMENTS: Spinal anesthesia** is accomplished by injecting a local anesthetic into the subarachnoid space. Addition of narcotics to the local anesthetic does not influence the spread of local anesthetic in cerebrospinal fluid unless a sufficient volume is added that changes the baricity of the local anesthetic solution. The degree of spread is determined primarily by the baricity of the solution and the patient's position. Baricity is the density of the local anesthetic solution in relation to the density of cerebrospinal fluid at normal body temperature. Local anesthetics are characterized as hyperbaric, hypobaric, or isobaric relative to cerebrospinal fluid. Normal lumbar lordosis and thoracic kyphosis of the spine also play a role in determining the final anesthetic level. The dose and specific type of local anesthetic agent used determine the duration of the resultant blockade, but not the spread. Relatively small volumes are used for spinal anesthesia and have little effect on the resultant neural blockade.

**ANSWER:**  B

8. Which of the following is true regarding malignant hyperthermia (MH)?

   A. Unusually low end-tidal carbon dioxide may be an early sign of MH.

   B. MH may be triggered by halogenated anesthetic agents, as well as by nitrous oxide.

   C. MH may be triggered by succinylcholine.

   D. Increased core temperature is an early sign of MH.

   E. MH is common and rarely results in significant morbidity.

*Ref.:* 1-5

COMMENTS: **Malignant hyperthermia** is a rare, potentially lethal condition. A fulminant episode is characterized by muscle rigidity, fever, tachycardia, respiratory and metabolic acidosis, severe hypermetabolism, arrhythmias, and eventual cardiovascular collapse. MH can occur minutes to several hours after the administration of triggering agents, such as succinylcholine or potent (halogenated) inhaled agents. The earliest, most sensitive, and most specific sign of MH is an unexplained rise in end-tidal $CO_2$ levels (with venous blood gas acidosis) followed by tachycardia, frequently with multifocal premature ventricular contractions. Increases in temperature are a relatively late finding.

Treatment involves cessation of the triggering anesthetics, administration of dantrolene, forced cooling of the patient, induction of saline diuresis to avoid renal dysfunction from myoglobinuria and widespread rhabdomyolysis, and monitoring of blood gas and potassium levels. MH is transmitted genetically, probably as an autosomal dominant trait with variable penetrance. Elevated serum creatinine phosphokinase levels can be seen in MH-susceptible patients, but this test is not useful for screening because of its poor specificity. Avoidance of triggering agents in patients suspected of MH susceptibility is the safest and easiest method of treatment.

**ANSWER:**  C

9. Which of the following statements regarding the toxicity of local anesthetics is false?

   A. Neurologic symptoms almost always precede those of cardiac toxicity.

   B. The site of injection is an important determinant of toxicity.

   C. The addition of a 1:100,000 epinephrine solution allows the administration of higher doses of local anesthetics.

   D. The relative toxicity of local anesthetics, in decreasing order, is procaine, lidocaine, bupivacaine, and tetracaine.

   E. Pregnancy reduces the risk for toxicity because hormones induce resistance to local anesthetics.

*Ref.:* 1-3, 5

COMMENTS: **Systemic toxicity from local anesthetics** primarily involves the CNS and the cardiovascular system. CNS toxicity usually occurs at doses well below those that result in cardiovascular toxicity. Manifestations of CNS toxicity include confusion, dizziness, tinnitus, somnolence, and seizures. The seizures are thought to be due to blockade of inhibitory pathways in the cerebral cortex. Cardiovascular toxicity is due to direct blocking effects on both cardiac and vascular smooth muscle and is generally manifested as cardiovascular collapse. Ventricular arrhythmias and asystole are the most common findings on the ECG.

Systemic absorption of local anesthetics is highly dependent on the vascularity of the injection site and the presence or absence of epinephrine. Epinephrine causes vasoconstriction and allows a higher maximum dose of local anesthetic to be safely administered without toxicity. Absorption of local anesthetics occurs most rapidly, with the highest serum levels, from the highly vascular intercostal space and is slowest, with the lowest serum levels, with infiltration of local subcutaneous tissue.

Pregnancy reduces the toxic threshold and the dose of local anesthetic needed for therapeutic purposes. The enlargement of the epidural veins seen with progressive enlargement of the uterus decreases the size of the epidural space and the volume of cerebrospinal fluid in the subarachnoid space. The decreased volume of these spaces facilitates the spread of local anesthetic. Biochemical changes of pregnancy, particularly progesterone, may also play a role in toxicity and spread of local anesthetics. It has been shown to have potent sedative effects.

**ANSWER:**  E

10. Which of the following statements regarding propofol is false?

    A. Induction and sedation doses for children are higher than those for adults after adjusting for weight.

    B. Propofol is a white, milky emulsion that may be contraindicated in patients with egg allergy.

    C. Unlike other induction agents, propofol does not suppress the respiratory system.

    D. The incidence of nausea and vomiting is lower with propofol-based anesthesia than with thiopental/isoflurane anesthesia.

    E. The hemodynamic changes seen with equianesthetic doses are frequently greater with propofol than with thiopental.

*Ref.:* 1, 2, 6

COMMENTS: **Propofol** is a nonbenzodiazepine, nonbarbiturate intravenous anesthetic with hypnotic properties. Stemming from its chemical structure as a substituted derivative of phenol, it is insoluble in water and is formulated as a 1% emulsion similar to parenteral lipid formulations. Persons allergic to eggs may have allergies to this formulation. Induction doses are higher for children and adolescents than for adults and should be reduced for elderly patients, hypovolemic patients, and those with poor cardiac reserve. Propofol produces profound dose-dependent respiratory depression that frequently leads to apnea in patients premedicated with other sedatives. After single-bolus administration, propofol is rapidly redistributed (in 2 to 8 minutes) and highly metabolized. For this reason, it is most commonly administered by continuous intravenous infusion. Emergence from anesthesia occurs rapidly after discontinuation of propofol, thus making it particularly suitable for short procedures. Nausea and vomiting are seen less frequently with a propofol-based anesthetic than with thiopental/isoflurane anesthesia, but the hemodynamic alterations are similar to or even greater than those seen with equianesthetic doses of thiopental.

**ANSWER:   C**

11. Which of the following statements regarding midazolam is true?

    A. Midazolam is a highly lipid-soluble agent that typically causes pain on injection.

    B. Midazolam is ten times as potent as diazepam.

    C. The respiratory depression caused by midazolam is usually minor but can be greatly exacerbated by the concomitant use of other sedatives or opioids.

    D. Midazolam has no active metabolites, which makes it ideal for use in outpatients.

    E. Midazolam is renally metabolized.

*Ref.:* 1, 2, 6

**COMMENTS:** Midazolam differs from other **benzodiazepines** in both structure and solubility. An imidazole side ring imparts stability and ease of rapid hepatic metabolism, and a water-soluble structure allows painless injection. Two active metabolites of midazolam exist and accumulate when continuous infusions are used. Like other benzodiazepines, midazolam potentiates respiratory depression (often synergistically) when administered with other sedatives or opioids. Benzodiazepines readily cross the placenta and have been associated with an increased incidence of cleft lip and palate when administered during the first trimester. Safety later in pregnancy has not been definitively established.

**ANSWER:   C**

12. Which of the following statements regarding neuromuscular blockade by nondepolarizing agents is false?

    A. The effects are prolonged by aminoglycosides.

    B. Vagolytic side effects occur with pancuronium.

    C. Nondepolarizing agents may trigger MH.

    D. Vecuronium undergoes mostly hepatic metabolism.

    E. Train-of-four monitoring effectively predicts the degree of blockade.

*Ref.:* 1, 2, 6

**COMMENTS:** Nondepolarizing muscle relaxants currently in clinical use include pancuronium, vecuronium, atracurium, cisatracurium, mivacurium, rocuronium, and doxacurium. Nondepolarizing muscle relaxants interfere with transmission at the neuromuscular junction by competing with acetylcholine for available receptor sites. These effects may be reversed by anticholinesterases, which prolong the half-life of acetylcholine to overcome the competitive inhibition of the muscle relaxant. The effect of nondepolarizing agents can be prolonged by aminoglycosides, clindamycin, tetracycline and other antibiotics, hypothermia, hypercapnia, and magnesium. Vagolytic activity is common with pancuronium and rocuronium but not with other agents. Except for mivacurium (which is metabolized by plasma cholinesterase) and atracurium/cisatracurium (which are metabolized by Hofman

elimination and nonspecific ester hydrolysis), the metabolism of nondepolarizing agents occurs in the liver, with varying amounts of biliary or renal metabolism and excretion. Train-of-four monitoring involves the administration of stimuli percutaneously to a peripheral nerve four times over a 1-second period and noting the distal muscular response. If fewer than two of the stimuli result in muscle contraction, more than 95% of the receptors are blocked.

**ANSWER:   C**

13. Which of the following statements regarding flumazenil is true?

    A. It is a benzodiazepine antagonist that acts by competitive inhibition.

    B. It has been used successfully to reverse the clinical effects of narcotic overdose.

    C. It is indicated for patients with suspected cyclic antidepressant overdoses.

    D. It reverses the respiratory depressant actions but not the sedative effects of all benzodiazepines.

    E. It is unlikely to improve the encephalopathy associated with hepatic failure.

*Ref.:* 1, 2, 6

**COMMENTS:** Flumazenil is a **benzodiazepine**-specific antagonist that competitively inhibits the activity of benzodiazepines at the benzodiazepine-receptor complex. Flumazenil does not antagonize the CNS effects of GABAergic-acting (leading to the secretion of γ-aminobutyric acid) drugs (ethanol, barbiturates, or general anesthetics), nor does it antagonize the effects of opioids. Flumazenil antagonizes the sedation, impaired recall, psychomotor impairment, and ventilatory depression produced by all benzodiazepines. Use of flumazenil is contraindicated in patients given benzodiazepines for life-threatening conditions (e.g., control of status epilepticus or ICP), patients showing serious signs of cyclic antidepressant overdose (because of an increased occurrence of seizures), and patients with known hypersensitivities. Case reports have demonstrated remarkable improvement in the encephalopathic changes associated with liver failure. Flumazenil should not be used as the only agent for treating hepatic encephalopathy but may be helpful in patients resistant to conventional medical therapy.

**ANSWER:   A**

14. Mechanisms of heat loss during general anesthesia include which of the following?

    A. Convection

    B. Radiation

    C. Conduction

    D. Evaporation

    E. All of the above

*Ref.:* 1, 2, 5

**COMMENTS: Heat loss** in the operating room (OR) is a complex problem involving all of the mechanisms mentioned. The contribution of each mechanism depends on the surrounding conditions in the OR. Radiative losses are often cited as the largest contributor to heat loss in the OR. Radiant energy is emitted by every body with a temperature higher than 0° K. Radiation requires no medium for transport because it is electromagnetic. Heat freely radiates from a body at a temperature of 37° C to a room at 25° C as long as the temperature gradient exists. Conductive heat loss requires that bodies be in direct contact with each other. Body heat is conducted to the OR table and other surfaces that come in contact with the patient. Heat is lost from the body by convection when OR air, which is circulated at a speed of approximately 3 cm/s, passes over the body. Finally, heat losses from the latent heat of vaporization (evaporation) occur during mechanical ventilation with dry air, during skin preparation with cold cleansing solutions, through sweating, and from large open wounds.

**ANSWER:** E

15. With regard to pulse oximetry studies, which of the following is true?

    A. Pulse oximetric analysis is unaffected by tissue perfusion.

    B. Methemoglobinemia results in a displayed arterial oxygen saturation of 85%.

    C. Oxygen saturation measurements may be artificially decreased in the presence of carboxyhemoglobin.

    D. A standard pulse oximeter measures light absorption at four wavelengths.

    E. Ambient light will not affect oximetric readings.

    ***Ref.:*** *1, 4, 6*

**COMMENTS:** The use of **pulse oximetry** studies has led to marked improvement in the care and safety of patients not only in the OR but also in the postanesthesia care unit and the intensive care unit. The concept of oximetry is based on Beer's law, which relates the concentration of a solute in suspension (in this case, hemoglobin) to the intensity of light transmitted through the solution. Pulse oximetric analysis measures the oxygen saturation only of pulsatile blood by using two wavelengths of light (red and infrared). The ratio of the pulse-added absorbencies of these two wavelengths is determined by the arterial oxygen saturation. Pulse oximetry may be difficult to perform in patients who are suffering from any type of shock or tissue hypoperfusion. Because both oxyhemoglobin and carboxyhemoglobin absorb red light similarly, the pulse oximeter reads the sum of the two hemoglobins and produces an artificially elevated reading of oxygen saturation. Direct measurement of saturation from an arterial blood gas sample is required to confirm the presence of carbon monoxide. Methemoglobinemia, a disorder that may occur with nitroglycerin toxicity or inhaled nitric oxide therapy, results in a displayed oxygen saturation of 85%. Methemoglobin does not absorb red light in the same manner as oxyhemoglobin or deoxyhemoglobin does. The absorbance of red and infrared light by methemoglobin is nearly equal and results in a displayed saturation of approximately 85%. Because ambient light can affect pulse oximeter readings, it is occasionally necessary to cover the probe to avoid artifactual readings.

**ANSWER:** B

16. While transporting an intubated patient from the OR to the intensive care unit, the pressure gauge on a completely filled size E compressed gas cylinder containing $O_2$ reads 2200 psi. How long can $O_2$ be delivered at a flow rate of 5 L/min from an E cylinder whose pressure gauge reads 1100 psi?

    A. 60 seconds

    B. 5 minutes

    C. 60 minutes

    D. 125 minutes

    E. 220 minutes

    ***Ref.:*** *1, 2*

**COMMENTS:** A full E cylinder reading 2200 psi contains approximately 625 L of $O_2$. Boyle's law states that for a fixed mass of gas at constant temperature, the product of pressure and volume is constant. Boyle's law allows estimation of the volume of gas remaining in a closed container by measuring the pressure within the container. When the pressure gauge reads 1100 psi, the volume of gas in the cylinder is half that of a full cylinder (or about 625 L ÷ 2 = 312.5 L). At a flow rate of 5 L/min, the cylinder in question will last approximately 1 hour. This information is important when portable sources of oxygen are being used during transport and diagnostic procedures remote from the OR.

**ANSWER:** C

17. After administration of epidural anesthesia to the T3 dermatome of a patient with severe lung disease who is undergoing open cholecystectomy, which of the following is least likely to occur?

    A. Increased heart rate

    B. Decreased venous return

    C. Decreased alveolar ventilation

    D. Systemic hypotension

    E. All of the above

    ***Ref.:*** *1, 2, 5*

**COMMENTS:** On average, after administration of epidural anesthesia, central neuraxial blockade to the T3 sensory dermatome is associated with sympathetic blockade two spinal segment levels higher and motor blockade two spinal segments lower. Blockade of the cardiac accelerator nerves (T1-4) and unopposed vagal activity result in relative bradycardia despite hypotension caused by the reduction in venous return secondary to vasodilation. In addition, motor nerve blockade of intercostal muscle function reduces alveolar ventilation and may precipitate respiratory embarrassment in a patient with underlying pulmonary disease, particularly if a significant fraction of intercostal muscle function is impaired.

**ANSWER:** A

18. Which of the following is least likely to occur in conjunction with a surgically induced stress response?

    A. Increased metabolic rate

    B. Hypercoagulability

    C. Suppression of the immune response

    D. Increased secretion of ACTH

    E. Increased secretion of thyroid-stimulating hormone

    ***Ref.:*** *7*

**COMMENTS:** Current evidence suggests that many adverse perioperative events can be attributed to the effects of the **stress response**. Somatic or visceral pain can trigger the systemic release of catecholamines and neuroendocrine hormones. Hormones released in response to stress include growth hormone, ACTH, vasopressin, prolactin, cortisol, glucagons, and renin-angiotensin-aldosterone. In contrast, secretion of thyroid-stimulating hormone is decreased by the stress response. The overall systemic effects of the stress response lead to increased metabolic activity, a hypercoagulable state, and a less effective immune response to infectious agents.

**ANSWER:** E

19. Preoperative noninvasive testing for the presence of inducible myocardial ischemia would be most appropriate for which of the following patients?

   A. A healthy 60-year-old man without historical cardiac risk factors scheduled for gastrectomy because of gastric carcinoma

   B. A patient with a history of MI 1 year previously and good exercise tolerance undergoing laparoscopic cholecystectomy

   C. A patient with diabetes and renal insufficiency undergoing inguinal hernia repair

   D. A patient with limited exercise tolerance and diabetes undergoing right hemicolectomy

   E. All of the above

*Ref.: 1*

**COMMENTS:** The need for **preoperative cardiac testing** is determined by assessing a patient's risk for **perioperative cardiac complications** and the likelihood that the surgical procedure will produce physiologic conditions that increase myocardial demand. Good exercise tolerance is an important prognostic determinant and can mitigate the need for cardiac testing if patients have known stable cardiac disease and are undergoing intermediate-risk surgery. Operations associated with large fluid shifts or high blood loss, along with vascular surgical procedures, are commonly cited as higher-risk operations. Patients at risk for cardiac complications will benefit from perioperative β-blocker therapy, and β-blockers should be given to all patients with cardiac risk factors unless contraindicated. Patients at high risk for cardiac complications undergoing intermediate- to high-risk surgical procedures (in reference to cardiac outcomes) should have noninvasive assessment of cardiac performance and possibly invasive testing if the noninvasive test results suggest significant cardiac risk. Since surgery in itself is not an indication for cardiac testing, the patient described in scenario A needs no further cardiac work-up.

**ANSWER:** D

20. A 67-year-old woman is scheduled for right hemicolectomy because of carcinoma of the colon. She has adult-onset diabetes and shortness of breath when climbing stairs. A 12-lead ECG shows signs of bradycardia with left bundle branch block. Her serum creatinine level is 2.1 mg/dL. What is the most appropriate next step?

   A. Conduct cardiac catheterization immediately.

   B. Proceed with surgery and evaluate risk status postoperatively.

   C. Administer an exercise ECG.

   D. Administer a dobutamine stress echocardiogram.

   E. Institute β-blockade.

*Ref.: 1*

**COMMENTS:** This patient has a number of intermediate risk factors for perioperative cardiac complications, including an elevated serum creatinine level, limited exercise tolerance, left bundle branch block, and diabetes. It is possible that perioperative risk can be altered by preoperative testing and subsequent interventions. Provocative cardiac tests such as a dobutamine stress echocardiography further stratify risk and help identify patients who need further cardiac work-up or interventions.

**ANSWER:** D

**REFERENCES**

1. Rogers MC, Tinker JH, Covino BG, et al, editors: *Principles and practice of anesthesiology*, ed 2, St. Louis, 1998, Mosby–Year Book.
2. Stoelting RK, editor: *Pharmacology and physiology in anesthetic practice*, ed 3, Philadelphia, 1999, JB Lippincott.
3. Sherwood ER, Williams CG, Prough DS: Anesthesiology principles, pain management, and conscious sedation. In Townsend CM, Beauchamp RD, Evers BM, et al, editors: *Sabiston textbook of surgery: the biological basis of modern surgical practice*, ed 18, Philadelphia, 2008, WB Saunders.
4. Dorian RS: Anesthesia of the surgical patient. In Brunicardi FC, Andersen DK, Billiar TR, et al, editors: *Schwartz's principles of surgery*, ed 9, New York, 2010, McGraw-Hill.
5. De Lanzac KS, Thomas MA, Riopelle JM: Anesthesia. In O'Leary JP, editor: *The physiologic basis of surgery*, ed 4, Philadelphia, 2008, Lippincott Williams & Wilkins.
6. Rutter TW, Tremper KK: Anesthesiology and pain management. In Mulholland MW, Lillemoe KD, Doherty GM, et al, editors: *Greenfield's surgery: scientific principles and practice*, ed 4, Philadelphia, 2006, Lippincott Williams & Wilkins.
7. Fleisher LA, Eagle KA: Clinical practice: lowering cardiac risk in noncardiac surgery, *N Engl J Med* 345:1677–1682, 2001.

# ACUTE AND CRITICAL CARE

# CHAPTER 8

# Acute Abdomen

*Nadine D. Floyd, M.D., and Theodore J. Saclarides, M.D.*

1. With regard to C fibers and visceral peritoneal innervation, which of the following statements is true?

   A. They are myelinated, polymodal nociceptors.

   B. They travel bilaterally with the sympathetic chains.

   C. Their stimulation is interpreted as localized, sharp pain.

   D. They conduct rapidly (<0.5 m/s).

   E. They refer pain to dermatomes.

   *Ref.:* 1-4

**COMMENTS:** See Question 2.

**ANSWER: B**

2. Which of the following is not a trigger of visceral pain?

   A. Ischemia

   B. Traction

   C. Distention

   D. Heat

   E. Inflammation

   *Ref.:* 1-4

**COMMENTS:** The visceral peritoneum is innervated by C fibers coursing with the autonomic ganglia. C fibers are unmyelinated, slow-conducting (0.5 to 5.0 m/s), polymodal nociceptors that travel bilaterally with the sympathetic and parasympathetic fibers. **Visceral pain** is a response to injury to the visceral peritoneum. Distention, stretch, traction, compression, torsion, ischemia, and inflammation trigger visceral pain fibers. Abdominal organs are insensate to heat, cutting, and electrical stimulation.

Visceral pain is typically vague and crampy and is perceived in the region of origin of the embryologically derived autonomic ganglia. Foregut organs (proximal to the ligament of Treitz) refer pain to the celiac chain, and the pain is felt in the epigastrium. Inflammation of the gallbladder may be perceived in both the epigastrium and the shoulder; the latter is typical for organs that reside in close proximity to the diaphragms. The organs of the midgut (small intestine and ascending colon) refer pain to the superior mesenteric chain (periumbilical pain) and those of the hindgut (transverse and descending colon, sigmoid colon, and rectum) to the inferior mesenteric ganglia and hypogastrium.

**ANSWER: D**

3. An 18-year-old man has a 12-hour history of vague, periumbilical abdominal pain, anorexia, and nonbilious vomiting. The pain has now localized to the right lower quadrant. On examination he is found to have tenderness over the McBurney point along with involuntary muscle rigidity. Which of the following best explains the localization of pain?

   A. Inflammation of the visceral peritoneum produces localizing pain.

   B. Pain over the McBurney point is caused by distention of the appendiceal lumen.

   C. Unmyelinated fibers carry pain signals with the thoracic and lumbar spinal nerves.

   D. Movement of the inflamed parietal peritoneum induces rebound tenderness.

   E. The somatic pain fibers course through spinal nerve roots L3-5.

   *Ref.:* 2-5

**COMMENTS:** Typically, early in the course of **appendicitis**, distention of the appendiceal lumen triggers the visceral nerves that course with the superior mesenteric artery ganglia and produces vague pain that is perceived in the periumbilical region. As appendiceal inflammation progresses and involves the parietal peritoneum, somatic pain fibers are triggered; these are thinly myelinated, fast-conducting fibers and course with the spinal nerve roots T7-L2. Movement of the inflamed parietal peritoneum will trigger these fibers and is the cause of "rebound tenderness." Muscle rigidity is involuntary spasm of the abdominal muscles in response to peritoneal inflammation.

**ANSWER: D**

4. Which of the following is not an ominous sign in a patient with abdominal pain?

   A. Diaphoresis

   B. Pallor

   C. Hypotension

   D. Patient lying still

   E. Jaundice

   *Ref.:* 2-4

**COMMENTS:** Initial evaluation of patients with **acute abdominal pain** should include assessment for signs of shock. Shock may be secondary to hypovolemia or a systemic inflammatory response. Signs include tachycardia, hypotension, pallor, dry mucous membranes, poor skin turgor, and slow capillary refill. Immediate intravenous access and resuscitation should be initiated. A patient writhing with colicky pain may have distention or obstruction of a hollow viscus (e.g., ureter or intestine), whereas a patient lying very still probably has diffuse peritoneal inflammation and a perforated viscus. A patient with right upper quadrant pain, fever, jaundice, and signs of septic shock may have ascending cholangitis requiring emergency decompression of the biliary tree. However, jaundice itself is not necessarily an ominous sign.

**ANSWER:** E

5. Regarding peritoneal fluids, which of the following statements is true?

   A. The abdominal cavity normally contains 150 to 200 mL (3 g/dL of isotonic fluid).

   B. The protein content of peritoneal fluid is 3 g/dL.

   C. Mesothelial cells absorb solutes via gradient-driven passive osmosis.

   D. Inflammation of the peritoneum decreases its permeability.

   E. Bacteria contaminating the peritoneum enter the systemic circulation through the subdiaphragmatic lymphatics.

*Ref.:* 2

**COMMENTS:** Normally, the peritoneum contains 50 to 100 mL of fluid, with solute concentrations being equal to those found in plasma. The protein content is less than that of plasma (3 g/dL). Fluid is absorbed by the mesothelial cells lining the peritoneum through endocytosis. Solutes with a molecular weight less than 30 kD are easily absorbed. Inflammation of the peritoneum increases its permeability. Gravity and the negative pressure created by exhalation under the diaphragm effect movement of the peritoneal fluid. The right paracolic gutter allows unhindered movement of fluid from the pelvis to the right subdiaphragmatic area, whereas the phrenicocolic ligaments obstruct flow through the left paracolic gutter. The **subdiaphragmatic lymphatics** play a major role in the absorption of peritoneal fluid and clearance of solutes and bacteria into the thoracic duct.

**ANSWER:** E

6. Which of the following will not alter the natural flow of peritoneal fluid?

   A. Fibrin

   B. Bowel obstruction

   C. Cirrhosis

   D. Positive pressure ventilation

   E. Previous appendectomy

*Ref.:* 2

**COMMENTS:** Adhesions, fibrin, paralytic ileus, and positive pressure mechanical ventilation all obstruct the normal **flux of peritoneal fluid**. Adhesions from previous surgery may create compartments within the abdominal cavity that are sequestered from the natural flow of peritoneal fluid. Fluid loss may occur in long-standing bowel obstruction that alters the dynamics of fluid secretion and absorption.

**ANSWER:** C

7. Regarding bacterial contamination of the peritoneal cavity, which of the following statements is not true?

   A. Bacterial contamination of the peritoneum triggers degranulation of mesothelial cells, which initiates the systemic inflammatory response.

   B. Once the systemic response is initiated, the endothelial cells increase their permeability to complement, opsonins, and fibrin.

   C. Serum levels of catecholamines decrease in feedback to mast cell degranulation.

   D. Ninety percent of the bacteria are cleared by phagocytosis and the reticular endothelial system.

   E. Intraabdominal bacteria enter the systemic circulation through the thoracic duct.

*Ref.:* 2

**COMMENTS:** Bacterial contamination triggers mast cells to degranulate, thereby initiating a local and systemic cascade of events. Locally, mesothelial and endothelial cells increase their permeability and allow products of complement, opsonins, and fibrin to enter the peritoneal cavity freely. This increased permeability depletes intravascular volume as fluid shifts into the peritoneal cavity. The **systemic inflammatory response syndrome** (SIRS) is initiated and consists of an increase in serum levels of catecholamines, glucocorticoids, aldosterone, and vasopressin. The combination of hypovolemia and SIRS causes hyperdynamic hemodynamics. After bacteria enter the abdomen, they circulate via the subdiaphragmatic lymphatics and enter the systemic circulation through the thoracic duct. Once circulating, more than 90% will be cleared by Kupffer cells and the reticuloendothelial system.

**ANSWER:** C

8. Regarding the initial assessment of a patient who comes to the emergency department because of acute abdominal pain, which of the following statements is not true?

   A. Performing thin-cut computed tomographic (CT) scanning with contrast enhancement is the first step in evaluating an acute abdomen.

   B. Absence of bowel sounds may be seen in cases of mechanical bowel obstruction.

   C. Hypoactive bowel sounds may suggest an intraabdominal infection.

   D. Plain radiographic studies can demonstrate abdominal free air, ascites, intraabdominal abscess, and intestinal pneumatosis.

   E. Ultrasound imaging permits diagnostic and therapeutic treatment of fluid collections.

*Ref.:* 2

**COMMENTS:** In a stable patient, a thorough history and physical examination are paramount in determining the potential cause of an **acute abdomen** and directing the initial work-up; CT scanning is not a substitute for doing so. Distention and high-pitched bowel sounds may represent an early mechanical bowel obstruction. Decreased or absent bowel sounds are suggestive of ileus secondary to an infectious process but may also be found in cases of long-standing obstruction. For a patient with a diffusely rigid abdomen, plain radiographs (upright chest radiograph or lateral decubitus films) may identify free air, which is suggestive of a perforated viscus. Plain radiographs can also demonstrate loculated extraluminal air-fluid levels (e.g., abscess), pneumobilia, portal vein air, pneumatosis intestinalis, or loss of the psoas shadow and fat lines (e.g., ascites). CT and ultrasound imaging can also demonstrate these abnormalities and more accurately characterize intraabdominal fluid or abscess. These modalities may also permit therapeutic percutaneous treatment of fluid collections.

**ANSWER:**  A

9. A 55-year-old man comes to the emergency department with a 6-hour history of acute, diffuse abdominal pain. On examination, his heart rate is found to be 115 beats per minute, his blood pressure 95/60 mm Hg, his respiratory rate 22 breaths per minute, and his pulse oximetric reading 93% on a 4-L nasal cannula. He has diffuse abdominal rigidity. Plain radiographic studies demonstrate extraluminal free air. Regarding resuscitation of the patient in the emergency department before transfer to the operating room, which of the following statements is true?

   A. Intravenous administration of antibiotics is the first priority.

   B. The initial intravenous access of choice is a central venous catheter.

   C. Two to 3 L of crystalloid should be administered intravenously.

   D. Endotracheal intubation should be established immediately.

   E. A CT scan of the abdomen should be ordered immediately

*Ref.:* 2, 3

**COMMENTS:** The initial evaluation of a patient with **abdominal pain** should include assessment for signs of hemodynamic instability, including tachycardia, hypotension, pallor, decreased skin turgor, and decreased urine output. Establishing intravenous access and starting intravenous hydration should be undertaken immediately, and for a patient with hypotension, boluses of crystalloid (lactated Ringer or normal saline solution) should be given. Routine pulmonary artery catheterization is not required unless there is a known history of serious cardiac disease or renal failure. However, if there is no evidence of active bleeding and the blood pressure does not improve after a minimum of 3 L of crystalloid has been infused, cardiac status should be reassessed and central venous pressure measurements considered. Not all patients require mechanical ventilation, but if there is evidence of rapid shallow breathing, impending ventilatory failure (hypercapnia, $Paco_2$ >50 mm Hg, pH <7.35), or a shunt refractory to oxygen failure (hypoxia, $Pao_2$ <60 mm Hg on an $Fio_2$ of 100%), endotracheal intubation and mechanical ventilation should be established.

**ANSWER:**  C

10. Regarding patients with a rigid abdomen and free air on plain film, which of the following statements is true?

   A. No further radiologic work-up is required.

   B. CT scanning with contrast enhancement is required to confirm the diagnosis.

   C. Bedside sonographic imaging is preferred over CT imaging to confirm the diagnosis of free air.

   D. Narcotics are contraindicated in patients with an acute abdomen.

   E. Preoperative prophylactic steroids are indicated in patients with free air.

*Ref.:* 2

**COMMENTS:** For a patient with a rigid abdomen and **free air** revealed by plain film imaging, no further radiographic work-up is required. Time would be unnecessarily wasted pursuing CT or sonographic imaging in a patient who needs prompt surgical exploration. Narcotics may be given after a patient has been adequately examined, a differential diagnosis established, and a treatment plan instituted. However, caution should be taken in administering narcotics to a hypotensive, incompletely resuscitated patient. There is no role for prophylactic steroid administration except for patients who take steroids chronically and are experiencing abdominal pain or an Addisonian crisis.

**ANSWER:**  A

11. A 35-year-old woman experiences an acute onset of epigastric and right upper quadrant pain several hours after a large dinner. She has had similar episodes in the past that resolved after a few hours. This episode persists, and she has fever and nonbilious vomiting. What is the most likely source of the abdominal pain?

   A. Perforated ulcer

   B. Acute appendicitis

   C. Perforation following bowel obstruction

   D. Cholecystitis

   E. Diverticulitis

*Ref.:* 2-4

**COMMENTS:** See Question 15.

**ANSWER:**  D

12. A 60-year-old man with chronic alcoholism awakens at 3:00 AM with severe, sharp epigastric pain that 3 hours later becomes diffuse abdominal pain. What is the most likely source of the abdominal pain?

   A. Perforated ulcer

   B. Acute appendicitis

   C. Perforation following bowel obstruction

   D. Cholecystitis

   E. Diverticulitis

*Ref.:* 2-4

**COMMENTS:** See Question 15.

**ANSWER:**  A

13. A 55-year-old man with a 2-day history of abdominal distention, vomiting, crampy abdominal pain, and obstipation is experiencing severe, diffuse abdominal pain. What is the most likely source of the abdominal pain?

   A. Perforated ulcer

   B. Acute appendicitis

   C. Perforation following bowel obstruction

D. Cholecystitis

E. Diverticulitis

*Ref.:* 2-4

**COMMENTS:** See Question 15.

**ANSWER: C**

14. A 22-year-old man awakens with periumbilical abdominal pain followed by nonbilious vomiting. What is the most likely source of the abdominal pain?

A. Perforated ulcer

B. Acute appendicitis

C. Perforation following bowel obstruction

D. Cholecystitis

E. Diverticulitis

*Ref.:* 2-4

**COMMENTS:** See Question 15.

**ANSWER: B**

15. A 65-year-old man with a history of chronic constipation has a 3-day history of abdominal distention without a bowel movement. He has fever and abdominal rigidity. What is the most likely source of the abdominal pain?

A. Perforated ulcer

B. Acute appendicitis

C. Perforation following bowel obstruction

D. Cholecystitis

E. Diverticulitis

*Ref.:* 2-4

**COMMENTS:** The examples in Questions 11 to 15 demonstrate the importance of a thorough history in determining a patient's diagnosis and tailoring the initial work-up in the management of an **acute abdomen**. Differentiating between patients who require immediate intervention and those who can undergo a more gradual work-up is also essential to avoid unnecessary delays in treatment. Biliary pain is typically midepigastric, with radiation to the right upper quadrant and right subscapular area. It often occurs after the intake of fatty food. It may be intermittent, crampy pain or constant, severe pain associated with nausea and vomiting.

Patients with a perforated ulcer will classically remember the exact moment when the perforation occurred. There may be an initial period of diminished pain followed by severe pain when diffuse chemical peritonitis sets in. Risk factors include a previous history of peptic ulcer disease, untreated *Helicobacter pylori* infection, use of medications such as steroids and nonsteroidal antiinflammatory drugs, and alcohol abuse.

When vomiting is part of the history, it is important to differentiate between patients with mechanical obstruction of the bowel, bile duct, or pancreatic duct and patients who have ileus in response to problems from a nonintestinal source. A patient with acute appendicitis and periumbilical pain may have one or two episodes of nonbilious emesis before localization of pain in the lower right quadrant. The early abdominal pain and vomiting

associated with appendicitis may resemble gastroenteritis. However, in appendicitis, pain is the predominant clinical feature and precedes diarrhea and vomiting in most instances. With gastroenteritis, the vomiting is typically more profuse and frequent and may be accompanied by profuse diarrhea as well.

A history of weight loss or new-onset obstipation and changes in stool patterns may suggest a colorectal malignancy. The duration of time over which these symptoms have developed and progressed may give insight regarding the urgency of the problem. A patient with a 3-day history of progressively obstructive symptoms (i.e., distention, crampy pain, and vomiting) and who has peritonitis and fever is more likely to have a complicated obstruction (e.g., ischemic, gangrenous, or perforated bowel) requiring immediate intervention. If the pain is diffuse, it may herald a free perforation causing diffuse contamination of the peritoneal cavity. If the pain is localized, it may represent a contained perforation, as can occur with diverticulitis. This type of pain typically occurs in the lower left quadrant. In contrast, weight loss, cachexia, a slow decrease in stool caliber, and mild cramping reflect a more gradual process that permits elective work-up and treatment.

**ANSWER: E**

16. A 65-year-old man with a history of chronic alcohol abuse has been experiencing epigastric and periumbilical pain associated with nonbilious vomiting for 1 day. He denies any melena or hematemesis. In the past he has had several episodes of similar pain that sometimes radiated to the back, and he was hospitalized for several days 2 months ago. He denies any previous surgery or medical problems. His blood pressure is 120/80 mm Hg, his pulse is 110 beats per minute, and his mucous membranes are dry. His abdomen is not distended and does not have any surgical scars. Bowel sounds are present but diminished. His abdomen is soft, and he exhibits voluntary guarding of the epigastrium. His serum amylase level is 550 units/100 mL. Regarding management of this patient, which of the following is the most reasonable initial step?

A. Establish intravenous access.

B. Conduct sonographic studies to demonstrate cholelithiasis.

C. Perform CT scanning to diagnose a pancreatic pseudocyst.

D. Perform esophagogastroduodenoscopy (EGD) to evaluate for varices and complications of cirrhosis.

E. Initiate a low-fat diet and antilipid treatment.

*Ref.:* 2, 6

**COMMENTS:** A patient with **pancreatitis** can have severe abdominal pain and rigidity. Surgery should be avoided except for complications (e.g., necrotizing pancreatitis or symptomatic pseudocyst). Initial management of a patient with acute pancreatitis should include bowel rest, intravenous resuscitation, parenteral nutrition, and monitoring in the intensive care unit when appropriate. Causes of pancreatitis should be investigated, including gallstones, hyperlipidemia, and drugs (i.e., thiazides). Alcohol abuse is a common cause of pancreatitis, but the fact that a patient abuses alcohol should not dismiss the necessity for a thorough work-up. After stabilization and resuscitation, diagnostic studies are conducted to define the pancreas and biliary tree. Sonographic studies can screen for stones but may not provide a good evaluation of the retroperitoneum because of overlying bowel gas. CT scanning with contrast enhancement and dedicated fine cuts through the pancreas reveals good pancreatic and retroperitoneal detail in most patients.

For patients with recurrent or chronic pancreatitis, a CT scan should be performed to look for complications of pancreatitis, such as a pancreatic pseudocyst, fistula, or mass. EGD is not generally used to make the diagnosis of pancreatitis. It may be a useful adjunctive diagnostic and potentially therapeutic tool during the evaluation of alcoholic patients experiencing upper gastrointestinal bleeding.

**ANSWER:** A

17. A patient with known diverticular disease of the colon has a 5-day history of worsening pain in the left lower quadrant. He now has fever and had diarrhea this morning. On examination he is found to have fullness in the lower left quadrant with guarding. What would the best management now include?

    A. Diagnostic laparoscopy

    B. Immediate operative exploration

    C. Air-contrast enema

    D. Colonoscopy

    E. CT scan of the abdomen and pelvis

*Ref.:* 2, 7

**COMMENTS:** In complicated cases, such as those involving fever, a mass, localized peritonitis, and leukocytosis, hospitalization with bowel rest, broad-spectrum intravenous antibiotics, and serial examinations should be initiated. CT scanning should be performed to differentiate cases of **diverticulitis** from phlegmon and abscess. The latter can be drained percutaneously. Elective resection and primary anastomosis can then be undertaken following successful nonoperative treatment of an abscess and after the inflammation has subsided. A patient who becomes hemodynamically unstable during a period of conservative management or does not improve with nonoperative measures will require prompt surgical exploration. In this setting, resection of the diseased segment is generally preferred, but the surgeon may elect to perform fecal diversion and drainage if the phlegmon is adherent and resection is too dangerous. Resection is more effective in treating the sepsis and reduces the number of operations needed to resolve the problem.

**ANSWER:** E

18. A 55-year-old man comes to the physician's office with complaints of left lower quadrant abdominal pain. He reports chronic constipation but denies any nausea or vomiting. He denies melena or bright red blood, fever, or anorexia. On examination, his abdomen is not found to be distended and exhibits no surgical scars. He has mild tenderness in the left lower quadrant without guarding. Of the following, which is the best management?

    A. Administer oral antibiotics and prescribe a clear liquid diet.

    B. Immediately conduct operative exploration.

    C. Begin bowel preparation for colonoscopy.

    D. Administer an air-contrast barium enema.

    E. Perform a CT scan of the abdomen.

*Ref.:* 2, 7

**COMMENTS: Diverticulitis** is a common source of abdominal pain that often does not require immediate intervention. Mild cases without evidence of peritonitis, fever, or leukocytosis can be treated on an outpatient basis with oral antibiotics. However, it is important to have a reliable and compliant patient who will return if worsening pain or fever develops. Once the episode subsides, a work-up, including colonoscopy or a barium enema (or both), should be performed to confirm evidence of diverticulosis and to rule out malignancy. However, these tests should not be performed during an acute exacerbation since the instrumentation and distention of the inflamed bowel entail a higher risk for perforation. CT scans of the abdomen are indicated for complicated cases (fever, leukocytosis, localized peritonitis) either at initial evaluation or if no improvement is seen within a short period.

**ANSWER:** A

19. Regarding peritonitis, which of the following statements is not true?

    A. Primary peritonitis is more common in children with nephrosis and adults with cirrhosis than in patients without such conditions.

    B. Primary peritonitis is usually monomicrobial.

    C. Chemical peritonitis often precedes bacterial contamination.

    D. Multiple organisms are commonly cultured from peritoneal dialysis catheters.

    E. Tuberculous peritonitis has an insidious onset.

*Ref.:* 2

**COMMENTS:** *Primary*, or **spontaneous**, **peritonitis** occurs in the absence of a known intraabdominal source. It is seen more often in children, and single microbes are isolated. The most commonly cultured organisms include pneumococcus and hemolytic streptococci. Among adults, patients with cirrhosis and ascites and those managed with peritoneal dialysis are at higher risk, and *Escherichia coli* and *Klebsiella* are more commonly cultured. **Secondary peritonitis** is more frequently encountered by the surgeon and implies inflammation secondary to a known intraabdominal source (e.g., perforated viscus). *Chemical* peritonitis is most commonly caused by sterile body fluids, including gastric contents, bile, urine, pancreatic fluid, and blood. Chemical peritonitis is often followed by bacterial contamination, as in the case of perforated peptic ulcer.

Patients with chronic peritoneal dialysis catheters are prone to peritonitis. These infections are monomicrobial and may respond to intraperitoneal and systemic antibiotics. If multiple organisms are grown from peritoneal fluid cultures, intestinal perforation should be suspected. *Tuberculous* peritonitis usually occurs in chronically ill or malnourished patients and may accompany pulmonary reactivation. Its onset is generally insidious, with several weeks of fever, weight loss, anorexia, ascites, and dull, diffuse abdominal pain.

**ANSWER:** D

## REFERENCES

1. Tavakkolizadeh A, Whang EE, Ashley SW, et al: Small intestine. In Brunicardi FC, Andersen DK, Billiar, TR, et al, editors: *Schwartz's principles of surgery*, ed 9, New York, 2010, McGraw-Hill.

2. Postier RG, Squires RA: Acute abdomen. In Townsend CM, Beauchamp RD, Evers BM et al, editors: *Sabiston textbook of surgery: the biological basis of modern surgical practice*, ed 18, Philadelphia, 2008, WB Saunders.

3. Silen W, editor: *Cope's early diagnosis of the acute abdomen*, ed 19, New York, 1996, Oxford University Press.

4. Martin RF, Rossi RL: The acute abdomen: an overview and algorithms, *Surg Clin North Am* 77:1227–1243, 1997.

5. Jaffe BM, Berger DH: The appendix. In Brunicardi FC, Andersen DK, Billiar TR, et al, editors: *Schwartz's principles of surgery*, ed 9, New York, 2010, McGraw-Hill.

6. Fisher WE, Andersen DK, Bell, RH, et al: Pancreas. In Brunicardi FC, Andersen DK, Billiar TR, et al, editors: *Schwartz's principles of surgery*, ed 9, New York, 2010, McGraw-Hill.

7. Bullard Dunn KM, Rothenberger DA: Colon, rectum and anus. In Brunicardi FC, Andersen DK, Billiar TR, et al, editors: *Schwartz's principles of surgery*, ed 9, New York, 2010, McGraw-Hill.

# CHAPTER 9

# Critical Care

*Crea Fusco, M.D., and José M. Velasco, M.D.*

1. A 76-year-old man with a medical history that includes hypertension, chronic renal insufficiency, and Child class A cirrhosis is admitted to the intensive care unit (ICU) after emergency exploratory laparotomy for ruptured appendicitis. His vitals signs are a temperature of 97.3° F, heart rate (HR) of 129 beats/min, blood pressure (BP) of 220/90 mm Hg, respiratory rate (RR) of 30 breaths/min, and oxygen saturation in arterial blood ($Sao_2$) of 90%. The patient is agitated and trying to pull his drains and nasogastric tube. He does not appear to respond to commands. Select the best choice to sedate this patient.

A. Lorazepam, 5 mg intravenously

B. Four-point restraints while trying to reason with the patient

C. Morphine delivered by patient-controlled anesthesia (PCA) with settings of 1 mg every 6 minutes and a 30-mg 4-hour lockout

D. Propofol and fentanyl drip

E. Placement of an epidural catheter for analgesia

*Ref.: 1-3*

**COMMENTS:** In the ICU, management of pain can be difficult and is often complicated by an inability to communicate with the patient and by the patient's physiologic instability, comorbid conditions, or delirium. Several methods have been developed to help assess **sedation**, including the **Riker Sedation-Agitation Scale** and the **Ramsay Scale**. This patient has both renal and hepatic dysfunction, which makes lorazepam an incorrect choice. It has a slow onset and intermediate half-life. In this situation, a faster-acting drug is preferable because the patient is obviously agitated. A propofol and fentanyl drip is the best answer because propofol is a general anesthetic agent with a rapid onset and ultrashort duration of action. Side effects with this medication include a risk for hypotension, high cost, pain on injection, and potential for hypertriglyceridemia. It has no analgesic effect and therefore additional medication is required to control the pain. Fentanyl is a better choice for analgesia because of the patient's renal failure and its rapid onset of action relative to morphine, which can take 5 to 10 minutes.

The use of four-point restraints without additionally sedating the patient is not a good option. Again, PCA is not a good option for a patient intubated and needing further sedation because of agitation. Moreover, morphine and its active metabolites (morphine-3-glucuronide and morphine-6-glucuronide) can accumulate in patients with renal insufficiency. Finally, placing an epidural catheter in an agitated patient would be difficult and dangerous to the patient and staff.

**ANSWER: D**

2. A 53-year-old man with a past medical history of coronary artery disease, Child class B alcoholic cirrhosis, and chronic renal insufficiency is admitted to the ICU after undergoing exploratory laparotomy and resection of necrotic small bowel from an incarcerated ventral hernia. Acute respiratory distress syndrome (ARDS) has developed in this patient. He has been intubated and placed on synchronized intermittent mandatory ventilation (SIMV). His ventilator settings are a fractional concentration of oxygen in inspired gas ($Fio_2$) of 90, RR of 24 breaths/min, tidal volume ($V_T$) of 400 mL, pressure support (PS) ventilation of 8 mm Hg, and positive end-expiratory pressure (PEEP) of 15 mm Hg. Arterial blood gas analysis revealed a pH of 7.59, $Pco_2$ of 20 mm Hg, $Po_2$ of 59 mm Hg, $HCO_3$ of 21 mEq/L, base deficit of −2, and $Sao_2$ of 88%. The nurse calls because the respirator alarms continue to go off. The patient is actually breathing at a rate of 43 breaths/min. After adequately sedating him, he is still dyssynchronous with the ventilator. A decision to paralyze him is made. Which paralytic agent is the most appropriate for this patient?

A. Pancuronium

B. Cisatracurium

C. Vecuronium

D. Succinylcholine

E. Rocuronium

*Ref.: 1*

**COMMENTS:** The best choice is cisatracurium, a nondepolarizing **neuromuscular blocker** and one of the most commonly used paralytics in the ICU. It, along with atracurium, is metabolized by plasma ester hydrolysis and Hofmann elimination and is therefore the best choice in this patient with both hepatic and renal dysfunction. Pancuronium is long acting but contraindicated in patients with coronary artery disease because it has a vagolytic effect and induces tachycardia. Vecuronium is intermediate acting (30 minutes) but is cleared by the kidney and liver. Rocuronium has a rapid onset and intermediate duration, thus making it a better choice for short procedures, as opposed to the needs of this patient, who must be sedated for a longer period.

**ANSWER: B**

3. Which of the following statements concerning radial artery cannulation is true?

A. Aortic systolic pressure is higher than radial systolic pressure.

B. The Allen test is an outdated mode of assessing collateral flow of the ulnar and radial arteries.

C. The incidence of infection is higher with catheters placed by surgical cutdown.

D. The catheter should be replaced every 3 days.

E. Intermittent flushing to keep the catheter free of clots is desirable.

*Ref.:* 4

**COMMENTS:** The incidence of complications after **arterial catheterization** seems to be operator independent, unlike the case with pulmonary artery (PA) catheterization. Known risk factors include intermittent punctures, age younger than 10 years, prolonged catheterization (>4 days), anticoagulant therapy, and use of a catheter larger than 20 gauge or made of polypropylene rather than Teflon. The radial artery is the site most frequently used for catheterization, provided that the ulnar artery and palmar arterial arch are patent. Therefore, the **Allen test** should be performed before attempting radial artery catheterization. A normal test result consists of a palmar blush within 7 seconds after the ulnar artery is released. Most patients with arterial thrombosis remain asymptomatic. Symptoms can be minimized by placing lines in arteries with good collateral circulation. Most thrombi (43%) are present at the time of catheter removal, and another 30% develop within 24 hours. A higher incidence of thrombosis occurs within the first 24 hours when surgical cutdown is performed (48% versus 23% with percutaneous placement), but the incidence of thrombosis at 1 week is the same for both methods of placement. Brachial artery cannulation has a high incidence of embolic occlusion of the distal arteries (5% to 41%) and should therefore be avoided. Infection remains the most common complication. Predisposing factors are prolonged catheterization, surgical cutdown, local inflammation, preexisting bacteremia, and failure to change the saline flush fluid, transducer, and flush tubing every 48 hours. The need for intermittent arterial catheter replacement is not established and indeed is controversial. The aortic mean arterial pressure (MAP) and diastolic arterial pressure are slightly higher than the radial MAP and diastolic arterial pressure. However, systolic pressure is consistently higher in the radial artery than in the aorta. This discrepancy increases with distal progression, smaller arterial caliber, and age and is explained by the reflection of pressure waves from capillary beds, which results in augmentation of the systolic and reduction of the diastolic values measured.

**A N S W E R :**   C

4. A 70-kg, 72-year-old man known to suffer from congestive heart failure (CHF), arthritis, diabetes mellitus, and a first-degree heart block is intubated in the ICU on postoperative day 2 after exploratory laparotomy for perforated sigmoid diverticulitis. His urine output has dropped to 10 mL/h for the last shift, and he is hypotensive despite several fluid boluses. A PA catheter is placed through the right internal jugular vein with some difficulty. As the line is advanced to 50 cm, the patient has a 14-beat run of ventricular tachycardia, which resolves when the catheter is pulled back. It is finally advanced to 62 cm and the balloon is inflated with 3 cc of air by the resident. As the line is being secured, a large amount of blood is noted in the endotracheal tube and the patient becomes hypotensive. Select the best intervention for this patient:

A. Place external pacing wires and administer lidocaine to treat the ventricular tachycardia.

B. Place a double-lumen endotracheal tube and occlude the appropriate bronchus with a Fogarty catheter.

C. Pull the PA catheter back 2 cm with the balloon inflated.

D. Suction the endotracheal tube while deflating the balloon by 2 cc of air.

E. Obtain a chest radiograph to confirm correct placement of the line.

*Ref.:* 5, 6

**COMMENTS:** The indications for **pulmonary artery catheters** and their value in patients with sepsis or hemodynamic instability are uncertain, but they may be useful in the management of patients unresponsive to the use of fluids and vasoactive agents. Dysrhythmias occur in 12% to 67% of patients undergoing catheterization but are usually self-limited, premature ventricular contractions. Complete heart block can develop in patients with preexisting left bundle branch block. A prophylactic pacing wire should be used in these patients. Prophylactic lidocaine and full inflation of the balloon may prevent ventricular ectopy. Hemoptysis in patients with a PA catheter suggests the diagnosis of perforation or rupture. Mechanisms involved in PA rupture include (1) overinflation of the balloon, (2) incomplete balloon inflation (<75%) with the exposed tip being forced through the wall, and (3) pulmonary hypertension. An "overwedge" pattern suggests eccentric balloon inflation, overdistention, or both. If hemoptysis develops, the catheter should be pulled back with the balloon deflated. Massive hemoptysis necessitates placement of a double-lumen endotracheal tube and occlusion of the bronchus on the side of the rupture with a Fogarty catheter. Emergency thoracotomy is needed. Looping or knotting of the catheter may occur in the right ventricle during insertion and can be avoided if no more than 10 cm of the catheter is inserted after a ventricular tracing is identified and before a PA tracing appears. Although catheter-related sepsis occurs in only up to 2% of insertions, bacterial colonization takes place in 5% to 35% of catheterizations. Infections are more common when the catheter is left in place for more than 72 hours or when it is inserted via an antecubital vein.

**A N S W E R :**   B

5. Which of the following statements is not correct with regard to cardiac output (CO)?

A. CO alone is not an indicator of myocardial contractility.

B. Ventricular end-diastolic volume (EDV), vascular resistance, and myocardial contractility determine stroke volume (SV).

C. Arterial blood pressure alone is an accurate indicator of CO.

D. CO varies directly with a pulse rate of up to 160 beats/min in sinus rhythm, after which it decreases.

E. Atrial contraction contributes up to 30% of EDV.

*Ref.:* 1, 7, 8

**COMMENTS:** Arterial blood pressure alone is not an accurate indicator of CO. **Cardiac output** is determined by preload, afterload, and contractility. In simplest terms, CO is equal to HR multiplied by SV, which is equal to EDV minus end-systolic volume (ESV). Therefore, $CO = HR \times (EDV - ESV)$. SV is a function of the extent of shortening of myocardial fiber, which depends on preload (initial volume), afterload (resistance to ventricular emptying), and contractility. The relationship between diastolic filling and SV is governed by Starling's law, which states that as muscle fiber length increases, so does the force of contraction. Increasing fiber length stretches the sarcomere toward the optimal 2.2-μm length. Therefore, CO alone is not an indicator of **myocardial contractility**. EDV, vascular resistance, and myocardial contractility are the primary determinants of SV. EDV is largely made up of passive ventricular filling during diastole. Diastolic filling time shortens as the pulse rate increases to 160 beats/min, but beyond this rate, CO decreases. Ventricular contractility depends on three interdependent variables: velocity of shortening, force of contraction, and length of displacement. Atrial contraction (the atrial kick) contributes 15% to 30% of EDV.

**ANSWER:** C

6. Which of the following factors is not a determinant of CO?

   A. End-diastolic pressure

   B. Afterload

   C. Contractility

   D. HR

   E. Ventricular interaction

*Ref.:* 8

**COMMENTS:** The four factors that determine cardiac output are **preload, afterload, contractility,** and **heart rate**. Preload is defined as end-diastolic sarcomere length, which is related to EDV. Left atrial pressure is correlated with left ventricular end-diastolic pressure in normal hearts. Pulmonary capillary wedge pressure (PCWP) is a reflection of left atrial pressure and is commonly used as an index of preload. The relationship between PCWP and EDV is not constant but is affected by changes in left ventricular compliance, wall thickness, HR, ischemia, and medications. Ventricular interaction also affects CO. Shifts of the interventricular septum, normally slightly convex toward the right ventricle, may compromise ventricular filling. In general, preload must be optimized before afterload manipulation. Afterload is the impedance to ventricular ejection and is estimated by systemic or pulmonary vascular resistance. An increase in afterload produces an increase in contractility. Contractility is an intrinsic property of the myocardium that is manifested as a greater force of contraction for a given preload. All the available inotropic agents increase contractility by increasing intracellular calcium concentrations and availability. HR may influence CO in a number of ways. Bradycardia and excessive tachycardia should be corrected. An increase in HR affects preload and increases contractility.

**ANSWER:** A

7. A 57-year-old man with a history of coronary artery disease, hypertension, and hyperlipidemia has complaints of severe abdominal pain, bloody diarrhea, and 20-lb weight loss in the last 3 months. An upright chest radiograph in the emergency department shows free air. The patient is admitted to the hospital. His vitals signs are a temperature of 97.1° F, HR of 119 beats/min, RR of 29 breaths/min, BP of 71/50 mm Hg, and $Po_2$ of 93 mm Hg. Laboratory studies showed a white blood cell (WBC) count of 17, 3/mm³, hemoglobin level of 7.0 g/dL, platelet count of 189,000/mm³, sodium concentration of 134 mEq/L, potassium concentration of 3.5 mEq/L, chloride concentration of 98 mEq/L, $CO_2$ level of 18 mEq/L, blood urea nitrogen (BUN) concentration of 24 mEq/L, and creatinine concentration of 1.5 mEq/L. The patient is intubated and placed on the ventilator. Blood gas analysis show metabolic acidosis. An echocardiogram shows no wall or valvular abnormalities. Which one of the following will not directly affect oxygen delivery ($Do_2$)?

   A. Rapid infusion of 2 L of saline solution

   B. Administration of three ampules of sodium bicarbonate to correct the acidosis

   C. Increasing PEEP by 2.5 units

   D. Transfusion of 2 units of packed red blood cells (PRBCs)

   E. Increasing $Fio_2$ to 60%

*Ref.:* 1

**COMMENTS:** See Question 8.

**ANSWER:** B

8. The patient is taken to the operating room (OR) and found to have perforated colon cancer with fecal peritonitis. On postoperative day 2 he becomes septic, acute renal failure (ARF) develops, and he has high $Fio_2$ requirements to keep $Sao_2$ greater than 90%. With regard to tissue utilization of oxygen, which one of the following statements is false?

   A. The brain requires 15% of the resting CO and 20% of the total basal oxygen consumption ($\dot{V}o_2$).

   B. The kidneys receive 25% of CO but can tolerate a reduction to a third of their normal blood flow for up to 1 hour.

   C. The heart extracts 70% of the available oxygen from its arterial supply.

   D. During acute hypoxia, blood is preferentially shunted to the heart and liver.

   E. The arterial-venous oxygen difference is a measure of the extent to which blood flow matches the metabolic demand for oxygen.

*Ref.:* 1

**COMMENTS:** $Do_2 = CO \times Cao_2$; $Cao_2 = [1.31 \times (Hgb)(Sao_2)] + [0.0031 \times Pao_2]$; $Cao_2$, content of arterial oxygen; $Hgb$, hemoglobin; $Pao_2$, partial pressure of oxygen. **Oxygen delivery** depends on the arterial content of oxygen and on CO. Increasing the proportion of CO to satisfy the continuous high requirements of the brain and heart, not the liver, for oxygen is crucial for survival during states of severe deficiency in oxygen transport, such as cardiac arrest. In general, organs with low **oxygen extraction ratios** tolerate decreased blood flow well. Because the kidneys extract only 10% of the oxygen available in the arterial blood supply, they tolerate decreased blood flow far better than does the heart or brain. Organs other than the heart tend to compensate for decreased blood flow by extracting more oxygen from their blood supply. The extent of this extraction can be estimated by the arterial-venous difference in oxygen content. Normally, the body consumes only 25% of its total oxygen supply. The normal mixed venous blood is 75% saturated, with a partial pressure of oxygen of 40 mm Hg. These values decrease in response to a fall in CO, which can be detected before changes in BP, pulse rate, or central venous pressure (CVP) are noted. Increased extraction is made possible by relaxation of the precapillary sphincters, which enlarges the available capillary beds for exchange of oxygen.

**ANSWER:** D

9. A 50-year-old man is admitted to the ICU because of lower gastrointestinal bleeding. He has experienced three episodes of hematochezia, a 20-lb weight loss in the last 4 months, dyspnea, and dizziness. His vitals signs are a temperature of 98.1° F, HR of 108 beats/min, BP of 80/63 mm Hg, and $Sao_2$ of 94%. His hemoglobin level is 9.1 g/dL. The patient receives several liters of crystalloid and his BP improves to baseline. CO remains elevated at 4.3 L/min. Which of the following is primarily responsible for the increase in CO in this patient?

A. Tachycardia

B. Increased contractility

C. Increased afterload

D. Decreased sympathetic nervous activity

E. Decreased blood viscosity

*Ref.:* 9

COMMENTS:

$$Do_2 = CO \times Cao_2; Cao_2 = [1.31 \times (Hgb)(Sao_2)] + [0.0031 \times Pao_2]$$

**Oxygen delivery ($Do_2$)** is maintained in patients with acute mild to moderate normovolemic anemia by the increased CO, which compensates for the reduction in oxygen-carrying capacity. Decreased blood viscosity is primarily responsible for the increased CO since it results in improved laminar flow. In blood, viscosity depends on particulate concentration and flow. A reduction in hematocrit by 50% produces an eightfold greater reduction in viscosity in the postcapillary venules than in the aorta. Because of the decreased viscosity in acute normovolemic anemia, decreased afterload, improved preload, and increased contractility are observed. Although increased cardiac sympathetic tone is seen during anemia, its direct effect on the heart is not primarily responsible for the increased CO.

**ANSWER:** E

10. All of the following are associated with an inaccurate estimation of hemoglobin oxygen saturation ($Sao_2$) by pulse oximetric analysis except:

A. Carboxyhemoglobin

B. Albinism

C. Septic syndrome

D. Nail polish

E. Hyperbilirubinemia

*Ref.:* 10

**COMMENTS: Pulse oximetric** analysis is based on placing a pulsating arterial vascular bed between a diode and a light detector (spectrophotometer with plethysmographic characteristics). It detects the oxygenated part of hemoglobin available for carrying oxygen ($Sao_2$), as opposed to the percentage of total hemoglobin that is oxygenated. An elevated carboxyhemoglobin level causes overestimation of $Sao_2$ by pulse oximetric analysis because its absorption coefficient is similar to that of oxygenated hemoglobin. Inaccurate readings are associated with the following: dark-pigmented skin (not albinos), low-flow states or venous congestion, nail polish, vital dyes (methylene blue or indocyanine green dyes), ambient light, anemia, hyperbilirubinemia, changes in the oxyhemoglobin dissociation curve, and cardiac arrhythmias.

**ANSWER:** B

11. A 60-year-old 80-kg patient is in a septic state and febrile when admitted to the ICU. Some measured values include the following: MAP, 50 mm Hg; hemoglobin concentration, 5.8 g/dL; CVP, 8 mm Hg; pH, 7.20; CO, 7 L/min; $Pco_2$, 52 mm Hg; temperature, 102.7° F; and $Pao_2$, 82 mm Hg. Which of the following values apply to this patient?

A. $P_{50}$ greater than 27

B. Alveolar-arterial gradient of 20

C. $P_{50}$ less than 27

D. Shift of the hemoglobin dissociation curve to the left

E. Oxygen-carrying capacity of 6.06 mL/g

*Ref.:* 11

**COMMENTS:** The **oxyhemoglobin dissociation curve** (Figure 9-1) is an important tool for understanding how the blood carries and releases $O_2$, in other words, hemoglobin's affinity for oxygen. The partial pressure of $O_2$ ($Po_2$) is on the x-axis and oxygen saturation ($So_2$) is on the y-axis, and the from the hemoglobin dissociation curve it can be seen that the amount of $O_2$ carried by hemoglobin increases rapidly up to a $Po_2$ of about 60 mm Hg. Above 60 mm Hg, the hemoglobin dissociation curve flattens out, and there is a much smaller change in hemoglobin saturation for the same change in $Po_2$. Conversely, in the peripheral circulation, hemoglobin can release large amounts of $O_2$ with decreasing hemoglobin saturation and yet maintain a relatively high $Po_2$, which is needed to maintain a gradient for diffusion into the peripheral tissues. The position of the oxyhemoglobin dissociation curve along the horizontal axis, termed the $P_{50}$ value, is the $Po_2$ at which 50% of the hemoglobin is saturated. The normal value is approximately 27 mm Hg. This patient has not only elevated $Pco_2$, which causes a rightward shift, but also metabolic acidosis secondary to low hemoglobin and low perfusion pressure. A rightward shift would be expected, and the resultant $P_{50}$ would be greater than 27. A right shift indicates a decreased affinity of hemoglobin for oxygen, thus making it easier for hemoglobin to release oxygen to tissues. Other answers are

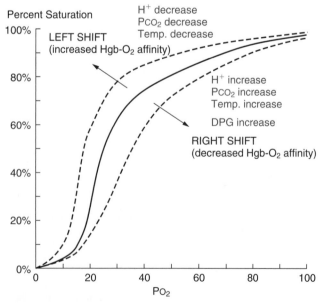

**Figure 9-1.** Oxyhemoglobin dissociation curve. DPG, diphosphoglycerate.

incorrect because the $O_2$ capacity in our patient is 8.06. (1.39 mL of $O_2 \times$ Hgb.) The alveolar-arterial (A-a) gradient is $P_{AO_2} = [F_{IO_2} \times (PB - PH_2O)] - PaCO_2$. *PB*, atmospheric pressure (760 mm Hg); *PH$_2$O*, vapor pressure of water (47 mm Hg); *PaCO$_2$*, alveolar pressure of $CO_2$, which can be calculated by dividing $PaCO_2$ by the respiratory quotient (normally 0.8). In our patient alveolar-arterial gradient is 5.23.

**ANSWER:  A**

12. A 53-year-old woman with a 2-year history of metastatic bronchogenic carcinoma is admitted to the ICU after right sleeve lobectomy with an HR of 104 beats/min, BP of 64/43 mm Hg, and RR of 34 breaths/min. After multiple fluid boluses the patient remains hypotensive, so a PA catheter is placed and secured at 43 cm. The following values were determined: PA pressure, 38/27 mm Hg; CVP, 26 mm Hg; pulmonary artery occlusion pressure (PAOP), 27 mm Hg; and cardiac index, 2.0 L/min/m$^2$. Which of the following explains the clinical scenario?

A. CHF from sepsis

B. Malignant pleural effusion

C. Cardiac tamponade

D. Hypovolemia

E. Pneumothorax

*Ref.:* 11

**COMMENTS:** There are many potential causes of **pericardial tamponade**, with bronchogenic carcinoma, renal failure, tuberculosis, breast carcinoma, and lymphoma and leukemia being among the most common. Hemodynamic monitoring with a PA catheter can help determine the diagnosis by showing equalization of right ventricular diastolic pressure, PA diastolic pressure, and PAOP within 2 to 3 mm Hg of each other, along with elevated mean right atrial pressure. With small effusions most patients are asymptomatic, but with fluid in excess of 500 mL, patients can experience the onset of dyspnea, cough, chest pain, tachycardia, and jugular venous distention. Pulsus paradoxus, hypotension, cardiogenic shock, and paradoxical movement of the jugular venous pulse are also signs to be noted. This patient has pericardial tamponade and is unlikely to improve with medical management. Pericardial drainage is recommended in all patients with large effusions because of recurrence rates in the 40% to 70% range. Administration of a fluid bolus is an appropriate measure but likely to be temporary. For immediate decompression, one can perform bedside pericardiocentesis. Definitive treatment of persistent symptomatic cardiac effusions is surgical pericardiectomy.

**ANSWER:  C**

13. Which of the following treatments of a hypotensive patient is correct?

A. Pericardiocentesis in a 54-year-old man after myocardial infarction (MI) with adequate volume status and hypotension refractory to inotropic agents

B. Cardiac pacing in a 73-year-old woman taking digitalis with atrial fibrillation on the electrocardiogram (ECG), a ventricular response rate of 40, and adequate volume status

C. Intraaortic balloon pump (IABP) in a 47-year-old woman with sepsis from pyelonephritis, good volume, and an echocardiogram showing no mechanical defects

D. Inotropic agents in a 68-year-old woman with metastatic breast cancer, distended neck veins, and PA catheter readings showing normalization of right and left heart pressure

E. Clamping of the infrarenal aorta in a patient with a gunshot wound to the chest and low right and left atrial pressure

*Ref.:* 1

**COMMENTS: Cardiogenic shock** most commonly occurs as a consequence of acute left ventricular infarction. However, it may also be due to right ventricular infarction, ruptured papillary muscle, ruptured ventricular wall, acute aortic valvular insufficiency, mitral regurgitation, and a ventricular septal defect. However, before assuming that the hypotension is caused by a cardiogenic mechanism, one must be sure that there is adequate blood volume. Therefore, a patient who is hypotensive with low right and left atrial pressure should undergo fluid administration as the initial management. If cardiac performance improves with fluid administration alone, cardiogenic shock is probably not present. If adequate filling pressures are attained and the hypotension persists in the absence of mechanical defects, arrhythmia, and sepsis, a primary pump problem probably exists and should be managed with inotropic agents. One form of cardiogenic shock is cardiac tamponade, which is seen in traumatized patients, postoperative cardiac patients, and those suffering from uremia and certain malignancies. Pericardial tamponade has a trend toward equalization of pressures in the right and left sides of the heart. In a patient who is overdigitalized or hypokalemic, a very low ventricular rate in response to atrial fibrillation or flutter may result in hypotension and should be managed with cardiac pacing. If a patient remains in cardiogenic shock despite adequate blood volume, appropriate HR, absence of a mechanical or valvular defect, appropriate administration of inotropic agents, and restoration of pressure and coronary blood flow, support via IABP counterpulsation may be needed. **Intraaortic balloon pump counterpulsation** is most beneficial in patients with severe left ventricular dysfunction. It assists in left ventricular systolic unloading by directly reducing stroke work, which in turn reduces myocardial oxygen consumption during the cardiac cycle, and in diastolic augmentation, which raises arterial BP and provides better coronary arterial perfusion during diastole and improved delivery of oxygen to the myocardium. Patients with hemodynamic compromise secondary to right ventricular MI require fluid resuscitation and inotropic support. Any preload reducers must be avoided. Afterload reducers in the presence of hypotension are not warranted.

**ANSWER:  B**

14. The alarm on the cardiac monitor continues to go off on a 73-year-old man with CHF and diabetes mellitus who was recently transferred to the ICU. He appears calm and is sitting up in bed watching a baseball game. His vitals signs are an HR of 155 beats/min, BP of 125/84 mm Hg, RR of 18 breaths/min, and SaO$_2$ of 96%. An ECG taken 7 days ago is normal. A most recent one, taken 24 hours previously, shows that his previously distinct P waves have been replaced with rapid, polymorphic, irregular P waves that are irregular and occurring at a rate greater than 300/min. The ECG is repeated and confirms the presence of an arrhythmia. At this point, which is the best initial intervention for this patient?

A. Anticoagulation with a heparin drip

B. Cardioversion with paddles and settings at 260 J up to 3 times

C. Repeat ECG in 48 hours

D. Restoration of sinus rhythm by pharmacologic means such as amiodarone or diltiazem

E. Morphine, 4 mg by intravenous push, to alleviate the pain

*Ref.:* 1, 12

**COMMENTS:** The most common sustained **dysrhythmia** is **atrial fibrillation**, which has a prevalence of 5% in persons older than 65 years. There are numerous causes that may trigger new-onset atrial fibrillation, including ischemia, MI, hypertension, electrolyte imbalance, pulmonary embolism (PE), and digoxin toxicity. Initially, an ECG should be obtained and if the arrhythmia is symptomatic, it should be treated aggressively. New-onset atrial fibrillation with a duration of less than 48 hours is a clear indication to restore sinus rhythm by either electrical or pharmacologic means. This can be performed with intravenous calcium channel blockers, amiodarone, or β-blockers, which are usually effective in rapid conversion. Cardioversion should be performed in patients who are hemodynamically unstable. Cardioversion in patients with atrial fibrillation for longer than 48 hours is contraindicated until they are fully anticoagulated. Acute intervention may not be necessary in patients with a history of well-tolerated arrhythmia.

**ANSWER: D**

15. A 58-year-old woman is found to have meningococcemia and sepsis. On examination, she is confused, agitated, and in respiratory distress. She is intubated and placed on assist/control mode (AC) ventilation. A central line is placed and several fluid boluses are given but she is still hemodynamically unstable. A continuous drip of a vasoactive drug is started. After administration, her HR remains at 105 beats/min, MAP rises to 70 from 45 mm Hg, CO drops to 2.8 from 3.3 L/min, and systemic vascular resistance increases to 1150 from 500 dynes•s/cm⁵. Based on the changes observed, which drug was most likely administered?

A. Dobutamine

B. Dopamine

C. Phenylephrine

D. Epinephrine

E. Milrinone

*Ref.:* 1

**COMMENTS: Inotropic agents** increase cardiac contractility by increasing the concentration and availability of intracellular calcium. **Catecholamines** act by binding to adrenergic receptors. Each type of receptor controls a particular cardiovascular function (Table 9-1). Epinephrine, norepinephrine, dopamine, and dobutamine are all catecholamines. The $\alpha_1$ **receptor** mediates arterial vasoconstriction by causing contraction of vascular smooth muscle, and the $\alpha_2$ **receptor** induces constriction of venous capacitance vessels. The $\beta_1$ **receptor** stimulates myocardial contractility, and the $\beta_2$ **receptor** causes relaxation of bronchial smooth muscle and relaxation of vascular smooth muscle in skeletal muscle beds. The **dopamine receptors** cause relaxation of vascular smooth muscle. The dopamine-1 receptor induces relaxation of renal and splanchnic vascular smooth muscle, and the dopamine-2 receptor inhibits uptake of norepinephrine at the sympathetic nerve terminal, which results in prolonged action of norepinephrine at the mother end plate. The effects of dopamine are unpredictable and the side effects might be significant, thus its use in ICU has been ebbing. The response to catecholamines in normal individuals is different

**TABLE 9-1    Hemodynamic Response Receptors**

| Drug | Dose (mcg/kg/min) | HR | MAP | CO | SVR | α | β₁ | β₂ |
|---|---|---|---|---|---|---|---|---|
| Dopamine | 5 | ↑ | ↑ | ↑ | | | + | |
| | 5-20 | ↑↑ | ↑↑ | ↑ | ↑↑ | ++ | ++ | |
| Dobutamine | 2-20 | ↑↑ | ↑ | ↑ | ↓ | | ++ | + |
| Epinephrine | 0.01-0.1 | ↑↑ | ↑↑ | ↑ | ↑↑ | ++ | ++ | + |
| Phenylephrine | 10-100 (mcg/min) | | ↑↑ | ↓ | ↑↑ | ++ | | |
| Norepinephrine | 1-20 (mcg/min) | ↑ | ↑↑ | ↑ | ↑↑ | ++ | + | |
| Milrinone | 0.3-1.5 | | | ↑↑ | ↓ | | | |

CO, Cardiac output; HR, heart rate; MAP, mean arterial pressure; SVR, systemic vascular resistance.
↑, increase
↓, decrease
+, positive

from that in critically ill patients. Receptor populations change over short periods , and upregulation and downregulation can occur, depending on the disease state. Because receptor numbers and affinities vary with the clinical setting, various and unexpected responses are seen. It is important that catecholamines be administered for a predetermined effect. If the effect is not attained with the particular catecholamine chosen, the dose should be adjusted or another agent used.

**ANSWER: C**

16. A 68-year-old woman, a known diabetic with chronic renal failure, a distant history of MI, and an inability to climb one flight of stairs because of shortness of breath, has a new 2-cm spiculated mass with multiple calcifications throughout the breast, found on routine screening mammography. On examination, she has a fixed, hard 2.5-cm mass at the 10-o'clock position with small, soft, palpable axillary lymph nodes. She has a sister and aunt who died of invasive breast cancer, so she is very anxious and wants to have her operation as soon as possible. What is the most appropriate answer to her in regard to scheduling her operation?

A. The comorbid conditions are not significant; therefore, the operation can be scheduled for tomorrow.

B. An ECG, chest radiograph, and blood work are needed first.

C. This is a surgical emergency, and β-blockers will be started and the operation performed in the morning.

D. Cardiac function should be evaluated first and then plans made for surgery.

E. Because the comorbid conditions are significant, she is not a surgical candidate.

*Ref.:* 1, 13

**COMMENTS:** Approximately 44 million patients undergo noncardiac surgery in the United States, and of those, 30% have or are at risk for coronary artery disease with a 2.8 times higher risk for **postoperative cardiac events.** The **American College of Cardiology/American Heart Association (ACC/AHA) Task Force on Practice Guidelines** published guidelines on perioperative cardiovascular evaluation in 1996 with an update in 2002. The proposed function of these guidelines was to identify high-risk patients, risk-stratify them, and perform preoperative testing as necessary. It also would help determine whether patients needed coronary revascularization before their nonemergency operation. This patient has three intermediate risk factors: diabetes, renal insufficiency, and a previous history of MI. These factors, along with her poor functional status, mandates noninvasive testing of cardiac function, so she should not be scheduled for surgery before these tests are performed. An ECG, chest radiograph, and blood work are a good start, but according to the guidelines, the patient requires a noninvasive cardiac stress test. She does have many comorbid conditions but is undergoing a low-risk operation (breast, endoscopy, cataracts) associated with less than 1% risk. Intermediate-risk surgeries include intrathoracic, major orthopedic, intraperitoneal, head and neck, and prostate surgery, and they have a cardiac risk of less than 5%. High-risk surgeries such as aortic, major vascular, and prolonged procedures with significant fluid shifts have a greater than 5% cardiac risk. If a patient has undergone coronary artery bypass grafting (CABG) or a percutaneous intervention in the last 5 years without return of symptoms, no further work-up is needed. In addition, if there has been a cardiac evaluation in the last 2 years with no change in symptoms, no further work-up is needed. Patients who will not need revascularization will need medical therapy aimed at minimizing perioperative risk. Multiple studies have been performed on the perioperative use of **β-blockers**, many of which have been inconclusive or have design flaws. It is generally accepted that high-risk patients should take β-blockers, with an HR goal of less than 60 beats/min. Currently, the 2006 recommendations from the ACC/AHA recognize that there are insufficient data available to advocate the use of β-blockade in patients with low cardiac risk who are undergoing intermediate- or high-risk surgery. The POISE trial (PeriOperative ISchemic Evaluation) is currently ongoing and is designed to evaluate the efficacy of 30 days of **metoprolol** and its effect on cardiac events.

**ANSWER:** D

17. Which of the following conditions is not usually associated with elevated dead space ventilation?

A. 42-year-old female after MI with CHF and a CO of 1.5 L/min

B. 28-year-old woman on partum day 1 with shortness of breath, a $PaO_2$ of 60 mm Hg, and segmental clots bilaterally in the pulmonary arteries

C. 52-year-old Hispanic immigrant with a long-standing ventricular septal defect and PA pressure of 80/52 mm Hg

D. 22-year-old man after multiple gunshot wounds, massive transfusions, and a mean arterial to inspired oxygen ratio ($PaO_2/FIO_2$) of 180

E. 62-year-old woman smoker with the following ventilator settings: controlled mandatory ventilation (CMV) at a rate of 12 breaths/min, $FIO_2$ of 60%, $VT$ of 600 mL, and PEEP of 5 cm $H_2O$

*Ref.:* 14, 15

**COMMENTS:** The most common causes of **increased dead space** in critically ill patients are decreased CO, PE, pulmonary hypertension, ARDS, and excessive PEEP, all of which directly cause decreased blood flow to the pulmonary vasculature. In dead space ventilation with a high ventilation/perfusion ($\dot{V}/\dot{Q}$) ratio, there is decreased blood flow to ventilated areas, which primarily affects elimination of carbon dioxide. In ARDS, some areas of lung are perfused but not ventilated. Alveoli may be filled with secretions, exudate, blood, or edema, thereby increasing the shunt fraction. Other areas of the lung may be ventilated but not perfused, which accounts for the dead space ventilation. **Positive end-expiratory pressure** can cause dead space ventilation by decreasing CO and stenting alveoli open, which causes the surrounding capillaries to collapse and thereby decreases alveolar perfusion. Carbon dioxide production and the dead space–tidal volume ratio ($VDS/VT$) determine minute ventilation. The anatomic dead space includes the volume of the airways to the level of the bronchiole (150 mL). Dead space can also include alveoli that are well ventilated but poorly perfused. When combined, the anatomic and alveolar dead space constitutes the physiologic dead space, which is essentially the volume of gas moved during each tidal breath that does not participate in gas exchange.

**ANSWER:** E

18. A 17-year-old asthmatic girl is brought to the OR for ruptured ectopic pregnancy. Postoperatively on the floor, she is found to be profoundly dyspneic and in acute respiratory failure. She is intubated and transferred to the surgical ICU, where her ventilatory settings are AC mode, RR of 18 breaths/min, $FIO_2$ of 0.80, $VT$ of 600 mL, and PEEP of 0 mm Hg. She was sedated and paralyzed for the intubation and is not breathing over the ventilator settings. After examining the patient and the flow pattern on the ventilator, changes in the ventilatory settings are made. Which change in ventilator setting would best limit intrinsic PEEP?

A. Increase $VT$

B. Decrease in the inspiratory flow rate

C. Increase in PEEP

D. Decreased RR

E. Change from AC mode to SIMV

*Ref.:* 16, 17

**COMMENTS: Intrinsic positive end-expiratory pressure** (commonly known as auto-PEEP) is a state at end exhalation in which there is incomplete gas emptying, which can elevate alveolar volume and pressure. It is the threshold pressure needed to be overcome to initiate inspiratory flow. Severe bronchospasm increases the expiratory time needed, and patients in status asthmaticus or severe chronic obstructive pulmonary disease (COPD) are at risk for intrinsic PEEP. If combined with narrowed airways, such as in asthma, and parenchymal noncompliance, the inspiratory work of breathing is increased. Therefore, there is an imbalance of respiratory muscle strength and work of breathing leading to respiratory failure.

During mechanical ventilation, when the expiratory time is insufficient to allow full exhalation of a ventilator breath, expiratory flow is still occurring when the next ventilator breath is delivered. To best limit intrinsic PEEP, one can decrease the RR, thereby giving the patient more time to exhale between breaths. In addition, decreasing $VT$ will allow minimal improvement. One should also limit the inspiratory time to leave more time in the respiratory cycle for exhalation. Avoidance of hyperinflation and overdistention at the expense of minute ventilation, otherwise known as permissive hypercapnia, is an important method of ventilatory management in asthmatics.

**ANSWER:** D

19. The intensivist in the ICU is called to evaluate multiple patients with respiratory difficulty. The respiratory therapist has been busy collecting data on each of them. Which of the following patients does not need urgent changes in management while ventilatory support is being provided for the others?

A. 47-year-old woman with bilateral pneumonia and an RR of 55 breaths/min

B. 72-year-old man after quadruple bypass with a $Paco_2$ of 67 mm Hg

C. 64-year-old mechanic after colectomy for ulcerative colitis with an alveolar-arterial oxygen difference of 390 mm Hg.

D. 61-year-old woman heavy smoker with ARDS and measured dead space ventilation ($Vds/Vt$) of 0.7

E. 28-year-old postal worker after a dog bite to the arm and fasciitis with a shunt fraction greater than 5%

*Ref.:* 18

COMMENTS: The indications for **respiratory support** include inadequate parameters of ventilation (RR >35 breaths/min, $Vds/Vt$ >0.6, $Paco_2$ >60 mm Hg), poor oxygenation (a-a $O_2$ difference and $Pao_2$), and impaired respiratory mechanics. Decreased **vital capacity** (VC = inspiratory reserve volume + $Vt$ + expiratory reserve volume) can lead to the need for intubation, and 15 mL/kg is life sustaining. Decreased inspiratory force, the force needed to create negative pressure in the lungs, can also indicate a need for respiratory support. In the absence of metabolic alkalosis or chronic hypercapnia, a $Paco_2$ greater than 60 mm Hg is abnormal. **Dead space ventilation**, the amount of $Vt$ that does not encounter perfused alveoli, is used as an indirect measure of ventilation-perfusion abnormality. It has been shown that increased physiologic $Vds/Vt$ (>0.6) is significantly associated with mortality in patients with ARDS ($Pao_2/Fio_2$ ratio of less than 200 mm Hg). The **shunt fraction**, or pulmonary venous mixture, can be defined as the amount of blood shunted around the lung as a fraction of CO. Shunt fraction is measured at the inspired oxygen concentration required to maintain adequate oxygenation ($Po_2$ of 60 to 70 mm Hg). A shunt fraction greater than 20% requires respiratory support.

ANSWER: E

20. With regard to ventilatory mechanics, which of the following statements is false?

A. The work of breathing at rest consumes 2% of total body oxygen consumption.

B. COPD is associated with an increase in the work of breathing as a result of increased inspiratory work.

C. The work of breathing may increase to 50% of total-body oxygen consumption in postoperative patients.

D. Airway pressure reflects the compliance of the chest wall and diaphragm, as well as that of the lungs.

E. Compliance is measured as the change in volume divided by the change in pressure.

*Ref.:* 19, 20

COMMENTS: For patients with **chronic obstructive pulmonary disease**, the work of breathing is increased because of increased expiratory work, not inspiratory work. It can be assessed by preoperative pulmonary function testing and optimized by preoperative chest physical therapy, bronchodilators, and antibiotics if infection is present. The work of breathing at rest consumes 2% of total-body $Vo_2$ and can be markedly increased, up to 50% of total $Vo_2$, in postoperative patients because of increased airway resistance and decreased compliance of the lung, chest wall, and diaphragm. The proper use of volume-cycled ventilators and PS ventilation can take over most of the work of breathing during the

postoperative period. **Compliance** is defined as the change in pressure associated with each milliliter increase in lung volume. Measuring airway pressure reflects the compliance of the chest wall and diaphragm, as well as that of the lungs. In relaxed patients this is of little importance, but in restless patients, intraesophageal or intrapleural pressure provides a more accurate measure of compliance. In acute respiratory failure, decreased compliance is usually associated with decreased **functional residual capacity**. Less compliant lungs need ventilatory management that maintains inflation of alveoli by the use of PEEP and recruits closed alveoli by elevating peak inspiratory pressure. However, because positive airway pressure may overdistend already ventilated alveoli, the peak inspiratory pressure should be kept below 40 cm $H_2O$.

ANSWER: B

21. A 53-year-old man suffers an MI, falls from a height of 4 m off the train tracks, and sustains a severe head injury. He has multiple long-bone fractures, severe heart failure, diffuse axonal injury, and ARDS. He is severely hemodynamically unstable and taking multiple vasopressors, and he had had an episode of asystole after bathing. His $Pao_2/Fio_2$ ratio is 95 and his peak airway pressure ranges from 42 to 47 cm $H_2O$ despite lung-protective ventilation. The family expresses the desire to "do everything." Which of the following is not a reasonable ventilation strategy for this patient?

A. Prone positioning

B. Inhaled nitrous oxide ($N_2O$)

C. Permissive hypercapnia

D. Pharmacologic paralysis

E. Partial liquid ventilation

*Ref.:* 1, 21

COMMENTS: In patients with severe lung disease, it can be a challenge to oxygenate and ventilate. Goals for adequate ventilation include an $Sao_2$ of greater than 90% and airway pressures of less than 35 to 40 cm $H_2O$. There are no definitive answers in a difficult-to-ventilate patient, but all the strategies listed are accepted maneuvers. Because of this patient's unstable BP and episode of asystole with bathing, **prone positioning** is not a reasonable strategy for him. It can also lead to loss of tubes and lines and the development of pressure ulcers if teams are unfamiliar with the procedure. When indicated, prone positioning can increase oxygenation by changing the dependent areas of the lung and realigning the distribution of inflated alveoli with pulmonary perfusion. Inhaled $N_2O$ is an endogenous compound with vasodilator properties that can improve oxygenation but is expensive and not always available. It has been shown to improve PA pressure and oxygenation in patients with acute lung injury and ARDS, but no overall decrease in mortality has been shown. **Permissive hypercapnia**, in which accumulation of $CO_2$ and respiratory acidosis are allowed, attempts to minimize barotrauma and volutrauma to the lung. Most centers accept a pH of 7.2 or above. Paralysis can allow synchronization of the ventilator and relax the chest wall musculature. It also decreases the work of breathing by allowing the ventilator to do all the work. Partial liquid ventilation partially fills the lung with perfluorocarbon, which carries respiratory gases and can preserve lung histology, compliance, and systemic oxygenation. Another option not listed, **extracorporeal membrane oxygenation (ECMO)**, bypasses the lungs, oxygenates the blood, and can protect the lungs from high $Fio_2$ and ventilator settings. It requires anticoagulation and is therefore a contraindication in this patient with a severe head injury.

ANSWER: A

22. A family meeting is called for a 69-year-old man who was intubated 6 days earlier for pneumonia and respiratory distress. He is now awake, alert, and asking for the tube to come out. His family wants to know when and whether he will be extubated. Which of the following characteristics of this patient does not meet conventional weaning criteria?

A. Negative inspiratory force of −10 cm $H_2O$

B. A respiratory frequency/tidal volume ($RF/V_T$) ratio of 105 or less

C. Correction of underlying pulmonary and nonpulmonary complications

D. Pulse oximetry reading of 92%

E. Vital capacity of 12 to 15 mL/kg and peak inspiratory pressure of less than 25 cm $H_2O$

*Ref.:* 22

**COMMENTS:** Many indices have been proposed to predict **weaning** outcome and success or failure of extubation. Most surgical patients (90%) are weaned from mechanical ventilation in less than 1 week. Conventional **weaning criteria** include (1) measurements of oxygenation with a pulse oximeter (best determined by arterial blood gas analysis, with an $SaO_2$ >90% and any $FIO_2$ usually being adequate for weaning) and (2) measurements of ventilation, such as an RR less than 24 breaths/min, $PaCO_2$ less than 50 mm Hg, peak inspiratory pressure below 30 cm $H_2O$, $V_T$ of at least 5 to 8 mL/kg, and a vital capacity double the $V_T$ value. Failure to satisfy these conventional criteria is associated with unsuccessful weaning in as many as 63% of patients. The rapid, **shallow breathing test** (**$RF/V_T$**) is performed by having the patient breathe room air for 1 minute as quickly as possible. When $RF/V_T$ is 105 or less, successful weaning occurs in 78% of patients, and when $RF/V_T$ is less than 80, the success rate is 95%. Conversely, an $RF/V_T$ value of 105 or higher is accompanied by a failure rate of 95%. Another method often described is the SOAP assessment: (1) ability to clear *secretions*, (2) adequate *oxygenation* ($PaO_2/FIO_2$ ratio >200 mm Hg, which requires an $FIO_2$ of 0.4 to 0.5 and PEEP <8 cm $H_2O$), (3) ability to protect the *airway*, and (4) adequate *pulmonary* function. Clinical judgment and correction of underlying pulmonary and nonpulmonary complications continue to be the best guide to successful weaning. In addition, helpful ventilation scores include an $FIO_2$ of less than 40%, **continuous positive airway pressure** (**CPAP**) of 3 cm $H_2O$, effective static compliance greater than 50 mL/cm $H_2O$, dynamic compliance greater than 40 mL/cm $H_2O$, ventilator minute ventilation of less than 10 L/min, and a triggered ventilatory rate of less than 20 breaths/min. The duration of ventilatory support is not correlated with survival rates at discharge. Forty-one percent of long-term ventilated patients survive. Because muscle atrophy is often present, a progressive ventilatory withdrawal plan designed to restore muscle function should be used. Intermittent mandatory ventilation, PS ventilation, and weaning by T-piece have been used effectively.

**A N S W E R :** A

23. A 29-year-old firefighter is intubated in the ICU after being exposed to smoke on the job. She has thick yellow secretions that require frequent suctioning along with the administration of bronchodilators. On hospital day 5, she has a percutaneous central venous catheter placed through the right internal jugular vein. Several hours later, she undergoes respiratory arrest. Her peak inspiratory pressure has risen from 24 to 41 cm $H_2O$, and her plateau pressure has stayed at 16 cm $H_2O$. Choose which of the following is the most likely reason for the respiratory arrest:

**TABLE 9-2 Patient's Respiratory Pressures**

|  | Day 1 | Day 2 | Day 3 | Day 4 | Day 5 |
|---|---|---|---|---|---|
| $FIO_2$ | 0.6 | 0.6 | 0.55 | 0.5 | 0.5 |
| PEEP | 10 | 10 | 8 | 5 | 5 |
| PIP | 25 | 23 | 24 | 32 | 41 |
| Plateau pressure | 17 | 18 | 18 | 17 | 16 |
| RR | 20 | 19 | 23 | 24 | 27 |
| $O_2$ Sat | 91 | 89 | 94 | 95 | 93 |

$FIO_2$, fractional concentration of oxygen in inspired gas; $O_2$ Sat, $O_2$ saturation; PEEP, positive end-expiratory pressure; PIP, peak inspiratory pressure; RR, respiratory reserve.

A. Tension pneumothorax

B. Flash pulmonary edema

C. pulmonary embolus (PE)

D. Endotracheal tube obstruction

E. Auto-PEEP with breath stacking

*Ref.:* 20

**COMMENTS:** This patient has an obstruction of the endotracheal tube. The key to identifying this problem is recognizing the components of the patient's respiratory pressure in Table 9-2, most importantly the **peak inspiratory** and **plateau pressures**. The peak inspiratory pressure is the pressure required to overcome the resistance in the endotracheal tube and airways, as well as the compliance of the airways. The inspiratory plateau pressure is the pressure generated to overcome the elastance of the lung parenchyma, pleural space, and chest wall. This patient had increasing peak inspiratory pressure, so her problem was related to the tube, not the lung itself. Tension pneumothorax and flash pulmonary edema are associated with increases in both peak inspiratory pressure and inspiratory plateau pressure. PE also does not change the inspiratory pressure.

**A N S W E R :** D

24. A 73-year-old woman weighing 60 kg is admitted to the hospital with acute pancreatitis. She is aggressively resuscitated with fluid but becomes hypotensive and has increasing work of breathing and $O_2$ requirements within the next 12 hours. The patient is transferred to the ICU and intubated. A PA catheter is placed and the wedge pressure is 8 cm $H_2O$. Arterial blood gas analysis shows values of a pH of 7.36, a $PaO_2$ of 62, a $PCO_2$ of 42, a serum bicarbonate of 21, and a base deficit of −2 with $SaO_2$ of 90%. Which of the following ventilation strategies is most appropriate for this patient?

A. Pressure control ventilation (PCV) with a pressure of 40 cm $H_2O$ and an inverse ratio ventilation of 3:1

B. SIMV with a $V_T$ of 720 mL and RR set to keep the pH at 7.4

C. AC ventilation with a $V_T$ of 600 mL and prone positioning

D. AC ventilation with a $V_T$ of 360 mL and RR to keep the pH above 7.2

E. SIMV with a $V_T$ of 600 and $FIO_2$ of 100%

*Ref.:* 23-25

**COMMENTS:** See Question 25.

**A N S W E R :** D

25. Which one of the following criteria is not included in the definition of ARDS?

    A. PA wedge pressure of 14 mm Hg

    B. Chest radiograph showing bilateral pulmonary infiltrates

    C. Infectious cause

    D. Onset of 6 hours

    E. $Pao_2/Fio_2$ ratio of 175

*Ref.:* 23-25

COMMENTS: Because the principal physiologic problem in **acute respiratory distress syndrome** is hypoxemia refractory to increasing $Fio_2$, therapy is centered on provision of mechanical ventilation to maximize oxygen delivery while minimizing lung injury. PEEP is used to improve oxygenation and lung compliance and should be optimized with the help of pressure-volume curves to facilitate the maintenance of open alveoli and diffusion of oxygen into the pulmonary capillaries. For a given $Fio_2$, $Pao_2$ usually increases on administration of **positive end-expiratory pressure** in patients with ARDS. However, excessive PEEP (>15 cm $H_2O$) can be hazardous and lead to pneumothorax from barotrauma and decreased venous return to the heart. Overdistention of alveoli can be prevented by keeping the peak inspiratory pressure below 35 cm of $H_2O$. Newer ventilatory methods attempt to enhance alveolar recruitment, maintain alveolar patency throughout the respiratory cycle, maintain an $Sao_2$ of greater than 90%, avoid dynamic hyperinflation (volutrauma), and reduce the risk for oxygen toxicity. Spontaneous, augmented low-volume ventilation, with PS ventilation being used as a primary ventilatory support mode, directs flow to regions of low ventilation/perfusion. Diuretics in cases of obvious fluid overload and cardiac decompensation and broad-spectrum antibiotics in cases of established pulmonary infection or other sources of sepsis may be useful for patients with ARDS. The consensus conference on ARDS (ARDSnet.org) showed that a volume-restricted ventilation strategy reduced mortality. In this well-accepted study, 861 patients were randomly assigned to either a traditional-volume ventilation strategy (12 mL/kg of ideal body weight with plateau pressures of <50 cm $H_2O$) or low-$V_T$ ventilation (6 mL/kg with plateau pressures <30 cm $H_2O$). The study was halted early because of significantly reduced overall mortality (31.0% versus 39.1%, $P < .0007$). Permissive hypercapnia was allowed and sodium bicarbonate was given to maintain pH higher than 7.2.

The patient developed ARDS, probably because of acute pancreatitis and systemic inflammatory response syndrome (SIRS). Criteria used to define ARDS include an acute onset, bilateral pulmonary infiltrates on chest radiographs, hypoxemia ($Pao_2/Fio_2$ ratio <200 mm Hg), and absence of cardiogenic pulmonary edema (i.e., PCWP <18 mm Hg) or no clinical evidence of left atrial hypertension. There does not have to be an infectious process for a patient to have ARDS. Acute lung injury is a milder form with a $Pao_2/Fio_2$ ratio of 201 to 300 mm Hg. The lung response can be divided into an exudative phase (24 to 96 hours), with leakage of proteinaceous fluid into the pulmonary interstitium and corresponding damage to the alveolar-capillary interface; an early proliferative phase (3 to 10 days), with proliferation of alveolar type II cells, cellular infiltration of the septum, and organization of hyaline membranes; and a late proliferative phase (7 to 10 days), with fibrosis of the alveolar septum, ducts, and hyaline membranes. Frequently, the radiographic changes can lag behind the clinical picture in ARDS considerably.

ANSWER: C

26. A 59-year-old woman with a long-standing history of gastroesophageal reflux disease (GERD) underwent a Nissen fundoplication that was complicated by 2 L of blood loss and hypotension in the OR. Her vitals signs are an HR of 103 beats/min, BP of 100/70 mm Hg, RR of 16 breaths/min, and $Sao_2$ of 96%. Her urine output was 15 mL of urine per hour over the last 4 hours. Laboratory results include a urine osmolality of 600 mOsm/kg, urine sodium concentration of 15 mEq/L, plasma sodium concentration of 140 mEq/L, urine creatinine concentration of 20 mg/dL, and plasma creatinine concentration of 1.5 mg/dL. What is the next step in management?

    A. Flushing the Foley catheter with 60 mL of normal saline

    B. Hemodialysis

    C. Nephrology consultation

    D. Decompressive laparotomy for abdominal compartment syndrome

    E. Administration of a 1000-mL fluid bolus of normal saline as a fluid challenge

*Ref.:* 26, 27

COMMENTS: **Acute renal failure** is a serious morbidity for postsurgical patients, with mortality rates greater than 50%. Renal failure can be prerenal, renal, or postrenal. The most common cause in surgical patients is hypovolemia, as is the case in this patient from blood loss in the OR. Some indicators for prerenal causes include urine osmolality greater than 500 mOsm/kg, fractional excretion of sodium ($FE_{Na}$) of less than 1%, and urine sodium concentration of less than 20 mEq/L, whereas an $FE_{Na}$ greater than 3% and urinary sodium concentration greater than 40 mEq/L are indicative of parenchymal or postrenal causes. Medications, intravenous contrast material–induced nephropathy, rhabdomyolysis, and transfusion reactions are all options to consider. This patient's $FE_{Na}$ is 0.8%.

ANSWER: E

27. A 46-year-old brittle diabetic and hypertensive woman is brought to the ICU after being found unresponsive in her bed. After undergoing a computed tomographic (CT) scan of her head, abdomen, and pelvis with intravenous contrast media, she is transferred to the ICU. The ICU team places a central line, orders an echocardiogram, and places a bladder catheter. Her urine output has been approximately 10 mL/h for the last 4 hours. Her $FE_{Na}$ is calculated to be 2.4%. Which of the following is not consistent with acute tubular necrosis (ATN)?

    A. Oliguria

    B. $FE_{Na}$ greater than 2%

    C. Urine osmolality of 200 mOsm/kg

    D. Creatinine clearance greater than 125 mL/min

    E. Sodium wasting

*Ref.:* 26, 27

COMMENTS: A **creatinine clearance** of 125 mL/min represents normal renal function. ATN is characterized by a rise in plasma creatinine concentration (decrease in creatinine clearance or glomerular filtration rate [GFR]), a urine volume that is reduced (oliguric) or normal, changes in the findings on urinalysis, and an $FE_{Na}$ greater than 1% to 2%. Oliguria, or urine output less than 500 mL/24 h, is a frequent but not an absolute feature of ATN. Whether oliguria occurs may depend on the severity of the renal injury or the relative reabsorption of filtrate at the tubular level.

Even if a patient's **glomerular filtration rate** falls to 10 L/day (normal, 180 L/day), urine output of 1 to 2 L/day would still will be normal as long as 8 to 9 L of filtrate was reabsorbed. In cases of well-preserved tubular function, as in prerenal forms of ARF, **fractional excretion of sodium** is low, consistent with the sodium-avid state. As tubular dysfunction progresses, the ability of nephrons to reabsorb sodium is disrupted, and a greater percentage of the filtered sodium is excreted in urine. As a result, $FE_{Na}$ will be greater than 1% to 2% because of inappropriate sodium wasting by altered tubular function. Loss of urinary concentrating ability is an early feature of ATN. A urine osmolality of less than 350 mOsm/L is consistent with ATN, whereas an osmolality greater than 500 mOsm/L suggests a prerenal cause of ARF. However, lower values can be seen during prerenal ARF, thus limiting the value of this test as a sole indicator of tubular function.

**ANSWER:** D

28. A 62-year-old man with peripheral vascular disease, diabetes, and bilateral tissue loss in the lower extremities is admitted for angiography of his lower extremities. He has chronic renal failure and his serum creatinine level is 5.0 mg/dL, which has been his baseline for the last 3 years. Which of the following agents is indicated to reduce the risk for intravenous contrast–induced nephropathy?

   A. Calcium channel blocker

   B. Aggressive diuresis

   C. Saline volume expansion before and after the procedure

   D. Acetylcysteine given only after exposure to contrast material

   E. Mannitol and saline hydration

*Ref.:* 26, 28

**COMMENTS:** In most cases, **radiocontrast agents** can lead to a reversible form of ARF. The pathogenesis is not well established, but two proposed mechanisms of injury are renal vasoconstriction and direct tubular toxic effects. The risk is minimal in patients with normal renal function, including those with diabetes, and the renal failure is nonoliguric and transient in most cases. Severe renal failure requiring short- or long-term dialysis is rare and most likely to occur in patients whose baseline creatinine level is greater than 4 mg/dL. Risk factors for the development of contrast-induced nephropathy include underlying chronic renal failure with a plasma creatinine level greater than 1.5 mg/dL, diabetic nephropathy with renal insufficiency, CHF, multiple myeloma, and a large volume of contrast material. Saline volume expansion in the precontrast and postcontrast period is the only preventive measure consistently shown to be of benefit. Hydration with furosemide may increase the risk for contrast-induced nephropathy when compared with saline alone. Furthermore, the use of saline solution and mannitol does not have any benefit over the use of saline alone. **Calcium channel blockers** given to minimize renal vasoconstriction after exposure to contrast media have not been conclusively shown to prevent renal failure. The role of **nonionic contrast agents** is not clearly defined. Studies seem to support the use of isosmolar nonionic agents in high-risk patients, especially those with diabetes. There are conflicting data on the role of **acetylcysteine** and sodium bicarbonate infusions in the prevention of contrast-induced nephropathy, but given its relatively safe side effect profile and the few series supporting its use, use of both can be justified, particularly in high-risk patients. A rational approach to preventing contrast-induced nephropathy in high-risk patients, such as the patient in question, would include acetylcysteine (600 mg orally twice daily the day before and on the

day of exposure to contrast material), saline volume expansion before and after the procedure, and an isosmolar nonionic contrast agent. Several recent meta-analyses have shown that **sodium bicarbonate infusion** can decrease the damage associated with contrast-induced nephropathy if given both before and after the procedure as well. The former may be more important for patients with renal dysfunction and diabetes.

**ANSWER:** C

29. Choose the situation that does not require immediate renal replacement therapy.

   A. 27-year-old bipolar patient, after running a half marathon, taking a prescribed lithium dose and found to have ataxia, confusion, and inverted T waves

   B. 68-year-old man after sigmoid colectomy with new-onset seizures and BUN of 150 mg/dL

   C. 58-year-old man after a motor vehicle collision with multiple long-bone fractures, BUN of 120 mg/dL, creatinine of 2.8 mg/dL, and diffuse bleeding

   D. 71-year-old woman with diabetes maintained on an insulin drip after total abdominal hysterectomy and bilateral salpingo-oophorectomy with an $FE_{Na}$ of 0.7% and urine output of less than 20 mL/h for last 7 hours

   E. 45-year-old man with respiratory distress after massive resuscitation for a septic episode, bilateral lung haziness on chest radiography, and coarse crackles who is unresponsive to diuretics

*Ref.:* 1, 29-31

**COMMENTS:** Indications for acute **dialysis** treatment include (1) persistent hyperkalemia refractory to medical management; (2) pulmonary edema unresponsive to conventional therapy; (3) severe acidemia; (4) symptoms of uremia such as anorexia, nausea, and vomiting; (5) uremic encephalopathy, seizures, asterixis, uremic pericarditis, and uremic bleeding; and (6) overdose with a dialyzable toxin such as lithium or ethylene glycol. **Renal replacement therapy** is needed in 1% to 2% of patients with ARF, and as many as 15% of patients may ultimately require dialysis at some point in their life. It may be indicated for symptomatic fluid overload, sepsis, uremic complications, and severe electrolyte or acid-base disorders. Frequently in the ICU, continuous renal replacement therapy is superior to intermittent hemodialysis or peritoneal dialysis, but in the United States, it is only used in 10% to 20% of ICU patients. Proponents of this method over others argue that it allows better hemodynamic stability and prevention of shifts in intracerebral water, minimizes the risk for infection, and provides continuous control of fluid status and acid-base abnormalities. Complications include the need for anticoagulation and a high level of nursing care.

**ANSWER:** D

30. A 68-year-old woman with history of a GERD, cholelithiasis, and coronary artery disease is seen in the emergency department with nausea, vomiting, and epigastric pain. Laboratory tests showed amylase and lipase values of 259 and 1782 units/L, leukocytosis of 18,300/mm³, and a prothrombin time (PT) and international normalized ratio (INR) of 47 seconds and 1.9 respectively. The patient received 6 L of crystalloid solution because of hypotension and required intubation. After 48 hours the hemoglobin has dropped by 2 g. What are the factors that have the strongest correlation with stress-related bleeding in critically ill patients?

A. Mechanical ventilation and hypotension

B. Coagulopathy and renal failure

C. Steroids and sepsis

D. Mechanical ventilation and steroids

E. Mechanical ventilation and coagulopathy

*Ref.:* 1, 32

**COMMENTS:** Risk factors for **stress-related mucosal lesions** are mechanical ventilation longer than 48 hours, coagulopathy, significant burns, and head injury. These lesions have been found in 25% to 100% of ICU patients within 48 hours of admission, but clinically significant bleeding occurs in only 5% to 10%. Patients with risk factors should receive prophylaxis until consuming an enteral diet of at least 50% of their caloric intake.

**ANSWER:   E**

31. One hour after prolonged transurethral resection of the prostate (TURP), a 70-year-old man with mild coronary artery disease, cirrhosis, and hypertension experiences bradycardia, hypertension, confusion, nausea, and headache. Findings on preoperative laboratory tests were normal, and his home medications included lactulose, atenolol, and alendronate (Fosamax). Over the last few hours he was given a 2-L bolus of 0.9% normal saline for hypotension. The patient is transferred to ICU, where on examination he is found to be sluggish and slurring his voice. He is afebrile with an HR of 93 beats/min, BP of 140/73 mm Hg, and RR of 14 breaths/min. He continues to be confused and lethargic and does not follow commands. What is the best explanation for his condition?

A. Hypotonic irrigating solution

B. Hyperkalemia

C. Isotonic saline solution

D. Atenolol

E. Hepatic encephalopathy

*Ref.:* 33, 34

**COMMENTS:** The patient is most likely suffering from **transurethral resection (TUR) syndrome**, which is caused by excessive absorption of irrigating solution and results in hyponatremia. The usual irrigation fluid is 1.5% glycine, which has an osmolarity of 200 mOsm/L, as compared with the normal serum osmolarity of 290 mOsm/L. Excessive systemic absorption of the irrigating solution can result in a **dilutional hyponatremia**, hypoproteinemia, and ultimately, decreased serum osmotic pressure. Extremely low sodium levels (<110 mEq/L) may result in severe cerebral edema and cause seizures. **Hyponatremia** (serum sodium concentration <135 mEq/L) is the most common electrolyte disorder seen in hospitalized patients. Severe hyponatremia (<115 mEq/L) has developed acutely in this patient and can lead to rapid redistribution of water from the extracellular to the intracellular fluid compartment. This shift can lead to increased intracranial pressure and cerebral edema. However, the neurologic symptoms (nausea, vomiting, headache) may all be attributed to other postsurgical problems, with the hyponatremia not being recognized until seizures occur. The first goal of therapy is to raise the serum sodium level sufficient to prevent cerebral herniation. Initially, hypotonic saline solution should be given to achieve a rate of correction not to exceed 8 to 10 mEq/L in a 24-hour period and less than 18 mEq/L at 48 hours. In severely symptomatic patients (e.g., seizures), this

rate can be raised to 2 mEq/L/h for the first few hours. Concurrent furosemide diuresis may be used to decrease the risk for pulmonary edema. Chronic asymptomatic hyponatremia may be seen in patients with heart and renal failure, which is associated with increased total body water and salt retention. Water restriction alone may be efficacious for chronic asymptomatic hyponatremia. Rapid correction of hyponatremia risks myelinolysis and poor neurologic outcomes. Treatment of TUR syndrome traditionally consists of terminating the procedure as rapidly as possible, administration of furosemide (Lasix) intraoperatively or postoperatively, and administration of a 0.9% NaCl (and in severe cases 3% NaCl) solution over a 3- to 6-hour period. Newer bipolar resecting equipment allows irrigation with 0.9% normal saline, which has drastically decreased the probability of TUR syndrome. However, these patients may still suffer from fluid overload as a result of absorption of isotonic fluid.

**ANSWER:   A**

32. A 37-year-old woman comes to the emergency department complaining of a severe headache. She undergoes an emergency head CT scan, which shows subarachnoid hemorrhage; an angiogram identifies an arteriovenous malformation, which is subsequently embolized. Four days later, her serum sodium concentration is 122 mEq/L. Which is the most correct statement regarding the syndrome of inappropriate secretion of antidiuretic hormone (SIADH) and cerebral salt wasting (CSW)?

A. SIADH and CSW share the same underlying pathophysiology and cannot be reliably distinguished.

B. SIADH and CSW can be differentiated by measuring urine sodium and serum uric acid concentrations.

C. SIADH and CSW can be differentiated by measuring urine osmolality and sodium concentration.

D. Assessment of extracellular fluid volume will best differentiate between SIADH and CSW.

E. Regardless of the diagnosis, treatment of the hyponatremia is the same.

*Ref.:* 33, 35

**COMMENTS: Hyponatremia** is common in the setting of central nervous system disease. Most often it results from **inappropriate secretion of antidiuretic hormone (ADH)**. With SIADH, the hyponatremia initially results from ADH-induced water retention. This volume expansion activates natriuretic mechanisms that induce the loss of sodium and water, with the patient typically being restored to a nearly euvolemic state. With chronic SIADH, the loss of sodium (and often potassium) is much more significant than the water retention. **Cerebral salt wasting** is characterized by hyponatremia and loss of extracellular volume from inappropriate sodium wasting in urine. Patients with CSW meet the laboratory criteria for SIADH: hyponatremia, elevated urine osmolality (>100 mOsm/kg), elevated urine sodium concentration (>40 mEq/L), and low serum uric acid concentration. However, they also have clinical evidence of hypovolemia (decreased skin turgor, elevated hematocrit, decreased weight, hypotension) rather than the nearly euvolemic state seen with SIADH. Furthermore, volume repletion with isotonic saline in patients with CSW will lead to a dilute urine (and eventual correction of the hyponatremia), whereas isotonic saline administration may worsen the hyponatremia of SIADH because the sodium is retained while the water is excreted. SIADH is usually treated by fluid restriction; however, this must be done with caution in patients with SIADH because of the risk of hypotension and cerebral infarction. Isotonic saline may be used but requires careful monitoring of the serum sodium concentration; if a further fall in serum sodium occurs, a switch to hypertonic saline may be necessary. CSW generally responds well to volume repletion with isotonic saline. Salt tablets and mineralocorticoids (such as fludrocortisones) may also be useful as adjunctive measures.

**ANSWER: D**

33. In which of the following patients is hypermagnesemia unlikely to be present?

    A. 38-year-old woman with metastatic breast cancer, anorexia, and an HR of 38 beats/min

    B. 56-year-old man with pancreatitis and tetany

    C. 73-year-old man after exploratory laparotomy for an incarcerated ventral hernia with an RR of 5 breaths/min

    D. 20-year-old woman with headache, elevated liver enzymes, and loss of the patellar reflexes

    E. 44-year-old woman with severe diarrhea and hypotension

    *Ref.:* 35

**COMMENTS: Hypermagnesemia** (>2.8 mg/dL) is associated with conditions characterized by depressed neuromuscular excitability, such as bradycardia, hypotension, respiratory depression, and loss of deep tendon reflexes; therefore, all of the patients except for the one in answer B are likely to be hypermagnesemic. It is rare but it can be caused by increased magnesium intake from antacids or laxatives or from renal insufficiency. **Hypomagnesemia** defined as less than 1.6 mg/dL and is associated with gastrointestinal and renal losses or malnutrition. It is typically manifested as hypocalcemia and leads to neuromuscular hyperexcitability and tetany. Other symptoms include anorexia, vomiting, weakness, depression, psychosis, seizures, ataxia, and ventricular arrhythmias, including torsades de pointes.

**ANSWER: B**

34. An 80-kg, 65-year-old woman with severe lupus is admitted to the ICU after exploratory laparotomy for sigmoid diverticulitis (Hinchey type IV). She is given a stoma and brought to the ICU intubated. Her vitals signs are a temperature of 97.5° F, HR of 105 beats/min, BP of 70/50 mm Hg, and $Sao_2$ of 96%. In the first hour her urine output is 20 mL; she has received 4 L of crystalloid and 1 unit of PRBCs, and her antibiotics have been redosed. Her CVP is 10 mm Hg but she remains hypotensive. Choose the next intervention that will be most beneficial?

    A. Additional 2 L of a normal saline bolus

    B. Hydrocortisone, 100 mg intravenously

    C. Administration of furosemide for low urine output

    D. Initiation of vasopressor therapy with norepinephrine or dopamine

    E. Aggressive rewarming

    *Ref.:* 36

**COMMENTS:** In a patient in septic shock who is adequately volume-resuscitated (shown by a CVP of 10 mm Hg) and is unresponsive to fluid challenges, vasopressor therapy should be started. Administration of **vasopressin** can quickly restore BP; in the **Surviving Sepsis Guidelines**, norepinephrine or dopamine administered centrally is the initial vasopressor of choice. Epinephrine,

phenylephrine, and vasopressin should not be administered as the initial vasopressor to patients in septic shock. Vasopressin may subsequently be added as a second-line therapy. Epinephrine can be used as the first alternative agent in septic shock when blood pressure is poorly responsive to norepinephrine or dopamine. **Dobutamine** should be used in patients with myocardial dysfunction as evidence by elevated cardiac filling pressures and low CO. In general, the rate of fluid administration should be reduced if cardiac filling pressures increase without concurrent hemodynamic improvement.

**ANSWER: D**

35. Norepinephrine therapy is started in the patient in Question 34. Later, vasopressin, 0.03 units/min, is added, but the patient remains hypotensive with a MAP below 55 mm Hg. Her hemoglobin concentration is 9.0 g/dL. After performing an echocardiogram, dobutamine infusion was started at a maximum of 20 mcg/kg/min; pH is 7.21 with a $Pco_2$ of 34 mm Hg. The patient remains hypotensive. What is the next step?

    A. Increase the cardiac index to predetermined supranormal levels.

    B. Administer hydrocortisone, 100 mg intravenously.

    C. Have a family discussion about withdrawing care.

    D. Perform an adrenocorticotropic hormone (ACTH) stimulation test.

    E. Switch the ventilatory mode to AC.

    *Ref.:* 37

**COMMENTS:** Although there is still much debate in the critical care literature about steroids, intravenous corticosteroids are recommended in patients with **septic shock** who despite adequate fluid replacement require vasopressor therapy to maintain adequate BP. Random cortisol levels may be helpful in determining a patient's benefit from steroid therapy, although it is not required. Consideration can be made to discontinue **corticosteroid therapy** in patients with a random cortisol level of greater than 25 mcg/dL. An ACTH stimulation test is not recommended to identify the subset of patients with septic shock who should receive hydrocortisone.

**ANSWER: B**

36. A 70-kg, 33-year-old woman who had not seen a physician in 10 years arrives at the emergency department with symptoms of dyspnea, fatigue, weight gain, diplopia, and dysphagia following an urgent laparoscopic cholecystectomy 10 days ago. On examination, she is awake and alert. She is afebrile with an HR of 80 beats/min, BP of 120/70 mm Hg, and RR of 29 breaths/min. Her heart sounds are normal and breaths are bilateral and shallow. She has ptosis and significant prominal muscle weakness in all extremities. She is drooling slightly and having difficulty swallowing. Her vital capacity is 500 mL and her laboratory tests are pending. Which of the following treatments is the most appropriate to initiate next?

    A. Administration of pyridostigmine

    B. Endotracheal intubation

    C. Administration of steroids

    D. Administration of intravenous immunoglobulin

    E. Administration of levothyroxine

    *Ref.:* 38

COMMENTS: This patient is having a **myasthenic crisis**, which is a consequence of an autoimmune attack on the acetylcholine receptor complex. There is clinical weakness that is most marked after prolonged muscle exertion and should be considered in any patient with respiratory distress and cranial nerve findings. Myasthenic crisis with respiratory failure develops in approximately 20% of patients and necessitates intubation. It can be precipitated by bronchopulmonary infections, sepsis, surgical procedures, tapering of steroid medications, pregnancy, and some drugs. Upper airway muscle weakness can lead to collapse of the airways and aspiration. Patients with marginal vital capacity (<15 mL/kg), weak cough or voice, and worsening negative inspiratory force should be considered for intubation.

ANSWER:  B

37. After the patient in Question 36 is treated for myasthenia gravis, the respiratory therapist asks you for the settings on a ventilator. While she is setting up, you think about the different types of modes. Which one of the following do you have correct?

A. AC ventilation provides full ventilatory support and is a good mode to use in an agitated, tachypneic patient.

B. SIMV allows breaths to be triggered by patients and avoids stacking breaths.

C. PCV is good because minute ventilation can be set and hypoventilation and apnea do not occur.

D. CMV allows patients to increase minute ventilation by triggering additional breaths.

E. AC ventilation, when triggered by the patient, gives only the $V_T$ that patients generate on their own.

*Ref.:* 1

COMMENTS: CMV, AC ventilation, and SIMV are **volume-cycled ventilator modes**. CMV is generally used only in the OR or in patients under anesthesia because it does not allow patients to trigger additional breaths. Patients receive a set number of fixed-volume breaths. AC ventilation is used for full ventilatory support; it gives a full-volume breath when triggered by a patient, which would lead to significant respiratory alkalosis in a patient who is agitated and tachypneic. SIMV synchronizes a patient's triggered breath with one that the ventilator is scheduled to deliver and avoids stacking. It is a useful mode when weaning a patient from the ventilator, especially with **pressure support** added. PCV is designed as a protective mode to prevent alveolar overdistention and epithelial injury. Its major advantages are lower mean and peak airway pressure and a decelerating flow pattern. It is patient-triggered, and therefore patients must have an intact respiratory drive. If not, apnea and decreasing minute ventilation can occur.

ANSWER:  B

38. A 50-year-old alcoholic man (40 kg) is brought to the ICU for monitoring of symptoms of alcoholic withdrawal. A nasogastric tube is inserted and tube feeding (1.0 kcal/mL) is initiated with a goal of 50 mL/h in 16 hours. Within 24 hours, he is awake, alert, and not exhibiting any signs of withdrawal and did not need any medications in the last shift. He is cooperative but dyspneic and tachypneic and has a witnessed respiratory arrest. Advanced cardiac life support is started and he is intubated with return of cardiac activity. On review of his morning laboratory results, he has a hemoglobin concentration of 12 g/dL, platelet count of 190,000/mm³, sodium concentration of 136 mEq/L, potassium concentration of 3.0 mEq/L, albumin

level of 1.8 g/dL, magnesium concentration of 1.7 mg/dL, and phosphate level of 1.0 mg/dL. What intervention could have been done to decrease the chance of respiratory arrest?

A. Administer two doses of naloxone (Narcan) before intubation.

B. Administer phosphate and recheck levels before giving a large carbohydrate load.

C. Administer total parenteral nutrition through a peripherally inserted central catheter line instead of enteric feeding.

D. Infuse an alcohol drip through a peripheral intravenous line on admission to the unit.

E. Administer 4 g of magnesium by intravenous piggyback before giving benzodiazepine.

*Ref.:* 1, 35, 39

COMMENTS: This patient had a respiratory arrest secondary to **refeeding syndrome. Hypophosphatemia** should be expected when a chronically malnourished patient has nutritional support started. When a carbohydrate load is given, a spike in insulin increases phosphate uptake into cells and causes a significant drop in serum phosphate concentration. Muscle contractility is very dependent on a normal phosphorus level, and diaphragmatic contraction can be limited in hypophosphatemic patients with respiratory failure. Severe hypophosphatemia (<1 mg/dL) is associated with significant morbidity, including acute respiratory failure, ventilator dependence, rhabdomyolysis, altered mental status, cardiomyopathy, and muscle weakness. This can be avoided by the slow introduction of nutritional support, especially carbohydrates, and continual monitoring of serum phosphate levels. This patient already had a low phosphate level, and very quick advancement of the tube feedings to the target rate drove the level even lower than the measured laboratory values. Administration of naloxone is the next reasonable choice, but the question states that he has not required any medications in the recent past and was awake and alert on examination. Oversedation is a risk with intubation, but in this case it is not the best answer.

ANSWER:  B

39. A 66-year-old woman who has been in the ICU for 2 weeks following total hip replacement complicated by massive infection and sepsis is complaining of right calf pain. A bedside ultrasound duplex study demonstrates deep venous thrombosis (DVT) in her right lower extremity. Which statement is correct concerning DVT?

A. Duplex bedside ultrasound has a sensitivity and specificity of 75%.

B. High-risk factors for DVT include hour-long thoracic procedures, hip fractures, and spinal cord injuries.

C. A protocol for determining the level of prophylaxis for DVT is not required for any ICUs.

D. All patients with DVT should receive an intravascular inferior vena cava filter.

E. Patients determined to have DVT do not require anticoagulation.

*Ref.:* 1, 40

COMMENTS: See Question 40.

ANSWER:  B

**40.** After her ultrasound, the patient from Question 39 gets out of bed to go to physical therapy, and severe dyspnea, tachycardia, and hypotension develop. She is taken back to bed, her pulse oximetry reading is 75%, and she is given oxygen. A CT angiogram shows bilateral clots in the pulmonary arteries. With regard to PE, which of the following is true?

  A. Early chest radiographic abnormalities are rarely present in patients with PE.

  B. A shunt abnormality is present early after the PE and a $\dot{V}/\dot{Q}$ abnormality becomes the mechanism for hypoxemia in later stages.

  C. Thrombolytic therapy has been shown to reduce mortality rates in comparison to heparin in patients with PE.

  D. Heparin should never be given until the diagnosis of PE is absolute.

  E. More than 33% of patients with PE have negative lower extremity duplex studies for DVT.

*Ref.:* 1, 40

**COMMENTS:** The prevalence of **pulmonary embolism** in the United States exceeds 600,000, with the incidence of nonfatal PE approaching 20 per 1000 inpatients. **Deep venous thrombosis** occurs in 30% of ICU patients and is monitored by governing bodies in the United States, and all ICUs should have a prevention protocol. High-risk factors are thoracic or general procedures requiring general anesthesia for longer than 30 minutes, neurosurgical procedures, CABG surgery, surgery for gynecologic cancers, CHF, and respiratory failure, along with long-bone fractures and spinal cord injuries. ICU patients almost always have at least one risk factor and need prophylaxis. Options include pharmacologic treatment with **low-molecular-weight heparin** (LMWH), unfractionated heparin, or pneumatic compression devices.

In regard to diagnosis, **duplex ultrasound** has a specificity and sensitivity greater than 95%. Many emboli can be silent, but symptoms of small to medium emboli are usually pulmonary (i.e., dyspnea, chest pain, and cough). Tachypnea and tachycardia are present as well. Massive PE often produces cardiovascular findings such as elevated PA pressure and right heart strain. Angiography is the definitive diagnostic technique for this disease, but a helical CT scan of the chest with infusion has shown excellent specificity. Even without pulmonary infarction, radiographic abnormalities appear as diaphragmatic elevation, atelectasis, and effusion. For treatment of DVT, heparin therapy over a period of 5 to 7 days with an overlap with warfarin constitutes the treatment of choice. Warfarin should be continued for 6 to 12 weeks for calf vein and large-vein thrombosis and up to 6 months for PE. **Thrombolytic therapy** has not been shown to reduce mortality rates in comparison to heparin in large prospective series.

**ANSWER:** E

**41.** A 56-year-old man with a past medical history of hypertension and diabetes mellitus is admitted to the ICU after right femoral-popliteal bypass surgery for neurovascular monitoring. In the morning during rounds, his signals are undetectable, and his right foot is cold and painful. He is taken back to the OR for revision of his bypass, and fasciotomies are performed in all four quadrants. An unfractionated heparin drip is started with a weight-based protocol to achieve a partial thromboplastin time (PTT) two times the normal value. His laboratory results immediately before return to the OR showed a WBC count of 11,000/mm$^3$, hemoglobin concentration of 10.2 g/dL, platelet count of 350,000/mm$^3$, potassium concentration of 4.1 mEq/L,

BUN of 30 mg/dL, and creatinine concentration of 2.1 mg/dL. A week later on rounds, the patient complains of left calf pain. Duplex ultrasound shows DVT in his left lower extremity. His WBC count is 12,300/mm$^3$ with a hemoglobin level of 9.1 g/dL, platelet count of 97,000/mm$^3$, potassium concentration of 4.6 mEq/L, BUN of 39 mg/dL, and creatinine level of 2.3 mg/dL. Which of the following treatments options is the best choice?

  A. Discontinuation of anticoagulation

  B. Discontinuation of unfractionated heparin and initiation of warfarin

  C. Discontinuation of unfractionated heparin and initiation of argatroban

  D. Discontinuation of unfractionated heparin and initiation of LMWH

  E. Bolus heparin drip and increase in the PTT goal to 2.5 times the normal value

*Ref.:* 1, 41

**COMMENTS:** See Question 42.

**ANSWER:** C

**42.** The patient from Question 41 tolerates his anticoagulation, but he has been continually oozing from his fasciotomy sites and his hemoglobin has drifted down in the past 3 days to a level of 7.8 g/dL. On review of his chart you see that in the preoperative clearance note from cardiology he had a hemoglobin level of 13.0 g/dL and no significant cardiac disease. His family is concerned about how pale he has been during this ICU stay. His vital signs are an HR of 86 beats/min, BP of 128/69 mm Hg, and Sao$_2$ of 96%. What is the appropriate answer regarding a blood transfusion for this patient at this time?

  A. Transfuse 5 units of PRBCs to reach the preoperative hemoglobin level of 13 g/dL.

  B. Check complete blood count (CBC) levels daily and hold transfusion until the hemoglobin level is lower than 9 g/dL.

  C. Start erythropoietin at 40,000 units daily.

  D. Transfuse PRBCs to a level greater than 10 g/dL.

  E. Check daily CBC levels and hold transfusion until the hemoglobin level is lower than 7 g/dL.

*Ref.:* 1, 41, 42

**COMMENTS:** Type II **heparin-induced thrombocytopenia** (HIT) has developed in this patient. Type I HIT occurs in 1% to 2% of patients and causes transient sequestration of platelets with a drop in the count to less than the normal range or a 50% fall in the platelet count within the normal range. In general, this is of little consequence. Platelet levels normalize in a few days after heparin is discontinued. Type II is more severe, and antiplatelet antibodies develop in 0.1% to 0.2% of patients exposed to heparin. It is associated with thrombotic complications in more than 30% of cases and should be suspected in a patient in whom resistance to anticoagulation, thromboembolic events, and a fall in the platelet greater than 30% or a count of less than 100,000/mm$^3$ develop. Once HIT is suspected, all sources of heparin, including LMWH, should be discontinued. Warfarin can actually worsen the prothrombotic state and should not be used before complete anticoagulation is achieved with either argatroban or lepirudin, both antithrombin agents.

**Anemia** is very common in critically ill patients; in the United States, approximately 85% of patients spending more than 1 week in the ICU receive 1 or more units of PRBCs in their first week. Blood is a scarce and expensive resource and is associated with morbidity, including transfusion reactions, infections, and worse outcomes. Historically, patients received transfusions if their hemoglobin level dropped below 10 g/dL. However, a multicenter prospective randomized clinical trial in 1999 showed that transfusion for a hemoglobin level of less than 7 g/dL had the same 30-day mortality rate as transfusion when the hemoglobin level was less than 10 g/dL (except in patients with significant cardiac disease). This patient had preoperative cardiac clearance and is not presently showing any signs of hemodynamic instability.

Patients with anemia of critical illness have been shown to have a blunted response to both endogenous and exogenous erythropoietin. A multicenter trial showed a mild increase in hemoglobin, but it is unclear in the literature whether this improves clinical outcomes.

Lepirudin undergoes renal elimination, which should be noted in situations such as this patient with renal insufficiency. **Argatroban** is metabolized hepatically and is the best choice in this situation.

**ANSWER:** E

43. The patient from Questions 41 and 42 wants to know whether there are any types of blood substitutes that could be given if he does need a transfusion. You discuss the options and characteristics of an ideal blood substitute. Which of the following is not a characteristic of an ideal substitute?

    A. Universal compatibility

    B. Long-term storage capability

    C. Decreases physiologic loading and unloading of $O_2$

    D. Capability of volume expansion

    E. Freedom from disease transmission

*Ref.:* 1, 43

**COMMENTS:** There is a worldwide shortage of blood, which has a limited shelf life, is expensive, and has multiple transfusion-associated morbidities. The scientific community has been working to develop an ideal blood substitute that should have the following characteristics: physiologic loading and unloading of $O_2$ (not minimizing it), capability of volume expansion, immediate availability, universal compatibility, no adverse physiologic effects, freedom from disease transmission, and long-term storage capability. Several products have been developed but have not been found to have any benefit in injured patients yet; most studies have involved those with acute blood loss and not long-term anemia.

**ANSWER:** C

44. A 24-year-old woman undergoes laparotomy for a class IV injury to her liver and during the procedure is transfused with 12 units of cold, stored PBRCs. Despite appropriate treatment of the liver injury, there is persistent bleeding from the raw surface of the parenchyma, the puncture sites of all intravenous lines, and the skin incision. In addition to aggressive resuscitation, which initial treatment is most appropriate at this time?

    A. Infusion of 10 mL of a 10% $CaCl_2$ solution

    B. 5 units of fresh frozen plasma and observation in the OR

    C. 2 units of platelets while applying compression on the liver

    D. Halting the operation and transferring to the ICU for correction of hypothermia

    E. 1 mg/kg of enoxaparin while remaining in the OR

*Ref.:* 44

**COMMENTS: Hypothermia**, **acidosis**, and **coagulopathy** are frequently encountered in trauma patients and are often referred to as the "**deadly triad**." This patient has had a massive transfusion, defined as the administration of more than 10 units of blood or more than one blood volume of the patient within 24 hours. All of the choices will probably be needed to correct the patient's coagulopathy, but rewarming is the best selection initially. The surgeon should control any surgical bleeding and terminate the procedure to allow warming of the patient and replacement of components in the ICU. Blood warmers, warm saline lavage, blankets, and heated inspired gases are useful adjunctive measures to prevent hypothermia. The known associated complications of **massive transfusions** include electrolyte and acid-base abnormalities, changes in hemoglobin-oxygen affinity, hypothermia, coagulopathy, and dysfunction of various organs. Coagulation proteins and platelets are consumed in the normal process to achieve hemostasis through clot formation. Despite low levels of factors V and VIII in blood stored for 14 to 21 days, dilutional coagulopathy is rare. Recommendations for combatting coagulopathy have included prophylactic administration of 1 or 2 units of fresh frozen plasma for anywhere from every 2 to 10 units of transfused blood. The indications for administration of calcium should be based on hemodynamic considerations because lowering the ionized calcium level by citrate to a level that blocks coagulation could lead to death from myocardial dysfunction and decreased peripheral vascular resistance. Hypothermia decreases clearance of citrate from the blood, thereby allowing a marked reduction in ionized calcium. The clotting system is impaired because of a decreased ability to form stable clots and decreased production of clotting factors. Enoxaparin is not indicated as the initial step in such a situation.

**ANSWER:** D

45. Choose the statement that is not true with regard to ECMO.

    A. ECMO is an appropriate treatment for patients without prohibitive risk of death from respiratory failure and without other lethal comorbid conditions.

    B. Low-flow ECMO can be used in patients with primary hypercapnic respiratory failure to improve removal of $CO_2$.

    C. Indications for ECMO include status asthmaticus and patients maintained on high ventilator settings for more than 7 days.

    D. Patients with a compliance of less than 0.5 mL/cm $H_2O$/kg and a $Pao_2/Fio_2$ ratio of less than 100 are good candidates for ECMO.

    E. Patients treated with ECMO usually have a 20% predicted survival rate without this bypass.

*Ref.:* 45-47

**COMMENTS: Extracorporeal membrane oxygenation** is considered a supportive nontherapeutic intervention that maintains adequate gas exchange and circulatory support while resting the injured lungs or heart (or both). Successful use of ECMO was first reported in 1972; it subsequently lost favor but has enjoyed a resurgence in the last two decades for coronary artery diseases. All of the answers are true except for C. ECMO can be used for patients with status asthmaticus or other forms of airway obstruction with hypercapnia, but it is contraindicated in patients with high ventilator settings for more than 7 days, incurable disease, age older than 70 years, poor neurologic status, and active bleeding because of the need for systemic anticoagulation. Indications are poor gas exchange, compliance of less than 0.5 mL/cm $H_2O$/kg, a $Pao_2/Fio_2$ ratio of less than 100, and a shunt fraction greater than 30%. A typical ECMO system has a membrane oxygenator, heat exchanger, roller or pump, circuit tubing, and access catheters. It removes $CO_2$ extracorporeally and gently oxygenates the lungs with low-flow ventilation. Overall, survival to discharge occurs in approximately 50% of patients treated by ECMO, and it is used as a last effort in patients with severe cardiopulmonary failure.

**ANSWER:** C

**46.** A 43-year-old alcoholic is admitted to the hospital with acute pancreatitis and severe abdominal pain. A central line is placed, she is given several liters of fluid resuscitation, and laboratory tests are ordered. Her vital signs are a temperature of 39° C, HR of 92 beats/min, BP of 102/53 mm Hg, RR of 24 breaths/min, and $Sao_2$ of 93%. Admission laboratory results included an amylase concentration of 400 units/L, lipase concentration of 1740 units/L, WBC count of 14,000/mm$^3$, and hemoglobin level of 14 g/dL. You are trying to decide whether she qualifies to be entered into a study for SIRS. You know that she needs two of several characteristics to qualify. Which of the following is not included in the definition of SIRS?

A. Temperature lower than 36° C or higher than 38° C

B. RR greater than 20 breaths/min

C. $Paco_2$ lower than 32

D. Hemoglobin level less than 10 g/dL

E. White blood cell count lower than 4000/mm$^3$ or higher than 12,000/mm$^3$

*Ref.:* 1, 48, 49

**COMMENTS: Systemic inflammatory response syndrome** is a generalized hyperinflammatory response to a number of different etiologic factors to the body. In 25% to 35% of patients it persists and can lead to multiple organ dysfunction syndrome, sepsis, and septic shock. This patient's clinical condition qualifies for SIRS because it has all the aforementioned qualifiers except for hemoglobin, which is not in the definition. SIRS does not occur de novo but in response to an instigating process that stimulates the inflammatory cascade of coronary artery disease. It can be caused by noninfectious insults such as trauma, nonseptic shock, drugs, and toxins and may continue even after the initial instigating factor is removed or successfully treated. In addition, it may be perpetuated by poor perfusion from subpar resuscitation.

**ANSWER:** D

**47.** A 54-year-old Hispanic man with uncontrolled diabetes comes to the emergency department because of scrotal edema and tenderness. He complains of fevers and chills but denies nausea, vomiting, or diarrhea. He has a foul odor on rectal examination, pus is expressed, and cellulitis of the skin is noted around his scrotum and anus. He has crepitus along his perineum and extending up along his inguinal crease. His vital signs are a temperature of 101.3° F, HR of 128 beats/min, BP of 90/62 mm Hg, and $Sao_2$ of 92%. Which of the following therapeutic strategies is most appropriate?

A. Emergency placement of a central line and administration of vancomycin with transfer to the ICU

B. Opening the wound in the ER and packing with iodoform gauze

C. Sending the patient for a CT scan with intravenous, oral, and rectal contrast media to evaluate the extent of the problem

D. Immediate surgical intervention with débridement of all devitalized tissue

E. Admission to the ICU with frequent checks on the cellulitis

*Ref.:* 36, 50

**COMMENTS:** See Question 48.

**ANSWER:** D

**48.** The patient in Question 47 has now been in the hospital for 6 hours, is requiring multiple vasopressors, and is showing signs of multiple organ failure (MOF). You just had a grand rounds on early directed-goal therapy. Which one of the goals is not included in the initial resuscitation recommended in the Surviving Sepsis Guidelines?

A. Target CVP of 8 to 12 mm Hg

B. Central venous $So_2$ greater than 70%

C. Institution of antibiotics within 12 hours of admission

D. MAP higher than 65 mm Hg

E. Urine output greater than 0.5 mL/kg

*Ref.:* 36, 50

**COMMENTS: Fournier gangrene** is a necrotizing fasciitis of the male genitalia and perineum that has a mortality reaching 50%. This disease travels along fascial planes and can spread rapidly. The best answer is immediate surgical débridement, and the area should be irrigated copiously. Both aerobic and anaerobic coverage should be started, with the most common organism being *Escherichia coli*. At times, diabetic patients do not feel much pain, so a detailed physical examination is important. CT scans can help distinguish the extent of the disease, but insertion of a rectal probe and contrast material in this patient would probably be impossible. In addition, he is hemodynamically unstable, and sending him to the radiology department without securing his airway or adequately resuscitating him would be very dangerous. Opening the wound in the emergency department would not be adequate débridement and unlikely to be tolerated by the patient. The Surviving Sepsis Guidelines, which outlines early goal-directed therapy, has been shown to reduce in-hospital mortality in patients with severe sepsis and septic shock. All of the answers except C are correct and are targeted for initial resuscitation in the first 6 hours in patients with hypotension or elevated serum lactate. If any of the interventions are not achieved, the guidelines published by Society of Critical Care Medicine recommend further fluid and transfusion of PRBCs to a hematocrit of higher than 30% or an infusion of dobutamine (or both). In addition, a targeted CVP of 12 to 15 mm Hg is recommended for mechanically ventilated patients or those with decreased compliance. Antibiotics should be given within 1 hour of recognizing severe sepsis or sooner if suspicion is high. Broad-spectrum agents with good penetration into the presumed source should be started. The guidelines suggest obtaining cultures and performing imaging studies promptly to determine infection if this does not delay the administration of antibiotics.

**ANSWER:** C

49. With regard to MOF, which of the following statement is false?

    A. Sepsis is the major risk factor.

    B. Injury to the microvascular endothelium is uniformly present.

    C. Neutrophil-mediated injury is dependent on adherence to the microvascular endothelium.

    D. There is a bimodal pattern to the development of MOF.

    E. An increase in the gastrointestinal barrier is often present.

*Ref.:* 1

**COMMENTS: Sepsis** is the major risk factor for the development of **multiple organ failure**. Injury to the microvascular endothelium causes a generalized inflammatory state, and early recognition and adequate treatment are essential if serious ischemia-reperfusion injury and MOF are to be prevented. Several components of the immune defense system are involved. Neutrophil-mediated injury is dependent on adherence to the endothelium and neutrophil aggregation. Platelet-activating factor, produced by various inflammatory cells, causes microvascular injury through ischemia and stasis. Breakdown of the intestinal mucosal barrier may allow ongoing bacterial translocation and stimulation of the immunoinflammatory reaction. There is a bimodal pattern of development of MOF. The first peak occurs within 72 hours of the initial insult, and late MOF is manifested at 6 to 8 days and is typically related to an infection.

**ANSWER:** E

50. A 22-year-old man involved in a motor vehicle accident is found to have a thoracic spine fracture (T6) and paraplegia. The patient is hypotensive with a systolic BP of 70 mm Hg, is bradycardic with a pulse of 48 beats/min, and is breathing comfortably. Which of the following would be the most appropriate initial treatment?

    A. Isotonic fluid administration

    B. Steroid administration within 24 hours of the injury

    C. Immediate intubation

    D. α-Agonist administration

    E. Immediate magnetic resonance imaging

*Ref.:* 51, 52

**COMMENTS: Neurogenic shock** refers to a condition characterized by hypotension and bradycardia that results from interruption of the sympathetic nervous system pathways within the spinal cord. Common causes include sensory stimulation, such as severe pain, exposure to unpleasant events or sights, high spinal anesthesia, and traumatic spinal cord injury. Clinical characteristics include a BP that is often low, as in other forms of shock. However, the pulse rate is usually slower than normal, and the skin is flushed, warm, and dry. CO is reduced secondary to decreased blood return to the heart because of the increased capacitance of the arterioles and venules. Since the heart receives sympathetic input, there is a difference between injuries above and below T4. The former depresses

cardiac function and decreases venous return. The bradycardia is caused by sympathectomy of the **spinal injury** above the level of T4 with no capacity for compensatory tachycardia. Treatment of neurogenic shock secondary to spinal cord injury is usually more complicated, not only because of more prolonged hypotension but also because of the presence of coincident hypovolemic shock resulting from associated injuries. Such patients often require ventilatory support as a result of decreased spontaneous respiration and loss of the accessory muscles for breathing. Aggressive fluid therapy should be instituted early under continuous cardiovascular monitoring. Persistent hypotension necessitates recognition of possible hemorrhagic shock, and a vasopressor such as ephedrine or phenylephrine may be needed. If the injury is below T4, a pure α-agonist may aggravate the reflex bradycardia. Thus, a drug with mixed chronotropic and inotropic effects (e.g., norepinephrine or dopamine) is preferred. A nasogastric tube should be inserted because gastric atony, dilation, and hypersecretion develop in these patients. Treatment of milder forms of neurogenic shock consists of removing the nociceptive stimulus. Neurogenic shock resulting from high spinal anesthesia can usually be treated with a vasopressor such as ephedrine or phenylephrine, each of which increases CO by direct effects on the heart and by increasing peripheral vasoconstriction. Although the administration of steroids remains controversial, their usefulness for blunt spinal cord injury has been suggested when they are given within 8 hours of injury and their administration is extended for 48 hours.

**ANSWER:** A

51. A 60-year-old man with renal failure who has been undergone dialysis for the past 2 years is admitted for cellulitis surrounding the fistula site on his right upper extremity. Antibiotics are started and the patient is observed. On hospital day 4, his fistula clots and he is taken to the OR for revision. On the following day, he is febrile, coughing up thick green sputum, and dyspneic despite having undergone dialysis that morning. A chest radiograph shows an infiltrate in his right lower lobe, and laboratory tests show a WBC count of 18,000/mm³. Which characteristic of nosocomial pneumonia listed below is not correct?

    A. Characterized by onset within 24 hours of hospital admission

    B. Purulent sputum

    C. Isolation of the pathogenic organism from blood or the lung

    D. Elevated WBC count

    E. Infiltrate on chest radiography

*Ref.:* 53, 54

**COMMENTS:** See Question 52.

**ANSWER:** A

52. What is the next step in treatment for the patient in Question 51?

    A. Hold antibiotic coverage until culture-proven infection is noted.

    B. Start empirical broad-spectrum antibiotics based on risk factors and an antibiogram of the ICU.

    C. Perform bronchoscopy daily until the secretions have cleared.

D. Start one antibiotic based on the most likely pathogen and escalate as needed.

E. Intubate and place the patient on a low-volume, lung-protective ventilation protocol.

*Ref.:* 53, 54

COMMENTS: **Hospital-acquired pneumonia** (HAP) is the second most common of all nosocomial infections in the United States. The Centers for Disease Control and Prevention's definition of **nosocomial pneumonia** is a clinical one that requires pneumonia to occur more than 48 hours after hospital admission and excludes any infections that are present or incubating at admission. The other two criteria include appropriate findings on physical examination *or* an infiltrate on chest radiography plus one of the following: purulent sputum, isolation of the pathogenic organism from blood or the lung, identification of a virus from the lower respiratory tract, or serologic or pathologic evidence of recent infection. Many clinical studies have shown that early, appropriate, and adequate antibiotic therapy can reduce the mortality rate from HAP, currently listed anywhere from 24% to 76%. The American Thoracic Society presumes that early-onset pneumonia is due to *Haemophilus influenzae*, methicillin-susceptible *Staphylococcus aureus*, *Streptococcus pneumoniae*, or anaerobes. Late-onset HAP occurs more than 4 days after admission and is usually caused by gram-negative organisms, especially *Pseudomonas aeruginosa*, *Acinetobacter*, Enterobacteriaceae (*Klebsiella*, *Enterobacter*, *Serratia*), or methicillin-resistant *S. aureus* (MRSA). Broad-spectrum antibiotics should be started early and deescalated, not escalated, when culture sensitivities are known. This patient does not require intubation at this time, and low-volume, lung-protective ventilation is best used for ARDS. Patients with HAP do not need bronchoscopy daily. Chest therapy, elevation of the head of the bed, and ambulation are all methods to improve pulmonary toilet.

**ANSWER: B**

53. A 27-year-old man who ingested 40 tablets of his brother's lithium, 4000 mg of ibuprofen, and two bottles of antifreeze during a suicide attempt has been in the ICU for 6 days. He was obtunded and on admission had a temporary dialysis catheter placed urgently in his right internal jugular vein and had been undergoing hemodialysis for the first 3 days after admission. What was the best method of gastric decontamination for this patient on initial admission at approximately 3 hours after ingestion?

A. Gastric lavage and activated charcoal

B. Whole-bowel irrigation

C. Intubation and gastric lavage

D. Activated charcoal

E. Syrup of ipecac

*Ref.:* 55

COMMENTS: See Question 54

**ANSWER: B**

54. He is now complaining of vague pains all over, anorexia, cough with thin white sputum, and malaise and has not had flatus or a bowel movement for 24 hours. Chest radiography shows bilateral haziness at the costophrenic angles. Physical

examination showed the patient to not be in acute distress. His lungs have some crackles in the bases bilaterally. His right arm is slightly swollen, and he has some redness around the right side of his neck and chest. His abdomen is soft, distended, tympanitic, and nontender. His vital signs include a temperature of 101.6° F, HR of 100 beats/min, BP of 128/75 mm Hg, and Sao$_2$ of 96%. Laboratory findings included a WBC count of 18,500/mm$^3$, sodium concentration of 140 mEq/L, potassium concentration of 4.3 mEq/L, BUN of 21 mg/dL, creatinine level of 0.8 mg/dL, aspartate/alanine aminotransferase (AST/ALT) levels of 54/49 units/L, and total bilirubin of 0.9 mg/dL. What is the most likely diagnosis?

A. Acalculous cholecystitis

B. HAP

C. Catheter-related bloodstream infection

D. Perforated peptic ulcer

E. Viral respiratory infection

*Ref.:* 54, 55

COMMENTS: **Gastric lavage** is not indicated in this patient and is not a proven benefit, even when used within 1 hour of ingestion. Complications can include aspiration, laryngospasm, and mechanical injury. Ipecac causes local irritation of the gastric mucosa, which induces reflex vomiting after 30 minutes of administration. Ipecac should not be used in routine poisoning cases; there is no evidence that it improves outcomes, and it can do more harm by exposing the esophagus to the poison again. Whole-bowel irrigation is not specifically indicated for any poisoning but at times can be used with medications that are sustained-release or enteric-coated drugs, such as lithium, which our patient ingested. Activated charcoal is best given within 1 hour of ingestion and can be considered if the patient has ingested a potentially toxic amount of poison. There is no evidence showing that activated charcoal improves outcomes.

The most likely diagnosis is a catheter-related bloodstream infection. He had a catheter placed on an emergency basis and is now experiencing fevers and malaise, with cellulitis evident in the right side of his neck. His infection can explain the anorexia, ileus, and elevated WBC count. Catheter-related bloodstream infection is seen in approximately 5% of patients with indwelling catheters and should be suspected if any erythema or purulence is identified at the catheter site. The subclavian vein is the preferred site for reduction of infection, over internal jugular or femoral locations. Once an infection is suspected, blood should be drawn through the line and peripherally for culture, and immediate removal of the catheter is suggested and the tip sent for culture. A catheter–peripheral colony-forming unit (CFU) ratio of 8 signifies line sepsis, and a **catheter tip culture** with 25 CFUs confirms a **catheter-related infection**.

**ANSWER: C**

55. A 45-year-old man is recovering from MOF after an operation for a perforated gastric ulcer. He has been afebrile for 48 hours and is not taking any antibiotics. His WBC count is normal, and his renal failure has resolved. His encephalopathy is improving, and his oxygenation is adequate on 30% oxygen and 5 cm H$_2$O PEEP. Attempts at weaning him off the ventilator have been unsuccessful. His negative inspiratory pressure is 10 cm H$_2$O. Neurologic examination shows a symmetrical quadriparesis with sparing of the face and depressed deep tendon reflexes. Spinal tap fluid is normal. What is the most likely diagnosis?

A. Guillain-Barré syndrome

B. Myasthenia gravis

C. Neuromuscular blockade

D. Primary myopathy

E. Critical illness polyneuropathy (CPU)

*Ref.:* 56

**COMMENTS:** See Question 56.

**ANSWER:** E

56. Which of the following statements is true concerning the condition described in the previous question?

A. A nerve biopsy often shows demyelinization or inflammation.

B. Failure to wean from the ventilator is due to phrenic nerve involvement.

C. Corticosteroids are the treatment of choice.

D. Serum antibodies against acetylcholine receptors are always present.

E. Plasmapheresis is the initial treatment of choice.

*Ref.:* 56, 57

**COMMENTS:** CPU is an **axonal motor sensory neuropathy** that accompanies sepsis with encephalopathy. It is due to primary axonal degeneration and affects motor fibers more than sensory fibers. Frequently, it is manifested as failure to wean a patient from the ventilator because of phrenic nerve involvement despite clinical improvement. Symmetrical quadriparesis with facial sparing and depressed deep tendon reflexes is characteristic, and electromyography confirms the diagnosis. Spinal fluid is normal, unlike the case in patients with **Guillain-Barré syndrome**. Facial involvement and detection of antibodies against acetylcholine are characteristic of myasthenia gravis. Nerve biopsy shows axonal degeneration without demyelinization or inflammation. Treatment is supportive and corticosteroids are contraindicated.

**ANSWER:** B

57. A 63-year-old man is admitted to the ICU following a Hartmann procedure for Hinchey type IV diverticulitis 5 days earlier. The patient is intubated and maintained on AC ventilation, is tachycardic, and is febrile to 101° F. The nurse has noticed an increase in tracheobronchial secretions that are purulent in character. A chest radiograph shows a new infiltrate in the right lung. Which of the following statements is false regarding this patient's condition?

A. The most likely organism involved is methicillin-sensitive *S. aureus.*

B. The frequency of ventilator circuit changes does not influence the incidence of this complication.

C. Kinetic beds and elevation of the head of the patient to 45 degrees decrease its incidence.

D. The risk for development of this complication is highest in the second week.

E. Qualitative cultures or secretions are preferred over quantitative culture techniques.

*Ref.:* 58

**COMMENTS: Ventilator-associated pneumonia** (VAP) has significant costs and a mortality of about 25%. The risk of acquiring VAP is highest in the first week (3% per day), thereafter decreasing to 2% per day in the second week and to 1% per day in the third week. VAP is generally categorized as early (<48 hours after intubation) or late (occurring after 5 to 7 days of intubation). Early-onset VAP is associated with bacteria that are normally sensitive to antibiotics (*S. aureus, H. influenzae,* and *S. pneumoniae*), whereas late-onset VAP is typically associated with antibiotic-resistant bacteria (MRSA, *P. aeruginosa, Acinetobacter,* and *Enterobacter* species). The major risk factors for VAP include trauma, burns, and stay in neurosurgical units as opposed medical ICUs. Known risk factors include patients older than 60 years who require prolonged (>48 hours) mechanical ventilatory support, aspiration, a nasogastric tube, failure to elevate the head of the bed, and endotracheal cuff pressures of less than 20 cm $H_2O$. Orotracheal intubation carries a lower incidence of VAP than does nasotracheal intubation. Because contamination of ventilator circuits is universal, the ventilator circuit change interval does not affect the incidence of VAP. Heat and moisture exchangers may be associated with a slightly lower incidence of VAP than heated humidifiers. Drainage of subglottic secretions is associated with a decreased incidence of VAP, especially early-onset VAP. Kinetic beds and positioning of patients at 45 degrees from horizontal are also associated with a decreased incidence. Previous exposure to antibiotics in a prolonged preoperative hospitalization exposes patients to health care–related infections. Selective digestive decontamination has been reported to be associated with a decreased incidence of VAP, yet these therapies should be time-limited to prevent the growth of resistant organisms. The suspicion for VAP in this patient with a prolonged period of ventilation and new onset of fever, leukocytosis, and purulent sputum should be high, particularly if the chest radiograph shows a new infiltrate. The diagnosis is best established by quantitative culture of secretions obtained from the lower respiratory tract. The two techniques used include **protected specimen brush** (PSB) **sampling** and **bronchoalveolar lavage** (BAL). A threshold of 1000 CFU/mL for PSB and 10,000 CFU/mL for BAL is currently recommended. The presence of less than 50% neutrophils in BAL fluid has also been used to exclude pneumonia. Even though the effect of these techniques on patient outcome is unclear, they have resulted in a significant reduction in the use of antibiotics.

**ANSWER:** D

**REFERENCES**

1. Adams CA, Biffl WL, Cioffi WG: Surgical critical care. In Townsend CM, Beauchamp RD, Evers BM, et al, editors: *Sabiston textbook of surgery: the biological basis of modern surgical practice,* ed 17, Philadelphia, 2008, WB Saunders.
2. Winters B: Analgesia and sedation in critical care medicine. In Cameron JL, editor: *Current surgical therapy,* ed 9, Philadelphia, 2008, CV Mosby.
3. Milbrandt EB, Ely EW: Agitation and delirium. In Fink MP, Abraham E, Vincent JL, et al, editors: *Textbook of critical care,* ed 5, Philadelphia, 2005, WB Saunders.
4. Moran SE, Pei KY, Yu M: Hemodynamic monitoring: arterial and pulmonary artery catheters. In Gabrielli A, Layon AJ, Yu M, editors: *Civetta, Taylor & Kirby's critical care,* ed 4, Philadelphia, 2009, Lippincott Williams & Wilkins.

5. Rhodes A, Grounds RM, Bennett ED: Hemodynamic monitoring. In Fink MP, Abraham E, Vincent JL, et al, editors: *Textbook of critical care*, ed 5, Philadelphia, 2005, WB Saunders.

6. Gaspardone A, De Luca L: ST elevation myocardial infarction (STEMI) contemporary management strategies. In Gabrielli A, Layon AJ, Yu M, editors: *Civetta, Taylor & Kirby's critical care*, ed 4, Philadelphia, 2009, Lippincott Williams & Wilkins.

7. Moran SE, Pei KY, Yu M: Hemodynamic monitoring: arterial and pulmonary artery catheters. In Gabrielli A, Layon AJ, Yu M, editors: *Civetta, Taylor & Kirby's critical care*, ed 4, Philadelphia, 2009, Lippincott Williams & Wilkins.

8. Marino PL: *Circulatory blood flow: the ICU book*, ed 2, Philadelphia, 1998, Lippincott Williams & Wilkins.

9. Marini JJ: Principles of Gas Exchange. In Fink MP, Abraham E, Vincent JL, et al, editors: *Textbook of critical care*, ed 5, Philadelphia, 2005, WB Saunders.

10. Kalet RH, Tang JF: Bedside monitoring of pulmonary function. In Fink MP, Abraham E, Vincent JL, et al, editors: *Textbook of critical care*, ed 5, Philadelphia, 2005, WB Saunders.

11. Schmalfuss CM: Pericardial disease. In Gabrielli A, Layon AJ, Yu M, editors: *Civetta, Taylor & Kirby's critical care*, ed 4, Philadelphia, 2009, Lippincott Williams & Wilkins.

12. Camm J, Savelieva I: Supraventricular arrhythmias. In Fink MP, Abraham E, Vincent JL, et al, editors: *Textbook of critical care*, ed 5, Philadelphia, 2005, WB Saunders.

13. Naik BI, Murfin D, Thannikary L: Preoperative evaluation of the high-risk surgical patient. In Gabrielli A, Layon AJ, Yu M, editors: *Civetta, Taylor & Kirby's critical care*, ed 4, Philadelphia, 2009, Lippincott Williams & Wilkins.

14. Marini JJ, Dries DJ, Perry JF: The lung structure and function. In Gabrielli A, Layon AJ, Yu M, editors: *Civetta, Taylor & Kirby's critical care*, ed 4, Philadelphia, 2009, Lippincott Williams & Wilkins.

15. Laghi F: Weaning from mechanical ventilation. In Gabrielli A, Layon AJ, Yu M, editors: *Civetta, Taylor & Kirby's critical care*, ed 4, Philadelphia, 2009, Lippincott Williams & Wilkins.

16. Corbridge TC, Corbridge SJ: Severe asthma exacerbation. In Fink MP, Abraham E, Vincent JL, et al, editors: *Textbook of critical care*, ed 5, Philadelphia, 2005, WB Saunders.

17. Katsaounou PA, Vassilakopoulos T: Severe asthma exacerbation. In Gabrielli A, Layon AJ, Yu M, editors: *Civetta, Taylor & Kirby's critical care*, ed 4, Philadelphia, 2009, Lippincott Williams & Wilkins.

18. Pinsky MR: Heart-lung interactions. In Fink MP, Abraham E, Vincent JL, et al, editors: *Textbook of critical care*, ed 5, Philadelphia, 2005, WB Saunders.

19. Caples SM, Hubmayr RD: Respiratory system mechanics and respiratory muscle function. In Fink MP, Abraham E, Vincent JL, et al, editors: *Textbook of critical care*, ed 5, Philadelphia, 2005, WB Saunders.

20. Marino PL: *Principles of mechanical ventilation: the ICU book*, ed 2, Philadelphia, 1998, Lippincott Williams & Wilkins.

21. Peters CW, Yu M, Sladen RN, et al: Acute lung injury and acute respiratory distress syndrome. In Gabrielli A, Layon AJ, Yu M, editors: *Civetta, Taylor & Kirby's critical care*, ed 4, Philadelphia, 2009, Lippincott Williams & Wilkins.

22. Rajan T, Hill NS: Noninvasive positive-pressure ventilation. In Fink MP, Abraham E, Vincent JL, et al, editors: *Textbook of critical care*, ed 5, Philadelphia, 2005, WB Saunders.

23. Ware LB, Bernard GR: Acute lung injury and acute respiratory distress syndrome. In Fink MP, Abraham E, Vincent JL, et al, editors: *Textbook of critical care*, ed 5, Philadelphia, 2005, WB Saunders.

24. Marino PL: *Acute respiratory distress syndrome: the ICU book*, ed 2, Philadelphia, 1998, Lippincott Williams & Wilkins.

25. Ventilation with lower tidal volumes as compared with traditional volumes for acute lung injury and the acute respiratory distress syndrome. The Acute Respiratory Distress Syndrome Network, *N Engl J Med* 342:1301–1308, 2000.

26. Bagshaw SM, Bellomo R: Acute renal failure. In Gabrielli A, Layon AJ, Yu M, editors: *Civetta, Taylor & Kirby's critical care*, ed 4, Philadelphia, 2009, Lippincott Williams & Wilkins.

27. Kulaylat MN, Dayton MT: Surgical complications. In Townsend CM, Beauchamp RD, Evers BM, et al, editors: *Sabiston textbook of surgery: the biological basis of modern surgical practice*, ed 18, Philadelphia, 2008, WB Elsevier.

28. Barrett BJ: Contrast dye-induced nephropathy. In Fink MP, Abraham E, Vincent JL, et al, editors: *Textbook of critical care*, ed 5, Philadelphia, 2005, WB Saunders.

29. Mullins RJ: Acute renal failure. In Cameron JL, editor: *Current surgical therapy*, ed 9, Philadelphia, 2008, CV Mosby.

30. Bellomo R, D'Intini V: Renal replacement therapy in the ICU. In Fink MP, Abraham E, Vincent JL, et al, editors: *Textbook of critical care*, ed 5, Philadelphia, 2005, WB Saunders.

31. Balogun RA, Okusa MD: Lithium. In Fink MP, Abraham E, Vincent JL, et al, editors: *Textbook of critical care*, ed 5, Philadelphia, 2005, WB Saunders.

32. Mendez-Tellez PA, Dorman T: Postoperative respiratory failure. In Cameron JL, editor: *Current surgical therapy*, ed 9, Philadelphia, 2008, CV Mosby.

33. Berl T, Taylor J: Disorders of water balance. In Fink MP, Abraham E, Vincent JL, et al, editors: *Textbook of critical care*, ed 5, Philadelphia, 2005, WB Saunders.

34. Popovtzer MM: Disorders of calcium and magnesium metabolism. In Fink MP, Abraham E, Vincent JL, et al, editors: *Textbook of critical care*, ed 5, Philadelphia, 2005, WB Saunders.

35. Huston JM, Eachempati SR, Barie PS: Preoperative and postoperative care. In Cameron JL, editor: *Current surgical therapy*, ed 9, Philadelphia, 2008, CV Mosby.

36. Dellinger RP, Levy MM, Carlet JM, et al: Surviving sepsis campaign: international guidelines for management of severe sepsis and septic shock, *Intensive Care Med* 34:17–60, 2008.

37. Annane D, Sebille V, Charpentier C, et al: Effect of treatment with low doses of hydrocortisone and fludrocortisones on mortality in patients with septic shock, *JAMA* 288:862–871, 2002.

38. Juel VC, Bleck TP: Neuromuscular disorders in the ICU. In Fink MP, Abraham E, Vincent JL, et al, editors: *Textbook of critical care*, ed 5, Philadelphia, 2005, WB Saunders.

39. Trzeciak S, Dellinger RP: Hypophosphatemia and hyperphosphatemia. In Fink MP, Abraham E, Vincent JL, et al, editors: *Textbook of critical care*, ed 5, Philadelphia, 2005, WB Saunders.

40. Banner MJ: Bedside assessment and monitoring of pulmonary function and power of breathing in the critically ill. In Gabrielli A, Layon AJ, Yu M, editors: *Civetta, Taylor & Kirby's critical care*, ed 4, Philadelphia, 2009, Lippincott Williams & Wilkins.

41. Pineo GF, Hull RD: Pulmonary embolism. In Fink MP, Abraham E, Vincent JL, et al, editors: *Textbook of critical care*, ed 5, Philadelphia, 2005, WB Saunders.

42. Hallal A, Schulman C, Cohn S: Anemia of critical illness. In Fink MP, Abraham E, Vincent JL, et al, editors: *Textbook of critical care*, ed 5, Philadelphia, 2005, WB Saunders.

43. Poole BD, Schrier RW: Acute renal failure. In Fink MP, Abraham E, Vincent JL, et al, editors: *Textbook of critical care*, ed 5, Philadelphia, 2005, WB Saunders.

44. Streiff MB: Coagulopathy in the critically ill patient. In Cameron JL, editor: *Current surgical therapy*, ed 9, Philadelphia, 2008, CV Mosby.

45. Warner, BW: Pediatric surgery. In Townsend CM, Beauchamp RD, Evers BM, et al, editors: *Sabiston textbook of surgery: the biological basis of modern surgical practice*, ed 18, Philadelphia, 2008, WB Elsevier.

46. Rowe SA, Bartlett RH: Extracorporeal life support. In Fink MP, Abraham E, Vincent JL, et al, editors: *Textbook of critical care*, ed 5, Philadelphia, 2005, WB Saunders.

47. Haft J, Bartlett R: Extracorporeal life support for respiratory failure. In Cameron JL, editor: *Current surgical therapy*, ed 9, Philadelphia, 2008, CV Mosby.

48. Jan BU, Lowry SF: The septic response. In Cameron JL, editor: *Current surgical therapy*, ed 9, Philadelphia, 2008, CV Mosby.

49. Reinhart K, Bloos F, Brunkhorst FM: Pathophysiology of sepsis and multiple organ dysfunction. In Fink MP, Abraham E, Vincent JL, et al, editors: *Textbook of critical care*, ed 5, Philadelphia, 2005, WB Saunders.

50. Olumi AF, Richie JP: Urologic surgery. In Townsend CM, Beauchamp RD, Evers BM, et al, editors: *Sabiston textbook of surgery: the biological basis of modern surgical practice*, ed 18, Philadelphia, 2008, WB Saunders.

51. Vitarbo EA, Levi ADO: Spinal cord injury. In Fink MP, Abraham E, Vincent JL, et al, editors: *Textbook of critical care*, ed 5, Philadelphia, 2005, WB Saunders.

52. Muehlschlegel S, Greer DM: Neurogenic shock. In Gabrielli A, Layon AJ, Yu M, editors: *Civetta, Taylor & Kirby's critical care*, ed 4, Philadelphia, 2009, Lippincott Williams & Wilkins.

53. Fagon JY, Chastre J: Nosocomial pneumonia. In Fink MP, Abraham E, Vincent JL, et al, editors: *Textbook of critical care*, ed 5, Philadelphia, 2005, WB Saunders.

54. Bohnen JMA: Antibiotics for critically ill patients. In Cameron JL, editor: *Current surgical therapy*, ed 9, Philadelphia, 2008, CV Mosby.

55. Seger D: Poisoning: overview of approaches for evaluation and treatment. In Fink MP, Abraham E, Vincent JL, et al, editors: *Textbook of critical care*, ed 5, Philadelphia, 2005, WB Saunders.

56. Leijten FS, de Weerd AW: Critical illness polyneuropathy: a review of the literature, definition and pathophysiology, *Clin Neurol Neurosurg* 96:10–19, 1994.

57. Valenstein E, Musulin M: Neuromuscular disorders. In Gabrielli A, Layon AJ, Yu M, editors: *Civetta, Taylor & Kirby's critical care*, ed 4, Philadelphia, 2009, Lippincott Williams & Wilkins.

58. Leroy OY, Alfandari S: Respiratory infections in the ICU. In Gabrielli A, Layon AJ, Yu M, editors: *Civetta, Taylor & Kirby's critical care*, ed 4, Philadelphia, 2009, Lippincott Williams & Wilkins.

# CHAPTER 10

# Trauma

*Edie Y. Chan, M.D., and Jamie Elizabeth Jones, M.D.*

1. A 44-year-old man suffers a gunshot wound to his abdomen. He is hemodynamically stable and taken to the operating room. On exploration, his injuries are found to be limited to two small bowel injuries 7 cm apart, each with destruction of 70% of the bowel wall, and a through-and-through injury to the ascending colon with destruction of 30% of the bowel wall. How should these injuries be managed?

A. Resection and anastomosis of the small bowel injuries and primary repair of the colon injury

B. Primary repair of both the small bowel and colon injuries

C. Primary repair of the small bowel injuries, primary repair of the colon injury, and creation of a diverting ileostomy

D. Resection of the small bowel injuries and exteriorization of the colon injury as a colostomy

E. Resection and anastomosis of all injuries

*Ref.: 1*

**COMMENTS:** Historically, all **colon injuries** were treated by diversion. However, with the progression of surgical technique, resuscitative and critical care, and antibiosis, many colon injuries can be repaired primarily. Patients who are hemodynamically stable and have injuries that involve less than 50% of the circumferential bowel and no vascular disruption can undergo primary repair. In regard to small bowel injury, resection is indicated for injuries involving greater than 50% of the wall circumference, multiple injuries in a short segment, or both.

**ANSWER:** A

2. A 27-year-old woman is brought to the emergency department awake and alert after sustaining a gunshot wound to her neck. The wound is anterior to the origin of the sternocleidomastoid muscle at the angle of the mandible. The patient is asymptomatic. All of the following are correct management choices except:

A. Cervical spine radiographic studies

B. Mandatory neck exploration

C. Four-vessel angiographic studies

D. Flexible esophagoscopic examination

E. Contrast-enhanced esophagographic examination

*Ref.: 2*

**COMMENTS:** See Question 3.

**ANSWER:** B

3. Soon after the patient in Question 2 arrives in the emergency department, left hemiparesis and aphasia develop. At this time, which of the following treatments should be provided?

A. Continued observation

B. Repair of the carotid artery injury

C. Ligation of the carotid artery injury

D. Repair of the vertebral artery injury

E. Systemic anticoagulation

*Ref.: 2*

**COMMENTS:** The patient in Question 2 has suffered an injury to zone III of the neck. Zone III is defined as the area anterior to the sternocleidomastoid between the angle of the mandible and the base of the skull. Even without hard signs of vascular injury or change in neurologic status, patients with zone III injuries should routinely undergo angiography. Physical examination alone cannot be relied on to diagnose carotid artery or aerodigestive injuries in this zone. Cervical spine radiographic studies are needed to rule out any associated fracture. In addition, the esophagus should be investigated with both esophagoscopy and contrast-enhanced imaging. In Question 3, the patient has a mild neurologic deficit consistent with a carotid artery injury. The current recommendation regarding **carotid artery injury** is surgical repair unless complete occlusion or hemodynamic instability is present.

**ANSWER:** B

4. The upper part of the abdomen of a 42-year-old man strikes the steering wheel during a motor vehicle accident. He is hemodynamically stable. Because of positive findings on diagnostic peritoneal lavage (DPL), he undergoes exploratory laparotomy, at which time complete transection of the pancreatic neck is found. What is the most appropriate management of this injury?

A. Distal pancreatectomy with oversewing and drainage of the proximal pancreatic stump

B. Roux-en-Y pancreaticojejunostomy to the distal end of the pancreas with oversewing and drainage of the proximal pancreatic stump

C. Primary repair and drainage of the pancreatic duct

D. Whipple operation

E. Total pancreatectomy

*Ref.: 3*

**COMMENTS:** Operative management of **pancreatic injuries** centers on the location of the injury and whether the duct is involved. Approximately 50% of the pancreas is located on either side of the superior mesenteric artery. For pancreatic wounds with an intact duct, drainage of the area with soft closed suction drains suffices. If the main pancreatic duct is injured to the left of the mesenteric vessels, as in this patient, distal pancreatectomy with drainage of the proximal stump is indicated. The proximal pancreatic duct should be individually ligated with nonabsorbable suture if possible and the parenchymal tissue oversewn or stapled across with a stapler. The spleen should be preserved if the patient's hemodynamic status allows. Roux-en-Y pancreaticojejunostomy to the distal end of the pancreas with oversewing of the proximal pancreatic stump carries a high rate of leakage. The Whipple procedure and total pancreatectomy would be reserved for injuries that involve extensive devitalization of the duodenum and head of the pancreas. Primary repair is technically difficult and does not address the transected pancreatic tissue.

**ANSWER:  A**

5. A 30-year-old man is brought to the emergency department after being involved in a Jet Ski crash. His vital signs are stable. A high-riding prostate is noted on rectal examination. On portable pelvic radiographs he is found to have bilateral pubic rami fractures. He has not yet voided since admission. Which of the following should be the next step?

   A. Wait for the patient to void freely before attempting transurethral bladder catheterization.

   B. Initially attempt gentle transurethral bladder catheterization, but stop if resistance is encountered.

   C. Obtain a urethrogram before attempting transurethral bladder catheterization.

   D. Insert a suprapubic cystostomy tube.

   E. Perform computed tomography of the pelvis with three-dimensional reconstruction.

   *Ref.:* 4

**COMMENTS:** Approximately 10% of all patients with a **pelvic fracture** have a concomitant urethral injury. Findings on physical examination, such as blood at the meatus, a freely movable prostate, and perineal hematoma, should raise suspicion for a **urethral injury**. If any of these signs are present or there is a significant anterior pelvic fracture, a urethrogram should be obtained to exclude an injury before transurethral catheterization is attempted. Bladder decompression plus drainage is the mainstay of treatment of urethral injuries, either via suprapubic cystostomy for complete disruption or a with a bridging transurethral catheter for partial tears.

**ANSWER:  C**

6. After a gunshot wound to the chest and the subsequent development of hemothorax, a 24-year-old man requires multiple blood transfusions, including fresh frozen plasma. On admission to the intensive care unit (ICU), the patient becomes increasingly tachypneic and begins to become hypoxic. After the airway is secured, a chest radiograph is obtained and reveals bilateral patchy infiltrates. Which of the following statements regarding this condition is true?

   A. This type of reaction usually develops approximately 12 to 24 hours after a transfusion.

   B. The mortality rate with this condition nears 50%.

   C. It is associated with elevated pulmonary capillary wedge pressure.

   D. Clinical improvement is typically seen within 2 to 8 days.

   E. This condition results from entrapment of activated platelets in the lung.

   *Ref.:* 5

**COMMENTS:**  This clinical manifestation is most consistent with **transfusion-related acute lung injury** (**TRALI**), which is similar to acute respiratory distress syndrome (ARDS) in its findings of hypoxemia, bilateral pulmonary edema, tachycardia, and hypotension. This reaction usually develops within 2 to 6 hours after the transfusion of blood products such as platelets or fresh frozen plasma and occurs once in every 2500 to 5000 units transfused. It does differ from ARDS, however, in that elevated pulmonary capillary wedge pressure is not seen and mortality rates are between 5% and 8% versus nearly 50% with ARDS. TRALI results from the transfusion of blood containing human leukocyte antigens or by activation of the patient's granulocytes by metabolites released during storage. Management is supportive and entails mechanical ventilation with small tidal volumes.

**ANSWER:  D**

7. A 44-year-old man suffers a gunshot wound to his left thigh that results in an injury to the superficial femoral artery. The injury is repaired with a saphenous vein interposition graft within 4 hours of the injury. Although the patient had equal pulses bilaterally and was neurologically intact, 5 hours postoperatively the left distal pulses diminish and he begins to experience pain with passive dorsiflexion and extension. The left anterior compartment of the lower part of the leg has a pressure of 30 mm Hg. Which of the following statements is true regarding compartment syndrome in an extremity?

   A. Fractures are the cause of approximately 30% of all compartment syndromes.

   B. The lateral compartment of the lower part of the leg is the most commonly affected.

   C. A compartment pressure of 25 mm Hg negates a need for fasciotomy.

   D. Paresthesias are an early clinical development.

   E. A four-compartment fasciotomy should be performed.

   *Ref.:* 6-8

**COMMENTS:  Compartment syndrome** of the extremity is an extremely important diagnosis to make as early as possible because of the significant risk for permanent limb dysfunction and potential loss. Causes of compartment syndrome include crush injury, reperfusion after a time of ischemia, and fractures, which account for 50% of cases. The anterior compartment of the lower part of the leg contains mostly type I (slow twitch) muscle fibers and is encased by dense fascia, thus making it most vulnerable to the development of ischemia. The diagnosis is largely clinical, with pain out of proportion to the findings on examination, pallor, paresthesias, diminished pulses, and tense compartments being the initial symptoms. However, because of the fact that for even after an hour of ischemia impulses can still be conducted through peripheral nerves, paresthesias are a late sign of compartment syndrome. In addition, even though compartment pressures of 30 mm Hg or higher are classically quoted, lesser pressures do not prove that there is adequate tissue perfusion, and if other signs or symptoms of compartment syndrome are present, fasciotomies should still be performed.

**ANSWER:** E

8. Regarding rhabdomyolysis:

   A. Acute renal failure occurs secondary to the release of myoglobin.

   B. An alkalotic environment promotes the formation of myoglobin casts in the renal tubules, thereby worsening the kidney damage.

   C. The renal failure from rhabdomyolysis typically resolves within 3 to 5 days.

   D. Severe hyponatremia is a frequent complication.

   E. Alkalinization to a pH between 8 and 9 is an important treatment goal.

   *Ref.:* 9

**COMMENTS:** Acute renal failure is the most significant complication of **rhabdomyolysis** and occurs when myoglobin casts are formed in the proximal renal tubules from the damaged muscle and then precipitate and form casts in the proximal renal tubules. This cast formation is thought to be inhibited by an alkalotic environment (goal pH of 6 to 7), which can be achieved by intravenous sodium bicarbonate treatment. A urine dipstick positive for blood, in conjunction with a lack of red blood cells on microscopic examination, points to a diagnosis of rhabdomyolysis. In addition, the presence of urine myoglobin and elevated serum creatinine phosphokinase is indicative of this diagnosis. Serial metabolic profiles should be obtained to monitor for hyperkalemia, the most significant and dangerous electrolyte imbalance. For patients who do suffer from acute renal insufficiency, the overall prognosis with early and aggressive volume resuscitation is good, with most patients recovering to baseline function within 2 weeks to 1 month.

**ANSWER:** A

9. An 18-year-old man is admitted to the ICU after undergoing emergency laparotomy and splenectomy. He received 12 units of red blood cells and 8 units of fresh frozen plasma. Over the course of the next 12 hours, his abdomen becomes increasingly distended and firm, and urine output decreases significantly. Which of the following statements is true regarding abdominal compartment syndrome?

   A. Pulmonary capillary wedge pressure is typically low.

   B. Functional residual capacity is increased.

   C. There is increased central venous return.

   D. Central venous pressure is increased.

   E. Cardiac output increases.

   *Ref.:* 10, 11

**COMMENTS: Abdominal compartment syndrome** is typically associated with elevated peak respiratory pressure, decreased urine output, hypoxia, and other deleterious physiologic effects. Overall, there is decreased venous return to the heart leading to decreased cardiac output and decreased visceral perfusion. In addition, because of the increased pressure in the abdomen, the diaphragm's ability to contract is lessened, and pulmonary compliance and functional residual capacity are reduced. This then leads to increased pulmonary vascular resistance, which is measured as increased pulmonary capillary wedge pressure. The diagnosis of abdominal compartment syndrome is achieved primarily by clinical evaluation of the patient (vital signs and physical examination) but can be corroborated by measurement of bladder pressure. To measure bladder pressure, 50 mL of sterile saline is inserted through the Foley catheter after the bladder has been completely drained, and the distal tubing port is clamped. A transducer needle is then introduced into the specimen collecting port. A pressure of 25 mm Hg or greater is consistent with intraabdominal hypertension. Operative treatment of abdominal compartment syndrome is prompt decompressive laparotomy with temporary abdominal closure.

**ANSWER:** D

10. A 25-year-old woman is the driver of an automobile involved in a high-speed motor vehicle accident. She is 30 weeks pregnant. She complains of abdominal pain but does not have peritoneal signs. Her vital signs are stable. Which of the following statements are true regarding trauma in a pregnant patient?

    A. Less than 5% of all pregnancies are affected by trauma.

    B. The uterus is protected by the bony pelvis until the beginning of the second trimester.

    C. A woman of 25 weeks' gestation will have a palpable fundal height at approximately the level of the umbilicus.

    D. Blood volume during pregnancy increases by approximately 30%.

    E. Hypotensive patients should be placed in the right lateral position.

    *Ref.:* 12, 13

**COMMENTS:** Trauma is the leading cause of death in women of childbearing age, and thus understanding the physiologic changes throughout the progression of **pregnancy** is imperative. However, since approximately 10% of pregnant patients are unaware of their pregnancy, a pregnancy test is recommended for all women of childbearing age early in their resuscitation. The most common cause of fetal death is, in fact, maternal death. Therefore, the focus of all initial resuscitative effort is directed toward the mother. Blood volume may increase by as much as 50% during pregnancy, which means that a patient may not have the tachycardia and hypotension usually associated with acute blood loss until almost 30% of total blood volume is lost. Although the primary and secondary surveys for a pregnant patient are virtually identical to those of a nonpregnant patient, it is important to perform a focused abdominal examination. The pelvis typically protects the uterus until about 12 weeks. At about 20 weeks' gestation, the fundal height of the uterus approximates the umbilicus and, for every week of gestation past this stage, raises the height by roughly 1 inch. During the advanced stages of pregnancy, the uterus causes compression on the inferior vena cava, thereby leading to decreased central venous return. Hypotensive patients should be placed in the left lateral position, which even in patients with suspected spinal injury can be accomplished by securing the patient firmly to the backboard, which can then be tilted to the left. Evaluation of the fetus is accomplished by fetal heart tone monitoring and pelvic ultrasound. Tachycardia, bradycardia, and decelerations with contractions are all signs of potential fetal distress.

**ANSWER:** B

**11.** A 28-year-old woman is an unrestrained driver in a motor vehicle crash. She has stable vital signs and left upper quadrant tenderness without signs of peritonitis. Select the most appropriate next step in management of the abdominal pain?

A. Computed tomographic (CT) scan of the abdomen and pelvis

B. Diagnostic peritoneal lavage (DPL)

C. Admission for observation and serial abdominal examinations

D. Abdominal ultrasound

E. Exploratory laparotomy

*Ref.: 4*

**COMMENTS:** Evaluation of any trauma patient should follow the advanced trauma life support (ATLS) principles, with a complete primary and secondary survey. It is during the secondary survey that a thorough abdominal examination, including inspection and palpation, is performed. CT is the best radiographic tool for diagnosing blunt abdominal injury; it has higher sensitivity than **focused assessment with sonography for trauma** patients (FAST) and is noninvasive, in contradistinction to **diagnostic peritoneal lavage**. In addition, CT is useful for evaluating the retroperitoneum, which DPL cannot. Absolute indications for immediate laparotomy in patients with **blunt abdominal trauma** are abdominal distention with cardiovascular instability despite resuscitation and the presence of peritonitis.

**ANSWER:** A

**12.** A 58-year-old man is a restrained passenger in a high-speed motor vehicle collision. On arrival at the emergency department his pulse is 118 beats/min with a blood pressure of 90/58 mm Hg. After 2 L of lactated Ringer solution is administered, his pulse decreases to 95 and blood pressure increases to 120/62. Abdominal CT is performed and shows an isolated splenic injury with a laceration 2 cm in parenchymal depth. Which of the following statements is true regarding this type of injury?

A. Approximately 60% of all splenic injuries in adults are successfully managed nonoperatively.

B. The type of injury in this patient has a 5% failure rate with nonoperative management.

C. This patient's age is associated with a higher failure rate with nonoperative management.

D. This patient's initial tachycardia and hypotension preclude him from nonoperative management.

E. Nonoperative management of a grade V splenic injury is associated with an approximate 25% success rate.

*Ref.: 4, 14*

**COMMENTS:** See Question 13.

**ANSWER:** E

**13.** The same patient as in Question 12 is admitted for observation and serial hemoglobin tests. On hospital day 2, the patient's heart rate increases to 120 beats/min and systolic blood pressure decreases to 100 mm Hg. His hemoglobin is now noted to be 7 g/dL. Select the next step in management.

A. Transfusion of 2 units of packed red blood cells and serial hemoglobin determinations

B. Angiography

C. Repeated CT

D. DPL

E. Immediate laparotomy

*Ref.: 4, 14*

**COMMENTS:** The spleen is the most commonly injured organ after **blunt abdominal trauma**. The patient described in this question has a grade II splenic laceration as diagnosed on CT (Table 10-1). Approximately 30% of all **splenic injuries** are treated operatively on arrival at the hospital. Of the remaining 60% to 70%, 80% to 90% of these are treated successfully with nonoperative management. Failure rates increase with the grade of injury, with a failure rate of 10% for grade I and II injuries, which increases to 75% for grade V injuries. Contraindications to conservative management include hemodynamic instability after adequate resuscitation, requirement for transfusion, and peritonitis. Independent risk factors for failure of nonoperative management include age older than 55 years, the presence of a pseudoaneurysm, and the amount of hemoperitoneum present on the initial CT. This patient fails conservative management because of continued hemodynamic instability and a requirement for transfusion. This necessitates laparotomy for splenectomy. The indication for angiography is the presence of an arteriovenous fistula or pseudoaneurysm on either initial or repeated CT, and it is usually performed 24 to 48 hours after admission with a splenic injury of grade III or higher.

**TABLE 10-1  Spleen Organ Injury Scale—1994 Revision by the American Association for the Surgery of Trauma**

| Grade | | Injury Description | AIS-90 |
|---|---|---|---|
| I | Hematoma | Subcapsular, <10% of surface area | 2 |
| | Laceration | Capsular tear, <1 cm in parenchymal depth | 2 |
| II | Hematoma | Subcapsular, 10% to 50% of surface area; intraparenchymal, <5 cm in diameter | 2 |
| | Laceration | 1-3 cm in parenchymal depth and does not involve a trabecular vessel | 2 |
| III | Hematoma | Subcapsular, >50% of surface area or expanding; ruptured subcapsular or parenchymal hematoma; intraparenchymal hematoma >5 cm or expanding | 3 |
| | Laceration | >3 cm in parenchymal depth or involving a trabecular vessel | 3 |
| IV | Laceration | Laceration involving the segmental or hilar vessels and producing major devascularization (>25% of spleen) | 4 |
| V | Laceration | Completely shattered spleen | 5 |
| | Vascular | Hilar vascular injury that devascularizes the spleen | 5 |

AIS, Abbreviated injury scale.

**ANSWER:** E

**14.** A 38-year-old car mechanic is taken to the emergency department after having been pinned underneath a car. On chest radiography, multiple rib fractures are noted, as well as an airfluid level consistent with the stomach being above the level of the left diaphragm (Figure 10-1). Which of the following statements regarding this injury is true?

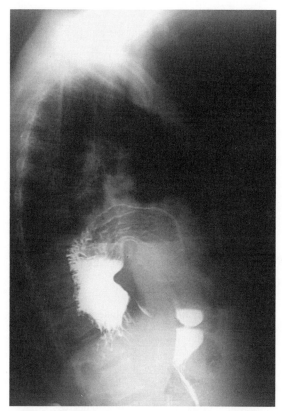

**Figure 10-1.** Lateral chest film showing herniation of the stomach into the left pleural cavity.

A. Right-sided diaphragmatic rupture is more common than left-sided rupture.

B. There is a 60% incidence of coexisting pelvic fractures.

C. The best initial radiographic assessment for this type of injury is FAST.

D. There is a 40% incidence of normal chest radiographic findings in patients with a documented diaphragmatic injury.

E. There is a 60% incidence of coexisting thoracic aortic injury.

*Ref.:* 15

**COMMENTS:** See Question 15.

**ANSWER:** D

**15.** For the patient in Question 14, what is the most appropriate next step in management?

A. FAST

B. Laparotomy

C. CT scan

D. Thoracotomy

E. Laparoscopy

*Ref.:* 15

**COMMENTS: Diaphragmatic injuries/**rupture occur in 3% to 5% of patients suffering major **blunt abdominal trauma.** Although this injury is uncommon, it is associated with a high incidence of coexistent injuries, including pelvic fractures (40%), hepatic and splenic injuries (25%), and rupture of the thoracic aorta (5%). The left side is affected three times more often than the right side. Chest radiography, despite a 40% incidence of negative findings in the face of known injury, is still the best initial diagnostic modality. The diagnostic accuracy of CT and FAST for detecting injury to the diaphragm is low. Once a diagnosis of diaphragmatic rupture has been made, treatment is operative. In this situation, in which diaphragmatic rupture is strongly suspected, laparoscopy is typically avoided because insufflation of the abdomen may cause tension pneumothorax. In the acute setting of diaphragmatic injury, laparotomy is the preferred operative approach. It allows reduction of any organs back into the abdominal cavity, as well as thorough inspection of all intraperitoneal contents. Diagnosing small diaphragmatic injuries can be difficult inasmuch as up to almost half of all patients will have normal findings on physical examination at initial evaluation. Missed diaphragmatic injuries tend to enlarge over time, which may lead to herniation and strangulation of abdominal organs. Primary repair is not usually feasible because of the rapid atrophy of diaphragmatic muscle fibers. A thoracotomy is generally performed for a chronic diaphragmatic hernia since it provides better access to the adhesions usually found in the chest.

**ANSWER:** B

**16.** A 30-year-old man suffers a stab wound to the right anterior aspect of his chest, approximately 3 cm inferior to the middle portion of the clavicle. Paramedics reported a weakly palpable pulse 5 minutes earlier in the ambulance, but on admission, no palpable pulses are present. His pupils are reactive. What is the initial surgical approach?

A. Median sternotomy

B. Right-sided clavicular incision

C. Right-sided anterolateral thoracotomy

D. Right-sided posterolateral thoracotomy

E. Left-sided anterolateral thoracotomy

*Ref.:* 4, 16, 17

**COMMENTS:** An **emergency department thoracotomy** differs from an emergency thoracotomy in that the patient is so unstable that transportation to the operating room is precluded. It is performed for a select group of patients, with the overall survival rate being dependent on the mechanism and ranging from 1.5% to 19%. It is least successful in patients with injuries caused by a blunt mechanism and is therefore usually reserved for those who initially have vital signs present but then lose these signs in the emergency department. In patients with a penetrating mechanism, emergency thoracotomy is indicated for those who lost their pulse and blood pressure either in the emergency department after initial evaluation or during transport to the emergency department. It is of highest use when cardiac tamponade or severe thoracic hemorrhage is suspected. The thoracotomy is performed via an anterolateral approach, regardless of the supposed side of injury, and allows release of pericardial tamponade, open cardiopulmonary resuscitation, and aortic cross-clamping. Injuries to the ascending aorta, innominate artery, proximal right subclavian artery, and either carotid are best managed with a median sternotomy. A right-sided clavicular incision is appropriate for a midsubclavian arterial injury. A right anterolateral approach is appropriate for injuries to the lung and chest wall. The right-sided posterolateral approach is the appropriate exposure for injuries to the trachea and midesophagus. A left posterolateral thoracotomy is used for exposure to the descending aorta and hilum.

**ANSWER: C**

17. A 17-year-old man arrives at the emergency department after having suffered a stab wound to the anterior aspect of his abdomen in the right upper quadrant. Entrance into the peritoneum is unclear on physical examination, and diagnostic peritoneal lavage (DPL) is performed. One liter of 0.9% normal saline is introduced into the abdomen, with 800 mL being retrieved. It is sent to the laboratory and returns with a value of 20,000 red blood cells/mm$^3$. What is the most appropriate next step in management?

   A. CT scan of the abdomen and pelvis

   B. Observation with serial abdominal examinations

   C. Suture repair of the stab wound

   D. Exploratory laparotomy

   E. Discharge home with wet-to-dry dressing changes for the stab wound

   *Ref.:* 4

**COMMENTS: Diagnostic peritoneal lavage** is a very sensitive but nonspecific test that can be used for either blunt or penetrating trauma. In this situation, DPL is used to determine intraperitoneal injury. It is performed by introducing a catheter into the abdomen via the Seldinger technique and then infusing 1 L of 0.9% normal saline. The fluid is then returned by gravity and sent to the laboratory for analysis. For penetrating injuries, a positive DPL is defined as one with greater than 10,000 red blood cells/mm$^3$, 500 white blood cells/mm$^3$, or the presence of bilious/particulate material. In this patient with a positive **diagnostic peritoneal lavage**, the next most appropriate step in management is exploratory laparotomy.

**ANSWER: D**

18. A 21-year-old man is taken to the emergency department with a gunshot wound to the right side of his chest. The first wound is located 2 cm lateral to the right nipple, and a second wound is present just medial to the tip of the right scapula. Vital signs on initial evaluation are a heart rate of 126 beats/min and a systolic blood pressure of 88 mm Hg. A right-sided chest tube is placed, with return of 1200 mL of blood. He is resuscitated with 2 L of lactated Ringer solution, and his vital signs return to within normal limits. His chest tube output is rechecked 4 hours later, and the total amount in the collection container is 2300 mL. What is the next most appropriate step in management?

   A. Chest CT

   B. Immediate complete blood count

   C. Thoracotomy

   D. Immediate arterial blood gas analysis

   E. Admission to the ICU for continuous cardiac monitoring and pulse oximetry

   *Ref.:* 4, 16

**COMMENTS:** This patient has a massive **hemothorax**, which is defined as greater than 1500 mL of blood loss on initial placement of tube thoracostomy or loss greater than 200 mL/h for 4 hours after the initial return. Emergency thoracotomy is indicated not only for massive hemothorax but also for cardiac tamponade, major injuries to the tracheobronchial system, and injuries to the esophagus.

**ANSWER: C**

19. The head and face of 45-year-old man were assaulted with fists and feet. He arrives at the emergency department with incomprehensible responses to questions, eyes opening to pain only, and a flexor response to pain. What is this patient's Glasgow Coma Scale (GCS) score?

   A. 5

   B. 6

   C. 7

   D. 8

   E. Not enough information given to calculate

   *Ref.:* 18

**COMMENTS:** See Question 20

**ANSWER: C**

20. For the patient in the previous clinical scenario, what is the next best step in management?

   A. CT scan of the head

   B. Continue to perform primary and secondary surveys

   C. Chest radiography

   D. Elevation of the head of the bed 30 degrees

   E. Endotracheal intubation

   *Ref.:* 19

**COMMENTS:** The first step in management for any trauma patient is assessment of the patient's airway. It is not appropriate to continue the primary survey until the airway has not only been assessed but also either deemed secure or made secure. This patient has a **Glasgow Coma Scale** score of 7 and is unable to protect his airway. In addition, hypoxia and hypercapnia develop in patients with severe head injury and have deleterious effects on intracranial pressure (ICP) and cerebral perfusion pressure (CPP). Obtaining a secure airway thus allows control of oxygenation and ventilation.

**ANSWER: E**

21. For the patient in Question 19, head CT shows a 2-cm subdural hematoma without a midline shift. The patient is taken to the operating room and the hematoma is evacuated. Postoperatively, he is admitted to the ICU intubated and sedated with an ICP monitor in place. Which of the following treatment measures can be used to maintain adequate CPP?

   A. Hyperventilation to a P$CO_2$ of 25 mm Hg

   B. Mannitol, 1 g/kg intravenously for 3 days

   C. Hydrocortisone, 100 mg intravenously every 8 hours for 3 days

D. Strict blood pressure control to a systolic range of 90 to 100 mm Hg

E. Reverse Trendelenburg positioning of the bed at all times

*Ref.:* 4, 18, 20

**COMMENTS:** The overall goal in treating patients with **traumatic head injury** is maintaining adequate cerebral blood flow. An estimate of this flow is obtained by calculating **cerebral perfusion pressure** (CPP = mean blood pressure – ICP). The goal CPP in an adult is 60 to 70 mm Hg. Therefore, patients should be aggressively volume-resuscitated to maintain adequate mean blood pressure. ICP monitors are indicated in patients with a GCS score of 3 to 8 and either (1) an abnormal finding on CT of the head or (2) any two of the following: (a) age older than 40 years, (b) posturing response to pain, or (c) systolic blood pressure less than 90 mm Hg. Overall, there is a 5% infection and 1% hematoma formation rate associated with ICP-monitoring catheters. Treatment measures used to decrease ICP include elevation of the head of the bed to 30 degrees or more, hyperventilation of patients to a $Pco_2$ of 30 to 35 mm Hg, barbiturates, and mannitol at a dose of 1 g/kg intravenously. $Pco_2$ should not be kept below 30 mm Hg to avoid worsening the cerebral ischemia. Steroids do not have a role in the treatment of acute traumatic head injury.

**ANSWER:** B

22. A 32-year-old construction worker is taken to the emergency department after having fallen off a roof 4 hours earlier. He has no neurologic function below cervical spine level 5. CT shows C5 and C6 anterior wedge fractures, with compromise of the spinal canal. Which of the following statements is true regarding this type of injury?

A. The current treatment standard is to administer methylprednisolone intravenously on arrival at the emergency department.

B. Approximately 50% of all spinal fractures occur in the cervical vertebrae.

C. Neurogenic shock is characterized by hypertension with bradycardia.

D. Only 15% of patients with neck pain have a true cervical spine injury.

E. Methylprednisolone therapy should be continued for 72 hours after the time that the injury occurred.

*Ref.:* 21

**COMMENTS:** Approximately 10,000 patients a year suffer a **spinal cord injury**. Of extreme importance in the early management of these patients is strict spinal immobilization. Seventy-five percent of all spinal fractures are located in the cervical spine. However, just 5% of patients with neck pain after trauma have a true cervical spine injury. Initial radiologic assessment is accomplished with anteroposterior, lateral, and open-mouth odontoid projections. If these films are equivocal or the C7/T1 interface is not well visualized, CT is a useful addition. In patients who do suffer a spinal cord injury, neurogenic shock can develop, which is caused by loss of sympathetic vascular tone and leads to hypotension and bradycardia. Corticosteroid use has been shown to be useful when initiated in less than 3 hours after the incident occurred. In this instance, it should be given initially as a 30-mg/kg bolus of methylprednisolone over a 1-hour period, followed by 5.4 mg/kg/h for 23 more hours. If the patient is seen, as in this case, between 3 and 8 hours after the incident, steroids should be continued for 48 hours. Steroids have not been shown to have a role in the treatment of penetrating injuries to the spinal cord.

**ANSWER:** A

23. Regarding pelvic fractures, which of the following statements is true?

A. Patients with a pelvic fracture have 30% mortality if hypotension is initially present.

B. A pubic symphysis diastasis of 3 cm doubles the volume of potential pelvic space for a hematoma.

C. When a laparotomy is performed in a patient with an unstable pelvic fracture, it is imperative to make a large surgical incision (xiphoid to symphysis) to allow better visualization in the pelvis.

D. The most common cause of death following an open pelvic fracture is overwhelming infection and sepsis.

E. The external iliac artery is commonly involved in severe pelvic fractures.

*Ref.:* 22, 23

**COMMENTS:** A **pelvic fracture** is diagnosed in approximately 10% to 20% of trauma patients. The overall mortality rate associated with a pelvic fracture is 10% to 15%, but this rate increases to almost 50% when hypotension, an open component, or both exist. The most common cause of death from open pelvic fractures is uncontrollable hemorrhage. The open component prevents tamponade within the pelvic space. After a pelvic fracture is diagnosed or suspected, a thorough examination of the perineum must be conducted to rule out an open component. Because a pubic symphysis diastasis of 3 cm doubles the potential space for a hematoma to form, early attempts to stabilize the pelvis are extremely important. Such stabilization can be performed through noninvasive means (wrapping the pelvis in a sheet, applying a pelvic girdle) or invasive means (external fixation, pelvic C-clamp). If a laparotomy is required because of an intraabdominal injury, a large incision below the semilunar line should be avoided. Once an incision is made below this level, the pelvic hematoma secondary to the fracture will decompress and lead to massive bleeding. If this does occur, after the other injuries have been addressed as quickly as possible, the pelvis should be packed tightly and the patient returned to the ICU for stabilization. Once stabilized, the patient can either undergo angiography or return to the operating room. The external iliac artery courses deep to the inguinal ligament and is rarely involved in pelvic fractures. The superior and inferior gluteal arteries, obturator artery, and internal pudendal artery, all branches of the internal iliac, are most frequently injured.

**ANSWER:** B

24. An 18-year-old man undergoes emergency laparotomy for multiple gunshot wounds to the abdomen. On entering the abdomen there is a large amount of hemoperitoneum. All four quadrants are packed and the packing is then removed. The injuries found are five small intestine enterotomies, a through-and-through injury to the transverse colon, and a 3-cm laceration of the infrarenal aorta. The best management of the aortic injury is:

A. Primary repair

B. Saphenous vein patch angioplasty

C. In situ placement of a polytetrafluoroethylene (PTFE) graft

D. Aortic ligation above the level of injury with a bilateral axillofemoral bypass

E. Aortobifemoral bypass with a PTFE graft

*Ref.:* 6

**COMMENTS:** Although it has been traditional teaching that artificial grafts not be used in an infected or contaminated field, this is one circumstance in which it is common practice. After débridement of the **aortic injury**, the large size of the defect prohibits primary repair or vein patch angioplasty. Axillofemoral and aortobifemoral bypasses are time-consuming operations that this patient will probably not tolerate. In situ placement of a PTFE graft is the preferred operation, and all care should be taken to thoroughly irrigate the abdomen before placement of the graft. In addition, the repair should be covered by omentum after completion.

**ANSWER:  C**

25. A 32-year-old woman is a restrained passenger in a high-speed motor vehicle collision. In the emergency room she is found to be nontachycardic with a systolic blood pressure of 110 mm Hg. Blood is drawn for determination of the hemoglobin concentration, which is noted to be 12.2 g/dL. On FAST, a moderate amount of fluid is seen in the right upper quadrant, between the liver, kidney, and diaphragm. What is the next most appropriate step in management?

A. Laparotomy

B. CT scan of the abdomen and pelvis with intravenous contrast enhancement

C. Angiography for embolization of the liver laceration

D. DPL

E. Observation with serial abdominal examinations

*Ref.:* 4, 24

**COMMENTS:** See Question 26.

**ANSWER:  B**

26. A grade IV liver laceration is diagnosed in the patient from Question 25 (Table 10-2). Her vital signs 6 hours after admission are a pulse of 100 beats/min and systolic blood pressure of 105 mm Hg. What is the next most appropriate step?

A. Exploratory laparotomy

B. Angiography

C. Repeated FAST

D. Diagnostic laparoscopy

E. Repeated hemoglobin determination

*Ref.:* 4, 24

**COMMENTS:** The overall success rate for nonoperative treatment of blunt **hepatic injuries** is about 90% for all levels of injury. Patients with grade IV and V injuries are able to be treated without surgery between 75% and 80% of the time. Requirements for nonoperative therapy include hemodynamic stability, no signs or symptoms of peritonitis, and a transfusion requirement of no more than 2 to 4 units of packed red blood cells. This patient is hemodynamically stable, and therefore further localization of the

intraabdominal injury with CT initially is warranted. The initial CT not only can localize the injury but, in the case of solid organ injuries, can also provide information regarding active hemorrhage. She should be closely monitored in an intensive care setting with serial abdominal examinations and hemoglobin determinations. Angiography is a helpful adjunct to nonoperative treatment, but it is usually reserved for situations in which active extravasation or a "blush" is seen on CT. Repeated CT is advised for patients who do experience a decrease in their hemoglobin to reevaluate the liver damage and look for any active extravasation that would be amenable to angiographic embolization.

**TABLE 10-2  Liver Injury Scale**

| Grade | Injury | Description of Injury |
|---|---|---|
| I | Hematoma | Subcapsular, <10% of surface area |
| | Laceration | Capsular tear, <1 cm in parenchymal depth |
| II | Hematoma | Subcapsular, 10% to 50% of surface area |
| | | Intraparenchymal, <10 cm in diameter |
| | Laceration | 1-3 cm in parenchymal depth, <10 cm in length |
| III | Hematoma | Subcapsular, >50% of surface area or expanding, ruptured subcapsular or parenchymal hematoma |
| | | Intraparenchymal, >10 cm or expanding |
| | Laceration | >3 cm in parenchymal depth |
| IV | Laceration | Parenchymal disruption involving >75% of the hepatic lobe or 1-3 Couinaud segments within a single lobe |
| V | Laceration | Parenchymal disruption involving >75% of the hepatic lobe or >3 Couinaud segments within a single lobe |
| | Vascular | Juxtahepatic venous injuries (retrohepatic vena cava, central major hepatic veins) |
| VI | Vascular | Hepatic avulsion |

From the American Association for the Surgery of Trauma, www.aast.org. Derived originally from Moore EE, Cogbill TH, Jurkovich GJ, et al: Organ injury scaling: spleen and liver, *J Trauma* 38:323–324, 1995.

**ANSWER:  E**

27. A patient with a grade V blunt liver injury is discharged home on hospital day 7 without needing operative intervention. She returns to the clinic 2 months after discharge with persistent dull continuous right upper quadrant pain. She denies any fevers or chills, and all laboratory studies, including a hepatic function panel, are within normal limits. CT of the abdomen and pelvis is performed and reveals a localized homogeneous fluid collection directly adjacent to the liver. What is the correct diagnosis and treatment?

A. Hemobilia; angiography with embolization

B. Biloma; CT- or ultrasound-guided percutaneous drainage

C. Biloma; exploratory laparotomy with external drainage

D. Hepatic necrosis; CT- or ultrasound-guided percutaneous drainage

E. Hepatic necrosis; exploratory laparotomy with wide débridement and drainage

*Ref.:* 4, 24

**COMMENTS:** Because of the increasing number of patients with **significant liver lacerations** being treated (successfully) nonoperatively, posttreatment complications are being encountered more often. Such complications include hemobilia, biloma, hepatic necrosis, and abscess. Hemobilia occurs when a connection exists between the biliary and arterial systems, and it is typically manifested as right upper quadrant pain, melena, and jaundice. Hemobilia can be diagnosed by CT with intravenous contrast enhancement or upper endoscopy and is usually treated by angiography with embolization. Patients with hepatic necrosis or abscess (or both) typically have right upper quadrant pain, fever, leukocytosis, and at times, localized peritonitis. It can be appreciated on CT with intravenous contrast enhancement as nonperfused liver parenchyma sometimes associated with a heterogeneous adjacent fluid collection. This condition warrants laparotomy with débridement. Bilomas occur as a result of leakage of bile and typically close spontaneously over time. The fluid collections themselves are best treated with radiologically guided percutaneous drainage when localized as it is in this patient. If the fluid collection is not amenable to percutaneous drainage, endoscopic retrograde cholangiopancreatography (ERCP) is recommended because biliary stents and sphincterotomy can reduce intrahepatic biliary pressure and increase healing.

**ANSWER:**  B

28. A 22-year-old man undergoes exploratory laparotomy for a transpelvic gunshot wound. A 2-cm partial-thickness laceration is found in the proximal portion of the intraperitoneal rectum. What is the appropriate surgical management of this injury?

   A. Hartmann procedure—end colostomy with oversewing of the distal rectal stump

   B. Primary repair with a diverting loop colostomy

   C. Primary repair with presacral drainage

   D. Presacral drainage only

   E. Primary repair only

*Ref.:* 4, 25

**COMMENTS:**  Repair of **rectal injury** largely depends on location (i.e. intraperitoneal versus extraperitoneal). The posterior rectum and distal third of the anterior rectum are not serosalized, and injury in these regions is considered extraperitoneal. Nondestructive lacerations that are less than 50% of the circumference of the rectal wall should be repaired primarily after débridement of any devitalized tissue in the absence of peritonitis. This therapy differs sharply from that of extraperitoneal rectal injuries, which should be treated chiefly by fecal diversion. Presacral drainage, which historically had been used rather routinely, has been decreasing in use and has not been shown to decrease the complication rate.

**ANSWER:**  E

29. All of the following are damage control treatment options for unstable patients with a ureteral injury except:

   A. Ligation of the injured ureter

   B. Percutaneous nephrostomy

   C. Ureteral drainage via luminal cannulation

   D. Transureteroureterostomy

   E. Placement of a bridging stent

*Ref.:* 4, 26

**COMMENTS:**  When a trauma patient is unstable on the operating room table and damage control has been initiated, time should

not be spent on primary repair of a **ureteral injury**, thus making transureteroureterostomy inappropriate at this time. Surgical options for this type of situation consist of simple ligation of the ureter, placing a percutaneous nephrostomy through the renal parenchyma into the renal pelvis, inserting a catheter into the proximal end of the damaged ureter and bringing it out through the wound, and placing a catheter or stent in the proximal and distal ends of a small-segment ureteral injury.

**ANSWER:**  D

30. Regarding orotracheal intubation in an injured patient, which of the following statements is true?

   A. Succinylcholine is a neuromuscular blocking agent that can cause hyperkalemia, but it can be used safely in spinal cord injury and burn patients within the first 72 hours after injury.

   B. During rapid-sequence intubation, preoxygenation should occur for 3 minutes via bag-valve-mask ventilation.

   C. Ketamine has a quick onset of action but can cause tachycardia and hypertension.

   D. Etomidate is contraindicated in patients with a suspected brain injury or open globe because of its side effect of increasing ICP.

   E. Cervical spine immobilization during intubation should be maintained with a rigid cervical collar.

*Ref.:* 4, 19

**COMMENTS:**  The most commonly used method for securing a trauma patient's airway is **orotracheal intubation**. Rapid-sequence intubation consists of preoxygenating the patient for 3 minutes with bag-valve-mask ventilation, maintaining in-line cervical stabilization, applying cricoid pressure, administering paralytic/induction agents, performing laryngoscopy, and then placing an endotracheal tube. In-line cervical stabilization should be maintained with the help of an assistant, not a rigid cervical spine collar. Etomidate is a common induction agent used in trauma victims. It has a quick onset of action and is indicated for patients with a suspected brain injury or open globe because it typically does not cause an increase in ICP. Two of ketamine's common side effects are tachycardia and increased blood pressure. However, it has a longer onset of action. Succinylcholine does cause a rise in the serum potassium concentration and can lead to severe hyperkalemia in patients with burns or spinal cord injury. However, this does not occur within the first 24 hours after the injury. Even though some studies have advocated safe use of succinylcholine following a major burn, most authors recommend avoiding its use beyond 24 hours.

**ANSWER:**  B

31. An 18-year-old man was involved in a high-speed motor vehicle collision and was ejected from the vehicle. He was found approximately 100 feet from the vehicle by emergency personnel. He arrives at the emergency department hemodynamically stable. CT of the chest, abdomen, and pelvis with intravenous contrast enhancement is performed approximately 5 hours after the time of the accident. Of note, the left kidney does not enhance. What is the most appropriate treatment at this time?

   A. Observation only

   B. Laparotomy with renal artery repair

C. Laparotomy with renal vein repair

D. Laparotomy with left nephrectomy

E. Angiography

*Ref.:* 26

**COMMENTS:** This patient has an ischemic kidney secondary to **injury** to the **renal** vasculature. Revascularization, if attempted, should be done within 4 hours of the time of injury. Since this patient is not a candidate for revascularization, angiography is not indicated. However, as in this case, when the kidney has a prolonged warm ischemia time, laparotomy is also not necessarily indicated. Avascular kidneys should not be resected if possible. Typically, they involute over time without complication and can sometimes regain some level of function. This patient should continue to be monitored, however, with serial abdominal examinations and for signs and symptoms of bleeding.

**ANSWER:** A

32. With regard to retroperitoneal hematomas, which of the following statements is true?

A. Zone 3 (pelvic hematoma) should be explored whether secondary to a blunt or penetrating traumatic injury.

B. A stable hematoma in zone 1 (midline) should not be explored because treatment of vascular injuries in this zone are best managed by embolization.

C. Zone 2 (perinephric hematomas) should be explored when the injury is due to a penetrating mechanism.

D. The Mattox maneuver allows the right-sided abdominal organs (right colon, duodenum, right kidney) to be reflected medially for exposure of the abdominal aorta.

E. All zone 1 injuries should be observed in patients with hemodynamic stability.

*Ref.:* 7

**COMMENTS:** The most important concept to learn regarding treatment of **retroperitoneal injuries** is the anatomy. Zone 1 is composed of the midline retroperitoneum and is divided into supramesocolic and inframesocolic segments, with the transverse mesocolon used as the dividing line. The perinephric spaces constitute zone 2, whereas the pelvic retroperitoneum is referred to as zone 3. All zone 1 injuries should be explored, regardless of mechanism, because of the major vascular structures located there. However, zone 2 and 3 injuries are treated similarly in that they should be explored only for a penetrating mechanism. Zone 3 hematomas are most commonly associated with pelvic fractures, and treatment is directed at fixation and angiographic embolization.

**ANSWER:** C

33. An 18-year-old college football player is struck in the chest during a game and sustained multiple anterior rib fractures. His vital signs are a heart rate of 98 beats/min and an irregular systolic blood pressure of 110 mm Hg. The initial work-up for a cardiac injury includes all of the following except:

A. Electrocardiogram (ECG)

B. Chest radiograph

C. FAST

D. Troponin levels

E. Echocardiogram

*Ref.:* 4, 27

**COMMENTS:** See Question 34.

**ANSWER:** B

34. Which of the following statements is true regarding blunt cardiac trauma?

A. The most commonly involved chamber of the heart is the left ventricle.

B. All patients suspected of having an injury should undergo transthoracic echocardiography.

C. Arrhythmias are the most common clinically significant symptoms.

D. The most common arrhythmia is ventricular fibrillation.

E. Approximately 5% of all patients with chest trauma have cardiac involvement.

*Ref.:* 4, 27

**COMMENTS:** Approximately 10% to 20% of all patients with **blunt chest trauma** have cardiac involvement. Arrhythmias are the most common clinically significant symptom, with ST-segment and T-wave changes being found most often. The right ventricle, which is the anterior-most chamber, is the most commonly involved. Evaluation of these patients includes FAST to rule out tamponade, an ECG, and troponin levels. The ECG and troponin levels should be obtained both on admission and 8 hours afterward. Transthoracic echocardiography is indicated only in patients with hemodynamic instability or the presence of arrhythmias (as in the patient described).

**ANSWER:** C

35. A 20-year-old woman is involved in a high-speed motor vehicle accident with significant damage to the front of the car. She arrives in the emergency department with a GCS score of 15, heart rate of 102 beats/min, respiratory rate of 18 breaths/min, and a systolic blood pressure of 108 mm Hg. A chest radiograph is obtained and demonstrates a 10-cm mediastinum and deviation of the left main stem bronchus. What is the most appropriate next step in management?

A. Observation

B. Left-sided chest tube

C. Repeated chest radiograph in 6 hours

D. CT angiogram of the chest

E. Transesophageal echocardiogram

*Ref.:* 28

**COMMENTS:** A widened mediastinum (>8 cm), deviation of the left main stem bronchus, tracheal deviation, an indistinct aortic knob, and apical caps are all signs of **aortic injury** on chest radiography. Although a transesophageal echocardiogram can visualize the proximal descending aorta, it is limited in evaluating the ascending aorta and its arch. In addition, this is an invasive procedure that requires some level of sedation. CT angiography is an excellent screening test for aortic injury with a high negative predictive value.

**ANSWER:  D**

---

**36.** A full-thickness injury to the aorta directly distal to the origin of the left subclavian artery is diagnosed in the patient in Question 35. What is the correct surgical approach for repair?

A. Left supraclavicular approach

B. Left infraclavicular approach

C. Median sternotomy

D. Left anterolateral thoracotomy

E. Left posterolateral thoracotomy

*Ref.:* 28

**COMMENTS:** A left posterolateral thoracotomy in the fourth intercostal space is the best operative approach for a **descending aortic injury**. Injuries to the ascending aorta, innominate artery, proximal right subclavian artery, and either carotid are best managed with a median sternotomy. A left-sided clavicular incision is appropriate for a midsubclavian arterial injury. A left anterolateral thoracotomy is used for emergency department thoracotomies because it provides access to the pericardium and thoracic aorta, thereby allowing open cardiac massage and aortic cross-clamping.

**ANSWER:  E**

---

**37.** Which of the following statements regarding blunt aortic injury is true?

A. It is estimated that patients with a contained rupture have a 1% per hour rate of rupture within the first 48 hours after injury.

B. The proximal descending aorta is the most commonly injured and involves approximately 80% of all cases.

C. Overall operative mortality after repair is between 30% and 40%.

D. Paraplegia occurs after operative repair in less than 5% of patients.

E. Approximately 20% of chest radiographs are falsely negative.

*Ref.:* 28

**COMMENTS:** It is estimated that 85% of all patients with a full-thickness **aortic injury** die at the scene of the injury. About 60% of aortic injuries occur in the proximal descending segment, at the origin of the left subclavian artery. Other less common locations are the ascending aorta, the arch, or the level of the diaphragm. Approximately 5% to 10% of patients with an aortic injury will have normal findings on chest radiography. Operative repair should be timely because there is a 1% per hour rupture rate within the first 48 hours after injury. Operative repair is associated with 5% to 25% mortality, and paraplegia occurs in 10% of patients postoperatively.

**ANSWER:  A**

---

**38.** A 14-year-old girl is an unrestrained passenger in a motor vehicle collision. She complains of right lower extremity pain. On examination, her knee is markedly swollen and has a notably limited range of motion. The foot is cool to the touch, and the dorsalis pedis and posterior tibialis pulses are absent. Radiographs of the right lower extremity show no fracture. What is the most appropriate next step in management?

A. CT of the right lower extremity

B. Ankle-brachial indices of both lower extremities

C. Angiography

D. Operative revascularization with four-compartment fasciotomy

E. Operative revascularization without fasciotomy

*Ref.:* 7

**COMMENTS:** Posterior knee dislocations are associated with a **popliteal artery injury** approximately 33% of the time. This type of dislocation occurs when a direct force is applied to a flexed knee. Because of the absence of extensive collateral flow around the knee joint, an injury to the popliteal artery is associated with a fairly high amputation rate, up to 20%. It is imperative to recognize and repair this type of injury early. In this patient, the lack of distal pulses warrants a direct trip to the operating room, without need for any further diagnostic testing. Because of the high rate of amputation for this type of injury, it is recommended that a fasciotomy be performed at the time of revascularization when a patient has evidence of ischemia, as in this clinical scenario.

**ANSWER:  D**

---

**39.** Select the correct statement regarding flail chest:

A. It occurs when three or more adjacent ribs are fractured in one place.

B. Work of breathing is increased secondary to paradoxical chest wall motion.

C. Patients with flail chest should be aggressively resuscitated because of the probable development of a pulmonary contusion.

D. Patients with this condition should be prophylactically intubated secondary to a high likelihood of respiratory failure.

E. If a patient does require mechanical ventilation, it is important to avoid the use of positive end-expiratory pressure.

*Ref.:* 4

**COMMENTS: Flail chest** occurs when three or more adjacent ribs are fractured in at least two places. This leads to a segment of chest wall that has the opposite movement with respirations and thereby increases the patient's work of breathing. Most often, this condition can be treated with vigilant pain control and aggressive pulmonary toilet. Pulmonary contusions often occur with flail chest and are not fully appreciated on chest radiographs until 24 to 48 hours after injury. Fluid resuscitation should be conservative so that any developing pulmonary contusions are not worsened further. However, if respiratory failure does develop and mechanical ventilation is needed, positive end-expiratory pressure is important to maintain functional residual capacity.

**ANSWER:  B**

---

**40.** An 8-year-old child hits a curb with his bicycle, which causes him to flip over the handlebars. He had no initial sequelae and was monitored at home by his parents. However, 2 days after the incident, he begins having nonbilious emesis. He is brought to the emergency department and undergoes CT of the abdomen and pelvis, which demonstrates a duodenal hematoma. What is the next step in management?

A. Initiation of nil per os (NPO) status and gastric decompression with a nasogastric tube

B. Esophagogastroduodenoscopy to assess for luminal compromise

C. Drainage of the hematoma via laparoscopy

D. Drainage of the hematoma via laparotomy

E. Resection of the injured portion of the duodenum with primary anastomoses

*Ref.:* 4, 29

**COMMENTS:** Blunt injuries to the duodenum can be difficult to diagnose. **Duodenal hematomas** typically occur up to 3 days after injury with a gastric outlet obstruction type of clinical picture. The duodenal lumen is narrowed because of the hematoma itself and the associated edema. CT with oral contrast enhancement and upper gastrointestinal studies are useful in diagnosing this condition. If no other indication exists for exploration, treatment is conservative and consists of placement of a nasogastric tube for decompression. Typically, these hematomas and their symptoms resolve within 7 to 15 days after injury. Operative exploration is reserved for patients in whom the symptoms do not resolve within this period.

**ANSWER:** A

41. Which of the following statements regarding FAST is true?

A. A 2.5-MHz convex-array transducer should be used.

B. The hepatorenal space, known as the Morison pouch, is viewed between the eleventh and twelfth ribs in the right midaxillary line.

C. The splenorenal space is evaluated between the ninth and eleventh ribs in the left midaxillary line.

D. The bladder should preferentially by emptied before examination to allow better visualization of fluid in the pelvis.

E. FAST is an important part of the primary survey.

*Ref.:* 30

**COMMENTS:** **Focused assessment for the sonographic examination of trauma patients** is performed as part of the ATLS secondary survey. A 3.5-MHz convex-array transducer is used to evaluate for the presence of fluid in the abdomen. Four areas are to be examined. The first is the pericardial window, which is viewed with the transducer placed subxiphoid. The hepatorenal space is evaluated in the right midaxillary line, between the eleventh and twelfth ribs. The splenorenal space is evaluated in the right posterior axillary line, between the ninth and eleventh ribs. The last area examined is the pouch of Douglas in the pelvis. This rectouterine/rectovesical space is evaluated with the transducer placed approximately 3 cm above the pubic symphysis. A full bladder actually helps elucidate the presence of blood in this space, and Foley catheters should be placed after FAST has been performed.

**ANSWER:** B

42. An 18-year-old man arrives at the emergency department with a stab wound in the right upper quadrant of his abdomen. His initial vital signs are a heart rate of 122 beats/min and mean arterial pressure of 50 mm Hg. Two liters of lactated Ringer solution is infused. On physical examination, his abdomen is distended and tender to palpation. After the 2 L of fluid, the patient's repeated vital signs are as follows: heart rate, 130; mean arterial pressure, 48. What is the next most appropriate step in management?

A. Transfusion of 2 units of packed red blood cells

B. DPL

C. CT scan of the abdomen and pelvis with intravenous contrast enhancement

D. Diagnostic laparoscopy

E. Exploratory laparotomy

*Ref.:* 1, 4

**COMMENTS:** This patient is hemodynamically unstable and has a **penetrating wound to the abdomen**. Hypotension despite initial resuscitation, evisceration, and peritoneal signs are all clear indications for emergency laparotomy in the setting of a penetrating injury. Further diagnostic testing at this time is unnecessary.

**ANSWER:** E

43. During exploratory laparotomy in a patient with multiple gunshot wounds to the abdomen, a through-and-through gunshot wound is noted in the left lobe of the liver. Brisk bleeding is seen from the bullet track. All of the following operative maneuvers for this injury are appropriate except:

A. Pringle maneuver

B. Tractotomy

C. Omental packing

D. Ligation of the proper hepatic artery

E. Large mattress sutures traversing the bullet track

*Ref.:* 4, 24

**COMMENTS:** In regard to **hepatic injuries**, there are three overall goals of treatment: (1) control of hemorrhage, (2) débridement of nonviable tissue, and (3) adequate drainage. Multiple operative techniques can be used to establish control of bleeding, and often a combination of these techniques are used. The Pringle maneuver is direct compression of the portal triad, either manually or with a vascular clamp. This takes a small amount of time and is helpful in identifying whether the bleeding source is from the triad, hepatic veins, or retrohepatic vena cava. It is important to keep note of how long compression is applied because these patients tend to be hypovolemic and hypothermic and as a rule do not tolerate hepatic ischemia well. Omental packing is performed by first creating a pedicle of omentum and then placing it across or in the defect. This creates a well-vascularized "packing" of the liver that also has its own natural hemostatic properties. Large mattress sutures have been used for quite some time and work by compressing the bullet track with the surrounding liver parenchyma. A tractotomy is the act of opening the already present wound to fully examine the track and identify the bleeding vessels. This then allows directed individual vessel ligation. Historically, selective hepatic artery ligation has been used and involves ligation of the hepatic artery branch to the involved lobe. Although this is still a viable option, it is associated with a fairly high rate of abscess formation and hepatic necrosis. The proper hepatic artery, however, should not be ligated.

**ANSWER:** D

**44.** A 58-year-old man is an unrestrained front seat passenger in a high-speed motor vehicle collision. In the emergency department he has stable vital signs, and the only finding on physical examination is a left leg that is flexed at the hip, adducted, and internally rotated. A radiograph is obtained and confirms posterior dislocation of the left hip. The next step in management is:

A. Immediate closed reduction, either in the emergency department or in the operating room

B. CT scan to diagnose intraarticular bone fragments

C. Admission to the hospital and splinting of the left hip and thigh

D. Placement of skeletal traction

E. Open reduction

*Ref.:* 23

**COMMENTS: Posterior hip dislocations** occur most commonly when direct force is applied to the knees of a person whose hips and knees are in a flexed position (i.e., sitting). Immediate closed reduction is imperative and can be performed with intravenous sedation in the emergency department or in the operating room under general anesthesia. The timing of the reduction is important to reduce risk for the development of further damage to the sciatic nerve and avascular necrosis of the femur. Avascular necrosis of the femoral head is a significant complication that often leads to total hip arthroplasty. After the hip is reduced, CT of the hip is recommended to evaluate the acetabulum and the intraarticular area for any fragments.

**ANSWER:** A

**45.** An 18-year-old man is involved in a boating accident and suffers a right open tibial fracture and an obvious arterial injury, with no detectable tibial nerve function. Which of the following statements about this situation is true?

A. The patient's age is a negative prognostic indicator in regard to the limb salvage rate.

B. If this patient were to undergo primary amputation, at least 10 cm of the proximal end of the tibia should be preserved to facilitate the use of a prosthesis.

C. A Mangled Extremity Severity Score (MESS) higher than 5 is a strong indicator that this patient would benefit from primary amputation.

D. A warm ischemia time of longer than 4 hours is an absolute indication for primary amputation.

E. Although the MESS is not specific in determining future functional limb status, it is highly sensitive in determining the need for primary amputation.

*Ref.:* 23

**COMMENTS: Mangled Extremity Severity Score** is composed of four categories: skeletal/soft tissue injury, ischemia, shock, and age (Table 10-3). A score higher than 7 generally warrants primary amputation. However, no single scoring system has been shown to be highly specific or sensitive in determining the success of limb salvage or future limb function. Older age, ischemia time longer than 6 hours, hypotension, poor nutritional status, and severe coexisting injuries all have a negative impact on the chance of limb salvage. For best prosthetic fitting, 10 cm of the proximal end of the tibia is recommended.

**TABLE 10-3  Mangled Extremity Severity Score**

| Component | Points |
| --- | --- |
| **Skeletal and Soft Tissue Injury** | |
| Low energy (stab, simple fracture, "civilian" gunshot wound) | 1 |
| Medium energy (open or multiplex fractures, dislocation) | 2 |
| High energy (close-range shotgun or "military" gunshot wound, crush injury) | 3 |
| Very high energy (same as above plus gross contamination, soft tissue avulsion) | 4 |
| **Limb Ischemia (Doubled When >6 h)** | |
| Pulse reduced or absent but perfusion normal | 1 |
| Pulseless; paresthesias, diminished capillary refill | 2 |
| Cool, paralyzed, insensate, numb | 3 |
| **Shock** | |
| Systolic blood pressure always >90 mm Hg | 0 |
| Hypotensive transiently | 1 |
| Persistent hypotension | 2 |
| **Age (yr)** | |
| <30 | 0 |
| 30-50 | 1 |
| >50 | 2 |

From Johansen K, Daines M, Howey T, et al: Objective criteria accurately predict amputation following lower extremity trauma, *J Trauma* 30:568–573, 1990.

**ANSWER:** B

**46.** Select the correct statement regarding radiation exposure:

A. Hematopoietic syndrome occurs after exposure to 5 to 10 Gy and is characterized by pancytopenia.

B. Exposure to 8 Gy is associated with a 50% mortality rate.

C. After exposure, the majority of radioactivity is contained in the patient's clothing.

D. Gastrointestinal syndrome occurs after exposure to 1 to 4 Gy and is characterized by nausea, vomiting, abdominal pain, and bloody diarrhea.

E. Leukemia and solid tumors are known long-term effects of total body irradiation and appear 7 to 10 years after the exposure.

*Ref.:* 31

**COMMENTS: Radiation exposure** is a rare but serious event. The effects of exposure are directly related to the dose. Exposure to less than 1 Gy typically produces no symptoms and is associated with 0% mortality. Exposure to greater than 8 Gy results in 100% mortality. Hematopoietic syndrome occurs after exposure to 1 to 4 Gy and is characterized by pancytopenia that develops within 48 hours of the event. Exposure to 8 to 12 Gy results in gastrointestinal syndrome, which is manifested as nausea and vomiting acutely and then, over a period of 1 to 2 weeks, as bloody diarrhea and death. Neurovascular syndrome is described after exposure to greater than 15 Gy and results in massive vasodilation, shock, and death.

**ANSWER:** C

**47.** An explosion occurs at a nearby construction site, and one worker near the blast is brought to the emergency department. He is covered in soot and has superficial partial-thickness burns on his left arm and hand (approximately 4% of total body surface area) and perforated tympanic membranes bilaterally. The remainder of his physical examination is negative. Select the correct statement regarding his injuries:

A. After the patient's burn wounds are cleaned and dressed and a hearing examination is performed, the patient is ready for discharge.

B. An initial chest radiograph should be performed.

C. An intestinal blast injury typically causes abdominal pain and occurs within the first 8 to 12 hours after the blast.

D. Tympanic membrane perforation is the most significant indicator of mortality in patients with a blast injury.

E. Blast lung injury occurs primarily because of air embolism induced by shock waves.

*Ref.:* 32

**COMMENTS:** Victims involved in a blast or explosion can suffer from a myriad of injuries caused by burn, blunt, and penetrating mechanisms. Therefore, these injuries are categorized as primary, secondary, tertiary, or quaternary according to mechanism. Primary **blast injury** refers to damage to hollow visceral organs secondary to the blast wave itself. An example is tympanic membrane perforation, which is also a good screening tool for significant blast injuries. The majority of patients with tympanic membrane rupture heal without intervention. Other examples of primary blast injuries involve the lung and intestine. Intestinal blast injuries are rare, can occur anywhere in the small or large bowel, and typically have a delayed clinical manifestation (>24 hours after the blast). Blast lung injury is the most significant indicator of mortality and is primarily due to disruption of the alveolar septa with subsequent edema and hemorrhage induced by the shock waves. Overall, this leads to a clinical picture similar to ARDS. This injury can be complicated by pneumothorax, air emboli, and bronchopleural fistulas. Because of the significant morbidity and mortality associated with blast lung injury, patients involved in a blast or explosion should be screened with chest radiographs and otoscopic examination. This patient, who does have perforated tympanic membranes, should not only undergo chest radiography but also be observed for at least 12 hours before discharge. Secondary blast injuries occur from objects propelled by the blast wave. When the victim is thrown and strikes an inanimate object, the injuries are categorized as tertiary. Quaternary injuries are a miscellaneous category and consist of burns and crush injuries.

**ANSWER:** B

48. A 79-year-old woman is taken to the emergency department after a fall from standing. She has an obvious deformity of her right humerus, palpable radial and ulnar pulses, and numbness of the dorsal aspect of her forearm and hand. Select the correct statement:

A. The nerve most likely injured is the median nerve.

B. The presence of palpable distal pulses precludes the need for angiography.

C. Patients with this nerve injury should not have their hand or wrist splinted because splinting can lead to markedly decreased range of motion.

D. Operative intervention is indicated only for patients with an open component.

E. The majority of the nerve injuries just described resolve without surgical intervention.

*Ref.:* 33

**COMMENTS:** This patient has a fracture of the **humerus**, which commonly occurs after falls or motor vehicle collisions. The nerve injury described in this woman involves the **radial nerve**, the most commonly injured nerve when the fracture occurs in the distal third of the humerus. Approximately 70% of patients with radial nerve injury associated with fracture of the humerus experience resolution without surgical intervention. However, these patients should have their hand and wrist splinted during recovery. Operative intervention in patients with humeral fractures is indicated for an open component, as well as an inability to achieve adequate alignment with closed reduction. Arterial injuries can occur, especially with proximal humeral fractures, and should always be suspected, even in patients with palpable distal pulses.

**ANSWER:** E

## REFERENCES

1. Britt LD, Rushing GD: Penetrating abdominal trauma. In Cameron JL, editor: *Current surgical therapy*, ed 9, Philadelphia, 2008, CV Mosby.
2. Sims CA, Reilly PM: Penetrating neck trauma. In Cameron JL, editor: *Current surgical therapy*, ed 9, Philadelphia, 2008, CV Mosby.
3. Ledgerwood AM, Lucas CE: Blunt abdominal trauma. In Cameron JL, editor: *Current surgical therapy*, ed 9, Philadelphia, 2008, CV Mosby.
4. Hoyt DB, Coimbra R, Acosta J: Management of acute trauma. In Townsend CM, Beauchamp RD, Evers BM, et al, editors: *Sabiston textbook of surgery: the biological basis of modern surgical practice*, ed 18, Philadelphia, 2008, WB Saunders.
5. Cushing NM, Ness PM: Blood transfusion therapy. In Cameron JL, editor: *Current surgical therapy*, ed 9, Philadelphia, 2008, CV Mosby.
6. Zarzaur BL, Croce MA: The management of vascular trauma. In Cameron JL, editor: *Current surgical therapy*, ed 9, Philadelphia, 2008, CV Mosby.
7. Hirschberg A, Mattox KL: Vascular trauma. In Townsend CM, Beauchamp RD, Evers BM, et al, editors: *Sabiston textbook of surgery: the biological basis of modern surgical practice*, ed 18, Philadelphia, 2008, WB Saunders.
8. Feliciano DV: The management of extremity compartment syndrome. In Cameron JL, editor: *Current surgical therapy*, ed 9, Philadelphia, 2008, CV Mosby.
9. Mullins RJ: Acute renal failure. In Cameron JL, editor: *Current surgical therapy*, ed 9, Philadelphia, 2008, CV Mosby.
10. Hojman H, Rabinovici R: Abdominal compartment syndrome. In Cameron JL, editor: *Current surgical therapy*, ed 9, Philadelphia, 2008, CV Mosby.
11. Adams CA, Biffle WL, Cioffi WG: Surgical critical care. In Townsend CM, Beauchamp RD, Evers BM, et al, editors: *Sabiston textbook of surgery: the biological basis of modern surgical practice*, ed 18, Philadelphia, 2008, WB Saunders.
12. Knudson MM, Wan JJ: Reproductive system trauma. In Feliciano DV, Mattox KL, Moor EE, editors: *Trauma*, ed 6, New York, 2008, McGraw-Hill.
13. Mikami DJ, Beery PR, Ellison EC: Surgery in the pregnant patient. In Townsend CM, Beauchamp RD, Evers BM, et al, editors: *Sabiston textbook of surgery: the biological basis of modern surgical practice*, ed 18, Philadelphia, 2008, WB Saunders.
14. Edmonds RD, Peitzman AB: Injury to the spleen. In Cameron JL, editor: *Current surgical therapy*, ed 9, Philadelphia, 2008, CV Mosby.
15. Rudloff U, Pachter HL: Diaphragmatic injuries. In Cameron JL, editor: *Current surgical therapy*, ed 9, Philadelphia, 2008, CV Mosby.
16. Manaker J, Scalea TM: Emergency department thoracotomy. In Cameron JL, editor: *Current surgical therapy*, ed 9, Philadelphia, 2008, CV Mosby.
17. Wall MJ, Huh J, Mattox KL: Indications for and techniques of thoracotomy. In Feliciano DV, Mattox KL, Moor EE, editors: *Trauma*, ed 6, New York, 2008, McGraw-Hill.
18. Weingart JD: Head injuries. In Cameron JL, editor: *Current surgical therapy*, ed 9, Philadelphia, 2008, CV Mosby.
19. Mackersie RC, Tang JF: Airway management in the trauma patient. In Cameron JL, editor: *Current surgical therapy*, ed 9, Philadelphia, 2008, CV Mosby.

20. Patterson JT, Hanbali F, Franklin RL, Nauta HJW: Neurosurgery. In Townsend CM, Beauchamp RD, Evers BM, et al, editors: *Sabiston textbook of surgery: the biological basis of modern surgical practice*, ed 18, Philadelphia, 2008, WB Saunders.

21. Pasquale M, Li M: Spine and spinal cord injuries. In Cameron JL, editor: *Current surgical therapy*, ed 9, Philadelphia, 2008, CV Mosby.

22. Cryer HG: Pelvic fractures. In Cameron JL, editor: *Current surgical therapy*, ed 9, Philadelphia, 2008, CV Mosby.

23. Browner BD, DeAngelis JP: Emergency care of musculoskeletal injuries. In Townsend CM, Beauchamp RD, Evers BM, et al, editors: *Sabiston textbook of surgery: the biological basis of modern surgical practice*, ed 18, Philadelphia, 2008, WB Saunders.

24. Sonnenday CJ: Liver injury. In Cameron JL, editor: *Current surgical therapy*, ed 9, Philadelphia, 2008, CV Mosby.

25. Weinberg JA, Fabian TZ: Rectal injuries. In Cameron JL, editor: *Current surgical therapy*, ed 9, Philadelphia, 2008, CV Mosby.

26. Brandes SB, Buckman RF: Retroperitoneal injuries: Kidney and Ureter. In Cameron JL, editor: *Current surgical therapy*, ed 9, Philadelphia, 2008, CV Mosby.

27. Haut ER: Blunt cardiac injury. In Cameron JL, editor: *Current surgical therapy*, ed 9, Philadelphia, 2008, CV Mosby.

28. Safi HJ, Estrera AL, Miller CC, et al: Thoracic vasculature with emphasis on the thoracic aorta. In Townsend CM, Beauchamp RD, Evers BM, et al, editors: *Sabiston textbook of surgery: the biological basis of modern surgical practice*, ed 18, Philadelphia, 2008, WB Saunders.

29. Rotondo MF, Newell MA: Pancreatic and duodenal injuries. In Cameron JL, editor: *Current surgical therapy*, ed 9, Philadelphia, 2008, CV Mosby.

30. Dente CJ, Rozycki GS: The surgeon's use of ultrasound in thoracoabdominal trauma. In Cameron JL, editor: *Current surgical therapy*, ed 9, Philadelphia, 2008, CV Mosby.

31. Lee JO, Herndon DN: Burns and radiation injury. In Feliciano DV, Mattox KL, Moor EE, editors: *Trauma*, ed 6, New York, 2008, McGraw-Hill.

32. Hirschberg A, Stein M: Trauma care in mass casualty incidents. In Feliciano DV, Mattox KL, Moor EE, editors: *Trauma*, ed 6, New York, 2008, McGraw-Hill.

33. Peterson SL, Lehman TP: Upper extremity injury. In Feliciano DV, Mattox KL, Moor EE, editors: *Trauma*, ed 6, New York, 2008, McGraw-Hill.

# CHAPTER 11

# Burns

*Steven D. Bines, M.D.; Thomas A. Messer, M.D.; and Stathis J. Poulakidas, M.D., F.A.C.S.*

1. Select the true statement regarding the epidemiology of burn injury:

   A. Most burn injuries occur in occupational environments.

   B. Young adult men are the most likely to suffer burn injury.

   C. The most common cause of death after admission for burn injury is airway occlusion.

   D. Scalding is the most common cause of burns in children younger than 5 years.

   E. Prevention has not has a significant impact on the incidence or mortality of burn injury.

   *Ref.:* 1-3

**COMMENTS:** Approximately 1 million injuries are caused by thermal trauma yearly in the United States. The majority of **burn injuries** occur in the home (43%). In general, 65% of burns occur in non–work-related accidents, 17% in work-related accidents, and 5% each in recreational or in assault or abuse cases. House fires contribute to 75% to 80% of deaths from burns. Burns occur in a bimodal distribution, with increased risk occurring in children younger than 4 years and adults 65 years and older. African Americans and Native Americans are disproportionately affected. Burns occur more frequently in vulnerable populations, including those with epilepsy, those with heavy alcohol use, the poor, and people living in substandard housing. Asphyxiation is a common cause of death at the scene of a fire, but the most common recorded cause of death in burn patients after admission is multiorgan failure. Other causes, in decreasing order of frequency, are shock, trauma, pulmonary failure or sepsis, cardiovascular failure, and burn wound sepsis. **Hot-water scald injuries** are the most common cause in children younger than 5 years, with flame burns becoming more frequent in those 5 years and older. Ordinances requiring water heaters to be set at no higher than 120° F have decreased the incidence of scald burns. Efforts at prevention have significantly decreased the number of burn injuries occurring in the United States, although disabled or impaired individuals are still at risk.

**ANSWER: D**

2. Which of the following regarding burn wound depth is true?

   A. First-degree burns heal rapidly but contribute significantly to the total body surface area (TBSA) burned in large, mixed-depth wounds.

   B. Second-degree burns characteristically cause erythema, pain, and blistering.

   C. Third-degree burns are generally painful and extremely sensitive to touch.

   D. Fourth-degree burns mandate amputation of the involved extremities.

   E. Superficial partial-thickness burn is the contemporary term for first-degree burns.

   *Ref.:* 1-3

**COMMENTS:** Skin consists of two layers: epidermis and dermis. The **epidermis** is composed of five progressively differentiated layers of keratinocytes, the outermost of which, the stratum corneum, is relatively impermeable. The epidermis provides barrier functions and protects against infection, absorption of toxins, exposure to ultraviolet (UV) light, and fluid and heat loss. The **dermis** is a cellular and extracellular layer that provides the skin with durability and elasticity. Within the dermis, fibroblasts synthesize mesenchymal proteins, and inflammatory cells are present and contribute to the inflammatory responses to injury. Dermal papillae interdigitate with the epidermal rete ridges to form the dermal-epidermal junction, a site affected by some exfoliative diseases of the skin. Superficial, or **first-degree**, burns involve only the epidermis and are erythematous and painful. The damaged epidermis will slough off within 3 to 4 days and be replaced by regenerating keratinocytes. Most sunburn is first-degree, and the treatment of superficial burns is similar to that of sunburn. **Superficial burns** do not contribute significantly to the systemic response to burn injury and are not counted in the percentage of TBSA (%TBSA) burned. **Partial-thickness burns** (**second-degree**) involve both the epidermis and dermis and are subdivided into superficial partial thickness and deep partial thickness, depending on the depth of dermal involvement. Superficial partial-thickness burns involve the papillary dermis. Blistering occurs within 24 hours of injury. The exposed underlying dermis is typically pink, blanching, moist, and tender to touch because the nerve endings are preserved. These burns heal within 2 to 3 weeks with little risk of scarring. **Deep partial-thickness burns** extend to the reticular dermis and may require more than 3 weeks to heal. These wounds blister and reveal mottled pink/white dermis. Sensation may be decreased, and the wounds may dry after initial observation. If deep partial-thickness wounds take longer than 3 weeks to heal, grafting may be required. **Full-thickness (third-degree) burns** extend through the entire dermis into subcutaneous tissue. Full-thickness burns may be dry, leathery, firm, and insensate. Even if mottled in appearance, they do not blanch and may be hemorrhagic. These wounds require excision of the burn eschar and skin grafting for closure. Intermediate-depth wounds may be difficult to judge by initial appearance. Their potential to heal should be determined with serial observations because the initial evaluation may be inaccurate, even by experienced clinicians. Light reflectance techniques, fluorescein, thermography, and magnetic resonance imaging have not proved useful with respect to serial clinical evaluation. Non-contact laser Doppler imaging can be helpful but has not gained widespread clinical use. **Fourth-degree burns** extend to muscle, bone, or other deep structures. They are particularly common with electrical injuries or burns with prolonged contact occurring in impaired patients. These very deep burns pose serious reconstructive challenges, and amputation may be required when the extremities or digits are involved.

**ANSWER:** B

3. Which of the following statements regarding the zones of injury in a burn wound is true?

   A. A zone of hyperemia inside a zone of stasis

   B. A zone of hyperemia superficial to a zone of stasis, with a deeper zone of coagulation beneath

   C. A zone of coagulation at the surface of a burn wound, a zone of stasis within the injured dermal layer, and a deep zone of hyperemia characterized by vasodilated subcutaneous vessels

   D. A zone of coagulation, surrounded by a zone of stasis, surrounded by a zone of hyperemia

   E. A zone of hemorrhagic burn that must be coagulated, a zone of stasis in which the depth of burn injury is already fixed, and a zone of hyperemia that may convert to coagulation

*Ref.:* 1

**COMMENTS: Jackson's classification of zones of injury** in 1953 referred to the varying depth of injury radiating outward from a burn wound and defined the pathophysiology of cutaneous thermal injury. The **central zone of coagulation** is necrotic and irreversibly damaged; it represents a full-thickness injury that will require excision and grafting. The zone of stasis refers to the surrounding region and is characterized by constricted vessels and hypoxia. Initially viable, this tissue may convert to coagulation or a full-thickness injury as a result of edema, infection, or shock with decreased perfusion. **The zone of stasis** may remain viable if adequately perfused. In a patient with a large TBSA burn, the viability of this zone may be critical in providing donor sites and reducing the total area that requires grafting. The **zone of hyperemia** is characterized by vasodilation as a result of inflammatory mediators, and the tissue is viable.

**ANSWER:** D

4. Select the most accurate statement regarding burn injury:

   A. Contact burns occur commonly and rarely require grafting.

   B. Intoxication is infrequently associated with deep burn injury.

   C. Circumferential burns on both feet are seen in accidental bathing injuries in children.

   D. Flash burns are generated by brief, intense heat, and articles of clothing are frequently protective.

   E. Electrical burns are deeper than they appear because of the high flash temperatures generated by arcing.

*Ref.:* 1

**COMMENTS:** The **mechanism of burn injury**, if known, may aid in assessing wound depth and predicting its capacity to heal. **Flash burns** are responsible for 50% of admissions to burn centers. Explosions caused by natural gas, propane, and gasoline vapors generate brief, intense heat. If not directly ignited, clothing is protective, with burns affecting only exposed skin. The depth of injury can be variable; many flash burns heal without grafting. **Flame burns** generally result in deep dermal or full-thickness injury because of the duration of exposure. Structure fires and ignition of bedding or clothing are common causes of flame burns, and burn depth is proportional to the time required to remove the burning or smoldering material from the victim. Intoxication or carbon monoxide (CO) poisoning occurring during a house fire increases the likelihood of deep flame burns. **Scald burns** are the second most common cause of burns in the United States. The depth of injury is related to water temperature and the duration of contact. At 140° F (60° C), water causes deep dermal injury in 3 seconds. Clothed areas may be scalded more deeply because of prolonged contact with wet fabric before removal. Young children and elderly patients will scald faster and at lower temperatures. If not cautious, diabetic patients may accidentally scald themselves when soaking neuropathic or insensate feet in hot water. These burns are frequently deep partial to full thickness, and such patients are likely to have impaired healing as a result of their comorbid conditions. **Hot oil** and **grease burns** tend to be deep partial or full thickness because of the very high temperatures reached while cooking or heating oil. **Contact burns** result from direct contact with a heat source and often occur in work environments. The hot presses used in industrial applications can cause particularly devastating combined crush/burn injuries that may result in poor functional outcomes. Deep contact burns in domestic environments occur in children or impaired individuals (drugs, alcohol). Palmar or plantar surface burns generally deserve a period of observation because of the propensity of the thicker dermis of these surfaces to heal and generally less optimal results in terms of sensation and function obtained with split-thickness skin grafting in these areas. **Electrical injuries** may cause deep tissue destruction that belies the surface wound when current flows through the patient, but flash burns from electrical arcing without direct contact are similar to flash burns from other sources.

**ANSWER:** D

5. Which of the following patients do not meet the criteria for referral to a burn center?

   A. A 50-year-old woman with a 1% TBSA partial-thickness burn on her left hand from a cooking accident

   B. A 30-year-old construction worker with pain and blistering bilaterally on the knees after kneeling in wet cement all afternoon

   C. A 25-year-old man with 7% TBSA partial-thickness burns on the chest

   D. A 42-year-old woman with no cutaneous injury, found lying down at the scene of a house fire, and noted to have carbonaceous sputum after intubation in the field

   E. An 18-year-old man in a motor vehicle collision with 30% TBSA burns on his chest and circumferential burns bilaterally on his arms

*Ref.:* 4

**COMMENTS:** The American Burn Association and the American College of Surgeons Committee on Trauma have published guidelines for **patient transfer to a burn center** for care: (1) partial-thickness burns on greater than 10% of TBSA; (2) burns that involve the face, hands, feet, genitalia, perineum, or major joints; (3) third-degree burns (any size) in any age group; (4) electrical burns, including lightning injury; (5) chemical burns;

(6) inhalation injury; (7) burn injury in patients with preexisting medical disorders that could complicate management, prolong recovery, or affect mortality; (8) any patient with burns and concomitant trauma (such as fractures) in which the burn injury poses the greatest risk for morbidity or mortality (in such cases, if the trauma poses the greater immediate risk, the patient's condition may be stabilized initially in a trauma center before transfer to a burn center); (9) burned children in hospitals without qualified personnel or equipment for the care of children; and (10) burn injury in patients who will require special social, emotional, or rehabilitative intervention. These criteria are not meant to be exclusive, and many centers will treat patients with wounds smaller than those mentioned in the guidelines. Many burn centers care for patients with exfoliative skin disorders, major wounds, necrotizing infections, and other diseases that require significant wound management and critical care.

### ANSWER: C

6. A 6-year-old girl suffers full-thickness flame burns on her forearm after playing with matches. Which of the following is correct regarding wound healing after her skin grafting?

   A. Capillary leakage results from inadequate cooling of burn wounds after injury.

   B. Epithelialization signals the end of burn wound healing.

   C. Diffusion allows skin grafts to survive before neovascularization.

   D. Routine exposure to UV light may help speed repigmentation of the healing burn wound.

   E. Epidermolysis is typical of excessive myofibrillar adhesion to the basement membrane.

*Ref.:* 1

COMMENTS: Burned tissues initially respond with coagulation and constriction of the microvasculature for **hemostasis**. In the coagulation pathways, including cleavage of fibrinogen by tissue factor, matrix is laid down so that cells can migrate into the wound bed. Inflammatory cells generate plasmin for clot resolution. Vasoconstriction is followed by the vasodilation and capillary leakage seen in the resuscitative phase of injury. Capillary leakage allows migration of cells into the wound but also extravascular leakage, which leads to pulmonary edema, compartment syndromes, and the potential for ischemic injury in tissues with marginal viability (zone of stasis). A great many **inflammatory mediators** are released, including interleukins, prostaglandins, and neuropeptides, and cause cellular adhesion, chemotaxis, and proliferation. Serotonin, histamine, bradykinin, and arachidonic acid metabolites allow continued vasodilation and vascular permeability. Signals and mediators from cutaneous cells contribute to the inflammation. Neutrophil margination may potentiate ischemia and contribute to reperfusion injury. Inhibition of these pathways is of interest but is currently not clinically useful. **Epithelialization** of full-thickness wounds occurs from the wound edges, whereas partial-thickness burn wounds heal from the epidermal appendages surviving in the wound bed. Formation of granulation tissue indicates the wound is able to be closed. **Skin grafts** survive by imbibition (diffusion) of nutrients and oxygen for several days after placement until neovascularization links capillaries in the graft to those in the wound bed (inosculation). Once epithelialized, the barrier functions of the outer skin are restored, and the inflammatory state of the wound may be altered. Basement membrane continues to develop after epithelialization, which explains why blistering and epidermolysis are commonplace early after wound closure. **Dermal** and **subcutaneous fibrogenesis** continues along with cellular migration and angiogenesis. Type III and type I collagen are deposited in a mat and result in dermal scar. Cross-linking of type I collagen fibrils increases breaking strength, albeit never to preinjury levels. Matrix metalloproteinases aid remodeling of the matrix and may prevent hypertrophic scar formation. Myofibroblasts aid wound closure by contraction, which may contribute to disability following burn injury. Melanocytes migrate from the wound edges and epidermal appendages after the epithelial cells. Protection from UV rays aids return of pigmentation. Hypertrophic scars have increased sensory nerves, thereby contributing to their sensitivity and pruritus.

### ANSWER: C

7. A 25-year-old man pulled from a house fire has burns on his right arm circumferentially, bilaterally on his legs, and on his perineum. What is the approximate %TBSA burned?

   A. 28%

   B. 36%

   C. 64%

   D. 46%

   E. 72%

*Ref.:* 1

COMMENTS: It is important to estimate the size of a burn initially to guide transfer to definitive care, fluid resuscitation, and caloric needs, as well as for prognostic information. This is generally expressed as the percentage of **total body surface area** burned. Initial estimation is often performed at facilities without experienced burn personnel. The "rule of nines" may be used to approximate the area of burn involvement before burn care; this rule describes body surface area by anatomic area as follows: head and neck, 9%; each upper extremity (front and back), 9%; anterior trunk, 18%; posterior trunk, 18%; anterior lower extremity (each), 9%; posterior lower extremity (each), 9%; and perineum/genitalia, 1%. More detailed tools, such as the Lund-Browder chart, analyze body surface area more accurately by smaller divisions and are adjusted for age (children have proportionally larger heads and smaller legs). Alternatively, small or scattered patches of burn can be estimated by using the surface of the patient's palm to represent 1% **total body surface area**.

### ANSWER: D

8. A 50-kg woman is burned in a house fire and suffers 60% TBSA partial- and full-thickness burn wounds. What is your initial fluid administration plan?

   A. 1000-mL bolus of lactated Ringer (LR) solution and then 750 mL/h

   B. 5% dextrose ($D_5$)/LR at 600 mL/h, with titration of fluid administration hourly to a urine output of 0.5 mL/kg/h

   C. 500-mL LR bolus, repeated as needed to bring central venous pressure (CVP) up to at least 10 cm $H_2O$; maintain fluid rate at 375 mL/h

   D. LR at 750 mL/h for 8 hours and then 375 mL/h for the following 16 hours

   E. LR at 800 mL/h for 12 hours and then 400 mL/h for 12 hours

*Ref.:* 1-3

**COMMENTS:** The **Parkland formula** is most commonly used to estimate the **fluid resuscitation requirements** for the first 24 hours after burn injury. This formula calls for 3 to 4 mL/kg/%TBSA burn to be given over a 24-hour period. Half of the volume should be given over the first 8 hours after injury and the remainder over the following 16 hours. For this 50-kg patient, fluid administration should begin with $4 \times 50\,kg \times 60\%$ TBSA = 12,000 mL crystalloid over the first 24 hours after injury. Half (6000 mL) should be given over the first 8 hours (6000 mL/8 h = 750 mL/h) and the remainder over the following 16 hours (6000 mL/16 h = 375 mL/h). In addition to the calculated resuscitation volumes, children less than 20 kg require maintenance fluids $(D_5/\frac{1}{2}N)$ to prevent hypoglycemia. The patient's response to resuscitation should be monitored and fluid administration adjusted accordingly. The most useful **marker of resuscitation** is adequate hourly urine output, defined as 30 to 50 mL/h in adult patients and 1 mL/kg/h in children in the absence of myoglobinuria. Crystalloid boluses should be avoided unless required because of hypotensive episodes (mean arterial pressure persistently less than 60 mm Hg) or to resuscitate blood loss from other traumatic injuries. Intravenous fluids are rapidly extravasated as a result of the capillary leakage that occurs in the first 48 hours. Decreased urine output for 1 to 2 hours would require increasing the hourly fluid rate. Adequate or excessive urine output may prompt reduction of fluid administration rates. Many burn centers use algorithm-driven fluid resuscitation protocols, and computer-assisted protocols have been designed. Intravenous fluid administration based on CVP or pulmonary artery catheter monitoring may lead to overresuscitation in many burn patients, but it may be necessary in those with cardiac failure, renal failure, or cardiogenic shock. It is important to decrease fluid administration if not required because the morbidity (abdominal and extremity compartment syndromes, pulmonary edema) from massive volumes of resuscitation fluid is not insignificant. **Colloid** administration once the capillary leak has closed, 12 to 48 hours after injury, may help restore intravascular volume in patients with persistent low urine output and hypotension despite adequate crystalloid administration. In such cases, 5% albumin (0.3 to 0.5 mL/kg/%TBSA burn) can be administered over a 24-hour period. **Plasmapheresis** also reduces intravascular fluid requirements in patients who do respond to standard crystalloid resuscitation. Indications for plasmapheresis include a sustained mean arterial pressure of less than 60 mm Hg and urine output of less than 30 mL/h in a patient whose ongoing fluid needs are more than twice the fluid volume estimates. Early plasmapheresis (12 to 24 hours after injury) appears to decrease the incidence of complications from the administration of excessive fluid, such as extremity compartment syndromes, abdominal compartment syndrome, and pulmonary edema.

**ANSWER:** D

9. Which of the following is correct regarding inhalation injury in burn patients?

   A. The admission chest radiograph is useful for ruling out inhalation injury on admission.

   B. Supraglottic inhalation injury may necessitate intubation even if gas exchange is initially unaffected.

   C. With proper pulmonary toilet, pneumonia is an unusual complication of smoke inhalation.

   D. Smoke inhalation is basically just a subset of acute respiratory distress syndrome (ARDS) seen in burn victims.

   E. Daily bronchoscopy is mandatory to monitor the evolution of inhalation injury.

*Ref.:* 1, 2

**COMMENTS:** **Inhalation injury** occurs in up to a third of major burns and significantly increases mortality in patients when combined with cutaneous burns. Conceptually, inhalation injury can be divided into three types, all of which can coexist within any given patient: CO poisoning (and other toxic inhalation), upper airway thermal injury, and lower airway injury. Upper airway burns occur as a result of thermal injury, as well as the toxic substances in smoke. The capacity for the oropharynx to absorb heat generally prevents thermal injury from extending lower into the airway. Oropharyngeal thermal injury can be diagnosed by direct laryngoscopy and, if significant, is an indication for prophylactic endotracheal intubation to control the airway before life-threatening airway edema develops, particularly after large-volume resuscitation ensues. Endotracheal tubes may be difficult to secure if the patient has facial burns. They are usually tied with cotton tape wrapped around the face in most units. Airway edema is maximal 12 to 24 hours after injury, and if airway protection is required, the patient may remain intubated for 72 hours. Short courses of steroids may be administered to patients without significant burns, but they are contraindicated in those with large burns because of infectious and wound complications. Extubation may be performed when the patient has met weaning parameters. Lower airway inhalation injury results from exposure of the respiratory epithelium to toxic irritants in smoke or steam. Chest x-ray findings on admission are typically normal because infiltrates and lung injury tend to develop in delayed fashion over the days following injury. Damage to the airway leads to inflammation, sloughing of mucosa, and impaired ciliary function, which results in edema, hemorrhage, bronchoconstriction, and bronchial obstruction. Pulmonary edema, **acute respiratory distress syndrome**, and pneumonia may complicate inhalation injury, with pneumonia occurring in up to 50% of patients. Lower airway inhalation injury is diagnosed most commonly by fiberoptic bronchoscopy, although nuclear medicine ventilation-perfusion scanning has been used. Treatment is primarily supportive and consists of aggressive pulmonary toilet, supplemental oxygen, and endotracheal intubation if required for either airway protection or oxygenation. Bronchoscopy may be used as an adjunct for pulmonary toilet if airway plugging leads to lobar collapse, but it is not always required for management. Aerosolized heparin is administered by some centers to aid mobilization of fibrin-rich casts, which contribute to airway obstruction. Laboratory and clinical research is ongoing for therapies dealing with smoke inhalation injury. Patients with severe inhalation injury may be extremely difficult to ventilate, and ventilatory strategies vary among burn centers. Low–tidal volume ventilation, high-frequency oscillatory ventilation, and even extracorporeal membrane oxygenation (ECMO) have been used by burn units.

**ANSWER:** B

10. Select the true statement regarding inhalation of toxic gases.

    A. Hydrogen cyanide is not a component of smoke in most house fires in the United States.

    B. Burn-injured patients with significant carboxyhemoglobin levels are best treated at a center with hyperbaric oxygen (HBO) capabilities.

    C. CO poisoning is best treated with amyl nitrate (available in antidote kits) if administered within 2 hours of injury.

    D. HBO can be administered via endotracheal tube by a high-pressure ventilator in a general intensive care unit bed at many facilities.

E. CO poisoning should be treated until carboxyhemoglobin levels are less than 10% and the patient is asymptomatic.

*Ref.:* 1, 3

**COMMENTS:** Many toxic compounds are present in **smoke**, depending on the materials combusted. **Carbon monoxide** poisoning is commonly seen in burn victims, as well as in nonburned patients exposed to exhaust in a variety of domestic and occupational environments. CO toxicity correlates with levels of arterial carboxyhemoglobin. Because of the higher affinity of the CO molecule than the oxygen molecule for hemoglobin, CO-bound hemoglobin is not available for oxygen transport to peripheral tissues. Carboxyhemoglobin levels of less than 10% are asymptomatic, levels up to 25% lead to headache and nausea, levels of 30% to 40% cause confusion and weakness, levels above 40% can result in coma, and levels greater than 60% lead to death. The treatment of CO toxicity is 100% oxygen, which shortens the half-life of carboxyhemoglobin from 4 hours to 45 to 60 minutes. **Hyperbaric oxygen** therapy has been used for isolated patients with CO poisoning and neurologic impairment without other injuries, but it is not generally practical for ventilated or burned patients because HBO chambers are typically small and patients are not accessible during dives. Patients should receive 100% oxygen until carboxyhemoglobin levels have decreased to less than 10%. **Hydrogen cyanide** is generated by combustion of the nitrogen- and carbon-containing substances found in a number of natural and synthetic household and industrial materials. Its characteristic bitter almond odor is difficult to detect at the scene of a fire. Cyanide hinders cellular respiration by inhibiting cytochrome *c* oxidase, which results in central nervous system (CNS) and cardiovascular dysfunction, as well as anion gap metabolic acidosis with elevated mixed venous oxygen saturation. Cyanide toxicity may be underappreciated and should be treated presumptively when suspected. Oxygen therapy is beneficial, and antidote kits in the United States contain amyl nitrate, thiosulfate, and sodium nitrite, which are methemoglobin generators. Methemoglobin chelates cyanide and will decrease oxygen-carrying capacity, so these treatments should be used with caution in a critical care setting only.

**ANSWER:**  E

11. Which of the following is correct regarding ARDS in burn patients?

   A. Hypercapnia is detrimental to healing of burn wounds.

   B. ARDS is a frequent cause of mortality from respiratory failure in burn patients.

   C. ARDS and pulmonary edema are due to massive fluid overload, which leads to left heart failure.

   D. ARDS is most likely to develop in burn-injured patients with combined cutaneous burns and smoke inhalation.

   E. ECMO is routinely used for burn-injured patients at risk for ARDS.

*Ref.:* 1, 2

**COMMENTS: Acute respiratory distress syndrome** may occur in burn-injured patients with or without inhalation injury and is an independent risk factor for death. Mortality in these cases tends to be due to sepsis and multiple organ failure rather than respiratory failure alone. ARDS is defined by acute onset, bilateral infiltrates on chest radiographs consistent with pulmonary edema, absence of clinical signs of left-sided heart failure (e.g., pulmonary artery wedge pressure of 18 mm Hg or less), and a $Pao_2/Fio_2$ ratio of

200 or lower. Clinical manifestations include pulmonary edema, hypoxemia, and altered lung compliance. Microscopic evaluation of the lungs reveals diffuse alveolar damage, microvascular permeability, infiltration of inflammatory cells into the lung parenchyma, interstitial and alveolar edema, and the formation of hyaline membranes. The pathologic changes in the lung eventually end in parenchymal fibrosis. **Inflammatory mediators** such as platelet-activating factor, interleukin-1 (IL-1), IL-2, IL-6, IL-8, prostaglandin, thromboxane, leukotrienes, hematopoietic growth factors (granulocyte colony-stimulating factor), intercellular adhesion molecules, vascular cell adhesion molecules, and nitric oxide are released locally and systemically after a burn injury. Tumor necrosis factor-$\alpha$ and IL-1 correlate with ARDS severity, and IL-2 promotes multisystem edema, sequestration of neutrophils in the lung, and platelet activation. Reactive oxygen intermediates are generated by macrophages, have been implicated in lung injury and ARDS, and may be exaggerated by combined burn and smoke injuries. One review of burn patients revealed a 73% incidence of respiratory failure and a 20% incidence of ARDS in patients with inhalation injury, as compared with a 5% incidence of respiratory failure and a 2% incidence of ARDS in patients without inhalation injury. ARDS is less likely to develop in patients with inhalation injury but without cutaneous burns. Advanced age is an additional risk factor for ARDS in burn patients. Ventilator management of ARDS in burn-injured patients may result in ventilator-induced lung injury, particularly if normalization of arterial blood gases is pursued. **Lung-protective ventilation**, as demonstrated by the ARDS Network, has been shown to decrease mortality in ARDS patients by 22% by limiting tidal volumes to 6 mL/kg present body weight (PBW) to maintain mean airway pressure at less than 30 cm $H_2O$. Hypercapnia may be tolerated to low pH values (7.15 to 7.20) to accomplish these goals, and respiratory rates into the 30s may be induced before becoming limited by auto-PEEP (positive end-expiratory pressure). Deep sedation may be required for ventilator synchrony. For patients deemed to be at high risk, implementation of low–tidal volume strategies may be warranted before the development of ARDS. Use of prone positioning, ECMO, high-frequency percussive or oscillatory ventilation (HFPV, HFOV), and nitric oxide has all been reported but has not gained widespread use.

**ANSWER:**  D

12. Select the true statement regarding infection in burn patients.

   A. A rim of erythema surrounding the wound signals invasive burn wound infection.

   B. A scheduled rotation of central line insertion sites significantly decreases the rate of catheter line sepsis.

   C. Selective decontamination of digestive flora reduces systemic infection.

   D. Gram-positive organisms are the most significant cause of delayed burn wound infection.

   E. Invasive infection may convert second-degree burn wounds to full-thickness injury and necessitate skin grafting for closure.

*Ref.:* 1, 2

**COMMENTS: Infection** is a frequent source of morbidity and mortality in burn patients and may occur in up to 80% of patients with large burns. Fevers and abnormal white blood cell counts are common in burn patients; physical examination is the most reliable means of diagnosing infections. Tetanus prophylaxis is indicated for burn wounds, as with other traumatic wounds; cases of tetanus are rare in patients who have been immunized in childhood. Though once practiced, the administration of **prophylactic systemic antibiotics** to patients with burn injuries has been shown to be unnecessary and, in fact, leads to the development of gram-negative and fungal infections. Clinical judgment, laboratory and radiologic examinations, and physical examination are important tools in the diagnosis of infection. Endogenous skin flora are killed by heat similar to skin cells, and an initial swab of burn wounds may be sterile. Bacteria in hair follicles and sebaceous glands may survive (as with epidermal cells), and quantitative skin cultures may reveal $10^3$ bacteria per gram of tissue (normal). A level of $10^5$ bacteria per gram is considered invasive burn wound infection. As bacterial cells increase in number following injury, they erupt from hair follicles and glands and colonize the dermal-subcutaneous boundary. Perivascular growth can result in thrombosis of vessels and necrosis of the remaining dermis, which could result in the conversion of a partial-thickness burns into full-thickness wounds. The infection progresses over days from gram positive to gram negative, and by 21 days after a burn, more than half of the wounds still open are colonized by resistant gram-negative bacteria. Routine burn wound care includes daily washing with soap and water and dressing with topical antimicrobials until wound closure, combined with monitoring of the wound site for signs of wound sepsis. Fever, erythema, increasing pain, and changes in wound drainage or odor may be signs of new infection. Burns seen early typically have a surrounding area of blanching erythema present, but burn wounds initially seen late are more likely to be infected. Significant erythema, swelling, and foul drainage are signs of infection and should be treated. Very superficial infections can be treated with cleansing and topical antimicrobials, but with significant cellulitis, systemic antibiotics are indicated. If deep infection is suspected, wounds should be excised. Burns greater than 20% to 30% TBSA add an immunosuppressive effect to the already significant risk for infection because of the large open skin surface. Early excision and coverage with autograft, homograft, or xenograft help reduce the risk for infection. Large burns initially seen late in the course may require even more aggressive débridement, even to a fascial level at times, in addition to topical agents and systemic antibiotics (in established infection) to gain control of wound sepsis and enable final skin graft closure of wounds. Frequent inspection of the wounds is important to monitor for infection, with changes in color, odor, or quantity of the exudate being suggestive of infection. Dark discoloration may be suggestive of fungal infection—this is best diagnosed on biopsy specimens. If questionable, quantitative tissue cultures may be performed to determine whether the wounds are appropriate for final autografting because graft survival rates may be greater than 90% when colony counts are less than $10^2$/g but only 60% when counts are greater than $10^5$/g. The antibiotic selected for perioperative prophylaxis and treatment of suspected wound infections should include coverage of both **gram-positive** and **gram-negative** organisms, and consideration should be given to highly resistant organisms or fungal infection if the patient does not respond to therapy. Early wound closure is the best preventive measure against sepsis in burn patients. Selective gut decontamination has failed to show benefit. The diagnosis of **sepsis in burn patients** is not always straightforward because many elements of (SIRS) are present in uninfected burn patients. Intravenous catheter infection is a serious problem in burn-injured patients. Unburned sites are preferred for insertion of peripheral and central venous catheters after initial resuscitation, and scheduled catheter rotation to new sites has not been shown to decrease rates of line sepsis. Current and old intravenous sites should be inspected when evaluating a patient for occult infection, and suppurative thrombophlebitis may require wide excision of infected veins.

**ANSWER:** E

13. An 8-year-old girl suffers 18% TBSA, patchy, indeterminate-depth burns as a result of scalding with hot water. Which of the following is most correct regarding the topical antimicrobial agents that may be used?

A. Mafenide acetate is an undesirable choice because metabolic alkalosis often contributes to narcotic-induced hypoventilation in pediatric burn patients.

B. A 0.5% aqueous solution of silver nitrate may be applied to burn wounds because of its effective antibacterial activity against staphylococci and gram-negative organisms.

C. Silver sulfadiazine should be discontinued if neutropenia occurs as a result of its use.

D. Silver sulfadiazine is the most commonly used topical agent in U.S. burn centers because of its effective penetration of burn eschar.

E. Elemental silver-impregnated dressings must be moistened frequently with normal saline to retain antimicrobial activity.

*Ref.:* 1

**COMMENTS:** Systemic antibiotics are not indicated for prophylaxis. **Topical antimicrobial agents** delay colonization and infection of wounds but have not changed mortality as much as early excision and grafting have. **Silver sulfadiazine** is the most commonly used agent for burns in the United States. Advantages include a broad spectrum of activity, soothing effect in most patients, and no significant metabolic activity. Silver sulfadiazine does not penetrate eschar, so it does not treat established wound infections. Many providers have implicated it as a cause of early postburn neutropenia, but this neutropenia is typically self-limited, and more current information suggests that it is more likely the result of margination of neutrophils rather than depletion by the topical agent. One other caution is the use of silver sulfadiazine in a sulfa-allergic patient. **Mafenide acetate** penetrates eschar and is therefore useful for the treatment of burn wound infections; it has broad spectrum of activity against gram-negative organisms; It may be applied as a cream or a solution and is often used after grafting. Mafenide acetate is a carbonic anhydrase inhibitor that may cause metabolic acidosis when used on large areas. It is also painful on application, particularly to partial-thickness burns. **Silver nitrate** has a broad spectrum of activity and may be used for burn wound dressings. Dressings need to be repeatedly impregnated with aqueous solution to prevent precipitation onto the wound. Concentrated silver nitrate may cause chemical burns and hyponatremia, along with the rare case of methemoglobinemia. Wounds, normal skin, linens, and the patient environment will be stained black by silver nitrate. Ointments of bacitracin, neomycin, and polymyxin B are commonly used for facial burns. **Mupirocin** has been used against methicillin-resistant *Staphylococcus aureus* (MRSA). **Acticoat** (Smith & Nephew, London, England) is a dressing impregnated with elemental silver that may be applied to burn wounds or grafts. Sheets of Acticoat are usually moistened in sterile water before application because sodium chloride will cause precipitation and inactivation of the silver ions. Silver disrupts bacterial cellular respiration, and silver dressings may be left in place for up to 7 days if necessary.

**ANSWER:** B

14. Which of the following is not true of nutritional support in burn-injured patients?

A. Caloric needs in burn-injured patients may be estimated as 25 kcal/kg/day + 40 kcal/%TBSA burned/day.

B. Serum albumin levels provide a useful marker of nutritional status after the patient has recovered from the initial period of burn shock and resuscitation.

C. The Harris-Benedict equation can be used but may overestimate caloric requirements.

D. Early excision and grafting will decrease caloric requirements after graft closure.

E. Urinary nitrogen losses are not generally helpful for assessment of protein loss in burn-injured patients.

*Ref.:* 1, 2

COMMENTS: **Thermal injury** causes a hypermetabolic state with an increased basal metabolic rate, increased oxygen consumption, negative nitrogen balance, and weight loss. Administration of increased calories is required for wound healing, immune function, and cellular function. **Nitrogen losses** are significant after major burns; urinary measurements do not account for losses from the wounds. The Harris-Benedict equation multiplies basal energy expenditure (BEE) by a factor of up to 2 for major burns. The formula for BEE varies by gender: for women, BEE = 65.5 + (9.7 × weight in kilograms) + (1.8 × height in centimeters) − (4.7 × age in years); for men, BEE = 66.5 + (13.8 × weight in kilograms) + (5.0 × height in centimeters) − (6.8 × age in years). Harris-Benedict calculations overestimate caloric needs for patients with moderate burn size. The Curreri formula overestimates needs for large burns and is best used for burns less than 40% TBSA. The Curreri formula to determine the calories needed daily is 25 kcal/kg/day + 40 kcal/%TBSA/day. Indirect calorimetry can be used to quantify oxygen consumption and carbon dioxide production to calculate nutritional requirements: kcal/day = (3.9 × $V_{O_2}$) + (1.1 × $V_{CO_2}$) × 1.44. The Fick equation can be used if the patient has a pulmonary artery catheter in place, but pulmonary artery monitoring is becoming less commonplace. Infection, ARDS, and donor sites increase catabolism. Likewise, healing and skin graft closure of wounds decrease the catabolic state, thus making reevaluation important to ongoing care. Serum albumin levels are not accurate markers of the **nutritional state**. **Prealbumin levels** correlate more closely with nutritional and catabolic status and may be monitored over the course of weeks during a patient's hospitalization. C-reactive protein may be used to monitor the patient's generalized inflammatory state. A variety of other markers have been investigated for similar purposes. Calories should be provided as oral or enteral feedings in virtually all cases. Inability to feed because of ileus is rare in burn patients; feedings should be instituted early after admission in all patients with large burns and interrupted as infrequently as possible. Interruption of enteral tube feedings occurs frequently as a result of the administration of medications, procedures, and tube occlusion or malposition and may lead to significant decreases in the calories delivered. Small burns generally require oral feedings only, whereas moderate or large burns are more likely to require supplemental enteral feedings in patients who are not intubated. Ventilated patients should have **enteral feedings** initiated early via nasogastric or nasojejunal tubes. Glucose levels should be monitored. The optimal range for glucose management in burn-injured patients has not yet been fully defined, but it is generally agreed that hyperglycemia should be avoided. Many nutritional and metabolic manipulations are the subject of research and are as yet unproven.

ANSWER: B

15. A 22-year-old man suffers partial- and full-thickness burns to 45% of TBSA in a gas explosion while at work. Which of the following is most correct regarding surgical management of his wounds?

A. Assessment of the depth of injury on admission is accurate enough for definitive surgery to be planned in more than 90% of cases.

B. Fascial excision allows grafts to be placed over a healthy muscle bed and is the preferred approach to burns on the hands and dorsal surface of the feet.

C. Sheet (unmeshed) grafting is preferred for areas subjected to repeated shear, thus making it the choice for extensive burns on dorsal surfaces.

D. The principle of early excision and grafting benefits burned patients by reducing the number of infections and, ultimately, the mortality with severe burns.

E. Widely meshed grafts minimize the degree of wound contraction associated with the use of split-thickness grafts.

*Ref.:* 1, 2

COMMENTS: **Early excision** plus grafting of burn wounds has led to a significant decrease in mortality in burn patients over the last 30 years. Length of stay, cost, and reconstructive surgeries have also decreased as a result. Excision of deep partial- and full-thickness burn wounds should be done after resuscitation is complete and the patient is stabilized, often by 3 to 4 days. When uneven burns or those of indeterminate depth are present, it is reasonable to delay surgery for 7 to 10 days and observe for healing to avoid grafting to portions of the wounds that will heal. Wounds that are expected to heal within 3 weeks are best treated with antimicrobial dressings, whereas full-thickness burns, as well as deep partial-thickness wounds with delayed healing, require grafting. **Fascial excision** refers to removal of burned skin and subcutaneous tissue down to the level of the fascia, frequently with electrocautery. This approach provides a bed that readily takes graft and is usually easy to define. However, such deep débridement often results in fragile, aesthetically displeasing grafts. **Tangential excision** involves sequentially cutting away eschar with a handheld knife with a depth guard until viable dermis or subcutaneous tissue is present as noted by diffuse punctuate bleeding. Experience is important in judging the depth of excision required to support a graft. Hemostasis may be achieved with a combination of electrocautery, suture ligature, thrombin spray, direct pressure, and dilute epinephrine solution in gauze pads. Skin grafts may be full thickness or split thickness, depending on the amount of dermis present when harvested. Harvesting is most commonly done with a dermatome. Thinner grafts will heal with greater contraction, but thicker grafts come at a cost of loss of dermis at the donor site, which leads to prolonged times until healing and increased donor site scarring. **Meshing of grafts** (ranging from 1 : 1 to 4 : 1) may be used to allow egress of fluid from the wound bed through the graft and to increase the area covered when donor sites are limited. Widely meshed grafts are associated with prolonged healing, increased scarring, and more contraction than are less meshed or sheet grafts. A variety of dressings may be placed over grafted areas, the goal of which is to maintain contact of the graft with the wound bed to allow graft survival, prevent shearing, and facilitate subsequent vascular ingrowth into the graft.

ANSWER: D

16. Which of the following is correct regarding the skin substitutes used in burn reconstruction?

A. Cultured epidermal autografts have dramatically increased survival in patients with nearly 100% TBSA burn injuries.

B. Allografting to burn wound sites is limited to temporary closure because of eventual rejection of the graft by the patient.

C. Porcine xenograft has the advantage of better early vascularization and engrafting after placement as a result of decreased antigenicity in comparison to most cadaveric human allografts.

D. Use of the Integra Dermal Regeneration Template is advantageous because of lower rates of wound infection than with early autografting in heavily colonized burn wounds.

E. Vascularization of porcine xenograft may be aided by use of low-dose cyclosporine, provided that the patient is free of infectious complications at the time of placement.

*Ref.:* 1, 2

**COMMENTS:** After débridement and excision of burn eschar, closure of the wound with immediate **autografting**, when possible, is preferred. **Full-thickness skin grafts** are the best possible cutaneous replacement, but they are not feasible for burns of significant size because the full-thickness donor site must be closed primarily. **Meshed split-thickness grafts** may be used to cover areas larger than the donor site harvested, but for large burns and patients with limited donor sites, even meshed autografts will not be able to cover all open wounds. Wounds not able to be autografted immediately may be covered with biologic dressings while awaiting donor site healing before reharvesting. **Human allograft** has been widely used as a temporary biologic dressing. It is usually meshed 1 : 1 to allow drainage of fluid and applied in a similar fashion to other skin grafts. Allograft will vascularize and engraft, provide wound closure for 2 to 4 weeks, and subsequently be rejected and need to be replaced with new allograft or autograft if available. Sheets of allograft may be placed over widely meshed autograft at the time of surgery to protect grafts as the interstices epithelialize. **Porcine xenograft** is cheaper and more easily stored before use, but it does not vascularize and engraft. It may be used similar to allograft for temporary biologic coverage of burn wounds, as well as for exfoliative diseases of the skin (e.g., toxic epidermal necrolysis). **Cultured epidermal autografts** grown from patient keratinocytes were initially promising as a skin substitute but have not significantly evolved in burn wound management at this time. **Dermal substitutes** such as the Integra Dermal Regeneration Template (Integra Lifesciences, Plainsboro, NJ) have seen more clinical use. The Integra dermal template is a bilaminate composed of an outer silicone film that provides barrier function and an inner layer of type 1 collagen and chondroitin sulfate. This inner layer serves as a template for the ingrowth of autologous fibroblasts, endothelial cells, and other mesenchymal cells. After vascularization of the Integra, the silicone film is removed, and very thin autografts may be applied to the neodermis. Reported advantages include neodermis architecture similar to that of uninjured dermis, which results in improved cosmetic and functional results, as well as rapid healing of thin autograft donor sites. Disadvantages include wound infection and increased length of time and immobilization before final autograft closure.

**ANSWER:** B

17. A 27-year-old factory worker has worsening pain and discoloration of the hands after working with an unknown cleaning agent yesterday. Which of the following is true regarding chemical injury?

A. The affected hands should be soaked in water for at least 30 minutes to dilute the concentration of the offending agent.

B. Phenol is absorbed systemically and may result in CNS toxicity with even small areas of cutaneous involvement.

C. Dry powders, such as concrete, should be moistened before removal from affected areas.

D. Initial treatment of a chemical burn wound includes the application of a neutralizing agent.

E. Alkali burns are frequently worse than acid burns because alkali creates a leathery, impermeable eschar at the surface of the skin.

*Ref.:* 1, 2

**COMMENTS:** Many agents used in household and occupational settings have the capacity to cause **chemical burns** on exposed skin. For virtually all chemicals, the immediate approach to treatment is the same. All affected clothing should be removed immediately to ensure cessation of exposure, and the burns should be flushed with copious amounts of water to dilute away the offending substance. Soaking in a tub or basin is undesirable because the affected body surface will continue to be bathed in the chemical, albeit at lesser concentrations. Dry powders causing chemical burns should be brushed away. Patient referrals are often accompanied by a request for neutralizing agents, but any delay in flushing wounds may result in deepening of the burns, and neutralizing agents may actually cause exothermic reactions and further skin injury. Unlike thermal injury, chemical burns cause progressively deepening damage to skin until the chemicals are inactivated by reaction with tissues or are diluted away by flushing with water. Acid burns are usually more self-limited because the action of acids tans the skin and forms a barrier to deeper penetration of the acid. Alkali (e.g., drain cleaners, cement), in contrast, combines with cutaneous lipids to form soaps that continue to dissolve skin until neutralized. Chemical burns are often seen late in the course because they appear superficial at first and may progress from a mild discoloration to sloughing over a period of days. Treatment of the skin wounds is similar to that for other burns—partial-thickness injuries heal with topical antimicrobials, and full-thickness injuries will require skin grafting. In addition to cutaneous injury, some chemical agents may be absorbed and result in systemic illness. Anhydrous ammonia may cause severe pulmonary injury and ARDS. Chromic acid may result in renal and hepatic failure, as well as anemia, even with small areas of cutaneous exposure. Formic acid causes metabolic acidosis, hemolysis, and hemoglobinuria. Phenol (carbolic acid), a disinfectant, can cause CNS depression, vomiting, respiratory distress, and seizures despite the superficial skin injury. **Hydrofluoric acid** is unique in that it is a very strong acid that allows fluoride ions to enter tissues and chelate calcium and magnesium, thereby resulting in severe local tissue destruction and the systemic effects of severe hypocalcemia, including cardiac dysrhythmias. Conventional treatment includes the application of calcium gels (often calcium gluconate mixed with water-soluble lubricant) to arrest progress of the agent, as well as monitoring and correction of serum calcium levels. Direct injection of calcium gluconate has been used but should be done cautiously in already edematous tissues, especially the digits. Intraarterial injection of dilute calcium gluconate has been performed with success at some centers. **Hot tar burns** are seen in roofing workers. These injuries are actually thermal in nature, but adherent tar will continue to burn until cooled and may complicate assessment of wound depth until removed. Citrus-based solvents are effective if available; otherwise, petrolatum-based ointments may be placed over adherent tar to aid in removal.

**ANSWER:** B

18. A 22-year-old utility company employee is found down at a job site at the base of the ladder. He has a charred wound in

the left temporal region with palpable shards of skull present. His left arm is waxy and fixed in flexion. There are full-thickness burns on his left flank, the lower part of his left leg is firm, and the toes of his left foot are burned and missing. Which of the following is the correct statement regarding electrical injury?

A. The cause of the dark, reddish urine noted in the urinary catheter will most likely be revealed by computed tomography of the abdomen.

B. Signs concerning for compartment syndrome should prompt urgent escharotomy of the affected limbs.

C. Neurologic deficits that develop in a delayed fashion, weeks to months after the injury, have a better prognosis.

D. Early fascial decompression of the extremities may be important in preserving limb function.

E. Myoglobinuria is addressed by maintaining an hourly urine output of 0.5 mL/kg in adults and 1 mL/kg in children less than 20 kg.

*Ref.:* 2

COMMENTS: **Electrical injuries** are classified in the medical literature into low-voltage, high-voltage (>1000 V), and lightning injuries (also termed ultra-high voltage). Patients injured by electricity may, in fact, have injuries by any of three mechanisms: **flash burns** from the very high temperatures generated when high-voltage current arcs through the air, **flame burns** because of ignition of clothing, and **true electrical injury** as a result of conduction of electrical current through the patient's body. Low-voltage injuries may cause local tissue injury but rarely lead to systemic injury. **High-voltage injuries** may cause unpredictable patterns of local injury, including deep tissue destruction belied by the small size of the skin wounds, full-thickness cutaneous wounds at entry/exit sites and areas where arcing occurs across joints or flexor surfaces, and musculoskeletal injuries from severe tetanic contractions of the paravertebral and other muscle groups. Patients with electrical injury are at particularly high risk for associated traumatic injuries because electrical exposures frequently occur in occupational settings and may involve falls from a height. In fact, the tetanic muscle contractions caused by alternating current tend to cause "hanging up" by workers who grasp an electrical source and pull themselves in; patients who hang up and survive often do so because they subsequently fall and break contact with the current, but they suffer other injuries as a result. Evaluation of patients suffering high-voltage electrical injury includes full examination for **traumatic injury**, radiographic studies, electrocardiogram, and bladder catheterization. Patients with no loss of consciousness at the scene, no history of arrhythmias during transport, and a normal admission electrocardiogram do not require cardiac monitoring unless the severity of the injury would otherwise require it. Deep tissue damage secondary to high-voltage current may result in unseen muscle swelling and necrosis. Neurovascular examination should document the extent of disability present at admission, and progressive deterioration in extremity function should prompt consideration of compartment release by **fasciotomy**. **Compartment pressures** may be measured if the patient is not likely to need compartment release, but fasciotomy should be prompted by clinical grounds if significant concern exists. Escharotomy refers to the division of bandlike circumferential full-thickness burn eschars through to subcutaneous fat only. Fixed deficits or mummified extremities may not benefit from compartment release. Pigmented urine suggestive of **myoglobinuria** should be treated by fluid resuscitation sufficient to produce a urine output of 100 mL/h. Fasciotomies or even early débridement or amputation of necrotic muscle can be performed to avoid renal failure. Urine myoglobin assays are often not immediately available, but urine that is heme positive by dipstick with no red blood cells on microscopic examination may be presumed to be myoglobinuria resulting from rhabdomyolysis; hematuria found on urinalysis should additionally prompt reconsideration of occult genitourinary trauma. Toddlers may suffer electrical burns to the mouth from chewing on appliance cords. **Full-thickness oral burns** are typically treated conservatively with attention to preserving mouth opening, and families should be counseled about the possibility of delayed facial artery bleeding after the eschar softens and falls off. High-voltage injuries may result in progressive demyelinating injury and lead to sensory or motor loss weeks or months after the injury. Early cataract formation has been associated with high-voltage electrical exposure.

ANSWER: D

REFERENCES

1. Mulholland MW, Lillemoe KD, Doherty GM, et al, editors: *Greenfield's surgery: scientific principles and practice*, ed 4, Philadelphia, 2006, Lippincott Williams & Wilkins.
2. Souba WW, Fink MP, Jurkovich GJ, et al, editors: *ACS surgery: principles and practice*, ed 6, New York, 2007. WebMD. Available at http://www.acssurgery.com.
3. Herndon DN, editor: *Total burn care*, ed 3, Philadelphia, 2007, WB Saunders.
4. *Guidelines for the operation of burn centers: resources for optimal care of the injured patient*, 2006, pp 79-86. Committee on Trauma, American College of Surgeons. Available at http://www.ameriburn.org/Chapter14.pdf.

# SOFT TISSUE, HERNIA, AND BREAST

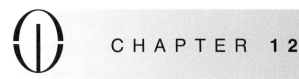

# CHAPTER 12

# Skin and Soft Tissue

*Tina J. Hieken, M.D.*

1. With regard to ultraviolet (UV) radiation, which of the following statements is true?

   A. Most of the UV radiation that reaches the earth is type B (UVB, wavelength of 290 to 320 nm).

   B. Type A UV (UVA) radiation is responsible for most of the sun damage to human skin.

   C. UVA is within the photoabsorption spectrum of DNA, whereas UVB is not.

   D. The melanin content of skin is the single best intrinsic factor for protecting skin from the harmful effects of UV radiation.

   E. UV radiation acts as a tumor promoter but not a tumor initiator.

   *Ref.:* 1-3

**COMMENTS:** **Ultraviolet radiation** comprises the middle of the electromagnetic spectrum and is divided into UVA (320 to 380 nm), UVB (290 to 320 nm), and UVC (240 to 290 nm), whereas visible light has a wavelength of 400 to 700 nm. UVC is virtually eliminated by stratospheric ozone and oxygen. Only 5% of solar UV emission is UVB, but it is the most carcinogenic part of the spectrum and is responsible for sunburn. Since UVB is partially eliminated by stratospheric ozone, a 1% decrease in stratospheric ozone increases UVB flux at the earth's surface by about 3%. More than 95% of the sun's UV radiation that reaches the earth's surface is UVA. Sunbeds for indoor recreational tanning emit predominantly UVA. UV light acts both by inducing direct DNA damage and by other mechanisms, such as alteration of cellular immunity and DNA repair mechanisms. Although UVB and UVC radiation is within the photoabsorption spectrum of DNA, UVA radiation contributes to the development of skin cancers mainly via non-DNA targets. It penetrates more deeply and affects dermal fibroblasts, which results in photoaging. Recent data suggest that UVA may also directly affect DNA; experimental studies have shown UVA-induced development of the characteristic carcinogenic photoproduct (cyclobutane pyrimidine dimer) seen classically with DNA damage secondary to UVB. **Melanin** is the most important factor in protecting the skin from the harmful effects of UV light. Tightly woven clothing, sunscreen use, and avoidance of the sun also offer protection against the harmful effects of UV radiation. **Ultraviolet radiation** can act as both a tumor initiator and a tumor promoter.

**ANSWER:** D

2. Which of the following statements regarding genetic predisposition to skin cancer is not true?

   A. About 10% of cases of malignant melanoma are familial.

   B. Familial melanoma is characterized by an earlier age at onset, multiple primary tumors, and a frequent association with multiple dysplastic nevi.

   C. The *p16/CDKN2A* tumor suppressor gene, located on chromosome 9, is implicated in 90% of cases of familial melanoma.

   D. Mutations of *PTC*, a tumor suppressor gene, are responsible for most cases of basal cell nevus syndrome.

   E. The penetrance of *p16/CDKN2A* gene mutations exhibits geographic variation.

   *Ref.:* 2, 4, 5

**COMMENTS:** Approximately 10% of melanoma patients have a family history of **melanoma**. Factors that increase the risk for melanoma include the presence of **dysplastic nevus syndrome** (familial atypical mole and melanoma syndrome or atypical nevus syndrome), a clinical syndrome distinguished by the presence of numerous large dysplastic nevi usually over the trunk, xeroderma pigmentosum (characterized by mutations in genes responsible for the fidelity of DNA repair), familial retinoblastoma, and a family history of melanoma. Individuals at high risk include those with two or more first-degree relatives with melanoma, two relatives of any degree if one exhibits signs of dysplastic nevus syndrome, and those with three relatives of any degree with melanoma. As with other familial cancers, **familial melanoma** is characterized by earlier age at onset and multiple tumors. Germline mutations in the *CDKN2A* gene, which encodes the proteins p16/INK4A and p14ARF, are the most common cause of inherited risk for melanoma with high penetrance and may be identified in up to 40% of all melanoma families with three or more affected individuals. The penetrance of this gene is variable and varies significantly with geography, with melanoma penetrance of 0.13 (0.58) in Europe, 0.5 (0.76) in the United States, and 0.32 (0.91) in Australia by the age of 50 (80). Although commercial testing is available, testing may be premature at this time because the risk for other cancers in *CDKN2A* families and factors that modify penetrance are not yet well described. In addition, the lack of correlation between *CDKN2A* gene carriers and the phenotypic dysplastic nevus syndrome may falsely reassure family members. Mutations of the *CDK4* gene have been identified in a few melanoma kindreds. The most frequently identified gene that predisposes to melanoma is the *MC1R* gene associated with red hair and freckles. Variations in this gene are associated with an elevated risk for melanoma, even in patients without red hair, but such variations impart a weak susceptibility to melanoma (low penetrance) in white populations. The deleterious effect of *MC1R* variations is amplified by high sun exposure. Mutations in *PTC*, the human homologue of the *Drosophila* patched gene, have been identified in most patients with **basal cell nevus (Gorlin) syndrome**. Mutations have also been identified in a few sporadically occurring basal cell carcinomas.

ANSWER: C

3. A 25-year-old woman is evaluated for a left axillary abscess. She states that she has had problems with recurrent infections in this location over the past few years. On examination of the axilla she has a 3-cm fluctuant area with overlying erythema and a few adjacent pustules. Which of the following is not true regarding her condition?

A. It is an infection of the apocrine glands.

B. Staphylococci and streptococci are the predominant organisms isolated.

C. The axilla, areola, groin, perineum, perianal, and periumbilical areas are usually involved.

D. The lesions begin with slight subcutaneous induration and progress to suppuration and cellulitis.

E. Definitive treatment necessitates radical excision with split-thickness skin grafting or open wound packing.

*Ref.:* 6

COMMENTS: **Hidradenitis suppurativa** is an acneiform infection that involves the apocrine glands and occurs most frequently in the axillae and groin. The initial symptoms may be suppuration and cellulitis or a chronic condition characterized by coalescing cutaneous nodules with a surrounding fibrous reaction. Successful treatment varies with the individual. In some patients, cure is achieved with improved hygiene. Others respond to high doses of oral or topical antibiotics. Incision and drainage of an acute abscess may be required. Occasionally, in extensive and chronic cases, radical excision and reconstruction with split-thickness skin grafts, flaps, or open-wound packing are required. In older patients this disease is uncommon, and neoplasm should be excluded.

ANSWER: E

4. Which of the following is true regarding benign cystic lesions of the skin?

A. An epidermal inclusion cyst lacks a fully mature epidermis with a granular cell layer.

B. The wall of a trichilemmal cyst, usually located on the scalp, is characterized by an epidermal lining that includes a granular cell layer.

C. The most common location of a ganglion cyst is on the dorsal aspect of the wrist.

D. Malignant degeneration may occur in a dermoid cyst.

E. A pilonidal cyst results from infection in a congenital coccygeal sinus.

*Ref.:* 7-9

COMMENTS: A number of **cystic lesions** occur in the skin. Complete excision of each of the lesions listed is curative, whereas incomplete excision may lead to recurrence. When infection is present, primary incision plus drainage with secondary excision is preferred. The diagnosis can often be determined from the history and location of the cyst. **Epidermal inclusion cysts**, the most common type of cutaneous cyst, have a completely mature epidermis with a granular layer. The creamy material in the center of these cysts is keratin from desquamated cells. The wall of a **trichilemmal cyst**, the second most common type and often found on the scalp, does not have a granular layer. **Ganglions** are composed of connective tissue from the synovial membrane of a joint or tendon sheath and contain thick jellylike mucinous material similar in composition to synovial fluid. Ganglions commonly occur over the tendons of the wrist, hands, and feet and may be congenital, related to trauma, or a result of arthritic conditions. They are more common in females. Sixty percent of ganglions occur on the dorsal aspect of the wrist and arise in the region of the scapholunate ligament. Asymptomatic ganglions may be treated expectantly. If treatment is needed, the initial approach can be aspiration with a large-bore needle, with or without steroid injection. Failure of this approach necessitates surgical excision, which should include removal of the pedicle of the ganglion from its origin at the involved joint or tendon sheath. **Dermoid cysts** are found along the body fusion planes and usually occur over the midline abdominal and sacral regions, over the occiput, and on the nose. Malignant degeneration has not been reported. Although in the past it was thought that **pilonidal cysts** result from penetration of a congenital coccygeal sinus by an ingrown hair, which sets the stage for infection and cyst formation, most now believe that pilonidal cysts are acquired. They result from embedded hairs in the intergluteal cleft but may occur at other locations and are more common in hirsute persons. They are two to four times more common in males than females.

ANSWER: C

5. A 32-year-old man has multiple soft tissue masses over his trunk and extremities. He is noted to have axillary freckling and café au lait spots. Which of the following is not true regarding his condition?

A. It is associated with an increased risk for the development of central nervous system (CNS) tumors and lymphoma.

B. A malignant peripheral nerve sheath tumor (PNST) will develop in 50% of affected individuals.

C. Malignant PNSTs in these patients are more often multiple and occur at a younger age than do their sporadically occurring counterparts.

D. The gene responsible for this disorder is inherited in an autosomal dominant fashion.

E. It is associated with an increased risk for the development of nonneurogenic soft tissue sarcomas.

*Ref.:* 10-12

COMMENTS: **Neurofibromatosis** (NF) is a multisystem genetic disorder with characteristic cutaneous, neurologic, and bony manifestations. **Neurofibromatosis type 1** (NF1, von Recklinghausen disease) is an autosomal dominant disorder estimated to affect 1 in 3000 individuals. The NF1 gene, located on chromosome 17q11.2, encodes a protein, neurofibromin, that is important in neuroectodermal differentiation and cardiac development. NF1 patients may have café au lait spots (six or more spots >5 mm in children younger than 10 years or >15 mm in adults); neurofibromas (two or more); axillary or inguinal freckling; Lisch nodules (iris hamartomas, two or more); optic nerve gliomas; sphenoid dysplasia or long-bone abnormalities; cutaneous, subcutaneous, and visceral plexiform neurofibromas; and a first-degree relative with NF1. The presence of two or more of these eight characteristics confirms the clinical diagnosis of NF1. The most common tumor is a neurofibroma (a benign PNST), and benign schwannomas and neurilemomas may also be present. Although about half of malignant PNSTs develop in patients with NF1, affected individuals have a 3% to

15% lifetime risk for the development of malignant tumors, including CNS tumors, Wilms tumor, soft tissue sarcomas, and lymphomas, as well as malignant PNSTs. These tumors often occur in association with major peripheral nerve trunks. Malignant tumors appear as enlarging soft tissue masses, variably associated with pain and other neurologic symptoms. NF1-associated malignant PNSTs may be multiple and tend to occur at a younger age than do their sporadic counterparts. Positron emission tomography (PET) may help differentiate benign neurofibromas and schwannomas from malignant tumors.

**ANSWER:** B

6. Risk factors for the development of soft tissue sarcoma include all of the following except:

   A. Retinoblastoma

   B. Li-Fraumeni syndrome

   C. von Hippel-Lindau syndrome

   D. Lymphedema

   E. External beam radiation

*Ref.:* 12-15

**COMMENTS:** Inherited syndromes, including retinoblastoma (also associated with osteosarcoma), **Li-Fraumeni syndrome** (also leukemia and brain, breast, and adrenocortical cancers), and neurofibromatosis, confer an increased risk for **soft tissue sarcoma**. Ionizing radiation is a risk factor for soft tissue sarcomas, and such tumors tend to behave in an aggressive fashion. Chronic lymphedema also predisposes to soft tissue sarcoma in the affected extremity, predominantly angiosarcoma. **von Hippel-Lindau syndrome** is associated with renal cell carcinoma, as well as pheochromocytomas and hemangioblastomas (benign CNS tumors).

**ANSWER:** C

7. A 42-year-old woman has a mass in the posterior aspect of the upper part of her arm that was first noted 3 months earlier. It is not painful and she has no associated symptoms. Magnetic resonance imaging (MRI) demonstrates a 5-cm neoplasm arising from the triceps. The best next step in the management of this patient is:

   A. PET–computed tomography (CT)

   B. Fine-needle aspiration (FNA) biopsy

   C. Percutaneous core needle biopsy

   D. Incisional biopsy

   E. Excisional biopsy

*Ref.:* 13, 14, 16, 17

**COMMENTS:** See Question 8.

**ANSWER:** C

8. After biopsy, a high-grade malignant fibrous histiocytoma is diagnosed in the patient in Question 7. Which of the following is true regarding this condition?

   A. Postoperative adjuvant radiotherapy improves outcome.

   B. Preoperative chemotherapy improves outcome.

   C. Lymph node dissection should be performed at the time of definitive surgical treatment.

   D. Grade is a more important predictor of outcome than tumor size and location.

   E. Muscle compartment resection is necessary to maximize the chance for cure.

*Ref.:* 13, 14, 16, 17

**COMMENTS:** **Soft tissue sarcomas** account for less than 1% of adult and 15% of pediatric malignancies. Estimates of the incidence of soft tissue sarcoma in the United States in 2009 are 10,660 new cases and 3820 deaths. The extremities are the most common site (>40%). There are more than 50 histologic types of soft tissue sarcoma, with liposarcoma, malignant fibrous histiocytoma, and leiomyosarcoma being the most common. With expert pathologic review, 80% to 90% of extremity soft tissue sarcomas can be diagnosed by percutaneous core needle biopsy. For lesions smaller than 3 cm, complete excision is an appropriate diagnostic procedure. When an **incisional biopsy** is necessary to achieve a diagnosis or when excising smaller tumors, it is important to plan the incision properly and avoid unduly contaminating tissue planes to not interfere with definitive surgical treatment. An incision oriented on the long axis of the limb is preferred and should be carried out so that the incision and remainder of the surgical field may be completely resected at the time of definitive surgical treatment. For the majority of soft tissue sarcomas in adults, complete surgical resection is the mainstay of treatment. Principles of surgical treatment include resection with approximately 2-cm margins of normal tissue (except vital structures) and avoidance of enucleation. Excision and amputation of muscle groups are no longer primary treatment modalities for most patients. Sarcomas rarely metastasize to lymph nodes. **Postoperative adjuvant radiotherapy** is beneficial in improving local control in patients with high-grade, large and deep tumors, whereas it is probably unnecessary for patients with small (<5 cm), superficial, low-grade tumors treated by complete resection (microscopically negative margins). **Preoperative radiotherapy** permits a lower administered dose with a smaller treated field but is associated with a higher incidence of postoperative wound complications, and treatment proceeds without knowledge of the final surgical histopathology. Preoperative radiotherapy is preferred for patients with marginally resectable, very large, high-grade tumors to maximize the chance of a microscopically margin-negative resection and functional preservation of the limb. With the exception of rhabdomyosarcoma and Ewing sarcoma, **neoadjuvant chemotherapy** is not generally beneficial. Limited data suggest that neoadjuvant chemotherapy may be justified in carefully selected high-risk patients with large, high-grade tumors. In terms of distant recurrence and disease-specific survival, tumor size and tumor grade are equally important independent predictors of outcome.

**ANSWER:** A

9. With regard to basal cell carcinoma, which of the following statements is true?

   A. It originates from the deep dermal appendages.

   B. Intermittent intense exposure to UV light is a greater risk factor than exposure at a low dose per episode of a similar total dose.

   C. Fifty percent occur on the head and neck.

   D. The risk for a second basal cell carcinoma is lower for men with index tumors on the trunk.

   E. Superficial basal cell carcinoma is the most common type.

*Ref.:* 18, 19

COMMENTS: **Basal cell carcinoma** is the most common malignancy in the United States and accounts for about 80% of all skin cancers. Basal cell carcinoma originates from the pluripotential basal keratinocytes of the epidermis and from hair follicles, not from the dermis. Exposure to UV radiation is a major risk factor for basal cell carcinoma, especially recreational exposure to the sun during childhood and adolescence. Although **cutaneous squamous cell carcinoma** appears to be strongly related to cumulative sun exposure, the relationship between exposure to UV radiation and risk for basal cell carcinoma, like melanoma, is more complex. The timing, pattern, and amount of exposure are significant. Other risk factors are fair skin, light-colored hair and eyes, topical arsenic exposure, and immunosuppression. Eighty percent occur on the head or neck. The most common type of basal cell carcinoma is the nodular form, which accounts for 60% of cases, and it appears as a classic domed, pearly papule with surface telangiectasia (E-Figure 12-1; E-Figures throughout this chapter are available online at www.expertconsult.com). Other types of basal cell carcinoma include superficial (15%), which usually appears as a minimally raised pink-red patch or papule, and morpheaform (sclerosing, infiltrative), which appears as a white scarlike plaque with indistinct margins. Some basal cell carcinomas are pigmented. Basal cell carcinomas rarely metastasize, but if they are neglected or recurrent, they can be locally destructive and require extensive local treatment and reconstruction. After an initial diagnosis of basal cell carcinoma, the risk for a second tumor is elevated tenfold. Male gender, truncal carcinomas, and older age increase risk for the development of subsequent basal cell carcinomas.

**ANSWER: B**

10. A 75-year-old man has a newly noted, raised 1.5-cm pearly nodule with surface telangiectasia on the cheek. What is the next most appropriate step in his care?

   A. Punch biopsy

   B. Topical imiquimod

   C. Curettage

   D. Surgical excision

   E. Radiation therapy

*Ref.:* 18, 19

COMMENTS: **Basal cell carcinoma** may be treated surgically or nonsurgically. Surgical approaches include curettage, electrodesiccation, cryosurgery, excision, and Mohs micrographic surgery. The latter two have the benefit of histologic evaluation of the excised tumor. The cure rate after surgical excision is greater than 99% for primary lesions of any size on the neck, trunk, and extremities. Surgical excision is less efficacious for larger lesions of the head unless frozen section control of margins or **Mohs surgery** (fixation in vivo with repeated horizontal frozen section and excision to microscopic negative margins) is performed. Although recent randomized trial data show no significant difference in recurrence with primary or recurrent facial tumors, Mohs surgery is often used for these tumors and is probably beneficial for larger, poorly defined lesions in anatomically critical areas of the face. Treatment without histologic evaluation is acceptable for small low-risk lesions. Nonsurgical approaches include radiotherapy, topical and injectable therapy, and photodynamic therapy. **Radiotherapy** is useful for tumors in difficult-to-treat locations and unresectable tumors, but it is potentially carcinogenic, has inferior cosmesis and efficacy, and is best avoided in patients younger than 60 years. Topical therapy includes 5-fluorouracil and imiquimod. Imiquimod, a nonspecific immune response modifier,

was approved by the Food and Drug Administration (FDA) in 2004 for the treatment of superficial basal cell carcinomas smaller than 2.0 cm in nonimmunocompromised adults. Therapy 5 days per week for 6 weeks results in histologic clearance rates of greater than 80%.

**ANSWER: D**

11. A fair-skinned 68-year-old woman has a sharply demarcated 2-cm ulcerated skin lesion in an old burn scar on her forearm. What is the most appropriate treatment for this patient?

   A. Topical chemotherapy

   B. Topical biologic therapy

   C. Surgical excision with frozen section

   D. Mohs micrographic surgery

   E. Radiotherapy

*Ref.:* 2, 18

COMMENTS: **Cutaneous squamous cell carcinoma** appears most frequently on sun-exposed areas, with two thirds occurring on the head or neck; typical locations include exposed portion of the ears, the lower lip at the vermillion border, the paranasal areas, the maxillary skin, and the dorsum of the hands (E-Figures 12-2 and 12-3). Risk factors include fair skin and light eyes, prior actinic keratosis, xeroderma pigmentosum, and exposure to nitrates, arsenicals, and hydrocarbons, as well as chronic excessive sun exposure, immunosuppression, previous trauma, and burns. The aggressiveness of these cancers is related to the underlying cause, location, and size of the lesion and is increased in lesions arising in areas of previous burns (Marjolin ulcer) or trauma and in lesions of the lips and perineum. Excision of cutaneous squamous cell carcinoma, generally with margins of 4 to 5 mm, should be accompanied by frozen section evaluation of the surgical margins. These tumors are radiosensitive. Surgery is preferred for tumors arising in scarred, traumatized, or previously irradiated skin. Large lesions may require adjuvant radiotherapy after surgical excision. Mohs surgery may be used for lesions with clinically indistinct margins. Regional lymph node dissection for squamous cell carcinoma is performed for clinically evident (palpable) disease.

**ANSWER: C**

12. Which of the following is a potential premalignant precursor of melanoma?

   A. Keratoacanthoma

   B. Actinic keratosis

   C. Seborrheic keratosis

   D. Dysplastic nevus

   E. Bowen disease

*Ref.:* 2, 18

COMMENTS: **Keratoacanthomas**, characterized by rapid growth, rolled edges, and a crater filled with keratin, can mimic either squamous or basal cell carcinoma in appearance (E-Figure 12-4). Although they often grow rapidly and then involute over a period of several months, biopsy is usually performed. **Actinic (solar) keratosis** and **cutaneous horns** are premalignant lesions found on the sun-exposed areas of skin in fair-skinned individuals, more commonly in those with prolonged exposure to the sun or to carcinogens (E-Figure 12-5). These lesions may be treated with cryotherapy or topical agents. Raised lesions or lesions resistant to this treatment should be excised, although some may involute spontaneously. The likelihood of progression to squamous cell carcinoma is low (estimated to be 1 in 1000), with an associated lifetime risk of 5% to 10%. **Bowen disease** is cutaneous squamous cell carcinoma in situ. About 10% of these lesions progress to invasive squamous cell carcinoma. They should be excised completely to negative margins. The presence of dysplastic nevi confers an increased risk for the development of melanoma. In addition, some dysplastic nevi represent true precursors of melanoma and may progress to invasive melanoma if untreated. They are usually reddish to brown, have scalloped edges and variegated pigmentation, are generally larger than 6 mm in diameter, and often appear on the trunk and other non–sun-exposed regions of the body.

**ANSWER:** D

13. A 65-year-old man has a rapidly growing red-blue nodule on his left forearm. The remainder of his physical examination is normal. Biopsy demonstrates Merkel cell (neuroendocrine) carcinoma of the skin. Appropriate care for this patient includes all of the following except:

A. Chest radiograph

B. Wide local excision with 2- to 3-cm margins

C. Sentinel lymph node biopsy with selective lymph node dissection

D. Axillary lymph node dissection

E. Postoperative adjuvant radiotherapy

*Ref.:* 2, 18, 20

**COMMENTS: Merkel cell** (neuroendocrine) carcinoma of the skin is derived from neuroectoderm and is manifested as a rapidly growing pink to red to blue to violaceous firm nodule, often in elderly patients. This tumor is histologically indistinguishable from small cell carcinoma of pulmonary origin, and a chest radiograph should be obtained to exclude metastases from a lung primary. After biopsy confirmation of the diagnosis, primary treatment consists of wide excision with 2- to 3-cm margins and histologic confirmation of negative margins. Although approximately 30% of patients initially have palpable regional lymph nodes, up to 70% of the remainder relapse in the regional lymph nodes within 2 years of diagnosis without nodal treatment. Current National Comprehensive Cancer Network (NCCN) guidelines recommend sentinel lymph node biopsy with selective lymph node dissection for patients with clinically node-negative Merkel cell carcinoma; approximately 30% of patients will be found to have occult metastatic disease. Immunohistochemistry with pancytokeratin AE1/AE3, cytokeratin 20, and chromogranin A helps detect micrometastatic disease. This approach improves locoregional disease control, and sentinel node status is a significant indicator of prognosis. Adjuvant radiotherapy is usually given to the primary site and may include the draining lymphatics and regional nodal basin for patients with node-positive disease. This improves locoregional control over surgical treatment alone, and some studies have suggested a survival benefit as well. Overall survival is poor, with mortality rates of 50% to 80% overall and 30% at 5 years after diagnosis.

**ANSWER:** D

14. Regarding the epidemiology of melanoma, which of the following is not true?

A. The incidence of melanoma is increasing more rapidly than that of any other solid tumor.

B. The increased incidence of melanoma is mainly due to an increased diagnosis of early lesions, whereas the incidence of thicker tumors is declining.

C. The death rate from cutaneous melanoma is increasing.

D. Before the age of 45 years, the incidence of melanoma is greater in females than in males.

E. More than 20% of melanomas are diagnosed in individuals younger than 40 years.

*Ref.:* 2, 16, 20-22

**COMMENTS:** For past several decades, the incidence of **melanoma** has been increasing more rapidly than that of any other solid tumor. Analysis of recent Surveillance, Epidemiology, and End Results (SEER) data shows a continued increasing incidence of 3% to 6% per year in the United States, with the death rate from melanoma increasing as well, although at a lower rate of less than 1% per year. The greatest increase continues to be in older men. This increase applies to all thickness groups, including tumors greater than 4 mm, and to all histologic types, thus implying that the increase in incidence is not just due to increased screening and that surveillance and early detection efforts have not led to a measurable reduction in the incidence of unfavorable melanomas. While the age of the U.S. population continues to increase, with the median age at diagnosis increasing from 40 to older than 50 years over the past generation, melanoma is still diagnosed in a substantial proportion of patients at a young age. Melanoma is second only to adult leukemia among cancers in terms of years of productive life lost. Melanoma is more common in women younger than 40 to 45 years and more common in men thereafter.

**ANSWER:** B

15. Which of the following is not a risk factor for melanoma?

A. Total nevus count

B. Fair skin

C. Natural red or blonde hair

D. Prior blistering sunburn

E. Cigarette smoking

*Ref.:* 2, 3, 21

**COMMENTS:** In addition to the well-established risk associated with solar UV radiation in susceptible individuals, especially intense intermittent exposure, blistering childhood sunburns also elevate the risk for development of **melanoma**. Constitutional **risk factors** include fair skin, red or blonde hair, blue or green eye color, the presence of many nevi, raised nevi, and dysplastic nevi. Patients with xeroderma pigmentosum have an elevated risk for the development of both melanoma and nonmelanoma skin cancer, as do immunocompromised patients and those with a previous history of nonmelanoma skin cancer and individuals with a family history of melanoma.

**ANSWER:** E

**16.** The preferred diagnostic biopsy method for pigmented skin lesions is:

A. Punch biopsy

B. Incisional biopsy

C. Shave biopsy

D. Excisional biopsy

E. Excision with 0.5-cm margins

*Ref.:* 2, 21, 23

**COMMENTS:** Information from **diagnostic biopsy guides** treatment and provides important prognostic and staging information for patients with newly diagnosed **melanoma**. A properly performed diagnostic biopsy is of crucial importance. **Excisional biopsy** (with 1 mm of normal surrounding skin) to remove the entire visible lesion is recommended. The excision should not be extended to permit more cosmetic closure because this may lead to unnecessarily extensive subsequent surgery. Ideally, the biopsy scar should be oriented to be most compatible with definitive treatment should the lesion prove to be melanoma (usually in the longitudinal axis for extremity lesions and perpendicular to the underlying muscle fibers for truncal and head and neck lesions). Excisional biopsy is not always performed or possible. **Shave biopsy** is discouraged for the diagnosis of pigmented lesions because the deep margin is often positive. **Punch or incisional biopsy** may be performed for large lesions or those in anatomically constrained areas and should include the full thickness of the skin and the most elevated and the darkest portions of the lesion. Patients in whom the diagnosis is made by less than excisional biopsy may require additional treatment and should be counseled that the final diagnosis may differ from that arrived at by biopsy. Regardless of the biopsy type, pathologic review by a dermatopathologist with an interest in pigmented lesions improves diagnostic accuracy, minimizes diagnostic error, and facilitates optimal patient care. The biopsy report should include tumor thickness (millimeters), histologic type, presence or absence of ulceration, Clark level, mitoses per square millimeter, peripheral and deep margin status, tumor location, and comments on the presence or absence of regression, tumor-infiltrating lymphocytes, vertical growth phase, angiolymphatic invasion, neurotropism, and microsatellitosis.

**ANSWER:** D

**17.** Which of the following is a component of current American Joint Commission for Cancer (AJCC) tumor staging for melanoma:

A. Presence or absence of regression

B. Presence or absence of lymphovascular invasion

C. Level of invasion

D. Tumor diameter

E. Tumor mitotic rate

*Ref.:* 24

**COMMENTS:** Adoption of mitotic rate in the classification of thin melanomas is one of the key changes in the new (2009, effective January 2010) AJCC **staging system** for cutaneous **melanoma**. The level of invasion is no longer used in AJCC tumor staging, except when the **mitotic rate** (described per square millimeter of tissue) cannot be obtained. Melanomas 1 mm or less in thickness are now classified as "a" for lesions with fewer than

1 mitosis/mm$^2$ that are nonulcerated and as "b" for lesions with 1 or more mitoses/mm$^2$ or ulceration. Previously, melanomas 1 mm or less in thickness but level IV or V, as well as ulcerated melanomas, were categorized as T1b. As in the last staging iteration, ulceration differentiates "a" from "b" lesions in all other thickness categories. The AJCC recommends that the mitotic count per square millimeter of tissue be enumerated on the standardized pathology report for review by clinicians and reported by cancer registrars to national databases because the mitotic rate has prognostic significance as a continuous variable.

**ANSWER:** E

**18.** The most common histologic type of melanoma is:

A. Superficial spreading

B. Nodular

C. Lentigo maligna

D. Acral lentiginous

E. Desmoplastic

*Ref.:* 2

**COMMENTS: Superficial spreading melanoma** is the most common type; it accounts for 70% of melanomas and is characterized by some degree of radial growth (E-Figure 12-6). **Nodular melanoma**, the next most common type, accounts for about 15% of melanomas and is characterized by vertical growth with a minimal to absent radial growth phase (E-Figure 12-7). **Lentigo maligna melanoma**, about 10% of melanomas, is characterized by an extensive radial growth phase, most commonly occurs on sun-exposed body areas in older patients, and is generally diagnosed at a thinner stage (E-Figure 12-8). **Acral lentiginous melanoma** is the most common type of melanoma in nonwhite individuals and is usually darkly pigmented (E-Figure 12-9). The prognosis depends on the thickness of the lesion, not the histologic subtype per se.

**ANSWER:** A

**19.** Adverse prognostic factors for clinically localized (stage I and II) melanoma include all of the following except:

A. Older age

B. Male gender

C. Increasing tumor thickness

D. Tumor regression

E. Tumor ulceration

*Ref.:* 2, 25

**COMMENTS:** Older age is a predictor of poorer **survival** as established in numerous studies and verified in retrospective reviews of recent clinical trials. Male patients fare worse than females. Tumor site (extremity better than the trunk or head or neck) is also prognostic. Tumor thickness is the most important predictor of outcome in patients with clinically localized melanoma, followed by ulceration (Figure 12-1). Although approximately half of **melanomas** show some degree of regression, the influence of regression on outcome is unclear; reports are variable regarding its significance, with some suggesting a favorable and others an adverse influence on outcome.

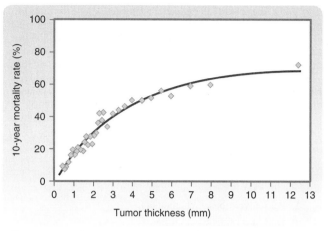

**Figure 12-1.** Observed (*diamonds*) and predicted (*solid line*) 10-year mortality rate in patients with clinically localized melanoma. This is based on a mathematical model derived from the American Joint Committee on Cancer melanoma database of 15,230 patients. (*From Balch CM, Soong SJ, Gerschenwald JE, et al: Prognostic factors analysis of 17,600 melanoma patients: validation of the American Joint Committee on Cancer melanoma staging system, J Clin Oncol 19:3622–3634, 2001.*)

**A N S W E R :**   D

20. A 33-year-old woman has a 2.1-mm-thick, nonulcerated nodular melanoma on her right thigh. The results of physical examination are otherwise normal. What is the most appropriate treatment?

A. Wide local excision with 1.0-cm margins

B. Wide local excision with 2.0-cm margins

C. Wide local excision with 2.0-cm margins and sentinel lymph node biopsy

D. Wide local excision with 2.0-cm margins, sentinel lymph node biopsy with frozen section, and possible inguinofemoral lymph node dissection

E. Wide local excision with 3.0-cm margins, sentinel lymph node biopsy with frozen section, and possible inguinofemoral lymph node dissection

*Ref.:* 2, 20, 21, 23, 24

**COMMENTS:** Treatment of **melanoma** involves complete excision of all skin and subcutaneous tissue down to the underlying fascia for a defined distance from the biopsy site, scar, or margins of the pigmented lesion, depending on tumor thickness. Recommended margins, based on data from five randomized clinical trials, are 0.5 cm for melanoma in situ, 1.0 cm for thin melanomas, and 2.0 cm for melanomas thicker than 1.0 mm. Wider margins are considered for lesions thicker than 4 mm and those with satellite lesions. Margins may be adjusted for concerns regarding cosmesis and function (Table 12-1). **Lymphatic mapping** (lymphoscintigraphy), **sentinel lymph node** biopsy, and selective lymph node dissection are recommended for patients with melanomas greater than 1.0 mm in thickness. Sentinel lymph node biopsy may be recommended for thicker melanomas, mainly those 0.76 mm or thinner, Clark level IV or V, ulcerated, diagnosed by incomplete biopsy, exhibiting regression, with a high mitotic rate, and occurring in younger patients. The likelihood of finding a positive sentinel lymph node is most strongly predicted by tumor thickness, with minimal risk for melanomas thinner than 0.76 mm, 5% for

melanomas 0.76 to 1.0 mm, 8% to 10% for melanomas 1.01 to 1.5 mm, 18% to 30% for melanomas 1.51 to 4.0 mm, and 30% to 40% for melanomas thicker than 4.0 mm. Although use of the mitotic rate to classify thin melanomas as T1b was based on survival data, some data suggest that the likelihood of occult nodal disease increases with increasing mitotic rate. The use of immunohistochemistry (with at least one melanoma-specific marker such as HMB-45, Melan-A, or MART-1) will increase the sentinel lymph node positivity rate by approximately 10% over hematoxylineosin staining alone. Nomograms that incorporate patient age, site, thickness, level, and ulceration have been developed to help predict the likelihood of a positive sentinel lymph node. The current AJCC melanoma staging committee states that "sentinel node staging [is] encouraged for standard patient care" and that "staging with sentinel node technology should be required as entry criterion for all melanoma patients presenting with clinical stage IB and II disease before entry into clinical trials involving new surgical techniques or adjuvant therapy." Frozen section examination of melanoma sentinel lymph nodes has been abandoned because of its low sensitivity (50%) and concern that tissue destruction may preclude an accurate diagnosis from permanent sections.

**TABLE 12-1   Recommended Margins for Wide Local Excision of the Primary Site**

| Thickness | Margin | Note |
| --- | --- | --- |
| Melanoma in situ | 5 mm | Head and neck: consider preoperative margin assessment |
| Melanoma <1 mm | 1 cm | |
| Melanoma 1-4 mm | 2 cm | 1 cm acceptable in limited anatomic locations |
| Melanoma >4 mm | 2 cm | Consider 3 cm if easily obtained |

**A N S W E R :**   C

21. The patient in Question 20 is found to have metastatic melanoma in an inguinal sentinel lymph node. Which of the following statements regarding her condition is incorrect?

A. On completion lymphadenectomy, the likelihood of nonsentinel lymph node metastases is 10% to 30%.

B. Completion lymph node dissection should be performed.

C. Adequate inguinofemoral lymph node dissection implies removal of a minimum of seven to eight lymph nodes.

D. Adjuvant radiation therapy is beneficial for patients with more than three involved lymph nodes and when there is breach of the nodal capsule with bulky nodal disease.

E. Completion lymph node dissection is unnecessary for micrometastatic disease (<0.2-mm tumor within the sentinel lymph node).

*Ref.:* 2, 20, 21, 23, 26-28

**COMMENTS:** As yet there have been no prognostic factors or nomograms that accurately and reproducibly identify a subset of sentinel lymph node–positive **melanoma** patients without risk of harboring additional metastatic lymph nodes. **Completion lymph node dissection** should be performed for all sentinel node–positive patients. The goals of surgery include control of regional disease and improved survival. The majority of patients who undergo completion lymph node dissection will not be found to have additional positive lymph nodes. However, examination of these nonsentinel lymph nodes is by necessity less rigorous than the stepwise examination of the sentinel lymph node, so small foci of disease may be missed. Unlike breast cancer, there is no lower limit of the size of metastatic **melanoma** within a lymph node that defines a positive lymph node. Retrospective studies suggest that patients with nodal disease less than 0.1 mm are at substantially increased risk for relapse versus sentinel node–negative patients. Standard surgical oncology teaching defines complete lymph node dissections on the basis of anatomic boundaries. Recommendations based on expert opinion have suggested a minimum number of lymph nodes per region to define a complete lymph node dissection. A recent review by the Sidney Melanoma Unit based on more than 2000 regional lymph node dissections for melanoma suggested following standard anatomic guidelines consisting of minimum (and target mean) **lymph node counts** of 10 (21) for the axilla, 7 (14) for inguinal and ilioinguinal dissections, and 20 (39) for cervical dissections involving four or more levels . The 2010 NCCN guidelines recommend complete lymph node dissection based on proper anatomic boundaries, which they recommend be dictated into the operative note, but they do not set a target number of lymph nodes. A recent meta-analysis of **sentinel lymph node biopsy**–guided selective lymph node dissection versus observation with therapeutic lymph node dissection for nodal relapse demonstrated a significantly higher risk for death (hazard ratio of 1.6) for patients in the therapeutic lymph node dissection group. **Adjuvant radiotherapy** is considered for most patients with multiple cervical lymph node metastases and for those with bulky, large (metastatic nodes >3 cm in size) or extracapsular disease at any site. Even though no published randomized trials have compared surgery alone with surgery and postoperative radiotherapy, retrospective single-institution studies suggest improved regional control and disease-free survival.

**ANSWER:** E

22. Whether a deep (pelvic) lymph node dissection is performed with inguinofemoral lymph node dissection may be based on all of the following except:

    A. Findings on pelvic CT or PET-CT

    B. Palpable versus micrometastatic nodal disease

    C. The number of positive nodes in the superficial compartment

    D. Primary tumor ulceration

    E. The status of Cloquet's node

*Ref.:* 20, 21, 23, 27, 29

**COMMENTS:** The appropriate extent of **groin dissection** in patients with metastatic **melanoma** to the lymph nodes remains controversial. Isolated pelvic nodal disease is seen in the absence of superficial inguinal lymph node involvement and should be sought on lymphoscintigraphy performed for sentinel node identification, but this is uncommon. Some surgical oncologists perform radical ilioinguinal lymph node dissection for all patients deemed candidates for inguinal node dissection, whereas others take a selective approach. Proponents of routine radical ilioinguinal lymph node dissection note that a third of patients have additional disease only in the iliac and obturator nodes with no further inguinal nodal disease and that there are no clear indicators to help the surgeon select patients who will not benefit from pelvic lymph node dissection. Selective addition of deep pelvic lymph node dissection is based on the likelihood of finding involved nodes, which is increased when dissection is performed for macrometastatic inguinal disease and when a greater number of inguinal nodes are involved. Preoperative imaging results (CT or PET-CT) may also be used in conjunction with the clinical findings to help guide the extent of dissection. Cloquet's node is the most inferior node in the iliac chain; evaluation of this node may be used to determine the potential value of deep pelvic node dissection that encompasses the obturator and hypogastric nodes in addition to the iliac nodes up to the level of bifurcation of the common iliac vessels. Complications of either procedure include seroma, lymphocele, lymphatic fistula, and lymphedema. There is no evidence that the more extensive operation carries greater morbidity.

**ANSWER:** D

23. Adjuvant systemic therapy for node-positive melanoma patients may include any of the following except:

    A. Adriamycin-based chemotherapy

    B. High-dose interferon alfa-2b

    C. Enrollment in a clinical antiangiogenic agent trial

    D. Enrollment in a clinical immunotherapy trial

    E. Observation

*Ref.:* 2, 20, 30

**COMMENTS:** Numerous randomized clinical trials of **chemotherapy**, nonspecific immune stimulants, and **vaccines** for high-risk stage II and stage III **melanoma** have been conducted, but most have been underpowered and yielded negative results. The FDA-approved adjuvant therapy for node-positive melanoma patients is high-dose **interferon** alfa-2b, 20 million $IU/m^2$ 5 days per week intravenously for 4 weeks, followed by 10 million $IU/m^2$ subcutaneously 3 days per week for 48 weeks. Although randomized controlled clinical trials have demonstrated improved disease-free survival with adjuvant interferon alfa-2b, there is a very modest effect on overall survival, and associated side effects of the treatment are significant. Newer agents under study in the adjuvant setting include antiangiogenic therapy such as bevacizumab and the anti–CTLA-4 antibody ipilimumab. Because of the lack of effective adjuvant therapy with low toxicity, observation, either as a control arm of a clinical trial or in the absence of clinical trial enrollment, is acceptable. Doxorubicin (Adriamycin) is not effective for the treatment of **melanoma**.

**ANSWER:** A

24. Which of the following is the most significant prognostic factor for patients with node-positive (stage III) melanoma?

    A. Nodal size

    B. Number of involved lymph nodes

    C. Tumor thickness

    D. Tumor ulceration

    E. Patient gender

*Ref.:* 23-25

**COMMENTS:** The most significant prognostic factor for patients with **node-positive melanoma** is the number of involved lymph nodes. The next most significant prognostic factor is nodal tumor burden (microscopic or clinically occult versus macroscopic or clinically apparent), followed by primary tumor ulceration and thickness. Nodal size is not a component of staging, nor has it been shown to have significant independent prognostic value. Gender does not have a significant effect on outcome in patients with node-positive melanoma.

**ANSWER:** B

25. A 52-year-old man is evaluated for a palpable left inguinal lymph node 7 years after wide local excision of a thin melanoma on the ipsilateral right calf. No sentinel lymph node biopsy or other staging was done at the time of his initial diagnosis. What should be the next step in the care of this patient?

   A. Excisional biopsy

   B. Excisional biopsy with frozen section examination followed by immediate inguinofemoral lymph node dissection

   C. Total-body PET-CT per melanoma protocol

   D. FNA biopsy (cytology)

   E. Measurement of serum S-100 protein and lactate dehydrogenase (LDH)

*Ref.:* 2, 31

**COMMENTS:** Recurrence in the **regional lymph node** basin is the most common site of initial recurrence after treatment by wide local excision alone and can occur even in patients with thin primary **melanomas** and many years after the initial diagnosis. Evaluation of clinically palpable lymph nodes is most expeditiously performed by FNA, with or without ultrasound guidance. Core needle biopsy or excisional biopsy can be done if the FNA is negative or nondiagnostic. Frozen section evaluation of lymph node metastases of melanoma has low sensitivity, and freezing the tissue may destroy areas with metastatic disease; the diagnosis is generally deferred to evaluation of the permanent section. **Complete regional lymphadenectomy** will lead to durable long-term survival in approximately half of such patients. Once the diagnosis of nodal melanoma recurrence is established, given that the remainder of the patient's physical examination is unremarkable, a metastatic work-up that includes liver function tests, PET-CT, and MRI of the head is appropriate before surgery to exclude the presence of clinically unsuspected metastatic disease. In this clinical scenario, evaluation with PET-CT is estimated to change treatment in 15% to 30% of patients.

**ANSWER:** D

26. Which of the following is not indicated for the initial treatment of in transit metastasis from cutaneous melanoma?

   A. Excision

   B. Injection

   C. Laser treatment

   D. Heated limb perfusion

   E. Amputation

*Ref.:* 2, 21, 23, 24, 32

**COMMENTS: In transit metastases** develop in about 2% of patients with cutaneous **melanoma** and appear as visible dermal or subcutaneous tumor nodules between the primary site and regional draining nodal basin. They arise from intralymphatic tumor spread. After evaluation for metastatic disease, treatment depends on the extent of disease. Limited in transit metastases amenable to excision may be treated by wide excision with 1-cm margins. Other local therapy options include laser ablation with

healing by secondary intention and local immunotherapy with bacille Calmette-Guérin (BCG) or interferon alfa injection or topical application of imiquimod cream. Injection results in a response in approximately 80% of lesions, sometimes in neighboring lesions as well, and the toxicity is predominantly local (erythema, edema, ulceration). For extensive disease, **isolated limb perfusion** with a pump oxygenator circuit and regional chemotherapy (most commonly melphalan and sometimes the addition of tumor necrosis factor-α), with or without concomitant regional lymph node dissection, has limited indications but may be useful for locoregional control of disease. This involves surgical placement of arterial and venous cannulas in the affected extremity, which is excluded from the general circulation with a tourniquet. The reported complete response rate is 40% to 80%, but the toxicity may be considerable and includes lymphedema, compartment syndrome, and neuropathy. Responses may not be durable, with 50% recurrence rates 18 months after infusion. Recently, isolated limb infusion with percutaneously placed cannulas has been proposed as an alternative, less morbid therapy with complete responses rates of approximately 30%. With these available therapies, major amputation is rarely required as primary therapy for in transit disease. As secondary treatment, amputation may provide palliation, or regional control, for unmanageable progressive recurrences when other approaches fail. Indications are usually intractable pain with loss of limb function (often associated with tumor fungation, bleeding, infection, gangrene, and severe lymphedema) in patients whose life expectancy is at least 3 months and who have reasonable performance status otherwise. In the absence of nodal metastases, patients with in transit disease have 5- and 10-year overall survival rates of 69% and 52%, whereas those with concomitant regional nodal metastases have diminished 5- and 10-year overall survival rates of 46% and 33%.

**ANSWER:** E

27. A 37-year-old man is evaluated for a 4-month history of anemia and intermittent abdominal discomfort and distention 7 years after treatment of a stage I melanoma on his right forearm. The results of physical examination are normal, colonoscopy is negative, and CT demonstrates an area of invaginated jejunal mesentery with an adjacent dilated loop of small bowel. What is the next most appropriate step in the management of this patient?

   A. Exploration and small bowel resection

   B. Video capsule endoscopy

   C. Systemic biochemotherapy

   D. Whole-body PET-CT

   E. Air contrast small bowel barium study

*Ref.:* 2, 21, 23, 24, 32

**COMMENTS:** The small intestine is the most common site of **gastrointestinal tract metastases** from cutaneous **melanoma,** which are present in a high proportion of patients with melanoma at autopsy. Symptomatic patients most commonly have abdominal pain, chronic gastrointestinal bleeding, obstruction, and weight loss. Polypoid tumors arising from the submucosa may act as the lead point for an intussusception, as in this case. Surgical resection of solitary and even multiple small intestinal metastases is associated with improved survival over nonoperative therapy and is effective treatment of associated obstruction. With complete resection of small intestinal disease, median survival times of 4 years are reported. Since this patient is symptomatic without evidence of other disease by physical examination or CT of the abdomen and pelvis, further preoperative radiologic work-up is unlikely to alter the need for or benefit of surgery. Although the disease recurs in most patients at multiple sites and they are best treated with systemic therapy, those who are suitable candidates for resection of limited metastatic disease may experience long-term disease-free survival. In general, for stage IV melanoma the site of the metastatic disease and the serum LDH level correlate with prognosis. One-year survival rates for those with cutaneous, subcutaneous, or distant nodal metastases (M1a) versus those with lung metastases (M1b) versus those with any other visceral metastases or any metastasis with an elevated serum LDH level (M1c) are estimated to be 62%, 53%, and 33%, respectively. Factors reported to be associated with improved outcome after resection of **melanoma metastases** include initial disease stage, disease-free interval after treatment of the primary melanoma, initial site of metastasis, solitary site of disease, and complete resection. Even when not performed with curative intent, palliative surgical treatment of metastatic melanoma may be beneficial for the treatment of symptomatic patients.

**ANSWER:** A

## REFERENCES

1. Tran TT, Schulman J, Fisher DE: UV and pigmentation: molecular mechanisms and social controversies, *Pigment Cell Melanoma Res* 21:509–516, 2008.
2. Urist MM, Soong S-J: Melanoma and Cutaneous Malignancies. In Townsend CM, Beauchamp RD, Evers BM, et al, editors: *Sabiston textbook of surgery: the biological basis of modern surgical practice*, ed 18, Philadelphia, 2008, WB Saunders.
3. Tyrrell RM: Ultraviolet protection. In Lejeune FJ, Chaudhuri PK, Das Gupta TK, editors: *Malignant melanoma: medical and surgical treatment*, New York, 1994, McGraw-Hill.
4. Bishop DT, Demenais F, Iles MM, et al: Genome-wide association study identifies three loci associated with melanoma risk, *Nat Genet* 41:920–925, 2009.
5. Bishop DT, Demenais F, Goldstein AM, et al: Geographical variation in the penetrance of CDKN2A mutations for melanoma, *J Natl Cancer Inst* 94:894–903, 2002.
6. Velasco AL, Dunlap WW: Pilonidal disease and hidradenitis, *Surg Clin North Am* 89:689–701, 2009.
7. Netscher D, Fiore N: Hand surgery. In Townsend CM, Beauchamp RD, Evers BM, et al, editors: *Sabiston textbook of surgery: the biological basis of modern surgical practice*, ed 18, Philadelphia, 2008, WB Saunders.
8. Cole P, Heller L, Bullocks J, et al: The skin and subcutaneous tissue. In Brunicardi FC, Andersen DK, Billiar TR, et al, editors: *Schwartz's principles of surgery*, ed 9, New York, 2010, McGraw-Hill.
9. Rakinic J: Modern Management of Pilonidal Disease. In Cameron JL, editors: *Current surgical therapy*, ed 9, Philadelphia, 2008, CV Mosby.
10. Benz MR, Czernin J, Dry SM, et al: Quantitative F18-fluorodeoxyglucose positron emission tomography accurately characterizes peripheral nerve sheath tumors as malignant or benign, *Cancer* 116:451–458, 2010.
11. Pletcher BA: Neurofibromatosis Type 1. In eMedicine Clinical Knowledge Base, Neurology. Updated December 2009. Available at www.emedicine.com. Accessed January 31, 2010.
12. Das Gupta TK, Chaudhuri PK, editors: *Tumors of the soft tissues*, ed 2, Norwalk, Conn, 1998, Appleton & Lange.
13. Singer S, Canter RJ: Soft tissue sarcoma. In Cameron JL, editor: *Current surgical therapy*, ed 9, Philadelphia, 2008, CV Mosby.
14. Singer S: Soft tissue sarcomas. In Townsend CM, Beauchamp RD, Evers BM, et al, editors: *Sabiston textbook of surgery: the biological basis of modern surgical practice*, ed 18, Philadelphia, 2008, WB Saunders.
15. Hieken TJ: Genetic testing for cancer susceptibility. In Saclarides TJ, Millikan KW, Godellas CV, editors: *Surgical oncology: an algorithmic approach*, New York, 2003, Springer-Verlag.
16. Jemal A, Siegel R, Ward E, et al: Cancer statistics, 2009, *CA Cancer J Clin* 59:225–249, 2009.
17. Hueman MT, Thornton K, Herman JM, et al: Management of extremity soft tissue sarcomas, *Surg Clin North Am* 88:539–557, 2008.
18. Kazin R, Shermak MA: Skin and soft tissue. In Cameron JL: *Current surgical therapy*, ed 9, Philadelphia, 2008, CV Mosby.
19. Rubin AI, Chen EH, Ratner D: Basal-cell carcinoma, *N Engl J Med* 353:2262–2269, 2005.
20. Hieken TJ: The role of sentinel node biopsy in skin cancer, ed 3. In eMedicine Clinical Knowledge Base, Dermatology. Updated March 2009. Available at www.emedicine.com. Accessed January 31, 2010.
21. Faries MB, Morton DL: Cutaneous Melanoma. In Cameron JL, editor: *Current surgical therapy*, ed 9, Philadelphia, 2008, CV Mosby.
22. Criscione VD, Weinstock MA: Melanoma thickness trends in the United States, 1988-2006, *J Invest Derm* 130:793–797, 2010.
23. Lange JR, Balch CM: Cutaneous melanoma. In Cameron JL, editor: *Current surgical therapy*, ed 8, Philadelphia, 2004, CV Mosby.
24. Balch CM, Gershenwald JE, Soong SJ, et al: Final version of 2009 AJCC melanoma staging and classification, *J Clin Oncol* 27:6199–6206, 2009.
25. Balch CM, Soong SJ, Gershenwald JE, et al: Prognostic factors analysis of 17,600 melanoma patients: validation of the American Joint Committee on Cancer melanoma staging system, *J Clin Oncol* 19:3622–3644, 2001.
26. Ollila DW, Ashburn JH, Amos KD, et al: Metastatic melanoma cells in the sentinel node cannot be ignored, *J Am Coll Surg* 208:924–930, 2009.
27. Spillane AJ, Cheung BL, Stretch JR, et al: Proposed quality standards for regional lymph node dissections in patients with melanoma, *Ann Surg* 249:473–480, 2009.
28. Pasquali S, Mocellin S, Campañá LG, et al: Early (sentinel lymph node biopsy-guided) versus delayed lymphadenectomy in melanoma patients with lymph node metastases: personal experience and literature meta-analysis, *Cancer* 116:1201–1209, 2010.
29. Santinami M, Carbone A, Crippa F, et al: Radical dissection after positive groin sentinel biopsy in melanoma patients: rate of further positive nodes, *Melanoma Res* 19:112–118, 2009.
30. Eggermont AMM, Testori A, Marsden J, et al: Utility of adjuvant systemic therapy in melanoma, *Ann Oncol* 20(Suppl 6):vi30–vi34, 2009.
31. Brady MS, Akhurst T, Spanknebel K, et al: Utility of preoperative (18) F fluorodeoxyglucose–positron emission tomography scanning in high-risk melanoma patients, *Ann Surg Oncol* 13:525–532, 2006.
32. Wargo JA, Tanabe K: Surgical management of melanoma, *Hematol Oncol Clin North Am* 23:565–581, 2009.

# CHAPTER 13

# Hernia

*Norman Wool, M.D., and José M. Velasco, M.D.*

1. Components of the Hesselbach triangle have included the following anatomic landmarks except:

   A. Femoral vein

   B. Medial border of the rectus sheath

   C. Cooper ligament

   D. Inguinal ligament

   E. Inferior epigastric vessels

   *Ref.:* 1-3

**COMMENTS:** The inferior epigastric vessels serve as the superolateral border of the **Hesselbach triangle**. The medial border of the triangle is formed by the rectus sheath, and the inguinal ligament serves as its inferior border. Physical examination often cannot accurately distinguish between direct and indirect inguinal hernias. Hernias occurring within the Hesselbach triangle are considered direct hernias, whereas hernias occurring lateral to the triangle are indirect hernias. The original description of the Hesselbach triangle defined the inferior border as the ligament of Cooper (pectineal ligament). The borders were subsequently modified, with the inguinal ligament being substituted for the Cooper ligament to allow easier identification of the area by surgeons who use the traditional anterior approach for herniorrhaphy.

**ANSWER:** A

2. Which of the following statements is false regarding the iliopubic tract?

   A. Extends from the anterior superior iliac spine to the pubis

   B. Is a condensation of the transversalis fascia

   C. Is of anatomic interest but has little clinical significance

   D. Runs underneath the shelving portion of the Poupart ligament

   E. Many branches of the lumbar plexus run inferior to the iliopubic tract

   *Ref.:* 1-3

**COMMENTS:** The transversalis fascia is the portion of the endo-abdominal fascia that underlies the transversus abdominis muscle. It has several thickenings, the most important of which is the **iliopubic tract**, which arises from the iliopectineal arch, inserts on the anterior superior iliac spine, and extends over the femoral vessels to the pubis. Proper utilization of the transversalis fascia during repair of an inguinal hernia is important to the success of operations not using prosthetic material. The iliopubic tract has particular significance because of its importance as a landmark to laparoscopic surgeons. Many of the branches of the lumbar plexus run inferior to the tract, and damage to these nerves may be the result of aggressive dissection or the placement of tacks or staples to affix a prosthesis below this structure.

**ANSWER:** C

3. Which of the following statements is false regarding the incidence of abdominal wall hernias?

   A. Two thirds of all inguinal hernias are classified as indirect.

   B. Femoral hernias are more common in females than in males.

   C. Indirect hernias are common in females.

   D. Hernias generally occur with equal frequency in males and females.

   E. Premature babies have a 10% incidence of inguinal hernia.

   *Ref.:* 1-3

**COMMENTS:** Approximately three fourths of all abdominal wall hernias occur in the inguinal region, and roughly two thirds of them are indirect inguinal hernias. **Groin hernias** are considered to be at least 25 times more common in males than in females. The incidence of inguinal hernias is increased by prematurity. The most common hernia in each gender is an indirect inguinal hernia. Femoral hernias are rare in men and direct hernias are uncommon in women. It has been estimated that inguinal hernias develop in 25% of males and 2% of females during their lifetime. Hernias therefore constitute a significant economic problem in terms of loss of time from work.

**ANSWER:** D

4. According to the Nyhus classification of groin hernias, which of the following statements are true?

   A. A type II indirect hernia has a dilated internal ring and extends into the scrotum.

   B. A type IIIa hernia is a classically described indirect hernia.

   C. A femoral hernia is classified as type IIIc.

   D. Type IV hernias are pantaloon-type hernias.

   E. Type V hernias are spigelian hernias.

   *Ref.:* 2

**COMMENTS: Groin hernias** may be primary or recurrent. They are classified as inguinal and femoral, with inguinal hernias being further subdivided into direct and indirect hernias. The Lloyd **Nyhus classification** further subdivided groin hernias according to their characteristics. Type I hernias are indirect hernias with a normal-size internal ring and typically occur in infants, children, and small adults. Type II hernias are indirect hernias with a dilated internal ring and an intact posterior wall and do not extend into the scrotum. Type III hernias are posterior wall defects. Type IIIa hernias are direct hernias regardless of size. Type IIIb consists of indirect hernias with a dilated internal ring encroaching on the Hesselbach triangle (massive scrotal, sliding, or pantaloon type). Type IIIc hernias are femoral hernias. Type IV consists of recurrent hernias of the direct, indirect, femoral, or a combined type. There are no type V hernias according to the Nyhus classification.

**ANSWER: C**

5. Which of the following statements is false regarding direct inguinal hernias?

   A. The most likely cause is destruction of connective tissue as a result of physical stress.

   B. Direct hernias should be repaired promptly because of the risk for incarceration.

   C. A direct hernia may be a sliding hernia involving a portion of the bladder wall.

   D. A direct hernia may pass through the external inguinal ring.

   E. An indirect hernia may be present as well.

*Ref.:* 1-3

**COMMENTS:** Destruction of connective tissue as a result of the physical stress of intraabdominal pressure, smoking, aging, connective tissue disease, and systemic illnesses reduces the strength of the transverse aponeurosis and fascia. **Direct inguinal hernias**, therefore, are acquired from the "wear and tear" of daily life, including straining to urinate or defecate, chronic coughing, and heavy lifting. A decrease in the content of hydroxyproline in the aponeurosis of patients with hernias has been demonstrated, as well as alterations in the ultrastructure of collagen. Large direct hernias may weaken the floor of the Hesselbach triangle and result in a functional direct component. Because there is generally diffuse weakness in the area of the Hesselbach triangle without a narrow-necked sac, the risk for incarceration is low. Rarely, incarceration results when the direct hernia passes through the external ring posterior to the cord structures. Involvement of the urinary bladder as a sliding component on the medial wall of a direct hernia sac does not usually cause a problem because the sac can simply be reduced unopened. The spermatic cord should be explored to rule out the presence of an indirect sac.

**ANSWER: B**

6. A sliding inguinal hernia on the left side is likely to involve which of the following?

   A. Ileal mesentery composing the lateral wall of the sac

   B. Ovary and fallopian tube in a female infant

   C. Omentum

   D. Bladder composing the posterolateral wall of the sac

   E. Cecum composing the anteromedial wall of the sac

*Ref.:* 1-3

**COMMENTS:** A **sliding hernia** is one in which the visceral peritoneum of an organ makes up part of the wall of the hernia sac. If the hernia is indirect, it most commonly involves the cecum on the right or the sigmoid colon on the left. The urinary bladder may also be a sliding component. In females, especially infants and children, portions of the female genital tract are often involved. Although most sliding hernias are indirect, they may also be femoral or direct. Recognition of the presence of a sliding hernia and the position of the visceral component is important to avoid injury to the involved organs during repair.

**ANSWER: B**

7. Which of the following statements is true regarding femoral hernias?

   A. Femoral hernias should not be repaired through an infrainguinal approach.

   B. Femoral hernias are more common in males than in females.

   C. Femoral hernias are more common than inguinal hernias in females.

   D. Large femoral hernias should always be repaired by the insertion of prosthetic material.

   E. Femoral hernias could lead to bowel obstruction, frequently as a Richter type of hernia.

*Ref.:* 1-4

**COMMENTS:** Although **femoral hernias** are found more often in females than in males, inguinal hernias are still more common than femoral hernias. Femoral hernias with small orifices in women are repaired from below the inguinal ligament with a few sutures or plugged with a cone of polypropylene mesh because they are rarely associated with hernias above the inguinal ligament. Large femoral hernias can be repaired with the McVay Cooper ligament procedure or even better with a preperitoneal permanent prosthesis placed either laparoscopically or from an open preperitoneal approach. Femoral hernias should be repaired promptly because incarceration is common. Viability of the intestine must be ensured since incarceration of the antimesenteric border of the intestine (Richter hernia) could result in infarction. The presence of bloody fluid in an otherwise empty sac mandates careful examination of the intestine to rule out ischemia. The McVay repair may be preferred with incarcerated femoral hernias to avoid infection of prosthetic mesh.

**ANSWER: E**

8. Correct statements regarding the management of an incarcerated groin hernia include all of the following except:

   A. Immediate or urgent surgical repair is always required for incarcerated groin hernias.

   B. Evaluation of the contents of the hernia sac is a step required in the repair of an incarcerated hernia.

   C. The contents within an incarcerated hernia can be omentum, intestine, or an ovary.

   D. A hydrocele may mimic an incarcerated hernia.

   E. Inadvertent reduction of incarcerated hernia contents during induction of anesthesia does not ensure bowel viability.

*Ref.:* 1-3

**COMMENTS:** Incarceration with potential resultant strangulation of small bowel is a serious complication of groin hernias. If the patient has an **incarcerated inguinal hernia** and strangulation is not suspected, an attempt at reduction by using sedation, Trendelenburg positioning, and gentle sustained pressure over the groin mass is appropriate. Reduction en masse refers to the persistent nature of incarcerated tissue frequently through the external ring despite an apparently successful reduction. If there is any indication of strangulation, reduction should not be attempted preoperatively. Rather, the sac should first be opened before reduction to inspect the viability of the contents. The presence of bloody fluid in the peritoneal cavity should raise the question of intestinal viability. Delayed repair following successful reduction may permit resolution of edema. A hydrocele can mimic an incarcerated hernia. Should physical examination fail to establish the diagnosis, a hydrocele will transilluminate clearly but a hernia will not. Ultrasound can confirm the presence of a hydrocele. The contents of an incarcerated inguinal hernia may be omentum, intestine, or an ovary. In patients with a suspected strangulated hernia, spontaneous reduction of the hernia's contents could occur. However, the surgeon should not assume that the bowel is viable. Examination of the abdominal contents is thus mandatory.

**ANSWER:** A

---

9. Which of the following statements about the management of inguinal hernias in infants and children is true?

   A. Repair should be delayed until a child reaches school age since most inguinal hernia defects close spontaneously.

   B. Repair usually requires a Bassini procedure.

   C. The distal sac should be removed to prevent the formation of a secondary hydrocele.

   D. Contralateral inguinal exploration is indicated routinely because of the high risk for bilaterality.

   E. Intubation of the clinically apparent hernia sac with a laparoscope is one method of examining the contralateral side.

*Ref.:* 1-3

**COMMENTS: Inguinal hernias in infants** and children are nearly always indirect and result from failure of obliteration of the processus vaginalis. Effective treatment requires only high ligation and transection of the sac with or without excision of the distal component. Repair need not be delayed unless the infant has associated medical problems. In fact, bowel obstruction and gonadal or intestinal infarction as a result of strangulation are most likely to occur during the first 6 months of life. Therefore, repair should be performed soon after the diagnosis is made. Exploration of the opposite side in children with a unilateral inguinal hernia is controversial. The incidence of a contralateral hernia following unilateral inguinal herniorrhaphy in children has been reported to be 10% to 30%. Contralateral exploration should be performed routinely in the subset of patients most likely to have a clinically occult hernia: children younger than 2 years, girls younger than 3 years (higher bilateral rate), patients with ventriculoperitoneal shunts, and children younger than 2 years with a left-sided hernia. This last recommendation is based on the fact that most (60%) pediatric hernias are right sided. Intubation of the clinically apparent hernia sac with a laparoscope is one method of examining the contralateral side.

**ANSWER:** E

---

10. Which of the following statements is false regarding the preperitoneal or posterior approach to repair of groin hernias?

   A. It may be appropriate for repair of both direct and indirect hernias.

   B. It may be appropriate for repair of femoral hernias.

   C. It is the preferred approach for repair of obturator hernias.

   D. The preperitoneal approach is not indicated for bilateral or recurrent hernias.

   E. Laparoscopic hernioplasty is an extension of the preperitoneal approach.

*Ref.:* 1-3

**COMMENTS:** The **preperitoneal approach**, which involves a transverse skin incision three fingerbreadths above the pubic tubercle, has been especially successful in the repair of femoral hernias. Both direct and indirect inguinal hernias can also be approached in this manner, although many surgeons have reported higher recurrence rates for direct hernias when using this approach. **Cooper ligament repair** is carried out in the same way as for an anterior approach. The ligament is approximated to the transversus abdominis aponeurosis medially with a transition suture between the transversus aponeurosis, the iliopubic tract, and the Cooper ligament, with completion laterally by approximation of the iliopubic tract and transversus aponeurosis. This approach as originally described has not achieved widespread use, largely because of increased recurrence rates believed to be due to tension. Modifications of the preperitoneal approach consisting of the use of prosthetic material have made it more popular, particularly for repair of bilateral, obturator, and recurrent hernias. General or regional anesthesia is necessary. Postoperative paralytic ileus is not infrequent. Laparoscopic hernioplasty is an extension of the preperitoneal concept. In most laparoscopic repairs, the prosthesis is placed in the preperitoneal space.

**ANSWER:** D

---

11. Which of the following statements is true regarding mesh-plug hernioplasty?

   A. It cannot be performed with the patient under local anesthesia with intravenous sedation.

   B. It is associated with a 7% to 10% recurrence rate.

   C. It may be appropriate for indirect, direct, femoral, and recurrent hernias.

   D. A 21-day recovery period is necessary before patients can assume normal daily activities.

   E. Manual labor is restricted for 6 weeks postoperatively.

*Ref.:* 4, 5

**COMMENTS:** In the 1990s, I. M. Rutkow and A. W. Robbins introduced the **mesh-plug hernioplasty**. In more than 3000 reported hernioplasties, a 1% overall recurrence rate has been documented for all varieties of inguinal hernias. Although Rutkow and Robbins perform the mesh-plug hernioplasty with epidural anesthesia, subsequent reports have described the procedure being performed with local anesthesia and intravenous sedation. In more than 1000 mesh-plug hernioplasties reported by K. W. Millikan and coworkers, a 0.1% recurrence rate was documented, with 96% of patients returning to normal activities within 3 days. In this series, all manual laborers returned to work without restriction on postoperative day 14. During the last decade, mesh-plug hernioplasty has become the most popular prosthetic hernia repair in the United States.

**ANSWER:** C

**12.** All of the following statements concerning the Lichtenstein repair are true except:

A. It is performed with local anesthesia in an outpatient setting.

B. Polypropylene is the most common prosthetic material used for repair.

C. The medial edge of the mesh is sutured to the transversalis fascia, and the lateral edge is sutured to the inguinal ligament.

D. To reduce recurrence rates, the most cephalad tails of the mesh should extend 2 to 4 cm beyond the internal ring.

E. To reduce recurrence rates, the most caudal aspect of the mesh should extend at least 2 cm over the pubic tubercle.

*Ref.:* 1-3, 6

**COMMENTS:** As commonly performed, the open herniorrhaphy technique is the tension-free repair popularized by Irving L. Lichtenstein and colleagues. The **Lichtenstein repair** is routinely performed in an outpatient setting with local anesthesia. Polypropylene mesh is most commonly sutured medially to the transversus abdominis arch, with the internal oblique being overlapped by approximately 2 cm. The latter edge of the mesh is sutured to the inguinal ligament. To reduce recurrence rates, Parviz Amid has described overlapping the mesh at least 2 cm over the pubic tubercle and 2 to 4 cm lateral to the internal ring. Lichtenstein encouraged patients to resume activities rapidly. The Lichtenstein repair was one of the first prosthetic repairs to achieve approximately an overall 1% or lower recurrence rate in the United States.

**ANSWER:** C

**13.** Which of the following is false with regard to the McVay Cooper ligament repair?

A. It is appropriate for indirect and direct hernias but not for femoral hernias.

B. Exposure of the Cooper ligament and the medial border of the femoral sheath is accomplished by incising the transversalis fascia.

C. A relaxing incision is mandatory.

D. The conjoined tendon is sutured to the Cooper ligament from the pubic tubercle laterally to the femoral canal.

E. With a transition stitch, the surgeon sutures the conjoined tendon to the inguinal ligament lateral to the femoral canal.

*Ref.:* 1-3

**COMMENTS: Cooper ligament hernioplasty** is used to repair the three most vulnerable areas for herniation in the myopectineal orifice—the deep ring, the Hesselbach triangle, and the femoral canal—and is therefore indicated for the three common types of hernia of the groin. In the McVay repair, the conjoined tendon is sutured to the Cooper ligament laterally. Exposure of the Cooper ligament is accomplished by incising the transversalis fascia and entering the preperitoneal space. A relaxing incision is mandatory because there is otherwise too much tension on the suture line. A transition stitch is necessary to suture the conjoined tendon to the inguinal ligament beyond the femoral canal. The internal inguinal ring is recreated with adequate laxity to allow easy passage of the tip of a Kelly clamp adjacent to the cord structures.

**ANSWER:** A

**14.** Which of the following hernias is most likely to recur after primary repair?

A. Epigastric hernia

B. Spigelian hernia

C. Indirect hernia

D. Femoral hernia

E. Incisional hernia

*Ref.:* 1-3

**COMMENTS:** Primary repair of **incisional hernias** can be associated with a 30% to 50% or higher **recurrence rate**, depending on the size of the hernia. Except for small incisional hernias, prosthetic mesh is necessary to reduce recurrence rates to 10% or possibly less. Patients with incisional hernias usually have predisposing factors, such as obesity, chronic debilitating illness, diabetes, advanced age, and smoking. The predisposing factors also play a role in the failure of primary repair. Recurrence rates after the other listed hernia repairs should all be 5% or less.

**ANSWER:** E

**15.** Which of the following developments has not led to a decrease in recurrence rates after groin hernia repair?

A. Modifications of the Bassini repair

B. Routine use of prosthetic material

C. Widespread acceptance of the "tension-free" concept

D. Use of the preperitoneal space for hernia repair

E. Use of laparoscopy in hernia repair

*Ref.:* 1-3

**COMMENTS: Recurrence rates for groin hernias** vary from less than 1% to 30%. True recurrence rates are difficult to establish because of inadequate patient follow-up. The Bassini repair and its modifications (Shouldice and McVay) all create tension at the suture line and have been found to have recurrence rates between 10% and 30% when performed outside specialized centers. Several developments in the latter half of the twentieth century have significantly influenced the currently accepted level of a recurrence rate of less than 5%. The routine use of prosthetic material to perform a tension-free hernia repair became accepted by surgeons after being popularized by Lichtenstein in the 1980s. Others, such as Rutkow, Robbins, R. D. Kugel, A. Gilbert, G. Wantz, R.E. Stoppa, and Nyhus, have used multiple prosthetic materials and approaches to continue to reduce the recurrence rate to below 1%. The most popular prosthetic materials are polypropylene, polyester fiber mesh, and polytetrafluoroethylene. Use of the preperitoneal space also helped lower recurrence rates by allowing larger pieces of prosthetic material to be used and incorporating intraabdominal pressure to aid in keeping the mesh in place. Laparoscopy by itself has not helped lower recurrence rates below those achieved with open tension-free mesh repairs, but it has given the surgeon another option for accessing the preperitoneal space.

**ANSWER:** A

**16.** Which of the following is not true regarding laparoscopic hernia repair?

A. Local anesthesia with sedation is the most common form of anesthesia used.

B. It could lead injury to the genitofemoral nerve and the lateral femoral cutaneous nerve.

C. Transabdominal preperitoneal or total extraperitoneal approaches are commonly used.

D. Fixation devices for the mesh should not be placed below the iliopubic tract.

E. It is best suited for recurrent and bilateral hernias.

*Ref.:* 1-3, 7

**COMMENTS: Laparoscopic techniques** for repair of inguinal hernias were introduced in the 1990s and have gained mild to moderate acceptance, with less than 10% of all inguinal hernia repairs being performed via these approaches. The repairs are usually performed with the patient under general anesthesia, and cost is considerably higher than an open approach with local anesthesia and sedation. Although there is controversy regarding its use for unilateral, newly diagnosed hernias, it seems ideally suited for recurrent and bilateral hernias, where the disability and technical difficulty associated with open (conventional) repairs cannot be overlooked. Laparoscopy can be performed totally extraperitoneally by dissecting within the preperitoneal space or transabdominally. In either case, a preperitoneal repair is performed. Mesh fixation devices placed below the iliopubic tract risk injury to the genitofemoral nerve and the lateral femoral cutaneous nerve. Placement of fixation devices is also avoided below the internal inguinal ring in an area known as the "triangle of doom." This triangle is bordered laterally by the spermatic vessels and medially by the vas deferens. Located within this triangle are the external iliac artery and vein and the femoral nerve.

**ANSWER:** A

17. Indications for preperitoneal laparoscopic repair of groin hernias include all of the following except:

A. Pregnancy

B. Irradiation

C. Prior open mesh repair

D. American Society of Anesthesiologists Physical Status II (ASA II)

E. Bilaterality

*Ref.:* 1, 8

**COMMENTS:** Pregnancy is a contraindication to elective **laparoscopic repair of a groin hernia**. Irradiation of the lower abdominal wall is a relative contraindication to preperitoneal repair. A previous low midline incision from prostate or bladder surgery or irradiation may make it difficult to enter and dissect the preperitoneal space. The latter two contraindications may dictate an open anterior approach. Bilaterality and failed open mesh repair are indications for laparoscopic preperitoneal repair. Even though laparoscopic repair could be performed with the patient under local or regional anesthesia, it is usually best done under general anesthesia. Therefore, patients with severe risk factors are not candidates for it.

**ANSWER:** A

18. Which of the following is a true statement regarding umbilical hernias?

A. They are the embryonic equivalent of a small omphalocele.

B. Repair in infants is usually deferred until approximately 1 years of age.

C. Repair in adults is generally indicated.

D. The "vest-over-pants" type of repair is stronger than simple approximation of fascial margins.

E. They are most common in white infants.

*Ref.:* 1-3

**COMMENTS: Umbilical hernias** are the result of a patent umbilical ring, whereas an omphalocele is the result of failure of abdominal wall closure in the midline during early intrauterine life. Umbilical hernias are said to be present in 40% to 90% of African-American infants. Incarceration is rare in infants. Unless the defect is large, most surgeons defer repair until the child is approximately 4 years of age because spontaneous closure does occur. In adults, however, repair should be carried out promptly because of the risk for incarceration. There is no convincing evidence that a "vest-over-pants" type of repair is structurally superior to simple approximation of the fascial margins. Repair in adults may benefit from the use of prosthetic material, such as polypropylene, if the fascial defect is large or tension is present. There are several variations of mesh repairs with no evidence-based consensus of choice at this time.

**ANSWER:** C

19. Which of the following hernias represent incarceration of a limited portion of the small bowel?

A. Spigelian hernia

B. Grynfeltt hernia

C. Petit hernia

D. Richter hernia

E. Littre hernia

*Ref.:* 1-3

**COMMENTS:** Spigelian, Grynfeltt, and Petit hernias are abdominal or lumbar hernias in unusual anatomic locations. A **spigelian hernia** occurs at the lateral border of the rectus at the linea semicircularis. A Petit hernia occurs at the inferior lumbar triangle bordered by the latissimus dorsi, external oblique, and iliac crest. A Grynfeltt hernia occurs at the superior lumbar triangle where the internal oblique inserts on the twelfth rib. Richter and Littre hernias represent incarceration of a limited portion of the small bowel. A Littre hernia has an incarcerated Meckel diverticulum or the appendix as its contents. A Richter hernia is characterized by noncircumferential incarceration of the small bowel, usually only the antimesenteric portion. It is important to recognize Richter and Littre hernias because vascular compromise may occur without evidence of intestinal obstruction.

**ANSWER:** D

20. Which of the following statements is false with regard to the Kugel mesh repair for inguinal hernias?

A. Less than a 1% recurrence rate has been documented.

B. The mesh is placed in the preperitoneal space.

C. The mesh is usually sutured to the conjoined tendon and the inguinal ligament.

D. The repair can be performed on all varieties of inguinal hernias.

E. The procedure is best performed with the patient under local anesthesia.

*Ref.: 9*

COMMENTS: The minimally invasive **Kugel mesh hernia repair** is a preperitoneal hernia repair. The procedure is usually performed with local or epidural anesthesia through an oblique skin incision approximately 2 to 3 cm above the internal ring. A pocket is developed in the preperitoneal space, and oval mesh with a semirigid ring is placed so that it covers the femoral, direct, and indirect defects of all varieties of inguinal hernias. The mesh is not usually sutured in place, but occasionally a suture may be placed in the Cooper ligament for large direct hernias. In a series of 808 repairs, Kugel reported a 0.62% recurrence rate over a 54-month period. This repair has not gained as wide use as the Lichtenstein or plug-and-patch technique.

ANSWER: C

21. Which of the following items represents the optimal convalescent period required before returning to manual labor after inguinal mesh herniorrhaphy?

A. 6 to 8 weeks

B. 4 to 5 weeks

C. 2 to 3 weeks

D. 1 week

E. Less than 1 week

*Ref.: 1-4*

COMMENTS: Traditionally, patients who engage in strenuous activities have been allowed periods of 6 to 8 weeks to recuperate after traditional open herniorrhaphy. Studies have shown that collagen maturation and tensile strength in a hernia wound require months to reach maximal states. Tension-free repair using prosthetic material has allowed patients to return to normal activities sooner. These repairs, including the mesh-plug, Kugel, and laparoscopic procedures, have allowed patients to perform any activity that they choose as soon as they feel comfortable, which is usually within 2 to 3 weeks. In a study of mesh-plug repairs, 465 manual laborers **returned to work** without restriction on postoperative day 14. Studies have demonstrated longer recovery when workers' compensation is involved.

ANSWER: C

22. Which of the following statements is not true with regard to incisional ventral hernias?

A. Primary repairs are associated with a 30% to 50% recurrence rate.

B. The incidence of incisional hernias is between 2% and 11% after laparotomy.

C. Prosthetic mesh repairs have reduced the recurrence rate to 20% or less.

D. Bilayer mesh can be placed safely in the intraabdominal cavity.

E. Comorbid conditions, such as diabetes, hypertension, and obesity, are uncommon in patients with incisional hernias.

*Ref.: 3, 10, 11*

COMMENTS: In the United States, approximately 2 million laparotomies are performed each year, with a reported **incisional ventral hernia** rate of between 2% and 11%. The population of patients in whom wound dehiscence occurs tends to be obese and they frequently might have one or more of the following: comorbidities of a smoking history, hypertension, and diabetes. Primary incisional ventral hernia repairs have been associated with recurrence rates of up to 50%. Prosthetic mesh repairs have lowered the recurrence rates to less than 10%. Recently, it has been found that a bilayer prosthesis composed of both polypropylene and polytetrafluoroethylene can be placed safely in the abdominal cavity without the development of bowel obstruction or enterocutaneous fistulas. Intraabdominal placement of the mesh allows the greatest underlay of the fascial defect, thereby enabling the greatest amount of tissue ingrowth to occur. When polypropylene alone is placed in the intraabdominal cavity, bowel obstruction, enterocutaneous fistula, and difficult reentrance to the abdomen occur with an unacceptable frequency.

There is increasing evidence of less recurrence with laparoscopic incisional hernia repair with mesh. This is typically an inlay with considerable overlap over the fascial defect. Postoperative discomfort and local wound problems seem to be decreased. Lighter synthetic mesh is gaining in popularity. Again, expertise and experience in this advanced laparoscopic procedure are necessary to achieve low recurrence rates and avoid serious complications. A frequent but easily treated complication of laparoscopic repair is **seroma**, which can occur in up to 30% to 50% of patients. It is usually self-limited. The use of drains to avoid seroma formation is controversial, and it has not been associated with a decrease in its incidence. Aspiration of seromas is best accomplished under image guidance if they are symptomatic or concern about infection exists.

ANSWER: E

23. Inguinal hernias:

A. Are best treated with laparoscopic techniques

B. Should always be repaired

C. Benefit from the use of mesh in reducing recurrence later

D. Are associated with a high incidence of strangulation

E. Are rare in females

*Ref.: 11, 12*

COMMENTS: Open **anterior mesh repairs** are the most frequently used repairs for inguinal hernias, with plug-and-patch and Lichtenstein repairs being the most common. The benefit of laparoscopic repair is still controversial, however. Most recurrence rates are slightly higher for laparoscopic repair and are more dependent on surgeon expertise and experience. Laparoscopic repair requires general anesthesia. Most agree that laparoscopic approaches are preferred for recurrence of hernias treated by anterior mesh repair and for bilateral hernias.

A recent study by Fitzgibbons prospectively studied the nonoperative management of small, asymptomatic hernias. The overall results were comparable in those in the nonoperative group who ultimately underwent repair later. Although defending surgery may make subsequent repair of larger hernias more difficult, implantation of mesh, infection, and chronic pain are avoided as well and have minimized morbidity in the asymptomatic group. The incidence of strangulation in inguinal hernias is 1% to 2%, and that in femoral hernias is as high as 20%.

Inguinal hernias are the most common hernias in females, although direct inguinal hernias are rare.

ANSWER: C.

**24.** The separation-of-components technique:

    A. Is best for hernias with fascial defects of 3 cm or less

    B. Has a recurrence rate of approximately 10%

    C. May be used when there is contamination or bowel surgery is required

    D. Is contraindicated for recurrent incisional hernias

    E. Ideally it avoids the use of mesh

*Ref.:* 13

**COMMENTS:** Although primary suture repair with mesh has acceptable recurrence rates for small incisional hernias, recurrence rates are disappointing when these techniques are used for very large hernias. In addition, more complications are associated with mesh repair of very large hernias either by open or by laparoscopic technique.

    The **separation-of-components technique** has demonstrated improved results in the repair of massive incisional hernias, with recurrence rates of approximately 20%. This technique can be used when there is contamination or bowel surgery is required, thereby avoiding the dreaded complication of mesh infection.

    The separation-of-components technique can be used for failed mesh repairs. In selected cases the addition of soft synthetic mesh has improved success with the technique.

**A N S W E R :** C

**25.** A 75-year-old man is seen in the emergency department with a 2-hour history of incarcerated femoral hernia. He takes warfarin for a past history of atrial fibrillation and has an international normalized ratio (INR) of 3.1. Which of the following are correct treatments:

    A. Admit the patient for correction of the INR and repair the hernia in the morning.

    B. Perform emergency laparoscopic repair of the hernia.

    C. Perform emergency open repair of the hernia.

    D. Attempt a reduction of the hernia in the emergency department after sedation.

    E. Use of mesh in the repair is recommended.

*Ref.:* 1, 3

**COMMENTS:** The risk for strangulation in **incarcerated femoral hernias** is reported to be as high as 20% to 40%. It is believed that the window for successful treatment to avoid bowel resection is 4 to 6 hours. This clinical condition is considered a surgical emergency, and fresh frozen plasma can be administered just before and during surgery. Laparoscopic repair can be challenging with an incarcerated hernia, and in addition there is concern for increased bleeding in the patient. Laparoscopic repair also requires the use of mesh, which may become infected. Although mesh decreases recurrence in femoral hernias, it is probably not advisable in this setting. An open approach is probably preferred and can be a tissue-to-tissue repair. Any attempt at reduction is probably contraindicated because of the high potential for strangulation. If the bowel drops into the abdomen during an open approach, insertion of a scope into the hernia sac may be useful in evaluating the integrity of the affected bowel.

**A N S W E R :** C

**26.** Chronic groin pain following inguinal hernia repair may be the result of:

    A. Division of the nerves during the surgical procedure

    B. Postoperative scar tissue

    C. Use of mesh

    D. Injury from the use of tacks or staples

    E. All of the above

*Ref.:* 1

**COMMENTS:** **Groin pain** following **inguinal hernia repair** is much more common than recurrence and has occurred at incidence as high as 29% to 76% in several series. Transient pain with mild numbness inferior to the incision is common and often transient. Intense pain and loss of sensation that persists suggest nerve injury or entrapment. In open repair, the ilioinguinal, iliohypogastric, or genital branch of the genitofemoral nerve is most commonly involved. Injury to the lateral femoral cutaneous and genitofemoral nerves in laparoscopic repairs may occur from tack placement. **Mesh inguinodynia** has been reported to result from an inflammatory response to mesh or resultant scar tissue, or both. Although nerve blocks may be diagnostic or therapeutic, exploration may be necessary along with neurectomy, removal of mesh, or tack removal.

    Nerve division at the time of the original surgery has not proved to be efficacious.

    This frustrating problem is best prevented by meticulous identification and avoidance of entrapment of the aforementioned nerves in open repair and avoidance of tack placement, particularly in the triangle of doom in laparoscopic procedures.

**A N S W E R :** E

**27.** A 55-year-old man who runs marathons has a recurrent inguinal hernia. Which statement is correct?

    A. The previous type of repair has no significance in the treatment plan.

    B. A Shouldice repair is recommended.

    C. He will have to stop running marathons after repair.

    D. Repair can be performed with the patient under local anesthesia with a high likelihood of success.

    E. Laparoscopic repair, if the previous repair was performed in open manner with mesh, is an evidence-based choice.

*Ref.:* 11

**COMMENTS:** **Repair of recurrent inguinal hernia** can be challenging in terms of preventing recurrence and avoiding morbidity such as chronic pain. Tissue-to-tissue repairs may be repaired with an anterior mesh repair such as the Lichtenstein or plug-and-patch repair. Obtaining a prior operative report is strongly recommended to facilitate selection of the appropriate current repair. Laparoscopic repair for recurrence of a hernia after open anterior mesh repair is supported by prospective trials. The caveat is that such results require expertise and experience in laparoscopic repair. The Shouldice repair is not generally recommended for recurrent hernias. Repair by an expert surgeon should allow resumption of all normal activity and is recommended for active individuals. Repair can be deferred if asymptomatic in selected patients.

**A N S W E R :** E

**28.** A 55-year-old man with liver failure and ascites has an enlarging umbilical hernia. The ascites is refracting to diuretic therapy. The correct therapy is:

A. Open repair with waterproof mesh

B. High-volume paracentesis immediately before repair

C. Deferring hernia repair until correction of the ascites by transjugular intrahepatic portosystemic shunting (TIPS) or liver transplantation

D. Laparoscopic repair with inlay mesh

E. Repair of the hernia and use of abdominal binder after the operation

*Ref.:* 3

**COMMENTS:** Repair of any **hernia** in a patient with **ascites** is a challenging problem. In general, any consideration of elective repair should be deferred until the ascites is controlled. If there is slow breakdown and leakage of ascites, urgent repair may be necessary to prevent peritonitis. Frequent paracentesis may be helpful in this difficult scenario with assorted high morbidity.

**ANSWER:** C

# REFERENCES

1. Malangoni MA, Rosen MJ: Hernias. In Townsend CM, Beauchamp RD, Evers BM, et al, editors: *Sabiston textbook of surgery: the biological basis of modern surgical practice*, ed 18, Philadelphia, 2008, WB Saunders.

2. Richards AT, Quinn TH, Fitzgibbons RJ: Abdominal wall hernias. In Mulholland MW, Lillemoe KD, Doherty GM, et al, editors: *Greenfield's surgery: scientific principles and practice*, ed 4, Philadelphia, 2006, Lippincott Williams & Wilkins.

3. Sherman V, Macho JR, Brunicardi FC: Inguinal hernias. In Brunicardi FC, Andersen DK, Billiar TR, et al, editors: *Schwartz's principles of surgery*, ed 9, New York, 2010, McGraw-Hill.

4. Robbins AW, Rutkow IM: Mesh plug repair and groin hernia surgery, *Surg Clin North Am* 78:1007–1023, 1998.

5. Millikan KW, Cummings B, Doolas A: The Millikan modified mesh-plug hernioplasty, *Arch Surg* 138:525–530, 2003.

6. Amid PK: How to avoid recurrence in Lichtenstein tension-free hernioplasty, *Am J Surg* 184:259–260, 2002.

7. Millikan KW, Deziel DJ: The management of hernia: considerations in cost effectiveness, *Surg Clin North Am* 76:105–116, 1996.

8. Hernia Section. In Cameron JL, editor: *Current surgical therapy*, ed 9, Philadelphia, 2008, CV Mosby.

9. Kugel RD: Minimally invasive nonlaparoscopic preperitoneal and sutureless inguinal herniorrhaphy, *Am J Surg* 178:298–302, 1999.

10. Millikan KW, Baptista M, Amin B, et al: Intraperitoneal underlay ventral hernia repair utilizing bilayer expanded polytetrafluoroethylene and polypropylene mesh, *Am Surg* 69:287–292, 2003.

11. Itani KMF, Hur K, Kim LT, et al: Comparison of laparoscopic and open repair with mesh for the treatment of ventral incisional hernia: a randomized trial, *Arch Surg* 145:322–328, 2010.

12. Itani KM, Fitzgibbons R Jr, Awad SS, et al: Management of recurrent inguinal hernias, *J Am Coll Surg* 209:653–658, 2009.

13. Ko JH, Wang EC, Salvay DM, et al: Abdominal wall reconstruction: lessons learned from 200 "components separation" procedures, *Arch Surg* 144:1047–1055, 2009.

# CHAPTER 14

# Breast

*Steven D. Bines, M.D.; Thomas R. Witt, M.D.;*
*Katherine Kopkash, M.D.; and Andrea Madrigrano, M.D.*

1. A 35-year-old woman visits her physician after her initial mammogram, which was normal, and asks what her lifetime chance for the development of breast cancer is. She has no personal or family history of breast disease. Her menarche occurred at age 13, and her first child was born when she was 22. She has never taken oral contraceptives. Which is not a factor in estimating the Gail risk?

   A. Age

   B. History of previous breast biopsy

   C. Prior history of radiation exposure

   D. Age at menarche

   E. Age at first live birth

   *Ref.:* 1-5

**COMMENTS:** The American Cancer Society (ACS) in 2008 estimated that there would be 179,920 new cases of breast cancer in the United States and 40,730 deaths. The lifetime probability for the development of breast cancer is now estimated to be 1 in 8 (12.5%). After continuously increasing for more than 2 decades, breast cancer incidence rates in women decreased by 3.5% per year from 2001 to 2004, probably due in part to a slight decline in mammography utilization and a reduction in the use of hormone replacement therapy.

The **Gail model** is a validated breast cancer risk assessment tool that is primarily based on nonmodifiable breast cancer risk factors. It is a multivariate statistical model that uses age, age at menarche, age at first live birth, family history of breast cancer, and number of breast biopsies to estimate breast cancer risk in individuals without a previous history of breast cancer. It has been shown to accurately estimate the proportion of woman in whom breast cancer will develop when used in large groups. However, it performs poorly in discriminating between individual women in whom breast cancer will and will not develop. Although previous thoracic radiation therapy does increase breast cancer risk, it is not part of the Gail model. Other significant risk factors for breast cancer in women include previous biopsy specimens revealing atypical hyperplasia or lobular carcinoma in situ (LCIS), personal history of breast cancer, family history of breast cancer, and being a known carrier of a mutation in the *BRCA1* or *BRCA2* genes or a first-degree relative of an individual with a mutation.

**ANSWER:** C

2. With regard to the natural history of breast cancer, which of the following statements is true?

   A. On average, a 1-cm breast cancer has been present subclinically for approximately 1 year.

   B. Dimpling of the skin occurs as a result of glandular fibrosis and shortening of the Cooper ligaments.

   C. Skin edema in breast cancer is only a result of direct skin invasion by tumor.

   D. Lymph node metastasis first occurs in levels II and III of the axilla up to 20% of the time.

   E. Ipsilateral lung involvement occurs most often as a result of direct chest wall invasion.

   *Ref.:* 6

**COMMENTS:** Most breast cancers are estimated to have **volume-doubling times** of 2 to 12 months, thus suggesting that the average 1-cm tumor has been present for at least 5 years before clinical detection. Neither skin dimpling nor edema requires direct skin invasion. These conditions can result from fibrosis (with shortening of the Cooper ligaments) and lymphatic blockage in the subdermal tissues, respectively. The most common site of initial axillary lymph node metastasis is level I, which is inferior to the axillary vein and lateral to the pectoralis minor muscle. All forms of distant metastases, including ipsilateral lung involvement, are due to hematogenous spread. Lymph node metastasis first occurs in level II or III in 2% to 3% of patients, the so-called **skip metastasis**.

**ANSWER:** B

3. With regard to the natural history of breast cancer, which of the following statements is true?

   A. Virtually all patients with untreated breast cancer die within 2 years of their diagnosis.

   B. The likelihood of distant metastasis is related to the size of the primary tumor and involvement of the axillary nodes.

   C. The most common initial site for distant metastasis is the liver.

   D. Stage for stage, the survival rate for breast cancer in males is lower than that in females.

   E. Survival is longer in patients who undergo mastectomy than in patients who undergo breast conservation for stage I and II breast carcinoma.

   *Ref.:* 5, 6

**COMMENTS:** Breast cancer is a disease of wide biologic variability, and although the **median survival** in untreated patients is 2.7 years, nearly 20% of untreated patients survive 5 years and some as long as 15 years. The 5-year relative survival rate for stage 0 disease (carcinoma in situ with no regional node involvement or distant metastasis) is nearly 100%, whereas the 5-year survival rate for stage IV disease (distant metastasis) is 20%. There is an increased chance for distant metastasis in those with positive axillary nodes and large tumors. Therefore, adjuvant systemic therapy is recommended for these high-risk patients. The lung is the most common site of distant disease in patients dying of disseminated breast cancer. However, bone is the most common initial site of distant metastasis, followed by the lung, soft tissues, liver, and central nervous system. **Male breast cancer** accounts for 0.8% of all breast cancers, and the majority are invasive ductal carcinomas. When matched for age and stage, survival is similar to that in women. Multiple large randomized prospective trials (with follow-up now longer than 35 years) have shown that there is no survival advantage for mastectomy over breast conservation; however, the risk for local recurrence is slightly higher in those choosing breast conservation.

**ANSWER: B**

4. A 55-year-old woman is found on examination to have a 3-cm breast mass with palpable axillary lymph nodes. A modified radical mastectomy is performed, and pathologic evaluation reveals a 3.2-cm infiltrating ductal carcinoma with 5 of 15 axillary nodes positive for metastasis. Her review of systems is otherwise negative and findings on laboratory studies and basic imaging are normal. What is her tumor-nodes-metastasis (TNM) stage?

A. T2N1M0

B. T1N2M1

C. T2N2M0

D. T4N1M0

E. T3N2M0

*Ref.:* 5

**COMMENTS:** Breast cancer stage is determined by the results of pathologic evaluation of surgical resection specimens and imaging studies. It is classified with the **tumor-nodes-metastasis classification system**, which is based on a description of the primary tumor (T), the status of regional lymph nodes (N), and the presence of distant metastasis (M). The most widely used system is that of the American Joint Commission for Cancer (AJCC). T1 designates tumors up to 2 cm in size, T2 is used for those between 2 and 5 cm, T3 indicates tumors larger than 5 cm, and T4 is used for tumors of any size with extension to the chest wall or skin. N1 indicates metastasis to 1 to 3 axillary nodes or clinically occult internal mammary nodes (or both); N2 includes metastasis to 4 to 9 axillary nodes or clinically positive internal mammary nodes (without axillary metastasis); and N3 is used for metastasis to 10 or more axillary nodes, a combination of axillary and internal mammary nodes, or paraclavicular nodes. M1 designates evidence of distant metastasis.

**ANSWER: C**

5. A 58-year-old woman has a chronic erythematous, oozing, eczematoid rash involving her left nipple and areola. There are no palpable breast masses, and the findings on a recently obtained mammogram are normal. Which of the following recommendations is appropriate?

A. Referral to a dermatologist

B. Oral vitamin E and topical aloe and lanolin

C. Biopsy

D. Encouragement of the patient to buy a nonallergenic brassiere

E. Routine clinical and mammographic follow-up in 1 year because findings on the current mammogram are normal

*Ref.:* 5, 6

**COMMENTS: Paget disease** accounts for 1% or less of breast malignancies and is characterized clinically by nipple erythema and irritation with associated itching and may progress to nipple crusting and ulceration. A manifestation of this sort is very concerning, and therefore biopsy of the nipple is necessary. Delay in diagnosis of Paget disease of the breast is common because of the mistaken presumption that the findings represent a benign dermatologic condition. Pathologically, Paget cells are large, pale-staining cells with round or oval nuclei and large nucleoli and are located between the normal keratinocytes of the nipple epidermis. More than 97% of patients with Paget disease have underlying ductal carcinoma in situ (DCIS) or invasive breast carcinoma, but there is an accompanying mass in only 54% of patients. Treatment of Paget disease includes mastectomy with axillary staging or wide excision of the nipple and areola to achieve clear margins, possibly axillary staging, and radiation therapy.

**ANSWER: C**

6. Which of the following is not a characteristic of medullary breast cancer?

A. Lymphocytic infiltrate

B. Benign appearance on ultrasound

C. High rate of lymph node metastasis

D. Statistically better than average prognosis

E. Usually manifested as a palpable mass

*Ref.:* 5, 6

**COMMENTS: Medullary breast cancer** accounts for approximately 5% of breast cancers. It is usually manifested as a palpable mass with smooth borders on imaging that can mimic benign conditions. On ultrasound, medullary carcinoma often has smooth contours, homogeneous interior echogenicity, and posterior enhancement, which are the same findings that one would expect with a fibroadenoma. These tumors are characterized by an infiltrate of small mononuclear lymphocytes, are less likely to be associated with axillary node metastasis, and have a better than average prognosis.

**ANSWER: C**

7. A 34-year-old woman underwent wide local excision, axillary dissection, and radiation therapy (5000 cGy over a 5-week period) in her left breast for a node-positive, estrogen receptor (ER)-negative, 2-cm infiltrating ductal carcinoma 3 years earlier. She received four cycles of adjuvant chemotherapy with cyclophosphamide (Cytoxan) and doxorubicin (Adriamycin) at that time. The surgeon now performs a biopsy of a new 2-cm mass in the same breast, and it shows infiltrating ductal carcinoma. She has no other evidence of local, regional, or distant disease on imaging studies and clinical examination. Which of the following treatment plans is most appropriate?

A. Left total mastectomy without axillary exploration

B. Reexcision to free margins, sentinel lymph node biopsy, and a 5000-cGy "boost" to the breast

C. A 5000-cGy "boost" to the breast and combination 5-fluorouracil–based chemotherapy

D. Taxane-based chemotherapy alone

E. Bilateral total mastectomy

*Ref.: 5, 7, 8*

**COMMENTS:** The **National Surgical Adjuvant Breast and Bowel Project (NSABP) B-06 trial** found that approximately 8.8% of patients treated by lumpectomy, axillary dissection, radiation therapy, and chemotherapy had a local recurrence by 10 years after initial treatment. A "**salvage**" **mastectomy** is usually required in these situations and results in long-term survival similar to that of patients who had a mastectomy performed as the primary operation. In the absence of palpable nodes, a second surgical axillary evaluation is unnecessary and hazardous. The effects of ionizing irradiation are cumulative and do not diminish with time, so additional radiation would lead to excessive toxicity in normal tissue in the irradiated area. Because local control is needed for this tumor, chemotherapy alone would be an inappropriate treatment option. Right total mastectomy is not indicated at this time based on the information provided.

**ANSWER:** A

8. Which characteristic of a positive axillary sentinel lymph node is not associated with additional positive nodes and distant recurrence?

A. Node diameter greater than 1 cm

B. Firmness on palpation

C. Isolated tumor cells

D. Nodal micrometastases

E. Grossly irregular nodal border

*Ref.: 9*

**COMMENTS:** Metastasis to regional lymph nodes is the most important prognostic factor in breast cancer patients. **Sentinel lymph node biopsy** has become a standard diagnostic procedure in clinically node-negative breast cancer patients. The standard nodal analysis includes both staining with hematoxylin and eosin and immunohistochemistry. **Nodal micrometastases** are considered to be 0.2 mm to 2 mm, whereas isolated tumor cells are less than 0.2 mm. A recently published prospective breast cancer study found that sentinel node micrometastases, but not isolated tumor cells, were associated with additional positive nodes and distant recurrence. Clinical evidence of lymph node involvement at the time of sentinel node surgery, whether by size, texture, or irregular borders, is associated with an increased likelihood of other nodes being involved. These data suggest that in the future, axillary lymph node dissection may be unnecessary in patients with isolated tumor cells but should be considered in patients with sentinel lymph node micrometastases.

**ANSWER:** C

9. A 39-year-old woman has an ill-defined 2-cm mass in the upper outer quadrant of her right breast. Mammography and ultrasound confirm this solid lesion. Ultrasound-guided fine-needle aspiration is performed, and cytologic evaluation reveals a highly cellular, monomorphic pattern. There are poorly cohesive intact cells, nuclear "crowding" with variation

in nuclear size, radial dispersion and clumping of the chromatin, and prominent nucleoli. What is the diagnosis?

A. Benign cyst contents

B. Fibroadenoma

C. Phyllodes tumor

D. Carcinoma

E. Fat necrosis

*Ref.: 5*

**COMMENTS:** Fine-needle aspiration has become a routine part of the pathologic diagnosis of breast masses. The fluid and cellular material from the aspirate are either submitted in physiologically buffered saline or fixed immediately on slides in 95% ethyl alcohol. Cyst fluid is usually turbid and dark green or amber and can be discarded if the mass totally disappears and the fluid is not bloody. **Fibroadenomas** are benign solid tumors characterized by a proliferation of connective tissue and a variable component of ductal elements that may appear compressed by the swirls of fibroblastic growth. **Phyllodes tumors** are histologically similar to fibroadenoma, but the whorled stroma forms larger clefts lined by epithelium that resemble clusters of leaflike structures. Invasive carcinomas are recognized by their lack of overall architecture, by the infiltration of cells haphazardly into a variable amount of stroma, or by the formation of sheets of continuous and monotonous cells without respect for form and function of a glandular organ. **Fat necrosis** will histologically show a lesion composed of lipid-laden macrophages, scar tissue, and chronic inflammatory cells.

**ANSWER:** D

10. A 42-year-old woman underwent lumpectomy and axillary dissection for a 2-cm, moderately differentiated, ER-negative infiltrating ductal carcinoma. Pathologic examination revealed adequate margins, and 1 of 19 lymph nodes was found to be positive for carcinoma. Which of the following treatment plans is most appropriate?

A. Radiation alone

B. Single-drug chemotherapy and radiation therapy

C. Multidrug chemotherapy and radiation therapy

D. Multidrug chemotherapy, radiation therapy, and tamoxifen

E. Multidrug chemotherapy alone

*Ref.: 5-7*

**COMMENTS:** Multiple randomized prospective studies have shown both disease-free and overall survival benefit for **adjuvant chemotherapy** in node-positive premenopausal women, the greatest advantage occurring in those with one to three positive nodes. Postmenopausal node-positive women have generally shown a more modest benefit. Multiple-drug therapy has consistently been more effective than single-drug therapy. Adding **tamoxifen** to the chemotherapy for node-positive premenopausal patients confers additional benefit when the cancer is ER positive, but it is not beneficial in ER-negative cancers. The use of radiation therapy in conjunction with surgery has allowed dramatic reductions in the extent of surgery required for local control of breast cancer. At 20 years of follow-up, local recurrence rates are approximately 8.8% for lumpectomy plus radiation as compared with 44% for lumpectomy alone.

**ANSWER:** C

**11.** Which of the following is not an indication for postmastectomy radiotherapy?

A. T3 tumors

B. Multicentric DCIS larger than 6 cm

C. Four or more positive axillary lymph nodes

D. Inflammatory breast cancer

E. Gross extranodal extension

*Ref.:* 5, 7

**COMMENTS:** For most patients with breast cancer, mastectomy provides effective local control and radiation therapy is not required. However, certain subsets remain at increased risk for local and regional recurrence and benefit from the ability of radiation to control any microscopic residual tumor. **Adjuvant radiation therapy** after mastectomy does decrease local-regional recurrences by up to two thirds, and some studies have shown an improvement in overall survival. Radiation therapy has many potential side effects as a result of irradiation of the chest wall, including skin ulceration, arm edema, rib fracture, radiation-induced pneumonitis, chest wall sarcoma, and cardiac toxicity. Therefore, most centers now recommend chest wall and nodal irradiation after mastectomy only for patients at increased risk for recurrence. This category includes those with multiple positive lymph nodes (more than four), patients with large cancers (>5 cm), aggressive histology (diffuse vascular invasion), and extranodal extension of breast cancer. Other indicators include positive surgical margins, **inflammatory breast cancer**, or involvement of the skin, fascia, or skeletal muscle. Extensive DCIS is not an indication for radiation therapy, provided that the margins of the mastectomy specimen are not involved.

**A N S W E R :  B**

**12.** Which of the following 5-year survival rates by stage for treated breast cancer is incorrect?

A. Stage I: 95% to 100%

B. Stage II: 80% to 90%

C. Stage III: 50% to 70%

D. Stage IV: 1% to 5%

E. Stage Tis: 98% to 100%

*Ref.:* 5

**COMMENTS:** The wide range of **survival rates** in patients with the same stages of breast cancer reflects the wide range of staging criteria used by various investigators, as well as the variability in biologic behavior among the differing subtypes of breast cancer within a given stage. Because of increasingly effective systemic therapies, patients with stage IV disease now have up to a 20% 5-year relative survival rate.

**A N S W E R :  D**

**13.** Which is not true regarding chronic granulomatous mastitis?

A. Tuberculosis is a common granulomatous infection of the breast.

B. Chronic granulomatous mastitis includes variants of ductal ectasia.

C. It can be recognized on frozen section.

D. It may be a sign of a systemic disorder.

E. This classification is considered to be a descriptive diagnostic term.

*Ref.:* 7

**COMMENTS: Chronic granulomatous mastitis** is a broad descriptive designation that includes variants of ductal ectasia, granulomatous infectious diseases, and idiopathic granulomatous conditions. It may be difficult to distinguish chronic granulomatous mastitis from ductal ectasia or from infectious granulomatous mastitis. Specific granulomatous infections such as tuberculosis may occur in the breast, although this is very uncommon; tuberculosis is responsible for approximately 0.025% to 0.1% of all surgically treated diseases of the breast. Recognition of granulomatous inflammation at the time of frozen section should prompt a search for the etiologic agent through culture. Granulomatous mastitis may be the initial sign of a systemic disorder such as **Wegener granulomatosis**. **Sarcoidosis** is another diagnostic consideration when granulomas are found in the breast. These conditions are often treated with corticosteroid therapy, with promising results.

**A N S W E R :  A**

**14.** A 75-year-old woman has a 1.2-cm mass in her right breast on physical examination that is found to be an infiltrating ductal carcinoma, ER/progesterone receptor (PR) positive, on core biopsy. Her axilla is clinically negative, as is her review of systems. She has multiple medical problems and wants to have as little done as possible. Which factor is not significantly associated with lymph node metastasis in elderly patients?

A. Age

B. Tumor location

C. Tumor size

D. Lymphovascular invasion

E. Human epidermal growth factor receptor-2 (HER-2)/neu status

*Ref.:* 10

**COMMENTS:** Nodal evaluation in elderly women with breast cancer remains controversial. The risk associated with lymph node evaluation must be balanced with the benefit of staging and local control. A recent large prospective multicenter trial found that on multivariate analysis, patient age, tumor size, and lymphovascular invasion were significant factors predicting **lymph node metastasis**. Patient race, palpable tumor, tumor grade, histologic subtype, and tumor location were not found to be significant. These findings suggest that some **elderly breast cancer** patients with a low likelihood of lymph node metastasis may be spared lymph node evaluation. HER-2/neu status is not an indicator of lymph node status.

**A N S W E R :  B**

**15.** A 42-year-old woman with no family history of breast cancer has an ill-defined thickening in the upper outer quadrant of her left breast. Her mammogram shows only a minimal increase in the fibroglandular markings in that area. Ultrasound examination reveals no mass lesion. One month later, the thickening is slightly more prominent, and the surgeon performs a biopsy of the area in question. The pathologic diagnosis is "stromal fibrosis," with the comments describing increased fibrosis, ductal ectasia, periductal inflammation, and microcyst formation with no epithelial hyperplasia. What is the increase in likelihood that breast cancer will subsequently develop?

A. Essentially none

B. Three times

C. Five times

D. Ten times

E. Twenty times

*Ref.:* 7

**COMMENTS: Stromal fibrosis** has not been shown to increase the incidence of breast cancer. The presence of proliferative lesions, such as **papillomatosis** (multiple tiny ductal papillomas) or hyperplasia of the usual variety, very slightly increases the risk for breast cancer. **Atypical hyperplasia** increases the risk fourfold unless it accompanies a strong family history of breast cancer, in which case the risk is increased ninefold.

**ANSWER:** A

16. A 24-year-old woman who is 9 months postpartum has a tender, fluctuant area in her right breast near the areolar border. She denies fever or chills and has no other medical problems. What is the most appropriate treatment?

A. Surgical incision and drainage

B. Needle aspiration

C. Multidrug antibiotics

D. Core needle biopsy to exclude malignancy

E. Needle aspiration and antibiotics

*Ref.:* 5, 11

**COMMENTS:** Infections of the breast fall into two general categories, **lactational infections** (such as in this patient) and **chronic subareolar infections** associated with **ductal ectasia**. Lactation-related infections are thought to arise from entry of bacteria through the nipple and into the duct system and are characterized by erythema, tenderness, and less often, fever and leukocytosis. They are most frequently due to *Staphylococcus aureus*. In the past, these abscesses were often drained surgically, but the more recent literature supports antibiotics and needle aspiration of the abscess.

**ANSWER:** E

17. With regard to breast development, which of the following statements is true?

A. Breast enlargement in male neonates is indicative of an underlying estrogen-secreting adrenal tumor.

B. Accessory nipples can be found anywhere from the axilla to the groin.

C. Extramammary breast tissue is not under the influence of the hormonal status of the patient.

D. Inverted nipples in children suggest underlying breast cancer.

E. Gynecomastia in a prepubertal boy requires excision.

*Ref.:* 5, 6

**COMMENTS:** If the embryologic mammary ridge extending from the axilla to the groin fails to involute fully, accessory nipples (**polythelia**) can appear along this route. Accessory breast tissue (**polymastia**) is also seen frequently in the axilla and may enlarge during pregnancy and lactation, as well as during the response to normal fluctuations in the patient's hormonal status during her menstrual cycle. **Accessory breast tissue** can be detected on mammography and may present differential diagnostic difficulties for both the mammographer and the clinician. Shortly after birth, both males and females may exhibit unilateral or bilateral breast enlargement, which is attributed to high levels of circulating maternal estrogen. These changes regress spontaneously during the neonatal period. In female infants, failure of one or both nipples to evert following birth and into adulthood leads to functional problems related to future breastfeeding but is unrelated to future breast cancer. **Gynecomastia** in prepubescent boys is usually a transient condition.

**ANSWER:** B

18. Which of the following is not true regarding magnetic resonance imaging (MRI) for evaluation of breast abnormalities?

A. It is useful for finding the primary breast lesion in patients with positive axillary nodes but no mammographic evidence of a breast tumor.

B. It is more accurate than mammography in diagnosing invasive lobular cancer.

C. It is more accurate than mammography in assessing tumor extent in older women.

D. Its sensitivity in detecting invasive cancer is greater than 90%.

E. Its use as a screening tool is still under investigation.

*Ref.:* 5

**COMMENTS: Magnetic resonance imaging** is increasingly being used for the evaluation of breast abnormalities. It is useful in finding the primary breast lesion in patients with malignant axillary nodes but no palpable or mammographic evidence of a primary breast tumor. MRI may be more accurate than mammography in assessing the extent of the primary tumor, particularly in young women with dense breast tissue, and in diagnosing invasive lobular cancer, and it may help determine eligibility for breast conservation. Use of MRI as a screening tool is still under investigation, but it appears promising for early detection of malignancy in patients with *BRCA* gene mutations. The sensitivity of MRI for invasive cancer is greater than 90%, but it is only 60% or less for DCIS.

**ANSWER:** C

19. With regard to current therapy for stage I and stage II breast cancer, which statement is true?

A. The Halstead radical mastectomy has resulted in a cure rate superior to that of other surgical treatment options.

B. Lumpectomy and radiation therapy are associated with a local recurrence rate of 25%.

C. Oncotype DX assists in making decisions regarding chemotherapy in node-negative, ER-positive, HER-2/neu–negative cancers.

D. Node-negative patients who undergo modified radical mastectomy have a survival advantage over those who choose lumpectomy, sentinel lymph node biopsy, and radiation therapy.

E. There is no role for skin-sparing mastectomy in the treatment of invasive cancers.

*Ref.:* 6-8, 12

**COMMENTS:** The two most commonly used modalities of definitive therapy for stage I and II breast cancer are (1) **modified radical mastectomy**, which preserves the pectoralis major muscle while excising all breast tissue, including the nipple and axillary nodal basin, and (2) wide local excision of the breast tumor (**lumpectomy**) and axillary evaluation (**sentinel lymph node biopsy** or **axillary dissection**, or both) in conjunction with post-operative whole-breast irradiation. A number of large randomized trials have shown no significant disease-free survival advantage for the more radical (pectoralis-removing) Halsted mastectomy. Lumpectomy plus radiation therapy is associated with a local recurrence rate of 14%. **Oncotype DX** is increasingly being used to determine how aggressive certain cancers are and can therefore help guide decisions regarding adjuvant therapy. **Cyclin D1** has been implicated as an important oncogene in breast cancer, and overexpression of it correlates with the expression of ER, yet it has not yet been shown to have independent prognostic significance. There is consensus that **p53 expression** in breast cancer correlates with high tumor grade, indices of proliferation such as S-phase fraction and proliferating cell nuclear antigen staining, aneuploidy, and absence of ER and PR and therefore correlates with poor prognosis. In general, **B cell lymphoma-2 expression** is associated with a phenotype that has a favorable prognosis and correlates with the presence of ER, whereas **B cell lymphoma-$X_L$** overexpression has an association with axillary lymph node positivity and high tumor grade. The **National Surgical Adjuvant Breast and Bowel Project B-06 trial** showed that regardless of nodal status, there was no difference in overall survival between patients undergoing modified radical mastectomy and those undergoing lumpectomy with surgical axillary staging and radiation therapy. A skin-sparing mastectomy can be performed for invasive cancer if immediate reconstruction is planned, and it does not have a detrimental effect on long-term survival or local recurrence rates.

**ANSWER:  C**

20. Which of the following clinical characteristics of breast masses on physical examination is more suggestive of malignant than benign disease?

    A. Indistinct borders blending into surrounding breast tissue

    B. Excessive mobility within breast tissue

    C. Tenderness over a soft mass

    D. Tethering to underlying muscular structures

    E. Variability through the menstrual cycle

*Ref.:* 5, 6

**COMMENTS:** Although there are many exceptions to the classic physical findings of breast cancer, the typical breast carcinoma is hard and has fairly distinct borders. Fixation to deeper structures is highly suggestive of malignancy. A smooth, rubbery, mobile mass is more suggestive of **fibroadenoma**. **Fibrocystic disease** may be manifested as a disk-like or polynodular thickening, with one or more of the borders blending indistinctly into the surrounding breast tissue. Tenderness over a soft breast mass is often found with breast cysts. Variability over the **menstrual cycle** is a benign feature.

**ANSWER:  D**

21. Which of the following is not true regarding skin-sparing mastectomy?

    A. Involves the removal of 30% to 50% of breast skin

    B. May be appropriate for a central tumor that would require removal of the nipple/areola complex

    C. May be used for multifocal, minimal breast cancers

    D. Includes skin excision with 1-cm margins around the previous biopsy site or scar overlying the index neoplasm

    E. Requires skin excision (marginal only) of the nipple/areola complex

*Ref.:* 7

**COMMENTS:** Wide skin excision is used routinely in every radical and modified mastectomy and often includes excision in excess of 30% to 50% of the breast skin. **"Skin-sparing" mastectomy**, or limited skin excision, can be defined as excision of the nipple/areola complex, the skin around the biopsy site, and the skin within 1 to 2 cm of the tumor margin. This technique usually sacrifices only 5% to 10% of the breast skin, and the excision is usually closed primarily or in association with breast reconstruction. The extent of breast skin excision required with mastectomy has decreased as locoregional control measures have improved over the last 60 years. Patients who are not candidates for lumpectomy and postoperative radiation therapy but are candidates for skin-sparing mastectomy include those with multicentric disease, invasive carcinoma associated with an extensive intraductal component, T2 tumors with a difficult-to-interpret mammograms, and central tumors that would require removal of the nipple/areola complex. The skin-sparing mastectomy may include sentinel lymph node biopsy as indicated and, if histologically positive, axillary lymph node dissection to be completed synchronously.

**ANSWER:  A**

22. With regard to phyllodes tumors of the breast, which statement is incorrect?

    A. It is histologically characterized by epithelial cystlike spaces.

    B. Examination reveals a firm, mobile, well-circumscribed mass.

    C. Ten percent to 15% are malignant.

    D. The benign version can grow aggressively and recur locally.

    E. It commonly metastasizes to lymph nodes.

*Ref.:* 5-7

**COMMENTS:** Although only approximately 10% of all **phyllodes tumors** (also called cystosarcoma phyllodes) are malignant, they are still the most common primary sarcoma of the breast. The benign variant of **cystosarcoma** is considered by many to be a "giant fibroadenoma" and, accordingly, is usually manifested clinically as a solitary, discrete, mobile mass within the breast (generally quite a bit larger than the average fibroadenoma). The diagnosis of malignancy in phyllodes tumor is at times difficult because of the poor correlation between histologic features and clinical behavior. The benign and malignant varieties may be differentiated by counting the number of **mitoses** seen per high-power field, in addition to observing other features. If the tumor is histologically benign, wide local excision is considered adequate treatment. Even when benign, phyllodes tumors have a high frequency of local recurrence, and therefore careful long-term follow-up is essential. In the malignant variety, lymph node involvement is uncommon because these tumors usually metastasize through the bloodstream, most often to the lung. Therefore, **total mastectomy** without axillary dissection may be indicated; although for small malignant lesions, wide excision with 2-cm margins may be appropriate.

Malignant cystosarcoma has no significant incidence of multicentricity within the breast (unlike ductal or lobular carcinoma).

**ANSWER:** E

23. With regard to breast carcinoma in men, which statement is true?

   A. It is detected most commonly in men 60 to 70 years old.

   B. Gynecomastia is a risk factor.

   C. It is commonly associated with a mutation in the *BRCA1* gene.

   D. The prognosis is worse stage for stage than for women.

   E. Sentinel lymph node biopsy is contraindicated.

*Ref.:* 5

**COMMENTS: Breast cancer** infrequently occurs in **men**; it accounts for just 0.8% of all breast cancers and less than 1% of all newly diagnosed cancers in men. The median age at diagnosis is 68 years, 5 years older than in women. Risk factors include increasing age, radiation exposure, factors related to abnormalities in estrogen and androgen balance (testicular disease, infertility, obesity, and cirrhosis), and genetic predisposition, including **Klinefelter syndrome**, family history, and ***BRCA2* gene mutations**. Ninety percent of male breast cancers are **invasive ductal carcinomas**. The majority of men with breast cancer have a breast mass, and when matched for age and stage, survival is similar to that in women. Treatment of carcinoma in the male breast is similar to that in the female breast, and prognostic factors include nodal involvement, tumor size, histologic grade, and hormone receptor status.

**ANSWER:** A

24. With regard to breast cancer screening, which of the following is not a current recommendation of the ACS?

   A. Monthly breast self-examinations are strongly encouraged and should be performed the week before menses.

   B. Screening mammograms should be performed yearly in women older than 40 years.

   C. Women 20 to 30 years of age should undergo clinical breast examinations at least every 3 years.

   D. Women with greater than a 20% lifetime risk for the development of breast cancer should undergo MRI and mammographic screening yearly.

   E. Women 40 years and older should have yearly clinical breast examinations.

*Ref.:* 1

**COMMENTS:** Research has shown that routine **breast self-examination** plays only a small role in breast cancer detection in comparison to being detected by chance or by physician examination or breast imaging. Therefore, breast self-examination should be discussed with patients as an option once they are in their 20s but is not a recommendation at this time. Women 40 years and older should undergo screening mammography every year and should continue to do so for as long as they are in good health. Women in their 20s and 30s should have a **clinical breast examination** as part of a periodic health examination by a health professional at a minimum of every 3 years. After the age of 40, women should have a breast examination by a health professional every year. Women at high risk (>20% lifetime risk) should undergo **magnetic resonance imaging** and **mammography** yearly. Women

at moderately increased risk (15% to 20% lifetime risk) should talk with their doctors about the benefits and limitations of adding MRI screening to their yearly mammogram. Yearly MRI screening is not recommended for women whose lifetime risk for breast cancer is less than 15%.

**ANSWER:** A

25. Modern therapy for breast cancer focuses on molecular markers to help guide treatment strategies. Which of the following statements is correct?

   A. Carriers of the *BRCA2* mutation are more likely to have triple-negative cancers.

   B. HER-2–positive cancers are unlikely to respond to treatment with trastuzumab.

   C. ER-positive/HER-2–negative patients should be treated with endocrine therapy.

   D. All breast cancers are sensitive to endocrine therapy.

*Ref.:* 5

**COMMENTS:** Before discovery of the ER, all breast cancers were thought to be sensitive to endocrine therapy. Clinical trials and laboratory research established that only cancers containing ER (ER-positive cancers) respond to endocrine treatments. Furthermore, because binding of **estrogen** to its receptor induces **progesterone receptor** expression, the presence of PRs correlates with response to endocrine therapy. The presence of both receptors in a tumor is associated with an almost 80% chance of favorably responding to hormone blockade. Recently, the uniqueness of tumors that are ER negative, PR negative, and HER-2 negative has been investigated, and these **triple-negative cancers** express proteins in common with myoepithelial cells at the base of mammary ducts and therefore are also called **basal-like cancers**. Women who carry a disease-associated mutation in ***BRCA1*** (but not *BRCA2*) are much more likely to contract a *basal-like cancer* than other subtypes. **Human epidermal growth factor receptor-2** (or the ***erb*-B2/neu protein**) is a product of the *erb*-B2 gene and is amplified in about 20% of human breast cancers. Trastuzumab is a humanized antibody directed against the extracellular domain of the surface receptor and is effective treatment of HER-2–positive breast cancer.

**ANSWER:** C

26. A 57-year-old woman with a 1.5-cm infiltrating ductal carcinoma is found to be ER negative, PR negative, and HER-2/neu positive. She comes to your office to discuss treatment options. What would you recommend?

   A. Modified radical mastectomy alone

   B. Wide local excision, radiation therapy, and tamoxifen

   C. Simple mastectomy, sentinel lymph node biopsy, trastuzumab (Herceptin), and tamoxifen

   D. Modified radical mastectomy and adjuvant chemotherapy

   E. Wide local excision, sentinel lymph node biopsy, radiation therapy, and adjuvant chemotherapy with trastuzumab

*Ref.:* 5

**COMMENTS:** In current practice, **lumpectomy** (wide local excision) is considered in cases in which the tumor can be excised to clear margins and leave an acceptable cosmetic result. Randomized trials have studied breast conservation for tumors up to 5 cm in size. Patients who undergo lumpectomy followed by radiation therapy have the same survival rate as do those who undergo modified radical mastectomy. **Sentinel lymph node biopsy** is an acceptable method of staging the axilla in breast cancer patients without clinically suspicious lymph nodes. Because the patient is ER and PR negative, she would not derive any benefit from treatment with tamoxifen. However, she is HER-2/neu positive and would therefore benefit from treatment with **tratuzumab**. Recent studies have shown that the addition of trastuzumab to conventional chemotherapy significantly reduces the rate of recurrence (almost a 50% reduction).

**A N S W E R :**  E

27. A 64-year-old woman underwent modified radical mastectomy without reconstruction 10 years earlier for a 3-cm, node-positive, ER-negative, infiltrating ductal carcinoma. She comes to you with a 2-cm immobile nodule in her scar. Which of the following statements is false?

   A. The patient should be restaged to detect any distant disease.

   B. Wide local excision followed by radiotherapy is appropriate if no distant disease is detected.

   C. There is level I evidence supporting a survival advantage in all age groups if chemotherapy is given.

   D. Local recurrence following mastectomy occurs in approximately 5% of patients.

   E. If metastatic disease is found, chemotherapy is favored over wide local excision alone.

*Ref.: 7*

**COMMENTS: Local recurrence of breast cancer** following mastectomy occurs in approximately 5% of patients. Local excision plus irradiation is appropriate treatment for this patient. In older patients, the benefits of **chemotherapy** are generally less, and the ability to deliver optimal therapy is made more difficult by the presence of other impairments. In elderly patients, the decision to administer adjuvant chemotherapy is made on an individual basis since there are no firm results from clinical trials. **Chest wall recurrence** in this setting is often eventually accompanied by metastatic disease, even though initial evaluation may not detect it.

**A N S W E R :**  C

28. A 32-year-old woman who is 10 weeks pregnant has a palpable 2.5-cm mass in the upper outer quadrant of her right breast. The mass is not visualized on ultrasound. Which of the following management options is appropriate?

   A. Reassurance of the patient that this is probably benign in nature

   B. Reexamination 1 month after delivery

   C. Cyst aspiration and, if no fluid is obtained, reassurance of the patient

   D. Palpation-guided core needle biopsy

   E. Simple mastectomy

*Ref.: 5, 7*

**COMMENTS:** See Question 29.

**A N S W E R :**  D

29. Core needle biopsy in the pregnant patient in Question 28 demonstrates an infiltrating ductal carcinoma, grade 3, ER negative, HER-2/neu negative. Further evaluation reveals a suspicious, palpable 1.5-cm right axillary mass that is positive on fine-needle biopsy. What is the most appropriate next step in her treatment?

   A. Chemotherapy and radiation therapy

   B. Modified radical mastectomy followed by chemotherapy

   C. Lumpectomy, axillary dissection, and radiation therapy

   D. Simple mastectomy with sentinel lymph node biopsy and chemotherapy

   E. Lumpectomy, axillary dissection, and immediate radiation therapy

*Ref.: 5, 7*

**COMMENTS:** Stage for stage, the **prognosis of breast cancer** is the same in pregnant as in nonpregnant women. However, the overall prognosis for **pregnant women** is worse because they tend to initially be seen with a more advanced stage. Reluctance to evaluate breast masses in pregnant women on the part of both the patient and her physician is a contributing factor. The evaluation and treatment of breast masses must not be delayed because of pregnancy. Diagnostic mammograms can be performed safely in pregnant women with proper shielding of the uterus. However, radiation therapy, even with proper shielding, is associated with a significant incidence of fetal injury and is contraindicated. Mastectomy is usually appropriate during early and middle pregnancy. During the third trimester, breast preservation may be considered if early delivery after confirmation of fetal maturity would facilitate prompt commencement of whole-breast irradiation. This patient has a suspicious axillary node and is therefore not a candidate for sentinel lymph node biopsy. It is worth noting that there have been no reported consequences to either the mother or the fetus from injections of technetium sulfur colloid or isosulfan blue, which are the two agents that may be injected during sentinel lymph node biopsy. This does not imply that there is no risk, simply that none have been reported to date. Chemotherapy has been given safely to patients in the second trimester. For patients in the second and third trimester in whom breast cancer is diagnosed, breast conservation therapy can be an option, with radiation therapy being delayed until after delivery.

**A N S W E R :**  B

30. A 40-year-old woman has a mammogram showing extensive microcalcifications involving the entire upper aspect of her right breast. Stereotactic biopsy is performed, and pathologic analysis reveals grade 3 DCIS with comedo features. What is the appropriate management?

   A. Total mastectomy with sentinel lymph node biopsy

   B. Wide local excision alone

   C. Modified radical mastectomy

   D. Wide local excision with radiotherapy

   E. Radiotherapy alone

*Ref.: 5, 6*

**COMMENTS:** See Question 31.

**A N S W E R :**  A

**31.** In the patient in Question 30, the operating surgeon performed a total mastectomy. Final pathologic review of the breast showed extensive DCIS and multiple foci of infiltrating ductal carcinoma, with the largest foci being 1.5 cm, ER positive, and HER-2/neu negative with a negative sentinel node. What is the next best step in the management of this patient?

A. Sentinel lymph node biopsy

B. Chemotherapy

C. Tamoxifen alone

D. Axillary dissection

E. Radiotherapy

*Ref.:* 5

**COMMENTS: Ductal carcinoma in situ** is a heterogeneous lesion morphologically, and pathologists recognize four broad categories: **papillary**, **cribriform**, **solid**, and **comedo**. DCIS is recognized as discrete spaces surrounded by basement membrane that are filled with malignant cells and usually with an identifiable, basally located cell layer made up of presumably normal myoepithelial cells. The solid and comedo types of DCIS are generally higher-grade lesions and probably invade over a shortened natural history. DCIS frequently coexists with invasive cancers. In current practice, reasons to select total mastectomy for the treatment of DCIS include the following: diffuse suspicious mammographic calcifications suggestive of extensive disease, inability to obtain clear margins on wide excision, likelihood of a poor cosmetic result after wide excision of involved tissue, patient not motivated to preserve her breast, and contraindications to radiation therapy. Sentinel node biopsy is currently recommended when mastectomy is performed for DCIS because up to 10% of patients with DCIS on diagnostic biopsy will be found to have invasive cancer in their mastectomy specimen. The addition of sentinel lymph node biopsy to mastectomy adds minimal morbidity, and because sentinel node mapping is no longer possible after mastectomy, it may avoid the need for axillary dissection if invasive cancer is identified later. If the axillary lymph nodes are found to be positive for cancer, this patient should undergo chemotherapy. Because her tumor is ER positive, she is also a candidate for adjuvant endocrine therapy, such as tamoxifen.

**ANSWER: D**

**32.** A 44-year-old woman has a tender, movable mass in the 12-o'clock position of her left breast. A mammogram shows a 2.5-cm, well-circumscribed density in the palpable area of concern. Ultrasound shows an anechoic, well-circumscribed mass with increased through-transmission. What is the appropriate first step in treatment?

A. Excisional biopsy

B. Ultrasound-guided core needle biopsy

C. Tamoxifen

D. Fine-needle aspiration

E. Magnification and compression mammographic views of the lesion

*Ref.:* 5

**COMMENTS: Cysts** within the breast are fluid-filled, epithelium-lined cavities that may vary in size from microscopic to large, palpable masses. A palpable cyst develops in at least 1 in every 14 women. Cysts are influenced by ovarian hormones, a fact that explains their variation with the menstrual cycle. Most cysts occur in women older than 35 years. A palpable mass can be confirmed to be a cyst by aspiration or ultrasound. Cyst fluid can be straw colored, opaque, or dark green and may contain flecks of debris. On **ultrasound**, cysts are round with smooth borders, have a paucity of internal sound echoes, and exhibit increased through-transmission of sound with enhanced posterior echoes. If the palpable mass disappears completely after aspiration and the cyst contents are not grossly bloody, the fluid need not be sent for cytologic analysis. If the cyst recurs, sending fluid for cytologic evaluation is justified. Surgical removal of a cyst is usually indicated if the cytologic findings are atypical or suspicious for malignancy or if the cyst continues to recur.

**ANSWER: D**

**33.** A 53-year-old woman with no family history of breast cancer detects a well-defined, 2-cm mass in the upper outer quadrant of her right breast. Mammography reveals only dense breast tissue, and findings on ultrasound are unremarkable. What is the next step in the management of this patient?

A. Mammography and ultrasonography are extremely sensitive, so you can reassure her that the lesion is benign.

B. Advise her to return for reevaluation in 3 months.

C. Perform a core needle biopsy in the office.

D. Order a breast MRI.

E. Schedule her for an excisional biopsy.

*Ref.:* 7, 13

**COMMENTS:** Most patients with breast cancer do not have a family history, so any **palpable mass** requires investigation. Either needle aspiration or core needle biopsy of a solid mass would be acceptable as an initial diagnostic step. A major goal of modern breast medicine is to minimize the number of patients with benign lesions who undergo open surgical breast biopsy for diagnosis. There are relatively few patients for whom excisional biopsy should be the initial procedure for diagnosis. For patients with a diagnosis of breast cancer, the goal is to make the diagnosis with a needle and to go to the operating room one time for definitive treatment. A definitive diagnosis of breast cancer made from a minimally invasive **needle biopsy** specimen permits optimal preoperative work-up, patient counseling, and surgical planning. Percutaneous histologic tissue acquisition techniques include large-core biopsy (typically 12 to 14 gauge), vacuum-assisted biopsy (typically 7 to 11 gauge), and larger-tissue acquisition methods. Dense breast tissue decreases the diagnostic sensitivity of mammography and can easily obscure a carcinoma. The absence of mammographic visualization in the presence of a palpable mass does not diminish the need for tissue diagnosis. In fact, up to 10% of breast cancers are found in women with a "negative" mammogram. Delaying evaluation of a well-defined mass for 3 months is ill advised. **Magnetic resonance imaging** is a very sensitive diagnostic tool, but at this point in evaluation of this lesion, a negative MRI result would not obviate the need for biopsy.

**ANSWER: C**

**34.** A 33-year-old asymptomatic woman is referred to the clinician with abnormal findings on a mammogram. No masses are palpable in either breast. The mammogram shows a tight cluster of microcalcifications at the 2-o'clock position in her left breast. Magnification compression views show at least 20 tiny, irregular calcifications in a 2-cm area that vary in shape and density with no associated mass lesion. There are no other calcifications present in either breast. Which of the following is the most likely diagnosis?

A. LCIS

B. Fibroadenoma

C. Infiltrating ductal carcinoma

D. DCIS (intraductal)

E. Fibrocystic changes

*Ref.:* 7, 14

COMMENTS: **Mammographic calcifications** are a hallmark of early breast cancer, particularly DCIS, but the common causes of calcifications identified on mammography are varied. Specific patterns have been identified that are often associated with and predictive of these pathologic processes. Parenchymal calcifications (i.e., those indicative of a pathologic breast process) occur in the lobar ductal system and in the terminal ductal lobular unit. Certain patterns of ductal calcification are almost pathognomonic of **ductal carcinoma in situ**, as is a specific bilateral pattern seen with **plasma cell mastitis**. One mammographic feature common to both high-grade DCIS and plasma cell mastitis is the appearance of calcium in a linear, branching pattern. Evenly scattered calcifications, more often than not bilateral, are indicative of a lobular process. This pattern is the one most commonly encountered and is indicative of either active or involutional fibrocystic change. **Clustered calcifications**, whether single or multiple, present a diagnostic dilemma because of the varied pathologic processes that give rise to this pattern. Close scrutiny of these areas on magnification views is required to delineate the finer characteristics of the calcifications. Coarse, granular-appearing calcifications are seen with partially calcified fibroadenomas and papillomas, fibrocystic change, and low- to intermediate-grade DCIS. Powdery calcifications are seen with sclerosing adenosis, with or without atypia, and low-grade DCIS. Large, coarse calcifications (popcornlike) are classically associated with a degenerating fibroadenoma and are readily discernible on mammography. **Lobular carcinoma in situ** and **invasive lobular carcinoma** are often mammographically featureless. The clustered geographic distribution and characteristics of the calcifications described in this scenario make a diagnosis of DCIS more likely than that of an invasive carcinoma, which often has an associated mass lesion seen on mammography.

ANSWER: D

35. A 47-year-old woman with a history of breast pain has a recent onset of nonspontaneous, bilateral, green nipple discharge from multiple ducts. She has generalized bilateral tenderness and no palpable mass on breast examination. The discharge is Hemoccult negative. Findings on mammography and ultrasound are unremarkable. Which of the following is the most appropriate first step in management?

A. Schedule MRI.

B. Perform an ultrasound-guided core biopsy.

C. Reassure the patient.

D. Obtain a galactogram.

E. Excise the major retroareolar ducts.

*Ref.:* 7

COMMENTS: **Nipple discharge** and breast tenderness are common complaints associated with **mammary duct ectasia** and **fibrocystic change**. Bilateral versus unilateral, multiple duct versus single duct, expressible (nonspontaneous) versus spontaneous, and colored (nonbloody) versus clear or bloody fluid are all strongly suggestive of a benign cause of the discharge. Accordingly, surgery would be inappropriate in this case. Reassurance is the appropriate management decision in this context, particularly in light of the clinical characteristics of the nipple discharge and the negative mammographic and physical examination findings. If the drainage is bloody, serous, or watery, further diagnostic work-up is indicated to determine the cause of the discharge. Although such discharges demand evaluation, the cause is often benign (commonly an intraductal papilloma or papillomatosis). Even though some surgeons prefer a preoperative contrast-enhanced radiograph of the involved duct (a **galactogram**) as a guide, the blood-distended duct is usually identifiable and can be removed through a circumareolar incision or lacrimal probe-guided terminal duct excision. If either preoperative or intraoperative ultrasound imaging is available, this modality can be used in real time to facilitate identification of the distended duct and to precisely map the area of operative excision. More recently, **ductoscopy** has been added as a tool for the evaluation of clinically worrisome nipple discharge.

ANSWER: C

36. With regard to pure tubular carcinoma, which of the following is true?

A. Lymph node involvement is seen in 25% of cases.

B. It is a highly aggressive, frequently fatal carcinoma.

C. It tends to be ER negative.

D. Neoadjuvant chemotherapy should be strongly considered.

E. Stage for stage, it has a more favorable prognosis than other forms of ductal carcinoma.

*Ref.:* 7

COMMENTS: When **tubular carcinoma** is present in its pure form, distant metastatic potential is highly unlikely. The diagnosis is made when characteristic angulated tubules, composed of cells with low-grade nuclei, constitute at least 90% of the carcinoma. Tubular carcinoma has a better prognosis than other varieties of infiltrating ductal cancer, and one classic study showed that all patients studied whose carcinoma was composed purely of the characteristic low-grade, angulated tubules survived at least 15 years, regardless of tumor size. Tubular carcinoma represents only about 3% to 5% of all invasive carcinomas, has the biologic correlates of a low-grade cancer (ER positive, diploid, low S phase, no expression of c-erbB-2), and is more likely to occur in older patients. The survival of patients with tubular carcinoma is generally similar to that of the general population, and systemic adjuvant therapy may be avoided in these patients. For selected cases of pure tubular carcinoma removed with an adequate negative margin, mastectomy, radiation therapy, or even axillary lymph node staging may be unnecessary.

ANSWER: E

37. A 39-year-old woman with no family history of breast cancer underwent excisional biopsy of a 2-cm breast mass. Histologic sections showed fibrosis, ductal ectasia, atypical lobular hyperplasia, and multiple foci of LCIS present at the medial, superior, and inferior margins. Which of the following statements is false?

A. At a minimum, she needs to undergo reexcision to achieve negative margins.

B. Tamoxifen can decrease risk for the future development of invasive cancer by 50%.

C. If breast cancer develops, it would most likely be a ductal carcinoma.

D. LCIS is typically not visible on mammography but is discovered incidentally on biopsy.

E. LCIS is often multicentric and bilateral.

*Ref.:* 5, 7

**COMMENTS: Lobular carcinoma in situ** is a histologic finding that is usually seen in tissue from a biopsy specimen of some other lesion. It represents a risk marker that predicts up to a ninefold increase in the chance for the development of breast cancer. **Atypical lobular hyperplasia** alone increases the risk fourfold. Acquisition of free margins is not necessary since LCIS is now not considered to be a malignant lesion but more of a risk factor for the development of breast cancer. Either infiltrating lobular or infiltrating ductal carcinoma may develop in this patient, with infiltrating ductal carcinoma being the more likely type. Less aggressive management is typically performed for this kind of lesion and consists of close follow-up with periodic physical examination and bilateral mammograms or the use of tamoxifen as chemoprevention, which has resulted in a nearly 50% reduction in risk for the development of breast cancer. LCIS is usually multicentric and often found in both breasts.

**ANSWER:** A

38. Which of the following statements is true regarding breast conservation surgery?

A. Sixty percent of locally recurrent breast cancers develop at or near the site of the original breast cancer.

B. Intraoperative radiotherapy (IORT) targeted to the tumor bed permits breast-conserving surgery and radiotherapy to be completed in one sitting.

C. IORT is significantly more expensive than MammoSite balloon catheter brachytherapy.

D. One known disadvantage of delivering radiotherapy at the time of breast cancer resection is increased toxicity to adjacent tissues.

E. IORT can be repeated as needed.

*Ref.:* 15

**COMMENTS:** The **TARGIT trial** (targeted intraoperative radiation therapy) is a phase III, prospective, randomized trial comparing single-fraction targeted **intraoperative radiotherapy** with conventional whole-breast external beam radiotherapy for the management of early-stage invasive breast cancer. Inclusion criteria for the trial include age 35 years and older and operable invasive breast cancer (T1-3, N0-1, M0) suitable for breast-conserving surgery. The principal objective of the trial is to determine whether single-fraction IORT targeted to the tumor bed provides equivalent local control as conventional therapy. In June 2010, the first phase initial results showed that IORT was equally effective at controlling recurrence. Toxicity was lower in the target group. However, the trial was limited to patients older than 45 and the tumor size was 3 cm or less. Randomized trials have shown that approximately 90% of locally recurrent breast cancers develop at or near the site

of the original breast cancer. IORT is a form of accelerated partial-breast irradiation in which the entire radiotherapy dose is given intraoperatively, typically at the time of tumor removal. Spherical applicators are used that conform the breast tissue around the radiation source to permit delivery of a uniform field of radiation to a prescribed tissue depth. Chest wall and skin can be protected by tungsten-impregnated silicone barriers, which provide 93% shielding and minimize pulmonary, cardiac, and skin toxicity. Other advantages of IORT include convenience in that breast-conserving surgery and radiotherapy are completed in one sitting while the patient is still under anesthesia, accurate dose delivery because the radiation dose is directed to the surgical margins, and lower cost (IORT is a third the cost of MammoSite balloon catheter brachytherapy). Important limitations of IORT are the possible need for additional radiotherapy (repeated IORT is not permitted, so if inadequate surgical margins are found after IORT, external beam therapy may be required), lack of pretreatment pathologic review, and concern that this modality may be subtherapeutic and leave patients at elevated risk for local recurrence.

**ANSWER:** B

39. With regard to asymptomatic, nonpalpable, mammographically detected breast masses, which of the following statements is true?

A. The mass should be excised if it is found in a woman older than 40 years.

B. Unless the mass is painful, it can be followed with a mammogram in 6 months.

C. Ultrasound is helpful in further defining breast lesions.

D. Imaging-guided biopsy is contraindicated.

E. Masses with a small, well-defined border and a "halo" sign around them are always benign.

*Ref.:* 5, 7

**COMMENTS:** Mammographic abnormalities that cannot be detected by physical examination include clustered microcalcifications and areas of abnormal density (masses, architectural distortions, and asymmetries). The **Breast Imaging Reporting and Data System (BI-RADS)** is used to categorize the degree of suspicion of malignancy for a mammographic abnormality. To avoid unnecessary biopsies for low-suspicion mammographic findings, probably benign lesions are designated BI-RADS 3 and are monitored with a schedule of short-interval mammograms over a 2-year period. **Imaging-guided biopsy** is performed only for lesions that progress during follow-up; this can be done by image-guided core needle biopsy or image-guided wire localization followed by surgical excision. **Ultrasound** is useful in establishing whether a lesion detected by other modalities is solid or cystic and in determining the contour and internal properties of a lesion. Smooth, rounded masses cannot be assumed to be benign even if previous mammograms demonstrate a stable appearance over a long period. Some malignant tumors, including mucinous and medullary carcinoma or cystosarcoma phyllodes, can have a benign appearance on both ultrasound imaging and mammography.

**ANSWER:** C

40. A 38-year-old asymptomatic woman with normal findings on examination comes to see you after a stereotactic biopsy. She was not given any results, but she brought her pathology slides with her (Figure 14-1). What is the best surgical procedure for her condition?

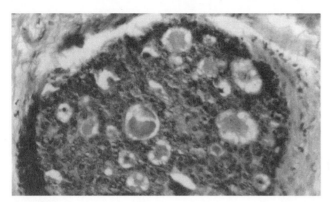

**Figure 14-1.**

A. Modified radical mastectomy

B. No surgical intervention necessary

C. Bilateral total mastectomy without axillary dissection

D. Lumpectomy and sentinel lymph node biopsy

E. Lumpectomy alone

*Ref.:* 5- 7

**COMMENTS:** The **hyperchromatic nuclei** in a fairly uniform population of neoplastic-appearing cells filling and distending the ducts, along with sharply defined punched-out (Swiss cheese) spaces, are typical of a **cribriform intraductal carcinoma**. In contrast to a comedo pattern of intraductal carcinoma, this lesion can often be treated by excision to free margins and close follow-up. However, if free margins are not obtained, the rate of recurrence is high. Even if free margins are achieved, the lesion occasionally recurs in an invasive form. If the patient is unwilling to accept that small chance, total mastectomy or irradiation is appropriate, even though it may be overtreatment. Axillary dissection is unnecessary, and the long-term survival rate following mastectomy is essentially 100%.

**ANSWER:** E

41. Assuming that it is the same patient as listed in Question 40, how would your recommendations change if instead the slide in Figure 14-2 were the one she presents to you?

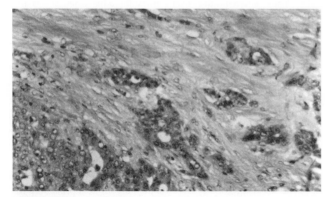

**Figure 14-2.**

A. Total mastectomy

B. No surgical intervention necessary

C. Bilateral total mastectomy with axillary dissection

D. Lumpectomy and sentinel lymph node biopsy

E. Lumpectomy alone

*Ref.:* 5-7

**COMMENTS:** The nests of epithelial cells invading the stroma in random fashion, with a suggestion of **tubule formation**, are typical of **infiltrating ductal carcinoma**. **Lumpectomy** with sentinel lymph node biopsy followed by breast irradiation is the most appropriate treatment of those listed. Total mastectomy or lumpectomy alone fails to assess the axilla for staging, and bilateral total mastectomies with axillary dissection would be considered overtreatment.

**ANSWER:** D

42. Which of the following factors does not influence the choice of systemic adjuvant therapy for invasive breast cancer?

A. Tumor size

B. DNA ploidy

C. HER-2/neu

D. Axillary node status

E. ER status

*Ref.:* 5

**COMMENTS:** **Metastatic disease** is the primary cause of death from breast cancer. Patients who benefit from chemotherapy or hormonal therapy do so because metastasis is prevented, cured, or delayed. Currently, the recommendation for adjuvant systemic therapy is based on consideration of tumor size, HER-2/neu status, nodal status, ER status, and age or menopausal status. In patients with **node-negative cancer**, certain groups may suffer higher relapse rates, and the absolute benefits of chemotherapy are greater. **Poor prognostic signs** include tumor size greater than 2 cm, poor histologic and nuclear grade, absence of hormone receptors, high proliferative fraction, and overexpression of certain oncogenes such as HER-2/neu. When **trastuzumab (Herceptin)** is used in patients with HER-2–positive breast cancers, there is a 50% reduction in recurrence. In general, all **node-positive** tumors require chemotherapy. In women with ER-positive breast cancer, 5 years of tamoxifen or an **aromatase inhibitor** after surgical treatment nearly halves their recurrence rate and reduces breast cancer mortality by a third. Oncotype DX is a diagnostic test that assesses the tumor tissue and estimates the likelihood that invasive breast cancer will return or recur after treatment. This test looks at a group of 21 genes within a woman's tumor sample—16 cancer genes and 5 control genes—to see how they are expressed or how active they are. The results of the test are reported as a quantitative **Recurrence Score**, which is a score between 0 and 100 that correlates with the likelihood of a woman's chance of having her cancer return and the likelihood that she will benefit from adding chemotherapy to her hormonal therapy.

**ANSWER:** B

43. Which of the following is not a germline mutation associated with a higher incidence of breast cancer?

A. *APC*

B. *BRCA1*

C. *BRCA2*

D. *p53*

E. *PTEN*

*Ref.:* 7

**COMMENTS:** All of the choices are **germline mutations**. A germline mutation is a mutation that exists in every cell of the body and is therefore capable of being passed to the offspring via the sperm or egg. The *APC* gene is involved in regulation of cell growth and, when inherited in mutated form, leads to familial adenomatous polyposis and an increased incidence of colon cancer; it does not increase the risk for breast cancer. The predominant genes responsible for hereditary breast cancer are *BRCA1* and *BRCA2*. Women who carry a germline mutation in either of these genes have about an 85% likelihood of breast cancer developing by the age of 70, although most cancers occur before 50 years of age. Women with these mutations also have an increased risk (30% to 60%) for the development of ovarian cancer. Inherited mutations of the *p53* gene result in **Li-Fraumeni syndrome**, which is associated with the development of a number of malignancies, including breast cancer, sarcomas, brain tumors, adrenocortical carcinomas, and leukemia. Germline mutations in the *PTEN* gene are associated with **Cowden disease**, which is a hereditary disorder (also known as **multiple hamartoma syndrome**) that is inherited as an autosomal dominant trait and is characterized by distinctive mucocutaneous lesions and cancer of the breast, thyroid, and female genitourinary tract.

**ANSWER:**  A

44. A germline mutation in *BRCA1* or *BRCA2* is associated with all of the following characteristics except:

   A. Autosomal dominant transmission

   B. High incidence of breast and ovarian cancer in women

   C. Higher than average incidence of breast cancer in men

   D. Incomplete penetrance

   E. Late-onset breast cancer

*Ref.:* 7

**COMMENTS:** Mutations in *BRCA1* or *BRCA2* result in a higher incidence of breast and **ovarian cancer**. The risk for breast cancer is about 85% in individuals who carry the mutation and have a family history of breast cancer. The risk for ovarian cancer is about 40% with *BRCA1* mutations and 20% with *BRCA2* mutations. Breast cancer will develop in about 10% of males with *BRCA2* mutations. These genes are incompletely penetrant; that is, some mutation carriers can live to old age without the development of cancer. The mutation is autosomal dominant, so a mutation in only one of the pair of chromosomes usually produces the disease. Although postmenopausal breast cancer can develop in women who carry germline mutations of these genes, cancer will develop in most of these carriers at a younger age.

**ANSWER:**  E

45. A 45-year-old woman had a recent stereotactic biopsy revealing atypical ductal hyperplasia. What is the next most appropriate step in her management?

   A. Bilateral prophylactic mastectomies

   B. Tamoxifen

C. Wire-localized excisional biopsy of the area

D. *BRCA* mutation testing

E. Mammography in 6 months

*Ref.:* 5

**COMMENTS:** Certain forms of benign breast disease can be important risk factors for the eventual development of breast cancer. The classification scheme for **benign breast disease** usually includes **nonproliferative lesions**, proliferation of breast epithelium without atypia (**hyperplasia**), and **proliferation with atypia**. The relative risk for cancer in women with either atypical ductal hyperplasia or atypical lobular hyperplasia is between four and five times the risk for development of breast cancer in a control population of women. If there is a positive family history with the existence of atypical hyperplasia, the risk is increased to nearly nine times that of the general population. **Tamoxifen** (20 mg/day for 5 years) is considered a preventive option in women found to have atypical hyperplasia. This patient should undergo wire-localized excisional biopsy of the area because there is up to a 15% chance of having a higher-stage lesion in the area (such as DCIS) when the surrounding tissue is examined.

**ANSWER:**  C

46. Which of the following statements regarding the human epidermal growth factor receptor-2 (HER-2) gene is false?

   A. It controls normal cell growth.

   B. It is amplified in 25% of breast cancers.

   C. Trastuzumab is an antibody against the HER-2/neu receptor.

   D. It is an independent predictor of poor outcome in breast cancer.

   E. HER-2 status is hereditary.

*Ref.:* 7, 16

**COMMENTS:** HER-2/neu (**c-erbB-2**) is a protooncogene that is found on the surface of some normal cells in the body; however, it is overexpressed or amplified in 25% of all breast cancers. It is a member of the **epidermal growth factor** family and is a transmembrane receptor with **tyrosine kinase** activity. Studies have shown that HER-2/neu overexpression is found in more aggressive cancers and is a negative prognostic factor. Women with node-negative but HER-2/neu–positive breast cancer seem to have an increased risk for recurrence in comparison to node-negative HER-2/neu–negative patients. Trastuzumab is a humanized murine monoclonal antibody raised against the erb-B2 or HER-2 surface receptor. HER-2 status is not considered a hereditary trait.

**ANSWER:**  E

47. Which of the following is false regarding breast reconstruction following mastectomy for breast cancer?

   A. The cosmetic result of immediate reconstruction is enhanced by preserving the maximum amount of breast skin during performance of the mastectomy.

   B. Immediate reconstruction has a detrimental effect on local recurrence rates.

   C. Reconstruction is often delayed in patients who might require postmastectomy radiation therapy.

D. Multiple factors are considered when choosing reconstruction procedures, including age, obesity, smoking history, concomitant disease, and the patient's psychological/emotional state.

E. Autogenous tissue usually provides better symmetry than an implant.

*Ref.:* 12

**COMMENTS: Breast reconstruction** may be performed as immediate reconstruction (same day as mastectomy) or as delayed reconstruction (months or years later). Immediate reconstruction is facilitated by preserving the maximum amount of breast skin, and it offers the advantages of combining the recovery period for both procedures and avoiding a period without reconstruction. In a recent study, 75% of reconstructions were performed immediately. Clinical trials have shown that there is no increased risk for cancer recurrence and no increased difficulty with surveillance for recurrence of breast cancer after immediate reconstruction. Reconstruction may be delayed in patients who might require postmastectomy radiation therapy and is usually delayed in patients with locally advanced cancer. Reconstructive options can be divided into two main types: those that use autogenous tissue and those that require alloplastic material. In general, autogenous tissue will usually provide better symmetry than an implant. One study showed that only 35% of **transverse rectus abdominus myocutaneous (TRAM) flap** reconstructions required a symmetry procedure versus 55% of **implant** reconstructions.

**ANSWER: B**

48. Which patient would not benefit from postmastectomy radiotherapy?

A. 49-year-old with inflammatory breast cancer

B. 25-year-old with 6 cm of DCIS

C. 57-year-old with a T1N2 infiltrating ductal carcinoma

D. 48-year-old with a 2.5-cm breast mass involving the underlying pectoral muscle

E. 42-year-old with a 3.0-cm primary tumor and one lymph node positive that has extracapsular extension

*Ref.:* 5

**COMMENTS:** Three large prospective randomized trials have addressed the role of **postmastectomy irradiation**, and in addition to the expected benefit of reducing local-regional recurrences, it also resulted in significant improvement in overall survival in all three studies. Postmastectomy irradiation has been found to reduce the risk for local or regional recurrence by approximately two thirds and to reduce breast cancer–specific mortality. Most centers now recommend chest wall and nodal irradiation after mastectomy for patients with multiple positive nodes (more than four positive nodes), for patients with large cancers or very aggressive histology (diffuse vascular invasion), and for extranodal extension of breast cancer. Other indications include positive surgical margins, inflammatory breast cancer, or involvement of the skin, pectoral fascia, or skeletal muscle. Radiation therapy is not indicated after mastectomy for DCIS, regardless of its size.

**ANSWER: B**

49. Which of the following patients is considered an appropriate candidate for breast-preserving therapy with lumpectomy followed by radiation therapy?

A. A 40-year-old woman with a history of active scleroderma and a T1N0 infiltrating ductal carcinoma of her right breast

B. A 45-year-old woman with a T1N1 infiltrating ductal carcinoma of her left breast after lumpectomy, negative surgical margins, and axillary lymph node dissection with 2 of 12 lymph nodes positive

C. A 37-year-old woman with a T2N0 infiltrating ductal carcinoma of her right breast who has a history of Hodgkin disease treated with 36 Gy to a mantle field 15 years earlier

D. All of the above

E. None of the above

*Ref.:* 17, 18

**COMMENTS:** The **National Surgical Adjuvant Breast and Bowel Project B-06 trial** demonstrated that lumpectomy followed by radiation therapy to the breast is appropriate treatment for patients with primary tumors 4 cm or less in diameter and either positive or negative axillary lymph nodes. Several other trials have confirmed these results for patients with stage I and II breast cancer. The 20-year results from the NSABP B-06 trial show equal overall survival and disease-free survival for all patients whether they were treated by breast preservation or mastectomy. However, the cohort of patients treated by lumpectomy alone without irradiation suffered a 35% recurrence rate in the ipsilateral breast. This recurrence rate is considered unacceptably high when compared with the 10% risk for **ipsilateral breast recurrences** in patients who underwent radiation therapy of the breast following lumpectomy. Several series have shown that patients with certain collagen vascular diseases may incur increased toxicity from radiation therapy. Although excessive complications have not been consistently shown with all types of collagen vascular disorders, severe fibrosis and soft tissue necrosis have been associated with scleroderma, thus suggesting that patients with scleroderma may be better served with a mastectomy. Patients with active **systemic lupus erythematosus** and **rheumatoid arthritis** may also be at increased risk for toxicity from radiation therapy. Mastectomy is recommended for patients who have had previous radiation therapy to the chest or to a mantle field (which includes the neck, axilla, mediastinum, and pulmonary hila) because the radiation tolerance of regional normal tissues may be exceeded and result in excessive toxicity.

**ANSWER: B**

50. A 15-year-old girl is brought to the office by her mother because of asymmetrical breast development. Physical examination reveals normal breast development on the left and a hypoplastic breast on the right, with hypoplasia of the pectoralis major muscle also seen on the right. What should the clinician explain to the mother?

A. This is a normal situation in this age group since breast tissue often develops at different rates and is slightly asymmetrical during adolescence.

B. This is an example of Poland syndrome.

C. This is an example of Li-Fraumeni syndrome.

D. This is an example of amazia.

E. This is an example of fragile X syndrome.

*Ref.:* 19

**COMMENTS:** This patient is demonstrating **Poland syndrome**, which is characterized by unilateral hypoplasia of the breast, pectoral muscles, and chest wall. **Li-Fraumeni syndrome** is one of the inherited breast cancer syndromes in which there is an increased incidence of breast cancer, soft tissue sarcoma and osteosarcoma, brain tumors, adrenocortical cancer, and leukemias in the same family. Nearly 30% of the tumors in these families occur before the age of 15. **Amazia** refers to a condition in which the nipple is present but the breast mound is absent.

**ANSWER: B**

51. A 13-year-old girl is referred to a breast surgeon for breast asymmetry secondary to a rapidly growing right breast mass. Physical examination reveals an 8-cm central right breast mass. She underwent menarche 1 year ago. Breast cancer was diagnosed in her mother at age 38. What is the appropriate next step?

    A. Mastectomy

    B. Incisional biopsy

    C. Mammogram

    D. Ultrasound

    E. Reassurance to the patient and her mother that this is normal breast development

    *Ref.:* 7

**COMMENTS:** See Question 52.

**ANSWER: D**

52. Regarding the patient in the Question 51, ultrasound reveals an 8-cm hypoechoic solid mass with rounded edges. What is the next appropriate step in the management of this patient?

    A. Excisional biopsy

    B. Mastectomy

    C. Cyst aspiration

    D. Bilateral mastectomies

    E. Reassurance to the patient and mother

    *Ref.:* 7

**COMMENTS:** This young woman most likely has a **juvenile fibroadenoma**. Fibroadenoma may be regarded as a generic term and refers to any benign, confined tumor of the breast that has a mixture of glandular and mesenchymal elements; juvenile fibroadenoma is considered a variant. These lesions tend to occur in women in the younger age range and are characterized by increased cellularity of stroma or epithelium. Juvenile fibroadenomas are notable for their rapid growth and large size and tend to occur around the time of menarche. They often have a common ductal pattern of epithelial hyperplasia and defining stromal hypercellularity. The initial imaging modality for a young woman is ultrasound because it is accurate in evaluating the dense breast tissue common in younger women, involves no radiation exposure, and is essentially painless. A rounded hypoechoic solid mass on ultrasound is indicative of fibroadenoma, and excisional biopsy would be considered appropriate treatment at this time.

**ANSWER: A**

53. Which statement is false regarding radial scars?

    A. Usually detected as a stellate lesion on mammography

    B. Extensive elastosis is common

    C. May be associated with or contain atypical ductal hyperplasia or DCIS

    D. Increases the risk for the future development of breast cancer by 40%

    E. Benign proliferative disease of the breast

    *Ref.:* 20

**COMMENTS: Radial scars** are benign breast lesions of uncertain etiology and behavior. They have a characteristic low-power stellate architecture with cystically dilated glands encircling the periphery. The mostly acellular core is composed of connective tissue and elastin surrounded by radiating bands of compressed ducts and lobules that demonstrate dual myoepithelial and epithelial layers. Proliferative epithelial lesions, including sclerosing adenosis, hyperplasia, and papillomas, are often seen within radial scars. One large review study found that radial scars do not confer an increased risk for subsequent breast cancer over that of other proliferative lesions, although there is a slightly increased association between radial scars and atypical hyperplasia. The growth pattern in radial scars can resemble a malignancy and is difficult to distinguish from invasive carcinoma on mammography, which prompts biopsy of these lesions.

**ANSWER: D**

54. A 45-year-old woman has an abnormal diagnostic mammogram revealing a cluster of indeterminate microcalcifications in the upper outer quadrant of her left breast. Physical examination reveals normal findings. The patient denies any risk factors for breast cancer. Which of the following is most appropriate for initial management?

    A. Stereotactic-guided core needle biopsy

    B. Ultrasound-guided core needle biopsy

    C. Reassurance and continuation of yearly mammography

    D. Excisional biopsy

    E. Repeat mammography of the left breast in 6 months

    *Ref.:* 13

**COMMENTS:** One of the goals of modern breast medicine is to reduce the number of unnecessary open surgical breast biopsies for benign lesions. Imaging-guided **percutaneous needle biopsy** is the diagnostic procedure of choice for imaging-detected breast abnormalities. It should be readily available to all patients with imaging-detected lesions. The presence of **indeterminate microcalcifications** is a suspicious finding on mammography that warrants a tissue diagnosis; therefore, reassurance or close follow-up is not an appropriate management option. Ultrasound is the preferred biopsy guidance method for sonographically visible lesions, but this lesion was found on mammography, and therefore stereotactic guidance would most likely be the initial choice for biopsy.

**ANSWER: A**

55. A 57-year-old woman undergoes imaging-guided biopsy of a 1.5-cm spiculated, centrally dense mass. Pathologic review shows benign breast parenchyma. Which of the following is the most appropriate recommendation at this point?

    A. Routine screening mammography in 1 year

    B. Additional imaging with contrast-enhanced MRI

    C. Short-term follow-up in 4 to 6 months

D. Wire-localized excisional biopsy

E. Tamoxifen

*Ref.: 19*

COMMENTS: When mammographic changes are highly suspicious for malignancy but a **negative core biopsy** is obtained, these results must be viewed with caution because the possibility of sampling error must always be considered. Definitive wide excision with wire localization in such circumstances would then be warranted. The reasons for the initial core biopsy in such suspicious cases are multiple and include the value of having a tissue diagnosis (rather than just a "suspicion") when discussing diagnosis and management options with the patient. Negative MRI findings would not preclude additional biopsy of this mammographically suspicious lesion.

ANSWER: D

56. A 47-year-old woman undergoes a modified radical mastectomy for a T2N2 infiltrating ductal carcinoma. She arrives at her first postoperative visit complaining of hypoesthesia of the upper posteromedial aspect of the ipsilateral arm. What might explain this finding?

A. Lymphatic fibrosis

B. Medial pectoral pedicle injury

C. Second intercostal brachial cutaneous nerve injury

D. Axillary vein thrombosis

E. Thoracodorsal pedicle injury

*Ref.: 19*

COMMENTS: A number of neurovascular structures are identified and dissected during axillary dissection that are at risk for injury. The axilla is rich in lymphatic vessels draining the ipsilateral arm. Some of these lymphatics are disrupted during axillary dissection, but continued fibrosis of the remaining lymphatics, especially in cases in which the dissected axilla has been irradiated, may lead to progressive **lymphedema** of the arm, which can begin years after therapy. The possibility of unsightly and disabling **lymphedema** occasionally developing has led to a generally more conservative surgical approach toward axillary dissection for breast cancer in recent years. The medial pectoral pedicle contains the principal motor nerve and partial blood supply to the **pectoralis major** muscle. Injury leads to atrophy but not ischemia because the blood supply to this muscle is derived from many different sources. The second intercostal **brachial cutaneous nerve** provides sensation to the upper lateral chest wall and medial and posterior aspect of the upper part of the arm. It passes transversely across the axilla about 1 to 2 cm caudal to the axillary vein. In the past, it was routinely sectioned to allow cleaner en bloc removal of the axillary contents, but many surgeons now choose to preserve it in cases in which it is not in close proximity to clinically suspicious lymph nodes. The **axillary vein** can be narrowed or ligated as a result of surgical error during the procedure or can undergo acute spontaneous thrombosis during the immediate postoperative period. Because collateral channels have not had a chance to develop, the resulting swelling of the ipsilateral arm is usually acute and painful. The **thoracodorsal** pedicle contains the motor nerve and the principal artery and vein serving the **latissimus dorsi** muscle. Injury to the nerve leads to atrophy, but this is rarely clinically significant, except in athletes. Loss of the vascular pedicle distal to its branch to the serratus muscle, however, would lead to ischemic loss of the latissimus dorsi myocutaneous rotation flap,

one of the principal sources of autologous tissue for breast reconstruction and for closure of soft tissue deficits of the chest wall. The **long thoracic nerve** is also at risk for injury during axillary surgery; such injury can cause loss of function of the serratus anterior muscle and in turn lead to winging of the scapula.

ANSWER: C

57. What is the incidence of lymphedema after axillary node dissection (levels I and II)?

A. 5%

B. 10%

C. 20%

D. 40%

E. 50%

*Ref.: 7*

COMMENTS: The incidence of **lymphedema after axillary node dissection** ranges from 15% to 30%, depending on the definition used. The probability of lymphedema increases with greater dissection and level of nodes removed, the tumor burden in the axilla, the presence of lymphedema before surgery, and whether radiation is applied to the field after surgery. With the advent of sentinel lymph node biopsy, the rate of lymphedema has been shown to be much lower, in the range of 2% to 4%.

ANSWER: C

58. Radiation delivered to the breast after right lumpectomy and sentinel lymph node biopsy for a 1.2-cm node-negative infiltrating ductal carcinoma is likely to be associated with which of the following?

A. Decreased risk for systemic recurrence

B. Can be used in lieu of chemotherapy in early-stage breast cancers

C. Increased risk for lymphoma

D. Decreased risk for local recurrence

E. Cardiac toxicity

*Ref.: 7*

COMMENTS: The addition of **breast irradiation** after **breast conservation** has been shown in multiple randomized trials to decrease the incidence of local tumor recurrence but is considered controversial in terms of survival benefit. Radiation is used for local control, and chemotherapy is a modality for systemic control; the decision for chemotherapy is made independently and based on the presence of tumor factors and risk for distant disease. Lymphoma is not associated with breast irradiation. The risk for cardiac toxicity in right-sided lesions with modern techniques of radiation therapy planning and dosimetry is very low.

ANSWER: D

59. For which patient described below is an aromatase inhibitor, such as anastrozole (Arimidex) or letrozole (Femara), considered to be useful?

A. A 57-year-old woman with T1N0 ER-positive breast cancer

B. A 35-year-old woman with LCIS

C. A 65-year-old woman with T2N1, ER-negative breast cancer

D. A 42-year-old woman with DCIS

E. A 45-year-old woman who is a known carrier of the *BRCA* mutation

*Ref.:* 7, 19

**COMMENTS: Aromatase inhibitors** are useful only in the **postmenopausal** setting for women with invasive cancers. In postmenopausal women, the ovaries stop producing estrogen, but low levels of estrogen remain because aromatase converts other steroid hormones into estrogen in the peripheral fat. The **ATAC trial** (Arimidex, tamoxifen, alone or in combination) showed that in postmenopausal women with invasive breast cancer, taking **anastrozole** led to a lower recurrence rate, a lower chance for the development of a new primary, and less toxicity than in women taking tamoxifen. A subset analysis of this trial showed that the advantage of anastrozole was seen only in women with steroid receptor–positive breast cancer. **Tamoxifen** may be indicated for chemoprevention in high-risk patients, such as those with LCIS or DCIS or those carrying a *BRCA* mutation. Aromatase inhibitors, however, are not currently approved for chemoprevention.

**ANSWER:** A

60. What additional treatment should a 42-year-old patient with a 2-cm focus of ER-positive DCIS transected at the margin by lumpectomy receive?

A. Radiation therapy alone

B. Tamoxifen alone

C. Surgical reexcision alone

D. Surgical reexcision and tamoxifen alone

E. Surgical reexcision, radiation therapy, and tamoxifen

*Ref.:* 7, 19

**COMMENTS:** If ductal carcinoma has been transected at the margin of resection, its rate of recurrence is unacceptably high in both the noninvasive and invasive forms. **Reexcision** to clear margins is the standard of care. Subsequent radiation therapy significantly reduces local recurrence and is recommended for all but the smallest of tumors. The addition of tamoxifen has been shown to further decrease the incidence of recurrent DCIS and new invasive breast cancer. Recent studies have shown that this benefit is best seen in women with ER-positive DCIS.

**ANSWER:** E

61. Which of the following is associated with the appearance of invasive lobular carcinoma on mammography?

A. Discrete bilateral masses

B. Partially cystic appearance

C. Indistinct mass with poorly defined borders

D. Masses with microcalcifications

E. Branching pleomorphic microcalcifications

*Ref.:* 5

**COMMENTS:** When compared with invasive ductal carcinoma, **invasive lobular carcinoma** tends to be more indistinct and

difficult to visualize on mammograms. The extent of the tumor is often underestimated on the mammogram and may be more accurately appreciated by ultrasound imaging or **magnetic resonance imaging**. Nonetheless, recurrence and survival rates for invasive lobular carcinoma are equivalent to those for ductal carcinoma, stage for stage.

**ANSWER:** C

62. In which population is the incidence of *BRCA* mutations highest?

A. Ashkenazi Jews

B. Patients with a history of radiation therapy for Hodgkin disease

C. Patients with a first-degree relative with breast cancer

D. A woman with a Gail score of 2.3%

E. A woman with a prior diagnosis of uterine cancer

*Ref.:* 7

**COMMENTS:** The *BRCA* mutation rate is highest in **Ashkenazi Jews** and ranges from 1% to 3%. The incidence of breast cancer in those who underwent mantel irradiation for Hodgkin disease is five times that of the general population. A person with a first-degree relative with postmenopausal breast cancer has a relative risk 1.8 times that of the general population. **Ovarian cancer** increases the risk for breast cancer in a woman, but uterine cancer has not been linked to breast cancer.

**ANSWER:** A

63. What is the approximate false-negative rate for sentinel lymph node biopsy?

A. 1%

B. 8%

C. 15%

D. 20%

E. 25%

*Ref.:* 7, 19

**COMMENTS:** The sentinel lymph node biopsy technique has a learning curve of approximately 30 cases before proficiency is attained. In experienced hands, the false-negative rate ranges from 4% to 12%. The use of tracer **blue dye** versus **technetium-labeled sulfur colloid**, or both, has not been shown to affect the detection rate or false-negative rate if the surgeon is proficient. **Isosulfan blue** dye, however, is associated with a small incidence of anaphylactoid reactions.

**ANSWER:** B

64. In which patient should MRI be used as an adjunct to mammography for breast cancer screening purposes?

A. A 27-year-old woman in whose mother breast cancer was diagnosed at age 52

B. A 52-year-old woman with dense breasts

C. A 72-year-old woman with a history of DCIS

D. A 31-year-old woman whose sister carries the *BRCA* mutation but has declined genetic testing for herself

E. A 55-year-old woman who received radiation treatments at age 50 for uterine cancer

*Ref.:* 21

**COMMENTS: Magnetic resonance imaging** uses magnetic fields to produce detailed cross-sectional images of tissue structures and provides very good soft tissue contrast. The ACS has recommendations for breast MRI screening as an adjunct to mammography based on certain levels of evidence. The ACS recommends annual MRI screening (based on evidence from nonrandomized screening trials and observational studies) for patients with the *BRCA* mutation, those with first-degree relatives who are *BRCA* carriers but are themselves untested, and those with a lifetime risk of 20% to 25% or greater for the development of breast cancer, as defined by BRCAPRO or other models that are largely dependent on family history. The ACS recommends annual MRI screening (based on expert consensus opinion and evidence of lifetime risk for breast cancer) for those with irradiation of the chest between 10 and 30 years of age, patients and their first-degree relatives with **Li-Fraumeni syndrome**, and patients and their first-degree relatives with **Cowden disease** and **Bannayan-Riley-Ruvalcaba syndrome**. There is insufficient evidence to recommend for or against MRI screening in the following subgroups: those with a lifetime risk of 15% to 20%, as defined by BRCAPRO or other models that are largely dependent on family history, those with LCIS or atypical lobular hyperplasia, patients with atypical ductal hyperplasia, women with heterogeneously or extremely dense breasts on mammography, and women with a personal history of breast cancer, including DCIS. The ACS recommends against MRI screening for women with less than a 15% lifetime risk for breast cancer.

**ANSWER:** D

**65.** Which of the following has typically been associated with breast pain?

A. Breast cancer

B. LCIS

C. DCIS

D. Sclerosing adenosis

E. Breast cysts

*Ref.:* 5, 7

**COMMENTS:** Although **breast pain** may be the most common initial breast symptom, it is rarely associated with carcinoma. Normal ovarian hormonal influences on breast glandular elements frequently produce **cyclic mastalgia**. Occasionally, a simple cyst may cause noncyclic breast pain, and aspiration of the cyst ends the evaluation. Frequently, lifestyle and dietary changes result in improvement of **mastalgia**. Decreasing caffeine intake and the use of bras with better support are the first steps in the management of breast pain. Medications such as **danazol**, **primrose oil**, and nonsteroidal antiinflammatory drugs have been shown to occasionally be effective in refractory cases. In many cases, patients report a lessening of the pain after being reassured that the pain is not associated with cancer.

**ANSWER:** E

**66.** An ultrasound image of a patient's breast reveals a 2-cm simple cyst. Aspiration yields clear straw-colored fluid, and there is complete resolution on postprocedure ultrasound imaging. What should the clinician's next step be?

A. Order repeat ultrasound imaging in 3 months.

B. Have the fluid sent to the laboratory for Hemoccult testing, cytologic studies, and assessment for tumor markers.

C. Perform wire-localized excision of the cavity.

D. Prescribe antibiotics for the patient.

E. Advise the patient to continue with routine clinical breast examinations and mammograms.

*Ref.:* 19

**COMMENTS:** A simple **cyst** that completely resolves after aspiration of straw-colored fluid needs no further diagnostic or surgical evaluation. Routine follow-up with clinical examination and scheduled mammograms is indicated. If the cyst recurs, especially in the postmenopausal setting, surgical excision should be considered.

**ANSWER:** E

## REFERENCES

1. American Cancer Society, 2008. Available at www.cancer.org.
2. DevCan: Probability of developing or dying of cancer software, Version 6.2.1, Statistical Research and Applications Branch, NCI, 2007. Available at http://surveillance.cancer.gov/devcan/.
3. National Cancer Institute: Surveillance, epidemiology, and end results program, delay-adjusted incidence database: SEER incidence delay-adjusted rates, 9 Registries, 1975–2004, 2007.
4. Gail MH, Brinton LA, Byar DP, et al: Projecting individualized probabilities of developing breast cancer for white females who are being examined annually, *J Natl Cancer Inst* 81:1879–1886, 1989.
5. Iglehart JD, Smith BL: Diseases of the breast. In Townsend CM, Beauchamp RD, Evers BM, et al, editors: *Sabiston textbook of surgery: the biological basis of modern surgical practice*, ed 18, Philadelphia, 2008, WB Saunders.
6. Hunt KK, Newman LA, Copeland EM, et al: The breast. In Brunicardi FC, Anderson DK, Billiar TR, et al, editors: *Schwartz's principles of surgery*, ed 9, New York, 2010, McGraw-Hill.
7. Bland KI, Copeland EM, editors: *The breast: comprehensive management of benign and malignant disorders*, ed 3, St. Louis, 2004, WB Saunders.
8. Fisher B, Jeong JH, Anderson S, et al: Twenty-five-year follow-up of a randomized trial comparing radical mastectomy, total mastectomy, and total mastectomy followed by irradiation, *N Engl J Med* 347:567–575, 2002.
9. Reed J, Rosman M, Verbanac KM, et al: Prognostic implications of isolated tumor cells and micrometastases in sentinel nodes of patients with invasive breast cancer: 10-year analysis of patients enrolled in the prospective East Carolina University/Anne Arundel Medical Center Sentinel Node Multicenter Study, *J Am Coll Surg* 208:333–340, 2009.
10. Chagpar AB, McMasters KM, Edwards MJ: Can sentinel node biopsy be avoided in some elderly breast cancer patients? *Ann Surg* 249:455–460, 2009.
11. Tan SM, Low SC: Non-operative treatment of breast abscesses, *Aust N Z J Surg* 68:423–424, 1998.
12. Wilhelmi BJ, Phillips LG: Breast reconstruction. In Townsend CM, Beauchamp RD, Evers BM, et al, editors: *Sabiston textbook of surgery: the biological basis of modern surgical practice*, ed 18, Philadelphia, 2008, WB Saunders.
13. The American Society of Breast Surgeons, 2008. Available at www.breastsurgeons.org.
14. Tabar L, Dean PB: *Teaching atlas of mammography*, New York, 2001, Thieme.
15. Holmes DR, Baum M, Joseph D: The TARGIT trial: targeted intraoperative radiation therapy versus conventional postoperative whole-breast radiotherapy after breast-conserving surgery for the management of early-stage invasive breast cancer (a trial update), *Am J Surg* 194:507–510, 2007.
16. Slamon DJ, Godolphin W, Jones LA, et al: Studies of the HER-2/neu proto-oncogene in human breast and ovarian cancer, *Science* 244:707–712, 1989.

17. Fisher B, Anderson S, Redmond CK, et al: Reanalysis and results after 12 years of follow-up in a randomized clinical trial comparing total mastectomy with lumpectomy with or without irradiation in the treatment of breast cancer, *N Engl J Med* 333:1456–1461, 1995.
18. Perez CA, Taylor ME: Breast: stage Tis, T1 and T2 tumors. In Perez CA, Brady LW, editors: *Principles and practice of radiation oncology*, ed 3, Philadelphia, 1998, Lippincott-Raven.
19. Harris J, Lippman M, Morrow M, et al: *Diseases of the breast*, Philadelphia, 2004, Lippincott Williams & Wilkins.
20. Berg JC, Visscher DW, Vierkant RA, et al: Breast cancer risk in women with radial scars in benign breast biopsies, *Breast Cancer Res Treat* 108:167–174, 2008.
21. Saslow D, Boetes C, Burke W, et al: American Cancer Society guidelines for breast screening with MRI as an adjunct to mammography, *CA Cancer J Clin* 57:75–89, 2007.

# ENDOCRINE SURGERY

# CHAPTER 15

# Head and Neck

*Phillip S. LoSavio, M.D.*

1. Which of the following statements is true regarding the anatomy of the upper aerodigestive tract?

   A. The oral tongue lies posterior to the circumvallate papillae.

   B. The soft palate is a subsite in the oral cavity.

   C. The supraglottic and glottic regions of the larynx are divided by a transverse plane through the laryngeal ventricles.

   D. The false vocal cords are a part of the glottic region of the larynx.

   E. The floor of the mouth contains the openings of the sublingual, submandibular, and parotid glands.

   ***Ref.:*** 1-3

**COMMENTS:** The oral tongue lies anterior to the circumvallate papillae. The soft palate is a subsite of the oropharynx, not the oral cavity. The false vocal cords are a part of the supraglottic larynx. The floor of the mouth contains openings for the sublingual (ducts of Rivinus) and submandibular glands (Wharton duct), but not the parotid glands. The ducts for the parotid glands (Stensen duct) exit into the oral cavity adjacent to the upper second molar.

For staging and treatment purposes of head and neck cancer, it is important to understand the anatomic definitions of the different subsites of this region as they are defined by the American Joint Commission for Cancer (AJCC). **Oral cavity** subsites include the lips, oral tongue (anterior two thirds), buccal mucosa, floor of the mouth, upper and lower alveolar ridge, retromolar trigone, and hard palate. The oral cavity begins at the skin-vermillion junction anteriorly. Posterior boundaries include the circumvallate papillae as it relates to the tongue, the anterior tonsillar pillars, and the junction of the hard and soft palate. **Oropharynx** subsites include the base of the tongue, tonsils, soft palate, and pharyngeal wall lying between the soft palate and pharyngoepiglottic fold. **Hypopharynx** subsites include the piriform sinuses, postcricoid region, and posterior pharyngeal wall between the pharyngoepiglottic fold down to the upper esophageal sphincter.

The **larynx** is divided into three parts: supraglottis, glottis, and subglottis (Figure 15-1). Each has its own lymphatic drainage patterns and pathways of oncologic spread. These differences are a consequence of the different embryologic origins of the supraglottic and glottic larynx. The **supraglottic larynx** includes the epiglottis, aryepiglottic folds, arytenoids, ventricle, and false vocal cords. The **glottis** consists of the true vocal cords and the anterior and posterior commissures. It is divided from the supraglottis by a transverse plane passing through the ventricle. The **subglottis** starts inferior to the glottis and extends to the inferior border of the cricoid cartilage. It has no subsites.

**ANSWER: C**

2. Which of the following statements is true regarding the anatomy of the salivary glands?

   A. The paired submandibular glands are the largest of the major salivary glands in the head and neck and are located in the submandibular triangle just inferior to the body of the mandible.

   B. The retromandibular vein lies deep to the deep lobe of the parotid gland.

   C. Anatomic landmarks used for identifying the main trunk of the facial nerve during parotid surgery include the tympanomastoid suture line, the tragal pointer, and the posterior belly of the digastric muscle.

   D. The three major nerves most at risk for direct injury during surgery on the submandibular gland include the hypoglossal nerve, spinal accessory nerve, and lingual nerve.

   E. Injury to the greater auricular nerve during surgery on the parotid gland may lead to sensory deficits of the lower lip area on the affected side.

   ***Ref.:*** 1, 2

**COMMENTS:** The **parotid glands**, not the submandibular glands, are the largest of the major glands in the head and neck. The **retromandibular vein** can usually be well visualized as it passes between the superficial and deep lobe of the parotid on computed tomography (CT). The three major nerves most at risk for injury during surgery on the submandibular gland include the hypoglossal, marginal mandibular, and lingual nerves. The parotid gland is encased in a capsule of parotid fascia. The facial nerve (cranial nerve [CN] VII) is identified in reference to various anatomic structures. The tympanomastoid suture line is considered to be a reliable landmark. The main trunk of the nerve is located just deep and medial to this anatomic marker. The nerve also lies about 1 cm deep and inferior in reference to the tragal pointer, although this landmark is less reliable. The posterior belly of the digastric muscle provides a reference regarding the approximate depth of the nerve. As a last option, the nerve could be identified by following the peripheral buccal branches, although this should never be considered the standard approach to dissecting the nerve. The submandibular gland sits in the submandibular triangle of the neck. The marginal mandibular nerve (branch of CN VII) lies just deep to the superficial layer of the deep cervical fascia, which lies below the platysma. The gland wraps around the mylohyoid muscle, which is retracted anteriorly during surgery for exposure. The lingual nerve provides innervation to the gland through the submandibular ganglion. CN XII also lies deep to the gland. The greater auricular nerve supplies sensation to the earlobe, as well as to the preauricular and postauricular skin. The lower chin and lip region receive sensory innervation from

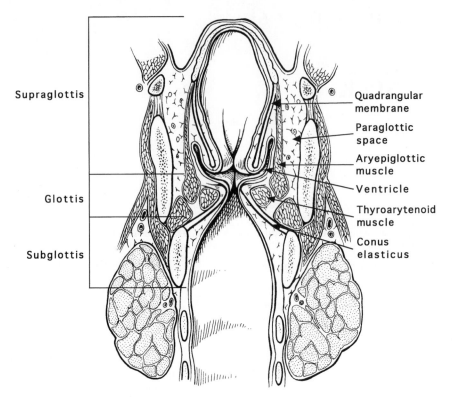

**Figure 15-1.** Coronal view of the larynx.

the mental nerve, a branch of the third division of the trigeminal nerve (V3).

**ANSWER: C**

3. Which statement is most accurate regarding the histology of the head and neck?

A. The pharynx is lined exclusively by nonkeratinizing stratified squamous epithelium.

B. The minor salivary glands lie in the submucosa of the oral cavity and pharynx.

C. The Waldeyer ring consists of only two structures: the palatine tonsils and adenoids.

D. The adenoids have crypts lined by stratified squamous epithelium.

E. The nasal cavity consists entirely of ciliated respiratory epithelium.

*Ref.:* 1, 2

**COMMENTS:** The pharynx is lined by both nonkeratinizing stratified squamous epithelium and ciliated respiratory epithelium. The **Waldeyer ring** consists of the palatine tonsils, adenoids, and the lingual tonsils, which lie along the base of the tongue. The palatine tonsils have crypts lined by stratified squamous epithelium. The adenoids are covered by pseudostratified ciliated columnar epithelium with surface folds but, unlike the tonsils, do not have crypts. The tonsillar crypts are designed to trap foreign antigens for presentation to the lymphoid follicles. The nasal cavity is composed primarily of respiratory epithelium but also contains specialized sensory olfactory epithelium along the roof. Hundreds of minor salivary glands lie in the submucosa of the oral cavity and pharynx.

**ANSWER: B**

4. A 56-year-old man with T2N0M0 squamous cell carcinoma (SCC) of the lateral oral tongue is scheduled for partial glossectomy with selective lymph node neck dissection—levels I, II, and III in the ipsilateral neck. Which of the following statements is true regarding the anatomic classification of cervical lymphatic nodal basins?

A. Level IA contains the submandibular gland.

B. Tumors of the larynx most commonly metastasize to level I.

C. Level II is bounded superiorly by the cricoid cartilage.

D. The posterior border of level III is the anterior edge of the sternocleidomastoid (SCM) muscle.

E. Level IV is bounded anteriorly by the strap muscles.

*Ref.:* 1

**COMMENTS:** Level I is subdivided into two parts (Figures 15-2 and 15-3). Level IA contains mostly fibroadipose/lymphatic tissue with no major neurovascular structures. Level IB contains the submandibular gland. Tumors of the larynx most commonly metastasize to levels II, III, and IV. Level II is bounded superiorly by the skull base and inferiorly by the hyoid bone. Level IV is bounded superiorly by the cricoid cartilage. The posterior border of level III is the posterior edge of the SCM muscle.

C. The RLN supplies all the muscles of the larynx except the posterior cricoarytenoid muscle.

D. The vagus nerve exits the skull through the carotid canal.

E. The RLN enters the larynx through the thyrohyoid membrane to innervate the larynx.

*Ref.:* 1

**COMMENTS:** The left **recurrent laryngeal nerve** separates from the vagus in the mediastinum, wraps around the aortic arch at the ductus arteriosus, and then ascends back along the tracheoesophageal groove toward the larynx. The right RLN divides off the vagus and passes around the right subclavian artery to travel to the larynx. The RLN supplies all the muscles of the larynx except the cricothyroid muscle, which is innervated by the external branch of the superior laryngeal nerve. The superior laryngeal nerve also has an internal branch that supplies sensation to the larynx above the true vocal cords. The RLN provides sensation below this area. The vagus nerve exits the skull base on both sides through the jugular foramen, not the carotid canal. The internal branch of the superior laryngeal nerve, not the RLN, enters the thyrohyoid membrane. The RLN travels along the tracheoesophageal groove and enters the larynx just superior to the cricoid cartilage. Nonrecurrent nerves occur most commonly on the right side in up to 1% to 2% of patients and can be associated with a retroesophageal right subclavian vein.

**ANSWER:**   B

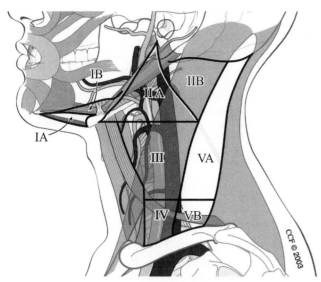

**Figure 15-2.**   Diagram of cervical lymph node levels I through V. Level II is divided into regions A and B by the spinal accessory nerve. (© Cleveland Clinic Foundation, 2003.)

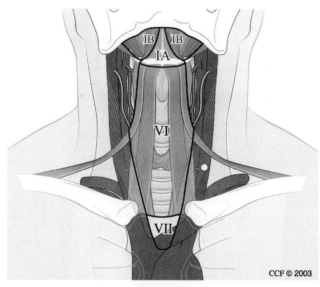

**Figure 15-3.**   Diagram of anterior lymph node levels I, VI, and VII. Though large in area, the majority of level VI lymph nodes are confined to the paratracheal region. (© Cleveland Clinic Foundation, 2003.)

**ANSWER:**   E

5. A 68-year-old woman is evaluated for a 1-month history worsening dyspnea and hoarseness. Fiberoptic laryngoscopy demonstrates left vocal cord paralysis with full mobility of the right true vocal cord. Findings on physical examination are otherwise unremarkable. CT of the chest demonstrates a large mediastinal mass. Which of the following statements is most accurate?

A. The left recurrent laryngeal nerve (RLN) branches off of the vagus nerve and passes around the left subclavian artery back to the larynx.

B. A nonrecurrent RLN can be associated with a retroesophageal right subclavian artery.

6. Which of the following statements is true regarding head and neck carcinogenesis and molecular therapy?

A. A synchronous second primary tumor is defined as one developing within 1 year of the initial cancer.

B. Human papillomavirus (HPV) has been shown to be a factor in the development of certain head and neck cancers.

C. Cetuximab (IMC-C225) is a monoclonal antibody therapy targeted against transforming growth factor-β.

D. p53 is commonly underexpressed in head and neck cancer.

E. The most frequently mutated tumor suppressor gene in head and neck cancer is cyclin D1.

*Ref.:* 1, 2

**COMMENTS:** Head and neck carcinogenesis is a complex process with multiple etiologic factors and a wide variety of genetic alterations that have been identified. The incidence of second primary tumors in head and neck cancer is not insignificant (3% to 7%), and they should be surveyed for in the upper aerodigestive tract, esophagus, and lung at the time of initial diagnosis. **Synchronous** versus **metachronous** lesions are defined in relation to the time of diagnosis from initial discovery of the tumor; synchronous lesions are found within 6 months, with metachronous lesion being diagnosed after 6 months. In recent years, **human papillomavirus** has been identified as an etiologic factor in certain head and neck cancers, specifically the oropharynx. Protooncogenes are genes that produce proteins involved in normal cell regulation and function. Mutation of these genes, including those for epidermal growth factor receptor (EGFR), cyclin D1, and vascular endothelial growth factor (VEGF), occurs in head and neck cancer. Tumor suppressor genes such as p53 and p16-ARF encode proteins that halt tumor growth and carcinogenesis. **Cetuximab** is novel monoclonal antibody therapy that has been designed to target EGFR. Trials are ongoing regarding its efficacy in combination with standard treatments such as radiotherapy and chemotherapy. Mutated p53 is poorly degraded and therefore commonly overexpressed in head and neck cancer. It is the most commonly altered tumor suppressor gene in human cancers, with p16-ARF being the most commonly altered gene locus in head and neck cancer.

**ANSWER: B**

7. A 75-year-old man with a long history of tobacco use comes to the office with a newly discovered tongue mass. A 3-cm ulcerated lesion is noted on the right anterior aspect of the tongue. Biopsy of the lesion demonstrates SCC. CT of the neck with intravenous contrast enhancement shows an enlarged 2-cm lymph node in the level II region on the left side. Findings on chest radiography are clear. How would you stage this patient's disease?

A. T1N1M0

B. T2N1M0

C. T1N2cM0

D. T2N2bM0

E. T2N2cM0

*Ref.:* 1, 3

**COMMENTS:** The **T classification** as defined by the AJCC refers to the primary tumor. Carcinoma of the oral cavity is staged according to size. T2 lesions are 2 to 4 cm, as in this patient. Oral cavity T staging is as follows: T1, less than 2 cm; T2, 2 to 4 cm; T3, greater than 4 cm; and T4, invasion of adjacent structures. Clinical staging of the neck has been made more accurate by high-resolution imaging (CT). Had this node been ipsilateral, it would have been staged as N1. However, since it is contralateral to the primary disease, it is classified as N2c. Table 15-1 applies to primary tumors of the oral cavity, oropharynx, hypopharynx, and larynx.

**TABLE 15-1   Regional Lymph Nodes (N)**

| | |
|---|---|
| NX | Regional lymph nodes cannot be assessed |
| N0 | No regional lymph node metastasis |
| N1* | Metastasis in a single ipsilateral lymph node, 3 cm or less in greatest dimension |
| N2* | Metastasis in a single ipsilateral lymph node, more than 3 cm but not more than 6 cm in greatest dimension; or in multiple ipsilateral lymph nodes, none more than 6 cm in greatest dimension; or in bilateral or contralateral lymph nodes, none more than 6 cm in greatest dimension |
| N2a* | Metastasis in a single ipsilateral lymph node more than 3 cm but not more than 6 cm in greatest dimension |
| N2b* | Metastasis in multiple ipsilateral lymph nodes, none more than 6 cm in greatest dimension |
| N2c* | Metastasis in bilateral or contralateral lymph nodes, none more than 6 cm in greatest dimension |
| N3* | Metastasis in a lymph node more than 6 cm in greatest dimension |

*Note: A designation of "U" or "L" maybe used for any N stage to indicate metastasis above the lower border of the cricoids (U) or below the lower border of the cricoids (L). Similarly, clinical/radiological ECS should be recorded as E- or E+, and histopathologic ECS should be designated EN, EM, or Eg.

Used with the permission of the American Joint Committee on Cancer (AJCC), Chicago, Illinois. The original source for this material is the *AJCC Cancer Staging Manual, Seventh Edition (2010)* published by Springer Science and Business Media LLC, www.springer.com.

**ANSWER: E**

8. A 42-year-old nonsmoking man is evaluated at the office because of a new left-sided neck mass. He has no recent history of illness. On examination, he is afebrile with stable vital signs. The mass measures approximately 3 cm, and it is fixed and located on level II. It is nontender and nonpulsatile and does not exhibit any overlying skin changes. The rest of his head and neck examination is unremarkable, including flexible fiberoptic examination of the larynx and hypopharynx. CT of the neck with intravenous contrast enhancement demonstrates an isolated enlarged 3-cm lymph node at level II with no other masses or abnormalities detected. Select the most appropriate next step.

A. Bone marrow biopsy to evaluate for suspected lymphoma

B. Positron emission tomography (PET)

C. Excisional biopsy of the lymph node

D. Fine-needle aspiration (FNA) of the lymph node

E. Magnetic resonance imaging (MRI) of the neck with and without gadolinium contrast enhancement

*Ref.:* 1, 2, 4

**COMMENTS:** A new-onset enlarged cervical lymph node in an adult with no previous history of infection is highly suggestive of metastatic cancer until proved otherwise. The next most appropriate step in diagnosis is to perform a **fine-needle aspiration** biopsy. This is the most useful diagnostic step in the work-up of a cervical neck mass. Bone marrow biopsy would be useful in staging after establishing the diagnosis of a hematologic malignancy such as lymphoma. The role of PET in head and neck cancer is still being elucidated. It may be useful to assist in searching for the site of an unknown primary lesion. Other current uses of PET include assessment of a patient's response to treatment and staging and metastatic surveillance. MRI would probably not add any additional useful diagnostic information. **Excisional biopsy** is not suitable as the initial diagnostic step since it may compromise appropriate definitive therapy such as neck dissection and has been shown to increase local cervical recurrence. Excisional biopsy is indicated when FNA suggests the diagnosis of lymphoma and further subtyping and classification are needed, if initial and repeat FNA biopsies are inconclusive, or if the FNA results are benign but there is high clinical suspicion for malignancy.

**ANSWER: D**

9. A 67-year-old man has a 2-month history of a new-onset right level II neck mass. FNA biopsy is performed and demonstrates SCC. Office examination of the head and neck fails to demonstrate a primary tumor site. CT confirms the enlarged node with no additional information. PET also shows increased uptake at the site of the lymph node with no other activity noted. What is the next most appropriate step in management?

A. Endoscopy under anesthesia with guided biopsies and bilateral tonsillectomy

B. Neck dissection

C. Irradiation of the neck and upper aerodigestive tract

D. Excisional node biopsy

E. Repeated FNA

*Ref.:* 1, 2

**COMMENTS:** A large number of patients with metastatic **cervical lymphadenopathy of unknown origin** will have their primary tumors identified during the office examination. For patients such as this one, in whom the primary site is not apparent, endoscopy of the upper aerodigestive tract under anesthesia should be performed. If no obvious mucosal lesion is detected, one should proceed with directed biopsies of the most likely primary sites. The site of the metastatic node can give some insight into the location of the primary tumor. Oropharyngeal cancers drain to the level II region and would be an area of concern in this patient. Nodes in the lower neck region might raise suspicion for a tumor below the clavicles. The work-up should proceed with a biopsy of the tonsils by tonsillectomy, with additional biopsy samples taken of the base of the tongue, piriform sinuses, and nasopharynx. These are the most common locations for a primary site of an unknown SCC of the head and neck. CT and PET were appropriate but did not add any additional clinical information. Neck dissection or radiation therapy (or both) may be the eventual therapy in this patient, but not before a thorough investigation for the primary site is performed. Excisional node biopsy would be appropriate only if FNA has been inconclusive. Repeated FNA is not needed since the diagnosis has already been established.

**ANSWER:** A

10. Which of the following has not been shown to be a risk factor for the development of head and neck cancer?

    A. Tobacco use

    B. Alcohol abuse

    C. Inhalation of heavy metal dust

    D. Plummer-Vinson syndrome

    E. High-fat diet

*Ref.:* 1, 3

**COMMENTS:** The two largest risk factors for the development of **squamous cell carcinoma** of the head and neck are **tobacco** and **alcohol abuse**. **Occupational exposure** to heavy metals and wood dust has been shown in some studies to increase the risk for sinonasal cancers. Exposure to ultraviolet light is associated with an increased risk for cutaneous malignancies of the head and neck, as well as lip cancer. Intake of salted fish and exposure to **Epstein-Barr virus** (EBV) have been associated with the development of nasopharyngeal carcinoma. Dietary and nutritional factors have a link with certain head and neck malignancies. Iron deficiency, as seen in **Plummer-Vinson syndrome**, has been linked to an increased risk for oral cavity and hypopharyngeal carcinoma. Although there may be a connection between fat intake and head and neck cancer, such an association has yet to be shown in any evidence-based medical studies. HPV infection has been studied extensively in regard to its relationship with cervical cancer. Recently, there has been great interest in its association with head and neck cancers, especially oropharyngeal cancer, as well as oral cavity and laryngeal cancers.

**ANSWER:** E

11. A 75-year-old man with T2N0M0 SCC of the lower lip undergoes primary resection of the tumor, with full-thickness resection resulting in a defect involving about 55% of the central lower lip but not involving the oral commissure. Which of the following is the best option for reconstruction of the defect?

    A. Primary closure

    B. Abbe two-stage cross-lip transfer flap

    C. Radial forearm free flap transfer

    D. Nasolabial transposition flap

    E. Estlander flap

*Ref.:* 1, 2

**COMMENTS:** The lip begins at the vermillion border and is a subsite of the oral cavity. Risk factors for lip carcinoma include sun exposure and tobacco use. The lower lip is by far the most common site of tumor development, with **squamous cell carcinoma** being the most common pathology. **Basal cell carcinoma** is the most frequent pathology found on diagnosis for upper lip cancers. Initial evaluation should include testing for mental nerve involvement, evaluation for mandibular invasion, and examination of the cervical lymphatics. CT can be useful, especially in staging the mandible and cervical nodes.

Treatment of early-stage disease can consist of either primary external beam radiation or surgical resection. Primary excision is typically the favored treatment. Elective lymph node neck dissection for a clinically negative neck is performed in patients with advanced T stage disease or in the setting of deep tumor invasion in which the risk for occult cervical lymph node disease is elevated. Therapeutic neck dissection is appropriate in patients with positive nodal disease. Indications for postoperative irradiation include advanced T stage, positive margins, perineural/perivascular invasion, multiple or bulky nodal disease, and invasion of bone. Fortunately, given its location, many lip cancers are detected early and can be treated with a high success rate. Stage I and II lesions have a 90% 5-year survival rate. The survival rate drops to about 50% in patients with cervical lymph node involvement.

Reconstructive options following excision of carcinoma of the lip generally depend on the location of the lesion (medial versus lateral with involvement of the oral commissure) and the size of the defect. Smaller lesions that involve less than a third to half of the lip can be closed primarily with local advancement of the tissue. Larger defects involving between half and two thirds of the lip will probably require donated tissue such as a pedicled two-stage cross-lip transfer flap. An **Abbe flap** is used for central defects, whereas **Estlander**-style flaps are used for lateral defects. Larger defects can be repaired with local advancement techniques, local rotational flaps, or distal free flaps.

**ANSWER:** B

12. A 55-year-old male smoker, otherwise healthy, has a 3-cm ulcer on the left lateral border of the anterior aspect of his tongue with no involvement of the floor of the mouth or mandible. Biopsy demonstrates SCC with a 6-mm depth of tumor invasion. CT of his neck shows no evidence of cervical lymphadenopathy. His remaining metastatic work-up is negative. Which of the following choices is the best option for treatment?

    A. Concomitant chemotherapy and external beam radiation

    B. Partial glossectomy with left supraomohyoid neck dissection

    C. Total glossectomy with left supraomohyoid neck dissection

    D. Primary chemotherapy with 5-fluorouracil and cisplatin

    E. Total glossectomy with bilateral modified radical neck dissection

*Ref.:* 1, 3

**COMMENTS:** The **oral tongue** is the most common site for cancer of the oral cavity. Most tongue cancers develop on the lateral border, as in this example. SCC is by far the most common pathology, but other malignancies may also occur. **Verrucous carcinoma** is a variant of SCC; it is described as having pushing borders with a very low propensity toward metastasis. Other nonepidermoid malignancies can include adenoid cystic carcinoma, Kaposi sarcoma, lymphoma, and melanoma. Cancer of the tongue is staged according to the same system as used for other oral cavity malignancies: T1, less than 2 cm; T2, 2 to 4 cm; T3, greater than 4 cm; and T4, invasion of adjacent structures.

Treatment of the primary site for early-stage (T1/T2) tongue cancer can consist of either primary surgical excision or radiation therapy. Advanced cancers are generally treated with multimodality therapy involving surgery and postoperative radiotherapy with or without chemotherapy. **Chemotherapy** alone has very poor results and is not a standard option for care. Primary excision with partial glossectomy or **hemiglossectomy** leaves a defect that requires some type of reconstruction. Smaller defects can usually be repaired by either primary closure or secondary intention. Larger defects may require a split-thickness skin graft. Large resection involving a majority of the tongue may need a regional (e.g., pectoralis major) or distant flap (e.g., radial forearm). Postoperative **radiation therapy** is indicated for patients with positive margins, advanced-stage tumors, extracapsular nodal spread, perineural/perivascular invasion, bulky or multiple nodal involvement, and deep muscular/bone invasion.

Therapeutic neck dissection is indicated for grossly positive nodal disease. Since patients with oral tongue cancer have a high rate of occult cervical metastases, even in a clinically N0 neck, elective neck dissection may be indicated for early-stage T1 tumors. Rates higher than 20% have led to a recommendation for limited supraomohyoid dissection—levels I, II, and III—in almost all patients. Factors that increase the risk for occult metastases include the depth of invasion, with depths greater than 4 to 5 mm showing an increased risk for occult metastatic disease. Sentinel lymph node biopsy is currently under investigation for its role in the treatment of N0 stage necks in patients with cancer of the oral cavity.

**ANSWER: B**

13. A T4N0M0 SCC in the midline anterior floor of the mouth is recently diagnosed in a 72-year-old man. The tumor is approximately 2.3 cm in diameter but is invading anteriorly into the cortical bone of the mandible. What is the best option for treatment in this patient?

A. Local resection with curettage of involved bone

B. Composite tumor resection with total mandibulectomy and bilateral radical neck dissection

C. Primary external beam radiation therapy

D. Composite tumor resection with segmental mandibulectomy and bilateral selective neck dissection

E. Primary chemotherapy

*Ref.:* 1, 3

**COMMENTS:** The **floor of the mouth** is a subsite of the oral cavity. The staging system used is the same as for all other cancers of the oral cavity. In this patient, although the size (2 to 4 cm) would stage it as a T2 cancer, invasion into cortical bone qualifies as T4 disease. The floor of the mouth is defined anatomically as extending from the lower alveolar ridge to the ventral surface of the tongue. Posteriorly, it is bounded by the anterior tonsillar pillars. Overall, treatment of cancer in the floor of the mouth is primarily surgical. Radiation therapy is less effective in patients

with deep invasion of bone or muscle, as in the patient in this example. Primary radiation treatment of the mandible also carries the risk of osteoradionecrosis. All patients undergoing radiation therapy that will encompass the oral cavity should receive a pretreatment dental evaluation so that any carious teeth that would predispose to this complication can be removed. In regard to surgical treatment of the floor of the mouth, **primary composite resection** of the involved area with 1-cm margins is usually appropriate. In oral cavity cancers, the mandible can prevent surgical access to the tumor, or it may be involved by tumor. For surgical access, mandibular osteotomy or visor flaps may be needed. When tumor approaches the bone but does not directly invade it, marginal resection of the inner or outer cortex of the bone can be done. The periosteum itself serves as a barrier to tumor invasion and can be considered a margin of resection. When direct cortical invasion has occurred, en bloc segmental resection is required. Surgical resection involving the floor of the mouth, tongue, and mandible is classically referred to as a "composite" or "commando" resection. The neck is treated similar to that for other tumors of the oral cavity. Grossly positive metastatic disease is treated by therapeutic modified radical neck dissection. Elective neck dissections are recommended for clinical N0 disease in most tumors, especially if advanced stage or deeply infiltrative. Radiotherapy as a primary treatment can be used when there is a significant contraindication to surgery. It is also used in the postoperative adjuvant setting for advanced-stage disease. Overall survival rates range anywhere from 64% to 95% for stage I disease to 6% to 52% for stage IV cancer. This patient has significant involvement of bone with direct invasion and requires a composite resection. The neck is clinically negative (N0) for metastatic disease, so bilateral elective supraomohyoid neck dissection is indicated for treatment. Radical neck dissection would be performed in the case of bulky metastatic cervical disease. External beam radiation can be used for early-stage tumors but is probably not the favored option, especially in light of the deep bone invasion. Primary chemotherapy has not been shown to be effective in treating cancer of the floor of the mouth.

**ANSWER: D**

14. A 62-year-old woman is seen in your office with a 1-cm painless mass involving the hard palate. You develop a differential diagnosis. Which of the following diagnoses is least likely in this location?

A. SCC

B. Granular cell tumor

C. Necrotizing sialometaplasia

D. Adenoid cystic carcinoma

E. Lipoma

*Ref.:* 1, 3

**COMMENTS:** There is no fat pad in this subsite of the oral cavity, unlike the buccal space and other areas of the head and neck, and therefore a **lipoma** should not be on the differential diagnosis. All the other diseases listed commonly occur in this area and should be considered when confronted with a mass in this area. Biopsy is usually warranted for diagnosis. Many benign lesions can mimic cancer of the hard palate. **Necrotizing sialometaplasia** is a self-limited inflammatory disease of the minor salivary glands that can be mistaken for carcinoma given its ulcerative appearance. No treatment is required. The palate is the most common site of Kaposi sarcoma in the oral cavity and should be considered in any patient with immunosuppression. Minor salivary gland tumors and SCC are both common malignancies in this region. Cancer at this site is rare in the United States, where it accounts for 0.5% of oral cavity malignancies. It is much more common in India because of the high incidence of betel nut chewing. Treatment of cancer of the hard palate usually involves local resection. Typically, surgery is favored over radiation therapy for early-stage lesions given the risk for **osteoradionecrosis**. More advanced tumors may require partial or total maxillectomy. It is generally thought that the incidence of occult metastatic cervical disease is low with hard palate tumors, so elective neck dissection is not indicated in most cases. Advanced-stage tumors generally receive combined-modality therapy consisting of surgery and adjuvant radiation therapy.

**A N S W E R :**  E

15. Which of the following statements is true regarding cancer of the oropharynx?

   A. HPV is a risk factor.

   B. Oropharyngeal cancer commonly metastasizes to level I of the neck.

   C. Concurrent treatment with chemotherapy and radiation therapy has little role in the management of advanced-stage oropharyngeal cancer.

   D. Subsites of the oropharynx include the base of the tongue, tonsils, soft palate, and adenoids.

   E. Extensive resection of the base of the tongue increases the possibility of postoperative velopharyngeal insufficiency.

*Ref.:* 1, 3, 5

**COMMENTS:** The **oropharynx** consists of several subsites, including the base of the tongue, tonsils, soft palate, and posterior pharyngeal wall. The adenoids are located in the nasopharynx. The oropharynx serves an important functional role in **speech** and **swallowing**. Extensive surgical resection in this area can lead to severe deficits. Besides the universal risk factors of tobacco and alcohol use, recent evidence has begun to suggest a role for HPV in the development of some oropharyngeal carcinomas. Most tumors of the oropharynx are SCC, but lymphoma and salivary gland neoplasms can also arise in this region. Cancers of the oropharynx most commonly metastasize to levels II, III, and IV of the neck, as well as the retropharyngeal nodes. Bilateral metastases are common, especially with lesions on the base of the tongue and palate. Many patients with oropharyngeal cancer may initially have a neck mass from an unknown primary site. Especially if this node is located in the level II region, the base of the tongue and tonsil should be highly suspected as the primary site. Cystic neck masses in an adult should always arouse concern for a possible metastatic oropharyngeal cancer and not be assumed to be a branchial cleft anomaly. Treatment of oropharyngeal cancer has evolved over the years. Traditional surgical approaches have included transcervical, transpharyngeal, and transmandibular routes for advanced tumors. More recently, transoral laser microsurgery has been introduced as a treatment option and has shown some promising early results. Concurrent treatment with chemotherapy and radiotherapy has been used as primary management of advanced disease with good results. There are no conclusive data to date regarding the superiority of surgery with postoperative radiation therapy over concurrent chemotherapy and radiation therapy. This is especially true in light of the rapidly advancing field of transoral laser surgery. Patients who do undergo more traditional surgical approaches can have large surgical defects requiring advanced reconstruction, including regional and distal flaps. In addition, external beam radiation can cause changes in the tissue and musculature that leave the patient with permanent oropharyngeal dysphagia. The soft palate is important in preventing regurgitation of food and liquids into the nose, as well as in contributing to normal speech that does not sound hypernasal. Patients who undergo resection of the soft palate can be fitted with a prosthesis called an obturator to allow improved **velopharyngeal function**.

**A N S W E R :**  A

16. Which of the following statements is most accurate regarding treatment of SCC of the larynx?

   A. The most common location of carcinoma in the larynx is the subglottis.

   B. Advanced-stage bulky tumors are best treated with transoral laser microscopic surgery.

   C. Vocal cord fixation qualifies a tumor as a T4 carcinoma.

   D. Patients undergoing open conservation laryngeal surgery should be assessed preoperatively for adequate pulmonary function.

   E. T2 cancers of the glottis are most commonly treated with multimodality therapy.

*Ref.:* 1, 3

**COMMENTS:** **Laryngeal carcinoma** is an extensive topic with a complex set of treatment approaches. It is the second most common noncutaneous head and neck cancer after cancer of the oral cavity. **Glottic** cancer is the most frequent, followed by **supraglottic**, with **subglottic** cancers being relatively uncommon. Hoarseness and otalgia are common initial symptoms. The diagnosis is made by **flexible laryngoscopy** in the office, with confirmatory biopsy of the tumor usually done in the operating room (OR). CT of the neck assists in staging, in addition to evaluation of the chest with either CT or bronchoscopy. The lungs are the most common site of distant metastases. Nodal metastases are much more common in supraglottic than in glottic cancer. The most frequent areas of spread are levels II, III, and IV. Elective neck dissection is usually recommended for T3 glottic and T2 supraglottic cancers. T staging of laryngeal tumors is complex. A general overview is as follows: T1, limited to one subsite; T2, extends to a second subsite; T3, vocal cord fixation; and T4, extralaryngeal spread. **Squamous cell carcinoma** is the most common pathology, as with other sites in the head and neck. Malignancies can arise from any type of tissue origin in the larynx, including salivary, cartilage, neuroendocrine, and lymphoid tissue. **Verrucous carcinoma** differs from invasive SCC in that it has pushing rather than invasive margins. The larynx is the second most common site after the oral cavity. It has an extremely low propensity for spread to the cervical lymphatics. Treatment of the primary site in laryngeal cancer is based on the subsite involved, extent of tumor involvement, and individual patient factors. Early-stage tumors (T1 and T2) are treated in most cases with single-modality therapy consisting of either surgery or radiation therapy. Advanced lesions (T3 and T4) are treated with multimodality therapy, with the two main options being either chemoradiation therapy or surgery with postoperative radiation therapy. In regard to early-stage lesions, the decision to proceed with radiation therapy versus surgery is based on multiple factors, including patient preference, medical stability for surgery, anticipated voice quality after surgery, and the patient's ability to comply with a 6-week course of radiation therapy. Early-stage tumors are commonly treated today with endoscopic transoral laser techniques. Laser excision of early-stage glottic lesions has a high cure rate, with reports in the 80% to 100% range for T1 and T2 lesions. Traditionally, advanced cancer of the larynx was treated by **total laryngectomy** with postoperative radiation therapy. Given the profound disability, social stigmatization, and negative psychological impact of this operation, laryngeal preservation with maintenance of the three functions of the larynx (respiration, phonation, and airway protection) is preferred. **Conservation laryngeal surgery** consists of both endoscopic and open techniques. Candidates for open conservation laryngeal surgery need to undergo a thorough preoperative evaluation of their pulmonary and cardiac function since these procedures will place the patient at an increased risk for aspiration. Traditional open conservative treatment of supraglottic cancers consists of a horizontal partial laryngectomy. Organ preservation in patients with advanced tumors is possible with nonsurgical therapy without any difference in survival. Total laryngectomy is indicated for patients with bulky advanced T4 disease, as salvage for failed conservative therapy, and in patients with a benign nonfunctional larynx after conservative treatment with repeated severe aspiration.

**ANSWER: D**

17. Which of the following statements is most accurate regarding the management of SCC of the hypopharynx?

    A. Hypopharyngeal carcinoma is most commonly initially seen at an early stage.

    B. The hypopharynx includes the piriform sinuses, posterior pharyngeal wall, and arytenoid cartilages.

    C. Ten percent of patients with hypopharyngeal carcinoma have palpable lymphadenopathy.

    D. Surgical therapy for advanced-staged hypopharyngeal carcinoma usually consists of total laryngopharyngectomy.

    E. Overall survival rates for patients with hypopharyngeal carcinoma compare favorably with those in patients with carcinoma of the glottis.

*Ref.:* 1, 3, 6

**COMMENTS: Hypopharyngeal cancers** have a poor prognosis overall in comparison to other head and neck cancers. These cancers tend to initially be seen at later stages with early lymphatic spread. About 70% to 80% of patients have cervical metastatic disease. The subsites of the hypopharynx include the piriform sinus, posterior pharyngeal wall, and postcricoid region. Staging is similar to larynx cancer: T1, one subsite; T2, more than one subsite; T3, hemilarynx fixation; and T4, invasion of adjacent structures. Risk factors besides tobacco use include iron deficiency anemia, as seen in Plummer-Vinson syndrome. Conservation surgery—partial pharyngectomy without laryngectomy—is indicated in the absence of cartilage invasion and extension to the piriform apex in patients with a mobile vocal cord. Any further involvement is an indication for either partial or total laryngectomy, in addition to pharyngectomy. Transoral laser microsurgery shows promising results. However, total open laryngopharyngectomy with bilateral neck dissection is still indicated in many cases as treatment given the advanced stage in most patients. Routine assessment of esophageal involvement is mandatory. Organ preservation with chemoradiation therapy is also commonly used at many institutions as a first line of therapy.

**ANSWER: D**

18. A 47-year-old male immigrant from southern China has a complaint of right-sided hearing loss for the past 3 weeks. He has no history of a recent upper respiratory infection or chronic ear disease. His clinical history is otherwise unremarkable.

Serous otitis media is noted in his right ear. In addition, a 1.5-cm level V lymph node is palpated in the left side of the neck. The rest of the physical examination is within normal limits. What is the next step in management?

    A. Treatment with amoxicillin for 10 days

    B. Flexible nasopharyngoscopic examination

    C. Ototopical antibiotic drops

    D. Oral and topical decongestants for 2 weeks with reexamination

    E. Observation with follow-up in 2 weeks if the symptoms do not resolve

*Ref.:* 1-3, 7

**COMMENTS:** Any adult patient with a new onset of unilateral middle ear effusion and no related history of recent upper respiratory illness should undergo evaluation of the nasopharynx. Another clinical clue in this patient is the presence of a level V node, which is a common location for cervical metastasis from **nasopharyngeal cancer.** This is especially true in this patient given his history of a southern Chinese background. This area, particularly the Guangdong Province, has an increased incidence of nasopharyngeal carcinoma. The etiologic factors are multifactorial and include genetic and environmental factors. Infection with **Epstein-Barr virus** has been shown to have an etiologic role. In addition, dietary factors, including the intake of salted fish, have a strong association with the development of this disease. Nasopharyngeal carcinoma is divided by the World Health Organization into two groups, keratinizing versus nonkeratinizing carcinoma, with the second group including both differentiated and undifferentiated subtypes. The diagnosis of nasopharyngeal carcinoma is done by nasopharyngoscopy and biopsy. High serologic levels of IgA to EBV viral capsid antigen and early antigen are seen in patients with this disease. It has been advocated as a screening tool in high-risk populations based on a study showing a 5.4% diagnosis rate of subclinical nasopharyngeal cancer in patients with elevated IgA levels to EBV who live in the Guangdong Province. Treatment consists mainly of chemotherapy and radiation therapy. Surgery has a limited role in treating nasopharyngeal cancer in patients with limited primary site recurrence and nodal recurrence.

**ANSWER: B**

19. Which of the following statements is true regarding salivary gland tumors?

    A. Approximately 80% of submandibular gland tumors are malignant.

    B. The most common location for adenoid cystic carcinoma is the parotid gland.

    C. Treatment of a pleomorphic adenoma of the parotid gland usually involves radical parotidectomy.

    D. Adenoid cystic carcinoma has a high rate of lymphatic spread.

    E. The most common malignant salivary gland neoplasm is mucoepidermoid carcinoma.

*Ref.:* 1, 3

**COMMENTS:** The study of **salivary gland neoplasms** begins with a review of anatomy. The salivary glands consist of major and minor glands. The major glands include the parotid, submandibular, and sublingual glands. Minor glands are scattered throughout the upper aerodigestive tract. The majority of neoplasms (70% to 80%) overall arise in the parotid gland, followed by the submandibular and minor glands. Nearly 80% of parotid tumors are benign. There is an approximately equal distribution of submandibular tumors, with minor gland tumors having an opposite distribution consisting of about 80% being malignant. Initial diagnosis of a salivary gland neoplasm can involve FNA biopsy and CT, although some advocate proceeding directly with excision. Warning signs of a possible malignancy include pain, rapid growth, nodal enlargement, and facial nerve paralysis.

The most common neoplasm overall in the parotid gland is a **pleomorphic adenoma**. It represents about two thirds of all salivary gland neoplasms. Treatment consists of resection via parotidectomy. Most lesions arise in the tail of the parotid, and lateral lobe parotidectomy is typically required for treatment. A **Warthin tumor** (papillary cystadenoma lymphomatosum) is the second most common benign tumor that arises in the parotid gland. Up to 10% of tumors are bilateral, with smoking shown to be a risk factor for the development of these lesions. They are noted to concentrate technetium-99m, which can aid in diagnosis. The most frequent malignant tumor overall is **mucoepidermoid carcinoma**, and it is the most common malignancy in the parotid gland. It is graded from low to high, with higher-grade lesions behaving very aggressively, similar to SCC. Treatment consists of total parotidectomy. Radical parotidectomy with resection of the facial nerve is typically indicated only in patients with gross nerve invasion and loss of function. Elective treatment of the neck is advocated in patients with advanced T stage or high-grade disease. Adenoid cystic carcinoma is the malignancy found most frequently in the submandibular and minor salivary glands. Its most common primary location is the oral cavity. These tumors are notorious for perineural spread, and they also commonly metastasize to the lung. Because these distant metastases can develop decades in the future, a yearly chest radiograph is recommended. Treatment consists of excision, but elective treatment of the neck is unnecessary given the low incidence of cervical spread.

**ANSWER:** E

20. Which of the following statement is most accurate regarding the use of chemoradiation therapy for head and neck cancer?

A. Chemotherapy can be used as single-modality primary therapy with intent to cure in many head and neck cancers.

B. Induction chemotherapy plus radiation therapy had superior overall survival results when compared with surgery plus radiation therapy for the treatment of advanced-stage laryngeal cancer.

C. Postoperative concomitant chemotherapy with radiation therapy improves overall survival in comparison to postoperative radiation therapy alone in high-risk locally advanced head and neck cancer.

D. Chemotherapy has no role in the palliative setting for metastatic head and neck cancer.

E. Chemotherapy in the postoperative adjuvant setting in conjunction with radiation therapy has the advantage of improving survival while not increasing mucosal toxicity.

*Ref.:* 1, 8-12

**COMMENTS:** Chemotherapy has developed an increasing role over the past two decades in the treatment of head and neck SCC. For early-stage patients, treatment consists of either radiation therapy or surgery, with chemotherapy having little to no role in treatment. It is never used as a primary single-modality treatment

for head and neck cancer with intent to cure. For patients with advanced metastatic or recurrent disease, chemotherapy can be used in the palliative setting to inhibit tumor growth for a limited effective period. Its main role is in the treatment of locoregionally advanced stage III/IV cancer. A second role in this group of patients is for organ preservation. Patients with advanced primary T stage are best served by total laryngectomy. For advanced-stage **unresectable tumors**, concurrent chemoradiation therapy, in comparison to radiation therapy alone, has shown improved locoregional control with questionable overall survival benefit.

**ANSWER:** C

21. A 34-year-old woman is seen in the office with a 3-month history of a left-sided neck mass and pain with mastication. On examination, a 3-cm nontender mass is present at level II; it moves laterally but not in the craniocaudal direction. CT with intravenous contrast enhancement demonstrates a 3.5-cm mass at the carotid bifurcation. A follow-up angiogram is obtained:

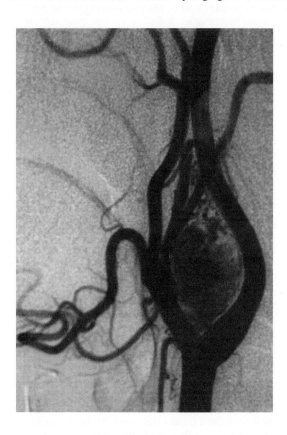

Which of the following statements is most accurate regarding this case?

A. It represents the most common paraganglioma in the head and neck.

B. The rate of malignancy is about 30%.

C. The majority of these lesions show functional secretion of catecholamines.

D. FNA biopsy is indicated to rule out malignancy.

E. Radiation therapy is the most effective treatment of these lesions.

*Ref.:* 1, 2

**COMMENTS:** A carotid **body tumor** is the most common **paraganglioma** in the head and neck. Other paragangliomas that occur in this region include the vagal and jugulotympanic types. The majority of paragangliomas are solitary and nonfamilial. Multicentricity is reported in about 10% of cases, with about a 6% rate of malignancy. Only about 1% to 3% of them are considered functional and can be evaluated with a 24-hour urine collection for analysis of catecholamines. The "**Fontaine sign**" refers to mobility in only the lateral direction on palpation, whereas pain occurring with chewing is called "**first-bite syndrome.**" Histopathologic evaluation of this tumor demonstrates two types of cells: type I, chief cells/granular cells; and type II, sustentacular supporting cells. Unlike most head and neck tumors, malignancy is not diagnosed by the presence of dysplastic changes in the primary tumor. The presence of metastatic disease either to the regional cervical lymphatics or to distant sites is the only diagnostic criteria. Imaging is the major modality for primary diagnosis since needle biopsy is contraindicated. CT will show a hypervascular mass at the carotid bifurcation, with MRI demonstrating a classic "salt and pepper" appearance on T2-weighted sequences because of hemorrhage and flow voids. On angiography, the internal and external carotid arteries will be bowed apart, a finding referred to as a "**lyre sign.**" These tumors are best treated surgically, and vascular reconstruction may be necessary. Radiation therapy can stop the growth of these lesions but not shrink their size. Patients should be aware of the potential risk of injury to the vagus.

**ANSWER: A**

22. A 66-year-old man with T3N2bM0 SCC on the base of the tongue undergoes concomitant chemotherapy and external beam irradiation for a total of 6 weeks. At the end of treatment he is noted to have a persistently enlarged, left neck level II lymph node about 5 cm in size, for which salvage surgical therapy and standard radical neck dissection are planned. Which of the following is true?

    A. The phrenic nerve is commonly injured during surgery.

    B. Radical neck dissection includes removing the internal jugular vein, SCM muscle, and vagus nerve.

    C. The patient will probably need postoperative physical therapy for his shoulder.

    D. Resection of the internal carotid artery is a common component of this surgery.

    E. Level VI is part of a radical neck dissection.

*Ref.:* 1, 2, 13

**COMMENTS:** **Neck dissection** involves removal of the cervical lymphatic tissue and related structures for the treatment of head and neck cancer. **Radical neck dissection** involves removing all of the cervical lymphatic tissue in neck levels I through V, in addition to removing the internal jugular vein, SCM muscle, and spinal accessory nerve. A **modified radical neck dissection** is performed for the same clinical indications as a radical neck dissection. The differentiating feature is that it preserves at least one of the following: the internal jugular vein, SCM muscle, or spinal accessory nerve. Level I through V lymph nodes are removed as for a traditional radical neck dissection. However, it is frequently possible to preserve one of the major structures just listed, especially when it is not involved with tumor. Particularly in the case of the spinal accessory nerve, this is preferable to prevent postoperative shoulder dysfunction from denervation of the trapezius muscle. The patient in this scenario will most certainly need postoperative physical therapy because of sacrifice of CN XII with his surgery.

**Selective neck dissection** is used for removing a limited number of lymph node levels, as opposed to resecting levels I through V. Furthermore, the internal jugular vein, SCM muscle, and CN XII are preserved. The philosophy behind performing this type of dissection is to remove the clinically uninvolved lymphatic groups thought to be most at risk for future metastatic disease. Therefore, the type of dissection is predicated on where the primary tumor is located. Oral cavity cancers typically metastasize to levels I, II, and III. These levels would be included in what is termed a **supraomohyoid selective neck dissection**. Laryngeal, hypopharyngeal, and oropharyngeal cancers commonly spread to levels II, III, and IV, which would be incorporated into a **lateral selective neck dissection**. **Posterolateral neck dissection** (levels II, III, IV, and V) is most commonly used in the setting of cutaneous malignancies involving the posterior region of the scalp.

**Sentinel lymph node biopsy** is under investigation for its efficacy in SCC of the head and neck. It is currently used in the management of cutaneous melanoma of the head and neck. The internal carotid artery, however, is not considered a standard part of routine neck dissection, and there is controversy regarding the utility and benefit of resection. The phrenic nerve is at risk when dissecting along the floor of the neck. A level VI or central compartment dissection is not part of a standard radical neck dissection. It is typically used in patients with thyroid tumors, tracheal tumors, or laryngeal cancers with extensive subglottic extension.

**Therapeutic neck dissection** has been used to treat positive metastatic cervical disease (N+) through either a radical or a modified radical neck dissection. Currently, some surgeons are beginning to advocate for the use of more limited selective neck dissection if the patient has limited N1 disease. In addition to being used as primary treatment, it also can be used as salvage treatment after failed nonsurgical therapy, such as external beam radiation. For patients with clinically negative disease in the neck (N0), **elective neck dissection** can be performed to target the most likely sites of metastatic drainage. Such dissection is based on the primary site of the tumor. Sentinel lymph node biopsy in the treatment of SCC of the head and neck is currently under investigation and not yet advocated widely as a proven standard of care.

**ANSWER: C**

23. A 65-year-old man is seen in the emergency department with angioedema of the tongue. Flexible laryngoscopy demonstrates a severely edematous larynx with no visible glottic space. Worsening stridor, severe agitation, and panic develop, and the patient begins to desaturate with a nasal trumpet in place and a 100% O₂ nonrebreather mask. What is the next step in management?

    A. Emergency beside tracheostomy or cricothyrotomy

    B. Transfer of the patient immediately to the OR for urgent tracheostomy

    C. Mild sedation of the patient with midazolam, an attempt at direct laryngoscopy with intubation, and if unsuccessful, proceeding with tracheostomy at the bedside

    D. Flexible fiberoptic intubation

    E. Racemic epinephrine nebulizer treatment

*Ref.:* 1

**COMMENTS:** Creation of a **surgical airway** or "**tracheostomy**" is one of the most fundamental skills in the management of upper airway pathology. There are three major indications for a tracheostomy: upper airway obstruction, chronic respiratory failure, and management of poor pulmonary toilet. The timing of a tracheostomy can be categorized into three groups. **Emergency** tracheostomy or cricothyrotomy is required in patients with imminent airway obstruction, as in this example. A cricothyrotomy is the most rapid form of surgical airway control but does require conversion to a formal tracheostomy because of the high risk of subglottic stenosis developing. This patient has no evidence of an identifiable airway on fiberoptic examination and therefore cannot be intubated fiberoptically, but he is beginning to desaturate secondary to his airway obstruction and will probably decompensate at any moment; therefore, there is no time to make arrangements in the OR. An **urgent** tracheostomy done in the OR setting is always preferable if possible. Sedating the patient will inhibit spontaneous ventilation, promote further upper airway collapse, and worsen an already precarious airway scenario. Direct intubation will also probably be unsuccessful because of the patient's tongue edema. Racemic epinephrine can decrease laryngeal/subglottic edema but will be of little immediate help in this setting.

An **elective** tracheostomy is commonly done for chronic respiratory failure and for improving pulmonary toilet. In patients with chronic respiratory failure, a tracheostomy decreases anatomic dead space ventilation, allows improved pulmonary toilet, and decreases the risk for laryngeal stenosis and the formation of granulation tissue from pressure by the endotracheal tube. Percutaneous tracheostomy has become an alternative to conventional tracheostomy in carefully selected patients. Bronchoscopic monitoring augments the safety of the procedure, which is frequently done in the intensive care unit. A smaller incision and the use of a dilator facilitate introduction of the cannula. Many surgeons still prefer an open traditional tracheostomy in all cases. Once the patient's medical status has stabilized and the initial indication for tracheostomy is resolved, decannulation can be considered after evaluation of the larynx to confirm good function of the vocal cords and a patent airway.

**ANSWER:**   A

24. A 68-year-old woman with chronic respiratory failure underwent a tracheostomy for long-term ventilator support. The procedure went uneventfully and the patient was discharged to a long-term care facility after an initial tracheostomy tube change 1 week later. The patient is readmitted 2 weeks later with a report at the nursing facility of a 1-minute episode of brisk bright red bleeding from the tracheostomy site that resolved without intervention. Her hemoglobin concentration is 10.2 g/dL, and coagulation studies are normal. What is the most likely diagnosis?

   A. Pneumonia

   B. Tracheitis

   C. Bleeding of granulation tissue in the stoma

   D. Tracheoinnominate fistula

   E. Bleeding from the anterior jugular vein

*Ref.:* 1, 2

**COMMENTS:** This is a case of classic "**sentinel**" **bleeding** that occurs before full rupture of the **innominate artery**. It can occur with a low tracheostomy or high innominate artery with erosion of the anterior tracheal wall as a result of pressure necrosis. Fiberoptic examination of the area should be performed to evaluate the situation. If there is obvious evidence of erosion, the patient might need a sternotomy and mediastinal exploration. If the index of suspicion is lower or the examination is inconclusive, diagnostic imaging with high-resolution CT or angiography (or both) may be appropriate. This complication carries an extremely high mortality

rate if blowout occurs. Attempts to control active bleeding can consist of direct digital pressure or inflation of a cuffed tube directly over the area for tamponade. Any of the other choices would not cause rapid-onset bright red bleeding. Bleeding from the anterior jugular veins usually occurs immediately in the postoperative setting if they were not ligated adequately during surgery. Other complications of tracheostomy in the early period include infection, pneumothorax, bleeding, and tube obstruction. Later complications can include wound breakdown, formation of granulation tissue, tracheal stenosis, tracheoesophageal fistula, and **tracheoinnominate fistula,** as just described.

**ANSWER:**   D

25. A 61-year-old man with T3N2cM0 SCC of the supraglottic larynx undergoes total laryngectomy with left radical neck dissection/right modified radical neck dissection and primary pharyngeal closure without any intraoperative complications. Tube feeding is started on postoperative day 2. On day 3 the patient is noted to have increasingly high output of yellow/cloudy fluid from the left neck drain recorded to be 400 mL over the past 24 hours. The hemoglobin concentration and white blood cell count are stable. The patient is afebrile with no signs of infection at the surgical site. What is the next most appropriate step in management?

   A. Immediate reexploration and closure of the pharyngeal fistula

   B. Thoracotomy with clamping of the thoracic duct

   C. Closed wound drainage, pressure dressings, and tube feeding consisting of medium-chain triglycerides

   D. Continuation of the current postoperative management

   E. Removal of the left neck drain with a pressure dressing applied to the wound

*Ref.:* 2

**COMMENTS:** This patient has a **chylous fistula**. The initiation of tube feeding provided lipids to the lymphatic system, which increased the volume of chyle flow. Pharyngeal fistulas do not generally develop this early in the postoperative course and do not usually have such extremely high drain output. However, it is always something to consider after a pharyngeal repair. Chylous fistulas typically occur in the left side of the neck during radical neck dissections when dissecting low in the level IV/V region. The incidence is about 1% to 2%. If recognized at the time of surgery, they should be repaired immediately with ligature. If they occur in delayed fashion, such as in this patient, they can usually be initially managed conservatively, as stated in choice C. The rationale for using **medium-chain triglycerides** is that they are absorbed directly through the portal circulation and not the lymphatic system. Another nutritional alternative in more severe cases is the use of total parenteral nutrition. In regard to deciding on surgical management, a general guideline accepted by many physicians is greater than 600 mL of output over a 24-hour period. Reexploration with control of the leak can be very difficult given the delicate nature of lymphatic tissue.

**ANSWER:**   C

26. A 71-year-old female tobacco user undergoes a salvage total laryngectomy with bilateral radical neck dissection and primary closure of her pharynx. This was performed after failed treatment with primary concurrent chemotherapy and external beam radiation. On postoperative day 6, breakdown of the wound occurs with a resulting 1- by 2-cm defect, just lateral to the

stoma, and salivary drainage from the wound. Initial treatment consists of culture-directed intravenous antibiotic therapy, local wound care, and use of a Penrose drain for control of the drainage. Later on that same day, bright red blood is noticed on the wound dressing. Which of the following factors is most important in the development of these complications?

A. Age of the patient

B. Tobacco use

C. Bilateral versus unilateral neck dissection

D. Previous radiation therapy

E. Carotid injury during dissection of the neck

*Ref.:* 2

**COMMENTS:** A postoperative **pharyngocutaneous fistula** has developed in this patient, along with probably carotid artery rupture secondary to local infection and breakdown of the vessel wall. Although age and tobacco use are important factors in wound healing, a previous history of external beam radiation therapy in a patient undergoing total laryngectomy places that individual at much higher risk for a postoperative pharyngocutaneous fistula. Rates of postoperative fistula formation have been reported to be anywhere from 30% to 60% in patients with a history of radiation therapy. The general medical status of the patient needs to be evaluated in regard to nutrition and underlying medical problems such as diabetes so that these factors can be optimized as much as possible before surgery. A vascularized tissue flap should be considered in these patients. **Carotid blowout** is a deadly and feared complication of neck dissection. A salivary fistula with wound infection is a strong predisposing factor. Again, the use of vascularized tissue flaps can aid in preventing fistulas. This clinical scenario is highly suggestive of an evolving carotid blowout. Immediate management includes the application of direct pressure to the wound, administration of fluids and blood products as needed, and surgical exploration. In the case of a large infected field, a segment of the carotid artery may need to be resected.

**ANSWER:** D

27. A 55-year-old man with advanced-stage SCC of the larynx is undergoing total laryngectomy with bilateral modified radical neck dissection. While dissecting on the right side you inadvertently enter the internal jugular vein and proceed to clamp the vessel with the intention of ligating it for hemostatic control. Shortly thereafter, the patient is noted to be hypotensive. Bilateral breath sounds are auscultated, but a mill wheel murmur is heard over the precordium. What is the next step in management?

A. Place the patient in the left lateral decubitus position and insert a central venous catheter.

B. Place the patient in the right lateral decubitus position and insert a central venous catheter.

C. Place the patient in the reverse Trendelenburg position.

D. Call for an intraoperative chest radiograph.

E. Pack the wound and place the patient in the prone position.

*Ref.:* 14

**COMMENTS:** This patient has **venous air embolism** as a result of the internal jugular vein being inadvertently opened. With all surgeries above the heart there is a risk for air embolism. This is

especially true in neurosurgical procedures, where there is significant elevation of the wound relative to the heart. In head and neck surgery, patients are typically placed in the reverse Trendelenburg position, which places them at additional risk for entrance of air into the venous system. A "**mill wheel murmur**" is the traditional finding on cardiac examination and may be detected on precordial Doppler ultrasound. The clinical manifestations can include cardiovascular, pulmonary, and neurologic findings. Cardiac findings can include tachyarrhythmias, right-sided heart strain, and myocardial ischemia. Pulmonary findings can include hypercapnia with decreased $O_2$ saturation. Decreased cardiac output results in decreased cerebral perfusion, but direct air embolism to the central nervous system can occur through a patent foramen ovale. Initial treatment involves placing the patient in the **left lateral decubitus position** (**Durant position**) to try to force the air to stay in the right side of the heart in an attempt to prevent it from traveling into the pulmonary circulation. Placement of a central venous catheter with aspiration of air from the right atrium can also be attempted. Other supportive efforts may need to include cardiopulmonary resuscitation if the situation deteriorates. Hyperbaric oxygen therapy has been shown to be of benefit in some studies.

**ANSWER:** A

28. A 22-year-old man is brought to the emergency department by ambulance with a 2-day history of lower tooth pain and neck swelling. He was prescribed antibiotics by his primary care physician yesterday, but his condition had not improved overnight. This morning he felt his "throat beginning to close" and called the emergency medical service. He is febrile at 102° F with a heart rate of 105 beats/min, blood pressure of 110/70 mm Hg, and respiratory rate of 20 breaths/min. His white blood cell count is 38,000/mm³. On examination he is noted to have firm tender swelling of the submental region with skin erythema. In addition, severe edema of the floor of the mouth and tongue is present. His $Sao_2$ is 100% on 40% $O_2$ by face tent, and the patient is ventilating well, anxious, and sitting forward drooling. Flexible laryngoscopy shows no laryngeal edema. What is the next appropriate step in management?

A. Intravenous antibiotics and steroids with close observation of the airway in the intensive care unit

B. High-resolution CT of the neck with dye

C. Immediate cricothyrotomy in the emergency department under local anesthesia

D. Immediate transfer to the OR for awake fiberoptic intubation and be prepared for tracheostomy if needed

E. Incision and drainage of a suspected neck abscess at the bedside

*Ref.:* 2

**COMMENTS:** This patient has **Ludwig angina**, probably secondary to an odontogenic infection given the history of tooth pain. This condition involves a rapidly evolving soft tissue cellulitis that spreads through the fascial planes of the sublingual space, submandibular space, and anterior aspect of the neck. It can cause severe swelling of the floor of the mouth and tongue and possibly airway obstruction. Initial management in this patient should involve securing his airway. Emergency cricothyrotomy would be appropriate in the emergency department if the patient was currently decompensating and exhibiting obstruction and needed an airway immediately. He is ventilating well but drooling and posturing forward. This patient should be taken to the OR expediently to perform fiberoptic intubation and possible tracheostomy under controlled circumstances. At that point CT could be performed to evaluate for an abscess collection. Exploration of the neck at the bedside, especially without securing the airway, is unsafe and not appropriate. Tonsillitis is the most frequent cause of deep tissue neck infections in children with odontogenic sources, and intravenous drug injection is a more common cause in adults. **Peritonsillar abscesses** are the most commonly encountered. Classic signs and symptoms include drooling, hot potato voice, otalgia (from irritation of CN IX), and unilateral swelling of the soft palate with uvular deviation to the opposite side. Treatment includes drainage by transoral needle aspiration or incision and drainage with a scalpel blade. A **parapharyngeal space abscess** can be manifested in similar fashion to a peritonsillar abscess as severe throat and neck pain but without the appearance of soft palate/peritonsillar swelling. The tonsil may appear deviated medially. It is adjacent to many of the other spaces and can allow spread along the carotid sheath ("Lincoln Highway of the neck") or damage to CNs IX to XII. Drainage is generally performed in a transcervical fashion if necessary. **Retropharyngeal space abscesses** are more common in young children and require some clinical suspicion to detect. Initial signs may include fever, lack of appetite, cervical adenopathy, and torticollis. This area can usually be approached transorally if the infection is limited but may require transcervical drainage. CT is mandatory to define its extent and to aid in planning access. The retropharyngeal space extends from the skull base to the mediastinum. The retropharyngeal space has a midline raphe that causes unilateral shifting, whereas the prevertebral space does not, with these collections appearing more midline.

**ANSWER:** D

---

29. A 15-year-old boy is taken to the emergency department with a 1-month history of recurrent right-sided epistaxis. He has had almost daily episodes, with some noted to be very difficult to stop with local pressure. He is currently bleeding from his right nostril and coughing up blood clots. The bleeding is able to be controlled with an 8-cm nasal pack. His vital signs are stable, he is resting comfortably, and blood is drawn for a complete blood count, which shows a hemoglobin level of 8.0 g/dL. What is the next step in management?

A. Discharge the boy home with follow-up in 2 to 3 days for removal of the packing.

B. Transfuse 2 units of packed red blood cells given the concern for possible further bleeding.

C. Remove the packing, perform diagnostic nasal endoscopy, and cauterize the bleeding site in the emergency department.

D. Admit overnight and remove the packing at the bedside in the morning.

E. Perform CT of the sinuses with or without intravenous infusion.

*Ref.: 2*

**COMMENTS:** Severe new-onset unilateral epistaxis in an adolescent boy should always raise suspicion for a **juvenile nasal angiofibroma**. This is a benign neoplasm arising around the region of the pterygopalatine fossa. It is almost exclusively found in adolescent boys. Treatment includes mainly surgery via either open or endoscopic approaches. Radiation therapy is used in only limited circumstances, especially since this is a benign lesion. The patient's bleeding is currently controlled, and although his hemoglobin

content is lowered, he is not showing any signs indicating a need for transfusion such as tachycardia or hypotension. The packing should remain in place until further diagnostic testing is performed given the suspicion for a possible neoplasm. In this case, CT of the sinuses with or without intravenous infusion is the next appropriate step given the suspicion for an underlying angiofibroma.

**Epistaxis** most commonly occurs from the **Kiesselbach space** along the anterior nasal septum. Bleeding from this site does not usually require more than simple pressure applied to the area or a small amount of anterior nasal packing. Cauterization can be done in the office setting under direct visualization if needed. Bleeding from the posterior nasal cavity typically arises from the **sphenopalatine artery**; it is less common but can be more severe. It may require control with posterior nasal packing, which can include a balloon device for tamponade. Any patient with such posterior packing in place should be monitored in the hospital because posterior packing has been shown to cause alterations in oxygen saturation. This is especially true in elderly patients and those with cardiopulmonary disease.

**ANSWER:** E

---

### REFERENCES

1. Lorenz RR, Netterville JL, Burkey BB: Head and neck. In Townsend CM, Beauchamp RD, Evers BM, et al, editors: *Sabiston textbook of surgery: the biological basis of modern surgical practice*, ed 18, Philadelphia, 2008, WB Saunders.
2. Cummings CW, Haughey BH, Thomas JR, et al: *Cummings otolaryngology: head and neck surgery*, ed 4, Philadelphia, 2005, CV Mosby.
3. Myers EN, Suen JY, Myers JN, et al: *Cancer of the head and neck*, ed 4, Philadelphia, 2003, WB Saunders.
4. McGuirt WF, McCabe BF: Significance of node biopsy before definitive treatment of cervical metastatic carcinoma, *Laryngoscope* 88:594–597, 1978.
5. Camp AA, Fundakowski C, Petruzzelli GJ, et al: Functional and oncologic results following transoral laser microsurgical excision of base of tongue carcinoma, *Otolaryngol Head Neck Surg* 141:66–69, 2009.
6. Steiner W, Ambrosch P, Hess CF, et al: Organ preservation by transoral laser microsurgery in piriform sinus carcinoma, *Otolaryngol Head Neck Surg* 124:58–67, 2001.
7. Al-Sarraf M, LeBlanc M, Giri PG, et al: Chemoradiotherapy versus radiotherapy in patients with advanced nasopharyngeal cancer: phase III randomized Intergroup Study 0099, *J Clin Oncol* 16:1310–1317, 1998.
8. The Department of Veterans Affairs Laryngeal Cancer Study Group: Induction chemotherapy plus radiation compared with surgery plus radiation in patients with advanced laryngeal cancer, *N Engl J Med* 324:1685–1690, 1991.
9. Forastiere AA, Goepfert H, Maor M, et al: Concurrent chemotherapy and radiotherapy for organ preservation in advanced laryngeal cancer, *N Engl J Med* 349:2091–2098, 2003.
10. Bernier J, Domenge C, Ozsahin M, et al: Postoperative irradiation with or without concomitant chemotherapy for locally advanced head and neck cancer, *N Engl J Med* 350:1945–1952, 2004.
11. Cooper JS, Pajak TF, Forastiere AA, et al: Postoperative concurrent radiotherapy and chemotherapy for high-risk squamous-cell carcinoma of the head and neck, *N Engl J Med* 350:1937–1944, 2004.
12. Bailey BJ, Johnson JT, Newlands SD: *Head and neck surgery: otolaryngology*, ed 4, Philadelphia, 2006, Lippincott Williams & Wilkins.
13. Patel RS, Clark JR, Gao K, et al: Effectiveness of selective neck dissection in the treatment of the clinically positive neck, *Head Neck* 30:1231–1236, 2008.
14. Mirski MA, Lele AV, Fitzsimmons L, et al: Diagnosis and treatment of vascular air embolism, *Anesthesiology* 106:164–177, 2007.

# CHAPTER 16

# Thyroid

*Tricia Moo-Young, M.D., and Richard A. Prinz, M.D.*

1. A 45-year-old woman has a newly diagnosed posterior pharyngeal neck mass found on magnetic resonance imaging performed for chronic neck pain (see image of transoral examination). The next step in appropriate management of this patient is:

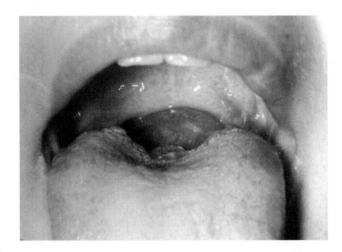

A. Computed tomography CT)

B. Fine-needle aspiration (FNA) biopsy

C. Excisional biopsy

D. Radioiodine uptake scan

E. Observation

*Ref.:* 1, 2

**COMMENTS:** The most likely diagnosis in this patient is a **lingual thyroid**. This abnormality arises when the thyroid fails to descend normally into the standard cervical position. In some patients this may be the only thyroid tissue present. It originates from the base of the tongue in the region of the foramen cecum. The diagnosis is best made with a radioactive uptake scan that demonstrates uptake of iodine within the mass. Cervical ultrasound demonstrating an absence of thyroid tissue is also highly suggestive of a lingual thyroid. If the gland is enlarged, patients may have obstructive symptoms such as dysphagia, choking, or airway obstruction. Management of these patients is typically excision.

**ANSWER:** D

2. With regard to the recurrent laryngeal nerve (RLN), which of the following is true?

A. The left RLN loops around the subclavian vein and ascends medially into the neck.

B. The right RLN loops around the inferior thyroid artery, ascends laterally to medially, and enters the cricothyroid membrane.

C. The laryngeal nerve is nonrecurrent in 0.5% of patients.

D. The RLNs innervate the true vocal cords and the cricothyroid muscles.

E. The medial branch of the RLN is primarily sensory.

*Ref.:* 1, 2

**COMMENTS:** The **recurrent laryngeal nerve** arises from the vagus nerve after it has already passed into the mediastinum. The left RLN loops around the aortic arch and then travels medially in the neck within the tracheoesophageal groove. The right RLN loops around the subclavian artery, passes posterior to the artery, and travels laterally to medially toward the tracheoesophageal groove. Once in the central aspect of the neck, the RLN nerve can branch into medial and lateral components. The medial branch typically carries the motor fibers and is at risk for injury along its course toward the cricothyroid membrane if not identified as a separate structure relative to the lateral sensory branch. The laryngeal nerves can be **nonrecurrent** in approximately 0.5% of patients. In this case the nerve originates from the cervical position of the vagus nerve. The risk for injury during cervical procedures is higher when the nerve is nonrecurrent because instead of running parallel to the tracheoesophageal groove, it travels perpendicular. It is more common on the right and is most often associated with the presence of aberrant cervical vascular anatomy such as a retroesophageal subclavian artery. The RLN innervates all the intrinsic muscles of the larynx except the cricothyroid muscles.

**ANSWER:** C

3. With regard to thyroid anatomy, which of the following statements is incorrect?

A. The inferior thyroid artery arises directly from the external carotid artery.

B. The thyroidea ima artery arises directly from the aorta in 1% to 4% of patients.

C. The ligament of Berry is located near the entry point of the RLN.

D. Venous drainage of the thyroid gland is via the superior, middle, and inferior branches.

E. The superior and middle thyroid veins drain into the jugular vein.

*Ref.:* 1, 2

**COMMENTS:** The **arterial blood supply** of the thyroid gland is provided by two main arterial branches. The superior thyroid artery arises from the external carotid artery and gives off multiple branches that are collectively referred to as the superior pole vessels. The inferior thyroid artery is given off as a branch of the thyrocervical trunk, which originates from the subclavian artery. The ligament of Berry is a condensation of the thyroid capsule located on the posterior surface of the gland. It is a tough band of tissue that passes either anterior or posterior to the course of the RLN as it travels into the cricothyroid membrane. The thyroid gland is drained by the superior, middle, and inferior thyroid veins, which eventually terminate in the jugular vein. The distal end of the thyroglossal duct persists in approximately 50% of people. This remnant is anatomically referred to as the pyramidal lobe.

**ANSWER:** A

4. Routine work-up of thyroid function includes all of the following except:

A. Thyroid-stimulating hormone (TSH)

B. Total thyroxine ($T_4$)

C. Free triiodothyronine ($T_3$)

D. Thyroglobulin

E. $T_3$ resin uptake

*Ref.:* 1, 2

**COMMENTS:** The initial work-up of **thyroid dysfunction** involves measurement of TSH. Thyroid production of $T_4$ is assessed by measuring both free and total $T_4$. Total $T_4$ is the amount of both free and protein-bound hormone. In cases in which free $T_4$ testing is unavailable, $T_3$ resin uptake can be measured. This test indirectly assesses competitive binding between radiolabeled $T_3$ and circulating unbound $T_3$ hormone. At high levels of free $T_4$, much of the resin is bound by circulating hormone and a smaller percentage by radiolabeled $T_3$. The product of the percent uptake and total serum $T_4$ concentration is equal to the free $T_4$ index. This value reflects the amount of free $T_4$ present in the circulation. Thyroglobulin is not routinely measured as part of the initial assessment of thyroid function.

**ANSWER:** D

5. With regard to thyroid hormone synthesis, which of the following is true?

A. Iodine trapping involves endocytosis of circulating iodine particles.

B. In the euthyroid state, $T_3$ is the main hormone produced by the thyroid.

C. Thyroid peroxidase is responsible for the peripheral conversion of $T_4$ to $T_3$.

D. Thyroglobulin is a glycoprotein synthesized in the rough endoplasmic reticulum of the thyrocyte.

E. The primary site of peripheral deiodination of $T_4$ to the active form $T_3$ occurs in the adrenal gland.

*Ref.:* 1, 2

**COMMENTS:** Synthesis of thyroid hormone consists of several steps. It begins with iodine trapping via adenosine triphosphate–dependent transport across the basement membrane of the thyrocyte. **Thyroglobulin**, a glycoprotein synthesized in the rough endoplasmic reticulum, then becomes iodinated by an intracellularly located catalytic enzyme called thyroid peroxidase. Two diiodotyrosines are coupled to form $T_4$. Peripherally, $T_4$ is converted to the active thyroid hormone $T_3$. In the euthyroid state, $T_4$ is the predominant hormone produced by the thyroid gland. Peripheral deiodination of $T_4$ to the active form $T_3$ occurs in the liver, muscle, kidney, and anterior pituitary. $T_3$ is transported in the serum bound to circulating carrier proteins such as thyroxine-binding globulin (TBG) and albumin.

**ANSWER:** D

6. Calcitonin is produced by the parafollicular cells of the thyroid gland. Measurement of calcitonin is essential in what disease process?

A. Graves disease

B. Follicular thyroid cancer

C. Hashimoto disease

D. Medullary thyroid cancer

E. Papillary thyroid cancer

*Ref.:* 1, 2

**COMMENTS:** **Calcitonin** is produced by the parafollicular cells of the thyroid gland. This 32–amino acid polypeptide is the principal hormone responsible for lowering serum calcium levels during states of hypercalcemia. The action of calcitonin takes places on the surface receptors of osteoclasts. They work to inhibit bone resorption and thus reduce serum calcium levels. **Medullary thyroid cancers** are tumors of the parafollicular cells that produce calcitonin. The resulting hypercalcitoninemia seen in these patients can be a measure of tumor burden.

**ANSWER:** D

7. With regard to thyroid hormone metabolism and drug effects, which of the following is true?

A. Iodine given in large doses stimulates the release of thyroid hormone.

B. Corticosteroids inhibit peripheral conversion of $T_4$ to $T_3$.

C. β-Blockers potentiate the effects of thyroid hormone through adrenergic stimulation of thyroid receptors.

D. The Wolff-Chaikoff effect involves the reflex release of thyroid hormone in response to loading with antithyroid medications such as methimazole.

E. Propylthiouracil (PTU) is safe for use in the treatment of hyperthyroidism in pregnant patients.

*Ref.:* 1, 2

**COMMENTS:** When given in concentrated doses, iodine can inhibit the release of thyroid hormone. This process of "thyroid stunting" is referred to as the **Wolff-Chaikoff effect**. It is sometimes seen in patients who have a diagnostic radioactive iodine scan and then demonstrate minimal uptake of radioactive iodine when the therapeutic dose is given. In preparing hyperthyroid patients for surgery, administration of potassium iodide solutions has been shown to treat hyperactivity. This stunting effect is transient and is thus not used for the long-term management of hyperthyroid patients. Concentrated potassium iodide (**Lugol solution**) should be used with caution in this setting since it will aggravate the hyperthyroidism after its initial effect wears off. β-Blockers do not directly inhibit synthesis of thyroid hormone but do counteract some of the peripheral effects of its action on the cardiovascular system. Corticosteroids not only inhibit peripheral conversion of $T_4$ to $T_3$ but also suppress the production of TSH. In **acute severe hyperthyroid** states corticosteroids can help in the initial treatment.

**A N S W E R :** B

8. A 25-year-old woman at 10 weeks gestation has increasing shortness of breath and anxiety. The clinician wishes to screen her for hyperthyroidism. Which of the statements is relevant to the interpretation of thyroid function in pregnant patients?

   A. TBG is decreased and thus levels of total $T_4$ and $T_3$ are increased.

   B. Decreased renal iodine clearance causes a reciprocal decrease in total $T_3$.

   C. Increased plasma volume decreases the total $T_4$ and $T_3$ levels measured in serum.

   D. A first-trimester increase in human chorionic gonadotropin (hCG) causes a reciprocal decrease in TSH levels.

   E. Thyrotoxicosis is relatively common in the first and second trimesters of pregnancy.

*Ref.:* 1, 2

**COMMENTS: Thyrotoxicosis** occurs in approximately 0.1% to 0.4% of pregnancies in the United States. If not recognized and treated promptly, severe complications can arise in both the mother and fetus. The hormonal changes and fluctuating metabolic demands during pregnancy have an important impact on thyroid physiology. These changes can make interpretation of laboratory tests of thyroid function in pregnant patients extremely challenging. During pregnancy there is a rise in **thyroxine-binding globulin,** which in turn causes an increase in total serum $T_4$ and $T_3$. The degree of change in TBG levels is dependent on the particular trimester. By 16 to 20 weeks, serum TBG levels have in most cases risen to double the nonpregnant values. Additionally, hCG shares structural similarity with TSH and has been shown to have weak thyroid-stimulating activity. This fact may explain why thyroid nodules often increase in size during pregnancy. The mimicked activity of TSH allows hCG to provide negative feedback in such a way that TSH levels during pregnancy are always lower than is reflective of the true thyroid functional state. Thus, if normal ranges of TSH that are specific to pregnancy are not used, hyperthyroidism can be inappropriately diagnosed. Additionally, in pregnancy renal clearance of iodine is increased, and thus patients will have increased baseline 24-hour radioactive iodine uptake when compared with nonpregnant patients. The increased renal clearance has no direct effect on circulating levels of total $T_3$. In fact, pregnant patients have increased $T_4$ and $T_3$ levels because of their increased total plasma volumes.

**A N S W E R :** D

9. All of the following are extrathyroidal manifestations of Graves disease except:

   A. Vitiligo

   B. Pretibial myxedema

   C. Exophthalmos

   D. Hypercalcemic paralysis

   E. Myasthenia gravis

*Ref.:* 1, 2

**COMMENTS:** See Question 10.

**A N S W E R :** D

10. Which of the antibodies is diagnostic of patients with Graves disease?

   A. Antithyroglobulin (anti-TGAb)

   B. Antithyroid peroxidase (anti-TPOAb )

   C. Anti-DNA antibodies (antinuclear)

   D. TSH receptor antibody (anti-TSAb)

   E. Anticardiolipin antibodies

*Ref.:* 1, 2

**COMMENTS: Graves disease** is an example of an organ-specific autoimmune disease. It has been associated with other autoimmune diseases such as pernicious anemia, vitiligo, alopecia, angioedema, and myasthenia gravis. The **extrathyroidal manifestations of Graves disease** include exophthalmos, pretibial myxedema, periodic hypocalcemic paralysis, and vitiligo. The common feature of autoimmune thyroid disease is the presence of immunoreactivity toward specific thyroid antigens. More than 90% of patients will express elevated **thyroid-stimulating hormone receptor antibodies** (TSAbs), which is considered diagnostic of Graves disease. Antithyroid peroxidases and **antithyroglobulin** (anti-TGAb) antibodies are present in 80% and 50% of patients, respectively. Rarely in Graves disease do patient have antinuclear antibodies such as anti-Ro, anti-dsDNA, or anticardiolipin antibodies.

**A N S W E R :** D

11. A 42-year-old woman complains to her physician of symptoms associated with hyperthyroidism. On examination she has a palpable nodule but no evidence of exophthalmos. She does have pretibial myxedema. Her laboratory work-up reveals a suppressed TSH level with elevated free $T_3$. What is the next step in the management of this patient?

   A. Radioactive $^{123}$I uptake scan

   B. Neck ultrasound

   C. PTU

   D. FNA

   E. Cervical ultrasound

*Ref.:* 1, 2

**COMMENTS:** See Question 12.

**A N S W E R :** A

12. Which of the following is not an acceptable indication for surgical treatment of hyperthyroidism in the patient in Question 11?

A. A nodule confirmed or suspicious for malignancy

B. Multinodular goiter

C. Noncompliance with medical management

D. Age younger than 15 years

E. Severe Graves ophthalmopathy

*Ref.:* 1, 2

**COMMENTS:** A diagnosis of **thyrotoxicosis** is suspected in this patient. Of the tests listed in Question 11, the one most likely to yield a diagnosis is a radioactive uptake scan. Elevated uptake with a diffusely enlarged gland confirms the diagnosis of **Graves disease** and assists in differentiating it from other forms of hyperthyroidism. In this patient the palpable mass on examination could instead be a toxic nodule, and the radioactive uptake scan would illustrate a "hot" nodule in the setting of a suppressed gland. A **thyroid uptake scan** is useful in determining whether the patient has a toxic nodular goiter as a potential explanation of her hyperthyroid state. Cervical ultrasound depicts thyroid anatomy but does not indicate thyroid function. A measurement of reverse triiodothyronine ($rT_3$) does not directly reflect the presence of hyperthyroidism but instead serves as a marker of $T_3$ turnover. The most useful test in the initial screening of patients for hyperthyroidism is TSH since suppression of TSH below normal is a sensitive indicator of excess circulating thyroid hormone. It would not be appropriate to initiate therapy for hyperthyroidism until a diagnosis is confirmed. Biopsy by FNA would be appropriate if the nodule were found to have no uptake on radioiodine uptake scan. Treatment of hyperthyroidism includes medical therapy, radioactive iodine, and surgical resection. Presently, the majority of patients with thyrotoxicosis are treated with pharmacologic agents or, alternatively, ablation with radioactive iodine. Surgical treatment is recommended for patients who have (1) a large goiter with low radioiodine uptake, (2) noncompliance with medical management, (3) suspicion of malignancy, (4) severe exophthalmos, (5) pregnancy, and (6) age younger than 15 years (because of the risks associated with exposure to radiation).

**ANSWER:** B

13. With regard to the pharmacologic treatment of hyperthyroidism, which of the following is not true?

A. PTU works by inhibiting organic binding of iodine and coupling of iodotyrosines.

B. PTU is associated with agranulocytosis.

C. PTU is the preferred treatment in pregnant patients.

D. Methimazole can worsen exophthalmos in patients with Graves disease.

E. Methimazole has longer half-life and requires once-daily dosing.

*Ref.:* 1, 2

**COMMENTS:** The two most commonly prescribed antithyroid medications in the treatment of Graves disease are **methimazole** and **propylthiouracil**. Both agents work by blocking organic binding of iodine and coupling of iodotyrosines. PTU additionally inhibits peripheral conversion of $T_4$ to $T_3$. Both have a side effect profile that includes hepatotoxicity and reversible granulocytopenia. Methimazole is favored since it requires once-daily dosing

because of its longer half-life. Both cross the placenta during pregnancy, but PTU appears to exhibit less transplacental transfer and has a lower toxicity profile. Radioactive iodine therapy, an alternative to surgery or medical therapy, can worsen **exophthalmos** following treatment, but neither antithyroid medication alters the degree of the eye findings associated with Graves disease.

**ANSWER:** D

14. Preoperative preparation of patients with Graves disease should include all of the following except?

A. Thyroid ultrasound

B. Preoperative β-blockade

C. Achievement of a euthyroid state through the use of antithyroid drugs

D. Administration of supersaturated potassium iodide (SSKI) 7 to 10 days before surgery

E. Lithium

*Ref.:* 1, 2

**COMMENTS:** Preoperatively, patients with Graves disease should have their **thyrotoxic state** controlled through the use of **antithyroid medications**. Without this, induction of anesthesia can induce a thyroid storm. Ultrasonography should be preformed to document whether there are any associated suspicious nodules that warrant further work-up before surgery. If a diagnosis of malignancy is made, the extent of surgery (subtotal versus complete versus lymph node dissection) can be determined preoperatively. Presently, many endocrine surgeons advocate giving patients a 7- to 10-day preoperative course of either **Lugol solution** or SSKI to help diminish the hypervascularity of the gland and minimize operative blood loss, although more recent studies have shown that preoperative administration of concentrated iodide preparations can also induce hypertrophy of the gland and should possibly be avoided in patients with diffusely enlarged toxic goiters. **β-Blockers** are not routinely administered to all patients with Graves disease preoperatively unless they exhibit signs of thyrotoxic-induced tachycardia. Hypothyroidism can be associated with a number of pharmacologic therapies, the most frequent being lithium. The mechanism involves blockage of the cyclic adenosine monophosphate–dependent pathway of hormone synthesis. It is also seen with other agents, including amiodarone, cytokines, and antithyroid medications. No relationship has been demonstrated between hypothyroidism and cimetidine.

**ANSWER:** B

15. With regard to Hashimoto thyroiditis, which of the following is true?

A. The majority of patients are transiently hypothyroid but with time return to a euthyroid state.

B. It is primarily treated surgically.

C. Radioactive iodine is useful in the treatment of Hashimoto thyroiditis.

D. Thyroid microsomal antibodies are detected in the serum of patients.

E. The incidence of hypothyroidism in Hashimoto thyroiditis is higher in women than in men.

*Ref.:* 1, 2

**COMMENTS: Hashimoto disease** is a type of autoimmune thyroiditis. Histologically, the gland exhibits a dense lymphocytic infiltrate associated with dense fibrosis. When the disease is active, patients can experience symptoms associated with either hypothyroidism or hyperthyroidism. The natural progression of the disease is the eventual development of a multinodular goiter associated with hypothyroidism. Surgery is rarely indicated except in the setting of (1) debilitating symptoms of thyroid dysfunction, (2) compressive symptoms from multinodular goiter, and (3) suspicion of malignancy. The presence of nodular disease mandates FNA to rule out lymphoma or papillary cancer. For reasons that are unclear, hypothyroidism in patients with Hashimoto thyroiditis is more common in men than in women.

**ANSWER: D**

16. A 24-year-old man has an incidentally discovered thyroid mass on CT performed during a recent visit to the emergency department for work-up of a fall at work. The patient undergoes neck ultrasonography. Which of the following features is most consistent with a benign mass?

    A. Incomplete halo

    B. Peripheral calcifications

    C. Hypoechoic lesion

    D. Irregular margins

    E. Size smaller than 2 cm

    *Ref.:* 1, 2

**COMMENTS:** The initial work-up of a thyroid nodule should not include a **thyroid uptake scan** unless the patient exhibits signs or symptoms of **hyperthyroidism**. In a clinically euthyroid patient the first test of choice should be ultrasound followed by **fine-needle aspiration** for any suspicious nodules discovered on clinical or radiographic examination. FNA has a false-negative rate of approximately 5% and a false-positive rate of 6%. A TSH level should be ordered to document thyroid function. Not all calcifications on thyroid ultrasound are associated with a malignant lesion. Typical benign cystic lesions will exhibit a complete halo (intact capsule) and peripheral calcifications. Size is not generally thought to be a consistent predictor of malignancy. However, lesions greater than 1 cm are believed to be amenable to fine-needle biopsy. Table 16-1 lists some of the **ultrasonographic** features associated with benign and malignant disease.

**TABLE 16-1  Ultrasonographic Features of Thyroid Nodules**

| Variable | Benign | Malignant |
| --- | --- | --- |
| Margins | Smooth, well-defined | Irregular, distinct |
| Calcifications | Peripheral and coarse | Punctuate and fine |
| Echogenicity | Anechoic or hyperechoic | Hypoechoic |
| Size | <1 cm | >1 cm |
| Peripheral halo | Complete halo | Incomplete halo |

**ANSWER: B**

17. The patient in Question 16 is found to have a 2-cm dominant nodule located in the right thyroid lobe. Cytologic evaluation of an FNA biopsy specimen reveals "follicular neoplasm associated with degenerative colloid." All of the following are appropriate steps in her management except:

    A. Right lobectomy with intraoperative frozen section

    B. Subtotal thyroidectomy

    C. Total thyroidectomy

    D. Ultrasound repeated in 6 months with FNA biopsy

    E. Preoperative evaluation of the vocal cords

    *Ref.:* 1, 2

**COMMENTS:** A finding of follicular features on **fine-needle aspiration** carries an approximately 10% to 20% risk of harboring a malignancy. Because **follicular neoplasms** cannot be diagnosed as malignant or benign without microscopic examination of the nodule capsule, surgical excision is necessary. At a minimum, the patient should undergo right lobectomy with or without frozen resection. In patients who have additional risk factors for thyroid cancer (e.g., family history, exposure to radiation), total thyroidectomy should be strongly considered to avoid the need for reoperative surgery if the nodule is found to be malignant. Patients with indeterminate pathology such as a "follicular neoplasm" should not be offered the option of observation and repeated imaging in 6 months. Preoperative evaluation of vocal cord function should be considered in patients scheduled for a thyroid operation.

**ANSWER: D**

18. Which of the following statements regarding Hürthle cell carcinoma is false?

    A. It represents a subtype of follicular thyroid cancer.

    B. Hürthle cell carcinoma accounts for 3% of all thyroid malignancies.

    C. It is more likely than follicular cancer to be multifocal.

    D. It demonstrates poor radioactive iodine uptake.

    E. Lymph node dissection is indicated for all patients.

    *Ref.:* 1, 2

**COMMENTS: Hürthle cell carcinoma** is considered a subtype of follicular carcinoma and, similarly, is characterized by vascular or capsular invasion. Of all thyroid malignancies, Hürthle cell cancers account for about 3%. Different from follicular carcinoma, Hürthle cell cancers are more often multifocal and bilateral, have a higher rate of local nodal metastases, and demonstrate poor radioactive iodine uptake. In part because of these features, Hürthle cell carcinomas have also been associated with higher mortality than follicular cancers. Previous radiation exposure has been correlated with an increase in bilateralism and multicentricity of Hürthle cell neoplasms, as well as an increased incidence of contralateral non–Hürthle cell malignant thyroid lesions. The 10-year survival rate of patients with Hürthle cell carcinoma is 70%. Approximately 10% to 20% of patients have lymph node metastasis when initially seen.

**ANSWER: E**

19. All of the following are considered an increased risk factor for cancer in a patient with a thyroid mass except:

    A. Age younger than 25 or older than 60 years

    B. Rapid growth

    C. Family history

D. Hot nodule on thyroid uptake scan

E. Male gender

*Ref.:* 3

**COMMENTS:** There is an associated increased risk for thyroid malignancy in patients with thyroid nodules and any of the following features: radiation exposure, rapid growth during observation, family history of thyroid cancer, cold nodule on radioactive uptake scan, male gender, and age younger than 25 or older than 60 years. **Hot nodules** on a thyroid uptake scan generally indicate hyperfunctioning growth associated with such conditions as toxic multinodular goiter or Graves disease.

**ANSWER:** D

20. Overall, papillary thyroid cancer carries a very favorable prognosis. Of the following, which factor is not considered a prognostic indicator in standard thyroid staging systems?

A. Age

B. Grade

C. Thyroglobulin level

D. Extrathyroidal spread

E. Size

*Ref.:* 1, 2

**COMMENTS: Risk stratification** is a fundamental aspect of how treatment and surveillance algorithms are developed. In addition to standard staging systems such as **TNM**, the most frequently used are **age, grade, extrathyroidal extension, and size** (AGES), **MACIS** (metastases, age, complete resection, extension, size), and **AMES** (age, metastases, extension, size). Although each of these staging systems does a reasonable job of predicting cancer-specific survival, none have any prognostic value in assessing risk for recurrence. Thyroglobulin levels are not a part of any present staging system.

**ANSWER:** C

21. Recent studies have shown that the incidence of thyroid cancer has nearly doubled in the last 2 decades. Plausible explanations given by epidemiologists include all of the following except?

A. Childhood radiation exposure

B. Iodine deficiency

C. Estrogen hormone

D. Increased used of diagnostic imaging modalities

E. Increased incidence of Hashimoto thyroiditis

*Ref.:* 1, 2

**COMMENTS:** According to the International Agency for Research on Cancer, a component of the World Health Organization, the average rate of increase in thyroid cancer was 58% between 1973 and 2002. The increase observed was most pronounced in females (67%, mainly papillary thyroid cancer) and in specific regions such as Australia (178%). The reason for the increased incidence of thyroid cancer is unclear. Current evidence supports the fact that the increase is most likely multifactorial, including radiation exposure; environmental, hormonal, and genetic factors; and the increased use of diagnostic studies. Iodine

status does appear to influence the subtype of thyroid cancer that populations are at risk for. There is a reported increased risk for thyroid cancer in iodine-replete areas, mainly papillary cancer, whereas iodine-deficient areas show a slightly increased incidence of follicular thyroid cancer. To date, no corollary has been drawn between the incidence of thyroiditis and an increased **incidence of thyroid cancer**.

**ANSWER:** E

22. A 35-year-old man with a newly diagnosed thyroid nodule is found to have elevated calcitonin and findings on FNA consistent with medullary thyroid cancer (MTC). In regard to the management of this patient, all are true except:

A. Preoperative ultrasound for lymph node mapping of the lateral and central compartments should be preformed routinely.

B. Biochemical screening for associated endocrinopathies (e.g., hyperparathyroidism or pheochromocytoma) is part of the preoperative work-up.

C. Treatment consists of total thyroidectomy.

D. Measurement of carcinoembryonic antigen (CEA) is a useful marker of disease burden.

E. Genetic counseling and screening should be offered to his immediate family members.

*Ref.:* 1, 2

**COMMENTS: Medullary thyroid cancer** arises from the parafollicular cells of the thyroid. Its serum tumor marker is **calcitonin**. Patients with diffuse and advanced disease can have symptoms of calcitonin excess (diarrhea, flushing, and abdominal cramping). More than 80% of cases of MTC are sporadic and thus have no hereditary association. That being said, every patient in whom MTC is newly diagnosed should be referred for genetic counseling and evaluation for a *RET* protooncogene mutation because there are identifiable genetic mutations that predict the prognosis and aggressiveness of the disease. The overall survival of patients with MTC is determined largely by the completeness of resection and the presence of persistent disease. Thus, surgical treatment of MTC tends to favor aggressive therapy. In patients with palpable MTC, more than 75% will have central lymph node involvement. All patients with biopsy-confirmed MTC and no evidence of nodal or distant metastases should undergo at a minimum **total thyroidectomy with central node dissection**. Whether lateral compartment dissection is preformed is dependent on whether there is radiographic or operative evidence of gross disease. Current 2009 American Thyroid Association guidelines for MTC recommend that all patients with findings on FNA or a calcitonin level suggestive of MTC should undergo preoperative neck ultrasonography for evaluation of lymph node metastases. Biochemical screening for associated manifestations (e.g., hyperparathyroidism, pheochromocytoma) should also be performed by obtaining a serum calcium level and measurement of either plasma metanephrines or 24-hour urine catecholamines. CEA and calcitonin are useful tumor markers in predicting disease burden and recurrence in patients with MTC.

**ANSWER:** C

23. A 34-year-old woman has recently undergone total thyroidectomy for a diagnosis of papillary thyroid cancer. Her current TNM stage is T1 (lesion <2 cm), NX's, MX's. Which of the following surveillance regimens is required 6 months after surgical and adjuvant radioactive iodine treatment?

A. Clinical examination, cervical ultrasound, and an unstimulated thyroglobulin level

B. Diagnostic whole-body scan (WBS) 6 months after the administration of recombinant TSH

C. Clinical examination, cervical ultrasound, and diagnostic WBS

D. Clinical examination, cervical ultrasound, WBS, and stimulated thyroglobulin level

E. Diagnostic WBS every 6 months until the thyroglobulin level is less than the upper limit of normal

*Ref.:* 1, 2

**COMMENTS:** Considerable controversy exists over exactly what surveillance algorithm is best for monitoring patients with **well-differentiated thyroid cancer** (WDTC) for recurrence. The options include clinical examination, ultrasound, measurements of thyroglobulin, CT/positron emission tomography (PET), and diagnostic WBS. Little controversy exists regarding whether or not serial thyroglobulin measurements should be a part of standard surveillance schemes for patients with WDTC. **Thyroglobulin** can be measured in a unstimulated (normal TSH) or stimulated (elevated TSH) state. Stimulated thyroglobulin is a much more sensitive measure of whether residual or recurrent disease is present. Patients who have undetectable stimulated thyroglobulin after therapy are unlikely to have residual disease. By contrast, if a patient has an unstimulated thyroglobulin level that is undetectable, there is 20% chance that this patient will have a rise in thyroglobulin when repeated in a stimulated setting. These patients in subsequent follow-up can be considered low risk and monitored with unstimulated thyroglobulin levels. Current American Thyroid Association guidelines recommend that all patients, regardless of risk level, should undergo baseline ultrasonography 6 or 12 months following surgery. **Whole-body scans** are reserved for high-risk patients to document the completeness of treatment and in patients who have elevated thyroglobulin antibodies, which makes thyroglobulin levels difficult to interpret.

**ANSWER:** A

24. A patient is undergoing planned total thyroidectomy for bilateral thyroid nodules, of which the right nodule was shown to be a follicular neoplasm with Hürthle cell features. During initial mobilization of the gland on the right side, an inadvertent injury to the right RLN occurs. Although the nerve is structurally intact, there is no evidence of signal with the use of intraoperative RLN monitoring. What is the next appropriate step in the management of this patient?

A. Perform direct fiberoptic laryngoscopy to inspect the status of the right vocal cord.

B. Perform a frozen section of the contralateral nodule and proceed with total thyroidectomy only if the biopsy specimen suggests malignancy.

C. Perform complete right lobectomy only.

D. Perform left subtotal lobectomy.

E. Perform complete right lobectomy with nodulectomy of lesions located on the left.

*Ref.:* 1, 2

**COMMENTS:** Injury to the **recurrent laryngeal nerve** occurs in less than 1% of patients. The risk is higher with low-volume surgeons, **reoperative surgery**, irradiated necks, and invasive cancers. Transient **neurapraxia** can occur as a result of excessive stretch on the nerve but typically recovers following the procedure. There can be loss of signal with intraoperative nerve monitoring, just as would be seen if the nerve were completely transected. Intraoperative laryngoscopy is of no use because the patient is unresponsive, and functional vocal cord evaluation is very limited while the patient is still intubated. If this problem is encountered in a patient such as this one in whom the intended operation is not yet complete, the best decision is to terminate the procedure on the side where the gland is already mobilized. After the recovery period, the patient should undergo formal vocal cord evaluation and have a lengthy discussion regarding the risks and benefits of proceeding with the subsequent portion of the operation.

**ANSWER:** C

25. With regard to the pathologic features of thyroid cancer, which of the following is true?

A. Psammoma bodies are a feature of MTC.

B. Hürthle cell cancer represents a subtype of anaplastic thyroid cancer.

C. Amyloid deposits are a characteristic of papillary cancer.

D. Medullary cancer typically spreads hematogenously.

E. Nuclear grooves and inclusions are a characteristic feature of papillary thyroid cancer.

*Ref.:* 1, 2

**COMMENTS:** The pathologic characteristics of **papillary thyroid cancer** include nuclear grooves and inclusions. **Psammoma bodies** are also pathognomonic of papillary thyroid cancer. MTC spreads via the lymphatics initially. Amyloid deposits represent collections of calcitonin within the thyroid specimen. **Hürthle cell cancer** is a subtype of follicular thyroid cancer that has a more aggressive phenotype.

**ANSWER:** E

26. A 62-year-old man undergoes total thyroidectomy for a left thyroid nodule. On preoperative ultrasound, malignant calcifications were noted. FNA was consistent with a follicular neoplasm. Final pathologic evaluation reveals follicular carcinoma with an insular component. With regard to his overall prognosis, which of the following statements is not true?

A. Insular thyroid cancer carries a worse prognosis than do other subtypes of WDTC.

B. Patients with insular thyroid cancer should routinely undergo prophylactic central neck dissection.

C. The insular component subtypes of follicular carcinoma demonstrate poor uptake of radioactive iodine.

D. Disease-free survival is shorter in patients with insular thyroid cancer than in those with stage-matched follicular and papillary thyroid cancer.

E. The death rate is higher in patients with insular thyroid cancer.

*Ref.:* 1-3

**COMMENTS:** Follicular or papillary thyroid cancers with an **insular component** have a far worse prognosis than do those with other subtypes of WDTC. Most notably, these patients have a higher rate of extrathyroidal extension and distant metastases. Disease-free survival is shorter, and there is a higher rate of tumor-related deaths. Additionally, these tumors tend to exhibit poor radioactive iodine uptake when compared with other WDTC types. Because of its aggressive biology, some clinicians consider the insular component subtype a separate entity from classic papillary or follicular carcinomas that do not have this feature. Despite their more aggressive nature, no studies to date have shown that patients with insular thyroid cancer should undergo prophylactic central neck dissection.

**ANSWER:  B**

27. A 72-year-old woman with Hashimoto thyroiditis is evaluated for a rapidly enlarging neck mass. The patient takes levothyroxine replacement. Despite no change in her medication dosage, she has been experiencing fevers, night sweats, and weight loss. Ultrasound revels a 4-cm left thyroid mass and a pseudocystic pattern. FNA is nondiagnostic. What is the next step in the management of this patient?

    A. Nonsteroidal antiinflammatory drugs

    B. Repeated FNA

    C. Radioactive iodine

    D. Open or core biopsy

    E. Increased dose of levothyroxine with follow-up ultrasound in 6 months

*Ref.:* 1, 2

**COMMENTS:** Primary **thyroid lymphoma** is rare (<1% of all thyroid malignancies). There is an increased association between lymphoma and Hashimoto thyroiditis. The initial work-up of a newly diagnosed thyroid mass should be completed. FNA can be diagnostic, but flow cytometry is needed to establish the diagnosis. On ultrasound, the thyroid will classically have a pseudocystic pattern. In the current patient, the presence of Hashimoto thyroiditis, a rapidly enlarging mass, and constitutional symptoms is highly suggestive of primary thyroid lymphoma. If FNA fails to yield a diagnosis on first attempt, it has been shown that repeated FNA is unlikely to be diagnostic in subsequent attempts. Observation is not an appropriate step in the management of any patient with a rapidly enlarging neck mass, and placing patients on a high-dose levothyroxine regimen has been shown to do nothing as far as halting the growth of thyroid nodules. Performing open or core biopsy is a feasible option in these circumstances and would more likely provide an adequate cell yield to complete flow cytometry and establish monoclonality. Treatment varies between chemotherapy and surgical ablation. Resection is typically reserved for patients who fail to respond to chemotherapy or have completed their course of adjuvant therapy and demonstrate incomplete regression of disease. If surgery is planned, total thyroidectomy should be performed, followed by chemotherapy.

**ANSWER:  D**

28. Which of the following genes has been associated with a less favorable prognosis in patients with papillary thyroid cancer?

    A. *RET* protooncogene

    B. *Ras*

    C. *BRAF*

    D. *Menin*

    E. *p53*

*Ref.:* 1, 2

**COMMENTS: Papillary thyroid cancer** is the most common type of thyroid cancer. Patients have an overall predicted 5-year survival rate that approaches 95% to 99%. Several clinical factors are currently used as prognosticators of a patient's clinical outcome. **B-type RAF** (BRAF) is a part of the Raf kinase family and plays a fundamental role in the classic intracellular signaling mitogen-activated protein kinase (MAPK) pathway. *BRAF* mutations are associated with an increased risk for lymph node metastasis, extrathyroidal invasion, and advanced tumor stages. BRAF as a therapeutic target is currently being investigated. ***RET*** is the gene found to be mutated in patients with MTC, and *menin* is mutated in patients with multiple endocrine neoplasia type I. Both *p53* and *RAS* have not been identified as genetic prognosticators in patients with papillary thyroid cancer.

**ANSWER:  C**

29. A 65-year-old man underwent treatment of renal cell carcinoma 10 years earlier. On routine PET he was found to have a mass in his left thyroid lobe with increased uptake suggestive of a malignancy. With regard to thyroid metastases, which of the following malignancies most commonly spreads to the thyroid?

    A. Renal cell carcinoma

    B. Breast cancer

    C. Colon cancer

    D. Lung cancer

    E. Melanoma

*Ref.:* 1, 2

**COMMENTS: Metastases to the thyroid** are rare. The most common metastases to the thyroid are from renal cell carcinoma, and they can develop several years after the initial diagnosis. Other types of cancer that metastasize to the thyroid include lung and breast cancer. Management depends on the state of the primary disease in other locations and predicted overall survival.

**ANSWER:  A**

**REFERENCES**

1. Hanks JB, Salomone LJ: Thyroid. In Townsend CM, Beauchamp RD, Evers BM, et al, editors: *Sabiston textbook of surgery, the biological basis of modern surgical practice,* ed 18, Philadelphia, 2008, WB Saunders.
2. Lal G, Clark OH: Thyroid, parathyroid and adrenal. In Brunicardi FC, Andersen DK, Billiar TR, et al, editors: *Schwartz's principles of surgery,* ed 9, New York, 2010, McGraw-Hill.
3. Hall SF, Walker H, Siemens R, et al: Increasing detection and increasing incidence in thyroid cancer, *World J Surg* 33:2567–2571, 2009.

# CHAPTER 17

# Parathyroid

*Tricia Moo-Young, M.D., and Richard A. Prinz, M.D.*

1. With regard to calcium homeostasis, which of the following statements is false?

   A. Calcium is the most abundant cation in human beings.

   B. Approximately 50% of calcium is free or ionized and is metabolically active.

   C. Hypoalbuminemia can make the measured total calcium concentration appear artificially low.

   D. Hypoventilation can decrease ionized calcium levels and thus exacerbate symptoms of hypocalcemia.

   E. Calcium is bound to citrate and is biologically inactive.

   *Ref.:* 1, 2

**COMMENTS: Calcium** is the most abundant cation in the human body. As much as 99% is stored in the musculoskeletal system. The remainder is present in serum and exists in three forms: (1) 45% is bound to albumin and is biologically inert, (2) 50% is ionized and metabolically active, and (3) a small percentage is complexed with citrate and also is biologically inactive. Hypoalbuminemia means that more of the total serum calcium will be free and metabolically active. Although total serum calcium may be low, the patient may not be metabolically hypocalcemic. Ionized calcium levels are inversely affected by the pH of blood. A 1-unit rise in pH will decrease the ionized calcium level by 0.36 mmol/L. Hypoventilation would cause a drop in pH and thus a subsequent rise in the ionized calcium level.

**ANSWER: D**

2. Vitamin D synthesis begins in the skin keratinocytes. What is the next step of activation in vitamin D synthesis?

   A. Hydroxylation in the kidney to yield 1,25-dihydroxyvitamin D

   B. Hydroxylation in the liver to yield 25-hydroxyvitamin D

   C. Decarboxylation in the liver to yield 25-hydroxyvitamin D

   D. Decarboxylation in the kidney to yield 25-hydroxyvitamin D

   E. Decarboxylation in the periphery to yield 25-hydroxyvitamin D

   *Ref.:* 1, 2

**COMMENTS: Vitamin D synthesis** begins in the keratinocytes of the skin. Subsequently, hydroxylation occurs in the liver to yield 25-hydroxyvitamin D. The final step in conversion of vitamin D to its active form occurs in the kidney, where a second hydroxylation reaction takes place to yield **1,25-dihydroxyvitamin D**. Sunlight plays a key role in the initial synthesis step in the skin. Persons who are not exposed to sunlight require supplemental vitamin D through dietary intake.

**ANSWER: B**

3. Calcitonin helps mediate calcium homeostasis by which of the following actions?

   A. Stimulates osteoblast-mediated bone formation and inhibits renal resorption of calcium and phosphate

   B. Directly inhibits secretion of parathyroid hormone (PTH)

   C. Inhibits intestinal absorption of calcium

   D. Stimulates hydroxylation of vitamin D

   E. Stimulates osteoclast-mediated bone resorption

   *Ref.:* 1, 2

**COMMENTS:** In humans, the **parathyroid** glands are derived from the branchial pouches. The superior parathyroid arises from the fourth **branchial pouch**, and the inferior parathyroid originates from the third. The percentage of patients with ectopic glands ranges between 2.5% and 22%. The position of the superior parathyroid is most consistent. By contrast, the inferior gland can be located in the thymus up to 15% of the time. The inconsistent position of the inferior gland is believed to be the result of its longer migratory path from the third branchial pouch. An undescended inferior parathyroid can be located above the superior gland at the base of the skull or angle of the mandible. The frequency of intrathyroidal glands is relatively rare (0.5% to 3%). **Calcitonin** is produced by the parafollicular cells (C cells) of the thyroid gland. It helps lower ionized calcium levels in primarily two ways. First, it inhibits osteoclast-mediated bone resorption. Second, it inhibits resorption of calcium and phosphate by the kidney. Calcitonin has no direct effects on intestinal absorption or osteoblast-mediated bone formation.

**ANSWER: A**

4. With regard to PTH, which of the following statements is incorrect?

   A. PTH directly stimulates increased intestinal absorption of calcium.

   B. PTH stimulates osteoclast resorption of calcium and phosphate.

   C. PTH cells express G protein–coupled calcium-sensing receptors.

D. PTH inhibits calcium excretion at the distal convoluted tubule of the kidney.

E. PTH enhances renally mediated hydroxylation of 25-hydroxyvitamin D.

*Ref.:* 1, 2

**COMMENTS: Parathyroid hormone** has a variety of actions and targets to help increase serum calcium levels. The parathyroid cells express a G protein–coupled membrane receptor that senses serum calcium levels. When calcium levels fall below appropriate levels, the receptor stimulates the release of PTH into the circulation. PTH has a half-life of about 2 to 4 minutes in the circulation. Before its rapid clearance, it first targets osteoclasts and stimulates them to resorb calcium and phosphate from bone. In the kidney, PTH blocks calcium excretion at the distal convoluted tubule. It *indirectly* promotes intestinal absorption of calcium by enhancing the renally mediated activation of vitamin D.

**ANSWER:** A

5. All of the following conditions can cause hypercalcemia in patients with normal parathyroid function except:

   A. Malignancy

   B. Sarcoidosis

   C. Lithium

   D. Cirrhosis

   E. Tuberculosis

*Ref.:* 1, 2

**COMMENTS:** A number of conditions can cause **hypercalcemia**, including granulomatous disorders such as sarcoidosis, tuberculosis, and histoplasmosis. Medications can falsely elevate the serum calcium level. Examples include thiazide diuretics, lithium, and vitamin A or D. Other conditions include Paget disease, immobilization, and malignancy. In hospitalized patients, malignancy is the most common cause of hypercalcemia.

**ANSWER:** D

6. Routine work-up of a patient with suspected primary hyperparathyroidism (PHPT) includes all of the following except:

   A. Serum 1,25-dihydroxyvitamin D levels

   B. 24-hour urine calcium

   C. Intact PTH (iPTH)

   D. Serum calcium level

   E. Detailed physical examination and history

*Ref.:* 1, 2

**COMMENTS:** In a patient with suspected PHPT, the minimum testing that should be performed includes **intact parathyroid hormone**, serum calcium, blood urea nitrogen, creatinine, and vitamin D levels. It is not necessary to measure PTH-related protein (PTHrp) unless metastatic cancer is suspected. It is important to document normal renal function before the interpretation of parathyroid function tests. Urinary calcium measurements need not be done routinely, except in patients who have a family history of hypercalcemia and no previous history of normal calcium levels.

In these patients, 24-hour urine calcium excretion should be measured to exclude benign **familial hypercalcemia hypocalciuria.**

**ANSWER:** B

7. All of the following are consistent with the diagnosis of secondary hyperparathyroidism except:

   A. Elevated serum phosphate level

   B. Normal serum calcium level

   C. Vitamin D deficiency

   D. Elevated PTH level

   E. Calcitonin is the drug of choice for initial treatment

*Ref.:* 1, 2

**COMMENTS: Secondary hyperparathyroidism** most commonly occurs in patients with a history of chronic renal failure. The pathophysiology of this condition is multifactorial but it is believed to be the result of chronic hyperphosphatemia and deficiency in active vitamin D because of loss of renal tissue. Patients will commonly have an elevated PTH level and normal serum calcium. In such a setting, vitamin D levels should be measured and, if low, treated for a minimum of 6 weeks with supplemental vitamin D. Some of these patients are managed medically with the use of **calcimimetic** agents such as cinacalcet. This medication works by binding the calcium-sensing receptors on the chief cells of the parathyroid gland and increasing its sensitivity to extracellular calcium. Calcitonin has no pharmacologic role in treating secondary hyperparathyroidism.

**ANSWER:** E

8. All of the following are indications for surgical treatment of secondary hyperparathyroidism except:

   A. Calcium-phosphate product of less than 70

   B. Uremic pruritus

   C. Osteitis fibrosa cystica

   D. Calciphylaxis

   E. Tumoral calcinosis

*Ref.:* 1, 2

**COMMENTS: Secondary hyperparathyroidism** is most commonly managed medically with the use of **calcimimetic** agents, phosphate binders, adequate calcium intake, and vitamin D replacement. Surgical treatment is indicated in patients with (1) renal osteodystrophy, (2) **calciphylaxis**, (3) calcium-phosphate product of greater than 70, (4) soft tissue calcium deposition and tumoral calcinosis, and (5) calcium level greater than 11 mg/dL with an inappropriately high level of PTH. **Renal osteodystrophy** is a major issue in hemodialysis patients. The aluminum present in the dialysate bath accumulates in bone and contributes to the development of osteomalacia. **Osteitis fibrosa cystica,** a type of renal osteodystrophy, is characterized by marrow fibrosis and increased bone turnover. Bone cysts, osteopenia, and decreased bone strength develop. To halt progression of this disease process, these patients with secondary hyperparathyroidism are treated surgically. Calciphylaxis is a rare vascular disorder in which calcium is deposited in the media of small to medium-sized arteries. As a result, ischemic damage to the dermal and epidermal structures develops. The ulcerated lesions are extremely painful and can become infected with subsequent sepsis and eventually death. Patients with early signs of calciphylaxis should undergo urgent parathyroidectomy, although there is some evidence that aggressive management of serum calcium and parathyroid levels with cinacalcet may be beneficial. Care should be taken in wound care management because aggressive débridement can lead to chronic nonhealing wounds since wound healing is very poor in these patients. Uremic pruritus is characterized by severe itching that is thought to result from increased deposition of calcium salt in the dermis without the visible lesions of calciphylaxis. Parathyroidectomy seems to alleviate these symptoms and halts progression to the more serious skin and vascular complications seen with calciphylaxis.

**ANSWER: A**

9. With regard to PHPT, which of the following statements is true?

   A. PHPT is more common in men than in women.

   B. A common feature of PHPT is polyuria.

   C. A history of nephrolithiasis is present in 80% of patients with PHPT.

   D. Five percent of patients with PHPT can have multiple glands affected.

   E. Familial hypercalcemic hypocalciuria is associated with PHPT.

*Ref.:* 1, 2

**COMMENTS: Primary hyperparathyroidism** is a relatively common disorder that affects 0.3% of the human population, most commonly women. The exact cause of PHPT is unknown. In 80% of patients only a single adenoma is present, but multiple adenomas or hyperplasia can be present in up to 15% to 20%. Patients with PHPT can have symptomatic or "asymptomatic" disease. Some degree of renal dysfunction is present in up to 80% of patients. **Nephrolithiasis**, however, is far less common, with an incidence of approximately 20% to 25%. The clinical manifestations of PHPT vary widely across patients, but if a detailed history is taken, many will complain of polydipsia and polyuria from the calciuresis associated with the disease. Although PHPT occurs sporadically in the majority of patients, in a small percentage it is part of a familial syndrome. **Multiple endocrine neoplasia** type I (MEN-I) results from a germline mutation in the *menin* gene located on chromosome 11q12-13. Patients with MEN-I are susceptible to the development of pancreatic neuroendocrine tumors, pituitary adenomas, and PHPT. MEN-IIA is an autosomal dominantly inherited condition caused by a germline mutation on chromosome 11 that is associated with PHPT, pheochromocytoma, and medullary thyroid cancer. Patients with familial jaw tumor syndrome have a higher risk for the development of parathyroid carcinoma. **Familial hypercalcemic hypocalciuria** is associated with elevated calcium levels and low urinary excretion of calcium. The primary defect is abnormal sensing of calcium in blood by the parathyroid gland and the renal tubules, which causes inappropriate secretion of PTH and excessive renal reabsorption of calcium.

**ANSWER: B**

10. In 2002, the National Institutes of Health (NIH) released a consensus statement outlining indications for the surgical treatment of patients with asymptomatic hyperparathyroidism. All of the following are part of the criteria for surgical treatment except:

   A. Creatinine clearance reduced by greater than 30% in comparison to age-matched subjects

   B. PHPT in a patient younger than 50 years

   C. Calcium elevated to greater than 1 to 1.6 mg/dL above normal

   D. Osteitis fibrosa cystica

   E. 24-hour urinary calcium excretion greater than 150 mg/day

*Ref.:* 1, 2

**COMMENTS: The 2002 National Institutes of Health Consensus Conference** defined "**asymptomatic**" **hyperparathyroidism** as the absence of bone, neurologic, gastrointestinal, or renal complaints associated with the disease. In their statement they outlined criteria for surgical referral in patients with "asymptomatic" disease (Box 17-1).

---

**BOX 17-1    National Institutes of Health Criteria for Parathyroidectomy**

Serum calcium >1-1.6 mg/dL above normal
Nephrolithiasis
Creatinine clearance reduced by 30% with age-matched control
Age <50 yr
History of life-threatening hypercalcemia
Neuromuscular symptoms (ataxia, proximal muscle weakness, hyperreflexia)
Reduction in bone mass >2 standard deviation below matched controls
24-hour urine calcium excretion elevated to >400 mg/day

---

**ANSWER: E**

11. A 54-year-old woman has proximal muscle weakness, polyuria, and a depressed mood. Laboratory work-up reveals a serum calcium level of 11.2 mg/dL and a PTH level of 110 ng/L. Which of the following is the least sensitive preoperative localization study to identify an abnormal parathyroid gland?

   A. Magnetic resonance imaging (MRI)

   B. Single-photon emission computed tomography (SPECT)

   C. Technetium-99m–labeled sestamibi scan

   D. Neck ultrasound

   E. Standard computed tomography (CT)

*Ref.:* 1, 2

**COMMENTS:** Although all of the these imaging studies have been used to identify the location of a parathyroid adenoma, **magnetic resonance imaging** is the least sensitive of those listed. Routine preoperative localization in patients with PHPT includes **neck ultrasound** and technetium-99m–labeled sestamibi scan. Sestamibi scan has a reported sensitivity as high as 90%. Ultrasound is slightly less sensitive (75%), but the ease of in-office use makes it a useful tool for the general surgeon. SPECT, when used with planar **sestamibi**, is very good at locating potential ectopic glands such as those in the mediastinum. MRI is the least sensitive of the other listed modalities but, when used along with CT, can be helpful in locating ectopic glands.

**ANSWER: A**

12. Of the following, which patient is the least likely to have multigland disease?

   A. A 65-year-old lady with a PTH level of 110 ng/L and calcium level of 10.5 mg/dL

   B. A 22-year-old woman with a PTH level of 140 ng/L, a calcium level of 10.1 mg/dL, and MEN-I

C. A 75-year-old man with a 10-year history of renal failure

D. A 44-year-old woman with a diagnosis of secondary hyperparathyroidism

E. A 39-year-old woman 6 years after a gastric bypass for morbid obesity

*Ref.:* 3, 4

**COMMENTS:** No study has yet identified a reliable predictor of which patients with sporadic hyperparathyroidism will have **multigland disease**. The exception is in familial, secondary, and tertiary hyperparathyroidism. Because of the nearly uniform incidence of four-gland hyperplasia, all these patients are managed with bilateral neck exploration and either total parathyroidectomy with **autotransplantation** or three-and-a-half gland parathyroidectomy. Although some surgeons believe that patients with higher preoperative PTH or calcium levels (or both) are more likely to have multigland disease, this has not proved to be true in clinical studies. Intraoperative PTH (IOPTH) monitoring is used to determine whether all hyperfunctioning tissue has been removed. Several different criteria for the interpretation of IOPTH have been published (Table 17-1). Studies comparing these various criteria and their ability to predict multigland disease have been controversial. The pitfalls of the various criteria include false-positive results that lead to unnecessary bilateral neck exploration versus false-negative results in which the presence of multigland disease is not recognized. The best clinical marker of single-gland disease is concordant preoperative imaging in combination with appropriate correction of IOPTH levels.

**TABLE 17-1  Criteria for Parathyroid Hormone Monitoring to Predict Operative Success**

| | |
|---|---|
| Miami Criteria | ≥50% decline from the highest (either preincision or preexcision) value within 10 minutes of gland removal |
| Vienna Criteria | ≥50% decline from the preincision value within 10 minutes of gland removal |
| Halle Criteria | Decay into the low normal range (PTH ≤35 ng/L) within 15 minutes |
| Rome Criteria | ≥50% decline from the highest preexcision level, and/or PTH concentration within the reference range at 20 minutes after excision, and/or ≤7.5 ng/L lower than the value at 10 minutes after excision |

**ANSWER:  A**

13. A 55-year-old woman with a diagnosis of hyperparathyroidism wishes to undergo minimally invasive parathyroidectomy (MIP). Which of the following would preclude a patient from being a candidate for this approach?

A. PHPT

B. Lack of preoperative localization

C. Preoperative imaging of a solitary lesion on only one of two localization studies

D. Previous neck surgery

E. Secondary hyperparathyroidism

*Ref.:* 1, 2

**COMMENTS: Minimally invasive parathyroidectomy** is the preferred approach in patients who have a solitary lesion that is imaged conclusively by ultrasound, sestamibi, or a combination of both scans. It is advisable to use **intraoperative parathyroid hormone determination** to document an appropriate drop in PTH levels after removal of the suspected gland. Previous neck surgery or lack of concordant imaging on two types of studies is not a contraindication to attempting MIP. Patients in who no localization has been successful should not generally be offered MIP. Patients suspected of having multigland disease are managed by four-gland exploration, although surgeons at some centers are advocating exploration via a minimally invasive approach.

**ANSWER:  B**

14. A pregnant mother in her first trimester comes to her clinician's office with a diagnosis of PHPT. What is the correct management?

A. Parathyroidectomy during the second trimester

B. Parathyroidectomy during the third trimester

C. Prescribing a calcimimetic agent to help reduce hypercalcemia until after delivery, when definitive surgery can be offered safely

D. Close observation and parathyroidectomy following delivery

E. Weekly injections of calcitonin until delivery, when definitive surgery can be offered safely

*Ref.:* 1, 2

**COMMENTS: Hyperparathyroidism during pregnancy** is often unrecognized and is associated with a 3.5-fold increase in miscarriage. Loss of the pregnancy most often occurs during the late second trimester. The incidence of hyperparathyroidism in pregnancy is 0.7%. Maternal complications include hyperemesis, nephrolithiasis, and pancreatitis. Fetal complications include spontaneous abortion and growth retardation. In those who reach delivery, neonatal complications include hypocalcemic crisis within the first few days of life. Calcimimetic medications have not been used in the setting of hyperparathyroidism in pregnancy. Calcitonin has no role in the management of hyperparathyroidism.

**ANSWER:  A**

15. A patient is undergoing directed exploration for PHPT. A single large parathyroid gland is found adjacent to the left superior thyroid pole. The preincision PTH level was 300 ng/L, and the pre–pedicle clamp level was 400 ng/L. Five and ten minutes after removal of the gland, the PTH level is measured to be 200 ng/L. All are appropriate next steps in the management of this patient except:

A. Repeated PTH measurement

B. Frozen section confirmation of the removed parathyroid gland

C. Four-gland exploration

D. Drawing blood from the contralateral jugular vein to determine the PTH level

E. Conclusion of the operation given the 50% drop from the highest pre-removal level

*Ref.:* 1, 2

**COMMENTS:** Although this patient did experience a 50% drop from the highest pre-removal level, 200 ng/L is still quite elevated. When the surgeon is going to accept a 50% drop, the final level should either approach normal or be following a kinetic trend toward normal. A preexcision level that is within a few-fold elevation of the upper limit of normal should demonstrate normal kinetics and rapidly approach normal levels within two to three half-lives of the hormone after the adenoma is removed. The first steps in this situation should be to repeat the PTH level 15 to 20 minutes following gland removal and send off a frozen section for confirmation of the candidate gland removed. At this point it would be appropriate to either await the results of these two tests or proceed with four-gland exploration. The use of **intraoperative parathyroid hormone** monitoring has revolutionized how parathyroid surgery is performed. It has allowed surgeons to perform directed operations and, before leaving the operating room, document whether biochemical cure has been achieved with relative certainty. There is wide variability in the literature on what constitutes appropriate use and interpretation of IOPTH monitoring. The most commonly used criteria include determination of a preincision PTH level, a stimulated (pre–pedicle ligation) level, and subsequent postremoval levels at 5-minute intervals until a normal level is achieved. Alternatively, some surgeons require only greater than a 50% drop in the PTH level from the highest pre-removal level (preincision or pre–pedicle ligation level). They do not require that the final level determined be within the normal range. In patients with **secondary** or **tertiary hyperparathyroidism** and stimulation levels as high as 2000 ng/L, a 90% decrease has been suggested as being indicative of cure.

**ANSWER:** E

16. The patient in Question 15 has a repeated PTH value of 200 ng/mL. Frozen section of the removed left superior candidate gland shows "hyperplastic parathyroid tissue." On further exploration, no gland can be identified in the left inferior location. The right side is explored, both glands are located, and "hyperplastic parathyroid tissue" is confirmed by frozen section. Blood is drawn from the left internal jugular vein to determine the PTH level, which is found to be 600 ng/L. All of the following include appropriate steps in the management of this patient except:

    A. Cervical thymectomy

    B. Exploration of the left carotid sheath

    C. Left thyroid lobectomy

    D. Left lateral neck dissection

    E. Exploration of the retroesophageal space

*Ref.:* 1, 2

**COMMENTS:** The left inferior parathyroid gland has not been identified in this patient. Frozen section has confirmed "**hyperplastic parathyroid tissue**" in the three identified glands. Failure to find a normal parathyroid gland among those identified should alert the surgeon that the patient probably has four-gland hyperplasia. Failure to find the remaining gland places the patient at high risk for persistent hyperparathyroidism. Most lower parathyroid glands are found in proximity to the lower thyroid pole. If not found in this location, the thyrothymic ligament and thymus should be explored. If the IOPTH level does not normalize after this maneuver, **intraoperative ultrasound** of the left thyroid lobe versus left lobectomy should be performed. Finally, *central* neck dissection and exploration of the left carotid sheath are performed. The procedure is terminated after these steps, and further imaging and

localization studies should be undertaken if the patient has persistent hyperparathyroidism.

**ANSWER:** D

17. The most common location for a missed adenoma in patients undergoing reoperative parathyroid surgery is in:

    A. The thymus

    B. A normal upper position

    C. A normal lower position

    D. The tracheoesophageal groove

    E. The carotid sheath

*Ref.:* 5

**COMMENTS:** Based on review of a series of more than 200 patients undergoing **reoperative surgery** for a missed adenoma, the most common location in which the missing gland was found was the tracheoesophageal groove (27%). The remaining locations included the anterior mediastinum/thymus (18%), the normal upper position (13%), the normal lower position (12%), intrathyroidal (10%), **undescended parathyroids** (8%), and the carotid sheath (4%). Failure to identify parathyroid pathology during an operation can occur in various settings, including the presence of an intrathyroidal adenoma, failure of the surgeon to expose the abnormal gland in its standard position, failure to recognize **multigland disease**, and failure to recognize an intrathymic adenoma.

**ANSWER:** D

18. All of the following have been associated with an increased risk for hungry bone syndrome after parathyroidectomy except:

    A. Graves disease

    B. Tertiary hyperparathyroidism

    C. Preoperative PTH level

    D. Age

    E. Large single adenomas

*Ref.:* 1, 2

**COMMENTS:** "**Hungry bone syndrome**" is characterized by **postparathyroidectomy hypocalcemia** and **hypophosphatemia**. Patients most at risk are those with four-gland hyperplasia from secondary or tertiary hyperparathyroidism. The postoperative calcium level in these patients can drop critically low and necessitate intravenous calcium supplementation. During this period both serum calcium and phosphate levels must be monitored closely. In some patients it can take more than 4 to 5 days for serum calcium and phosphate levels to stabilize. Other patients shown to have increased risk for this condition are those who are older or have concomitant thyrotoxicosis or a large single adenoma. The preoperative PTH level has not been found to be an independent predictor of whether "hungry bone syndrome" will develop postoperatively.

**ANSWER:** C

19. A patient with chronic renal failure comes to the emergency department complaining of increasing confusion, muscle weakness, nausea, vomiting, and fatigue. The serum calcium level is 12.4 mg/dL. The first step in management of this patient should be:

A. Emergency parathyroidectomy

B. Aggressive intravenous hydration

C. Initiation of furosemide infusion

D. Continuous calcitonin infusion

E. Initiation of bisphosphonates

*Ref.:* 6

**COMMENTS:** The first step in the management of this patient with **hypercalcemia** should be aggressive immediate hydration. This should be done before giving loop diuretics. Along with intravenous hydration, salt loading should be initiated to help induce a natural diuresis. Table 17-2 lists therapies used to treat **hypercalcemic crisis**, along with the onset of action, advantages, and disadvantages of each treatment.

**TABLE 17-2  Management Options for Hypercalcemic Crisis**

| Treatment | Onset | Advantages | Disadvantages |
|---|---|---|---|
| Saline hydration | Hours | These patients are usually dehydrated | Volume overload in cardiac-sensitive patients |
| Diuretics | Hours | Rapid action | Should not be started if the patient is severely volume depleted |
| Bisphosphonates | 1-2 days | High potency | Medications may be tolerated poorly in some patients |
| Calcitonin | Hours | Rapid onset | Rapid tachyphylaxis |
| Intravenous phosphate | Hours | Rapid action, useful in patients with cardiac and/or renal decompensation | Can cause renal damage or fatal hypocalcemia |
| Glucocorticoids | Days | Oral therapy, good for chronic management | Side effects of glucocorticoids |
| Dialysis | Hours | Especially useful in patients with renal failure, immediate reversal of life-threatening hypercalcemia | Invasive |

**ANSWER:**  B

20. Which of the following is not a sign or symptom of hypocalcemia?

A. Shortened QT interval

B. Trousseau sign

C. Circumoral numbness

D. Anxiety

E. Laryngospasm

*Ref.:* 1, 2

**COMMENTS: Postoperative hypocalcemia** following parathyroidectomy is not unusual. The majority of patients are asymptomatic and identified only when routine postoperative laboratory tests are obtained. Symptomatic patients will most commonly complain of circumoral numbness and tingling in their extremities. These two features are early signs of hypocalcemia. On examination these patients may have carpopedal spasm elicited by occlusion of blood flow to the forearm (**Trousseau sign**) or contraction of the facial muscles elicited by tapping on the facial nerve (**Chvostek sign**). However nearly 20% of the general population has a positive Chvostek sign. If the condition is allowed to worsen, tetany, laryngeal stridor, or tonic-clonic seizures can develop, all of which can be fatal. These patients should be treated immediately with intravenous calcium. In asymptomatic patients, oral calcium and vitamin D should be initiated promptly.

**ANSWER:**  A

21. A 34-year-old woman has undergone three operations for hyperparathyroidism. She states that in each previous operation the surgeon has removed pathologically confirmed hyperplastic parathyroid tissue in the central portion of her neck and nodules within various muscles of her neck. Nonetheless, she continues to have elevated parathyroid levels associated with progressive bone loss. What is the most likely diagnosis in this patient?

A. Missed parathyroid adenoma

B. Multigland disease

C. Parathyromatosis

D. Familial hyperparathyroidism

E. Vitamin D deficiency

*Ref.:* 1, 2

**COMMENTS:** This scenario is a classic description of a patient with **parathyromatosis**. This rare condition is manifested clinically as recurrent or persistent hyperparathyroidism following multiple attempts at resection. On exploration, patients will have several small nodules of hyperfunctioning parathyroid tissue throughout the neck and possibly the mediastinum. It can be difficult to distinguish this condition from parathyroid carcinoma or an "atypical adenoma." Parathyromatosis is believed to result from either a low-grade parathyroid malignancy, fracture of the parathyroid adenoma capsule at the original procedure, or overgrowth of embryologic rests of parathyroid tissue. Management of these patients involves either serial debulking of the disease when it can be radiographically identified or pharmacologic treatment. Patients are rarely cured with surgery.

**ANSWER:**  C

22. A 54-year-old woman arrives for surgical evaluation with a PTH level of 280 ng/L and serum calcium level of 14.5 mg/dL. She has a past medical history of mild renal failure (creatinine, 1.9 mg/dL) and jaw tumor syndrome. The most likely diagnosis in this patient is:

A. Parathyromatosis

B. Missed adenoma

C. Parathyroid carcinoma

D. Secondary hyperparathyroidism

E. Tertiary hyperparathyroidism

*Ref.:* 1, 2

**COMMENTS:** A preoperative serum calcium level greater than 14 mg/dL, a palpable nodule, and adherence to surrounding tissues have all been found to be useful predictors of **parathyroid carcinoma**. Additionally, patients with familial hyperparathyroidism and jaw tumor syndrome have an increased risk for parathyroid cancer. Parathyroid carcinoma is rare and represents just 1% of all cases of PHPT. The prognosis is extremely poor, and most patients have advanced disease when initially seen. Parathyroid carcinoma should be suspected in a patient with a preoperative calcium level greater than 14 mg/dL or a serum PTH level two to three times the upper limit of normal. Intraoperatively, parathyroid cancers are typically large and less brown than a benign parathyroid adenoma. Invasion or adherence to the surrounding tissues should also raise suspicion for parathyroid carcinoma. Appropriate surgical management of this condition entails en bloc resection of the tumor with ipsilateral thyroid lobectomy. It is *not* necessary to perform a total thyroidectomy. A compartment-oriented lymph node dissection is necessary only if there is gross evidence of lymph node involvement.

**ANSWER:** C

23. Which of the following is not part of the standard work-up of a patient with persistent or recurrent hyperparathyroidism?

   A. Selective venous sampling

   B. SPECT

   C. Technetium-Tc-99m-sestamibi scanning

   D. Ultrasound

   E. Positron emission tomography (PET)

*Ref.:* 1, 2, 7

**COMMENTS: Persistent hypercalcemia** is defined as hypercalcemia that fails to correct after parathyroidectomy. Recurrent hyperparathyroidism occurs less frequently and is defined by the development of hypercalcemia following a 6- to 12-month period of normocalcemia. Preoperative localization is the mainstay of treatment algorithms for patients with persistent or recurrent hyperparathyroidism. The tests available can be divided into those that are noninvasive versus invasive. The noninvasive tests include **ultrasound**, **sestamibi scanning**, **single-photon emission computed tomography**, **magnetic resonance imaging**, and **computed tomography**. Of these, CT and MRI are the least useful and carry the lowest sensitivity. Invasive testing includes selective venous sampling and, more recently, intraoperative radioprobe guidance. Patients receive intravenous technetium-99m the morning of surgery, and then the radioprobe is used intraoperatively to identify the parathyroid gland. One limitation of this technology is a high background level, which can prevent identification of an intrathyroidal parathyroid gland. **Positron emission tomography** has yet to have any defined role in parathyroid localization.

**ANSWER:** E

**REFERENCES**

1. Sosa JA, Udelsman R: The parathyroid glands. In Townsend CM, Beauchamp RD, Evers BM, et al, editors: *Sabiston textbook of surgery: the biological basis of modern surgical practice*, ed 18, Philadelphia, 2008, WB Saunders.
2. Lal G, Clark OH: Thyroid, parathyroid and adrenal. In Brunicardi FC, Andersen DK, Billiar TR, et al, editors: *Schwartz's principles of surgery*, ed 9, New York, 2010, McGraw-Hill.
3. Riss P, Kaczirek K, Heinz G, et al: A "defined baseline" in PTH monitoring increases surigcal success in patients with multiple gland disease. *Surgery* 142:398–404, 2007.
4. Lombardi CP, Raffaelli M, Traini E, et al: Intraoperative PTH monitoring during parathyroidectomy: the need for stricter criteria to detect multiglandular disease, *Lagenbecks Arch Surg* 393: 639–645, 2008.
5. Jaskowiak N, Norton JA, Alexander HR, et al: A prospective trail evaluating a standard approach to reoperation for missed parathyroid adenoma, *Ann Surg* 224:308–320, 1996.
6. Fauci AS, Kasper DL, Longo DL, et al: *Harrison's principles of internal medicine*, ed 17, New York, 2008, McGraw-Hill.
7. Chen H, Sippel RS, Schaefer S: The effectiveness of radioguided parathyroidectomy in patients with negative technetium Tc 99m-sestamibi scans, *Arch Surg* 144:643–648, 2009.

# CHAPTER 18

# Adrenal

*Tricia Moo-Young, M.D., and Richard A. Prinz, M.D.*

1. Which of the following statements regarding the anatomy of the adrenal gland is false?

   A. The arterial supply arises from the inferior phrenic artery, the renal artery, and the aorta.

   B. The left adrenal vein, joined by the inferior phrenic vein, drains into the left renal vein.

   C. The right adrenal vein enters directly into the inferior vena cava.

   D. The arterial supply arises from the inferior phrenic and renal arteries.

   E. The adrenal vein is longer on the left side.

   *Ref.:* 1, 2

**COMMENTS:** The arterial supply of the adrenal gland arises from three sources. Superiorly, branches are given off by the **inferior phrenic artery**, whereas the middle branches originate from the aorta. Along the medial and inferior aspect of the gland are contributory branches given off by the ipsilateral renal artery. The venous drainage of the adrenal gland differs by side. The left adrenal vein is joined by the inferior phrenic vein before it drains into the left renal vein and can measure 2 cm long. Variably, the left inferior phrenic vein will drain separately into the left renal vein. On the right, the adrenal vein enters directly into the inferior vena cava posteriorly and is shorter and broader than the left one. This shorter configuration can make ligation technically more challenging for the adrenal surgeon.

**ANSWER:** D

2. What enzyme is responsible for the conversion of norepinephrine to epinephrine?

   A. Tyrosine hydroxylase

   B. Monamine oxidase

   C. Catechol *O*-methyltransferase

   D. Phenylethanolamine-*N*-methyltransferase (PNMT)

   E. Dopamine β-hydroxylase.

   *Ref.:* 1, 2

**COMMENTS:** Histologically, the adrenal gland is divided into two components: the centrally located **medulla** and the peripherally located **cortex**. The adrenal cortex arises from the mesoderm and accounts for approximately 90% of the total adrenal mass. Histologically, the cortex is made up of three zones, the glomerulosa, fasciculata, and reticularis. Each zone corresponds to the synthesis of mineralocorticosteroids, **corticosteroids**, and sex steroids. The medulla is composed of **chromaffin cells** derived from **ectodermal neural crest cells**. The chromaffin cells are innervated by sympathetic fibers traveling from the sympathetic chain. They secrete the vasoactive catecholamines epinephrine and norepinephrine. Norepinephrine is converted to epinephrine by the enzyme PNMT. This enzyme is exclusively located within the adrenal medulla and is not found in ectopic adrenal medullary tissue. Thus, ectopic pheochromocytomas are incapable of producing **epinephrine** since they lack this enzyme.

**ANSWER:** D

3. What is the rate-limiting enzyme of catecholamine synthesis?

   A. Tyrosine hydroxylase

   B. Monamine oxidase

   C. Dopamine β-hydroxylase

   D. Dopa decarboxylase

   E. PNMT

   *Ref.:* 1, 2

**COMMENTS:** Tyrosine hydroxylase is the rate-limiting enzyme in catecholamine synthesis. The first step in **catecholamine synthesis** involves the conversion of L-tyrosine into dihydroxyphenylalanine (L-dopa) by the enzyme tyrosine hydroxylase. Dopa decarboxylase then converts L-dopa into dopamine. Dopamine is subsequently converted to norepinephrine by the enzyme dopamine β-hydroxylase. PNMT is the enzyme located exclusively in the adrenal gland and is responsible for the conversion of norepinephrine into epinephrine.

**ANSWER:** A

4. Aldosterone secretion is under the control of all of the following except:

   A. Potassium

   B. Adrenocorticotropic hormone (ACTH)

   C. Angiotensin II

   D. Heparin

   E. Epinephrine

   *Ref.:* 1-3

**COMMENTS: Aldosterone synthesis** is under the control of angiotensin II, potassium, and to a lesser extent, ACTH. Its synthesis is inhibited by somatostatin, dopamine, atrial natriuretic factor, and heparin. **Aldosterone synthase** (CYP11B2) is restricted to the zona glomerulosa, where aldosterone is primarily synthesized. **Angiotensin II** and potassium stimulate aldosterone secretion by increasing the transcription of CYP11B2. ACTH increases aldosterone secretion by no more than 10% to 20% over baseline values and does so by stimulating the earlier pathways of adrenal steroidogenesis. Epinephrine plays no direct regulatory role in aldosterone synthesis.

**ANSWER: E**

5. Congenital adrenal hyperplasia (CAH) is most commonly caused by a deficiency of which of the following enzymes?

   A. 21-Hydroxylase

   B. 17α-Hydroxylase

   C. 11β-Hydroxylase

   D. 5α-Reductase

   E. 21β-Hydroxylase

   *Ref.: 1, 2*

**COMMENTS:** The most common form of **congenital adrenal hyperplasia** is due to mutations or deletions of *CYP21A2*, the gene that encodes for 21-hydroxylase. This enzyme defect accounts for more than 90% of cases of CAH. In most patients, it is manifested as a salt-wasting form in which lack of the 21-hydroxylase enzyme impedes downstream synthesis of aldosterone. Clinically, this becomes apparent within the first few months of life with the development of hypovolemia and hyperkalemia. There is excess production of ACTH because of the lack of negative feedback on steroid synthesis. Upstream precursors accumulate as a result of lack of the 21-hydroxylase enzyme and are then shunted into the sex steroidogenesis pathway. This leads to the presence of ambiguous genitalia in females. The diagnosis is made by finding elevated levels of 17-hydroxyprogesterone, the 21-hydroxylase substrate, and by genetic testing.

**ANSWER: A**

6. What is the most common cause of primary adrenal insufficiency (Addison disease)?

   A. Tuberculosis

   B. Kaposi sarcoma

   C. Cytomegalovirus

   D. Lymphoma

   E. Autoimmune disorder

   *Ref.: 1, 2*

**COMMENTS:** More than 150 years ago, Thomas Addison described a clinical condition that involved salt wasting, skin hyperpigmentation, and histopathologic destruction of the adrenal gland. In the 1850s, tuberculous adrenalitis was the most common cause of primary adrenal insufficiency. Because of the decreased incidence of advanced tuberculosis, the current most common cause is autoimmune **Addison disease**. Clinical symptoms of the disorder can include nausea and vague abdominal pain, musculoskeletal complaints, and postural dizziness. The most characteristic feature of Addison disease is hyperpigmentation of the skin and mucous membranes. Autoimmune Addison disease is typically associated with other autoimmune disorders such as type 1 diabetes mellitus.

**ANSWER: E**

7. A 55-year-old male patient is currently being treated in the surgical intensive care unit for ventilator-associated pneumonia following partial hepatectomy. His laboratory values are as follows: hemoglobin, 8 g/dL; white blood cell count, $8 \times 10^3$ cells/μl; and blood glucose, 34 mg/dL. In postoperative week 2, increasing pressor requirements develop suddenly in this patient, whose sepsis had been resolving despite broadening his antibiotic coverage and blood cultures being negative. You suspect adrenal insufficiency. What initial laboratory test can assist in making the diagnosis?

   A. Serum cortisol

   B. 24-hour urine cortisol

   C. Serum chemistry panel

   D. Cosyntropin stimulation test

   E. Serum troponin levels

   *Ref.: 1, 2*

**COMMENTS:** See Question 8.

**ANSWER: C**

8. The patient described in Question 7 has worsening hypotension despite escalation in intravenous norepinephrine. What should be the immediate next step in the management of this patient?

   A. Addition of vasopressin

   B. Intravenous fluids

   C. Cosyntropin stimulation test

   D. Hydrocortisone injection

   E. Blood transfusion

   *Ref.: 1, 2*

**COMMENTS: Acute adrenal insufficiency** is a life-threatening emergency. In the critically ill patient population it can develop in either the acute or chronic phase of the illness. In the intensive care setting, if acute hypotension refractory to pressor support and not demonstrated to be cardiogenic in origin develops suddenly, acute adrenal insufficiency should be excluded. Although the **cosyntropin stimulation test** is the definitive means of diagnosing adrenal insufficiency, this test can take up to 24 hours to return. Thus, in the acute setting, evidence of hyperkalemia, hyperglycemia, and refractory hypotension is sufficient to begin empirically treating these patients with steroids until the diagnosis can be confirmed. The first step in the management of a hypotensive patient suspected of having adrenal insufficiency is volume resuscitation followed by empirical steroid replacement. Corticosteroid replacement in patients with acute adrenal insufficiency should include the intravenous administration of either hydrocortisone, 100 mg every 6 to 8 hours, or dexamethasone, 4 mg every 24 hours. Dexamethasone is long acting and does not interfere with the administration of a cosyntropin stimulation test. Maintenance therapy in patients with chronic adrenal insufficiency can be achieved with oral prednisone, 5 mg daily, and the mineralocorticoid fludrocortisone, 0.1 mg/day. Blood transfusion will not reverse this patient's condition, and it is not generally recommended for patients with a hemoglobin level greater than 7 g/dL.

**ANSWER:** B

9. A 45-year-old woman with known Addison disease is due to undergo laparoscopic cholecystectomy. Which of the following is the correct stress corticosteroid dosage that she should receive preoperatively?

A. Hydrocortisone, 25 mg on the day of the procedure only

B. Hydrocortisone, 50 to 75 mg on the day of the procedure, followed by a 2-day taper to the maintenance dose

C. Hydrocortisone, 100 mg on the day of the procedure, followed by a rapid 5-day taper to the maintenance dose

D. Hydrocortisone, 100 mg on the day of the procedure only

E. Hydrocortisone, 50 to 75 mg on the day of the procedure, followed by a 6-week taper to the maintenance dosage

*Ref.:* 1, 2

**COMMENTS:** In patients with **adrenal insufficiency**, supplemental corticosteroids are required during physiologic stress such as illness, trauma, anesthesia, and surgical procedures. One standard dose should not be applied to all patients with adrenal insufficiency but should be individualized to the daily maintenance dose and the procedure or stress that they are undergoing. There is no benefit to excessive dosing (>200 mg/day of **hydrocortisone**) or an extended duration of dosing. In fact, deleterious effects secondary to undue corticosteroid exposure have been seen. In this patient, the appropriate dose, relative to the surgical procedure, is her daily maintenance dose that morning, 50 to 75 mg of hydrocortisone intravenously before induction of anesthesia, and her steroid dose tapered back to the maintenance dosage over the next 2 days.

**ANSWER:** B

10. The initial biochemical screening tests for incidentally discovered adrenal nodules include all of the following except:

A. ACTH

B. Low-dose dexamethasone test

C. Serum aldosterone

D. Serum renin

E. Late-night salivary cortisol level

*Ref.:* 1-3

**COMMENTS:** Work-up of an **incidental adrenal mass** includes screening and secondary confirmatory testing. Screening tests include (1) a low-dose **dexamethasone test** or 24-hour urine cortisol (or both), (2) a morning serum **aldosterone** and **renin level**, and (3) fractionated urine **metanephrines**. Confirmatory tests are done when the results of initial testing are equivocal and include but are not limited to a high-dose dexamethasone test, serum catecholamines, and salt-loading aldosterone suppression testing. Measurement of the serum ACTH level is performed once a diagnosis of hypercortisolism is established. Cortisol levels follow a circadian rhythm, which explains why random cortisol levels are not useful in the screening of these patients. When there is normal diurnal variation, cortisol should be at its lowest late at night. In patients suspected of having Cushing syndrome, an elevated serum cortisol level at 11 PM can be an early, albeit not definitive factor

in diagnosis of the condition. For its simplicity and relative accuracy, measurement of late-night salivary cortisol levels has gained popularity in recent years. It is more costly than standard testing and should be repeated over several evenings for improved accuracy. With repeated measurements, levels less than 1.3 ng/mL on radioimmunoassay exclude the diagnosis of **Cushing syndrome**.

**ANSWER:** A

11. A 32-year-old woman has a 5-year history of poorly controlled hypertension. She is taking three different medications, including a diuretic, β-blocker, and potassium supplements. What should be the next step in establishing the diagnosis of surgically correctable hypertension?

A. Computed tomography (CT) of the abdomen and pelvis

B. Urine catecholamines

C. Serum aldosterone and renin levels

D. Renal ultrasound

E. Saline suppression testing

*Ref.:* 1, 2

**COMMENTS:** The most likely diagnosis in this patient is **primary hyperaldosteronism**. There is general consensus that all patients with young age, poorly controlled hypertension, and a history of **hypokalemia** should undergo evaluation for an aldosterone-secreting adenoma. The initial step is measuring the aldosterone-to-renin ratio. This test should be performed after discontinuing such interfering medications as spironolactone. An aldosterone-to-renin ratio of greater than 25 to 30 (e.g., a serum aldosterone level of ≥15 ng/dL with a renin level of <0.5 ng/mL) is suggestive of the diagnosis. The diagnosis is then confirmed by doing a 24-hour urine aldosterone, sodium, and potassium test with the patient ingesting a high-salt diet. A 24-hour urinary aldosterone level greater than 12 mcg in 24 hours is considered positive. After establishing the biochemical diagnosis, the next step is to determine whether there is laterality of the disease. Only at this time should diagnostic imaging be ordered.

**ANSWER:** C

12. Biochemical testing confirms the diagnosis of primary hyperaldosteronism in the patient in Question 11. Diagnostic imaging reveals a 1.5-cm area of fullness in both adrenal glands. The next step in management should be:

A. Imaging repeated in 6 months

B. Long-term management with spironolactone

C. Bilateral cortical-sparing adrenalectomies

D. Selective venous sampling

E. Laparoscopic ultrasound

*Ref.:* 1, 2

**COMMENTS:** The next step to assist in localization is **selective venous sampling**. The test is done by performing simultaneous measurements of **serum cortisol** and **aldosterone** in the cannulated adrenal veins and the peripheral circulation. Confirmation of successful cannulation is established by documenting a greater than fivefold elevation in cortisol concentration relative to the peripheral circulation. Lateralization is confirmed by an unbalanced ratio of aldosterone to cortisol when comparing one side with the other. Typically, most authors recommend at least a fourfold difference between the two sides rather than an absolute value of elevation above normal. **Intraoperative ultrasound** can facilitate intraoperative localization of adrenal tumors, particularly via laparoscopy. However, an operation is not the next step in this patient.

**ANSWER: D**

13. The most common cause of hyperaldosteronism is:

A. Bilateral idiopathic adrenal hyperplasia

B. Aldosterone-producing adenoma

C. Familial hyperaldosteronism type I

D. Adrenocortical carcinoma

E. Unilateral adrenal hyperplasia

*Ref.:* 1, 2

**COMMENTS:** The most common cause of **hyperaldosteronism** is bilateral idiopathic **hyperplasia** (60% to 70%). The second most common cause is an aldosterone-producing **adenoma** (35%). The remaining subtypes include unilateral adrenal hyperplasia (2%), carcinoma (<1%), and **familial hyperaldosteronism** types I and II (<1%). It is important to distinguish which subtype of hyperaldosteronism that a patient has because some types, including bilateral idiopathic hyperplasia, are managed nonoperatively.

**ANSWER: A**

14. A patient being evaluated for hyperaldosteronism has elevated aldosterone and renin levels. What is the probable cause of this condition?

A. Cirrhosis

B. Aldosterone-secreting adenoma

C. Familial hyperaldosteronism type II

D. Metastatic renal cell cancer

E. Bilateral idiopathic hyperplasia

*Ref.:* 1, 2

**COMMENTS:** This patient has **secondary hyperaldosteronism** as a result of increased renin production by the kidney. This condition can result from reduced intravascular volume as is seen in congestive heart failure, cirrhosis, nephrosis, renovascular hypertension, Bartter syndrome, and pregnancy. Adrenal function is normal, and treatment is directed at the underlying condition.

**ANSWER: A**

15. The most common *endogenous* cause of Cushing syndrome is:

A. Adrenocortical carcinoma

B. ACTH-hypersecreting pituitary adenoma

C. Cortisol-hypersecreting adrenal adenoma

D. Ectopic ACTH-producing tumor

E. Adrenal hyperplasia

*Ref.:* 1, 2

**COMMENTS:** Overall, the most common cause of **Cushing syndrome** is the exogenous use of corticosteroids. Among the endogenous types of Cushing syndrome, an ACTH-hypersecreting

pituitary adenoma is the most common (70%). Adrenal adenomas and **ectopic adrenocorticotropic hormone**-producing tumors each account for 10% of the endogenous causes of Cushing syndrome.

**ANSWER: B**

16. A 55-year-old male smoker with no previous medical history comes to the surgical clinic after having recently undergone CT for nonspecific abdominal pain. A 2.5-cm left adrenal mass was identified on CT. What is the next step in management of the incidental adrenal mass in this patient?

A. Magnetic resonance imaging (MRI)

B. CT-guided fine-needle aspiration (FNA) biopsy

C. Biochemical work-up

D. Observation and follow-up CT in 6 months

E. CT of the lung

*Ref.:* 1, 2

**COMMENTS:** Despite no previous history suggesting an underlying biochemical syndrome, the first step in management of an **incidental adrenal lesion** is to complete a functional evaluation. If the lesion is nonfunctional, the next step in management is to distinguish benign from malignant disease. MRI can be useful in this regard, but most times an index of suspicion for a malignant process can be garnered from CT alone. Image-guided biopsy is *not* believed to be useful in helping differentiate benign from **malignant adrenal lesions**. According to the National Institutes of Health (NIH) State-of-the-Science Conference on the work-up of adrenal **incidentalomas**, FNA is recommended in patients with a history of malignancy and no other signs of metastases. Before percutaneous biopsy it is imperative that the presence of a pheochromocytoma be excluded since a life-threatening pheochromocytoma crisis can occur with this intervention. Metastatic lung cancer should be considered in the differential diagnosis, but CT of the lung should not be the initial step in this patient.

**ANSWER: C**

17. A 66-year-old woman has a 3.8-cm left adrenal mass noted on CT. On review of the CT scan, which of the following suggests a benign lesion?

A. Mass larger than 3 cm

B. Rapidity of washout of contrast material of less than 50% at 10 minutes

C. Unilateral lesions

D. Heterogeneous enhancement

E. Less than 10 Hounsfield units (HU)

*Ref.:* 1, 2

**COMMENTS:** In the evaluation of **nonfunctional tumors** there are a number of radiographic findings that can assist the clinician in determining whether a lesion is likely to be benign or malignant (Table 18-1). Measurement of Hounsfield units on **computed tomography** is a commonly used parameter and is associated with acceptable rates of specificity and sensitivity when other features such as size, shape, or growth are considered. Less than 10 HU on unenhanced CT is indicative of a benign lesion. When intravenous contrast material is administered and delayed imaging is performed, the rapidity of washout of the contrast agent can be measured. Typically, benign lesions have rapid washout, with more than 50% of the initial attenuation value lost at 10 minutes on delayed imaging. Less than 50% washout suggests malignancy or pheochromocytoma. The reported sensitivity and specificity of assessing lesions by Hounsfield units with washout percentages are 98% and 92%, respectively.

**TABLE 18-1   Adrenal Incidentalomas: Imaging Characteristics of Benign versus Malignant Lesions**

| Variable | Benign | Malignant | Metastasis |
|---|---|---|---|
| Size | Small, <3 cm | Large, >3 cm | Variable |
| Shape | Round, smooth | Irregular | Variable |
| Enhancement | Homogeneous | Heterogeneous | Heterogeneous |
| Hounsfield units (HU) | <10 HU | >20 HU | >20 HU |
| Rapidity of washout of contrast agent | >50% at 10 minutes | <50% at 10 minutes | <50% at 10 minutes |
| Magnetic resonance imaging | Isointense relative to the liver on T2-weighted images | Hyperintense relative to the liver on T2-weighted images | Hyperintense relative to the liver on T2-weighted images |
| Growth | Stable, <1 cm/yr | Rapid, >1 cm/yr | Variable |

**ANSWER:** E

18. The patient in Question 17 undergoes repeated CT in 1 year, followed by MRI. CT shows that the lesion has grown from 3.8 to 4.1 cm during that period. Characteristics on CT reveal a low-attenuation lesion with less than 10 HU. MRI shows a hyperintense lesion on T1-weighted in-phase MRI. What is the probable diagnosis in this patient?

   A. Adrenocortical adenoma

   B. Pheochromocytoma

   C. Adrenocortical carcinoma

   D. Myelolipoma

   E. Aldosteronoma

*Ref.:* 1, 2

**COMMENTS:** The imaging characteristics described are typical of **myelolipoma**. These lesions are composed of erythroid, myeloid, and an abundant amount of adipose tissue. On non–contrast-enhanced CT, they are low attenuation and consistent with nearly pure fat. On MRI they are hyperintense on T1-weighted in-phase images. On T2-weighted images, malignant lesions are typically hyperintense and benign lesions are isointense relative to the liver. Generally, myelolipomas are benign and slow growing. There is no indication to surgically remove these lesions unless they are causing symptoms of compression or pain.

**ANSWER:** D

19. A 58-year-man has ACTH-independent hypercortisolism from a 5-cm left adrenal mass. He is initially seen in acute hepatic failure associated with corticosteroid psychosis and abdominal peritonitis. In this acute setting which of the following pharmacologic agents will assist in the management of this patient?

   A. Etomidate

   B. Mitotane

   C. Erythromycin

   D. Vincristine

   E. Intravenous vitamin A

*Ref.:* 1, 2

**COMMENTS:** **Etomidate**, a commonly used induction agent for general anesthesia, is a potent inhibitor of the 11-hydroxylase enzyme. It is the only inhibitor of steroid synthesis that can be given parenterally. It is the treatment of choice for control of **hypercortisolism** in critically ill patients unable to take oral medications. Its onset of action is very rapid (<1 minute), and its half-life is only 3 to 5 hours. The drug is administered as a continuous infusion, with nonhypnotic doses ranging between 0.2 and 0.6 mg/kg/h. The infusion is titrated according to the decline in serum cortisol levels. Once the cortisol levels are brought within a physiologic range, some patients may require hydrocortisone supplementation to avoid the development of adrenal insufficiency. **Mitotane**, a multiple enzyme inhibitor of cortisol, is a derivative of the insecticide DDT (dichlorodiphenyltrichloroethane). Its onset of action takes several days to achieve, and its dose must be titrated slowly because of associated toxic side effects. It is available only in an oral formulation. For these three reasons, mitotane is not indicated in the acute treatment of critically ill patients with refractory hypercortisolism. The other drugs listed have no role in the management of hypercortisolism.

**ANSWER:** A

20. According to the most current recommendations, which size cutoff should be used to select patients with adrenal incidentalomas for surgery?

   A. 3 cm

   B. 4 cm

   C. 5 cm

   D. 6 cm

   E. 2 cm

*Ref.:* 3

**COMMENTS:** The 2002 NIH Consensus Conference suggests that surgical resection should be considered for any nonfunctional **incidentalomas** 6 cm or larger. It is estimated that lesions larger than 6 cm have a 25% risk of harboring a malignancy. Observation is appropriate for lesions 4 cm or smaller. The risk for malignancy in a lesion smaller than 4 cm is 2%. Management recommendations for lesions between 4 and 6 cm are controversial. In more current studies, evidence has started to emerge that a lower threshold of 4 cm is appropriate. With improved imaging and increased use of laparoscopy in adrenal surgery, current practice has shown that more benign tumors are being removed because of lowering of the size criteria.

**ANSWER:** D

21. What is the most likely diagnosis in a patient who has elevated free cortisol and plasma ACTH levels and both low- and high-dose dexamethasone administration fail to suppress cortisol production?

   A. Bilateral adrenal hyperplasia

   B. Pituitary tumor

   C. Adrenal adenoma

D. Ectopic ACTH-producing tumor

E. Exogenous corticosteroids

*Ref.:* 1, 2

**COMMENTS:** Failure to suppress cortisol production after the administration of high-dose dexamethasone concomitant with elevated plasma ACTH levels suggests that the hypothalamic-pituitary-adrenal axis is not intact. This scenario suggests the presence of an ectopic source of ACTH. **Ectopic adrenocorticortropic hormone**-producing tumors account for 10% to 15% of cases of Cushing syndrome. Thoracic tumors are more common than abdominal tumors as a cause of ectopic ACTH syndrome. Of those arising in the mediastinum, primary lung carcinoids are the most common. Following in frequency are small cell lung cancer and thymic tumors. In approximately 20% of patients the site of ACTH production is never found.

**ANSWER:** D

22. An increased risk for deep venous thrombosis has been associated with which of the following conditions?

A. Hyperaldosteronism

B. Pheochromocytoma

C. Primary adrenal insufficiency

D. Bilateral adrenal hyperplasia

E. Hypercortisolism

*Ref.:* 4

**COMMENTS:** There is a documented increased risk of 1.9% for deep venous thrombosis in patients with **Cushing syndrome** in the nonoperative setting. In postoperative Cushing patients, the risk for venous thromboembolism ranges between 0% and 5.6%. Chronic glucocorticoid excess produces a metabolic syndrome that is associated with increased morbidity and mortality. The elevated risk for venous thromboembolic disease is thought to in part be due to the increased prevalence of cardiovascular disease, glucose intolerance, and obesity. Some researchers have postulated that the **hypercortisolism** is associated with a hypercoagulable state independent of these associated risk factors.

**ANSWER:** E

23. Which of the following is not an associated feature of Cushing syndrome?

A. Dyslipidemia

B. Psychosis

C. Hyperkalemia

D. Nephrolithiasis

E. Facial plethora

*Ref.:* 1, 2

**COMMENTS:** Patients with **Cushing syndrome** can have a wide variety of symptoms. Classically, patients will have newly diagnosed or poorly controlled hypertension, glucose intolerance, and truncal obesity. Additional signs and symptoms include easy bruising, proximal muscle weakness, decreased libido, nephrolithiasis, and a static flushed facial appearance (facial plethora). Nephrolithiasis occurs in up to 50% of patients with Cushing syndrome.

The underlying pathogenesis is not yet clearly defined. There is evidence that patients with Cushing syndrome have elevated urinary uric acid secretion, which could contribute to increased stone formation. Hyperkalemia is not a feature of Cushing syndrome; in fact, *hypokalemia* is more likely to occur given the weak mineralocorticoid effect of cortisol.

**ANSWER:** C

24. Which of the following is not a clinical feature of pheochromocytoma?

A. Headache

B. Hypoglycemia

C. Anxiety

D. Pallor

E. Facial plethora

*Ref.:* 1, 2

**COMMENTS:** Pallor, headache, and a sense of impending doom are all relatively common symptoms of patients with **pheochromocytoma**. Hyperglycemia is also a relatively common feature in such patients. The insulin-producing islet cells of the pancreas are under inhibitory control by $\alpha_2$ receptors. Thus, with catecholamine excess, a relative hypoinsulinemia can develop and lead to hyperglycemia. Flushing, nausea, and fever can occur rarely.

**ANSWER:** B

25. A 22-year-old man with a history of multiple endocrine neoplasia type IIA (MEN-IIA) is found on biochemical surveillance to have elevated serum catecholamines. CT reveals a 1-cm left adrenal mass and right adrenal fullness but no discrete mass. What is not appropriate management of this patient?

A. Bilateral adrenalectomy

B. Left adrenalectomy with cortical-sparing right adrenalectomy

C. Left adrenalectomy

D. Bilateral cortical-sparing adrenalectomy

E. Observation

*Ref.:* 2

**COMMENTS:** Considerable controversy exists around the appropriate surgical management of **pheochromocytomas** in patients with MEN. If at initial evaluation only one side shows evidence of a mass and unilateral adrenalectomy is performed, the chance of a contralateral pheochromocytoma developing over an interval of 12 years is 52%. Patients with **multiple endocrine neoplasia type II** should not undergo prophylactic removal of the contralateral side if no mass or presence of pheochromocytoma is confirmed. When the laterality of the pheochromocytoma is at question and the patient's disease is relatively asymptomatic, observation in young patients has been the favored approach by some surgeons because nearly a fourth of patients will experience at least one episode of acute adrenal insufficiency requiring hospitalization. This is a special concern in young patients, in whom the reliability of taking medications regularly or adjusting for physiologic stressors is highly variable. Alternatively, surgeons have begun performing laparoscopic cortical-sparing procedures in these patients, in whom the success rate of avoiding exogenous steroid dependence is reported to be between 65% and 100%. Thus, in the patient described here, it would be appropriate to perform a left adrenalectomy, a left adrenalectomy with cortical-sparing removal of the right, or bilateral cortical-sparing adrenalectomy. **Adrenal vein sampling** in these patients preoperatively can be a useful adjunct to assess the prevalence of **bilateral pheochromocytomas** when imaging is not able to lateralize the side of active disease.

**ANSWER:** A

26. Which of the following biochemical tests for the work-up of pheochromocytomas has the highest sensitivity?

    A. Urinary norepinephrine

    B. Urinary vanillylmandelic acid

    C. Urinary total metanephrines

    D. Plasma free metanephrines and normetanephrine

    E. Urinary epinephrine

    *Ref.:* 1, 2

**COMMENTS:** Elevated plasma free **metanephrine** and **normetanephrine** levels have the highest sensitivity among all the tests listed. However, its specificity (risk for false-positive results) is lower than that of the others listed. The specificity of plasma free metanephrines can be improved by using a cutoff value of at least four times the upper limit of normal. Table 18-2 illustrates the specificity of the other biochemical tests performed for the evaluation of **pheochromocytoma**.

**TABLE 18-2  Biochemical Tests for Pheochromocytoma**

| Test | Sensitivity (%) | Specificity (%) |
| --- | --- | --- |
| Plasma free metanephrines and normetanephrines | 99 | 85-89 |
| Urinary total metanephrines | 71-77 | 93-99 |
| Urinary epinephrine | 29 | 99 |
| Urinary norepinephrine | 50 | 99 |
| Urinary dopamine | 8 | 100 |
| Urinary vanillylmandelic acid | 64 | 95 |

**ANSWER:** D

27. A 44-year-old man is due to undergo laparoscopic adrenalectomy for pheochromocytoma. Which of the following agents should not be given as the initial or only medication to help achieve appropriate preoperative adrenoreceptor blockade?

    A. Phenoxybenzamine

    B. Amlodipine

    C. Prazosin

    D. Atenolol

    E. Metyrosine

    *Ref.:* 1, 2

**COMMENTS:** Preoperative **catecholamine receptor blockade** is done to reduce the incidence and magnitude of intraoperative fluctuations in blood pressure and the development of arrhythmias.

A β-**blocker** such as atenolol should never be administered before the use of an α-blocker because β-blockade can cause severe vasoconstriction and hypertension from inhibition of the vasodilator action of epinephrine. **Prazosin** and **phenoxybenzamine** are both α-blockers and have been used routinely for preoperative α-blockade in patients with pheochromocytoma. Infrequently, calcium channel blockers can be used as a substitute or as an adjunct to an α-blocker. The benefit of these agents is that coronary vasospasm is reduced and, when given in conjunction with an α-blocker, they can reduce the dosage of α-blocker needed. **Metyrosine** is an inhibitor of catecholamine synthesis that is also not commonly used in the preparation of patients with pheochromocytoma for surgery. The main limitations of metyrosine are its lack of widespread availability and patient tolerance of associated side effects.

**ANSWER:** D

28. The patient in Question 27 demonstrates signs of confusion and complains of sweating and headache several hours following his operation. His blood pressure is 130/65 mm Hg, his heart rate is 100 beats/min, and his respiratory rate is 12 breaths/min. What is the most likely cause of his symptoms?

    A. Dehydration

    B. Postoperative bleeding

    C. Hypoglycemia

    D. Narcotic overdose

    E. Incomplete removal of the pheochromocytoma

    *Ref.:* 1, 2

**COMMENTS:** In the postoperative setting, patients with **pheochromocytoma** should be monitored closely for signs or symptoms associated with hypoglycemia. Profound hypoglycemia can develop in these patients as a result of the rebound **hyperinsulinemia** that occurs with removal of the inhibitory catecholamine effect. Liver glycogen stores may be severely depleted in these patients because catecholamines promote glycogen breakdown. Thus, the patient's ability to respond acutely to the hypoglycemia is impaired. It is unpredictable in which patients hypoglycemia will develop, so those with pheochromocytoma are usually administered a prophylactic dextrose infusion postoperatively.

**ANSWER:** C

**REFERENCES**

1. Lal G, Clark OH: Thyroid, parathyroid and adrenal. In Brunicardi FC, Andersen DK, Billiar TR, et al, editors: *Schwartz's principles of surgery,* ed 9, New York, 2010, McGraw-Hill.
2. Duh QY, Yeh MW: The adrenal glands. In Townsend CM, Beauchamp RD, Evers BM, et al, editors: *Sabiston textbook of surgery: the biological basis of modern surgical practice,* ed 18, Philadelphia, 2008, WB Saunders.
3. NIH state-of-the-science statement on management of the clinically inapparent adrenal mass ("incidentaloma"), *NIH Consens State Sci Statements* 19:1–25, 2002.
4. Van Zaane B, Nur E, Squizzato A, et al: Hypercoagulable state in Cushing's syndrome: a systematic review, *J Clin Endorinol Metab* 94:2743–2750, 2009.

# ALIMENTARY TRACT

# Esophagus

*Minh B. Luu, M.D., F.A.C.S., and Keith W. Millikan, M.D., F.A.C.S.*

1. Which of the following is true regarding the anatomy of the esophagus?

    A. The narrowest point of the esophagus is at the level of the bronchoaortic constriction.

    B. The Meissner plexus is located in the submucosa.

    C. The Auerbach plexus is located between the longitudinal muscle and the adventitia.

    D. The serosa is the strongest layer of the esophagus.

    E. The outer longitudinal layer is an extension of the cricopharyngeus muscle.

    ***Ref.:*** 1

**COMMENTS:** The esophagus is a two-layered muscular tube approximately 25 to 30 cm in length. The esophagus is unique from other parts of the alimentary tract in its lack of a serosal layer. The inner circular muscle is an extension of the cricopharyngeus muscle. Two nerve plexuses, the Meissner and Auerbach plexuses, are found in the submucosa and between the muscle layers of the esophagus, respectively. They are the intrinsic autonomic nerve system of the esophagus responsible for peristalsis. Three distinct anatomic constrictions of the esophagus occur at the level of the cricopharyngeal muscle (approximately 14 mm), left mainstem bronchus (15 to 17 mm), and the diaphragmatic hiatus (16 to 19 mm), in order of increasing diameter.

**A N S W E R :**  B

2. Which of the following is true of the esophageal sphincters?

    A. The upper esophageal sphincter (UES) is mainly composed of the inferior constrictor muscle.

    B. The mean resting pressure of the UES is approximately 20 to 30 mm Hg.

    C. The lower esophageal sphincter (LES) is approximately 2 to 5 cm in length.

    D. The LES can be identified by an area of hypertrophic muscle.

    E. LES resting pressure is between 6 and 26 mm Hg and can be overcome by normal peristalsis.

    ***Ref.:*** 1, 2

**COMMENTS:** The upper and lower **esophageal sphincters** are high-pressure zones rather than actual anatomic landmarks. The cricopharyngeus muscle is thought to be the main contributor to the upper high-pressure zone. On swallowing, UES pressure can reach 90 mm Hg and return to an average resting pressure of 60 mm Hg. The **lower esophageal sphincter** is characterized by a resting pressure zone of approximately 6 to 26 mm Hg that measures 2 to 5 cm in length. Vagal-mediated relaxation of the LES occurs during normal food transit. Gastrin and motilin increase LES pressure, whereas cholecystokinin and secretin decrease LES pressure.

**A N S W E R :**  C

3. Which of the following is not true regarding esophageal motility?

    A. Primary waveforms are initiated after swallowing and are peristaltic along the length of the esophagus.

    B. Primary waveforms can generate pressures from 40 to 80 mm Hg.

    C. Secondary waveforms are initiated by voluntary mechanisms and are peristaltic.

    D. Tertiary waveforms are nonprogressive and nonperistaltic.

    E. Tertiary waveforms represent uncoordinated contractions of smooth muscle and are responsible for esophageal spasm.

    ***Ref.:*** 1, 2

**COMMENTS:** There are three types of **esophageal contractions**: primary, secondary, and tertiary. Primary waveforms are propulsive, are initiated after swallowing, travel the entire length of the esophagus, and generate pressures of 40 to 80 mm Hg (Figure 19-1). Secondary waves are also propulsive but are initiated by the presence of food rather than voluntary swallowing. Tertiary waveforms are uncoordinated contractions that are nonperistaltic.

**A N S W E R :**  C

4. A healthy 45-year-old woman is seen with a 6-month history of worsening heartburn, regurgitation, and dysphagia. Over-the-counter antacids have resulted in mild improvement in her symptoms. Which of the following is least likely to contribute to her symptoms?

    A. Presence of a hiatal hernia

    B. Cigarette smoking and alcohol consumption

    C. High-protein diet

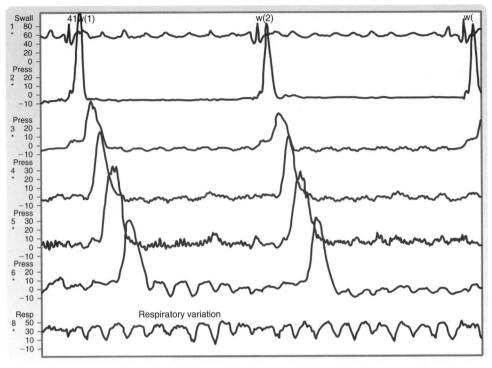

**Figure 19-1.** Normal esophageal peristalsis. *(From Bremner CG, DeMeester TR, Bremner RM, et al:* Esophageal motility testing made easy, *St. Louis, 2001, Quality Medical Publishing, p 35.)*

D. Obesity

E. Abnormal peristalsis

*Ref.:* 3, 4

**COMMENTS:** Reflux of gastric contents into the esophagus occurs once per hour in normal individuals without symptoms or signs of esophageal damage. **Gastroesophageal reflux disease** (GERD) is an imbalance of this normal physiology because of a defect in either the antireflux mechanism or esophageal protection. The presence of a hiatal hernia, obesity, consumption of alcohol, and tobacco smoking are associated with GERD. A high-protein diet is thought to increase LES pressure, thus decreasing the chance of GERD. After heartburn (80%), the most common symptom in a patient with GERD is regurgitation (54%). Abdominal pain, coughing, and dysphagia are present in less than 30% of patients. Wheezing is an atypical manifestation that occurs in less than 10% of patients with GERD.

**ANSWER:**  C

5. The patient from Question 4 consents to a laparoscopic Nissen fundoplication. Which of the following is the least important when performing a Nissen fundoplication for reflux disease?

A. Use of pledgets to prevent suture tears

B. Lengthening the intra-abdominal esophagus

C. Division of the short gastric vessels

D. Hiatal dissection and closure

E. Short and floppy fundoplication around the esophagus with a bougie

*Ref.:* 3

**COMMENTS:** The principles of **antireflux surgery** (ARS) that have been studied and accepted are hiatal dissection and closure, lengthening of the intra-abdominal esophagus, division of the short gastric vessels, creation of a short (2 cm) and floppy fundoplication, and the use of a bougie. Common techniques often used by many surgeons but not well established are fixation of wrap, use of pledgets, bougie size, and number of sutures used.

**ANSWER:**  A

6. Which of the following findings is a contraindication to ARS?

A. Presence of severe esophagitis on endoscopy

B. A DeMeester score of 55

C. Type III hiatal hernia seen on an esophagogram

D. Barrett esophagus with high-grade dysplasia

E. A shortened esophagus

*Ref.:* 2, 3

**COMMENTS:** The indications for **antireflux surgery** are severe esophageal injury, incomplete resolution of symptoms with medical therapy, patient preference against long-term pharmacologic therapy, or complications from a hiatal hernia. The success of ARS depends on the accuracy of diagnosing GERD, which can be enhanced by monitoring pH. The DeMeester score is used to assess the degree of abnormality (>14) of the pH study. The presence of a short esophagus requires a lengthening procedure such as a Collis gastroplasty in addition to fundoplication, but it is not a contraindication to ARS. The presence of high-grade dysplasia within a Barrett esophagus requires resection and is a contraindication to ARS.

**ANSWER:**  D

**7.** Seven years after her initial ARS, a patient undergoes a reoperation for recurrence of symptoms. During the reoperation, what is the most likely finding?

   A. Disrupted wrap

   B. Loose wrap

   C. Herniated wrap

   D. Slipped wrap

   E. Stricture

*Ref.:* 3, 5

**COMMENTS:** The long-term success rate of ARS approaches 90% with approximately a 1% per year failure rate. The most common operative finding on repeated **fundoplication** is a herniated fundoplication (33%) above the diaphragm, followed by a disrupted wrap (18%), a tight wrap (13%), and a slipped wrap (10%) onto the body of the stomach.

**A N S W E R :**   C

**8.** Which of the following endoluminal options for the treatment of GERD is no longer available?

   A. NDO full-thickness plicator

   B. Enteryx injection

   C. Bard Endocinch

   D. Stretta

   E. Esophyx

*Ref.:* 6-9

**COMMENTS:** The use of endoscopic techniques to treat esophageal reflux disease is an emerging field. The initial enthusiasm for an endoscopic method to augment the LES by suturing (NDO, Endocinch, **Esophyx**), radiofrequency energy (Stretta), or injection of a polymer (Enteryx) have been hampered by low success rates and lack of durability. Two reviews of the early experience with endoluminal therapy for GERD concluded that these procedures are safe and feasible but lack long-term durability. A recent report on the use of Esophyx showed that 82% of patients were not taking proton pump inhibitors, and 63% of patients had a normal pH study after 12 months. Following a death because of injection of polymer into the aorta, Enteryx was recalled by Boston Scientific in 2005.

**A N S W E R :**   B

**9.** Which of the following is not true of hiatal hernias and hernia repair?

   A. The hernia sac is usually excised.

   B. The use of mesh is associated with a lower recurrence rate than primary cruroplasty.

   C. Patients may initially be found to have iron-deficiency anemia.

   D. The gastroesophageal (GE) junction is above the diaphragm in type II hiatal hernias.

   E. An antireflux procedure is usually added to the hernia repair after extensive hiatal dissection.

*Ref.:* 3, 10

**COMMENTS:** A type II or **paraesophageal hernia**, in which the GE junction is below the diaphragm with the fundus of the stomach herniated into the chest, is the least common of the four types of hiatal hernia. Type I, also called a sliding hiatal hernia, is the most common hiatal hernia, and the GE junction is herniated into the chest. Type III is a combination of types I and II and involves herniation of the gastric fundus and body into the chest. Though not widely accepted, **type IV hiatal hernia** describes conditions in which the entire stomach and other intra-abdominal organs (e.g., colon, spleen) are herniated into the chest. Hiatal hernias are often the cause of anemia that resolves after surgical repair. The principles of hiatal hernia repair are excision of the hernia sac, lengthening of the intra-abdominal esophagus, primary cruroplasty with mesh reinforcement for defects larger than 5 cm, and the addition of a fundoplication or gastropexy.

**A N S W E R :**   D

**10.** A 55-year-old man is evaluated for dysphagia and chest pain. A barium esophagogram shows a 3-cm smooth filling defect in the distal end of the esophagus. Which of the following is true of his condition?

   A. Cystic transformation or central necrosis is often associated with these lesions.

   B. Patients often have hematemesis or chronic anemia because of ulceration.

   C. Endoscopic ultrasound (EUS) will show a hypoechoic mass in the submucosa.

   D. Endoscopic biopsy should be performed to rule out malignancy.

   E. Esophagectomy is recommended for lesions larger than 2 cm.

*Ref.:* 1

**COMMENTS:** Benign tumors of the esophagus are rare and represent less than 1% of esophageal neoplasms. **Leiomyomas** account for 60% of these lesions and are often found in the distal two thirds of the esophagus. Most of these tumors are asymptomatic. Pain and dysphagia are the most common complaints. They have a characteristic smooth filling defect on contrast-enhanced study and are described as a hypoechoic mass within the submucosa or muscularis propria on EUS. Recently, they have been classified as a gastrointestinal stromal tumor (GIST). Most of these tumors occur from mutations of the c-*KIT* oncogene. Leiomyomas are removed by enucleation, and biopsy should be avoided because of the increased risk for perforation.

**A N S W E R :**   C

**11.** Which of the following most likely contributes to GERD?

   A. Intra-abdominal LES length of 3 cm

   B. LES resting pressure of 12 mm Hg

   C. Thirty percent tertiary waveforms

   D. Total LES length of 5 cm

   E. Attachment of the phrenoesophageal ligament 4 cm above the GE junction

*Ref.:* 1-3, 10

**COMMENTS:** Factors that contribute to failure of the intrinsic antireflux mechanism are intra-abdominal **lower esophageal**

**TABLE 19-1  Manometric Features of Primary and Nonspecific Esophageal Motility Disorders**

| | Normal | Achalasia | Vigorous Achalasia | Hypertensive LES | Diffuse Esophageal Spasm | Nutcracker Esophagus | Ineffective Esophageal Motility | Nonspecific Esophageal Motility Disorder |
|---|---|---|---|---|---|---|---|---|
| Symptoms | None | Dysphagia Chest pressure Regurgitation | Dysphagia Chest pain | Dysphagia | Chest pain Dysphagia | Dysphagia Chest pain | Dysphagia Heartburn Chest pain | Dysphagia Chest pain |
| Esophagography | Normal | Bird's beak Dilated esophagus | Abnormal | Distal obstruction | Corkscrew esophagus | Normal progressive contractions | Slow transit Incomplete emptying | Slow transit Incomplete emptying |
| Endoscopy | Normal | Patulous esophagus | Normal | Normal | Hyperperistalsis | Hyperperistalsis | Nonspecific | Nonspecific |
| LES pressure | 15-25 mm Hg | Hypertensive (>26 mm Hg) | Normal or hypertensive | Hypertensive (>26 mm Hg) | Normal or slightly elevated | Normal | Normal or low | Normal |
| LES relaxation | Follows swallowing | Incomplete Residual pressure (<5 mm Hg) | Partial or absent | Normal | Normal | Normal | Normal | Incomplete (>90%) Residual pressure (>5 mm Hg) |
| Amplitude pressure | 50-120 mm Hg | Decreased (<40 mm Hg) | Normal | Normal | Normal | Hypertensive (>180 mm Hg) (>400 mm Hg) | Decreased (<30 mm Hg) | Decreased (<35 mm Hg) |
| Contraction waves | Progressive | Simultaneous Mirrored Pressurized | Simultaneous Repetitive | Normal | Simultaneous Repetitive | Long duration (>6 s) | Nontransmitted (>30%) | Nontransmitted (>20%) Triple-peaked, retrograde Prolonged (>6 s) |
| Peristalsis | Normal | None | None | Normal | None | Hypertensive peristalsis | Abnormal | Abnormal |

LES, Lower esophageal sphincter.

sphincter length less than 1 cm, LES resting pressure less than 6 mm Hg, the presence of esophageal dysmotility, LES total length less than 2 cm, and a low attachment of the phrenoesophageal ligament.

**ANSWER:  C**

12. A 35-year-old woman has complaints of dysphagia, regurgitation, and weight loss. Esophagography shows narrowing of the distal end of the esophagus, and manometry studies show significant tertiary waveforms. The LES has high residual pressure on swallowing. Which of the following has not been implicated as a possible cause of her disease?

A. *Helicobacter pylori* infection

B. Severe emotional stress

C. A parasitic infection

D. Drastic weight reduction

E. Degeneration of the Auerbach plexus

*Ref.:* 1, 11

**COMMENTS: Achalasia** is the most common motility disorder of the esophagus, and patients classically have dysphagia, regurgitation, and weight loss. The cause of achalasia is idiopathic; however, severe emotional stress, *Trypanosoma cruzi* infection causing destruction of the myenteric Auerbach plexus, and drastic weight loss have been implicated. No association between achalasia and *H. pylori* infection has been described.

**ANSWER:  A**

13. Which of the following manometric findings is not consistent with her disease?

A. LES pressure of 40 mm Hg

B. LES pressure of 10 mm Hg with deglutition

C. Esophageal body pressure above baseline

D. Significant aperistalsis

E. High-amplitude waveforms

*Ref.:* 1, 2, 11

**COMMENTS: Manometry** is the "gold standard" for the diagnosis of **achalasia** (Table 19-1). In typical achalasia, LES pressure is usually above 35 mm Hg and, more importantly, will fail to relax below 5 mm Hg with deglutition. Incomplete air evacuation will pressurize the esophagus and cause esophageal body pressures to be above baseline (Figure 19-2). Low-amplitude aperistaltic waveforms are often seen.

**ANSWER:  E**

14. A patient arrives at the emergency department 8 hours after balloon dilation of her esophagus with complaints of dysphagia and chest pain. She was found to be febrile, tachycardic, and normotensive. Esophagography showed "bird's beak" narrowing and a leak at the distal end of the esophagus with contrast material in the left side of the chest. After fluid resuscitation and antibiotics, which of the following is the most appropriate management?

A. Nasogastric tube decompression and observation

B. Endoscopic evaluation of the injury and stenting

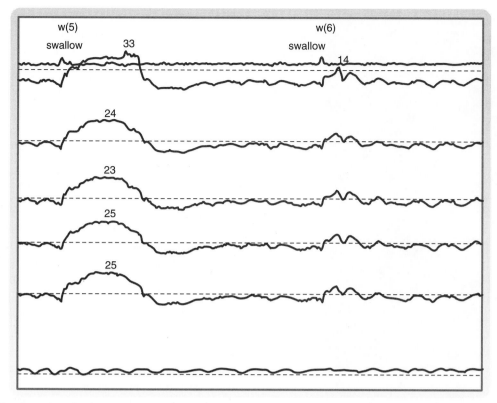

**Figure 19-2.** Esophageal motility in a patient with achalasia. *(From Bremner CG, DeMeester TR, Bremner RM, et al: Esophageal motility testing made easy, St. Louis, 2001, Quality Medical Publishing, p 75.)*

C. Left thoracotomy, primary repair, myotomy, and drain placement

D. Laparotomy, primary repair, and gastrostomy tube placement

E. Laparotomy, esophagectomy, and cervical esophagogastrostomy

*Ref.:* 1, 12

**COMMENTS:** The rate of esophageal perforation after **endoscopic pneumatic dilation** is low (4%). Early diagnosis plus treatment of esophageal perforation is associated with improved survival. In stable patients with a contained perforation, there is a role for nonoperative management consisting of nothing by mouth and intravenous antibiotics. If the perforation is because of an underlying pathology that causes distal obstruction (e.g., achalasia, esophageal cancer, or stricture), the operative treatment must address the underlying disease. A **myotomy** should be performed in patients with achalasia and esophagectomy considered only in those with a sigmoid esophagus or megaesophagus.

**ANSWER:** C

15. Which of the following is a true diverticulum consisting of all layers of the esophageal wall?

A. Zenker

B. Parabronchial

C. Epiphrenic

D. Pharyngoesophageal

E. Meckel

*Ref.:* 1, 13

**COMMENTS:** A parabronchial diverticulum (midesophageal diverticulum of the esophagus) is a true diverticulum caused by traction on inflamed mediastinal nodes. Historically, the inflamed nodes were caused by tuberculosis but now are more often seen with *Histoplasmosis* infection. A **Zenker** (pharyngoesophageal) diverticulum and an **epiphrenic diverticulum** are false diverticula caused by a pulsion mechanism.

**ANSWER:** B

16. A 40-year-old woman complains of chest pain and dysphagia. Manometric studies show simultaneous multipeaked contractions of 140 mm Hg, lasting 4 to 5 seconds and normal LES relaxation. Which of the following is true of her disease?

A. Esophagography will show a "corkscrew esophagus."

B. It can be caused by infection with *Trypanosoma cruzi.*

C. It is the result of fibrous replacement of esophageal smooth muscle.

D. It is also known as "vigorous" achalasia.

E. Bougie dilation is the first-line treatment.

*Ref.:* 1, 2

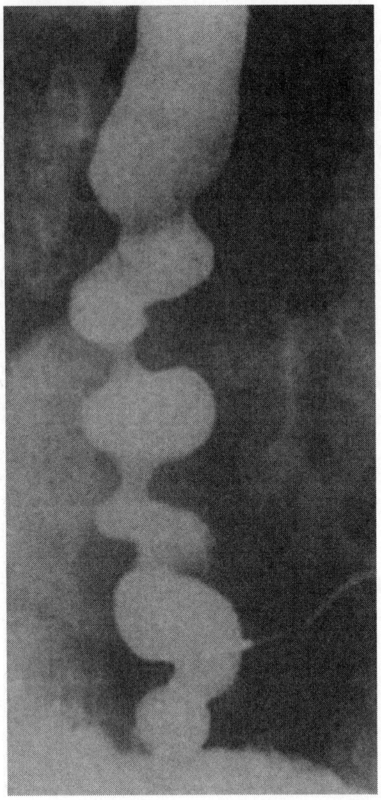

**Figure 19-3.** Barium esophagogram of diffuse esophageal spasm. *(Modified from Peters JH, DeMeester TR: Esophagus and diaphragmatic hernia. In Schwartz SI, Shires TG, Spencer FC, editors:* Principles of surgery, *ed 7, New York, 1999, McGraw-Hill, p 1129.)*

**COMMENTS: Diffuse esophageal spasm** is a poorly understood motility disorder of the esophagus. Chest pain and dysphagia are often present. The diagnosis is made by esophagography demonstrating a classic picture of a corkscrew esophagus (Figure 19-3). **Manometry** will show simultaneous multipeaked contractions similar to those seen in achalasia; however, the LES will have normal receptive relaxation. A variant of achalasia in which amplitude pressure is normal or elevated is also known as vigorous achalasia. Pharmacotherapy (nitrates, calcium channel blockers, phosphodiesterase inhibitors) aimed at smooth muscle relaxation is the first-line treatment of diffuse esophageal spasm. Bougie or pneumatic dilations are used with variable results for severe dysphagia with documented LES hypertension. Surgery, which involves a long **esophagomyotomy** from the level of the aortic arch to the LES, is reserved for patients who fail pharmacologic and endoscopic therapies.

**ANSWER:** A

17. A 65-year-old man has progressive dysphagia, halitosis, and regurgitation of undigested food. Esophagography shows a diverticulum at the level of the cricothyroid cartilage. Which of the following is not true of the disease?

　A. It is a false diverticulum.

　B. It is more commonly seen on the left side of the esophagus.

　C. It is the most common esophageal diverticulum.

　D. It is a traction diverticulum.

　E. It occurs in the Killian triangle.

*Ref.:* 1, 13

**COMMENTS:** See Question 18.

**ANSWER:** D

18. Which of the following is true of treatment options for the patient from Question 17?

　A. Observation is the first-line treatment in symptomatic patients.

　B. For diverticula 3 cm or smaller, surgical repair is superior to endoscopic repair in eliminating symptoms.

　C. For diverticula larger than 3 cm, endoscopic repair is superior to surgical repair in eliminating symptoms.

　D. Myotomy alone is usually sufficient to treat diverticula larger than 5 cm.

　E. Length of hospital stay and inanition are equivalent in endoscopic and surgical repairs.

*Ref.:* 1, 13

**COMMENTS:** A **Zenker diverticulum** can be treated with surgical or endoscopic approaches. Regardless of the method used, a myotomy of the cricopharyngeus muscle must be performed. Because of the difficulty of completing the **myotomy** in cases in which the diverticula are 3 cm or smaller, surgical repair is superior to endoscopic repair of these smaller lesions. For diverticula larger than 3 cm, the success rates are similar; however, recovery is shorter with the endoscopic method. A Zenker diverticulum is the most common diverticulum of the esophagus in older patients. It is a false diverticulum, with the mucosa and submucosa herniating between the oblique muscle fibers of the thyropharyngeus and cricopharyngeus muscles (Killian triangle).

**ANSWER:** B

19. A 65-year-old man with a 10-year history of heartburn undergoes endoscopy with distal esophageal biopsy, which showed intestinal columnar metaplasia. Which of the following is true of his condition?

　A. The metaplastic cells are more prone to reflux injury than the squamous epithelium.

　B. The condition is found in 50% of patients with GERD.

　C. *H. pylori* is associated with the condition.

　D. More than 70% of cases are found in men in their fifth and sixth decades.

　E. The condition is associated with a fivefold increase in risk for adenocarcinoma.

*Ref.:* 1

**COMMENTS:** Esophageal mucosal injuries result from reflux of gastric juice that may contain bile salts from the duodenum. Within a pH range of 2 to 6.5, bile salts are soluble and nonionized; they are therefore better absorbed by esophageal mucosa cells and cause the greatest cell damage. **Barrett esophagus** is a condition in which intestinal columnar epithelium replaces the esophageal squamous epithelium as a result of inflammation secondary to chronic reflux. The metaplastic cells are more resistant to injury from reflux but are more prone to malignant transformation. Barrett esophagus is found in 10% of patients with GERD, and more than 70% of cases are found in men aged 55 to 63 years. Patients with Barrett esophagus have a 40-fold increased risk for esophageal carcinoma.

**ANSWER:** D

20. The biopsy result of the patient in Question 19 also showed low-grade dysplasia. Which of the following is not an accepted treatment option?

A. Surveillance endoscopy

B. ARS

C. Radiofrequency ablation

D. Endoscopic mucosal resection

E. Esophageal resection

*Ref.:* 1

**COMMENTS: Endoscopic surveillance** is recommended for all patients with Barrett esophagus. In patients with **low-grade dysplasia**, endoscopy is recommended at 6-month intervals for the first year and yearly thereafter. Surveillance can be extended to every 2 to 4 years for individuals in whom there is no evidence of dysplasia on two consecutive yearly examinations. Antireflux, **ablative therapy** and mucosal resection are accepted options. Esophageal resection is recommended for patients in whom high-grade dysplasia is found. Ablative therapy for Barrett esophagus has been proposed for patients with high-grade dysplasia. Photodynamic therapy is the most common method used. Complications include persistent metaplasia (50%), as well as esophageal strictures (35%). Endoscopic mucosal resection has been used for the treatment of Barrett esophagus with low-grade dysplasia or as a tool for biopsy of the focus of Barrett esophagus with high-grade dysplasia. It is not recommended for long-segment **Barrett esophagus**.

**ANSWER:** E

21. An otherwise healthy 40-year-old man seeks treatment in the emergency department because of hematemesis after a night of binge drinking and retching. Which of the following is true of his condition?

A. It is caused by a pulsion diverticulum.

B. Endoscopy should not be performed because of the increased risk for perforation.

C. The bleeding is from an arterial source.

D. Surgical resection is often required.

E. *H. pylori* infection is a known risk factor.

*Ref.:* 14

**COMMENTS: Mallory-Weiss** tears are linear tears in the esophagogastric mucosa that cause bleeding in patients with repeated emesis. The diagnosis is made by endoscopy, and most bleeding stops spontaneously. Because the source of the bleeding is arterial, pressure tamponade is not helpful and may lead to perforation of the esophagus. For refractory bleeding, endoscopic injection or cautery can be used, but definitive treatment requires a gastrotomy and suture ligation.

**ANSWER:** C

22. A 60-year-old man has GERD and episodic dysphagia. An upper gastrointestinal contrast-enhanced study shows a type I hiatal hernia and thin bandlike narrowing of the distal end of the esophagus. Which of the following is true of his condition?

A. Oral dilation is the treatment of choice.

B. It is the result of hypertrophy of the circular muscle layer.

C. Endoscopic mucosal resection is recommended.

D. There is squamous mucosa above and below the narrowing.

E. Surgical resection is indicated.

*Ref.:* 1

**COMMENTS: Schatzki rings** are concentric constrictions of the distal end of the esophagus (Figure 19-4) occurring at the squamocolumnar junction; as a result, there is esophageal mucosa above and gastric mucosa below. The rings consist of muscularis mucosa, connective tissue, and submucosal fibrosis. Treatment involves oral dilation, which can provide relief for up to 18 months. Excision of the rings should be avoided, because the esophageal strictures that result from resection are much more difficult to manage.

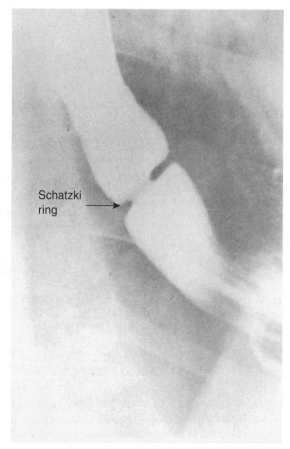

**Figure 19-4.** Barium esophagogram of a Schatzki ring. (*Modified from Wilkins EW Jr: Rings and webs. In Pearson FG, Cooper JD, Deslauriers J, et al, editors: Esophageal surgery, ed 2, New York, 2002, Churchill Livingstone, p 298.*)

**ANSWER:** A

23. With regard to squamous cell carcinoma of the esophagus, which of the following is not true?

 A. It affects mainly African-American men.

 B. Worldwide, it is the most common type of esophageal cancer.

 C. The male-to-female ratio is approximately 15 : 1.

 D. Alcohol and tobacco in combination are strong risk factors.

 E. Food additives such as nitrosamines have been implicated.

*Ref.:* 1, 15

COMMENTS: **Esophageal cancer** is the sixth most common malignancy and has an incidence of 20 per 100,000 in the United States. Worldwide, squamous cell carcinoma is the most common type; however, in the United States, adenocarcinoma accounts for up to 70% of patients with esophageal cancer. The male-to-female ratio is 3 : 1 for squamous cell carcinoma and 15 : 1 for adenocarcinoma. In addition, squamous cell carcinoma affects African-American men, whereas adenocarcinoma mainly affects white men. Alcohol and tobacco smoking increase the risk for esophageal cancer fivefold each and 25-fold to 100-fold in combination. Additives in pickled and smoked foods such as nitrosamines have been implicated in the risk for cancer.

ANSWER: C

24. A 75-year-old white man with a history of alcohol abuse, 40-pack-year tobacco use, and long-standing GERD controlled by antacids is evaluated for dysphagia and weight loss. Esophagography shows an apple core lesion at the distal end of the esophagus. Which of the following is true regarding further work-up?

 A. Endoscopic biopsy should be avoided because of the risk for perforation.

 B. Computed tomography (CT) is excellent for tumor staging.

 C. Positron emission tomography (PET) is an excellent tool for staging and can be used as a single diagnostic modality.

 D. Magnetic resonance imaging (MRI) is a poor imaging modality for liver metastasis.

 E. EUS is more sensitive than CT for evaluating the celiac lymph nodes.

*Ref.:* 1, 15

COMMENTS: Many imaging modalities are available for the characterization of esophageal cancers. Barium esophagography is a good first test for patients with dysphagia and a history suspicious for cancer. Although CT is accurate for M staging, it is only 57% accurate for T staging. PET is an excellent tool that can be used to evaluate N and M staging but should not be used as a single diagnostic modality. MRI is excellent for detecting metastatic and T4 lesions. **Endoscopic ultrasound** is the most important diagnostic tool in esophageal cancer staging. Tissue samples can be obtained from lymph nodes, as well as from the primary lesion. EUS is more sensitive and specific than CT in evaluating the celiac lymph nodes.

ANSWER: E

25. The patient in Question 24 underwent EUS that showed a T2 lesion. The biopsy specimen is positive for adenocarcinoma of the esophagus. His chance of having a positive lymph node is:

 A. 20%

 B. 40%

 C. 60%

 D. 80%

 E. 100%

*Ref.:* 1

COMMENTS: The risk of lymph node involvement is directly proportional to tumor depth or **T stage**. The incidence of positive lymph nodes is 18% for T1a intramucosa, 55% for T1b submucosa, 60% for T2 not beyond the muscularis propria, 80% for T3 with involvement of paraesophageal tissue but not adjacent structures, and 100% for T4 with involvement of adjacent structures.

ANSWER: C

26. The patient in Question 24 undergoes neoadjuvant chemoradiation therapy. Which of the following is true regarding multimodality therapy?

 A. A complete histologic response occurs in approximately 25% of patients.

 B. Squamous cell carcinoma and adenocarcinoma cell types have similar response rates to radiation therapy.

 C. Survival beyond 5 years has not been reported in patients with stage IV disease.

 D. Cisplatin-based combination therapy is no longer used because of the high rate of neuropathy.

 E. Radiation therapy alone is an option for stage I disease.

*Ref.:* 1, 16

COMMENTS: Treatment of esophageal cancer is complex, and multiple modalities are often necessary. The decision regarding treatment options depends on whether the intent is curative or palliative. **Squamous cell carcinoma** is much more radioresponsive than adenocarcinoma, although with the latter, a complete histologic response is seen in approximately 25% of patients undergoing neoadjuvant chemoradiation therapy. Neoadjuvant radiation therapy is limited to 4500 cGy to avoid the surgical morbidity associated with high-dose radiation. Cisplatin in combination with 5-fluorouracil and epirubicin is an established chemotherapy regimen, but the use of mitomycin C, etoposide, and paclitaxel as a third agent is gaining favor. Stage I disease is best treated with curative surgical resection.

ANSWER: A

27. The patient in Question 24 undergoes transhiatal esophagectomy. Which of the following is true of the procedure?

 A. Three incisions are required: cervical, thoracic, and abdominal.

 B. A gastric conduit is preferred, and the blood supply is based on the right gastroepiploic artery.

C. More lymph nodes can be harvested than with en bloc esophagectomy.

D. A substernal route of the replacement conduit is preferred because of the shorter route and improved function.

E. Cervical anastomotic leak rates are lower than thoracic leak rates but carry the same morbidity.

*Ref.:* 1, 15, 17, 18

**COMMENTS: Transhiatal esophagectomy** was first described by Wolfgang Denk in 1913 and popularized by Orringer in the 1980s. Incisions in the left side of the neck and abdomen are used and a thoracotomy is avoided. The esophagus is bluntly dissected, and the tubularized stomach is pulled through the posterior mediastinum to create a cervical esophagogastric anastomosis. The blood supply to the gastric conduit is based on the right gastroepiploic artery. A gastric pull-up procedure, based on the right gastroepiploic artery, in the posterior mediastinal position has the best functional result. Alternative routes (subcutaneous, substernal, or right pleural space) or conduits (colon or jejunum) can be used but result in inferior function.

**ANSWER:** B

28. Which of the following is not true of palliative therapy for dysphagia associated with advanced esophageal cancer?

A. Photodynamic therapy can provide relief for up to 10 months.

B. Dilation and stent placement carry a 10% risk for perforation.

C. Chemotherapy provides excellent relief with minimal morbidity.

D. External beam radiation therapy is a good option for high-risk patients.

E. Endoscopic laser therapy provides immediate relief of symptoms with low morbidity and mortality.

*Ref.:* 1, 15, 16, 18

**COMMENTS:** The goal of **palliative care** is to relieve suffering and improve overall quality of life by reducing tumor burden and restoring nutritional access. Chemotherapy, radiation therapy, photodynamic therapy, laser treatment, stenting, and feeding tubes are options for palliation. Dysphagia is the most common initial symptom of patients with esophageal cancer, especially in those with advanced disease. **Endoscopic laser** fulguration with the neodymium : yttrium-aluminum-garnet (Nd : YAG) laser is 75% to 80% successful in treating dysphagia, but multiple treatments may be required. **Photodynamic therapy**, an alternative form of laser therapy, is also an excellent tool for palliation in patients suffering from dysphagia. A photosensitizing drug (porfimer [Photofrin]) is injected intravenously before treatment and is selectively taken up by neoplastic cells. Activation of Photofrin with red light at 630 nm releases singlet oxygen, which kills the host cell. Chemotherapy will treat systemic disease and reduce overall tumor burden but needs to be administered with radiation therapy to control local disease.

**ANSWER:** C

29. A 45-year-old man arrives at the emergency department after ingesting lye in a suicide attempt. Which of the following is true?

A. Injury to the esophagus is the result of coagulative necrosis.

B. Endoscopy should not be performed within the first 72 hours because of the risk for perforation.

C. The lye should be neutralized with milk or egg whites if the patient is seen within the first hour of ingestion.

D. Before reepithelialization, dilations should be performed to decrease the long-term stricture rate.

E. For a long-segment interposition graft, the colon is the preferred conduit.

*Ref.:* 1, 18, 19

**COMMENTS: Caustic injury** to the esophagus can be attributed to the ingestion of acidic or alkaline liquids. Alkaline substances (lye) produce liquefactive necrosis of tissue and can cause deep tissue penetration. If diagnosed within the first hour of ingestion, half-strength vinegar or citrus juice can be used to neutralize the ingested alkali. After careful examination of the oropharynx, airway, chest, and abdomen, endoscopy should be performed to grade the burn. Serial esophagograms should be performed to evaluate for stricture formation rather than waiting for symptoms of obstruction to develop. Early stent placement or bougie dilation is effective in preventing long-term strictures; however, dilation should be performed only after reepithelialization has been confirmed with endoscopy. For long-segment strictures requiring resection, colonic interposition is the preferred graft.

**ANSWER:** E

**REFERENCES**

1. Maish M: Esophagus. In Townsend CM, Beauchamp RD, Evers BM, et al, editors: *Textbook of surgery: the biological basis of modern surgical practice*, ed 18, Philadelphia, 2008, WB Saunders.
2. Bremner CG: Esophageal function tests. In Cameron JL, editor: *Current surgical therapy*, ed 9, Philadelphia, 2008, CV Mosby.
3. Oelschlager BK, Eubanks TR, Pellegrini CA: Hiatal hernia and gastroesophageal reflux disease. In Townsend CM, Beauchamp RD, Evers BM, et al, editors: *Sabiston textbook of surgery: the biological basis of modern surgical practice*, ed 18, Philadelphia, 2008, WB Saunders.
4. Chung DH, Evers BM: The digestive system. In O'Leary JP, editor: *The physiologic basis of surgery*, ed 3, Philadelphia, 2002, Lippincott Williams & Wilkins.
5. Carlson MA, Frantzides CT: Complications and results of laparoscopic antireflux procedures: a review of 10,489 cases, *J Am Coll Surg* 193:428–439, 2001.
6. Poulose BK, Richards WO: Endoluminal approaches to gastroesophageal reflux disease. In Cameron JL, editor: *Current surgical therapy*, ed 9, Philadelphia, 2008, CV Mosby.
7. Fry LC, Monkenmuller K, Malfertheiner P: Systematic review: endoluminal therapy for gastro-oesophageal reflux disease: evidence from clinical trials, *Eur J Gastroenterol Hepatol* 19:1125–1139, 2007.
8. Torquati A, Richards WO: Endoluminal GERD treatments: critical appraisal of current literature with evidence-based medicine instruments, *Surg Endosc* 21:697–706, 2007.
9. Cadiere GB, Rajan A, Germay O, et al: Endoluminal fundoplication by a transoral device for the treatment of GERD: a feasibility study, *Surg Endosc* 22:333–342, 2008.
10. Smith CD: Paraesophageal hiatal hernia. In Cameron JL, editor: *Current surgical therapy*, ed 9, Philadelphia, 2008, CV Mosby.

11. Williams VA, Molena D, Peters JH: Achalasia of the esophagus. In Cameron JL, editor: *Current surgical therapy*, ed 9, Philadelphia, 2008, CV Mosby.

12. DeMeester SR: Esophageal perforation. In Cameron JL, editor: *Current surgical therapy*, ed 9, Philadelphia, 2008, CV Mosby.

13. Cohen JI: Management of pharyngoesophageal (Zenker's) diverticula. In Cameron JL, editor: *Current surgical therapy*, ed 9, Philadelphia, 2008, CV Mosby.

14. Harbison SP, Dempsey DT: Mallory-Weiss syndrome. In Cameron JL, editor: *Current surgical therapy*, ed 9, Philadelphia, 2008, CV Mosby.

15. Peyre CG, DeMeester TR: Management of esophageal tumors. In Cameron JL, editor: *Current surgical therapy*, ed 9, Philadelphia, 2008, CV Mosby.

16. Gibson MK: Neoadjuvant and adjuvant therapy of esophageal cancer. In Cameron JL, editor: *Current surgical therapy*, ed 9, Philadelphia, 2008, CV Mosby.

17. Orringer MB: Transhiatal esophagectomy without thoracotomy for carcinoma of the thoracic esophagus, *Ann Surg* 200:282–288, 1984.

18. Jobe BA, Hunter JG, Peters JH: Esophagus and diaphragmatic hernia. In Brunicardi FC, Andersen DK, Billiar TR, et al, editors: *Schwartz's principles of surgery*, ed 9, New York, 2010, McGraw-Hill.

19. Fischer AC: Chemical esophageal injuries. In Cameron JL, editor: *Current surgical therapy*, ed 9, Philadelphia, 2008, CV Mosby.

# CHAPTER 20

# Stomach and Duodenum

*Kamran Idrees, M.D., and John D. Christein, M.D.*

1. Which of the following statements is true with regard to the arterial blood supply of the stomach?

   A. The left gastroepiploic artery commonly arises from the left gastric artery.

   B. Ligation of the left gastric artery can result in acute left-sided hepatic ischemia.

   C. The stomach is extremely susceptible to ischemia because of poor collateral circulation.

   D. The inferior phrenic and short gastric arteries provide significant blood supply to the body of the stomach.

   E. A replaced right hepatic artery may originate from the left gastric artery.

   *Ref.:* 1, 2

**COMMENTS:** The arterial blood supply of the stomach is derived primarily from the **celiac artery**. The **left gastric artery** comes off of the celiac artery and supplies the stomach along the lesser curvature. An aberrant/replaced **left hepatic artery** originates from the left gastric artery (15% to 24%) and can represent the only arterial blood supply to the left hepatic lobe. This aberrant/replaced left hepatic artery runs in the gastrohepatic ligament. The **right gastric artery** typically arises from the common hepatic artery distal to the gastroduodenal artery. The **right and left gastroepiploic arteries** usually originate from the gastroduodenal artery and splenic artery, respectively. The short gastric arteries arising from the splenic artery and inferior phrenic arteries also contribute significant blood volume to the proximal part of the stomach. The stomach is well protected from ischemia and can easily survive with ligation of three of four arteries because of its rich collateral circulation.

**ANSWER:** B

2. After esophagectomy, the arterial blood supply of a gastric conduit is primarily based on which of the following vessels?

   A. Left gastroepiploic artery

   B. Left gastric artery

   C. Right gastroepiploic artery

   D. Right gastric artery

   E. Inferior phrenic arteries

   *Ref.:* 1, 2

**COMMENTS:** During gastric mobilization for esophageal replacement after **esophagectomy**, the left gastric artery and short gastric (vasa brevia) arteries are routinely divided. The major arterial source for the **neoesophagus** (gastric conduit) is derived from the **right gastroepiploic artery**.

**ANSWER:** C

3. Choose the correct type of vagotomy with the appropriate level of vagal transection from the pairs listed below:

   A. Truncal vagotomy/criminal nerve of Grassi

   B. Highly selective vagotomy/anterior and posterior vagal trunks below the celiac and hepatic branches

   C. Selective vagotomy/anterior and posterior vagal trunks above the celiac and hepatic branches

   D. Parietal cell vagotomy/terminal branches of the nerve of Latarjet

   E. Highly selective vagotomy/hepatic branches

   *Ref.:* 1, 2

**COMMENTS:** In the chest, the vagal trunks are situated to the right and left of the esophagus. At the level of the cardia, the left vagal trunk is found anterior and the right vagal trunk is found posterior secondary to embryonic gastric rotation. The anterior vagal trunk divides into hepatic and anterior gastric (anterior nerve of Latarjet) branches. The posterior vagus divides into the posterior nerve of Latarjet and celiac branches. One of the proximal posterior branches of the posterior vagal trunk is known as the **criminal nerve of Grassi** and is identified as a possible cause of recurrent ulcers if left undivided during selective vagotomy. **Truncal vagotomy** is conventionally performed at or just above or below the diaphragmatic esophageal hiatus before it gives off **celiac and hepatic branches**. In contrast, **selective vagotomy** is performed distal to this location and spares the celiac and hepatic branches. **Highly selective vagotomy** (also known as **proximal gastric or parietal cell vagotomy**) divides individual **terminal branches of the nerve of Latarjet** in the fundus and corpus of the stomach but spares the vagal branches to the antrum and pylorus, which control gastric motility and emptying—thus obviating the need for a drainage procedure.

**ANSWER:** D

4. Which cell type is matched with the appropriate secretory product?

   A. Parietal cell/ghrelin

   B. Chief cell/pepsinogen

   C. G cell/intrinsic factor

D. Delta cell/gastrin

E. Endocrine cell/somatostatin

*Ref.:* 1, 2

**COMMENTS:** See Question 5.

**ANSWER: B**

5. Which cell type is matched with the correct primary anatomic location?

A. Parietal cell/gastric cardia

B. Chief cell/gastric cardia

C. G cell/gastric antrum

D. Delta cell/duodenum

E. Endocrine cell/gastric corpus and fundus

*Ref.:* 1, 2

**COMMENTS:** The gastric mucosa consists of surface columnar epithelial cells and glands containing various cell types. The mucosal cells vary in their anatomic location and secretory function. Parietal and chief cells are located predominantly in the gastric fundus and corpus. **Parietal cells** produce **hydrochloric acid** and **intrinsic factors**, whereas **chief cells** secrete **pepsinogen**. The **G cells** of the antrum are the primary source of **gastrin**. **Somatostatin** is synthesized and stored in **delta cells** located in the gastric corpus and antrum. Mucus is secreted by gastric surface epithelial cells, neck cells, and the Brunner gland. **Ghrelin**, produced by **endocrine cells** of the gastric body, probably plays a role in the neuroendocrine response to changes in nutritional status and may be used to help in the treatment or prevention of obesity, or both, in the future.

**ANSWER: C**

6. Acid secretion is stimulated by the following parietal cell receptors except:

A. Acetylcholine

B. Secretin

C. Histamine

D. Gastrin

E. All of the above

*Ref.:* 1, 2

**COMMENTS:** See Question 7.

**ANSWER: B**

7. The final common pathway of acid secretion by parietal cells involves which of the following?

A. Protein kinase

B. Increased intracellular $Ca^{2+}$

C. Hydrogen-potassium adenosine triphosphatase ($H^+,K^+$-ATPase)

D. Phosphorylase kinase

E. Adenylate cyclase

*Ref.:* 1, 2

**COMMENTS:** It is important to have knowledge of the cellular basis for parietal cell acid secretion to understand the pharmacologic control of acid. The **parietal cell** has three specific plasma membrane receptors that stimulate acid secretion: **acetylcholine**, **histamine**, and **gastrin** receptors. All three receptors activate the $H^+,K^+$-**ATPase** pump, which results in secretion of hydrogen ion for potassium. Acetylcholine- and gastrin-stimulated secretion depends on specific membrane phospholipases and increases **intracellular calcium levels**, with subsequent **phosphorylase kinase**–induced phosphorylation and $H^+,K^+$-ATPase activity. Histamine activates **adenylate cyclase**, which in turn leads to protein phosphorylation via **protein kinase** and $H^+,K^+$-ATPase activation. **Somatostatin**, **cholecystokinin**, and **secretin** inhibit acid secretion.

**ANSWER: C**

8. All of the following stimulate gastric acid secretion except:

A. Gastric distention

B. Duodenal gastrin

C. Acetylcholine

D. Intraluminal protein

E. Somatostatin

*Ref.:* 1, 2

**COMMENTS:** Gastric acid secretion is regulated in three phases: cephalic, gastric, and intestinal. The **cephalic phase** is primarily mediated by the vagus nerve. **Vagal stimulation** (**acetylcholine**) directly releases acid from the parietal cells, in addition to releasing gastrin from the antrum. The **gastric phase** is initiated by **gastric distention**, **intraluminal peptides**, and **amino acids** and results in the release of gastrin. The majority of gastrin is released in the antrum with a small amount being secreted from the duodenal mucosa. The **intestinal phase** of gastric secretion accounts for only 10% of the total acid volume. **Duodenal gastrin** and the hypothetical peptide hormone enterooxyntin have been postulated to mediate the intestinal phase of acid secretion. Luminal acidity releases **secretin** and **somatostatin**, which inhibit acid secretion.

**ANSWER: E**

9. Which intestinal hormone is matched with the correct function?

A. Secretin/acts as a universal "on" switch

B. Gastrin-releasing peptide/acts as a universal "off" switch

C. Somatostatin/stimulates intestinal secretion and motility

D. Motilin/acts as a universal "on" switch

E. Vasoactive intestinal peptide (VIP)/stimulates intestinal secretion and motility

*Ref.:* 1, 2

**COMMENTS:** Gastrointestinal (GI) hormones are secreted by endocrine cells that are widely distributed and localized to specific GI mucosa. These hormones regulate GI secretion, motility, and absorption in a complex fashion. **Secretin** is released by S cells located in the duodenum and jejunum. The primary function of secretin is to induce the release of water and bicarbonate from pancreatic ductal cells. Secretin also inhibits the release of gastrin, gastric acid secretion, and gastric motility. **Gastrin-releasing peptide** (also known as **bombesin**) is found throughout the GI tract. It acts as the universal "on" switch by stimulating all GI hormones (except secretin), as well as GI secretions and motility. **Somatostatin** is produced by delta cells located primarily in the pancreas and gastric antrum. Because of its wide inhibitory action, somatostatin is known as the universal "off" switch of the intestinal tract. It inhibits the release of all GI hormones along with the inhibition of enteric water, electrolyte secretion, and motility. **Motilin**, secreted by M cells in the duodenum and jejunum, stimulates upper GI motility. **Erythromycin** is thought to increase GI motility through the activation of motilin receptors. **Vasoactive intestinal peptide** is present throughout the length of the intestinal tract and the central nervous system. It is a potent stimulator of intestinal secretion. VIP is the chief culprit in the watery diarrhea, hypokalemia, and achlorhydria syndrome (WDHA) associated with pancreatic endocrine tumors (also known as Verner-Morrison syndrome or VIPoma).

**ANSWER:** E

10. Which hormone is matched with the correct diagnostic/therapeutic function?

A. Cholecystokinin/treatment of esophageal variceal bleeding

B. Somatostatin/relief of spasm of the sphincter of Oddi

C. Gastrin/measurement of maximal gastric acid secretion

D. Glucagon/provocative test for gastrinoma

E. Secretin/stimulation of gallbladder contraction

*Ref.:* 1, 2

**COMMENTS:** GI hormones or their analogues have been used clinically as diagnostic or therapeutic agents. **Cholecystokinin (CCK)** is used to **stimulate gallbladder contraction**. This is useful in identifying patients with **biliary dyskinesia** or acalculous cholecystitis with the help of CCK cholescintigraphy. **Pentagastrin**, a **gastrin analogue**, is used to measure gastric acid secretion. **Somatostatin** or its analogues are used in various conditions as a result of their universal inhibitory function. Because they inhibit the release of GI hormones, somatostatin analogues are used for various endocrine neoplasms such as **Zollinger-Ellison syndrome**, **VIPoma, insulinoma,** and **carcinoid tumors**. They are also useful in patients with **pancreatic fistulas, pancreatic ascites,** and **enterocutaneous fistulas** by decreasing GI secretions. Additionally, they have been used as a treatment to decrease bleeding from the GI tract. **Glucagon** is used by endoscopists to **relax the Sphincter of Oddi** to facilitate endoscopic retrograde cholangiopancreatography (ERCP). **Secretin**, which inhibits acid secretion, causes a paradoxical increase in serum gastrin levels in patients with gastrinoma. **Pancreatic polypeptide** (PP) is predominantly secreted in the pancreatic head. PP serum levels drop following the Whipple procedure and may be related to the delayed gastric emptying observed after pyloric-preserving pancreatoduodenectomy. In addition, PP secretion necessitates intact vagal nerve function; thus, a blunt response to stimulation by sham feedings has been used to evaluate intact vagal nerve function, particularly in patients suspected of having iatrogenic vagus nerve injury.

**ANSWER:** C

11. With regard to regulation of gastric emptying, which of the following statements is true?

A. The greater the volume present in the stomach, the slower the gastric emptying.

B. Higher intake of lipids slows gastric emptying.

C. Emptying of solids is dependent on fundal tone.

D. Emptying of liquids is dependent on antral propulsion.

E. The lower esophageal sphincter regulates gastric volume.

*Ref.:* 1, 2

**COMMENTS: Gastric emptying** is regulated largely by neural and hormonal factors triggered by gastric volume and composition. Generally, the greater the volume, the faster the contents empty. Liquids empty faster than solids. The pattern of liquid emptying is exponential and is largely determined by **fundal tone.** Solids are reduced in size to particles 1 to 2 mm in diameter by **propulsive and retropulsive activity.** Gastric emptying is linear after an initial lag and depends on mechanical action of the **pyloroantral** region. Higher caloric intake, in the form of lipids, slows gastric emptying. The **lower esophageal sphincter** does not control gastric volume.

**ANSWER:** B

12. Which of the following clinical conditions is not associated with delayed gastric emptying?

A. Hypocalcaemia

B. Scleroderma

C. Hyperglycemia

D. Myxedema

E. Zollinger-Ellison syndrome

*Ref.:* 1-3

**COMMENTS:** Disorders of gastric emptying can be divided into rapid or delayed emptying, both of which can be significantly disabling conditions. **Delayed gastric emptying** is the more frequently encountered problem of gastric motility. Excluding mechanical obstruction, important causes of delayed gastric emptying include **metabolic derangements** (e.g., **myxedema** and **hyperglycemia**), **electrolyte abnormalities** (e.g., **hypokalemia** and **hypocalcaemia**), **drugs** (e.g., **narcotics** and **anticholinergics**), and **systemic diseases** (e.g., **diabetes mellitus** and **scleroderma**). Up to 40% of **postvagotomy** patients experience delayed gastric emptying. **Rapid gastric emptying** is less commonly observed. Causes of rapid gastric emptying include previous **gastric resection**, conditions with **impaired fat absorption** resulting in loss of the inhibition of gastric emptying (e.g., **pancreatic insufficiency** and **short bowel syndrome**), and conditions with **hypergastrinemia** such as **Zollinger-Ellison syndrome.**

**ANSWER:** E

13. Infection with *Helicobacter pylori* has been associated with all but which of the following conditions?

A. Duodenal ulcer

B. Gastric cancer

C. Mucosa-associated lymphoid tissue (MALT) lymphoma

D. Gastroesophageal reflux disease (GERD)

E. Chronic gastritis

*Ref.:* 1, 2, 4

**COMMENTS:** *H. pylori* is a curved or S-shaped, gram-negative microaerophilic motile bacterium whose natural habitat is the human stomach. *H. pylori* infection has been demonstrated to be associated with 90% of **duodenal ulcers** and 75% of **gastric**

**ulcers**. After eradication of the organism as part of ulcer treatment, recurrence of ulcer is extremely rare. In addition, *H. pylori* has been associated with **chronic atrophic gastritis**, which in turn leads to **gastric atrophy** and **intestinal metaplasia**, a suspected precursor of **gastric cancer**. *H. pylori* infection also increases the risk for low-grade **mucosa-associated lymphoid tissue lymphoma**; eradication of *H. pylori* results in resolution of MALT lymphomas in most cases. There appears to be a negative association between *H. pylori* infection and **gastrointestinal reflux disease**.

**ANSWER: D**

14. Which of the following tests is not appropriate for the initial detection of *H. pylori* infection in patients with peptic ulcer disease?

   A. Urea breath test

   B. Histologic examination of mucosa

   C. Rapid urease test

   D. Culture and sensitivity testing

   E. *H. pylori* serology

   *Ref.:* 1, 5, 6

**COMMENTS:** See Question 15.

**ANSWER: D**

15. Which of the following tests is best to document eradication of *H. pylori* infection in patients with peptic ulcer disease?

   A. Urea breath test

   B. Histologic examination of mucosa

   C. Rapid urease test

   D. Culture and sensitivity testing

   E. *H. pylori* serology

   *Ref.:* 1, 5, 6

**COMMENTS:** It is important to document the presence or absence of *Helicobacter pylori* to adequately treat patients with peptic ulcer disease. Both invasive and noninvasive tests are available for the diagnosis of *H. pylori* infection. **Invasive tests** require endoscopic mucosal biopsy and include **histologic examination**, the **rapid urease test**, and **culture**. **Noninvasive tests** include the **urea breath test** and **serology**. Histologic examination can accurately diagnose *H. pylori* with two biopsy specimens with high sensitivity and specificity (90%). The rapid urease test on a mucosal biopsy specimen uses a change in pH resulting from the breakdown of urea by a urease enzyme produced by *H. pylori*. This test is considered the initial test of choice because of its simplicity, accuracy, and rapid results. Culture of *H. pylori* has the most specificity (100%) but is difficult to perform and is currently not widely available. Cultures should usually be reserved for research purposes or patients with suspected antibiotic resistance. The urea breath test is a noninvasive test that analyzes breath for labeled carbon dioxide produced by bacterial urease from the conversion of ingested labeled urea. Because of its noninvasiveness plus high sensitivity and specificity (95%), the urea breath test is considered the test of choice for documentation of *H. pylori* eradication. Serologic tests are quick and inexpensive but cannot differentiate between active infection and previous exposure. Serology is useful for the initial diagnosis of *H. pylori* infection in patients in whom endoscopy is not indicated.

**ANSWER: A**

16. Which condition corresponds to the appropriate basal and pentagastrin-stimulated acid output?

   A. Duodenal ulcer/basal and pentagastrin-stimulated acid output is decreased

   B. Pernicious anemia/basal and pentagastrin-stimulated acid output is decreased

   C. Gastric cancer/basal and pentagastrin-stimulated acid output is decreased

   D. Zollinger-Ellison syndrome/basal and pentagastrin-stimulated acid output is increased

   E. Gastric atrophy/basal and pentagastrin-stimulated acid output is decreased

   *Ref.:* 1, 2

**COMMENTS:** The normal mean basal acid output is in the range of 1 to 8 mmol/h, and the response to pentagastrin-stimulated output ranges from 6 to 40 mmol/h. In patients with **duodenal ulcer** and **Zollinger-Ellison syndrome**, both **basal acid output** and **pentagastrin-stimulated acid output** are decreased. In contrast, adults with **pernicious anemia**, **gastric atrophy**, and **gastric cancer** are achlorhydric or have subnormal acid output. In these patients, maximal acid output remains decreased despite pentagastrin evaluation.

**ANSWER: A**

17. Elevated serum gastrin levels during fasting are typical in all but which of the following conditions?

   A. Short bowel syndrome

   B. Pernicious anemia

   C. Chronic gastritis

   D. Duodenal ulcer

   E. Gastric outlet obstruction

   *Ref.:* 1, 2, 6

**COMMENTS:** Conditions associated with **hypergastrinemia** and increased acid secretion include **Zollinger-Ellison syndrome**, **antral G-cell hyperplasia**, **retained antrum**, **renal failure**, **gastric outlet obstruction**, and **short bowel syndrome**. In contradistinction, an **elevated serum gastrin level with normal or diminished acid output** is seen in patients with **pernicious anemia**, **postvagotomy states**, **chronic gastritis**, and **gastric cancer** and in patients with **pharmacologic acid suppression**. Serum gastrin levels during fasting are normal in patients with **duodenal ulcer** but may be excessively elevated postprandially. The absolute level of an abnormally elevated serum gastrin level is not necessarily indicative of the cause. However, marked elevations (>1000 pg/mL) are often associated with Zollinger-Ellison syndrome. Ulcerogenic causes of **hypergastrinemia** resulting from elevated gastric acid secretion include **Zollinger-Ellison syndrome**, **antral G-cell hyperplasia**, **retained antrum**, **short bowel syndrome**, and **gastric outlet obstruction**. Zollinger-Ellison syndrome and antral G-cell hyperplasia are uncommon, but they must be differentiated to determine proper therapy. Both are associated with elevated gastrin and gastric acid levels. They can be differentiated on the basis of the serum gastrin response to several provocative tests. A pronounced increase in serum gastrin levels after the intravenous infusion of secretin is typically seen with Zollinger-Ellison syndrome. Elevations can occur with other conditions, but they are not as dramatic. In contradistinction, more marked increases in gastrin levels occur after stimulation by a protein in Zollinger-Ellison syndrome.

**ANSWER:** D

18. With regard to *H. pylori*–negative duodenal ulcer disease, all of the following statements are correct except:

   A. Nonsteroidal anti-inflammatory drugs (NSAIDs) are a major cause of duodenal ulcers in patients who are *H. pylori* negative.

   B. Because of the high prevalence of *H. pylori*–positive duodenal ulcers, patients should be treated for *H. pylori* without confirmatory testing.

   C. In contrast to *H. pylori*–positive duodenal ulcers, NSAID-induced ulcers are not frequently associated with chronic active gastritis.

   D. *H. pylori*–negative duodenal ulcers are usually large ulcers and multiple and are often associated with bleeding.

   E. Older age, multiple comorbid conditions, and sepsis are independently associated with *H. pylori*–negative duodenal ulcers.

*Ref.:* 1, 6

**COMMENTS:** Initial studies have demonstrated that *Helicobacter pylori* infection is present in more than 90% of patients with duodenal ulcers. However, more recently it has been shown that the prevalence of *H. pylori*–associated duodenal ulcers is only 75% and is found to be decreasing. Thus, it is important to first make the diagnosis of an active *H. pylori* infection rather than initiating **empirical therapy.** *Helicobacter pylori*–**negative duodenal ulcers** are independently associated with **nonsteroidal anti-inflammatory drug use, older age, multiple medical problems,** and **sepsis.** Use of NSAIDs is the major cause of duodenal ulcers in patients who are *H. pylori*–negative. **Bleeding** is the initial manifestation in these patients and they have large and multiple ulcers.

**ANSWER:** B

19. A 45-year old man requires surgery for an intractable duodenal ulcer. Which operation best prevents ulcer recurrence?

   A. Subtotal gastrectomy

   B. Truncal vagotomy and pyloroplasty

   C. Truncal vagotomy and antrectomy

   D. Selective vagotomy

   E. Highly selective vagotomy

*Ref.:* 1, 2, 6

**COMMENTS:** See Question 20.

**ANSWER:** C

20. Which operation for duodenal ulcer is least likely to produce undesirable postoperative symptoms?

   A. Subtotal gastrectomy

   B. Truncal vagotomy and pyloroplasty

   C. Truncal vagotomy and antrectomy

   D. Selective vagotomy

   E. Highly selective vagotomy

*Ref.:* 1, 2, 6

**COMMENTS:** The goal of surgical therapy for **duodenal ulcers** is to reduce acid production in a manner that is safe and has the fewest possible side effects. Acid can be reduced by eliminating vagal stimulation, removing the antral source of gastrin, and removing the parietal cell mass. Traditionally, subtotal two-thirds gastrectomy has carried the highest mortality rate. **Truncal vagotomy with antrectomy** has the lowest recurrence rate. Procedures involving antrectomy, pyloroplasty, or truncal vagotomy may be complicated by diarrhea, postprandial dumping, or bile reflux. **Selective vagotomy,** which preserves the hepatic and celiac vagal branches, has been associated with a lower rate of diarrhea than truncal vagotomy has. **Highly selective vagotomy,** also known as parietal cell vagotomy, aims to denervate the parietal cell–bearing portion of the stomach but preserve innervations to the pyloroantral region and thus maintain more normal gastric emptying. This operation carries the lowest mortality rate, the lowest incidence of side effects, but the highest recurrence rate, which ranges from 5% to 15%.

**ANSWER:** E

21. A 75-year-old man taking NSAIDs for arthritis has an acute abdomen and pneumoperitoneum. His symptoms are 6 hours old and his vital signs are stable after the infusion of 1 L of normal saline solution. What should be the next step in the management of this patient?

   A. Computed tomography of the abdomen

   B. Esophagogastroduodenoscopy (EGD)

   C. Antisecretory drugs, broad-spectrum antibiotics, and surgery if he fails to improve in 6 hours

   D. Antisecretory drugs, antibiotics for *H. pylori*, and surgery if he fails to improve in 6 hours

   E. Surgery

*Ref.:* 1, 2, 6

**COMMENTS:** See Question 23.

**ANSWER:** E

22. The patient in Question 21 is found to have a perforated duodenal ulcer. Which of the following best describes the required operation?

   A. Suture closure of the perforation

   B. Omental patch of the perforation

   C. Repair of the perforation and highly selective vagotomy

   D. Repair of the perforation and truncal vagotomy

   E. Repair of the perforation and gastric resection

*Ref.:* 1, 2, 6

COMMENTS: See Question 23.

ANSWER: B

23. If the patient in Question 21 were found to have a perforated gastric ulcer instead of a duodenal ulcer, what additional steps, if any, need to be performed at the time of operative intervention beside closure of the perforation?

    A. Feeding jejunostomy

    B. Gastrojejunostomy

    C. Gastrostomy tube placement

    D. Excision or biopsy of the ulcer

    E. Pyloroplasty

*Ref.: 1, 6*

COMMENTS: The preferred treatment of a **perforated duodenal ulcer** is resuscitation and prompt surgery. Nonoperative management is reserved for old contained perforations or for terminally ill patients who otherwise cannot undergo surgery. The diagnosis is a presumptive one based on clinical grounds and should not be excluded if pneumoperitoneum cannot be demonstrated, because about 20% of patients with perforations do not have this typical radiographic feature. Operative management requires closure of the perforation, which is generally best accomplished with an **omental (Graham) patch**. Closure of the perforation is usually sufficient in patients with duodenal ulcers; however, excision of the ulcer is necessary to rule out malignancy in patients with gastric ulcers before closure. Following simple repair alone, the traditional natural history has been that about one third of patients have no further ulcer problems, one third have ulcer recurrence amenable to medical management, and one third require a subsequent operation for ulcer disease. It is not clear how precisely this applies to patients with *H. pylori* infection or those with NSAID-induced ulcers. Definitive operations should be performed only in stable patients and those with documented failure after appropriate *H. pylori* eradication. **Truncal vagotomy** can be performed expeditiously but has a greater incidence of side effects. Highly selective vagotomy is an excellent choice but is time-consuming and requires a surgeon with the expertise to perform it. Resective procedures are generally avoided in the setting of perforation because of higher morbidity. Following surgery, ulcerogenic drugs should be withheld, and any concomitant *H. pylori* infection should be treated.

ANSWER: D

24. The most common cause of gastric outlet obstruction in adults is:

    A. Peptic ulcer disease

    B. Extrinsic neoplastic compression

    C. Cancer

    D. Primary lymphoma of the stomach

    E. Duodenal Crohn's disease

*Ref.: 1, 5, 6*

COMMENTS: With increased use of histamine receptor blockers and proton pump inhibitors in the medical management of peptic ulcer disease and effective treatment of *H. pylori* infection, malignancy is the most common cause of **gastric outlet obstruction**

instead of peptic ulcer disease. Among malignancies, primary adenocarcinomas of the pancreas, stomach, and duodenum (in decreasing order of frequency) are the leading cause of gastric outlet obstruction. Gastrointestinal stromal tumors (GISTs) of the stomach and duodenum and primary lymphomas of the stomach, duodenum, and pancreas are other causes of gastric outlet obstruction. Extrinsic compression from metastatic disease to the porta hepatis can also lead to obstruction. It is therefore important to have a high index of suspicion for a malignancy when a patient has gastric outlet obstruction rather than mistaking it for a benign obstruction from peptic ulcer disease.

ANSWER: C

25. A patient with gastric outlet obstruction and prolonged vomiting has which of the following metabolic abnormalities?

    A. Hypochloremic, hyperkalemic metabolic alkalosis

    B. Hyperchloremic, hypokalemic metabolic acidosis

    C. Hyponatremic, hypokalemic metabolic acidosis

    D. Hypochloremic, hypokalemic metabolic alkalosis

    E. Hyperchloremic, hyperkalemic metabolic acidosis

*Ref.: 1, 2*

COMMENTS: The classic metabolic abnormality resulting from gastric outlet obstruction and prolonged **vomiting** is **hypochloremic, hypokalemic metabolic alkalosis**. Initial loss of hydrochloric acid causes hypochloremia and mild alkalosis compensated for by renal excretion of bicarbonate. Therefore, in the early stages the urine is alkaline. Continued vomiting produces a severe extracellular fluid deficit and sodium deficit from both renal and gastric losses. The kidneys begin to conserve sodium and, in exchange, excrete hydrogen and potassium cations to accompany bicarbonate. The kidneys are the predominant site of potassium loss, and the urine is paradoxically acidic. Urine chloride content is reduced throughout and eventually absent. Serum ionized calcium levels are decreased because calcium is mildly alkaline and shifts to its nonionized form to reduce alkalosis. Treatment of this metabolic situation is accomplished primarily by the administration of isotonic saline solution, which replenishes the deficits in volume, sodium, and chloride. Potassium is replaced once renal function is optimized.

ANSWER: D

26. Which of the following endoscopic ulcer characteristics has the highest risk for recurrent bleeding?

    A. Oozing ulcer

    B. Clean based ulcer

    C. Nonbleeding "visible vessel"

    D. Nonbleeding ulcer with an overlying clot

    E. Dieulafoy ulcer

*Ref.: 6*

COMMENTS: **Esophagogastroduodenoscopy** is not only the diagnostic test of choice but can also be therapeutic in patients with **upper gastrointestinal bleeding**. EGD can localize the bleeding site and determine the risk for rebleeding based on the appearance of the ulcer bed. The endoscopic features of ulcers with a risk for **rebleeding** in decreasing order of frequency are active arterial bleeding (approaches 100%), nonbleeding "visible vessel" (≈50%), nonbleeding ulcer with an overlying clot (≈30% to 35%), oozing ulcer (≈10% to 27%), and a clean based ulcer (<3%). Dieulafoy ulcers are vascular malformations that bleed when superficial erosion into the vessel occurs. Unless actively bleeding, they are difficult to diagnose endoscopically.

**ANSWER:** C

27. During an operation for a bleeding duodenal ulcer, three-point "U" stitches are placed to ligate which of the following arteries after longitudinal pyloroduodenotomy?

    A. Common hepatic, right gastric, and gastroduodenal arteries

    B. Proximal and distal gastroduodenal and transverse pancreatic arteries

    C. Right gastric, gastroduodenal, and right gastroepiploic arteries

    D. Right gastric and anterior and posterior inferior pancreaticoduodenal arteries

    E. Common hepatic, gastroduodenal, and superior mesenteric arteries

    *Ref.:* 1, 2, 4, 6

**COMMENTS:** Massive bleeding is usually the result of posterior erosion of a duodenal ulcer into the gastroduodenal artery. Emergency surgical intervention is indicated when bleeding is refractory to endoscopic therapy or in the presence of hemorrhagic shock. After expeditious preoperative resuscitation, the abdomen is entered and a **longitudinal pyloroduodenotomy** is performed. Digital pressure is applied over the ulcer base to temporize the bleeding and allow resuscitation before suture control is obtained. Proper control of bleeding requires three-point suture ligation of the duodenal ulcer. These "U" stitches are placed superior and inferior to the site of penetration to ligate the proximal and distal **gastroduodenal artery**. A third suture is placed on medial aspect of the ulcer to control the **transverse pancreatic branch** coming off the gastroduodenal artery. After the bleeding is controlled, biopsy of gastric mucosa should be performed for histologic analysis for *H. pylori*. The longitudinal pyloroduodenotomy is then closed transversely (**Heineke-Mikulicz** or **Weinberg pyloroplasty**).

**ANSWER:** B

28. Which type of gastric ulcer corresponds with the correct anatomic location?

    A. Type I/prepyloric region

    B. Type II/lesser curvature of the stomach near the GE junction

    C. Type III/body of the stomach along the lesser curvature

    D. Type IV/lesser curvature of the stomach near the GE junction

    E. Type IV/prepyloric region

    *Ref.:* 1, 4, 6

**COMMENTS:** See Question 30.

**ANSWER:** D

29. Which type of gastric ulcer corresponds with the associated acid secretion?

    A. Type I/high acid secretion

    B. Type II/high acid secretion

    C. Type III/normal or low acid secretion

    D. Type IV/high acid secretion

    E. All of the above

    *Ref.:* 1, 4, 6

**COMMENTS:** See Question 30.

**ANSWER:** B

30. Which gastric ulcer corresponds with the correct recommended surgical management?

    A. Type I/Billroth I or II reconstruction

    B. Type II/truncal vagotomy and pyloroplasty

    C. Type III/Csendes gastrectomy with Roux-en-Y gastrojejunostomy or Pauchet gastrectomy and Billroth I reconstruction

    D. Type IV/Billroth I or II reconstruction with truncal vagotomy

    E. Type IV/total gastrectomy

    *Ref.:* 1, 4, 6

**COMMENTS:** Benign **gastric ulcers** have been classified in terms of their anatomic location. **Type I** ulcers are the most common (50%) and occur in the body of the stomach along the lesser curvature. These ulcers are associated with low to normal acid secretion. **Type II** gastric ulcers (25%) also occur in the body of the stomach but have associated duodenal ulcers. **Type III** gastric ulcers (20%) are located in the prepyloric region. Both type II and type III ulcers are associated with excessive acid secretion. **Type IV** ulcers are the least common (<10%) and occur near the GE junction along the lesser curve. Like type I ulcers, they are associated with low or normal acid secretion. Surgical intervention is indicated for patients who have failed maximal medical therapy (12 weeks), for those in whom complications develop, or for those in whom malignancy cannot be ruled out. Surgical therapy for benign gastric ulcers depends on the type of ulcer and its associated acid secretion. Type I ulcers are usually well treated with antrectomy or hemigastrectomy (including removal of the ulcer) without vagotomy. Type IV ulcers do not require vagotomy either. Type IV ulcers near the GE junction can be treated by modifications of distal gastrectomy that include ulcer excision. Distal gastrectomy with extension along the lesser curvature to include the ulcer (**Pauchet procedure**) and Billroth I reconstruction can be performed for ulcers that are 2 to 5 cm from the GE junction. For type IV ulcers at the GE junction, subtotal gastrectomy with Roux-en-Y jejunal reconstruction (**Csendes procedure**), a rotational **Tanner** gastrectomy, or a **Kahler-Muhlenberg** procedure should be performed. Because type II and type III ulcers are associated with acid hypersecretion, they are treated as duodenal ulcers. Truncal vagotomy with Billroth I or II reconstruction is the preferred surgical therapy because it accomplishes both goals of a decrease in acid secretion and excision of the ulcer.

**ANSWER:** A

**31.** Concerning the treatment of patients with Zollinger-Ellison syndrome, which of the following statements is true?

  A. Operative treatment of associated hyperparathyroidism takes precedence over abdominal surgery.

  B. Pancreatic tumors should not be removed by enucleation.

  C. Duodenal tumors usually require pancreaticoduodenectomy.

  D. Total gastrectomy is indicated if the tumor cannot be localized.

  E. Resection of liver metastases is not indicated.

*Ref.:* 1-3

**COMMENTS:** Treatment of **Zollinger-Ellison syndrome** is two pronged and aimed at both resecting the tumor when possible and protecting the gastric end-organ. Therapy must be individualized. Patients with known endocrine tumors should undergo careful evaluation for other potential endocrine tumors. In patients with **gastrinoma** and **hyperparathyroidism**, **parathyroidectomy** should be performed first to eliminate hypercalcemia. Abdominal surgery is not urgent with the current antisecretory medications. Although gastrinomas are often multiple and are usually metastatic, long-term survival is possible. Aggressive attempts to localize and resect tumors can provide cure in 5% to 20% of patients and can diminish gastrin secretion in others. Most gastrinomas can be found in the **triangle of Passaro**. Digital palpation through a duodenotomy and intraoperative ultrasound are useful operative adjuncts. Both pancreatic and duodenal gastrinomas can be resected by **enucleation** when appropriately located. Blind pancreatic resections are not generally indicated. When complete tumor removal is not possible, a gastric operation may be appropriate. Proximal gastric vagotomy may be useful, but **total gastrectomy** still provides the best long-term quality of life for some patients. Life-long pharmacologic treatment with antisecretory agents may control the ulcer diathesis in some patients, but problems with high doses, compliance, and side effects may occur. Resection or ablation of metastatic disease, although not curative, can provide important palliation and decrease the need for drug therapy.

**ANSWER:** A

**32.** With regard to the epidemiologic characteristics of gastric cancer, which of the following statements is false?

  A. The highest incidence is found in Japan.

  B. Gastric cancer is twice as common in males as in females.

  C. The incidence of gastric adenocarcinoma of the distal portion of the stomach has increased in the past several decades.

  D. There is a higher incidence in patients with blood group A.

  E. There is a higher incidence in patients who have undergone gastric resection for duodenal ulcer.

*Ref.:* 1, 6, 7

**COMMENTS:** The significant geographic variations in the incidence of **gastric cancer** are probably related to environmental and dietary differences that result in exposure to *N*-nitroso compounds, polycyclic hydrocarbons, and other potential carcinogens. The highest incidence is found in Japan, with lower rates in the United States and Western Europe. Gastric cancer occurs more frequently in males all over the world, and the incidence is higher in African-American men than in white men in the United States. The incidence of adenocarcinoma of the gastric cardia and GE junction has gradually increased, whereas that of the distal part of the stomach has decreased over the past few decades. Although most risk factors for gastric cancer are probably exogenous, genetic factors may also be involved, as exemplified by patients with pernicious anemia and by slightly increased risk in patients with blood group A. There is also an increased risk 10 to 15 years after gastric resection for benign disease, perhaps indicative of the role of bile reflux.

**ANSWER:** C

**33.** All of the following conditions are associated with gastric cancer except:

  A. Chronic atrophic gastritis

  B. *H. pylori* infection

  C. Hereditary nonpolyposis colorectal cancer

  D. Adenomatous gastric polyps

  E. Fundic gland polyps

*Ref.:* 1, 6, 7

**COMMENTS:** Certain gastric lesions have a significant association with gastric adenocarcinoma and can be considered precursors to malignancy. **Chronic atrophic gastritis**, of which several forms are recognized, underlies most gastric cancers. The epithelial changes of intestinal metaplasia and dysplasia are premalignant. Autoimmune chronic gastritis involves the body and fundus of the stomach. It is associated with pernicious anemia, achlorhydria, very high gastrin levels, and a high risk for cancer. Hypersecretory chronic gastritis involves the gastric antrum and is associated with peptic ulcer disease but not malignancy. *Helicobacter pylori* infection may be the most important risk factor for gastric adenocarcinoma worldwide. The IgG antibody positivity in various populations correlates with the local incidence of gastric cancer. **Hereditary nonpolyposis colorectal cancer** is an inheritable risk factor for gastric cancer. **Adenomatous gastric polyps** have malignant potential similar to colonic adenomatous polyps. The risk increases with increasing size of the polyp. **Fundic gland polyps** are benign and have no malignant potential.

**ANSWER:** E

**34.** With regard to the surgical treatment of gastric adenocarcinoma, which of the following statements is true?

  A. Total gastrectomy for antral lesions results in longer survival than does partial gastrectomy.

  B. Routine splenectomy does not improve survival rates.

  C. Extended lymph node dissection improves survival rates in patients with stages I and II lesions.

  D. Total gastrectomy for palliation is contraindicated.

  E. Linitis plastica should be resected to histologically negative margins.

*Ref.:* 1, 6, 7

**COMMENTS:** Gastric adenocarcinoma is preferably treated by resection, although resection usually proves to be **palliative**. The general strategy for curative resection is to remove as much of the stomach as necessary to obtain free margins and to perform limited node dissection. Although data from Japan support the benefit of extended nodal dissection (celiac, mesenteric, hepatic, and para-aortic), studies in the United States have not generally confirmed this benefit. Furthermore, these extended dissections can be associated with substantial morbidity. Most resections entail distal subtotal gastrectomy. Total gastrectomy is appropriate for locally extensive tumors, proximal tumors (to avoid esophageal anastomosis to the distal stomach remnant), and even palliation if necessary. Extending clear margins on a distal tumor by total rather than subtotal gastrectomy is of no benefit. Resections for **linitis plastica** are palliative, usually necessitate total gastrectomy, and are carried out to grossly negative margins only. **Splenectomy** is performed according to the location of gastric resection, but its routine performance does not improve the survival rate. The number of lymph nodes resected, the number of positive nodes, and the ratio of positive to the total number of lymph nodes have important staging implications. Furthermore, a minimum number of 15 lymph nodes should routinely be examined.

**ANSWER: B**

35. With regard to gastric volvulus, which of the following statements is true?

   A. Symptoms consist of severe nausea with an inability to vomit.

   B. The Borchardt triad includes acute epigastric pain, nausea, and bilious vomiting.

   C. It is frequently relieved simply by passage of a nasogastric tube.

   D. Gastric volvulus should always be managed conservatively.

   E. It is associated with an increased incidence of sigmoid volvulus.

*Ref.:* 1, 2

**COMMENTS: Gastric volvulus** is a serious complication of **paraesophageal hernia**. Two types of gastric volvulus may occur, depending on the axis of rotation. **Organoaxial** volvulus, the more common type, involves rotation around the axis of a line connecting the cardia and pylorus. With **mesenteroaxial** volvulus, the axis is approximately at a right angle to the cardiopyloric line. Combined types have also been described. Patients generally have severe pain and nausea but are unable to vomit. Gastric volvulus should be suspected in patients with the **Borchardt triad**, which includes acute epigastric pain, violent retching, and inability to pass a nasogastric tube. Strangulation can follow. Hence, acute gastric volvulus requires prompt surgical intervention. It is not associated with an increased incidence of sigmoid volvulus.

**ANSWER: A**

36. With regard to GISTs, which of the following statements is incorrect?

   A. A combination of cellular morphology on hematoxylin-eosin staining and KIT immunohistochemistry are required for the diagnosis of GIST.

   B. After the small intestine, the stomach is the second most common location for GISTs, followed by the colon and rectum.

   C. The majority of GISTs have an activating mutation in the *KIT* oncogene.

   D. GISTs are usually resistant to conventional chemotherapy and radiation therapy.

   E. Complete surgical resection is the standard of treatment.

*Ref.:* 1, 8

**COMMENTS: Gastrointestinal stromal tumors** are the most common mesenchymal neoplasms of the GI tract. The majority of these GISTs occur in the stomach (60%), followed by the small bowel (30%), esophagus (1% to 5%), and colon and rectum (5%). The diagnosis of GIST is based on the presence of characteristic pathologic findings on hematoxylin-eosin staining and expression of the **KIT receptor** on immunohistochemistry. Rarely, KIT might not be overexpressed, and in such cases molecular evaluation may be necessary. These tumors do not usually metastasize to lymph nodes. Complete surgical resection is the standard of treatment of primary, localized GISTs. The majority of GISTs have an activating mutation in the *KIT* protooncogene that can be effectively inhibited by tyrosine kinase inhibitors such as **imatinib mesylate (Gleevec)**. GISTs are resistant to conventional chemoradiation therapy. Laparoscopic resection is increasingly being used, provided that clean margins can be obtained. Both the size and number of mitoses per 50 high-power field have been used to categorize tumor aggressiveness. Tumor location may have prognostic implications in that extragastric tumors may carry a worse prognosis. Large or unresectable tumors that show KIT overexpression may initially be treated with Gleevec.

**ANSWER: B**

37. Which of the following statements is not true regarding gastric MALT lymphoma?

   A. Gastric MALT lymphomas result from the monoclonal proliferation of B cells as a result of stimulation of a specific infecting strain of *H. pylori*.

   B. Unresponsive gastric MALT lymphoma can usually be salvaged by gastric resection.

   C. Chromosomal translocations and genetic mutations can predict failure of *H. pylori* treatment.

   D. Less than 10% of gastric lymphomas have no associated *H. pylori* infection.

   E. External beam radiation is used to treat refractory MALT lymphoma.

*Ref.:* 1, 6

**COMMENTS: Gastric MALT lymphoma** is associated with chronic *Helicobacter pylori* infection in more than 90% of cases. This chronic infection with *H. pylori* results in monoclonal B-cell proliferation controlled by T lymphocytes. Treatment directed toward *H. pylori* eradication results in the resolution of MALT lymphomas in most cases. Certain chromosomal translocations and genetic mutations can predict resistance to *H. pylori* therapy and progression to a high-grade gastric lymphoma. Resistant gastric MALT lymphomas are usually salvaged with **radiation therapy**, cyclophosphamide-based chemotherapy regimens, monoclonal anti-CD20 antibody, or combinations of these treatments.

**ANSWER: B**

**38.** With regard to the diagnosis and treatment of MALT lymphoma, which of the following statements is correct?

   A. Upper GI endoscopy with gastric biopsy for determination of the presence of *H. pylori* and the histologic type of lymphoma is the diagnostic test of choice.

   B. Computed tomography of the abdomen, lymphangiography, chest radiography, and bone marrow biopsy are required for complete staging.

   C. *H. pylori* serology is sufficient to document remission.

   D. *H. pylori*–negative gastric MALT lymphoma should initially be treated with clarithromycin, amoxicillin, and a proton pump inhibitor.

   E. *H. pylori* Gram stain is sufficient to make the diagnosis alone.

*Ref.:* 1, 6

**COMMENTS: Upper endoscopy with biopsy** is the diagnostic test of choice. Gastric biopsies are used to evaluate for the presence of *H. pylori* and the histologic type of lymphoma. The depth of gastric wall invasion and the presence of nodal involvement can be determined with the help of **endoscopic ultrasonography**. Staging is completed with a chest radiograph, bone marrow biopsy, and computed tomography of the abdomen. Lymphangiography is not required for staging. Surveillance is achieved with upper endoscopy, biopsy, and endoscopic ultrasound every 3 months until histologic and radiographic resolution. Complete resolution is usually achieved in 3 to 6 months on average. *H. pylori*–negative gastric MALT lymphoma, which accounts for less than 10% of all gastric lymphomas, does not respond to bacterial eradication therapy.

**ANSWER: A**

**39.** All of the following statements are correct about high-grade gastric lymphoma except:

   A. Treatment usually requires combination chemotherapy and radiation therapy.

   B. Randomized clinical trials for early stages IE and IIE disease demonstrate nonsurgical therapy to be equivalent or superior to surgical treatment in regard to patient survival.

   C. Hemorrhage is a frequent complication of chemotherapy.

   D. Surgical treatment is usually reserved for patients with localized persistent lymphoma or complications associated with nonsurgical treatment.

   E. Perforation is very rare after chemotherapy.

*Ref.:* 1, 6

**COMMENTS: High-grade gastric lymphomas** require treatment with combination chemotherapy and the addition of radiation therapy for bulky or residual disease. Patient survival has been shown to be equivalent or better with nonsurgical treatment than with surgical treatment in several prospective clinical trials (randomized and nonrandomized). Complications were more frequent in the surgical groups than in the nonsurgical groups. Complications such as **perforation** and **hemorrhage** are very infrequent in patients undergoing chemotherapy or radiation therapy. Complications from chemoradiation therapy or persistent localized lymphoma are current indications for operative intervention in patients with gastric lymphoma.

**ANSWER: C**

**40.** A 23-year-old thin (92 lb) woman with a history of surgical correction of her scoliosis is evaluated for symptoms of postprandial epigastric pain, fullness, nausea, and vomiting. Her physical examination is unremarkable except for her thin physique/stature. Barium upper GI series showed a dilated duodenum and stomach with minimal flow of barium into the jejunum. Which of the following is the operative management of choice for this patient's condition?

   A. Segmental duodenectomy

   B. Pancreaticoduodenectomy

   C. Gastrojejunostomy

   D. Duodenojejunostomy

   E. Roux-en-Y hepaticojejunostomy

*Ref.:* 1

**COMMENTS:** The patient in this scenario has compression of the third portion of the duodenum by the superior mesenteric artery as it passes over it. This rare condition is known as **superior mesenteric artery syndrome** or **Wilkie syndrome**. This syndrome is usually seen in young asthenic females with predisposing conditions of weight loss, scoliosis or corrective surgery for it, supine mobilization, and placement of a body cast. The diagnosis is usually made with either a barium upper GI series or computed tomography, with oral and intravenous contrast enhancement demonstrating a dilated duodenum and stomach with abrupt or nearly complete cutoff of contrast agent at the third portion of the duodenum and minimal flow into the jejunum. Conservative management consisting of nutritional supplementation can be tried initially. In patients who fail medical management, the operative treatment of choice is **duodenojejunostomy**.

**ANSWER: D**

**41.** All of the following statements regarding Crohn's disease of the duodenum are correct except:

   A. Duodenal Crohn's disease accounts only for 2% to 4% of all patients with Crohn's disease.

   B. Because of its location, operative intervention is frequently needed for duodenal Crohn's disease.

   C. When an operation is required, a bypass such as gastrojejunostomy is performed rather than duodenal resection.

   D. In well-selected patients, strictureplasty can be carried out with good results.

   E. Adenocarcinoma is the leading cause of disease-specific death in patients with Crohn's disease.

*Ref.:* 1, 9, 10

**COMMENTS: Crohn's disease** of the duodenum is not common and is seen in only 2% to 4% of patients with Crohn's disease. Medical therapy remains the mainstay of treatment of duodenal Crohn's disease, with surgical intervention being reserved for patients who do not respond to medical therapy or in whom a complication develops such as obstruction or perforation. In patients who do need a surgical procedure, bypass is preferred over duodenal resection. In a few select patients, their anatomy might be amenable to **strictureplasty**.

Irrespective of the location of Crohn's disease, GI cancer remains the leading cause of death in patients with Crohn's disease.

**ANSWER: B**

**42.** With regard to adenocarcinoma of the small bowel, all of the following statements are correct except:

   A. Small bowel adenocarcinoma is found in decreasing order of frequency in the ileum, jejunum, and duodenum.

   B. Villous adenomas of the small bowel are commonly found in the duodenum around the ampulla of Vater.

   C. Adenocarcinoma of the duodenum usually occurs earlier than small bowel adenocarcinoma elsewhere in the jejunum and ileum.

   D. Villous adenomas of the duodenum are frequently associated with familial adenomatous polyposis.

   E. Operative resection is the treatment modality of choice and has curative potential.

*Ref.:* 1, 2, 6

**COMMENTS: Small bowel adenocarcinoma** accounts for the majority (35% to 50%) of small bowel malignant neoplasms, followed by carcinoid tumors, lymphomas, and sarcomas. Adenocarcinoma of the small bowel is more common in the duodenum, whereas **carcinoid tumors** and **lymphoma** are more frequently seen in the ileum. Small bowel adenocarcinoma is found in decreasing order of frequency in the duodenum, jejunum, and ileum. Although rare in the small bowel, **villous adenomas** are frequently found in the duodenum and are associated with **familial adenomatous polyposis syndrome** (31% to 92%). These villous adenomas have high malignant potential, especially if they are larger than 5 cm or are accompanied by bleeding or obstruction. Most patients have nonspecific symptoms initially; however, adenocarcinoma of the duodenum is manifested earlier with signs and symptoms of obstructive jaundice, gastric outlet obstruction, and abdominal pain. Operative resection (pancreaticoduodenectomy and local excision) is the treatment of choice, depending on the size and location of the adenocarcinoma, the patient's health, and the surgeon's expertise.

**ANSWER:** A

**43.** Concerning duodenal diverticula, all of the following statements are correct except:

   A. They are twice as common in women as in men.

   B. Duodenal diverticula are the second most common congenital diverticula of the intestine after Meckel diverticulum.

   C. The majority of duodenal diverticula are found in the periampullary region.

   D. Most of them are asymptomatic and found incidentally.

   E. They can result in cholangitis and pancreatitis from obstruction of the biliary or pancreatic ducts, respectively.

*Ref.:* 1

**COMMENTS: Duodenal diverticula** are false diverticula containing only mucosa and submucosa, as opposed to a true diverticulum, which contains all layers of the intestinal wall (e.g., Meckel diverticulum). Duodenal diverticula are the second most common cause of acquired diverticula after those in the colon. They are more commonly seen in women than in men (2:1) and usually occur later in life, similar to colonic diverticula. The majority of these diverticula (≈75%) are found within a 2-cm radius from the ampulla of Vater and generally protrude through the medial wall of the duodenum. These duodenal diverticula are rarely symptomatic, and symptoms are usually the results of hemorrhage, perforation, blind loop syndrome, cholangitis, or pancreatitis from obstruction of the biliary or pancreatic ducts. Juxtapyloric diverticula have been noted to be associated with choledocholithiasis. Their presence increases the difficulty of successful completion of ERCP.

**ANSWER:** B

**44.** Which of the following is the preferred treatment of a symptomatic duodenal diverticulum?

   A. Observation

   B. Broad-spectrum antibiotics

   C. Duodenal diverticulectomy

   D. Pancreas-sparing duodenectomy

   E. Pancreaticoduodenectomy

*Ref.:* 1

**COMMENTS:** As discussed earlier, most of the **duodenal diverticula** are asymptomatic and do not warrant any intervention. Surgery is reserved for patients in whom complications develop. They can cause abdominal pain, obstruction, perforation, bleeding, bacterial overgrowth, and pancreaticobiliary complications. When treatment is required, surgical excision (**diverticulectomy**) is recommended.

**ANSWER:** C

**REFERENCES**

1. Mercer DW, Robinson EK: Stomach. In Townsend CM, Beauchamp RD, Evers BM, et al, editors: *Sabiston textbook of surgery: the biological basis of modern surgical practice*, ed 18, Philadelphia, 2008, WB Saunders.
2. Dempsey DT: Stomach. In Brunicardi FC, Andersen DK, Billiar TR, et al, editors: *Schwartz's principles of surgery*, ed 9, New York, 2010, McGraw-Hill.
3. Rice-Townsend SE, Norton JA: Zollinger-Ellison syndrome. In Cameron JL, editor: *Current surgical therapy*, ed 9, Philadelphia, 2008, CV Mosby.
4. Winkleman BJ, Usatii A, Ellison EC: Duodenal ulcer. In Cameron JL, editor: *Current surgical therapy*, ed 9, Philadelphia, 2008, CV Mosby.
5. Fisher WE, Brunicardi FC: Benign gastric ulcer. In Cameron JL, editor: *Current surgical therapy*, ed 9, Philadelphia, 2008, CV Mosby.
6. Bland KI, Büchler MW, Csendes A, et al: *General surgery: principles and international practice*, ed 2, New York, 2008, Springer-Verlag.
7. Cho CS, Brennan MF: Gastric adenocarcinoma. In Cameron JL, editor: *Current surgical therapy*, ed 9, Philadelphia, 2008, CV Mosby.
8. Efron DT: Gastrointestinal stromal tumors. In Cameron JL, editor: *Current surgical therapy*, ed 9, Philadelphia, 2008, CV Mosby.
9. Mintz Y, Talamini MA: Crohn's disease of the small bowel. In Cameron JL, editor: *Current surgical therapy*, ed 9, Philadelphia, 2008, CV Mosby.
10. Tavakkolizadeh A, Whang EE, Ashley SW, et al: Small intestine. In Brunicardi FC, Andersen DK, Billiar TR, et al, editors: *Schwartz's principles of surgery*, ed 9, New York, 2010, McGraw-Hill.

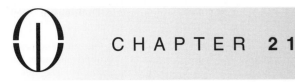

# CHAPTER 21

# Small Bowel and Appendix

*Jacquelyn Turner, M.D., and Theodore J. Saclarides, M.D.*

## A. Small Bowel

1. With regard to ileostomy physiology, which of the following statements is true?

   A. Daily output from an established ileostomy is approximately 1500 mL.

   B. Ileostomy output can increase by 50% at times of dietary indiscretion.

   C. With dehydration, the concentration of sodium output from the ileostomy rises.

   D. When compared with normal ileal fluid, ileostomy effluent contains a 100-fold increase in the number of aerobes and a 2500-fold increase in the number of coliform bacteria.

   E. The microbiologic flora of ileostomy output is similar to that of normal ileal fluid.

*Ref.: 1*

**COMMENTS:** The daily output from an established **ileostomy** is 500 to 800 mL. Although there is a great deal of variation in daily output among individuals, the output in a given patient varies only about 20% with changes in diet or with episodes of gastroenteritis. The usual **ileostomy sodium concentration** is 115 mEq/L, although the concentration rises and falls with changes in total body sodium. With dehydration, the sodium concentration falls and the potassium level rises as a result of the ability of the terminal ileum to conserve sodium in times of salt depletion. Normally, the sodium-to-potassium ratio is about 12:1. The microbiologic flora of ileostomy output is markedly different from that of normal ileal fluid. The total number of bacteria is 80 times greater, and there is a 100-fold increase in the number of aerobes, a 2500-fold increase in the number of coliform bacteria, and an increase in the number of total anaerobes.

**ANSWER: D**

2. Which of the following statements about small bowel motility is true?

   A. Oral feeding stimulates the production of migrating motor complexes (MMCs).

   B. If motility is impaired, absorption of nutrients is similarly affected.

   C. MMCs are peristaltic contractions occurring at 10- to 20-minute intervals.

   D. Vagotomy-induced diarrhea is the result of increased secretion secondary to denervation.

   E. Segmental bowel resection causes a temporary interruption of MMCs, but the clinical results are usually insignificant.

*Ref.: 2*

**COMMENTS: Migrating motor complexes** are propagated aboral peristaltic contractions occurring at 90-minute intervals. The activity fronts of MMCs usually originate high in the stomach, propagate distally, and end in the ileum, usually at the midileal level. Oral feeding inhibits MMCs, which results in irregular, non-propagating contractions throughout most of the small intestine. This postprandial inhibition may persist for 3 to 4 hours after a meal and is most pronounced with lipids. Although this motility pattern is disorganized, there is distal progression of chyme. Absorption is not affected by intestinal motility. Enteral feedings can therefore be used safely and efficiently in postoperative patients in whom motility may be altered.

Both gastric and small bowel motility can be affected by exogenous conditions. The small bowel is less sensitive than the stomach to general anesthesia and laparotomy, each of which decreases the frequency of MMCs. The frequency of MMCs returns to normal within 6 to 24 hours in the absence of peritonitis or abscess formation. The tone of the stomach is affected more than that of the small bowel by general anesthesia and laparotomy, at times taking longer than 24 hours to normalize. This may explain the occurrence of postoperative nausea and emesis. Vagotomy-induced diarrhea is a result of persistence of the sustained, organized wave of MMCs during the postprandial state.

Segmental small bowel resection or denervation temporarily reduces the frequency of MMCs, with a resultant temporary impairment of motility. Resection or denervation does not, however, produce long-term sequelae, provided that intestinal length is not sacrificed.

**ANSWER: E**

3. During an operation for presumed appendicitis, the appendix is found to be normal. The terminal ileum, however, is markedly thickened and feels rubbery to firm. Its serosa is

erythematous and inflamed, and several loops of apparently normal small intestine are adherent to it. The terminal ileum mesentery is thickened, with fat growing about the bowel circumference. Which of the following is the most likely diagnosis?

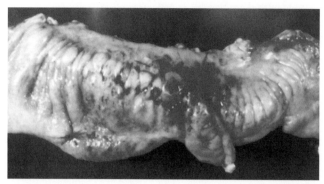

*(Courtesy of Mary R. Schwartz, M.D., Baylor College of Medicine.)*

A. Crohn's disease of the terminal ileum

B. Perforated Meckel diverticulum

C. Ulcerative colitis

D. Ileocecal tuberculosis

E. Acute ileitis

*Ref.:* 3, 4

**COMMENTS: Crohn's disease** is the most common primary disease of the small intestine that requires surgery. Its incidence is highest in the United States, England, and Scandinavia. Crohn's disease is three times more common in Jews than in non-Jews, more common in whites than in nonwhites, and slightly more common in males than in females. It occurs in all age groups but is most frequently diagnosed in young adults. The distribution of involvement is such that 30% of patients have disease limited to the small intestine and 20% to the colon. About 50% have both small and large intestinal involvement. Diseased segments may be separated by normal bowel (i.e., skip areas). Isolated involvement of the esophagus, stomach, or duodenum does occur but is rare. Crohn's disease can have an acute manifestation, and when it involves the terminal ileum, it may clinically resemble appendicitis. Involved segments of bowel may have a characteristic gross appearance. The mesenteric fat "creeps" over the serosa; the mesentery is thickened, dull, and rubbery; and it may contain lymph nodes as large as 4 cm in diameter. Not infrequently, partial obstruction of the involved segment can produce dilation of the proximal part of the bowel. Enteric fistulas to adjacent viscera may also be seen, such as to the bladder, vagina, or bowel. **Acute ileitis** may clinically mimic appendicitis and grossly appear as inflammation of the terminal ileum. The operative findings, however, do not resemble those of advanced Crohn's disease.

**Meckel diverticulitis** can mimic appendicitis clinically, but the inflammatory process is located approximately 50 cm proximal to the ileocecal valve, and the bowel wall and mesenteric changes seen with Crohn's disease are not present. **Tuberculosis of the terminal ileum**—rare in the United States—can produce scarring and stenosis of the distal ileum and enlargement of the mesenteric lymph nodes. Demonstration of caseation and acid-fast bacilli on biopsy of a mesenteric lymph node confirms the diagnosis. There may also be miliary seeding of the peritoneal cavity, seen as tiny disseminated white spots on the serosa and peritoneum. **Ulcerative colitis** is confined to the large bowel, and any associated pain can usually be distinguished from that of appendicitis.

**ANSWER:** A

4. During exploratory surgery for presumed appendicitis, the cecum and appendix are found to be normal. The terminal 50 cm of ileum, however, is inflamed, beefy red, and slightly edematous. It is soft, and there is no proximal ileal distention. Which of the following is the most appropriate operative choice?

A. Appendectomy

B. Resection of involved ileum and the appendix

C. Placement of irrigation catheters and appendectomy

D. Closure without appendectomy or ileal resection

E. Bypass ileo-ascending colostomy

*Ref.:* 3, 4

**COMMENTS:** When **acute regional enteritis** of the terminal ileum is encountered during exploration for presumed appendicitis, the appropriateness of **appendectomy** is somewhat controversial. The incidence of enterocutaneous fistula after surgery in patients with Crohn's disease is high, but the fistulas usually arise from the diseased ileum, not the appendiceal stump. In addition, 90% of patients in whom acute regional enteritis is found at surgery do not progress to chronic Crohn's disease. Symptoms resolve without sequelae. Therefore, if the stump of the appendix is not involved, most surgeons favor performance of an appendectomy. This step ameliorates the dilemma of the differential diagnosis if right lower abdominal pain develops at a later date. When acute regional enteritis is encountered, as in this clinical setting (i.e., without evidence of obstruction or fistula formation), the ileum should not be resected.

**ANSWER:** A

5. A 27-year-old man with a long-standing history of Crohn's disease is noted to have several of the extraintestinal manifestations of Crohn's disease, including erythema nodosum, arthritis, ankylosing spondylitis, anemia, and past episodes of pancreatitis. During evaluation of his right lower quadrant pain, he is found to have a segment of thickened ileum causing obstruction. Which of his extraintestinal manifestations of Crohn's disease would you not expect to subside after resecting the involved segment of bowel?

A. Erythema nodosum

B. Arthritis

C. Ankylosing spondylitis

D. Anemia

E. Pancreatitis

*Ref.:* 3

**COMMENTS:** The **extraintestinal manifestations of Crohn's disease** are listed in Box 21-1 but are not a primary indication for surgery in patients with this disease. Indications for surgery include obstruction, perforation, fistulas causing malabsorption, fistula to the urinary tract, cancer, and perianal disease. However, if the involved bowel was resected, most extraintestinal manifestations subside except for ankylosing spondylitis and hepatic complications. Bowel resection in patients with Crohn's disease should be

---

**Skin**

Erythema multiforme
Erythema nodosum
Pyoderma gangrenosum

**Eyes**

Iritis
Uveitis
Conjunctivitis

**Joints**

Peripheral arthritis
Ankylosing spondylitis

**Blood**

Anemia
Thrombocytosis
Phlebothrombosis
Arterial thrombosis

**Liver**

Nonspecific triad inflammation
Sclerosing cholangitis

**Kidneys**

Nephrotic syndrome
Amyloidosis

**Pancreas**

Pancreatitis

**General**

Amyloidosis

---

limited to the offending segment. If adjacent areas of bowel are affected but are not the cause of a complication such as perforation, obstruction, and fistula formation, that segment of the bowel should be spared. **Obstruction** is the most common indication for surgical therapy in patients with Crohn's disease. Options for obstructed segments of the bowel include segmental resection and primary anastomosis, strictureplasty, and bypass procedures. It should be kept in mind that repeated wide resections of small bowel could lead to short gut syndrome. Strictureplasty is beneficial in patients with multiple short areas of narrowing over long segments of bowel or in patients who have previously undergone small bowel resection. **Perforation** occurs in 15% to 20% of patients and usually results in the formation of a contained abscess, phlegmon, or an internal fistula to the bowel, bladder, or vagina. Enterocutaneous fistulas rarely occur in patients not previously operated on, but they are common after surgery. Free perforations into the peritoneal cavity are rare. When they do occur, they are generally on the antimesenteric border of the distal ileum, proximal to a stenotic lesion. Frank **hemorrhage** is rare, but it can occur if an ulcer erodes into a large blood vessel. Perirectal **abscesses** or **fistulas** develop in up to 30% of patients with Crohn's disease of the small bowel, usually without evidence of communication with the diseased segment of small bowel. Patients with Crohn's disease have an increased risk for the development of cancer in comparison with the general population, but the risk for colon cancer does not approach the level seen in patients with chronic ulcerative colitis. This difference may be related to the shorter period between diagnosis and colectomy for Crohn's disease than for ulcerative colitis. The risk, however, is not considered high enough to warrant prophylactic resection. Most cases of small bowel cancer associated with Crohn's disease have occurred in patients with long-standing disease and have appeared in a previously bypassed segment of bowel. They may also be formed at the site of a small bowel stricture.

**ANSWER:** C

---

6. Regarding the microscopic appearance of Crohn's disease, which of the following statements is true?

   A. The disease is confined to the mucosa.

   B. The disease is confined to the mucosa and submucosa.

   C. Granulomas demonstrating caseation without acid-fast bacilli confirm the diagnosis.

   D. Submucosal fibrosis occurs secondary to bacterial invasion.

   E. Marked lymphangiectasia is a prominent microscopic feature.

   *Ref.:* 3, 4

**COMMENTS:** Several microscopic features characterize but are nonspecific for **Crohn's disease**. These features progress from an early to a late phase of involvement and can be described as a granulomatous fibrotic inflammation progressing through all layers of the bowel wall. In the early phase, edema of the entire bowel wall is seen, accompanied by **lymphangiectasia** and hyperemia associated with an increased proportion of goblet cells in an otherwise normal mucosa.

In the intermediate phase, thickening is caused by fibrosis of the submucosal and subserosal areas of the bowel. Focal mucosal ulcers become numerous, and in 60% of patients, sarcoid-like granulomas appear, particularly in the submucosa, subserosa, and regional lymph nodes. These **granulomas** contain epithelioid giant cells, do not caseate, and do not contain acid-fast bacilli. The absence of granulomas does not exclude the diagnosis of Crohn's disease. Lymphangiectasia remains visible throughout the intermediate and late phases.

In the late phase, the dense fibrosis exceeds that expected from the simple healing of an inflammatory insult and produces a fixed stenosis and partial obstruction of the lumen. The mucosa is denuded over wide areas, with occasional islands of intact mucosal cells (pseudopolyps). Glands deep in the mucosa resemble those of the pyloric region and are termed aberrant pyloric glands or Brunner gland metaplasia. The ulcers can be deep, and progression through the bowel wall may occur, sometimes resulting in fistula formation.

**ANSWER:** E

---

7. A 17-year-old boy has persistent right lower quadrant pain as his only complaint. He has had intermittent cramping abdominal pain and normal bowel movements. He has undergone an appendectomy in the past. An upper gastrointestinal (GI) radiograph is shown in Figure 21-1. What is the next best step in his management?

   A. Nasogastric tube, steroids, and intravenous fluids

   B. Exploratory laparotomy with strictureplasty

   C. Exploratory laparotomy with ileocolic bypass

   D. Colonoscopy with intubation and biopsy of the terminal ileum

   E. Exploratory laparotomy with segmental resection

   *Ref.:* 3, 4

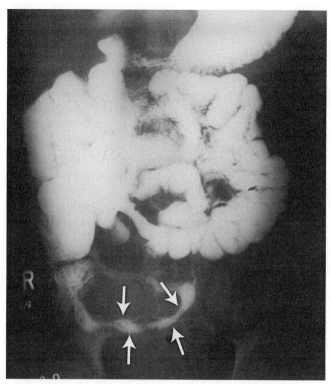

**Figure 21-1.** Upper gastrointestinal radiograph showing the classic string sign where luminal narrowing affects the passage of contrast material. Normal mucosal folds are not seen, and edema, or thickening, of the bowel wall separates the involved segment from the adjacent bowel.

**COMMENTS:** See Question 8.

**ANSWER:** E

8. The pathology from the patient in Question 7 reveals Crohn's disease. Which of the following statements is true of the etiology of this disease?

   A. The primary pathologic mechanism is progressive, obstructive lymphangitis.

   B. Crohn's disease is a form of sarcoidosis limited to the GI tract.

   C. A mouse footpad virus has been identified as the etiologic agent.

   D. The disease is the result of a local hypersensitivity reaction.

   E. The cause is unknown.

*Ref.: 3, 4*

**COMMENTS:** Despite extensive investigation, the cause of **Crohn's disease** is unknown. The possibility of a transmissible agent has emerged as a result of work demonstrating the development of granulomatous lesions in the mouse footpad following injection of intestinal homogenates obtained from patients with Crohn's disease. These results, however, have been difficult to reproduce, and their precise meaning requires further investigation. Although the granulomas associated with sarcoidosis and Crohn's disease are similar, Kveim test results, positive in 80% of patients with active sarcoidosis, are almost always negative in those with

Crohn's disease. It is generally thought that the immunologic alterations and psychosomatic manifestations seen in patients with Crohn's disease reflect responses to the disease rather than indicate its cause.

An **upper gastrointestinal series** of x-ray films with small bowel follow-through studies, as well as a barium enema with reflux into the terminal ileum, should be obtained when evaluating patients suspected of having Crohn's disease. **Barium enema** alone is not sufficient for determining the extent of disease. Luminal narrowing of the terminal ileum as a result of acute edema or chronic fibrosis of the bowel wall produces the string sign of Kantor seen on barium examination. Thickening of the bowel wall and mesentery increases the space between adjacent loops of bowel and may give the impression of extraluminal abscess formation. Fistulas may be seen but they are often obscured by adjacent loops of bowel. The mucosal pattern may be markedly distorted, and skip areas of diseased bowel with intervening normal bowel segments may also be detected.

Up to 90% of all patients with Crohn's disease ultimately need an operation. Because Crohn's disease is panintestinal and typically recurrent, surgery is not curative (all tissue at risk for Crohn's disease cannot be removed). Therefore, surgery is reserved for treating the complications of Crohn's disease, not to cure the disease. Whichever operation the surgeon chooses to perform, the foremost goal is preservation of intestinal length whenever possible. Most surgeons resect only grossly diseased bowel. Neither the use of frozen section microscopic examination to assess resection margins nor excision of involved mesenteric lymph nodes has been conclusively shown to improve the long-term course of the disease. Simple bypass and bypass with exclusion are no longer used routinely. The bypassed segment often continues to be a source of active disease, and it is prone to the development of bacterial overgrowth, obstruction, perforation, and possibly malignant transformation. **Bypass** is reserved for elderly or poor-risk patients, for patients with obstructive gastroduodenal disease (treated with gastrojejunostomy), for patients who have previously undergone extensive small bowel resection, and for instances in which resection would be too risky because of fixation to adjacent structures. Multiple fibrotic strictures in a patient who has undergone previous resections can be treated with **strictureplasty** in an attempt to conserve bowel length. In this patient, a diagnosis has not been established. He does not have evidence of bowel obstruction, so a nasogastric tube would be of little use. Recurrence of symptoms after surgery occurs in up to 50% of patients, and the yearly rate for reoperation remains constant at approximately 15%.

**ANSWER:** E

9. Regarding the clinical manifestations of Crohn's disease, which of the following statements is true?

   A. Most patients are initially seen in an acute stage with pain, nausea, and diarrhea.

   B. Bloody diarrhea is an infrequent symptom.

   C. Bloody diarrhea almost always produces anemia.

   D. Steatorrhea is present as a result of pancreatic involvement.

   E. Fever and signs of systemic toxicity are common.

*Ref.: 3, 4*

**COMMENTS:** Only 10% of patients with **Crohn's disease** are initially seen in an acute stage and with symptoms similar to those of **appendicitis**. In most instances, the onset is insidious, with intermittent pain or discomfort being the most frequent and sometimes the only symptom. The pain is often precipitated by a dietary indiscretion. With advanced disease, the pain may become associated with signs and symptoms of partial obstruction. Constant, localized pain, especially if associated with a palpable mass, suggests the presence of an abscess or bowel fistula.

Diarrhea is the next most frequent symptom, and unlike the diarrhea in patients with chronic ulcerative colitis, it rarely contains mucus, pus, or blood. Diarrhea is the result of several factors. The inflamed segment of small bowel has a decreased capacity to absorb intestinal contents. In addition, the obstruction produced by this involved segment alters the absorptive capacity of the proximal part of the bowel. Decreased absorption of bile salts in the terminal ileum leads to bile salt–induced damage to the absorptive cells of the colonic mucosa and produces a choleretic diarrhea.

One third of patients initially have fever and one half experience weight loss, weakness, and easy fatigability. Although the diarrhea is usually nonbloody, persistent occult loss of blood frequently produces anemia, which may be aggravated by deficiency of vitamin $B_{12}$. Hypoproteinemia occurs because of increased loss of protein from the inflamed bowel mucosa. Vitamin and mineral deficiencies are the results of decreased ingestion, altered metabolism, and decreased absorption.

**ANSWER:** B

10. A 26-year-old woman with a history of Crohn's disease is experiencing a Crohn's flare-up. She is 6 weeks pregnant. Which of the following is true regarding the use of corticosteroids in patients with inflammatory bowel disease?

   A. Corticosteroids are unsafe to use in pregnant patients with an acute flare-up of Crohn's disease.

   B. Corticosteroids effectively maintain remission of Crohn's colitis and ulcerative colitis.

   C. Corticosteroids used in enema (topical) form are not absorbed into the systemic circulation and therefore have no systemic side effects.

   D. Therapy every other day is effective in these patients.

   E. Intravenous corticosteroids and adrenocorticotropic hormone (ACTH) are equally effective in patients with acute severe ulcerative colitis that is refractory to oral treatment.

*Ref.:* 5

**COMMENTS:** The use of **steroids** in patients with an acute flare-up of **Crohn's colitis** or **ulcerative colitis** during pregnancy has been shown to be not only effective but also safe for the mother and fetus. The same statements apply to sulfasalazine.

Corticosteroids have never been shown to maintain remission of Crohn's colitis or ulcerative colitis. Sulfasalazine and the newer 5-acetylsalicylic acid (5-ASA) products, olsalazine and coated 5-ASA, are effective in maintaining remission of only ulcerative colitis.

Topical steroids in foam or enema preparations may be absorbed in small amounts (10% to 20%). Alternate-day dosing has not been effective in most patients with inflammatory bowel disease.

Intravenous ACTH is preferred instead of intravenous hydrocortisone by some, but controversy still exists regarding whether ACTH is more effective, even for previously untreated ulcerative colitis. An ACTH dose of 40 to 60 units over an 8-hour period appears to be as effective as 300 to 400 mg/day of hydrocortisone.

The duration of steroid therapy varies, depending on the severity of the disease, but it should always be tapered on an individual basis, with the goal of discontinuation. Many patients (10% to 15%) are kept on a low maintenance dose when complete elimination leads to flare-up. However, steroid therapy should not be continued as maintenance in patients who have achieved complete remission. Failure to achieve remission after 2 months of administering more than 15 mg of prednisone may be considered an indication for an operation.

**ANSWER:** E

11. For patients with inflammatory bowel disease refractory to medical treatment, nutritional support may influence the course of disease. Which of the following statements is true?

   A. Bowel rest and parenteral nutrition are the primary therapy for Crohn's colitis.

   B. Total parenteral nutrition (TPN) helps prevent the need for total colectomy in patients with ulcerative colitis.

   C. In patients with Crohn's ileitis, TPN is superior to enteral nutrition for providing adequate caloric replacement.

   D. In those with Crohn's disease and a high-output fistula, TPN promotes closure of the fistula.

   E. An elemental diet is the primary therapy for exacerbation of Crohn's disease.

*Ref.:* 6

**COMMENTS: Total parenteral nutrition** has no role as primary therapy for ulcerative colitis, but it may help maintain a satisfactory nutritional state during bowel rest. TPN does not prevent the need for colectomy in refractory cases. The role of TPN in patients with **Crohn's colitis** is not well established, but in those with Crohn's colitis and small bowel involvement, TPN may induce remission and promote fistula closure. Elemental diets have been shown by some to be effective in inducing remission of active Crohn's disease. The patient's tolerance may be poor, however, and the results are not superior to those obtained with corticosteroids and sulfasalazine. Peripheral intravenous alimentation rarely provides adequate caloric replacement and may induce venous sclerosis and phlebitis.

**ANSWER:** D

12. A 30-year-old woman has a bowel obstruction secondary to Crohn's disease. She has undergone multiple previous small bowel resections. At laparotomy, multiple strictures are noted throughout her bowel. Which of the following statements is true?

   A. Strictureplasty should be considered only for patients with an isolated stricture.

   B. Segmental bowel resections are preferable to strictureplasty for the current laparotomy.

   C. Anastomotic leakage and fistula formation following strictureplasty have been seen in 50% of cases.

   D. Restricture at the strictureplasty site has been seen in less than 5% of patients.

   E. Because residual disease is left behind, reoperation for Crohn's disease is more likely with strictureplasty than with bowel resection.

*Ref.:* 1

**COMMENTS: Strictureplasty** for **Crohn's disease** was first performed in 1981. Experience since then has shown it to be a safe alternative to resection in properly selected patients. Strictureplasty should be considered in any patient who has had extensive previous resections of diseased bowel and in whom further resection might create short bowel syndrome. Multiple strictures can be treated safely at a single laparotomy. The entire small bowel must be inspected to avoid overlooking strictures that are not obvious. This can be accomplished by passing, via a proximal enterostomy, a long intestinal tube with the balloon inflated to a diameter of 2 cm through the entire length of small bowel. Ideally, fibrotic rather than acute edematous strictures are treated. A longitudinal incision is made over the stricture and extended for 2 cm proximally and distally beyond the stricture. The enterotomy is then closed transversely. If a stricture is encountered at a patient's first surgery, resection rather than strictureplasty is preferable because it eliminates diseased bowel and establishes the diagnosis. Patients treated by strictureplasty have been compared with patients treated by resection. The need for reoperation at the original site is similar. Postoperative complications are infrequent. At the Cleveland Clinic, anastomotic leakage, abscesses, or fistulas have occurred in 9% of patients treated by strictureplasty. Restricture at the strictureplasty site occurred in only 2%.

**ANSWER:** D

13. A 54-year-old man is being assessed for colicky abdominal pain and occasional nonbilious emesis. He denies fevers and does not have leukocytosis. He has a history of melanoma that was resected from his arm 5 years earlier. His upper GI radiograph is shown in Figure 21-2. What is the next best step in this patient's management?

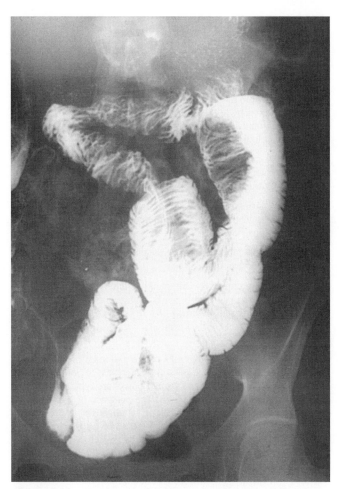

**Figure 21-2.** Upper gastrointestinal tract. *(Courtesy of Melvyn H. Schreiber, M.D., The University of Texas Medical Branch.)*

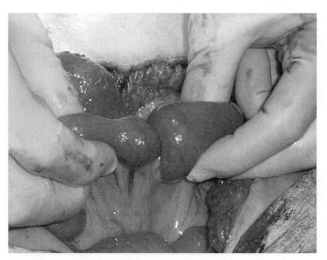

**Figure 21-3.** Intussusception. *(Courtesy of Steven Williams, M.D., Nampa, Idaho.)*

A. Barium enema with pneumatic decompression

B. Exploratory laparotomy and manual reduction

C. Exploratory laparotomy, manual reduction, and resection of the involved segment

D. Nasogastric tube placement, intravenous fluid, and a trial of nonoperative management

E. Exploratory laparotomy and intestinal bypass

*Ref.:* 3, 7

**COMMENTS: Intussusception** is the telescoping of one portion of an intestinal segment onto the lumen of an adjacent segment (Figure 21-3). It is commonly seen in children and is the most frequent cause of pediatric bowel obstruction. It is rare in adults, in whom it accounts for less than 5% of cases of bowel obstruction. Most cases of intussusception in adults are caused by a lead point, whereas only 8% to 20% are idiopathic. Causes of intussusception in adults include inflammatory bowel disease, adhesions, Meckel diverticulum, neoplasms, and intestinal tubes. Barium enema is useful for intussusception in children because it is diagnostic and therapeutic. However, barium enemas and pneumatic decompression are not useful in adults. Surgery is the mainstay for symptomatic adult intussusception. A formal bowel resection with oncologic principles is warranted when malignancy is suspected, such as in this patient with a history of melanoma. Melanoma can metastasize to the small intestine.

**ANSWER:** C

14. A 26-year-old man arrives at the emergency department with a complaint of recurrent, colicky, midabdominal pain. Physical examination reveals a palpable abdominal mass and several areas of increased pigmentation on his lips, palms, and soles. He states that his father had a colon polyp removed several years ago. Computed tomography (CT) of the abdomen was performed (Figure 21-4). Which of the following is the most likely diagnosis?

A. Familial polyposis with malignant degeneration

B. Gardner syndrome with intussusception

C. Peutz-Jeghers syndrome (PJS) with intussusception

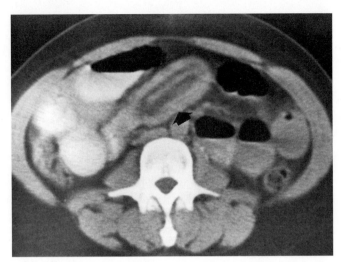

**Figure 21-4.** Abdominal computed tomographic scan.

D. Symptomatic Crohn's disease

E. Idiopathic intussusception

*Ref.:* 3, 4

**COMMENTS: Peutz-Jeghers syndrome** is an autosomal dominant familial disease characterized by intestinal polyposis and mucocutaneous hyperpigmentation. The polyps are hamartomas that are most frequently located in the jejunum and ileum, but they can also be found in the stomach, duodenum, colon, and rectum. It is generally believed that their malignant potential is extremely low. PJS can cause intussusception or hemorrhage. Up to one third of patients initially have abdominal pain and a palpable mass. Surgery is indicated for obstruction or bleeding and should be limited to conservative resection of the involved portion of bowel rather than attempt to resect all polyps.

**ANSWER:** C

15. A 60-year-old alcoholic man has a 24-hour history of nausea and vomiting, abdominal pain, distention, and decreased passage of stool and flatus. He underwent abdominoperineal resection of the rectum for cancer 18 months earlier, along with postoperative irradiation and chemotherapy. Examination reveals a distended, diffusely tender, tympanitic abdomen. Which of the following is the least likely diagnosis?

A. Pancreatitis with ileus

B. Adhesive bowel obstruction

C. Bowel obstruction caused by extrinsic compression

D. Bowel obstruction secondary to radiation injury

E. Alcoholic hepatitis with ascites

*Ref.:* 3, 4

**COMMENTS:** The classic manifestation of **bowel obstruction** is the triad of nausea and vomiting, cramping abdominal pain, and decreased passage of stool and flatus. However, nonobstructive conditions may have similar findings.

**Ileus** is temporary paralysis of the bowel caused by metabolic or neurologic factors. Electrolyte disorders (particularly hypokalemia) may cause paralytic ileus by disrupting the normal electrical activity of intestinal nerves and muscles. Neural reflexes that inhibit intestinal motor activity may be caused by distention of a hollow viscus (ureter), retroperitoneal processes (e.g., hemorrhage, pancreatitis, or spinal fracture), or peritonitis.

**Mechanical bowel obstruction** may be the result of a process extrinsic to the bowel wall, intrinsic to the bowel wall, or within the lumen of the bowel. Extrinsic lesions cause obstruction by kinking or compression of the lumen of the bowel. Intra-abdominal adhesions form in up to 90% of patients after abdominal surgery and may also follow intra-abdominal inflammatory conditions (e.g., diverticulitis or abscess). Adhesions may cause a fixed bend in the bowel or a tight band crossing a segment of bowel, or they can act as a focus for the bowel to twist on itself (volvulus). Adhesions are the most common cause of small bowel obstruction in adults. The other two major categories of extrinsic bowel obstruction are hernias and masses. Hernias may be external (inguinal, femoral, ventral, or perineal) or internal (caused by congenital or surgical defects in the mesentery). Obstructing masses may be neoplastic (primary malignancy, carcinomatosis, or desmoid tumor) or inflammatory (phlegmon or abscess). Intrinsic lesions may be congenital (atresia or duplication), anastomotic or inflammatory (Crohn's disease, radiation injury, or recovered ischemic bowel), or neoplastic (adenocarcinoma, melanoma, lymphoma, or sarcoma). Intraluminal lesions may cause bowel obstruction by acting as a lead point for intussusception or by acting as masslike intraluminal contents (large gallstone, bezoar, inspissated barium, stool, or foreign object).

Although abdominal distention may be because of ascites, its onset is much more gradual than 24 hours, and it is usually painless.

**ANSWER:** E

16. Which of the following statements is true regarding the radiographic appearance of small bowel obstruction?

A. Gas within the small bowel is distinguished from gas within the colon by luminal lines perpendicular to the bowel wall. The small bowel lines partially cross the lumen, whereas the colonic lines completely cross the lumen.

B. Ileus may be difficult to distinguish from small bowel obstruction, because both conditions can produce gaseous distention of the bowel with air-fluid levels.

C. The "string of pearls" sign refers to a series of radiolucent images in the small bowel representing the gallstones of gallstone ileus.

D. A gasless abdomen seen on plain films rules out small bowel obstruction.

E. The distinction between complete and partial small bowel obstructions during the early stages is made by assessing the colonic gas pattern.

*Ref.:* 3, 4

**COMMENTS:** Plain radiographs of the abdomen are useful for evaluating patients with a possible diagnosis of **small bowel obstruction**. Gas-filled loops of small bowel are typically seen in the central portion of the abdomen. The presence of both dilated (>4 cm) and normal-diameter (<2 cm) small bowel is typical of small bowel obstruction. Small bowel loops are recognized by the **valvulae conniventes (plicae circulares)**, which are visible as lines that completely cross the lumen. Colonic loops are usually located peripherally and have lines within them that only partially cross the lumen (**plicae semilunares** and **haustra**).

Air-fluid levels are seen with both small bowel obstruction and ileus. They are apparent only on upright or decubitus views, which allow gravity to be directed perpendicular to the x-ray beam, with pooling of intestinal fluid in the dependent portion of the bowel. The string of pearls sign is a series of small radiolucent circles seen when a small amount of air at the top of an air-fluid level is broken by several valvulae conniventes in a row.

A gasless abdomen may be seen in patients with small bowel obstruction. It may be the result of decompression of the obstructed proximal part of the bowel by emesis or nasogastric suctioning, or there may be completely fluid-filled bowel with no visible air.

Distinction between partial and complete bowel obstructions is important. A partial obstruction is present when the patient is able to pass some gas and liquid stool beyond the obstruction. Radiographically, this condition is recognized by gas seen in decompressed bowel distal to the transition point. In contrast, complete small bowel obstruction is manifested as an absence of flatus and stool (obstipation), and no gas is seen distal to the dilated proximal part of the bowel. Early, complete bowel obstruction may be confused with partial obstruction when distal gas and stool, present before the obstruction developed, have not yet been evacuated.

**ANSWER: B**

17. Which of the following is true regarding the initial treatment of patients with acute, complete small bowel obstruction?

A. Immediate surgery is warranted as soon as the diagnosis is made.

B. Nasogastric decompression for 24 hours allows spontaneous resolution of complete bowel obstruction in most patients.

C. The presence of fever, tachycardia, localized pain, or leukocytosis suggests strangulation and warrants prompt surgery.

D. All patients with complete small bowel obstruction require blood and plasma for resuscitation.

E. If a small bowel resection must be performed, a stoma and mucous fistula are necessary because an anastomosis is subject to nonhealing in the face of obstruction.

*Ref.:* 3, 4

**COMMENTS:** Timing an operation **for a small bowel obstruction** requires considerable clinical judgment. The duration of initial resuscitation must be balanced against the need to prevent gangrene by prompt intervention. Severe intravascular volume depletion can occur as a result of fluid sequestration (as much as 6 L) in the lumen of the bowel and peritoneal cavity. Sodium, chloride, and potassium depletion frequently accompanies bowel obstruction. Blood loss is unusual unless strangulation is present. Before induction of general anesthesia, fluid and electrolyte replacement should be instituted with isotonic saline solution to normalize the heart rate, blood pressure, and urine output. Potassium repletion should begin once adequate urine output is established. Surgery is delayed until the patient is stabilized. Nasogastric decompression is an important component of supportive therapy, nausea and vomiting are controlled by this measure, and the risk for aspiration is reduced. Swallowed air is evacuated, thus further limiting intestinal distention.

In patients with adhesive partial bowel obstruction and no signs of strangulation (i.e., fever, tachycardia, localized abdominal pain, or leukocytosis), a 24- to 48-hour period of bowel rest and nasogastric decompression is warranted. In most patients, the obstruction resolves spontaneously. Delay in surgical intervention for complete small bowel obstruction is not recommended (beyond

the period of resuscitation) because the possibility of strangulation is higher than with partial bowel obstruction.

There is no increase in the anastomotic leakage rate of small bowel anastomoses in urgent versus elective small bowel resections, provided that the segment of bowel used for the anastomosis is healthy. Therefore, a proximal stoma and mucous fistula are seldom necessary following small bowel resection for obstruction.

**ANSWER: C**

18. An 85-year-old woman has severe abdominal pain and abdominal distention. She is tachycardic, oliguric, and acidotic. She underwent abdominal radiographs, which showed pneumobilia and a mass (Figure 21-5). What is the best surgical management for this patient during exploratory laparotomy?

A. Resection of the mass

B. "Milking" the mass distally past the obstruction

C. Enterotomy and removal of the mass

D. Cholecystectomy, enterotomy, and removal of the mass

E. Hepaticojejunostomy

*Ref.:* 3

**COMMENTS:** This patient has **gallstone ileus**. Gallstone ileus accounts for 1% of all intestinal obstructions. It is caused by the passage of a large stone through a biliary enteric fistula, thus producing a bowel obstruction. The most common manifestation of

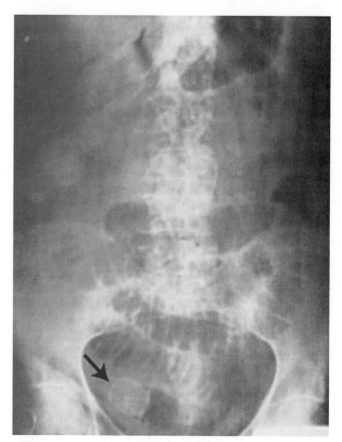

**Figure 21-5.** Abdominal radiograph showing pneumobilia and a mass (*arrow*).

gallstone ileus includes nausea, vomiting, and abdominal pain. About 50% of patients will have gallbladder-related symptoms. Plain abdominal radiographs can reveal pneumobilia, dilated loops of small bowel, and a calcified stone outside the gallbladder. The most common site of obstruction in patients with gallstone ileus is the terminal ileum because of the narrow lumen at the ileocecal junction.

Gallstone ileus is treated surgically. Obstruction is relieved by milking the stone in a retrograde fashion and removing it through a proximal enterotomy. The segment of bowel at the site of impaction should be inspected for evidence of ischemia and necrosis. If ischemic compromise has occurred, the ischemic bowel should be resected. Takedown of the biliary-enteric fistula and cholecystectomy can be done during the initial laparotomy. However, in patients who are not able to tolerate a prolonged operation, the fistula can be addressed at a second laparotomy.

**ANSWER: C**

19. A woman is undergoing open incisional hernia repair through a previous cesarean section incision. During the operation this structure (seen below) is noted about 60 cm from the ileocecal valve. What is true regarding this incidental finding?

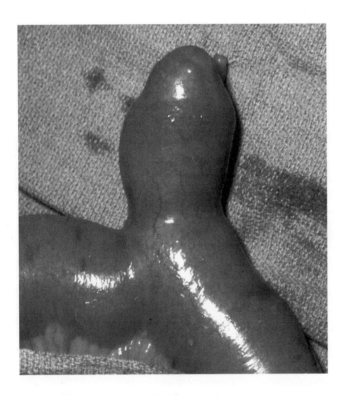

A. They are true diverticula.

B. They are found in various anatomic forms and clinical manifestations in 50% of the population.

C. Pancreatic tissue is the most common ectopic tissue found in this diverticula.

D. Most complications occur in the elderly.

E. Diverticulitis is the most common complication.

*Ref.: 3, 4*

**COMMENTS:** A **Meckel diverticulum**, the most frequently encountered diverticulum involving the small intestine, occurs in 2% to 4% of the general population. It is a true diverticulum and arises from the antimesenteric border of the ileum, 50 to 75 cm from the ileocecal valve. The diverticulum is a result of abnormal regression of the vitelline duct. Frequently, there is a persistent band of tissue extending from the tip of the diverticulum to the umbilicus.

The diverticulum may contain ectopic gastric mucosa capable of producing peptic ulceration and bleeding in adjacent ileal mucosa. This ectopic gastric mucosa can be visualized with $^{99m}$Tc-labeled scans. Gastric tissue is the most common ectopic tissue and is found in 50%. Pancreatic and colonic tissue may also be found in the diverticulum less commonly. Clinical problems are most often seen in the pediatric population. The most frequent complications are bleeding, intussusception, and obstruction. The latter is generally caused by volvulus or twisting around the persistent band. The least common complication is diverticulitis, which is clinically manifested as lower abdominal pain and is usually diagnosed as appendicitis. Therapy consists of diverticulectomy for uncomplicated diverticulitis and segmental ileal resection for bleeding or for complicated diverticulitis. **Prophylactic diverticulectomy** for an incidentally found Meckel diverticulum is controversial. Some clinicians report that diverticulectomy is not generally performed when a diverticulum is found incidentally unless there is evidence of ectopic gastric mucosa or the neck of the diverticulum is narrow. The rate of complications from a Meckel diverticulum is about 6.4% over a lifetime. Other clinicians argue that postoperative complications after prophylactic removal are low (<2%) and that it should therefore be removed.

**ANSWER: A**

20. Concerning duodenal, jejunal, and ileal diverticula, which of the following statements is true?

A. Duodenal diverticula are true diverticula.

B. Duodenal diverticula are often multiple, whereas jejunal diverticula are often solitary.

C. Asymptomatic duodenal diverticula should be resected to avoid potentially serious complications.

D. Asymptomatic jejunal diverticula do not require therapy.

E. Duodenal diverticula usually cause symptoms and are found during specific work-up.

*Ref.: 4*

**COMMENTS:** Most duodenal, jejunal, and ileum diverticula are asymptomatic and found incidentally. **Diverticula** of the duodenum, jejunum, and ileum are false (pulsion) diverticula and lack muscularis propria. Duodenal diverticula are usually solitary and project medially toward the head of the pancreas. Although most are asymptomatic, 10% of patients have nonspecific epigastric symptoms, such as bleeding and perforation. In instances of perforation, the local site should be drained. Gastrojejunostomy is the operation most often applicable, although biliary decompression is occasionally necessary. In instances of bleeding without inflammation, diverticulectomy is indicated, either from a dorsal approach using the Kocher maneuver or via a duodenotomy.

**Jejunal and ileal diverticula** are often multiple and project from the mesenteric border of the bowel into the leaves of the mesentery. This type of diverticulum is more common in the jejunum than in the ileum. The usual treatment of symptomatic diverticula in these areas is segmental resection. Asymptomatic diverticula of the duodenum, jejunum, or ileum do not require therapy.

**ANSWER: D**

**21.** What is the most common finding with small bowel tumors?

A. Hematemesis

B. Perforation

C. Abdominal pain

D. Intussusception

E. Anemia

*Ref.:* 3

**COMMENTS:** See Question 22.

**ANSWER:** C

**22.** What is the most common benign small bowel tumor?

A. Lipoma

B. Gastrointestinal stromal tumor (GIST)

C. Hamartoma

D. Hemangioma

E. Adenoma

*Ref.:* 3, 8

**COMMENTS:** The most frequent symptom of **small bowel tumors** is abdominal pain. Common benign lesions of the small intestine include **gastrointestinal stromal tumors**, **adenoma**, and **hemangioma**. The most common benign small bowel tumor is an adenoma. The most common *symptomatic* small bowel tumors are GISTs. Symptoms associated with small bowel tumors are often vague and nonspecific such as anorexia, dyspepsia, and abdominal pain. Patients may also have signs of obstruction that are usually related to intussusception. Occult bleeding is likewise a common initial symptom. When small bowel neoplasms are suspected, a barium small bowel follow-through study is indicated and is generally diagnostic.

GISTs arise from the interstitial cells of Cajal. They express CD117 and CD34. These tumors grow intramurally and can cause obstruction. At times, these tumors can reach considerable size and outgrow their blood supply, which results in GI bleeding. Mitotic rates higher than five per 50 high-power fields increase the risk for recurrence. Lipomas are included in the GIST category.

There are three types of **small bowel adenomas**: adenomatous polyps, villous adenomas, and Brunner gland adenomas. Most of these lesions are asymptomatic and found incidentally at the time of autopsy. Adenomas are usually manifested as bleeding or obstruction. The treatment of choice is segmental resection. Polypectomy may be performed in the duodenum if the tumor is histologically benign. Hamartomas of the small bowel are a part of PJS. Patients have 1- to 2-mm pigmented lesions located in the circumoral region of the face, buccal mucosa, palms, soles, and perianal region, as well as in the jejunum, ileum, and less commonly the stomach, colon, and rectum. The most common initial symptom is colicky abdominal pain, usually as a result of intermittent intussusception.

Hemangiomas are malformations consisting of a submucosal proliferation of blood vessels. They can occur anywhere along the GI tract, with the jejunum being the most common small bowel segment involved. Bleeding is the most frequent symptom. Angiography and $^{99m}$Tc-labeled red blood cell scanning are useful diagnostic studies.

When identified, small bowel tumors should be excised because of the risk for complications, to establish the diagnosis, and to exclude cancer. Very small lesions can be excised with an enterotomy and primary closure performed. Usually, segmental resection with primary anastomosis is needed.

**ANSWER:** E

**23.** What is the most common primary malignant small bowel tumor?

A. Leiomyosarcoma

B. Adenocarcinoma

C. Carcinoid

D. Lymphoma

E. GIST

*Ref.:* 3, 4

**COMMENTS:** See Question 24.

**ANSWER:** B

**24.** What is the most common finding in patients with malignant small bowel tumors?

A. Hematemesis

B. Perforation

C. Abdominal pain

D. Intussusception

E. Anemia

*Ref.:* 3, 4

**COMMENTS:** **Malignant tumors of the small bowel** account for 2% of all GI malignancies. The most frequent primary type is **adenocarcinoma**, followed in decreasing frequency by **carcinoid**, **GIST**, and **lymphoma**. Although adenocarcinoma occurs with equal frequency in the duodenum, jejunum, and ileum, the other types tend to occur most often in the ileum. In contrast to benign lesions, malignant lesions of the small intestine are usually accompanied by pain and weight loss. Other clinical manifestations may include diarrhea, obstruction, or chronic blood loss with anemia. Obstruction from malignant lesions is usually because of tumor infiltration and adhesion. The preferred therapy is wide resection with regional lymphadenectomy. For each entity, survival is dependent on a number of factors and is variable, but in general, GISTs have a 5-year survival rate that ranges from 7% to 56%, lymphomas have a 5-year survival rate of about 40%, and adenocarcinoma has the lowest (about 20%). Postoperative chemotherapy and radiation therapy can be useful in treating a patient with lymphoma but are not useful adjuncts for adenocarcinoma or sarcoma. Histiocytic lymphoma may develop in patients with long-standing celiac sprue and has a worse prognosis than do conventional small bowel lymphomas. The Mediterranean-type lymphoma, a variant associated with monoclonal alpha heavy chains and a dense plasma cell tumor infiltration, also carries a bad prognosis.

**ANSWER:** C

**25.** A 54-year-old man reports a 2-month history of abdominal pain and significant weight loss. He has undergone upper endoscopy, lower endoscopy, and CT, all of which had normal findings. On a barium upper GI study with small bowel follow-through, he was noted to have a mass in his midileum. At surgical exploration he is found to have a carcinoid tumor on frozen section in the midileum. Which statement is true regarding his condition?

A. The prognosis is related to tumor size, location, and histologic pattern.

B. The cell of origin is the Kupffer cell.

C. The rectum is the most common site of origin.

D. Carcinoid tumors are usually easily palpable on external physical examination of the bowel.

E. Resection is not indicated in patients with metastatic disease.

*Ref.: 2-4*

**COMMENTS:** The origin of **carcinoid tumors** is the Kulchitsky cell, which is thought to arise from the neural crest. Carcinoids can occur anywhere in the GI tract. The most frequent site is the appendix, followed by the ileum and rectum. Extraintestinal sites include the bronchus and ovarries. Small bowel carcinoid tumors tend to be multiple in 30% of cases, and a second GI tumor of another histologic type can be found in 30% of patients. The prognosis is a function of the size of the tumor and its site of origin. Ileal carcinoids tend to metastasize more commonly than do those that originate in the appendix.

The usual submucosal location of carcinoid tumors often makes them difficult to find on radiographic examination or with cursory palpation during exploratory laparotomy. The tumors may incite an intense fibrotic reaction in the surrounding soft tissue and mesentery, which can cause luminal narrowing. Mesenteric lymph node and liver metastases can be large in comparison with the primary tumor. Tumors less than 1 cm in diameter and without demonstrable metastases can be treated by excision or segmental resection. Those larger than 1 cm or with regional metastases should be excised widely. The excision should include right hemicolectomy for lesions of the distal ileum and appendix. For patients with metastases (local or distant) and in whom carcinoid syndrome is present, removal of the primary tumor and debulking of metastatic disease can provide considerable palliation.

**ANSWER:** A

26. A 54-year-old man reports a 2-month history of abdominal pain, diarrhea, flushing, palpitations, and significant weight loss. He underwent upper endoscopy and lower endoscopy, the findings of which were normal. CT demonstrated several hepatic lesions. Percutaneous biopsy of one of the liver lesions revealed carcinoid tumor. On a barium upper GI study with small bowel follow-through, he was noted to have a mass in his midileum. Which statement is true regarding his condition?

A. Cardiac manifestations occur early and primarily affect the mitral and aortic valves.

B. Cutaneous phenomena, such as flushing, are the most characteristic and frequently recognized manifestations.

C. Diarrhea is a significant complaint in less than 30% of patients.

D. The most useful diagnostic test for suspected carcinoid syndrome is determination of serum serotonin levels.

E. Carcinoid syndrome does not develop in patients with normal serotonin levels.

*Ref.: 2-4*

**COMMENTS:** Episodic manifestations of **carcinoid syndrome** include flushing, diarrhea, and asthma. The cutaneous manifestations are the most common and consist of episodes of flushing of the face, neck, arms, and upper part of the trunk, occasionally accompanied by vasomotor collapse. Diarrhea is significant in more than 80% of patients and is usually sudden in onset, watery, and accompanied by cramping pain and borborygmi. Asthmatic attacks occur in 25% of patients. Manifestations of long-standing involvement include the development of facial hyperemia with telangiectases on the cheeks, nose, and forehead; development of the cutaneous lesions of pellagra; and valvular heart disease. The valves most commonly involved are the tricuspid and pulmonic, although the mitral and aortic valves are sometimes affected. Peripheral edema is present in about 70% of patients and can occur in the absence of valvular disease.

Functioning carcinoid tumors divert up to 60% of dietary tryptophan into the production of serotonin, thereby contributing to the development of pellagra and protein deficiency. Serotonin is metabolized in the liver to **5-hydroxyindolacetic acid** (5-HIAA), which is excreted in urine. For this reason, the most useful diagnostic test in patients suspected of having a carcinoid tumor is determination of 5-HIAA levels in a 24-hour collection of urine. 5-HIAA is inactive and does not cause carcinoid syndrome. It is produced by release of serotonin into the systemic circulation either by liver metastases or by tumors located outside the portal distribution. Although it is generally believed that patients with carcinoid syndrome have tumors that produce serotonin, the role of serotonin in mediation of the syndrome is not clear. Not all patients with elevated production of serotonin have the syndrome. Some patients with the syndrome have normal levels of 5-HIAA in urine, and injection of pure serotonin does not create all of the manifestations of the disease. It is likely that carcinoid tumors have the capacity to produce a number of biologically active peptides, which accounts for the variability of the syndrome and discrepancies between a patient's serotonin levels and the clinical findings. Other substances produced by carcinoid tumors include histamine, dopamine, kallikrein, substance P, prostaglandins, and neuropeptide K. Treatment of carcinoid crisis include intravenous octreotide, intravenous antihistamine, and hydrocortisone.

**ANSWER:** B

27. On abdominal exploration for a suspected carcinoid tumor, a 2 cm mass is found at the terminal ileum. No liver lesions were detected on preoperative imaging or with intraoperative palpation. What is the best treatment option for this patient?

A. Segmental resection

B. Medical therapy with octreotide

C. Resection of the terminal ileum with preservation of the ileocecal valve

D. Right hemicolectomy with wide resection of the terminal ileum

E. Neoadjuvant therapy with streptozotocin and 5-fluorouracil

*Ref.: 3*

**COMMENTS: Treatment of small bowel carcinoid** is based on tumor size and the presence or absence of metastatic disease. Segmental resection is adequate for tumors smaller than 1 cm without regional lymph node metastasis. Wide excision is indicated for lesions larger than 1 cm, multiple tumors, or regional lymph node metastasis. Right hemicolectomy is indicated for lesions of the terminal ileum. Debulking is indicated for metastatic carcinoid tumors. This may involve liver resection. Hepatic artery ligation or percutaneous embolization has also produced good results in controlling the carcinoid symptoms produced by liver metastasis.

Medical therapy for patients with malignant carcinoid is directed at relieving symptoms. Octreotide, a somatostatin analogue, helps relieve symptoms in most patients. Regression of tumor with the use of octreotide has been reported. Interferon alfa has also been shown to relieve symptoms. Chemotherapeutic agents such as streptozotocin and 5-fluorouracil have had limited success in treating malignant carcinoid. They are used mostly in patients with metastatic disease who are symptomatic and unresponsive to other therapies.

**ANSWER:** D

28. Somatostatin has emerged as a safe and effective agent with a broad range of applications. Which of the following is true for patients with carcinoid tumors?

A. Somatostatin may be used as a provocative agent before measuring 5-HIAA levels.

B. Somatostatin receptor scintigraphy is more effective than CT or magnetic resonance imaging (MRI) in localizing primary and metastatic carcinoid tumors.

C. Somatostatin is ineffective for the management of carcinoid crisis.

D. Somatostatin therapy improves survival in patients with carcinoid syndrome.

E. Administration of somatostatin can be used as a provocative diagnostic test.

*Ref.:* 2, 3

**COMMENTS: Somatostatin** was first identified in 1973. Since then, a great deal of interest has been directed at characterizing and identifying its physiologic effects and the clinical utility of somatostatin and its analogues. Somatostatin is a 14–amino acid protein with several analogues of shorter lengths that maintain clinical effectiveness. The general effects of somatostatin are those of an inhibitory hormone. Several provocative agents may be used before conducting tests for neuroendocrine tumors, including pentagastrin, secretin, and calcium infusion. Somatostatin is not effective as a provocative agent.

**Somatostatin receptor scintigraphy** uses indium-111 and a gamma camera. This study has several advantages over conventional imaging (CT or MRI). Its sensitivity is higher (90% versus 70%) for metastatic disease, it is more effective in identifying the primary tumor site, and it visualizes the entire body to detect occult metastases. Carcinoid tumors visible by somatostatin receptor scintigraphy suggest that these particular tumors have somatostatin receptors and are therefore subject to the inhibitory effects of somatostatin.

**Carcinoid crisis** is a life-threatening episode that may develop during episodes of flushing, anesthesia, or surgery. Severe hypotension and bronchospasm may occur during carcinoid crises, and they may be refractory to the usual supportive care. The reported incidence of such crises is variable and ranges from 2% to 50%. Somatostatin may be administered preoperatively as a prophylactic agent or during a carcinoid crisis as a therapeutic agent. It is usually successful in reversing the condition.

Somatostatin has also been found to be highly effective in relieving the symptoms of carcinoid syndrome. It has even been suggested that chronic octreotide therapy results in longer survival in patients with carcinoid syndrome than in those treated with chemotherapy, but this hypothesis remains to be proved by randomized, controlled trials.

**ANSWER:** B

29. Which of the following conditions is not associated with an increased risk for small bowel malignancy?

A. Celiac disease

B. Crohn's disease

C. Scleroderma

D. Familial adenomatous polyposis

E. PJS

*Ref.:* 9

**COMMENTS: Cancer in the small intestine** is a relatively uncommon occurrence despite the fact that the small bowel contains approximately 90% of the surface area of the alimentary tract. Several conditions are associated with an increased risk for small bowel cancer. However, it is difficult to assess the magnitude of the increased risk, because small bowel cancers are uncommon and the number in any particular series is low.

**Celiac disease** is a chronic inflammatory condition of the small intestine. Lymphoma, esophageal carcinoma, and small bowel adenocarcinoma occur with increased frequency in patients with celiac disease. The majority of lymphomas occur in the small intestine, and adenocarcinoma is the next most frequent small bowel cancer in patients with celiac disease.

**Crohn's disease** is another chronic inflammatory condition that affects the small intestine. Risk factors associated with Crohn's disease and the development of adenocarcinoma in the small bowel include bypassed (rather than resected) segments of Crohn's disease, chronic fistulas, multiple strictures, long duration of disease in a particular segment of bowel, and male gender.

**Familial adenomatous polyposis** and **Peutz-Jeghers syndrome** are both inherited conditions. There is a strong propensity for the development of adenomas in patients with familial adenomatous polyposis and hamartomatous polyps in those with PJS. Both conditions are associated with an increased risk for adenocarcinoma of the small bowel.

**ANSWER:** C

30. A 62-year-old woman complains of abdominal pain and weight loss. She undergoes a small bowel follow-through study (Figure 21-6). Her past medical and surgical history includes a stable small right lung nodule, removal of a skin lesion on her right leg, and endoscopic polypectomy of a gastric polyp. She has a strong family history of breast cancer. If the lesion noted in the stomach is metastatic, what is the most likely primary cancer?

A. Squamous cell skin cancer

B. Lymphoma

C. Lung cancer

D. Breast cancer

E. Melanoma

*Ref.:* 3

**COMMENTS: Metastatic tumors** of the small bowel are more common than primary tumors. The most common metastases to the

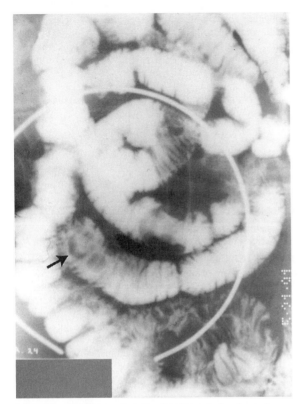

**Figure 21-6.** Small bowel study showing a lesion (*arrow*). (*Courtesy of Melvyn H. Schreiber, M.D., The University of Texas Medical Branch.*)

small bowel are primary tumors arising from other intra-abdominal organs. In these cases, small bowel involvement occurs by either direct extension or implantation of tumor cells. Extra-abdominal metastasis to the small bowel is rare. **Cutaneous myeloma** is the most common extra-abdominal source of metastasis to the small bowel. Other extra-abdominal sources include breast and lung cancers. Treatment is palliative resection or bypass if the metastatic tumor is not amenable to resection.

**ANSWER:** E

31. A 56-year-old woman underwent pelvic radiation therapy 5 years ago for cervical cancer. Now, 5 days after a right hemi-colectomy for villous adenoma of the cecum, her surgical wound is red and tender. The surgeon opens her wound, and the initial drainage is obviously purulent. The drainage persists as a continuous brown, liquid discharge. Which of the following is the most likely diagnosis?

    A. Simple wound infection

    B. Clostridial infection

    C. Anastomotic leakage with an enterocutaneous fistula

    D. Dehiscence

    E. Cellulitis

*Ref.:* 4

**COMMENTS:** Most **fistulas** are iatrogenic and result from **anastomotic leakage**, inadvertent injury to the bowel during the operation, laceration of the bowel during abdominal closure, or retained foreign bodies. Less than 2% of fistulas are the result of diseased bowel. When they are, the most common contributing factors are preoperative radiation therapy, intestinal obstruction, and inflammatory bowel disease. Although small bowel fistulas occasionally lead to generalized peritonitis, they most commonly produce a walled-off abscess manifested as an infection of the operative incision. The initial drainage may be purulent, but if the infection is caused by anastomotic leakage of the small bowel, the drainage becomes enteric within 1 to 2 days.

**ANSWER:** C

32. For the patient described in Question 31, which of the following is the most appropriate initial management?

    A. Packing of subcutaneous tissue with wet-to-dry dressings

    B. Packing of subcutaneous tissue with dry, absorbent dressings

    C. Immediate return to the operating room for exploration

    D. Protecting the skin around the fistula with Stomahesive karaya powder, aluminum paste, or zinc oxide and collecting the drainage fluid in an attached plastic bag

    E. Antibiotic and wet-to-dry dressing changes

*Ref.:* 4

**COMMENTS:** The initial management of a **small bowel fistula** includes the administration of appropriate intravenous fluids, proximal decompression with nasogastric suction, control and quantification of the output of the fistula, and protection of the surrounding skin. Fistulas are classified according to their locations and the volumes of their output. Proximal fistulas tend to have higher output and lead to more severe electrolyte and fluid imbalances. Nasogastric suction can be helpful in diminishing the output of proximal intestinal fistulas, but the output of those more distal in the gut may not be influenced by this maneuver. Sump catheters can provide a means of controlling and quantifying high-output fistulas, especially early in their formation. Maintaining proper position of the catheter in the wound can be problematic. Once the fistula tract is established, suction catheters should be promptly replaced with a stoma appliance fixed to the edges of the fistula. Enteric contents are highly corrosive, and the skin surrounding the fistula opening should be protected carefully. Gauze dressings are generally ineffective at absorbing all the drainage and protecting the skin. Therefore, their use is generally avoided. Most well-established fistulas do not produce sepsis, but in patients with persistent fever, systemic administration of antibiotics and a careful search for an undrained abdominal abscess are indicated.

Early in the work-up of this patient and before the GI tract has been filled with contrast material (from conventional GI radiographs), CT should be performed to look for areas of abscess formation or fluid accumulation. It may also identify the site of the fistula. If CT does not show the site, fistulography is helpful. If one is concerned about distal obstruction, a small bowel follow-through study may provide information if this issue was not satisfactorily answered by CT or fistulography.

**ANSWER:** D

33. Diagnostic work-up of the woman described in Question 31 reveals that she has a distal ileal fistula that is communicating with a small cavity. Which of the following is appropriate therapy?

    A. Prompt exploration and interruption of the fistula tract

    B. Prompt exploration and bypass of the fistula

C. Prompt exploration and resection of the portion of ileum involved in the fistula and primary reanastomosis

D. A 4- to 6-week trial of intravenous hyperalimentation

E. A 2-week trial of low-residue or elemental enteral alimentation

*Ref.:* 4

**COMMENTS:** Knowing the location of the **fistula** is of important prognostic and therapeutic value. The overall mortality rate for small bowel fistulas is 20%, and the rate is higher for jejunal fistulas and lower for those of the ileum. With proper supportive care, such as intravenous or enteral alimentation, and in the absence of distal obstruction, up to 40% of small bowel fistulas close spontaneously. **Enteral alimentation** has the advantage of avoiding the possible hepatic and septic complications associated with prolonged TPN. Even if there is a slight increase in fistula output after the start of enteral nutrition, the fistula may still close. Fistulas of the proximal jejunum may require transnasal insertion of a long tube through the stomach and duodenum and just beyond the fistula before starting enteral alimentation. Surgery should be avoided for 4 to 6 weeks to permit spontaneous closure and to allow the local inflammation to subside, thereby facilitating subsequent surgery. The preferred operation for correcting a persistent fistula is resection of the fistula in continuity with the segment of involved bowel, followed by primary anastomosis. Alternative therapies include complete or partial exclusion with primary anastomosis.

**ANSWER:**   E

34. One year after undergoing antrectomy and Billroth II reconstruction for peptic ulcer disease, a patient is being evaluated for anemia. The patient is also noted to have vague epigastric pain that is relieved by projectile bilious emesis without food particles. Which statement is true regarding this patient's condition.

A. Medical management with tetracycline and vitamin $B_{12}$ can definitively correct the condition.

B. Bacteria successfully compete for vitamin $B_6$, which may lead to megaloblastic anemia.

C. Bacterial deconjugation of bile salts can lead to steatorrhea.

D. The addition of intrinsic factor in the Schilling test causes urinary vitamin $B_{12}$ excretion to return to normal.

E. The addition of tetracycline in the Schilling test causes urinary vitamin $B_6$ excretion to return to normal.

*Ref.:* 3, 4

**COMMENTS:** The **blind loop syndrome** is caused by stasis of the intestinal contents with subsequent bacterial overgrowth. This stasis can be caused by a number of abnormalities, including stricture, stenosis, fistula, diverticulum, or the formation of a blind pouch (as noted in a Billroth II operation). The syndrome is characterized by steatorrhea, diarrhea, anemia, weight loss, abdominal pain, multiple vitamin deficiencies, joint pains, and occasionally neurologic disorders. The steatorrhea is the result of bile salt deconjugation in the stagnant fluid in the blind loop of bowel. Megaloblastic anemia is probably a result of successful competition by bacteria for vitamin $B_{12}$. The Schilling test reveals a type of urinary excretion of vitamin $B_{12}$ similar to that seen with pernicious anemia except that it is corrected, not by the addition of intrinsic factor, but by the use of oral tetracycline. Although the

administration of tetracycline and parenteral vitamin $B_{12}$ can correct megaloblastic anemia, only surgical correction of the cause of the bowel stasis is curative. Surgical correction includes converting the Billroth II to a Billroth I operation or the creation of Roux-en-Y limb gastrojejunostomy with a vagotomy to prevent marginal ulceration.

**ANSWER:**   C

35. With regard to short bowel syndrome, which of the following statements is true?

A. Resection of up to 70% of the bowel can be tolerated if the terminal ileum and ileocecal valve are preserved.

B. Diarrhea is best controlled by the administration of medium-chain triglycerides.

C. The administration of oral bile salts is of central importance in controlling steatorrhea.

D. Vagotomy/pyloroplasty and reversal of a segment of bowel are the two most important operations for the early management of short bowel syndrome.

E. Relative gastric hyposecretion, with increased intestinal pH in conjunction with interruption of the enterohepatic bile salt circulation, is the cause of steatorrhea.

*Ref.:* 3, 4

**COMMENTS:** As it pertains to **short bowel syndrome**, the entire jejunum can be resected without adverse nutritional sequelae. The entire ileum can be resected without harm as long as vitamin $B_{12}$ is replaced postoperatively. Up to 70% of the small bowel can be resected safely if the terminal ileum and ileocecal valve are left intact. If they are resected, however, loss of 50% to 60% of the small bowel can lead to severely compromised nutrition. The deficiencies created by extensive resection of the small bowel are **vitamin $B_{12}$ malabsorption**, altered fat absorption, and fluid and electrolyte problems. Vitamin $B_{12}$ malabsorption leads to vitamin $B_{12}$ deficiency and megaloblastic anemia. Altered fat absorption produces steatorrhea as a result of several factors. First, massive small bowel resection leads to gastric hypersecretion, because decreased bowel pH stimulates the intestine, thereby shortening transit time and interfering with the absorption of ingested fat. Second, interruption of bile salt resorption interferes with micelle formation. Third, the unabsorbed fats are irritating to the colonic mucosa, thereby increasing the diarrhea and steatorrhea associated with the syndrome. Fluid and electrolyte problems are a function of the shortened transit time and the diarrhea that results from loss of small bowel absorptive area.

Treatment of **short bowel syndrome** centers on control of diarrhea and parenteral maintenance of nutrition. With time (2 to 3 years), the mucosa of as little as 30 to 45 cm of small bowel may undergo enough hypertrophy to allow withdrawal of intravenous alimentation and the start of carefully modified oral feedings. Treatment with growth hormone, glutamine, and fiber has shown some promising results in terms of gut regeneration. Diarrhea can be controlled with agents such as Lomotil or codeine, which slow intestinal motility. Oral calcium carbonate is also useful and acts by neutralizing hydrochloric acid and free fatty acids. When oral intake is resumed, dietary fat is restricted to 30 to 50 g daily. Some patients benefit from the use of medium-chain triglycerides. Oral bile salts are tolerated and aid in the formation of micelles in some patients, whereas in others they cause increased diarrhea. Cholestyramine, an agent that sequesters bile acids, is useful in patients who have had less than 100 cm of small bowel resected. There is no standard approach to the resumption of oral intake, and the treatment must be highly individualized. Although some patients ultimately do well with a modified oral diet, others remain dependent on permanent parenteral nutrition. There are no operative procedures that reliably correct short bowel syndrome. Therefore, operative treatment should be considered only in patients who cannot maintain their body weight within 30% of normal without intravenous supplementation. **Operations** that may be useful are reversal of a segment of intestine, creation of a recirculating loop of small bowel, creation of an artificial sphincter, vagotomy and pyloroplasty, correction of bowel obstruction, and placing all bowel in continuity (i.e., reversal of preexisting stomas). Vagotomy and pyloroplasty have rarely been performed for short bowel syndrome since the introduction of H₂ blockers and proton pump inhibitors. Allotransplantation of small bowel in humans has been performed successfully but has a high failure rate and remains experimental.

**ANSWER: A**

36. With regard to tuberculous enteritis, which of the following statements is incorrect?

    A. Primary infection usually results from the ingestion of non-pasteurized milk contaminated with *Mycobacterium bovis*.

    B. Secondary infection results from the ingestion of bacilli contained in contaminated sputum.

    C. The duodenum is the site of involvement in 85% of patients.

    D. Infection may be indistinguishable from Crohn's disease or cancer.

    E. Approximately one half of the patients with colonic or ileo-colonic disease may be treated medically without surgery.

*Ref.:* 10

**COMMENTS: Primary enteral tuberculosis** is rare in the United States but is still common in underdeveloped countries where ingestion of nonpasteurized milk occurs more commonly. Usually, it causes minimal symptoms, but occasionally it results in stricturing and stenosis in the ileocecal area. The radiographic findings may be indistinguishable from those of carcinoma of the colon. Although it may be necessary to resect bowel because of high-grade obstruction, it is not appropriate to do so simply to establish the diagnosis. This can be accomplished with biopsy alone. Treatment with isoniazid, *p*-aminosalicylic acid, and strep-tomycin usually suffices.

**Ulcerative tuberculosis** is a form that develops secondary to pulmonary disease and is more common than the primary form of this disease in the United States. Symptoms are variable but most often consist of pain and diarrhea. The diagnosis is made by barium enema examination, and confirmation is obtained by documenting an appropriate response to antitubercular therapy, which may allow healing of the lesion. Surgery may be required for perforation, obstruction, or hemorrhage.

**ANSWER: C**

37. Regarding typhoid enteritis, which of the following statements is true?

    A. The diagnosis can be made by culturing *Salmonella typhi* from blood or stool.

    B. Chloramphenicol is the preferred treatment.

    C. Bleeding requiring operative intervention occurs in 10% to 20% of patients.

    D. Steroids have no use in treating typhoid enteritis.

    E. Hyperplasia and ulceration of Peyer patches and mesenteric lymphadenopathy are rare findings.

*Ref.:* 4

**COMMENTS: Typhoid enteritis**, a systemic infection caused by *S. typhi*, is accompanied by fever, headache, coughing, maculo-papular rash, abdominal pain, and leukopenia. Hyperplasia and ulceration of Peyer patches, mesenteric lymphadenopathy, and splenomegaly also occur. Chloramphenicol is not the drug of choice because of the emergence of resistant strains of bacteria and the risk for marrow toxicity. Currently, trimethoprim-sulfamethoxazole is preferred. Patients who remain in a toxic state after 1 week of therapy often benefit from a short course of prednisone. Bleeding occurs in 10% to 20% of patients and is usually treated by transfusion. Perforation through ulcerated Peyer patches occurs in 2% of patients and is most often free, solitary, and located in the terminal ileum. Operative closure and appropriate peritoneal toilet are required. Occasionally, the perforations are multiple, which necessitates intestinal resection with primary anastomosis.

**ANSWER: A**

38. Which of the following is true regarding small bowel endoscopy?

    A. Capsule endoscopy has replaced push enteroscopy for evaluation of the small intestine.

    B. Capsule endoscopy is available only in specialized centers participating in clinical trials.

    C. Intraoperative enteroscopy is a simple, safe technique that eliminates the need for the less sensitive technique of capsule endoscopy.

    D. Push enteroscopy is more sensitive and specific than capsule endoscopy in the area that can be examined by push enteroscopy.

    E. Push enteroscopy is usually able to examine all of the small bowel.

*Ref.:* 11

**COMMENTS:** Several techniques have been developed for **endoscopic examination of the small intestine.** Techniques currently in use include push enteroscopy, intraoperative enteroscopy, and capsule endoscopy. Push enteroscopy involves examination of the proximal jejunum by extending the depth of insertion during upper endoscopy with the use of either a colonoscope or an entero-scope. Push enteroscopy may also be used during colonoscopy after intubation of the ileocecal valve and further retrograde advancement of the colonoscope through the terminal ileum. The depth of examination is typically 30 to 50 cm in either direction, which does not allow evaluation of the majority of the central portion of the small intestine.

**Push enteroscopy** remains a commonly used technique for evaluating the small intestine. It is more sensitive and specific than capsule endoscopy over the length of intestine that can be examined by push enteroscopy. It also allows the performance of biopsies and therapeutic maneuvers. However, push enteroscopy is not able to examine the full length of the small intestine, as can be done with capsule endoscopy. Therefore, these two minimally invasive endoscopic examinations of the small intestine are complementary, and neither has made the other obsolete.

**Intraoperative enteroscopy** may be performed as described for push enteroscopy, but it is coupled with laparotomy or laparoscopy and surgical assistance in advancing the scope farther into the small intestine to reach greater depths for examination in either direction. In addition, intraoperative enteroscopy may be performed through an enterotomy in the small intestine, which further enhances the ability to completely examine the length of the small intestine.

**Capsule endoscopy** involves examination of the full length of the small intestine with a wireless camera contained in a capsule. It reaches the colon within 7 hours. The capsule is self-contained, with a lens of short focal length, a light-emitting diode, digital imaging technology, and a power source. The images are transmitted wirelessly to a recorder worn externally on a belt. The endoscopic images themselves are then viewed at a special workstation designed for processing and viewing the images acquired by the capsule and recorder. The plastic capsule weighs 3.7 g and measures 11 mm in diameter by 26 mm in length. Because of its small size and low weight, as well as it being completely self-contained, the capsule is well tolerated by patients and does not require hospitalization during conduct of the examination. The endoscopist is not able to control passage of the capsule and is unable to perform any therapeutic interventions with the capsule. One potential complication is bowel obstruction if the capsule becomes lodged at a narrow point in the GI tract. The capsule is disposable, and the battery is generally exhausted by the time that the capsule leaves the colon.

Although the entire small intestine may be examined endoscopically by both intraoperative enteroscopy and capsule endoscopy, these two procedures are also complementary. Intraoperative enteroscopy requires general anesthesia, laparotomy or laparoscopy, and complete mobilization of the small intestine from adhesions. It entails significantly higher morbidity than does capsule endoscopy. The findings on capsule endoscopy may provide the indication for intraoperative enteroscopy.

**ANSWER:** D

## REFERENCES

1. Gordon PH, Nivatvongs SH: *Principles and practice of surgery for the colon, rectum, and anus*, St. Louis, 1999, Quality Medical.
2. Memon MA, Nelson H: Gastrointestinal carcinoid tumors: current management strategies, *Dis Colon Rectum* 40:1101–1118, 1997.
3. Evers BM: Small intestine. In Townsend CM, Beauchamp RD, Evers BM, et al, editors: *Sabiston textbook of surgery: the biological basis of modern surgical practice*, ed 18, Philadelphia, 2008, WB Saunders.
4. Tavakkolizadeh A, Whang EE, Ashley SW, et al: Small intestine. In: Brunicardi FC, Andersen DK, Billiar TR, et al, editors: *Schwartz's principles of surgery*, ed 9, New York, 2010, McGraw-Hill.
5. Sleisenger MH, Fordtran JS: *Gastrointestinal and liver disease: pathophysiology, diagnosis, management*, ed 4, Philadelphia, 1989, WB Saunders.
6. Wilson JD, Braunwald E, Isselbacher KJ, et al: *Harrison's principles of internal medicine*, ed 12, New York, 1991, McGraw-Hill.
7. Marinis A, Yiallourou A, Samanides L, et al: Intussusception of the bowel in adults: a review, *World J Gastroenterol* 15:407–411, 2009.
8. Greenson JK: Gastrointestinal stromal tumors and other mesenchymal lesions of the gut, *Mod Pathol* 16:366–375, 2003.
9. Green PHR, Jabri B: Celiac disease and other precursors to small-bowel malignancy, *Gastroenterol Clin North Am* 31:625–639, 2002.
10. Corman ML: *Colon and rectal surgery*, ed 5, Philadelphia, 2005, JB Lippincott.
11. Rossini FP, Pennazio M: Small-bowel endoscopy, *Endoscopy* 34:13–20, 2002.

# B. Appendix

1. With regard to the location of the appendix, which of the following is true?

   A. The base of the appendix can always be found at the confluence of the cecal taenia.

   B. In the majority of the cases, the tip of the appendix is found in the pelvis.

   C. The appendix is often retrocecal and extraperitoneal.

   D. After the fifth gestational month of pregnancy, the appendix is shifted posteriorly and laterally by the gravid uterus.

   E. The position of the tip of the appendix in appendicitis does not determine the symptoms of the patient.

   *Ref.:* 1, 2

COMMENTS: The **appendix**, along with the ileum and ascending colon, is a derivative of the **midgut**. Following developmental rotation, the cecum becomes fixed in the right lower quadrant, and this determines the final location of the appendix. The appendiceal orifice and therefore the base of the appendix are always found at the antimesenteric confluence of the cecal **taeniae**. The anterior taenia, in particular, may be used as a landmark to find the appendix at surgery. Although the base of the appendix is found in a constant location, the position of the tip varies. The tip of the appendix is found retrocecally in the majority of patients (65%), in the pelvis in approximately 30%, and in a retroperitoneal position in approximately 7%. In **pregnancy**, the gravid uterus tends to push the appendix superiorly and the tip medially. The various locations of the tip of the inflamed appendix determine the location of physical findings produced by irritation of the parietal peritoneum, but the prodromal symptoms remain the same.

ANSWER: A

2. Which of the following regarding appendiceal innervation is correct?

   A. The innervation of the appendix is derived from both the autonomic and somatic nervous systems.

   B. In early appendicitis, the autonomic nervous system is responsible for poorly defined periumbilical pain.

   C. The somatic pain fibers are responsible for localization of pain in the periumbilical region.

   D. Both the autonomic and somatic nerve fibers follow a midgut embryologic origin.

   E. In the case of ruptured appendicitis, the somatic innervation is disrupted and the patient is often rendered pain free.

   *Ref.:* 1, 2

COMMENTS: The **innervation of the appendix** is derived from the autonomic nervous system, which follows a midgut embryologic origin. As with all visceral organs, no somatic pain fibers are found in the appendix. Early in the course of appendicitis, inflammation leads to poorly localized pain that is referred to the periumbilical region via the autonomic nerves. As the appendiceal inflammation worsens, irritation of the parietal peritoneum results in well-localized right lower quadrant tenderness through somatic nerves. There might be a temporary slight decrease in pain following rupture, but a truly pain-free interval is rare.

ANSWER: B

3. Which of the following statements regarding the pathogenesis of appendicitis is false?

   A. The antimesenteric border has the poorest blood supply and is usually the site of the perforation.

   B. Fecaliths are commonly responsible for appendicitis in children.

   C. Viral or bacterial infections can precede an episode of appendicitis.

   D. Obstruction of venous outflow and then arterial inflow results in gangrene.

   E. Obstruction of the lumen may occur as a result of lymphoid hyperplasia, inspissated stool, or a foreign body.

   *Ref.:* 1, 2

COMMENTS: In most instances of **appendicitis**, luminal obstruction leads to bacterial overgrowth, active secretion of mucus, and increased luminal pressure. Increased pressure leads to decreased venous return and, later, decreased arterial inflow, which results in gangrene, bacterial translocation, and perforation. The midportion of the antimesenteric border of the appendix has the poorest blood supply and most frequently shows evidence of perforation. The cause of the obstruction is usually lymphoid hyperplasia in younger patients and fecaliths in adults. Fecaliths are responsible for approximately 30% of cases in adults and have been identified in 90% of patients with gangrenous appendicitis with rupture. However, luminal obstruction does not occur in all cases, because the lumen of the appendix in some patients is found to be patent during radiologic, gross, and histologic examination. The pathogenesis in these cases remains unclear. It is thought that either viral or bacterial infection, such as *Salmonella*, *Shigella*, or infectious mononucleosis, can precede appendicitis, probably secondary to lymphoid hyperplasia in the appendix and subsequent obstruction.

ANSWER: B

4. A 27-year-old man has a 1-day history of right lower quadrant pain and leukocytosis. Probable nonperforated acute appendicitis is diagnosed. What is the best antibiotic and surgical management for this patient?

   A. Operate and then await the results of culture of peritoneal fluid obtained during the surgery and tailor the selection of antibiotics accordingly.

   B. Administer cefazolin perioperatively to reduce the risk for wound infection and then operate.

   C. Begin ceftriaxone and metronidazole (Flagyl) and monitor the patient with serial abdominal examinations, with surgery being reserved in the event that he fails to improve.

   D. Begin the administration of broad-spectrum antibiotics perioperatively such as ceftriaxone and Flagyl, and proceed with appendectomy.

   E. Begin clindamycin perioperatively, because *Bacteroides fragilis* is the most common organism involved in acute appendicitis.

*Ref.:* 1

**COMMENTS: Antibiotics** play an important role in the treatment of **appendicitis**. The flora of the normal appendix is similar to that of the colon. There is a mixture of aerobic (*Escherichia coli* most common) and anaerobic bacteria (*Bacteroides* most common). If early nonperforated appendicitis is suspected, an appendectomy is warranted. Perioperative antibiotics help prevent wound infection and should cover both anaerobes and aerobes. Of the choices of answers, ceftriaxone plus Flagyl is the antibiotic regimen that does the best. Peritoneal cultures in patients with acute nonperforated appendicitis are frequently negative. In addition, peritoneal cultures in patients with perforated appendicitis usually reveal colonic bacteria with predictable sensitivities. Therefore, antibiotic management should not rely on peritoneal cultures. Nonoperative treatment of appendicitis is controversial. Most agree that appendectomy is preferred for nonperforated cases. However, if perforation with a localized, walled-off abscess is diagnosed, percutaneous drainage and interval appendectomy may be considered.

**ANSWER:** D

5. With regard to the natural history of acute appendicitis, which of the following statements is true?

   A. Rupture occurs most frequently in adolescent girls because of the difficulty of establishing the diagnosis and the consequent delay in surgery.

   B. Perforation rates correlate with the severity of the initial illness.

   C. Acute appendicitis can resolve spontaneously.

   D. Early antibiotic treatment decreases the incidence of perforation.

   E. Nausea and vomiting precede the pain.

*Ref.:* 1, 2

**COMMENTS:** Some episodes of acute **appendicitis** apparently resolve spontaneously. The **natural history of acute appendicitis** is generally one of persistent obstruction leading to gangrene and perforation if left untreated. Perforation occurs more commonly in patients at either end of the age spectrum. Atypical abdominal pain

occurs in 45% of patients with proved appendicitis and is frequently found in elderly patients and those receiving steroids or chronic antibiotic therapy. Clinical manifestations of the disease do not always correlate with the risk for appendiceal rupture. Prompt appendectomy, therefore, is indicated when the diagnosis is made because it is the only certain way of preventing perforation and its attendant morbidity. Antibiotics are indicated for prophylaxis of infectious complications. Nevertheless, antibiotics do not alter the natural history of the disease. Anorexia is a fairly constant symptom, and the diagnosis should be questioned if it is not present. Vomiting occurs in 95% of patients and typically follows the onset of pain. This sequence has diagnostic significance because in 95% of patients, anorexia precedes the onset of pain and is followed by vomiting. Although many patients may experience vomiting, they usually have only one or two episodes. This is in contrast to the profuse and frequent vomiting seen in patients with gastroenteritis. Protracted diarrhea accompanied by vomiting is more suggestive of gastroenteritis than appendicitis.

**ANSWER:** C

6. A 27-year-old man is suspected of having acute appendicitis. On physical examination his abdomen is soft and nondistended. He does not have pain with coughing or reproduction of tenderness in the right lower quadrant when palpated in the left lower quadrant. He experiences abdominal pain during extension of the right thigh while lying on his left side. He does not have pain with passive rotation of his right hip in a flexed position. Where do you suspect the location of the tip of his appendix to be?

   A. Displaced to the right upper quadrant

   B. Extraperitoneal and lying anterior to the cecum

   C. In the pelvis

   D. In the left lower quadrant

   E. Retrocecal over the psoas muscle

*Ref.:* 1, 2

**COMMENTS:** Variations in the **location of the appendix** can account for variations in the classic location of somatic pain at the **McBurney point** (right lower quadrant, one third of the distance between the anterior superior iliac spine and the umbilicus). Pain exaggerated by coughing is called the **Dunphy sign** and is associated with peritoneal irritation. The **Rovsing sign** is elicited by palpating the left lower quadrant, which causes pain to be felt in the right lower quadrant, a finding suggestive of peritoneal irritation. The **psoas sign** is elicited by extension of the right thigh with the patient lying in the left lateral decubitus position. The stretched psoas muscle may irritate an inflamed overlying appendix and suggest retrocecal appendicitis. The **obturator sign** is elicited with passive external rotation of the flexed right hip. If positive, the obturator sign suggests that the inflamed tip is lying in the pelvis.

**ANSWER:** E

7. Which of the following imaging studies is not a proved adjunct for the diagnosis of appendicitis?

   A. Abdominal obstructive x-ray series

   B. Ultrasound imaging

   C. CT

D. Barium enema

E. Positron emission tomography (PET)

*Ref.:* 1-5

**COMMENTS:** The **diagnosis of acute appendicitis** is usually based on the history and findings on physical examination, particularly when substantiated by leukocytosis. Abdominal imaging studies are often performed in the evaluation of patients with acute abdominal pain. They are useful in terms of the differential diagnosis and to demonstrate complications of appendicitis but should not be considered mandatory. Plain abdominal films may show a fecalith, localized ileus in the right lower quadrant, or loss of the peritoneal fat strip. The use of **graded compression ultrasound** imaging has been applied successfully to the diagnosis of appendicitis in equivocal cases of right lower quadrant pain. The appendix is visualized, and pain is then assessed as gradually increasing pressure is placed on the area of the appendix with the ultrasound probe. An abnormal appendix is defined as a tubular, immobile, noncompressible image. On transverse imaging, it is seen as a target with an outer diameter of at least 6 mm, a wall thickness of at least 2 mm, or hyperechoic submucosa. With these criteria, graded compression ultrasound studies have high sensitivity (82%) and specificity (96%) with an overall accuracy of 88%. False-negative results are frequently associated with nonvisualization of the appendix. The advantages of this technique include wide accessibility, the ability to identify other pathologic conditions responsible for the pain, lack of ionizing radiation (for women of childbearing potential), and limited expense. Disadvantages include examiner variability and factors related to the patient that limit the study (e.g., obesity, bowel gas, or discomfort).

**Computed tomography** had been used more frequently in patients with an equivocal history, findings on physical examination, and laboratory test results. Currently, however, CT in patients with a presumptive diagnosis of appendicitis has evolved into a quick and accurate examination. Correlation between pathologic conditions and results on CT remains to be defined. CT is 90% sensitive, with an approximately 85% positive predictive value for the detection of intra-abdominal inflammation. Focused 5-mm cuts in the area of the appendix, along with intestinal or intravenous contrast enhancement (or both), aid in the radiographic diagnosis of appendicitis. The appendix is considered abnormal when it is thickened by more than 5 to 7 mm or filled with fluid. The wall is circumferentially thickened, and its appearance is referred to as the "target" sign. Periappendiceal inflammation along with fat stranding, fluid collections, or phlegmon is suggestive of appendicitis. Barium enemas were primarily used before the advent of ultrasound imaging and CT. A positive study result may show nonfilling of the appendix. However, a false-negative result, showing partial filling of the appendix, can occur in about 10% of patients, with equivocal findings seen in about 40%. Barium enema is no longer used routinely for the diagnosis of appendicitis. There is no defined role for PET in appendicitis.

**ANSWER: E**

8. A 9-year-old girl is sent home from school with a temperature of 39° C and complaints of abdominal pain. In the emergency department, ultrasound of the right lower quadrant was performed (Figure 21-7). The diameter of this tubular structure measured 11 mm with a thickened wall. Which statement is correct regarding her diagnosis?

A. Her disease is more common in adults because of the relatively larger diameter of the appendiceal lumen.

B. There is often a high rate of rupture because of commonly delayed diagnosis and more rapid progression of disease.

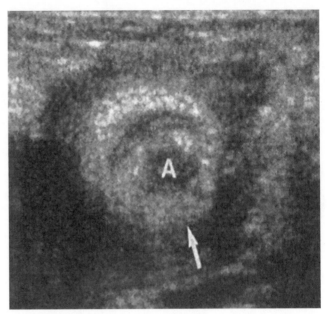

**Figure 21-7.** Abdominal ultrasound showing a thick tubular structure (*arrow*).

C. She probably has gastroenteritis and a normal appendix.

D. When rupture occurs, a localized periappendiceal abscess results more often than in adults.

E. Her disease is not usually associated with such high fever.

*Ref.:* 1, 2

**COMMENTS:** The diagnostic accuracy of acute **appendicitis in infants and young children** is lower than in adults. First, the patient is unable to give a precise history, and second, nonspecific abdominal pain in this age group is fairly common. Appendicitis is infrequent in infants (larger lumen of the appendix at its base versus the tip before differential growth of the cecum), and therefore it is less often considered a cause of abdominal pain. Vomiting, fever, and diarrhea are probable early complaints. On physical examination, abdominal distention is common. Leukocyte counts are not reliable. The presence of a fecalith on plain films of the abdomen in a child with suspicious symptoms should be enough to establish the diagnosis.

**Gangrene and rupture of the appendix** occur more commonly in children than in adults because of the delay in diagnosis, more rapid progression of the disease, and atypical findings. The rupture rate varies from 15% to 50%. In preschool children it is higher and ranges from 50% to 85%. Rupture of a gangrenous appendix in children is frequently followed by diffuse peritonitis and multiple intra-abdominal abscesses. The walling-off process is less efficient in children than in adults, partly because of the incompletely developed greater omentum. The mortality rate has traditionally been reported to be as high as 5%.

This patient has an **ultrasound** study consistent with appendicitis. Ultrasonography has a sensitivity of about 85% and a specificity of greater than 90% for the diagnosis of appendicitis. Ultrasound findings consistent with appendicitis include a noncompressible luminal structure, an appendicolith, an appendix dilated more than 7 mm, a thickened appendiceal wall, and the presence of periappendiceal fluid. Ultrasound is commonly used in children because it avoids exposure to radiation.

**ANSWER: B**

**9.** With regard to appendicitis in the elderly, which statement is false?

A. Elderly patients tend to initially be seen later in the course of the ailment.

B. Elderly patients have a higher rate of perforation because of omental atrophy.

C. Perforation has an associated mortality rate of 50%.

D. Appendicitis may mimic bowel obstruction.

E. Symptoms of appendicitis and the finding of anemia should raise suspicion for a concomitant cecal neoplasm.

*Ref.:* 1, 2

**COMMENTS:** Acute **appendicitis** in the **elderly** may not be accompanied by the typical signs and symptoms of appendicitis. Fever, leukocytosis, and right lower quadrant pain may be minimal or absent. Frequently, the absence of typical symptoms can lead to a delay in diagnosis and result in a 60% to 90% rupture rate. A mortality rate of approximately 15% has been reported for a ruptured appendix in elderly patients. The atrophic omentum is less capable of walling off a perforated appendix; consequently, diffuse peritonitis or a distant intra-abdominal abscess is more common than in younger patients. Physical examination is characterized by a paucity of findings. Abdominal distention is prominent, and symptoms and signs mimicking bowel obstruction such as nausea and vomiting are not uncommon. Occasionally, a patient has a painless palpable mass in the right lower quadrant because of a gangrenous appendix. Anemia, particularly in elderly patients, should raise suspicion for carcinoma of the cecum. This situation may necessitate a right hemicolectomy.

**ANSWER:** C

**10.** With regard to appendicitis in immunocompromised patients, which of the following statements is false?

A. Immunocompromised patients with appendicitis often have a fever, a normal white blood cell (WBC) count, and nonspecific abdominal pain.

B. Typhlitis often mimics acute appendicitis.

C. CT is particularly useful in immunocompromised patients.

D. Unusual infections such as those caused by mycobacteria, protozoa, and fungi do not usually mimic appendicitis.

E. Cytomegalovirus (CMV) infections and Kaposi sarcoma can occlude the appendiceal orifice and cause acute appendicitis.

*Ref.:* 1, 2

**COMMENTS:** Appendicitis in **immunocompromised** patients can be difficult to diagnose. The patient often has nonspecific findings on abdominal examination, fever, and a normal WBC count. The differential diagnosis in an immunocompromised patient with abdominal pain includes CMV enteritis, typhlitis, and unusual infections, including those caused by mycobacteria, protozoal species, and fungi. Typhlitis, or neutropenic colitis, often mimics appendicitis in these patients. CT can be particularly useful in helping establish the diagnosis. Acute appendicitis secondary to luminal obstruction in a patient with acquired immunodeficiency syndrome (AIDS) may be the result of a fecalith, CMV bodies, or Kaposi sarcoma. Approximately 30% of cases of acute appendicitis

in patients with AIDS is caused by conditions particular to AIDS.

**ANSWER:** D

**11.** A 32-year-old woman is 36 weeks pregnant. She is seen in the emergency department for fever, leukocytosis, nausea, vomiting, and right-sided abdominal tenderness. In terms of management, what is the next best step?

A. Treat with antibiotics in an attempt to avoid an operation.

B. Obtain an abdominal ultrasound.

C. Perform MRI.

D. Proceed with laparoscopy immediately.

E. Proceed with laparoscopy after delivery.

*Ref.:* 1, 2

**COMMENTS:** **Appendicitis** is the most common cause of an acute abdomen in **pregnant women** past the first trimester. Because the gravid uterus pushes the appendix to a more lateral and cephalad position and the appendiceal tip is more medial, the typical location of somatic pain is altered. Nevertheless, during the first 6 months of pregnancy, symptoms of appendicitis do not differ much from those in nonpregnant patients. Acute pyelitis and torsion of an ovarian cyst can be difficult to distinguish from appendicitis. The common occurrence of abdominal pain, nausea, and leukocytosis during the normal course of a pregnancy can also make the diagnosis more difficult. When the diagnosis is strongly suspected, prompt surgery is indicated. In this case, further work-up is needed for diagnosis. The next best step is to perform ultrasonography. MRI can also be performed but is more expensive and less readily available. It should be used if the ultrasound and history and physical examination are equivocal for appendicitis.

The incidence of appendicitis is not increased by **pregnancy**. Most cases occur during the second trimester. Appendicitis during the third trimester is associated with a higher incidence of rupture because of the delay in diagnosis. Furthermore, the omentum cannot wall off the inflamed appendix. Premature labor occurs in 50% of women in whom appendicitis develops during the third trimester. The fetal mortality rate is approximately 2% to 10% overall and rises to 35% with rupture. The prognosis of the fetus is related to the birth weight and the effects of sepsis. The maternal mortality rate is less than 0.5%

**ANSWER:** B

**12.** A 35-year-old woman complains of 5 days of abdominal pain mostly in the lower part of her abdomen. She has had occasional fevers with temperatures of 38.7° C. Her WBC count is 28,000/mm³. Urinalysis reveals moderate red blood cells and moderate WBCs without bacteria. She underwent CT (Figure 21-8). What is the best management of this patient?

A. Laparoscopic exploration and consideration of oophorectomy

B. Laparoscopic exploration and consideration of appendectomy

C. Intravenous antibiotics and nonoperative therapy

D. Colonoscopy

E. Transrectal drainage and intravenous antibiotics

*Ref.:* 1, 2

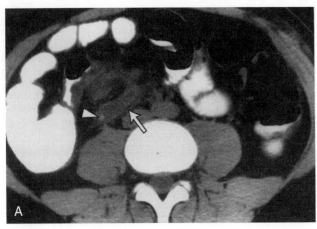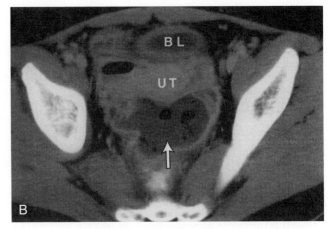

**Figure 21-8.** Abdominal computed tomographic scans. **A,** This image shows an inflamed tubular structure consistent with appendicitis *(arrow)* with a fecalith *(arrowhead)* at its base. **B,** This image shows a large pelvic abscess *(arrow)* containing fluid and gas. *BL,* Bladder; *UT,* uterus.

**COMMENTS:** A ruptured appendix may result in a localized **periappendiceal abscess**, diffuse peritonitis, or abscesses at other abdominal sites, notably in the pelvis, in the right subhepatic region, or between loops of bowel. Unrelenting obstruction of the appendix leads to gangrene and rupture of the organ. Because the patient is ill, the abdominal pain is more severe and diffuse and evidence of sepsis is apparent. Physical signs are more obvious after rupture, depending on the position of the appendix. With a periappendiceal abscess or **phlegmon,** a mass is usually felt, and its nature can be further clarified by ultrasound or CT.

A patient with a late manifestation of appendicitis (>48 hours) who is found to have an **appendiceal abscess** may benefit from nonoperative management. **Nonoperative management of an appendiceal abscess** reduces complications and overall hospital stay and can be accomplished through a percutaneous, transrectal, or transvaginal approach. Patients with abscesses larger than 4 to 6 cm benefit from abscess drainage, and those with a smaller abscess or phlegmon may be treated with antibiotics alone (Figure 21-9). Patients who are not improving with nonoperative treatment should be considered for operative drainage and appendectomy.

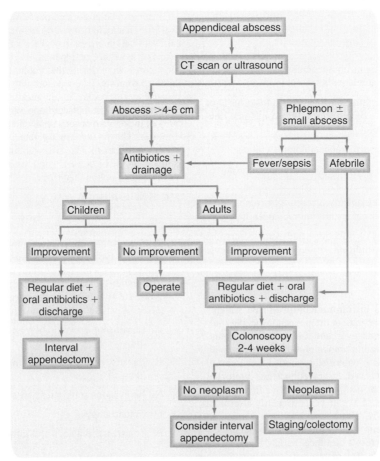

**Figure 21-9.** Treatment options for appendiceal abscess.

After the acute inflammation has subsided, adults should undergo colonoscopy or barium enema to evaluate for cancer. Elective performance of interval appendectomy in 6 to 8 weeks is controversial in adults and more commonly accepted in children.

**ANSWER:** E

13. For which of the following patients would nonoperative treatment of appendicitis be appropriate?

   A. A pregnant woman during the third trimester

   B. A 35-year-old patient with subsiding symptoms and a right lower quadrant mass

   C. An elderly patient with concomitant cardiac disease

   D. A 20-year-old woman with Crohn's disease

   E. A 20-year-old woman with a thickened appendiceal wall and right ovarian cyst noted on ultrasound

*Ref.:* 1, 2

**COMMENTS:** When the diagnosis of appendicitis is a strong consideration but not certain, in most instances surgery should be undertaken because delay involves a risk for rupture with its accompanying increased morbidity and mortality. Surgery should not be delayed during pregnancy because doing so increases the risk to both the mother and fetus. Nor should it be delayed for elderly patients because they face an increased risk for appendiceal rupture and death.

   The optimal timing of **surgery for a ruptured appendix** with an established periappendiceal abscess has been controversial. However, initial nonoperative therapy followed by interval appendectomy in 6 to 8 weeks may be considered for select patients whose symptoms are clearly subsiding and in whom a discrete right lower quadrant mass is palpable. Such expectant treatment consists of intravenous fluids and appropriate antibiotics. Vital signs, WBC count, and the size of the mass are watched closely. With these measures, most abscesses resolve, but prolonged hospitalization and antibiotic therapy are needed. Should progression occur, the abscess is drained. The manifestations of acute regional enteritis often mimic those of appendicitis. Acute ileitis should be distinguished from Crohn's disease because progression of the former to the latter occurs in only 10% of cases. If exploration reveals an acutely inflamed ileum and a normal appendix, an appendectomy may be performed, but only if the cecum is normal. Performance of an appendectomy in the face of cecal inflammation risks the formation of a fecal fistula.

**ANSWER:** B

14. A 20-year-old woman is operated on through a right lower quadrant incision for presumed appendicitis, but the appendix is normal. At this point, which of the following would be appropriate treatment?

   A. Proceeding with appendectomy if no other pathology is found

   B. Exploration and treatment of any associated pathologic condition, as indicated, without appendectomy

   C. Exploration and diverticulectomy if a Meckel diverticulum is present and is normal by inspection and palpation

   D. Exploration and, if no pathology is found, closure without appendectomy

   E. Exploration and ileal resection if the terminal ileum appears acutely inflamed

*Ref.:* 1, 2

**COMMENTS:** If appendicitis is not found at the time of surgery, careful exploration for other pathologic conditions must be carried out. The accuracy of the preoperative diagnosis should be 85%. In general, appendectomy is performed, except in some cases of Crohn's disease with extensive involvement of the ileum and cecum. The pelvic organs, gallbladder, colon, and gastroduodenal areas should be inspected to the extent possible. A laparoscopic approach may allow better evaluation of other areas than can be accomplished through a limited right lower quadrant incision.

   The differential diagnosis of appendicitis is basically that of an acute abdomen. The surgeon must be prepared to treat other pathologic entities should they be found on exploration for appendicitis. Such differential diagnoses include **acute mesenteric adenitis**, **gastroenteritis**, **diverticulitis**, **epiploic appendagitis**, and cancer.

   Acute mesenteric adenitis is most often confused with appendicitis in children. Frequently, an upper respiratory tract infection precedes or is present at the onset of diffuse abdominal pain. Generalized lymphadenopathy or relative lymphocytosis, when present, can be of help. At surgery, the mesenteric lymph nodes are assessed. If they are enlarged, a biopsy is performed. The lymph nodes are examined histologically for granulomas (including Crohn's disease), and tissue is cultured for mycobacteria and *Yersinia*. Infection with *Yersinia* causes mesenteric adenitis, ileitis, colitis, and acute appendicitis.

   Acute gastroenteritis is characterized by cramping pain followed by watery stools, nausea, and vomiting. Laboratory results are usually normal. Diagnosis of a specific bacterial infection (e.g., *Salmonella* or typhoid fever) is made by stool culture.

   The small intestine is inspected in a retrograde manner for evidence of inflammatory bowel disease or an inflamed Meckel diverticulum. The incidence of perforation or peritonitis with Meckel diverticulitis is about 50%. Resection of a Meckel diverticulum is indicated if diverticulitis is present. An asymptomatic Meckel diverticulum found incidentally during laparotomy in adults should not necessarily be removed. Diverticulitis of the cecum may be impossible to distinguish from acute appendicitis or cancer clinically. Both may be manifested as a right lower quadrant mass with evidence of infection and peritonitis. Sigmoid diverticulitis may also mimic appendicitis if a mobile, inflamed sigmoid colon is located in the right lower quadrant.

   Epiploic appendagitis results from infarction of the appendage secondary to torsion. The pain is short-lived and well localized, recovery is fairly rapid, and patients do not appear ill.

   If no pathology is found and a right lower quadrant incision is made, an appendectomy should be performed to eliminate potential confusion in the management of right lower quadrant abdominal pain in the future.

**ANSWER:** A

15. A patient suspected of having appendicitis underwent exploration. Crohn's disease was found. Which of the following is true?

   A. The normal appendix should always be removed.

   B. All grossly involved bowel, including the appendix, should be resected.

   C. An inflamed appendix, cecum, and terminal ileum should be resected.

   D. Perforated bowel and advanced Crohn's disease with obstruction should be resected.

   E. Only the tip of the appendix should be resected if the base is found to be involved.

*Ref.:* 1, 2

**COMMENTS:** If a **normal appendix** is found at the time of laparotomy, other causes should be sought. If **Crohn's disease** is encountered and the cecum and base of the appendix are normal, an appendectomy should be performed. If the base is involved with Crohn's disease, appendectomy should be avoided. If the areas involved with Crohn's disease are not complicated by perforation or obstruction, bowel resection is not indicated and medical therapy should be instituted. However, in the case of perforation or high-grade obstruction from a fibrotic segment, the involved bowel should be resected.

**ANSWER:** D

16. With regard to carcinoid of the appendix, which of the following statements is true?

A. The ileum is the most common location for GI carcinoids.

B. An appendectomy is sufficient for incidental carcinoid tumors less than 1 cm with positive lymph nodes.

C. Most carcinoid tumors occur at the tip of the appendix.

D. Right hemicolectomy is routinely indicated, regardless of nodal status.

E. Carcinoid tumors of the appendix are usually manifested as acute appendicitis.

*Ref.: 1, 2*

**COMMENTS:** The most common locations for GI carcinoids are the rectum, ileum, and appendix, in order of increasing frequency. **Appendiceal carcinoids** are usually solitary. About 75% of them occur at the distal tip and less than 10% occur at the base. They are usually an incidental finding and only rarely cause appendicitis. Carcinoids of the small bowel are multiple in approximately 30% of patients. Carcinoid syndrome usually occurs in patients with small bowel tumors that have metastasized to the liver. Appendiceal carcinoids less than 1 cm are generally considered biologically benign lesions, and only 3% metastasize. If the lesion is found at the tip of the appendix and is smaller than 1 cm, appendectomy is considered adequate treatment because these lesions have a lower risk for metastasis. Right hemicolectomy is indicated if tumor is present at the surgical margins, if there is nodal involvement, and if the lesion is larger than 2 cm. For tumors 1 to 2 cm in size, the decision to perform right hemicolectomy must be individualized because these patients have a substantial risk for metastasis. Chemotherapy with a combination of 5-fluorouracil and streptozocin has provided some palliation of carcinoid syndrome in patients with unresectable disease. Up to 25% of patients who undergo palliative resection survive for 5 years.

**ANSWER:** C

17. When a mucocele of the appendix is found at the time of surgery, which of the following is appropriate initial therapy?

A. Incisional biopsy with subsequent appendectomy if malignancy is confirmed by frozen section

B. Routine right hemicolectomy with lymph node dissection

C. Needle aspiration of cystic fluid for cytologic examination

D. Appendectomy

E. Closure and observation

*Ref.: 1, 2*

**COMMENTS:** Appendectomy is adequate treatment of a **mucocele**, but care must be taken to avoid rupture, because **pseudomyxoma peritonei** has been reported following rupture and peritoneal dissemination of the appendiceal contents even if the appendix was free of cancer. Histologically, mucoceles can be categorized as a benign type, which is the result of occlusion of the proximal lumen of the appendix, or a malignant type, which is a variant of a mucous papillary adenocarcinoma. Treatment of an appendiceal adenocarcinoma is right hemicolectomy.

**ANSWER:** D

18. Which of the following statements is true regarding laparoscopic versus open appendectomy?

A. Laparoscopic appendectomy is associated with less postoperative pain, shorter hospital stay, faster recovery, and lower wound infection rates.

B. Surgical costs for laparoscopic appendectomy are less.

C. The laparoscopic approach is contraindicated in morbidly obese patients.

D. Conversion from laparoscopic to open appendectomy occurs in approximately 50% of cases.

E. Laparoscopic appendectomy results in a lower intra-abdominal abscess rate in patients with advanced appendicitis.

*Ref.: 1, 2, 6, 7*

**COMMENTS: Laparoscopic appendectomy** has several advantages over the open technique, including a shortened hospital stay, faster recovery, and lower wound infection rates. The wound infection rate for laparoscopic appendectomy is less than one half that for open appendectomy. The major disadvantage of laparoscopic appendectomy is the use of disposable instruments, which can increase surgical cost; however, this may be offset by shorter length of stay. A laparoscopic approach may be preferable in the morbidly obese because of fewer wound-related difficulties. Rates of conversion are variable but occur approximately 10% of the time. For patients with advanced appendicitis at initial evaluation, there is a greater tendency for the formation of intra-abdominal abscesses with laparoscopic appendectomy than with an open technique.

**ANSWER:** A

### REFERENCES

1. Maa J, Kirkwood KS: The appendix. In: Townsend CM, Beauchamp RD, Evers BM, et al, editors: *Sabiston textbook of surgery: the biological basis of modern surgical practice,* ed 18, Philadelphia, 2008, WB Saunders.
2. Matthews JB, Hodin RA: Acute abdomen and appendix. In: Mulholland MW, Lillemoe KD, Doherty GM, et al, editors: *Greenfield's surgery: scientific principles and practice,* ed 4, Philadelphia, 2006, Lippincott Williams & Wilkins.
3. Galindo GM, Fadrique B, Nieto MA, et al: Evaluation of ultrasonography and clinical diagnostic scoring in suspected appendicitis, *Br J Surg* 85:37–40, 1998.
4. Roa PM, Rhea JT, Novelline RA, et al: Effect of computed tomography of the appendix on treatment of patients and use of hospital resources, *N Engl J Med* 338:141–146, 1998.
5. Raptopoulos V, Katsou G, Rosen MP, et al: Acute appendicitis: effect of increased use of CT on selecting patients earlier, *Radiology* 226:521–526, 2003.
6. Golub R, Siddiqui F, Pohl D: Laparoscopic versus open appendectomy: a metaanalysis, *J Am Coll Surg* 186:545–553, 1998.
7. Liu SI, Siewert B, Raptopoulos V, et al: Factors associated with conversion to laparotomy in patients undergoing laparoscopic appendectomy, *J Am Coll Surg* 194:298–302, 2002.

# CHAPTER 22

# Colon, Rectum, and Anus

## A. Colon and Rectum

*Jacquelyn Turner, M.D., and Theodore J. Saclarides, M.D.*

**1.** With regard to the anatomy of the colon and rectum, which of the following statements is true?

A. The colon has a complete outer longitudinal and an incomplete inner circular muscle layer.

B. The haustra are separated by plicae circulares.

C. The ascending colon and descending colon are usually fixed to the retroperitoneum.

D. The rectum is totally invested by three complete muscle layers.

E. The distal part of the rectum begins at the point where the taeniae merge.

*Ref.:* 1

**COMMENTS:** A thorough understanding of **anatomy** is integral to the surgical management of problems of the colon and rectum. The colon has two muscle layers: an outer longitudinal layer and an inner circular layer. The inner layer completely encircles the colon. The outer layer, unlike the case in the small intestine, is in the form of three grossly recognizable longitudinal strips, or taeniae coli, that do not cover the full circumference of the *colon*. At the rectosigmoid junction, the three taeniae coli become broad and fuse together, and the *rectum* is totally invested with two complete muscle layers. This explains why diverticula do not form in the rectum.

The plicae semilunares are spaced, transverse, crescentic folds that separate the tissue between the taeniae coli and form haustra. They produce a characteristic, intermittently bulging pattern that radiologically permits differentiation of the colon from the small intestine, which has circular mucosal folds known as plicae circulares or valvulae **conniventes**. In contrast to the plicae semilunares, the plicae circulares traverse the full diameter of the small bowel lumen, thereby facilitating radiographic distinction.

Usually, the ascending and descending portions of the colon are fused to the retroperitoneum, whereas the transverse and sigmoid portions are free. Developmental anomalies of fixation, as seen with malrotation and in some cases of volvulus, are not uncommon. Cecal volvulus, for example, could not occur unless incomplete fixation to the retroperitoneum makes it possible for a mobile cecum to rotate around a narrow mesenteric pedicle.

Surgeons have traditionally placed the upper border of the rectum at the peritoneal reflection. An alternative definition is the point at which the taeniae have completely merged. The rectum therefore lacks taeniae and appendices epiploicae. The distal end of the rectum is void of any peritoneal covering, the middle part of the rectum is covered by peritoneum ventrally, and the upper portion of the rectum is completely covered by peritoneum except for a thin strip dorsally, where the short mesorectum suspends the rectum to the presacral tissue.

**ANSWER:** C

**2.** Which of the following statements is true regarding colon physiology?

A. Transit time through the colon is independent of the fermentability of nonstarch polysaccharides such as lignin, cellulose, and pectins.

B. The left colon is the segment of colon where bacteria are the most metabolically active in the fermentation process. The right colon is the site of storage and dehydration of stool.

C. Fifty percent of the daily energy expenditure is obtained from the absorption of short-chain fatty acids by the colon; this energy is used to stimulate blood flow, regulate the pH of the colonic environment, and renew colonic mucosal cells.

D. Butyrate is a short-chain fatty acid and a bacterial fermentation product that is the main fuel for colonic epithelial cells.

E. Colonic epithelium can use various fuels, but it prefers glutamine over *n*-butyrate, glucose, or ketone bodies.

*Ref.:* 1, 2

**COMMENTS:** The colon plays an important role in the digestive process for fluids and electrolytes. In healthy subjects, the colon normally absorbs 1 to 2 L of water and up to 200 mEq of sodium and chloride per day. This absorptive capacity can increase up to 5 to 6 L/day, thereby protecting the person against severe diarrhea. The cecum and right colon absorb sodium and water the most rapidly, whereas the rectum is impermeable to sodium and water. Sodium is actively absorbed against chemical and electrical gradients in the colon. Butyrate plays a role in stimulating sodium absorption in the colon. Potassium and chloride are secreted by the colon through sodium-potassium adenosine triphosphatase ($Na^+,K^+$-ATPase) and $Na^+/K^+/Cl^-$ cotransportors. Chloride ions are actively absorbed at the expense of bicarbonate, which is secreted in exchange. Absence of luminal chloride inhibits secretion of bicarbonate. The main anions in stool include the short-chain fatty acids butyrate, acetate, and propionate. The host and colonic bacterial flora have a symbiotic relationship: the host promotes bacterial proliferation with energy substrates from the diet and cellular debris, whereas bacteria provide the host with **butyrate**, a bacterial fermentation product and short-chain fatty acid that fuels colonic epithelial cells. Nonstarch polysaccharides, or dietary fiber such as lignin, cellulose, and fruit pectins, are the main substrates for bacterial fermentation. Fermentation takes place mostly in the right colon, with the cecum being the colonic segment where bacteria are the most metabolically active. Colonic transit time and bulking of stool are dependent on the fermentability of nonstarch polysaccharides. The transit time of stool through the colon is also dependent on stool pH, the autonomic nervous system, and the gastrocolic reflex (postprandial increase in electrical activity and colonic tone).

**ANSWER:** D

3. A pregnant 32-year-old woman was admitted for severe abdominal pain and diarrhea. She was recently discharged from the hospital after having been treated for pyelonephritis. Plain films show a distended colon. She underwent flexible sigmoidoscopy, which reveals pseudomembranous colitis. Which statement is true regarding her condition?

   A. Diarrhea that begins 1 week after antibiotic use has been discontinued rules out pseudomembranous colitis.

   B. Pseudomembranous colitis does not occur in the absence of antibiotic therapy.

   C. Administration of oral vancomycin is appropriate treatment.

   D. There is a relapse rate of 50% after treatment.

   E. The use of alcohol-based hand gels by health care workers helps eliminate spread of this disease in a hospital.

*Ref.: 1, 3, 4*

**COMMENTS: Pseudomembranous enterocolitis**, first described by Theodor Billroth in 1867, has been seen with increased frequency and is associated with the use of many antibiotics. The disease has not been described with the use of vancomycin or with antimicrobials used to treat mycobacteria, fungi, or parasites. There is evidence that antibiotics change the intracolonic flora and allow overgrowth of *Clostridium difficile*, which then produces enterocolitis. There is also evidence, however, that pseudomembranous colitis is infectious and spread by patient-to-patient or staff-to-patient contact.

Pseudomembranous colitis should be suspected in any patient in whom diarrhea develops during or up to 3 weeks after the cessation of antibiotic therapy. The diagnosis is established endoscopically by visualizing the characteristic raised mucosal plaques or by a cytotoxic assay for **Clostroidium difficile exotoxin**, which usually has a positive result in patients with pseudomembranous colitis.

Therapy should begin with prompt cessation of the offending antibiotic. Oral vancomycin (125 mg four times a day for 10 days) or oral or intravenous metronidazole (250 to 500 mg four times a day for 7 to 14 days) has been used to treat this condition

successfully. *Oral* vancomycin is safe for use in pregnant women. The relapse rate is 20% with vancomycin and 23% with metronidazole. Most cases of *C. difficile* colitis can be successfully treated medically. Indications for surgery include signs of peritoneal inflammation, severe ileus, or toxic megacolon. Patients who benefit most from surgical intervention are those older than 65 years, the immunocompetent, those with severe leukocytosis, and those with lactic acidosis. Surgical treatment is a subtotal colectomy. The 30-day mortality rate after subtotal colectomy is approximately 53%. Independent predictors of 30-day mortality are leukocytosis greater than $50 \times 10^9$/L, lactate level greater than 5 mmol/L, age older than 75 years, immunosuppression, and shock requiring vasopressors.

**ANSWER:** C

4. With regard to amebiasis, which of the following statements is true?

   A. Most people in the United States are asymptomatic carriers.

   B. *Entamoeba histolytica* antibodies are detectable in the serum of more than 90% of those with active amebiasis.

   C. Acute amebic dysentery closely resembles fulminant ulcerative colitis and should be treated aggressively with steroids.

   D. Amebic abscess of the spleen is the most common complication of amebic colitis.

   E. Perforation of the colon with peritonitis occurs in approximately one half of the patients with an acute manifestation.

*Ref.: 1, 3*

**COMMENTS: Amebic colitis** is caused by the protozoan ***Entamoeba histolytica***, which infests primarily the colon and rectum and, secondarily, other organs such as the liver. It has been estimated that 10% of the American population are asymptomatic carriers. Transmission of the disease is through food or water contaminated with feces containing *Entamoeba* cysts. The disease can assume acute and chronic forms.

Acute amebic dysentery is seen with contamination of the water supply and has findings similar to those of acute ulcerative colitis (i.e., fever, cramps, and bloody diarrhea). Distinguishing between these two entities is important. Steroids are given routinely on a short-term basis to treat ulcerative colitis but are contraindicated in the treatment of amebic dysentery. The desired effect of steroids—muting of the inflammatory response—would mask the clinicopathologic progression of amebic colitis. In a typical case, proctosigmoidoscopy should reveal extensive ulceration of the intestinal epithelium, and a warm saline preparation of the stool usually demonstrates numerous trophozoites containing ingested erythrocytes. The diagnosis is strengthened by a serologic test for *E. histolytica* antibodies, which has a positive result in 90% of patients with active amebiasis. Perforation of the colon during the acute form of the disease is rare. Amebic abscess of the liver is the most common complication of amebic colitis, which may in turn rupture into the pleura, pericardium, or peritoneum. Treatment is metronidazole, 750 mg three times a day for 10 days.

**Chronic amebic dysentery** is more common than the acute form and is characterized by three to four foul-smelling bowel movements per day, along with abdominal cramping and fever. The diagnosis of chronic amebic dysentery is more difficult to establish because cysts or trophozoites are not always demonstrable in stool preparations and findings on sigmoidoscopy are normal in up to 30% of such individuals. *E. histolytica* antibodies, however, should be detectable. Treatment is diiodohydroxyquin, 650 mg three times a day for 20 days, and metronidazole or diloxanide furoate, 500 mg three times a day for 10 days.

**A N S W E R :**  B

5. Which disease is correctly matched to the appropriate treatment?

   A. Actinomycosis: penicillin and drainage

   B. Lymphogranuloma venereum: penicillin and steroids

   C. Tuberculous enteritis: isoniazid and colectomy

   D. *Yersinia* infections: metronidazole and appendectomy

   E. *Etamocha histolytica*: metronidazole and right hemicolectomy

*Ref.:* 1, 3, 5

**COMMENTS: Actinomycosis** is a suppurative, granulomatous disease caused by *Actinomyces israelii*, an anaerobic, gram-positive bacterium that produces chronic inflammatory induration and sinus formation. Although the causative organism is part of the normal oral flora, infections may occur in the cervicofacial area, thorax, or abdomen. The cecal region is the most frequent site of abdominal infection, with a pericecal mass, abscesses, and sinus tracts being produced. Rectal strictures have been reported as well. Treatment consists of surgical drainage and penicillin or tetracycline.

**Lymphogranuloma venereum** is a sexually transmissible disease caused by *Chlamydia trachomatis*. It occurs most frequently in men who have sex with men, in whom it starts as proctitis and produces tenesmus, discharge, and bleeding. Perianal and rectovaginal fistulas may develop, as may rectal strictures. The diagnosis is made with the Frei intracutaneous test when the test is available. Otherwise, the diagnosis may be confirmed by a complement fixation test. Tetracycline is curative, and steroids have been recommended.

**Tuberculous enteritis** is seen most commonly in the ileocecal region and occasionally leads to stenosis of the distal ileum, cecum, and ascending colon; the endoscopic and radiographic features produced may be indistinguishable from those of Crohn's disease. Surgery is reserved for patients with obstruction. Triple-drug therapy consisting of isoniazid, *p*-aminosalicylic acid, and streptomycin usually heals the intestinal lesions.

***Yersinia* infections** are caused by a gram-negative rod that is transmitted through food contaminated by feces or urine. It produces a clinical picture frequently indistinguishable from that of acute appendicitis. *Yersinia* may also cause acute gastroenteritis, which affects primarily the ileocecal region. *Yersinia* responds to treatment with tetracycline, streptomycin, ampicillin, or kanamycin.

**Amebic colitis** is caused by the protozoan *Entamoeba histolytica*, which infests primarily the colon and rectum and, secondarily, other organs such as the liver. It has been estimated that 10% of the American population are asymptomatic carriers. Transmission of the disease is through food or water contaminated with feces containing *Entamoeba* cysts. The disease can assume an acute or a chronic form. Treatment is metronidazole, 750 mg three times a day for 10 days.

**A N S W E R :**  A

6. With regard to ischemic colitis, which of the following statements is true?

   A. The most common symptoms are lower abdominal pain and bright red rectal bleeding.

   B. Occlusion of the major mesenteric vessels is responsible for producing the ischemia in most cases.

   C. The splenic flexure and hepatic flexure are the most vulnerable areas, although any segment of the colon may be involved.

   D. Nonoperative management is not justified because in a significant percentage of such patients, perforation and peritonitis eventually develop.

   E. The Griffith point is the vulnerable area at the rectosigmoid junction.

*Ref.:* 1, 3, 5, 6

**COMMENTS: Ischemic colitis** should be considered in the differential diagnosis of any elderly patient with left lower quadrant pain. It can also be found in individuals of any age in association with hypercoagulable states, periarteritis nodosa, systemic lupus erythematosus, rheumatoid arthritis, polycythemia vera, and scleroderma. Ischemic colitis may be manifested as three distinct clinical syndromes, depending on (1) the extent and duration of vascular occlusion, (2) the adequacy of the collateral circulation, and (3) the extent of septic complications. Ischemic colitis appears to be a disease of the small arterioles. Although this disease can occur in any segment of the large bowel, it is seen most commonly in the splenic flexure or distal sigmoid colon, a plausible explanation being the suboptimal blood flow in areas positioned between two vascular systems ("**watershed areas**") that rely on an intact but meandering artery for their blood supply. The Sudeck point is the area between the blood supply from the last sigmoid artery and the superior rectal artery. The clinical significance of the **Sudeck point** is questionable because of retrograde flow from the middle and inferior rectal arteries. The **Griffith point** is the vulnerable area at the splenic flexure that is positioned between areas perfused by the left branch of the middle colic artery and the ascending branch of the left colic artery. The diagnosis is made by endoscopic examination, which reveals cyanotic, edematous mucosa that may be covered with exudative membranes, or by barium enema, which may show the typical "thumbprinting" of the bowel wall. If gangrenous colitis is suspected on the basis of ominous physical findings, such as involuntary guarding and rebound tenderness, these studies are contraindicated and prompt laparotomy is mandatory.

Transient ischemic colitis usually responds to nonoperative management. Ischemic strictures may be resected electively with primary anastomosis after the initial ischemic episode has subsided. If surgery is needed for peritonitis and gangrenous colitis, resection with end colostomy is the preferred operation.

**A N S W E R :**  A

7. A 72-year-old woman with a history of hypertension, atrial fibrillation, and a recent hemorrhagic stroke is noted to have an episode of dark bloody stool. Her abdomen is diffusely tender on palpation. As a result of her stroke, her anticoagulation was discontinued 3 weeks earlier. The patient undergoes exploratory laparotomy, which reveals the presence of ischemia of the small bowel, cecum, and ascending colon and a normal distal colon and rectum. Which statement is most correct concerning intestinal blood flow?

   A. Ischemia of the colon is caused by lack of blood flow to the ileocolic, right colic, and middle colic arteries, which originate from the superior mesenteric artery.

   B. The rectum receives its blood supply from the superior and middle rectal arteries, which originate from the inferior mesenteric artery.

C. Approximately 20% of intestinal blood flow circulates to the mucosa and submucosa, and the remaining 80% passes to the serosa and muscularis layers.

D. The colon and small bowel are equally vulnerable to ischemic injury produced by acute reductions in blood flow.

E. An increase in functional motor activity of the colon is accompanied by a corresponding increase in blood flow.

*Ref.: 1, 7, 8*

**COMMENTS:** This patient probably has **mesenteric ischemia.** The mesenteric vascular anatomy has a vast amount of collateral blood flow. Collateral blood flow is especially noted when a patient has experienced chronic occlusion of one or more branches over time. However, sudden occlusion of a main branch may be poorly tolerated. The right and transverse sections of the colon are derived from the foregut and receive their blood supply from the **superior mesenteric artery** via its ileocolic, right colic, and middle colic branches. The left colon and sigmoid, derived from the hindgut, are supplied by the left colic and sigmoid branches originating from the inferior mesenteric artery. The rectum, a hindgut structure, is supplied by the superior hemorrhoidal artery, which originates from the inferior mesenteric artery, and by the middle and inferior hemorrhoidal arteries, which originate from the internal iliac artery or its internal pudendal branch. The venous and lymphatic drainage systems of the colon and rectum generally parallel the arterial supply, with the exception of the inferior mesenteric vein, which courses directly cephalad to empty into the splenic vein.

The total blood flow to the gastrointestinal tract is approximately 25 mL/kg/min, or 20% of cardiac output. During a meal, blood flow to the intestine rises to 50% above normal without a corresponding rise in cardiac output. Physical exercise, in contrast, doubles cardiac output with a 20% decrease in superior mesenteric arterial flow.

Approximately 80% of the blood flow to the wall of the colon reaches the mucosa and submucosa, and the remaining 20% supplies the muscularis. Despite the extensive collateral vessels to the colon, it receives only about 50% of the blood flow that the small intestine does. The colon is therefore more sensitive to ischemic injury during acute reductions in blood flow. In contrast to other areas of the body, an increase in functional motor activity of the colon does not result in a parallel increase in absolute colonic blood flow.

**ANSWER: A**

8. A 56 year old man is scheduled to undergo a laparoscopic segmental colectomy for a diagnosis of carcinoma of the descending colon. Which of the following statements is true concerning bowel preparation for colorectal operations?

A. Preoperative nonabsorbable oral antibiotics alone are effective in preventing postoperative wound infections.

B. Preoperative mechanical bowel cleansing alone is most effective in preventing postoperative wound infections.

C. Administration of broad spectrum antibiotic(s) should be administered in the immediate perioperative period.

D. Mechanical cleansing with sodium phosphate is preferred in patients with renal insufficiency, cirrhosis, ascites, and congestive heart failure.

E. Complete bowel obstruction and perforation are relative contraindications to mechanical cleansing but can still be used in select patients.

*Ref.: 1, 3, 9*

**COMMENTS:** The colon contains a higher concentration of bacteria, both aerobic and anaerobic, than any other area of the body, and infectious complications constitute the major morbidity of colorectal operations. Bacteroides is the most common anaerobic organism and Escherichia coli is the most common aerobic organism found in the colon. Mechanical cleansing of the colon has been a time-honored practice that can be achieved by the administration of a cathartic in combination with enemas, or by peroral lavage with a nonabsorbable polyethylene glycol-electrolyte solution administered the afternoon before surgery. Despite the widespread use of mechanical cleansing, the need of **mechanical bowel preparation** prior to colectomy has been recently questioned. Several small studies have suggested that its usage does not decrease the incidence of postoperative septic complications, and it may even be associated with increased morbidity. Oral and rectal Fleet Phospho soda (sodium phospate) has the benefit of mechanically cleansing the bowel with less volume. Yet, its use has been associated with significant complications so that sodium sulfate is no longer indicated for bowel cleansing. Polyethylene glycol is not contraindicated in patients with renal failure, cirrhosis, ascites, and congestive heart failure. Complete bowel obstruction and bowel perforation are absolute contraindications to mechanical bowel preparation. The combination of mechanical preparation and administration of nonabsorbable oral antibiotics effective against both aerobic and anaerobic colonic flora have never proved to decrease postoperative septic complications. Systemic antibiotics are often combined with lavage and oral antibiotics, but such a combination has not been conclusively demonstrated to confer an advantage over the use of lavage and oral antibiotics alone. The administration of systemic antibiotics in place of oral antibiotics is an effective **method of antibiotic prophylaxis,** and many surgeons have resorted to this regimen to avoid the nausea associated with some oral antibiotics. A broad-spectrum parenteral antibiotic should be administered within 30 minutes of the skin incision to provide adequate coverage against both aerobes and anaerobes.

**ANSWER: C**

9. Common causes of colorectal anastomotic breakdown include all of the following except:

A. Poor blood supply to the bowel edges

B. Short rectal stump

C. Inadequate bowel mobilization

D. Hand-sewn anastomosis

E. Poor technique

*Ref.: 1*

**COMMENTS: Anastomotic leaks** after a colorectal operation have a range of clinical findings (from postoperative tachycardia to fulminant sepsis) and consequences. The causes of anastomotic leaks can be divided into implicated and definitive factors. Implicated factors include the use of drains, advanced malignancy, shock, malnutrition, emergency surgery, smoking, steroid use, malnutrition, male gender (narrow pelvis), and technical reasons (i.e., tears from stapling devices). There are several definitive factors that contribute to anastomotic leaks. Poor blood supply to the anastomosis and tension on the suture line can contribute to leaks. Anastomoses that are below the peritoneal reflection and the length of the rectal stump are risk factors for leaks because of the increasing difficulty in performing the anastomosis. In addition, the environment of the anastomosis (such as radiation therapy, emergency operations, and contaminated fields) may also contribute to leaks.

Patients with Crohn's disease have a higher incidence of anastomotic leaks. There is no difference in the anastomotic leak rate between hand-sewn and stapled anastomoses.

**ANSWER:** D

10. Which of the following is the best initial management for acute colonic pseudo-obstruction (Ogilvie's syndrome)?

    A. Colonoscopy

    B. Rectal tube decompression

    C. Nasogastric tube decompression and correction of electrolytes

    D. Neostigmine

    E. Lower gastrointestinal and Gastrografin enema

*Ref.:* 1, 10

**COMMENTS: Ogilvie's syndrome** was first described by Sir William Heneage Ogilvie in 1948. This syndrome involves distention of the colon without evidence of mechanical obstruction and has been associated with the use of opiates and neuroleptic medications, diabetes, myxedema, scleroderma, uremia, hyperparathyroidism, lupus, Parkinson disease, retroperitoneal hematomas, and severe metabolic illnesses. Its pathophysiology is unclear. Ogilvie's syndrome is thought to involve an imbalance in neural input to the colon, distal to the splenic flexure, that results in contraction of the distal part of the colon and functional obstruction. Frequently, the right and transverse sections of the colon are dilated with a decompressed distal colon that contains some air on plain radiographs. The risk for ischemia rises when the cecal diameter reaches 12 cm or greater. Obstipation is present in up to 40% of patients with Ogilvie's syndrome. If the patient is hemodynamically stable, without peritonitis, and without a known mechanical obstruction, management includes hydration, mobilization, correction of electrolytes, avoidance of offending drugs such as opiates, placement of a nasogastric tube, tap water enemas, and serial abdominal examinations. Mechanical obstruction should be ruled out with a contrast-enhanced enema. Although **colonoscopy** is the initial management for **sigmoid volvulus** in that it can be both diagnostic and therapeutic, it is an alternative diagnostic tool to evaluate for mechanical obstruction when Ogilvie's syndrome is suspected, and it could be used therapeutically to decompress the colon if the aforementioned measures fail. Seventy percent of patients will improve with conservative treatment in the first 48 hours. **Neostigmine** and colonoscopy should be considered if conservative treatment fails to resolve the symptoms beyond 48 hours. Neostigmine is a cholinesterase inhibitor that can cause bradycardia. All patients receiving neostigmine must be placed on a cardiac monitor and atropine must be readily available if bradycardia were to occur. Placement of a rectal tube is rarely effective because the tube cannot be advanced blindly into the proximally distended colon. Patients who fail conservative therapy, neostigmine, and decompressive therapy should be considered for surgical treatment, options for which include cecostomy placement or resection if the cecum is ischemic or has been perforated.

**ANSWER:** C

11. In the United States, what is the most common cause of mechanical obstruction of the colon?

    A. Adhesions

    B. Diverticulitis

    C. Cancer

    D. Volvulus

    E. Inguinal hernia

*Ref.:* 1, 3

**COMMENTS:** Whenever a patient has signs and symptoms of intestinal obstruction, it is important to define the level of obstruction (i.e., small bowel or large bowel). **Colonic obstruction** is often suggested by the gas pattern on plain abdominal radiographs and can be confirmed radiographically by a carefully performed enema with water-soluble contrast medium. Barium used in this situation has potential hazards. One concern is causing peritonitis in the presence of a perforating lesion. Another is inspissation proximal to a partially obstructing cancer or diverticulitis, which effectively converts a partial obstruction to a complete one.

In the United States, colorectal cancer is by far the leading cause of large bowel obstruction. **Diverticulitis** is the next most common cause. In some parts of the world (e.g., Iran, Iraq, and Pakistan) where there is a high fiber content in the diet that results in large volumes of stool and an elongated colon, volvulus is the leading cause of obstruction. In the United States, sigmoid volvulus is rare and is usually seen in elderly, institutionalized patients. **Intussusception** is a common cause of colonic obstruction in infants and children but is unusual in adults unless a neoplasm has precipitated it. It is highly unusual to have obstruction of the large bowel secondary to adhesions or incarceration within an inguinal hernia, in contradistinction to obstruction of the small intestine. Other causes of large bowel obstruction include fecal impaction, especially in the elderly and infirm, and benign **strictures** secondary to ischemia or **inflammatory bowel disease**. A neglected obstruction from any mechanism can be fatal. Colon obstruction in the presence of a competent ileocecal valve creates a closed-loop phenomenon. Progressive distention of the colon between the point of obstruction and the ileocecal valve may lead to necrosis and perforation of the gut wall. **Volvulus** can behave in the same manner and have the same consequence.

**ANSWER:** C

12. A 74-year-old man was admitted to the hospital for abdominal pain and obstipation. Plain radiographs were taken (Figure 22-1). Which statement is true about this patient's diagnosis?

    A. This patient has a cecal bascule, which is usually caused by a twisting segment of bowel on a narrow mesentery.

    B. This patient has a cecal volvulus, which is treated by nonoperative reduction in 70% of patients.

    C. This patient has a cecal volvulus, which is commonly associated with signs of small bowel obstruction and is seen in elderly debilitated persons with psychiatric or neurologic diseases.

    D. This patient has a sigmoid volvulus, which is commonly associated with signs of small bowel obstruction and is seen in elderly debilitated persons with psychiatric or neurologic diseases.

    E. This patient has a sigmoid volvulus, which is initially treated by nonoperative reduction in up to 70% of patients.

*Ref.:* 1, 3, 6

**COMMENTS:** This patient has a sigmoid volvulus. The prerequisite for the development of sigmoid or **cecal volvulus** is a

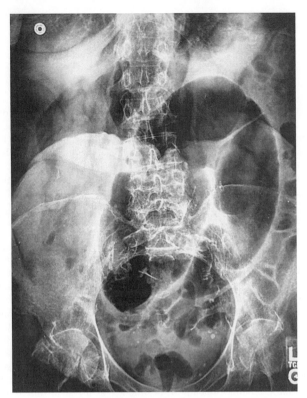

**Figure 22-1.** Abdominal radiograph.

mobile segment of bowel that can rotate around a mesentery whose points of fixation are in close proximity. Otherwise, there are surprisingly few similarities between sigmoid and cecal volvulus.

Volvulus of the cecum is found most frequently in persons 25 to 35 years of age, whereas it is unusual for **sigmoid volvulus** to occur in an active, otherwise healthy individual. Usually, it occurs in elderly, debilitated persons or in those with psychiatric or neurologic disorders in which immobility, medications that impair bowel motility, and loss of accessory defecatory muscles may lead to constipation and elongation of the colon.

Both types of volvulus typically cause abdominal distention and pain. With cecal volvulus, there may be radiographic evidence of small bowel obstruction. With sigmoid volvulus, the distended twisted loop has a fairly characteristic appearance of a "bent inner tube."

For sigmoid volvulus, endoscopic detorsion plus insertion of a rectal tube to evacuate the voluminous fecal contents is the preferred initial therapeutic approach but should be attempted only if the mucosa does not appear gangrenous. It should not be attempted if the patient has rebound abdominal tenderness or other signs of peritoneal inflammation. Although nonoperative detorsion is successful approximately 70% of the time, a recurrence rate of 33% to 60% mandates elective resection of the elongated colon if the patient is believed to have acceptable operative risk.

Nonoperative colonoscopic reduction of cecal volvulus is successful in only 25% of patients and should not be attempted in those with peritoneal inflammation. If a colonoscopy is unsuccessful or contraindicated (e.g., when there is tenderness), an operation is indicated as soon as the patient can be prepared. If gangrenous, the cecum must be resected. In the absence of vascular compromise, cecopexy with or without cecostomy is sufficient. The most important determinant of a patient's outcome is whether bowel gangrene is present, with mortality being highest if surgery is

performed for intestinal infarction or perforation. Mortality is also higher if operating for recurrent volvulus.

**ANSWER:** E

13. A 20-year-old healthy, active man with no previous medical problems is being evaluated for chronic constipation. His electrolyte levels are normal. He denies recent travel and is not currently taking any medications. Plain radiographs show a dilated colon. Transit studies are abnormal with slow transit times. What is the next best step in the management of this patient?

A. Flexible sigmoidoscopy

B. Modification of diet and antibiotics

C. Placement of a rectal tube proximal to the normal-caliber aganglionic bowel to decompress the dilated nondiseased bowel

D. Anal manometry, rectal biopsy, and barium enema

E. Exploratory laparotomy

*Ref.:* 1, 3

**COMMENTS:** This patient should be evaluated for **Hirschsprung disease**. **Megacolon** may be congenital or acquired. Both forms are characterized by dilation, elongation, and hypertrophy of the colon proximal to a segment of nonperistaltic collapsed bowel causing obstruction. Both are associated with increased risk for volvulus. Infection with *Trypanosoma cruzi*, Hirschsprung disease, and neuronal intestinal dysplasia should all be considered in a patient with slow transit constipation and megacolon.

Hirschsprung disease is caused by congenital absence of ganglion cells in the myenteric plexus of the bowel, which results in loss of peristaltic activity in that segment of intestine. The rectosigmoid region is most frequently involved, with variable extension of the disease proximally. There is a transition zone from normal bowel, which is dilated, to the abnormal bowel, which is aganglionic, aperistaltic, and of normal or decreased caliber. Although primarily a disease of infants and children, occasionally Hirschsprung disease does not appear until later in life if an ultrashort distal rectal segment is involved. In these cases, patients relate a history of constipation dating back to infancy. The diagnosis is apparent during the first 24 hours of life if the infant fails to pass meconium. A rectal biopsy is diagnostic. In adolescents and young adults, Hirschsprung disease can be diagnosed by anal manometric measurements. If the disease is present, normal relaxation of the internal sphincter, which is the expected response to rectal distention, is lost. Treatment of Hirschsprung disease is primarily surgical and involves the use of a coloanal anastomosis.

Acquired megacolon may be seen in patients with protozoal colon infections with *T. cruzi*, which is endemic in South and Central America. This condition has not been reported in North America. *T. cruzi* causes widespread destruction of the intramural nervous system. Acquired megacolon also occurs in patients with colonic dilation as a result of chronic constipation because of the loss of voluntary defecatory muscles (e.g., in paraplegia), extreme inactivity (e.g., in poliomyelitis), or voluntary inhibition of defecation (e.g., in psychotic disorders). Resection of the excessive redundant colon is occasionally justified in the latter group of patients. This patient does not relate a history of *T. cruzi* infection or neurologic disorder.

**ANSWER:** D

**14.** Which of the following is true regarding rectal prolapse?

A. The extruded mucosa has radially orientated folds.

B. Rectal prolapse occurs mostly in men with a male-to-female ratio of 6:1.

C. The Altemeier procedure involves full-thickness resection of the prolapsed rectum through a perineal incision.

D. Fecal incontinence is not a predominant symptomatic feature in rectal prolapse.

E. Rectal prolapse is commonly attributed to intussusception of the rectum as a result of a neoplasm forming a lead point.

*Ref.:* 1, 11

**COMMENTS: Rectal prolapse** is a pelvic floor disorder that is most commonly found in women with a 6:1 female-to-male ratio. This disorder has a bimodal distribution of incidence, with peak onsets within the first 3 years and after the seventh decade of life. There are varying degrees of prolapse—internal intussusception or occult rectal prolapse (or prolapse of the rectal wall without protrusion through the anus), **procidentia** (or complete protrusion of all layers of the rectum), and mucosal prolapse. Rectal prolapse is differentiated from incarcerated internal hemorrhoids by close examination of the mucosal folds. Incarcerated internal hemorrhoids have radially invaginated tissue, which distinguishes the hemorrhoidal cushion beds. Rectal prolapse has concentric folds. The pathophysiology of rectal prolapse is not clear. However, with the advent of defecography, Broden and Snellman have demonstrated that weakness in the pelvic floor results in full-thickness intussusception of the rectum through the anal canal. Recently, anorectal physiology studies have indicated that proximal pudendal nerve injury contributes to the pelvic floor weakness. Direct trauma, obstetric injury, neuropathic diseases such as diabetes, and neoplasms involving the sacral nerve root can all lead to pudendal nerve damage. Even though neoplasm is a common cause of adult small bowel intussusception, it is not usually the cause of the intussusception seen in rectal prolapse. The most common symptom is the sensation of an anal "mass" that reduces with manual pressure. Protrusion usually occurs with increased abdominal pressure such as during coughing or defecation. Fecal incontinence is a predominant symptom that is seen in 50% to 75% of patients with rectal prolapse. Other symptoms include tenesmus and rectal pressure. The operative repair for rectal prolapse can be done through an abdominal or perineal approach. The abdominal approach involves resection of redundant sigmoid colon and rectopexy. This approach is generally reserved for healthier patients who can tolerate abdominal surgery. Either an open or a laparoscopic approach can be used. The recurrence rate is low. The Altemeier procedure is a perineal approach that involves proctosigmoidectomy with full-thickness resection of redundant rectum while prolapsed. An anterior levatorplasty is also often performed with this procedure to correct the weakness of the pelvic floor muscles associated with this condition.

**ANSWER: C**

**15.** Which of the following is a common cause of massive colonic bleeding?

A. Cancer

B. Ulcerative colitis

C. Diverticulosis

D. Diverticulitis

E. Granulomatous colitis

*Ref.:* 3, 12, 13

**COMMENTS: Diverticulosis** and **angiodysplasia** are responsible for most cases of massive colonic bleeding. Although their relative frequency may vary from one institution to another, they are the two most common reasons for lower gastrointestinal hemorrhage. These two entities frequently coexist, and precise identification of the source of bleeding may require a combination of endoscopic, radiographic, and histologic methods. Before the advent of angiography, angiodysplasia was not recognized as a source of colonic hemorrhage. Its cause is not known, but it may be related to the degenerative changes associated with aging and to intramural muscular hypertrophy that obstructs the submucosal veins and leads to dilation and a propensity of these veins to bleed. Almost all cases of colonic angiodysplasia are located in the cecum and right colon. In contrast to diverticular disease, bleeding from angiodysplasia is venous and not as severe. Diverticulosis can also cause massive bleeding and is attributed to ruptured vasa recta at the apex or neck of a diverticulum. Diverticulitis can likewise cause bleeding as a result of superficial mucosal ulceration, but such bleeding is usually mild. **Ulcerative colitis** is more likely to cause mild to moderate bleeding and is frequently associated with diarrhea and systemic signs of a chronic illness, such as weight loss and failure to thrive. Cancer of the colon generally causes occult rather than massive gastrointestinal bleeding.

**ANSWER: C**

**16.** A 68-year-old man is admitted to the hospital after having passed three large maroon-colored stools. On arrival at the hospital, he passes more bloody stools as well as clots. He is pale, orthostatic, and tachycardic. Nasogastric aspirates are bilious. After resuscitation is begun, which of the following is the most appropriate initial test?

A. Angiography

B. Nuclear medicine red blood cell scan

C. Rigid proctoscopy

D. Colonoscopy

E. Barium enema

*Ref.:* 5

**COMMENTS:** Although all of the aforementioned tests may play a role in evaluating a patient with massive loss of blood through the rectum, **hematochezia proctoscopy** is the most appropriate initial test. Proctoscopy may reveal an anorectal source of the bleeding and a diffuse mucosal process, such as ulcerative proctitis.

Proceeding directly to a barium enema examination is ill advised because the barium obscures details if angiography is subsequently needed. Furthermore, finding sigmoid diverticula does not prove that they are the source of the bleeding. Mesenteric angiography is performed if the hemorrhage is brisk and persistent. A bleeding rate of approximately 1 to 5 mL/min is necessary to visualize the vessel responsible. The superior mesenteric artery should be injected first because most bleeding originates in the right colon. If no abnormalities are found, this step is followed by injecting the inferior mesenteric artery and finally the celiac axis. If a source of the bleeding is found, embolization may be performed with Gelfoam strips, coils, or autologous blood clots. Rebleeding following embolization occurs in approximately 25%

of cases. Embolization may occlude more than the single bleeding vessel and lead to ischemia and even colonic infarction, which occurs in approximately 5% of patients. Therefore, **embolization** should be reserved for patients who cannot tolerate surgery or vasopressin. **Vasopressin** may be selectively infused into the mesenteric vessel. Even though it stops the bleeding in many patients, it may also cause cardiac arrhythmias, heart failure, and hypertension. Cessation of vasopressin may precipitate further bleeding in 30% of patients. The use of vasopressin gives the physician time to complete resuscitation and address coexisting medical disorders.

**Sulfur colloid nuclear scanning** has also been used to assess lower intestinal bleeding. Unfortunately, the isotope is cleared rapidly by the reticuloendothelial system, and repetitive scanning is not possible. Alternatively, red blood cells may be tagged with technetium. This technique detects bleeding at a rate as low as 0.1 mL/min. Because this isotope is not cleared from the vascular system as rapidly, repeated scanning may be possible over an extended period. Sensitivity, specificity, and accuracy rates have varied widely among reported series, and the precise role of red blood cell scanning is controversial.

**Colonoscopy** has emerged as a valuable diagnostic and therapeutic tool for stable patients who are not bleeding briskly. No bowel cleansing is needed, but the examination must be done by an experienced endoscopist. Angiodysplastic lesions can be treated successfully by colonoscopic methods.

**ANSWER: C**

17. With regard to ulcerative colitis, which of the following statements is true?

  A. In at least one half of the patients, the entire colon is involved with skip areas.

  B. The characteristic histologic finding of crypt abscesses is the sine qua non of ulcerative colitis and is not seen with other inflammatory conditions of the bowel.

  C. The disease is most commonly a chronic relapsing one, with an acute and fulminant course seen in only 10% to 15% of patients.

  D. Cancers arising in association with ulcerative colitis tend to be located in the rectum and sigmoid colon, similar to cancers not associated with ulcerative colitis.

  E. Histologic demonstration of granulomas confirms the diagnosis.

*Ref.: 1, 3*

**COMMENTS: Ulcerative colitis** is usually limited to the mucosal and submucosal layers of the bowel. The rectum is almost always involved, with continuous proximal spread to varying lengths of colon. The entire colon is involved in at least one half of the patients. The characteristic **crypt abscesses**, which contain an infiltration of neutrophils and eosinophils, extend down into the bases of the crypts of Lieberkühn and the lamina propria. Although crypt abscesses may be seen with other inflammatory conditions of the colon, they are always present with ulcerative colitis and generally in greater number. In contrast to **Crohn's disease**, in which the supply of goblet cells is preserved, the microscopic appearance of ulcerative colitis characteristically reveals goblet cell depletion. Ulcerative colitis is most commonly chronic and relapsing in character, although in 10% to 15% of patients the disease runs an acute and fulminant course.

Cancers associated with ulcerative colitis are usually diagnosed later in their course because the signs and symptoms may be confused initially with an inflammatory relapse. For this reason, these cancers are associated with a poorer prognosis. Studies have shown that contrary to what has been believed, colitic cancers do not behave more aggressively than their noncolitic counterparts when similar stages are compared. When compared with noncolitic cases, cancers arising within a colitic colon are more evenly distributed throughout the colon, have a higher incidence of proximal involvement, and are frequently multiple. Granulomas found on histopathologic analysis are pathognomonic for Crohn's disease and are not usually seen in patients with ulcerative colitis.

**ANSWER: C**

18. A 39-year-old man with a history of mild long-standing ulcerative colitis controlled with sulfasalazine recently underwent routine colonoscopy that showed a lesion in the sigmoid colon. Pathologic evaluation reveals high-grade dysplasia. Which of the following is the best surgical option?

  A. Sigmoid colectomy, provided that the rectum is minimally involved

  B. Proctocolectomy, construction of an ileal reservoir, and ileoanal anastomosis

  C. Proctocolectomy with continent ileostomy (Koch pouch)

  D. Total proctocolectomy with Brooke ileostomy

  E. Polypectomy to reduce the risks associated with major abdominal surgery

*Ref.: 1, 3*

**COMMENTS: Proctocolectomy** with permanent end ileostomy is still an acceptable operation; however, healthy, motivated patients who require surgery for **ulcerative colitis** may be eligible for a sphincter-preserving procedure. Options include abdominal colectomy with ileorectal anastomosis, total proctocolectomy with **continent ileostomy** (Koch pouch), or the ileal pouch–anal anastomosis procedure. Ileorectal anastomosis does not eradicate the disease or remove mucosa at risk for malignant transformation. The continent ileostomy procedure may require revision surgery at a future date because of slippage of the nipple valve and is not considered the best operation for a patient with an intact, normally functioning sphincter. The combination of proctocolectomy, an **ileal reservoir** (J pouch), and ileoanal anastomosis offers advantages over proctocolectomy and permanent ileostomy because not only is the diseased mucosa eliminated, but so is the need for a permanent abdominal stoma. The operative technique was described by Mark Ravich and David Sabiston in 1947 and has undergone certain modifications, most notably construction of an ileal pouch proximal to the ileoanal anastomosis. The pouch may be S or J shaped, which increases intestinal storage capacity and decreases stool frequency. A temporary diverting ileostomy is usually required for 2 to 3 months while the pouch heals. The procedure is currently recommended for select patients with ulcerative colitis and those with familial polyposis. It is not indicated for Crohn's disease because of the risk for recurrence within the pouch, which may lead to complex fistulas and septic complications. Although advanced age is not an absolute contraindication, elderly patients with multiple comorbid conditions may be better served with a permanent ileostomy. Similarly, an ileoanal anastomosis should probably be avoided in patients with preexisting fecal incontinence from anorectal surgery or obstetric injuries. For appropriately selected patients, the functional results are good, with preservation of the autonomic innervation to the bladder and genitalia. Fecal sensation and continence are retained in most of these patients. This patient requires surgery because of dysplasia; total removal of mucosa at risk is essential. Polypectomy or segmental colectomy is not appropriate.

**ANSWER: B**

19. A 25-year-old woman has a history of repeated episodes of bloody diarrhea and general abdominal cramping along with lower abdominal pain and weight loss. The presumed diagnosis is ulcerative colitis. Which of the following is the correct management?

   A. A barium enema radiographic examination is done early to assess the extent and severity of her disease.

   B. Hydrocortisone has been shown to induce remissions, but such steroid-induced remissions are more likely than spontaneous remissions to be followed by a relapse.

   C. Total parenteral nutrition, if administered early as part of the treatment, may delay or even prevent the need for colectomy.

   D. Maintenance, low-dose steroids are effective in preventing relapse.

   E. If medical therapy fails and abdominal colectomy with an ileorectal anastomosis is performed, there is a 15% to 20% chance that carcinoma will develop in the rectal remnant during the next 30 years.

*Ref.: 3, 14*

**COMMENTS:** Endoscopy with biopsy is the most widely used method for diagnosing **ulcerative colitis**. Barium enema examinations can be performed but should be done with caution and avoided altogether during acute attacks because of the risk for perforation and precipitation of toxic megacolon. Prednisone or hydrocortisone is highly effective in treating acute phases of the illness. However, both drugs have side effects sufficiently adverse that the dose is tapered early when possible. Administration of low-dose steroids on a maintenance basis has not been shown to prevent relapses. The risk for relapse is the same whether it follows a steroid-induced remission or a spontaneous remission. The optimal role of **total parenteral nutrition** in the treatment of these patients has not been well defined, but it does not appear to delay the need for surgical intervention. It should not be used as primary treatment. **Infliximab** is used in patients with Crohn's disease, but it is also used in those with moderate to severe ulcerative colitis and an inadequate response to steroid treatment. Infliximab is an anti–tumor necrosis factor-α (TNF-α) antibody that blocks the TNF-α receptor, which in turns decreases inflammation. In general, it reduces signs and symptoms and maintains remission. Cancer develops in approximately 5% to 6% of patients with ulcerative colitis. Patients with pancolitis or disease of long-standing duration are at highest risk. When an ileorectal anastomosis is performed, lifetime proctoscopic surveillance for dysplasia or neoplasia is mandatory, because the risk for subsequent cancer is approximately 20% after 25 years. In addition to the risk for cancer, proctitis symptomatic enough to require proctectomy is another concern following ileorectostomy for ulcerative colitis. Approximately 50% of patients undergoing this operation require proctectomy because of cancer, dysplastic changes, or refractory proctitis.

**ANSWER: E**

20. An 18-year-old man with ulcerative colitis is admitted for an acute exacerbation of his disease. He is febrile and tachycardic with a heart rate of 135 beats/min. His blood pressure is stable. He is noted to have leukocytosis and colonic distention on plain radiographs. What is the next step in the treatment of toxic megacolon in this patient?

   A. Nasoenteric decompression, broad-spectrum antibiotics, and intravenous steroids

   B. Endoscopy

   C. Emergency total abdominal colectomy with ileostomy

   D. Nasoenteric decompression, broad-spectrum antibiotics, and infliximab

   E. Colostomy

*Ref.: 1, 6, 14, 15*

**COMMENTS: Toxic megacolon** is seen in patients with ulcerative colitis (1% to 13%) and less frequently in those with Crohn's colitis. Rapid fluid resuscitation plus transfusion of blood products is essential. A nasogastric tube should be inserted to help minimize the accumulation of swallowed air in the colon. Air usually gathers in the transverse colon, and such accumulation is promoted in patients lying supine. There is little need to confirm the diagnosis with endoscopy. In fact, intubation of the colon above the peritoneal reflection may cause perforation. In patients with a fulminant manifestation and no previous history of inflammatory bowel disease, a proctoscope, if inserted, should be advanced carefully to 10 to 15 cm and with little insufflation. It helps confirm suspected inflammatory bowel disease and rules out anorectal causes of blood per rectum, such as hemorrhoids. The diagnosis of toxic megacolon is based on the clinical findings of fever, tachycardia, and abdominal bloating, combined with radiographs of the abdomen showing colonic distention. Response to medical management is assessed with serial abdominal radiographs. Prompt administration of steroids is an important factor when inducing a response. Broad-spectrum antibiotics are also used. Even if medical therapy is successful, most patients do not have a satisfactory long-term outcome, and ongoing symptoms and even recurrent toxic colitis continue to be concerns. **Infliximab** is an anti–TNF-α antibody that blocks the TNF-α receptor, which in turns decreases inflammation. It is used to reduce the signs and symptoms of inflammatory bowel disease and maintain remission. Infliximab is not used in the setting of toxic megacolon related to inflammatory bowel disease.

Worsening colonic distention, fever, and leukocytosis are indications for surgery. In these instances, the operative choice is abdominal colectomy and ileostomy without proctectomy. This procedure allows sphincter-preserving surgery to take place once health has been restored.

**ANSWER: A**

21. A 22-year-old man in whom Crohn's disease has recently been diagnosed has just recovered from his first Crohn's flare-up. Currently, he has no perianal involvement. What medical therapy is not used as a first-line agent to maintain remission?

   A. 6-Mercaptopurine

   B. Metronidazole

   C. Mesalamine

   D. Infliximab

   E. Methotrexate

*Ref.: 1*

**COMMENTS:** Currently, there is no cure for Crohn's disease. Surgical and medical therapies are palliative. The goal of therapy is to relieve acute exacerbations or complications of the disease and control symptoms. Surgical therapy is reserved for obstruction, perforation, the rare instance of life-threatening bleeding, cancer, and complex fistulas.

Much of the treatment of **Crohn's disease** is medical. **Sulfasalazine** is commonly used for Crohn's disease. Its active component is 5-aminosalicylic acid (5-ASA). It has shown to be beneficial in patients with colitis and ileocolitis, but its effectiveness for Crohn's disease limited to the small bowel is controversial. Sulfasalazine alone has not been proved to maintain remission, but sulfasalazine in combination with a corticosteroid may be used to maintain remission. **Mesalamine**, a newer drug that also releases 5-ASA, is likewise used to maintain remission. Mesalamine is considered the first-line therapy for Crohn's disease and is also often used in combination with a corticosteroid. **Corticosteroids**, such as prednisone and budesonide, are useful in the induction of remission of active Crohn's disease. Corticosteroids alone are ineffective in maintaining remission. The mechanism of antibiotics in treating Crohn's disease is unclear. **Metronidazole** is the most commonly used antibiotic for Crohn's disease in the setting of perianal disease, enterocutaneous fistulas, or active colonic disease. **Infliximab** is an anti–TNF-α antibody that blocks the TNF-α receptor, which in turn decreases inflammation. It is used to reduce the signs and symptoms of inflammatory bowel disease and maintain remission. Infliximab has been useful in treating patients with Crohn's disease and fistulas but is not considered the first line of therapy for Crohn's disease. Other agents that have been shown to be effective for Crohn's disease but are not considered first-line agents include azathioprine and 6-mercaptopurine.

**ANSWER: D**

22. Which of the following statements is correct?

   A. Backwash ileitis is associated with ulcerative colitis.

   B. Diversion colitis is associated with ulcerative colitis and Crohn's colitis.

   C. Microscopic colitis is associated with *Yersinia* infection.

   D. Metronidazole is used to treat acute ileitis caused by *Yersinia* infection.

   E. Pseudomembranous colitis is associated with amebiasis.

*Ref.: 15*

**COMMENTS: Backwash ileitis** consists of nonspecific inflammation and dilation of the ileum in patients with **ulcerative colitis** involving the entire colon. There is no thickening or narrowing as seen in **Crohn's disease**. Its presence does not imply a pre–Crohn's disease condition, nor does it imply a poor outcome after the ileal pouch–anal anastomosis procedure.

**Diversion colitis** is found in segments of defunctionalized bowel. Instillation of short-chain fatty acids ameliorates this condition, thus supporting the concept that these substances (being primary nutrients for colonic mucosal cells) are deficient in this condition. Preliminary trials on idiopathic ulcerative proctocolitis have shown a response to short-chain fatty acid enemas. Following reversal of the fecal diversion, the endoscopic findings of diversion colitis usually resolve.

**Microscopic colitis** (also known as lymphocytic colitis) is characterized by a history of watery diarrhea and microscopic inflammation of colonic mucosa. The colitis often responds favorably to sulfasalazine. **Collagenous colitis** (which exhibits a collagenous band under the surface epithelium of the colon on microscopic examination) may be a variant of this condition because patients have similar symptoms and respond to sulfasalazine. Spontaneous remission of these two conditions is common.

Most of these patients have been incorrectly labeled for years as having irritable bowel syndrome. Colonoscopy with biopsy may yield the correct diagnosis.

Acute inflammatory ileitis causes right lower quadrant pain and is commonly confused with appendicitis or Crohn's disease. **Acute ileitis**, often attributable to *Yersinia enterocolitica* infection, is capable of producing a self-limited, acute ileitis and colitis, sometimes with a granulomatous reaction.

Antibiotic-induced colitis (also known as **pseudomembranous colitis**) is characterized by watery diarrhea, which is rarely bloody and is caused by proliferation of *C. difficile*. The diagnosis is best made by detecting *C. difficile* toxin in the stool. Either oral vancomycin or metronidazole is used to treat this condition. The latter is less expensive and is therefore used more often.

**ANSWER: A**

23. Pouchitis can frequently complicate the ileal pouch–anal anastomosis procedure. With regard to this condition, which of the following is true?

   A. It occurs with equal frequency in patients with familial polyposis and ulcerative colitis.

   B. It is found more frequently in patients with capacious S-shaped pouches than in those with J-shaped pouches.

   C. Most patients can be treated successfully with oral metronidazole.

   D. The pathogen responsible is usually *Bacteroides*.

   E. Recurrent persistent pouchitis invariably necessitates pouch excision.

*Ref.: 9*

**COMMENTS: Pouchitis** is a nonspecific inflammation of the ileal reservoir following the ileal pouch–anal anastomosis procedure. It occurs in up to 50% of patients. Its cause is not precisely known, but pouchitis is seen more frequently in patients with ulcerative colitis than in those with familial polyposis. Pouchitis is not related to pouch design, stasis within the pouch, or a specific aerobic or anaerobic bacterial pathogen. Pouchitis is manifested clinically as increased stool output and frequency, malaise, cramps, and arthralgias. Most cases respond to oral metronidazole and hospitalization, with pouch excision being required rarely.

**ANSWER: C**

24. A 21-year-old woman is noted to have persistent bloody diarrhea, abdominal cramps, and fever. Stool studies are negative for infectious diarrhea. Colonoscopy reveals friable mucosa in a continuous manner from the rectum to the sigmoid colon. No granulomas are found on biopsy. What statement is true regarding the most likely diagnosis in this patient?

   A. Pseudopolyps and cobblestoning are common colonoscopic findings.

   B. The patient is amenable to a curative operation.

   C. Rectal sparing is common with colonoscopy.

   D. Perianal fistulas are commonly seen on rectal examination.

   E. Small bowel involvement is common.

*Ref.: 3*

**COMMENTS: This patient probably has ulcerative colitis.** In ulcerative colitis, the anus is spared, whereas in **Crohn's disease**, anal or perianal disease is the first manifestation in 25% to 30% of patients. Anal disease ultimately develops in 50% to 70% of patients with Crohn's colitis. Rectal involvement can be seen with both of these inflammatory diseases of the colon but is more common in ulcerative colitis (95% versus 50%). The small bowel is extensively involved in approximately 50% of patients with Crohn's disease, whereas "backwash ileitis," a nonspecific dilation of the terminal ileum, occurs in perhaps only 10% of patients with ulcerative colitis and has no prognostic or physiologic implications.

The clinical features of these two entities are similar: chronic diarrhea, cramping, abdominal pain, and fever. Bloody stools, common with ulcerative colitis, are less frequent with Crohn's disease. Total proctocolectomy or colectomy, rectal mucosectomy, and ileal pouch–anal anastomosis eliminate ulcerative colitis, whereas there is no curative operation for Crohn's disease. Indeed, even after total proctocolectomy for pancolonic involvement of Crohn's disease, its recurrence rate may be as high as 50%. One third of patients require additional surgery for such recurrence. Toxic megacolon can be an emergency, life-threatening complication of either ulcerative colitis or Crohn's disease, although it occurs less frequently with the latter.

**ANSWER: B**

25. With regard to diverticular fistulas, which of the following statements is true?

A. Colocutaneous fistulas frequently occur spontaneously.

B. Patients with colovesical fistulas normally have urinary tract infections that may be accompanied by pneumaturia and fecaluria, and the diagnosis is best confirmed with a barium enema.

C. Coloenteric fistulas may be totally asymptomatic.

D. Surgical correction is best accomplished in stages.

E. Colonic fistula occurs in up to 30% of complicated cases of diverticulitis.

*Ref.:* 1, 3

**COMMENTS: Fistula** formation occurs in 5% of complicated cases of **colonic diverticulitis**. Fistulas are usually adjacent to viscera—the bladder, uterus, vagina, or small bowel. Colocutaneous fistulas rarely form spontaneously. They are most commonly seen as a postoperative complication in which they drain through operative incisions or drain tracts. **Colovesical fistulas** are most frequently the result of diverticular disease, followed in frequency by cancer, Crohn's disease, radiation-induced colitis, and foreign bodies. Their first symptoms (e.g., fecaluria and pneumaturia) are referable to the urinary tract. The patient may relate a history of abdominal pain and fever before development of the fistula. Although a barium enema may give information regarding the site and extent of involvement of the colon with diverticulosis, a fistula is demonstrated in only one half of the cases. Cystoscopy may demonstrate bullous (edematous) edema of the dome of the bladder, a finding consistent with a fistula. Computed tomography (CT) may reveal a constellation of findings, including air in the bladder, a thickened loop of bowel lying adherent to the bladder, and enteric contrast in the bladder (before intravenous contrast material has been administered). **Computed tomography** has become the diagnostic test of choice. Coloenteric fistulas may cause no symptoms or may be manifested as diarrhea, depending on which segments of bowel are involved with the fistula. The fistula can be corrected with a one-stage operation in most patients, which is the preferred treatment. If bowel preparation is inadequate or there is extensive

local inflammation or abscess formation beyond the immediate vicinity of the colon or its mesentery, staged procedures may be required.

**ANSWER: C**

26. Cecal diverticula are different from sigmoid diverticula in that:

A. Sigmoid diverticula are true diverticula.

B. Cecal diverticulitis is usually distinguishable from cancer.

C. Cecal diverticula are considered congenital in origin.

D. Asymptomatic cecal diverticula found on barium enema should be treated operatively because of the high incidence of complications.

E. In the presence of feculent peritonitis from perforation of a cecal diverticula, resection and primary anastomosis can be performed safely in most cases.

*Ref.:* 3

**COMMENTS: Sigmoid diverticula** lack a muscular component and thus are not considered true diverticula. Right-sided diverticula may occur as parts of diffuse colonic diverticulosis and are therefore pseudodiverticular and acquired. Occasionally, isolated, solitary, right-sided diverticula are found and possess all layers of the bowel wall. They are probably congenital in origin. **Cecal diverticulitis** is uncommon, and the correct preoperative diagnosis is rarely made because it is confused with acute appendicitis in 80% of patients and with cancer in approximately 5%. In patients with repeated attacks, the cecal inflammation and subsequent scarring and fibrosis may be indistinguishable from those associated with cancer. Similarly, an inflammatory mass of the sigmoid colon may resemble a cancer at laparotomy.

The surgical options depend on the extent of inflammation. If the inflammation are minimal and limited, segmental resection and anastomosis may be all that are necessary. If there has been perforation with frank feculent peritonitis, most surgeons hesitate to perform a primary anastomosis and instead resect the involved segment and divert the stool proximally. For both types of diverticula, surgical therapy is not required if the diverticulum is discovered incidentally and the patient is asymptomatic.

**ANSWER: C**

27. Which of the following disease processes warrants colonoscopy?

A. Determining the extent of ulcerative colitis in a patient in a toxic condition admitted to the hospital for an acute exacerbation

B. Management of patients with recurrent anal fistula and fissures

C. Evaluation of an equivocal finding on CT in a febrile patient with an acute exacerbation of diverticulitis

D. Evaluating gastrointestinal symptoms such as rectal bleeding and severe abdominal pain in a patient in an intensive care unit who recently underwent repair of an aortic abdominal aneurysm

E. Evaluation of the radiologic findings of a sigmoid colon cutoff sign and free air under the diaphragm in a patient with an acute abdomen

*Ref.:* 1, 5, 6, 15

**COMMENTS:** See Question 28.

**ANSWER:** B

28. Colonoscopy is indicated in the following group of patients except:

A. Patients with Crohn's colitis to monitor the efficacy of treatment

B. Patients with an 8- to 10-year history of ulcerative colitis involving the entire colon

C. Family members at risk for hereditary nonpolyposis colorectal cancer (HNPCC)

D. A patient with an adenomatous polyp found in the upper part of the rectum on sigmoidoscopy

E. Patients with colorectal cancer in a first-degree relative

*Ref.:* 1, 5, 6, 15

**COMMENTS:** Different colonic diseases have different indications for and contraindications to **colonoscopy**.

**Inflammatory bowel disease:** Endoscopy is essential for the diagnosis and management of inflammatory bowel diseases. It is not indicated simply for the purpose of monitoring response to medical therapy; this can be performed on a clinical basis alone. Patients with a history of ulcerative colitis for more than 8 to 10 years are at higher risk for adenocarcinoma of the colon and should undergo surveillance colonoscopy and biopsy of multiple sites for determination of dysplasia. This procedure should be done annually or every other year, even if the disease is in remission. Patients with inflammatory bowel disease appear to be at higher risk for cancer than those with limited left-sided disease, but the latter group should also undergo surveillance. For Crohn's disease, the risk for cancer and the indication for colonoscopy are less well understood. Patients with recurrent or multiple anal fistulas and fissures should undergo colonoscopy to exclude Crohn's disease. If the ileum is not intubated, a small bowel radiograph should be obtained. Colonoscopy should not be performed during acute manifestations of inflammatory bowel disease because of the potential for colonic perforation.

**Ischemic colitis/diverticulitis:** Colonoscopy is contraindicated in patients with acute peritoneal inflammation, such as acute diverticulitis, peritonitis, or perforation. Colonoscopy may be done after the acute inflammation has resolved to evaluate for cancer.

**Polyposis syndromes:** Some authors advocate flexible sigmoidoscopy for screening at-risk patients with a family history of familial polyposis. Because colonic polyps rarely develop in the absence of rectal polyps, it is probably not necessary to examine more proximal than the area normally covered by a flexible 60-cm sigmoidoscope.

**Hereditary nonpolyposis colorectal cancer:** Beginning at the age of 20 or 10 years younger than the earliest cancer case in the family, colonoscopy should be performed every 2 years in patients with HNPCC.

**Routine screening:** In general, colonoscopy is still the gold standard for screening for colon cancer. In the general population, screening can begin at the age of 50. For those at risk (i.e., strong family history), screening should begin at 40 years of age. Colonoscopy every 5 to 10 years is adequate for screening the asymptomatic population. CT colography (also known as virtual colonoscopy) is indicated for patients in whom fiberoptic colonoscopy was incomplete because of a tortuous sigmoid colon or pain. Colonoscopy may confirm or refute suspected or equivocal radiographic findings during a barium enema examination. If an adenomatous polyp or cancer is discovered during screening sigmoidoscopy, colonoscopy

is indicated to exclude the possibility of proximal synchronous polyps (30%) or cancer (4% to 8%).

**Volvulus/pseudo-obstruction:** Colonoscopy is indicated for patients with sigmoid volvulus and pseudo-obstruction of the colon, provided that there are no signs of peritoneal inflammation. Decompression of the distended colon can be achieved successfully with minimal patient preparation.

**ANSWER:** A

29. A 27-year-man after cholecystectomy has recently undergone colonoscopy for recurrent blood per rectum. His colonoscopic findings are seen in Figure 22-2. Which of the following is the most likely explanation for the endoscopic findings?

A. Diet high in fiber

B. Diet low in animal fat and protein

C. Ulcerative colitis

D. Familial polyposis

E. Previous cholecystectomy

*Ref.:* 1, 5

**COMMENTS:** In the United States, **colorectal cancer** is second only to lung cancer as the leading cause of death from cancer when both genders are considered. Environmental factors, particularly dietary habits, may explain the wide variation in the geographic distribution of colon cancer. This patient has **familial polyposis**. Genetic factors play a definite role in carcinogenesis, and mutational abnormalities have been identified in patients with familial polyposis and **hereditary nonpolyposis colorectal cancer** syndromes. Cancer develops in almost 100% of patients with familial polyposis, usually by the age of 40, if the colon is left untreated. In HNPCC, the lifetime risk for the development of colorectal cancer approaches 80%. Diets low in fiber and high in animal fats and protein are associated with an increased risk for colon cancer. The mechanisms may include alterations in intestinal transit time and an increase in the formation of carcinogenic compounds as a result of bacterial metabolism of dietary components. Gallstone

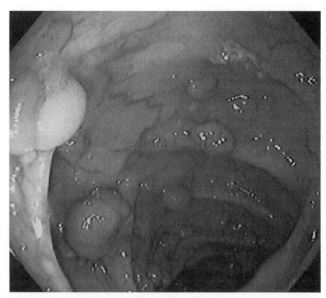

**Figure 22-2.** Post-cholecystectomy colonoscopic findings. *(From Pickhardt PJ: Differential diagnosis of polypoid lesions seen at CT colonography,* Radiographics *24:1535–1556, 2004.)*

disease appears to be more common in areas where colon cancer is prevalent. Some studies have suggested that cholecystectomy is associated with a higher incidence of subsequent colon cancer, particularly that involving the right colon. A proposed mechanism for this relationship is related to the carcinogenic potential of secondary bile acids, to which the intestinal mucosa is increasingly exposed after cholecystectomy as a result of increased enterohepatic cycling. Evidence supporting this association is conflicting, however, and any association that may exist is minimal.

Risk factors for the development of cancer in patients with ulcerative colitis include disease of long duration (the incidence increases 1% to 2% per year after 10 years) and total colonic involvement. An increased risk for cancer has also been seen in patients with **Crohn's disease** of both the small and large intestines, particularly in bypassed segments. The aforementioned notwithstanding, familial polyposis, HNPCC syndrome, and **ulcerative colitis** account for only a small percentage of the total cases of colorectal cancer; most colon cancers occur sporadically without a genetic or inflammatory predisposition.

**ANSWER:** D

30. Which statement is correct concerning intestinal polyposis syndromes?

   A. Hamartomas are found in patients with both juvenile polyps and Peutz-Jeghers syndrome.

   B. Familial polyposis syndrome often includes extraintestinal manifestations.

   C. Turcot syndrome often includes small bowel polyps.

   D. Peutz-Jeghers syndrome, Gardner syndrome, and Turcot syndrome are inherited in an autosomal recessive pattern.

   E. Familial polyposis and Turcot syndrome are benign conditions without malignant potential.

*Ref.:* 1, 3, 5

**COMMENTS: Hamartomas** are lesions in which normal tissue is found in an abnormal structural configuration. **Peutz-Jeghers syndrome** is transmitted as an autosomal dominant trait. The polyps are hamartomas and are found primarily in the jejunum and ileum, with involvement of the colon and rectum in one third and the stomach in one fourth of patients. The polyps may cause obstruction, intussusception, or bleeding. It is now generally accepted that there is an increased incidence of gastrointestinal cancers associated with Peutz-Jeghers syndrome, and polypectomy is therefore advised, particularly if the patient has recurrent colicky pain or anemia. Colonic lesions are usually treated by polypectomy, and colectomy is not generally needed. In addition to intestinal polyps, the syndrome is characterized by melanin spots on the oral mucosa, lips, palms of the hands, and soles of the feet. Juvenile polyps are solitary 70% of the time, and in 60% of cases they are located within 10 cm of the anal verge. Occasionally, a patient is found to have a syndrome of juvenile polyposis characterized by anemia, anergy, hypoproteinemia, and failure to thrive. Some clinicians have found a strong association between gastrointestinal malignancy and juvenile polyposis. In **Cronkhite-Canada syndrome**, the polyps, which are hamartomas, are dispersed throughout the gastrointestinal tract. This entity is characterized by hyperpigmentation of the skin, alopecia, and atrophy of the fingernails and toenails. **Familial adenomatous polyposis** by itself lacks extraintestinal manifestations. **Turcot** and **Gardner syndromes** are variants of familial polyposis associated with certain noncolonic manifestations. Turcot syndrome has the additional characteristic of central nervous system tumors. Small bowel polyposis is seen in all of the syndromes listed with the exception of Turcot syndrome.

In addition to the polyps, Gardner syndrome is typified by the presence of osteomas, exostoses, and desmoid tumors. The polypoid lesions observed with chronic ulcerative colitis are inflammatory "pseudopolyps," and the malignant potential of ulcerative colitis is not related to the presence of these lesions.

Of the conditions listed, Cronkhite-Canada syndrome is not inherited and does not have malignant potential. Familial polyposis, Turcot syndrome, and Gardner syndrome may represent different expressions of the same disease. Patients with familial polyposis, Turcot syndrome, or Gardner syndrome must undergo surveillance upper endoscopy at 3- to 5-year intervals. In the Cleveland Clinic Polyposis Registry, duodenal polyps were found in 33% of patients and gastric polyps in 28%, and although most gastric polyps were of the fundic gland type, all duodenal polyps were adenomas. Following colorectal cancer, the most common cause of death in these patients was cancer of the periampullary region. An autosomal dominant gene has been proposed for Peutz-Jeghers syndrome, familial polyposis, and Gardner syndrome, whereas it is believed that Turcot syndrome is caused by an autosomal recessive gene or an autosomal dominant gene with incomplete penetrance, and generations may be skipped.

**ANSWER:** A

31. With regard to the adenomatous polyposis coli syndromes, which of the following statements is true?

   A. Screening of family members at risk should begin at the age of 25 and consists of annual colonoscopy.

   B. Twenty-five percent of the offspring of an afflicted individual will have the disease.

   C. The risk for the development of colon cancer is approximately 50%.

   D. Abdominal colectomy and ileoproctostomy eliminate the risk for carcinoma.

   E. Periampullary tumors are an important cause of death.

*Ref.:* 1, 3, 6, 16

**COMMENTS:** Most reports of **polyposis syndromes** reflect experience in American and European populations, but these diseases have been identified in Africans and Asians as well. There is probably no race or geographic area that is exempt. The polyposis syndromes occur in approximately 1 in every 12,000 births. Thus, polyposis syndromes are diagnosed in 300 new patients each year in the United States. The disease is transmitted as an autosomal dominant trait, and therefore approximately 50% of the offspring of an afflicted individual have the disease. About 30% to 40% of patients do not have a family history of polyposis, and these cases represent spontaneous mutations at the polyposis locus.

The polyps are not present at birth but usually first appear at puberty and gradually increase in number so that by the age of 21, the colon and rectum are carpeted by thousands of polyps. If the polyps are left untreated, the risk for the development of cancer of the colon is approximately 100%, with death from colon cancer occurring at an average age of 41.5 years. Subtotal colectomy with ileoproctostomy has been advocated by some clinicians. If this procedure is performed, close surveillance of the rectal remnant is mandatory and is accomplished with proctoscopy performed at 6-month intervals. The incidence from rectal cancer after ileorectostomy varies widely among series, with one study reporting an incidence as high as 59% at 23 years. Other reports estimate the risk to be 5% to 15% and the chance of dying from rectal cancer extremely low. In fact, patients are less likely to die of rectal cancer than of periampullary tumors or desmoids. Nevertheless, the importance of surveillance proctoscopy cannot be overemphasized.

At the time of initial diagnosis, extensive carpeting of the rectum with more than 20 polyps should dissuade one from recommending ileorectostomy. The presence of *colon* cancer should also dissuade one from preserving the rectum. Mucosal proctectomy with ileo-anal anastomosis removes all neoplastic mucosa while avoiding the need for a permanent ileostomy.

For **familial adenomatous polyposis**, screening of asymptomatic family members at risk should begin at puberty and should include annual proctosigmoidoscopy. Upper gastrointestinal endoscopy should be done to verify involvement of the stomach and duodenum every 1 to 3 years beginning at the age of 20 to 25. If polyps are found, biopsy is recommended to verify the presence of adenomatous tissue. Alternatively, a family may choose genetic screening for members at risk. If genetic testing is negative, that individual may avoid annual flexible sigmoidoscopy.

**ANSWER:** E

32. The following statements are true about HNPCC syndrome (Lynch syndrome) except:

  A. It is inherited as an autosomal dominant trait.

  B. Most cancers in patients with HNPCC involve the right colon.

  C. Most patients are younger than 50 years.

  D. In up to 40% of patients who undergo segmental (rather than total) colectomy, metachronous colorectal cancers develop within 10 years.

  E. There is a high frequency of endometrial, ovarian, breast, and gastric cancers.

*Ref.:* 9, 17

**COMMENTS:** **Hereditary nonpolyposis colorectal cancer syndrome** occurs in two varieties: (1) site-specific colorectal cancer (Lynch syndrome I) and (2) colorectal cancer associated with other forms of cancer (e.g., endometrial, ovarian, breast, urothelial, biliary, and gastric; Lynch syndrome II). Accounting for approximately 5% to 6% of all colorectal cancers, HNPCC is caused by mutations in the mismatch repair genes that normally repair errors in DNA replication. It is inherited as an autosomal dominant trait and may affect multiple generations in succession. Afflicted individuals show a predominance of right-sided cancers (72.3%), are likely to have multiple carcinomas (18.1%), are usually young (mean age of 44.6 years), and often have metachronous colorectal cancers (40% risk over a 10-year period) following segmental colectomy. It is interesting to note that these individuals may have improved survival when compared with those with sporadic cancers. The Amsterdam criteria help identify suspected families with the 3-2-1-0 rule. There may be three successive generations affected by colorectal cancer, one affected person is a first-degree relative of the other two, one affected person is younger than 50 years, and there should be no evidence of familial polyposis. If this rule is satisfied, genetic studies or an endoscopic screening program for family members should be instituted.

Family members at risk should undergo biannual colonoscopy beginning at age 25 or 10 years younger than the age of an affected family member. Women should have an annual pelvic examination with transabdominal and transvaginal ultrasound to examine the ovaries and the thickness of the endometrial stripe. Serum markers for ovarian cancer should also be determined. Mammograms should be obtained earlier than usually advised. Alternatively, a family may choose to undergo genetic screening to identify members who have inherited the mutation.

If a new cancer is found in an HNPCC family, consideration should be given to subtotal colectomy because of the risk for metachronous tumors. If a woman has completed childbearing, hysterectomy and bilateral salpingo-oophorectomy may also be considered at the time of colectomy.

**ANSWER:** B

33. Match the gene in the left column with the applicable statement in the right column:

  A. Familial adenomatous polyposis

  B. *p53*

  C. *hMSH2*

  D. *DCC*

  E. K-*ras*

  a. Tumor suppressor gene (adenoma polyposis coli [*APC*]) located on chromosome 17

  b. Late-occurring alteration resulting in loss of cell-to-cell contact, thereby enhancing metastases

  c. Located on chromosome 5

  d. Most common mutation found in patients with HNPCC

  e. Oncogene that when mutated, codes for a protein that cannot regulate cell growth and differentiation

*Ref.:* 17

**COMMENTS:** The **adenoma polyposis coli** gene is located on chromosome 5, is large (consisting of approximately 15 exons), and encodes for a cytoplasmic protein of 2843 amino acids. *APC* mutations occur in patients with both sporadic colorectal cancers and **familial polyposis**, are frequent, are comparable in incidence with adenomas and carcinomas, and occur early in the development of cancer. The protein product of the *APC* gene is normally involved in maintaining cellular adhesion and suppressing neoplastic growth, but the mutant protein may not be capable of serving this function. The *APC* gene thereby acts as a tumor suppressor gene. Approximately 35% of patients with sporadic cancers and up to 75% of those with polyposis cancers have *APC* mutations that can occur at variable points within the gene. This may explain the various phenotypes associated with the polyposis syndromes.

The *p53* gene is a tumor suppressor gene located on chromosome 17. Mutations of this gene are the most common genetic abnormality found in various human cancers. The gene encodes for a nuclear phosphoprotein that regulates transcription and negatively influences cellular proliferation by binding at specific DNA sites. For example, cells damaged by ultraviolet light or radiation are kept from replicating by the wild-type (natural) p53 protein. Mutant p53 binds to wild-type p53, thereby preventing specific binding to DNA and permitting tumor growth.

**Mismatch repair genes** correct errors of DNA replication. Alterations in these genes have been implicated in the pathogenesis of HNPCC. The genetic sequences identified are (1) *hMSH2* on chromosome 2 (mutation of this gene may account for up to 40% of the genetic alterations seen in families with HNPCC); (2) *hMLH1* on chromosome 3, which may act as a tumor-suppressor gene; (3) *hPMS1* on chromosome 2; and (4) *hPMS2* on chromosome 7. Mutations of the latter two genes account for only 10% of the mutations seen in families with **HNPCC**. Germline mutations of the *hMSH2* and *hMLH1* genes by themselves are not enough to produce the HNPCC phenotype. A somatic mutation of the remaining wild-type allele is also necessary.

The *DCC* gene is located on chromosome 18 and encodes for a protein involved in cell-to-cell contact. Deletions of this gene have been found in 73% of patients with colorectal cancers but in only 11% of those with adenomas, thus suggesting that gene loss occurred late during tumorigenesis. Cancers with loss of the *DCC* gene are more likely to initially be seen as advanced disease (in comparison with tumors maintaining this gene), and patient survival is consequently compromised.

The K-*ras* gene, an oncogene found on chromosome 12, encodes for a plasma membrane–based protein involved in the transduction of growth and differentiation signals. Approximately 50% of patients with colorectal cancer have K-*ras* mutations. Large adenomas and adenomas with small areas of invasive cancer have nearly the same incidence of K-*ras* mutations, thus suggesting that genetic alterations in the K-*ras* gene occur early (but not as early as *APC* mutations) during tumorigenesis. It has yet to be proved whether K-*ras* mutations have any prognostic significance.

**ANSWERS:** A-c; B-a; C-d; D-b; E-e

34. With regard to colorectal polyps, which of the following is not considered precancerous?

   A. Hyperplastic polyp

   B. Tubular adenoma

   C. Tubulovillous adenoma

   D. Villous adenoma

   E. Adenomatous polyp

*Ref.:* 1, 3

**COMMENTS:** See Question 35.

**ANSWER:** A

35. Which of the following statements is true regarding colorectal polyps?

   A. Tubular adenoma is the most common type of colon polyp, and mitosis occurs at the surfaces of crypts.

   B. Hyperplastic polyps are the most common type of colon polyp, and mitosis occurs at the depths of crypts.

   C. Tubular adenomas are usually pedunculated and differentiate into mature goblet cells.

   D. The malignant potential of colorectal polyps is related to both size and location of the polyp.

   E. The most common location for hyperplastic polyps is the ascending colon.

*Ref.:* 1, 3

**COMMENTS:** Polypoid colorectal lesions can be classified as neoplastic or non-neoplastic. Non-neoplastic polyps include hyperplastic polyps, pseudopolyps, and hamartomas. Neoplastic polyps include tubular adenomas, tubulovillous adenomas, and villous adenomas. **Hyperplastic polyps** are the most common type of all polyps. They result from an imbalance between cell division and cell exfoliation. They are small, multiple, and sessile, and they occur most frequently in the rectosigmoid area. Although hyperplastic polyps are non-neoplastic and have no malignant potential, they are nonetheless removed to differentiate them from neoplastic polyps (adenomas), which have varying malignant potential, depending on their size, histologic pattern, and degree of cellular atypia. Hyperplastic polyposis (multiple lesions scattered throughout the colon) may be associated with a higher risk for colon cancer, especially if the polyps are large and located proximally.

Distinction between hyperplastic polyps and **adenomatous polyps** (**tubular**, **tubulovillous**, or **villous**) is readily made based on the histologic characteristics of cellular differentiation and

location of cell division. In normal colonic mucosa and hyperplastic polyps, cell division is limited to the depths of the crypts of Lieberkühn, and differentiation into mature cells occurs as the cells migrate up the crypt to the surface. In adenomatous polyps, cell division occurs at all levels of the crypt, including the surface, and differentiation is incomplete.

Neoplastic polyps may be classified by histologic characteristics (tubular versus villous) and morphologic features (sessile versus pedunculated). Tubular adenoma is the most common type of neoplastic polyp, and it constitutes approximately 75% of this group. Generally, tubular adenomas are asymptomatic, pedunculated, less than 1 cm in size, and (as with all colon polyps) found most commonly in the rectosigmoid region. The likelihood that a neoplastic polyp contains cancer is directly related to its size and configuration. Tubular adenomas less than 1 cm in diameter rarely harbor malignancy. Those 1 to 2 cm in diameter are likely to be malignant in 10% of cases, with a 30% malignancy rate for larger lesions. Sessile adenomas, of all histologic types, are more likely than pedunculated ones to harbor an occult cancer (Figure 22-3). Villous adenomas account for approximately 10% of neoplastic colon polyps. They are generally sessile and, when compared with tubular adenomas, are larger and more likely to cause symptoms such as rectal bleeding, mucous discharge, or diarrhea. They also have a significantly higher risk for malignancy. Overall, approximately 40% to 50% of villous adenomas contain cancer, and one half of those are invasive.

Below is Haggitt's classification of cancer-containing colorectal polyps:

• Level 0: Carcinoma does not invade the muscularis mucosae (carcinoma in situ or intramucosal carcinoma).
• Level 1: Carcinoma invades through the muscularis mucosae into the submucosa but is limited to the head of the polyp.
• Level 2: Carcinoma invades the level of the neck of the polyp (junction between the head and stalk).
• Level 3: Carcinoma invades any part of the stalk.
• Level 4: Carcinoma invades into the submucosa of the bowel wall below the stalk of the polyp but above the muscularis propria. These lesions should be considered an invasive colorectal cancer.

**ANSWER:** B

36. A pedunculated 1.5-cm tubular adenoma is removed endoscopically from the sigmoid colon and found to contain well-differentiated adenocarcinoma extending to but not beyond the muscularis mucosae. The margin of resection is free of tumor. Select the best therapeutic option.

   A. Observation only

   B. Endoscopic fulguration of the polypectomy site

   C. Operative colotomy and excision of the polypectomy site

   D. Sigmoid colectomy

   E. Laparoscopic segmental colectomy

*Ref.:* 1, 3, 18, 19

**COMMENTS:** By definition, this lesion is classified as carcinoma in situ and is treated adequately by **endoscopic polypectomy**. Because a lymphatic plexus exists just below the muscularis mucosae, lymphatic dissemination is possible only when invasion beyond this structure has occurred. The muscularis mucosae of the colon wall may extend for a variable distance into the stalk of the polyp and may not even reach the head. Pedunculated polyps

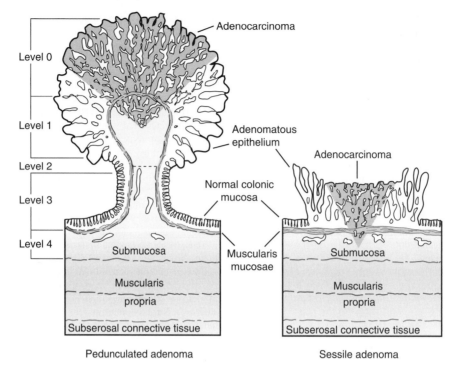

**Figure 22-3.** Anatomic landmarks of pedunculated and sessile adenomas. *(From Haggitt RC, Glotzbach RE, Soffer EE, et al: Prognostic factors in colorectal carcinoma arising in adenomas: implications for lesions removed by endoscopic polypectomy,* Gastroenterology *89:328–336, 1985.)*

consist of four anatomic levels: level 1 is the head itself, level 2 is the interface between the head and the stalk, level 3 is the stalk, and level 4 is the junction between the stalk and the colonic wall. Endoscopic polypectomy should be considered adequate treatment for a polyp containing invasive cancer at level 1, 2, or 3, if the carcinoma is well differentiated and does not exhibit invasion of the veins or lymphatics and the resection margins are free of cancer. For example, endoscopic polypectomy would be sufficient for a tubular adenoma with a well-differentiated cancer extending to level 3 as long as there was no evidence of venous or lymphatic invasion and the margin of resection was free of disease. A poorly differentiated cancer extending to level 2, however, would require formal segmental resection either laparoscopically or by open means. Similarly, any polyp with cancer extending to level 4 requires segmental resection, regardless of differentiation or vascular invasion. **Laparoscopic colectomy** is now becoming a widely accepted operation for curative colon cancer. The Clinical Outcomes of Surgical Therapy (COST) Study Group performed a randomized controlled trial comparing open colectomy with laparoscopically assisted colectomy and found no difference in intraoperative complications, reoperations, survival, and tumor recurrence. This patient, however, does not need any further treatment other than observation and endoscopic surveillance of the polypectomy site.

**ANSWER:** A

**37.** A biopsy specimen of a villous lesion of the rectum beginning 4 cm from the anal verge and extending proximally for 5 cm exhibits cellular atypia. Transrectal ultrasound shows that the muscularis propria is not involved. No suspicious lymph nodes are seen. Which of the following steps is the most appropriate for management?

A. Repeated biopsy

B. Fulguration

C. Transanal excision

D. Abdominoperineal resection (APR)

E. Intracavitary radiotherapy

*Ref.:* 1, 3

**COMMENTS:** A **villous adenoma** with the dimensions given has a 30% to 50% chance of harboring cancer. A sigmoidoscopic biopsy represents a limited sample size and is not adequate proof of the lesion's precise histologic characteristics. In this instance, the finding of atypia suggests a high probability of cancer elsewhere in the adenoma. Complete full-thickness transanal excision of the lesion should be performed so that if a carcinoma is present, its depth of penetration can be assessed accurately. If there is no invasive cancer, the patient is monitored by interval endoscopic examinations because the risk for recurrence is approximately 10%, even though the initial lesion was benign. If invasive cancer is found, the need for further treatment is determined on the basis of the depth of penetration. A stage T1 cancer is adequately treated by transanal excision, provided that the tumor is well differentiated, it lacks vascular or lymphatic invasion, and the margins of excision are clear. A stage T2 cancer should be treated by radical resection. Alternatively, irradiation with or without chemotherapy may be appropriate, but long-term studies are needed to determine the efficacy of such treatment. Fulguration of the lesion can be performed in elderly or poor-risk patients in whom precise histologic staging is not essential. This is not the standard of care for good-risk patients. If there is a local recurrence after transanal excision of a benign lesion, endoscopic fulguration, argon plasma coagulation, or repeated transanal excision may be considered. APR is rarely indicated for benign polyps because there are so many treatment options that are less radical. Intracavitary radiotherapy is reserved for superficial malignant lesions and is not the preferred treatment in this case.

**ANSWER:** C

**38.** With regard to screening for colorectal cancer, which of the following is true?

   A. Barium enema alone is the most cost-effective means of screening asymptomatic patients.

   B. Screening in the general population should begin at 60 years of age.

   C. Fecal occult blood testing (FOBT) is an adequate screening tool for colon cancer.

   D. When combined with flexible sigmoidoscopy, FOBT is an acceptable screening option in average-risk individuals.

   E. For patients with familial polyposis, colonoscopy should be performed every 6 months beginning at the age of 20.

*Ref.:* 9

**COMMENTS: Screening** asymptomatic, low-risk patients for colorectal cancer must be accomplished with a cost-effective means that encourages patients' compliance. The test that easily accomplishes these goals is annual examination of the stool for occult blood (**fecal occult blood testing**). This test uses the peroxidase-like activity of hemoglobin. Stools are collected on three separate occasions and smeared on filter paper impregnated with guaiac solution. Hydrogen peroxide is added, and if hemoglobin is present to catalyze the reaction, the colorless guaiac is oxidized to a blue-colored quinone. Prolonged storage of the test slides may interfere with proper performance of the test. Normal blood loss in stool is 2 mg of hemoglobin per gram of stool. FOBT requires fecal blood loss of 10 mg of hemoglobin per gram of stool to obtain a positive result.

Mass screening programs yield positive results in 1% to 8% of patients. The positive predictive value of a positive test result is 10% for cancer and 30% for adenoma. These programs diagnose a higher percentage of early localized cancers than may be expected otherwise, a fact that lends support to performing FOBT as a matter of routine. FOBT is not a perfect test. For example, small adenomas and cancers not actively bleeding may not yield a positive result. In fact, in patients with a known cancer, the sensitivity of FOBT is 50% to 85%. Furthermore, it is not clear whether the mortality from colorectal cancer is reduced by FOBT alone. When annual FOBT is combined with periodic **flexible sigmoidoscopy**, there is evidence to suggest that cancer mortality is reduced. When used as a screening tool, barium enema is combined with sigmoidoscopy and is performed every 5 years. Alternatively, colonoscopy may be performed every 10 years.

Current screening practices for asymptomatic patients endorsed by the American Cancer Society consist of the following: annual digital rectal examination with FOBT beginning at the age of 40 and flexible sigmoidoscopy at 50 years of age. If the findings are normal, sigmoidoscopy is repeated at 3 to 5 years. If a polyp is found, the remainder of the colon must be examined with **colonoscopy**. Alternative screening tests for asymptomatic patients include colonoscopy or the combination of flexible sigmoidoscopy and barium enema.

Screening is not a term that applies to high-risk conditions such as familial polyposis and HNPCC. For these conditions, the high likelihood of finding neoplastic lesions, coupled with the increased risk to the patient if the tumors are not found, mandate tests in addition to FOBT. Beginning at puberty, patients at risk for familial polyposis should be examined at yearly intervals with flexible sigmoidoscopy. If the disease does not become apparent by the age of 40, the patient probably does not have it. Patients at risk for HNPCC should undergo colonoscopy beginning at 25 years of age. Alternatively, genetic testing can be performed. If an at-risk individual tests negative, that person can be spared the intense endoscopic surveillance programs and instead undergo screening used for the general population.

**ANSWER:** D

**39.** Which of the following is the most common site of colon metastasis?

   A. Brain

   B. Lymph nodes

   C. Direct organ extension

   D. Peritoneal dissemination

   E. Incisional implantation

*Ref.:* 1, 3, 19

**COMMENTS:** Of the various mechanisms by which colon cancer may spread, the lymphatic route to regional **mesenteric lymph nodes** is the most common. This fact has surgical importance because it dictates the extent of resection necessary when operating with curative intent. Hematogenous spread from colon cancer is primarily via the portal circulation to the liver. Cells that escape this effective filter can reach the lungs and rarely the brain.

Rectal cancers can metastasize to the spine via the Batson plexus. Because the rectum has dual venous drainage—through the portal vein and the inferior hemorrhoidal veins into the iliac veins—malignant cells may reach the liver or the lungs. Distal rectal cancers may spread to the lungs without entering the portal circulation. Direct extension to adjacent structures can occur with or without distant metastases.

If the colon cancer has broken through the serosal surface, implantation on the peritoneal surface, locally or widely, can result and thus accounts for metastatic deposits in the rectovesical pouch (Blumer shelf), in the peritoneum under the umbilicus (Sister Mary Joseph nodule), and in the ovary (Krukenberg tumor, originally described for metastases from the stomach to the ovary). Incisional implantation is a rare form of tumor recurrence. Tumor implantation in surgical wounds seems to occur with equal frequency whether the operation was performed with laparoscopic or open techniques and may reflect widespread intra-abdominal disease.

**ANSWER:** B

**40.** Which of the following is the most important prognostic determinant of survival after treatment of colorectal cancer?

   A. Lymph node involvement

   B. Transmural extension

   C. Tumor size

   D. Histologic differentiation

   E. DNA content

*Ref.:* 1, 3, 5, 20

**COMMENTS:** Of the many variables that affect the cure of patients with colon cancer, the status of the **lymph node**s has consistently remained the most important. The long-term **survival** of node-positive patients is approximately one half that of node-negative patients. The extent of nodal disease also has an impact on the **prognosis**. Patients with four or more positive lymph nodes have a lower 5-year survival rate than do patients with three or fewer positive nodes.

Tumor size in and of itself has no bearing on metastatic potential or prognosis. The DNA content of colorectal tumors has been studied extensively, and aneuploidy seems to correlate well with histologic differentiation, transmural penetration, and the presence of nodal metastases. DNA content, however, has not been shown conclusively to be an important independent prognostic indicator. Microsatellite instability has also not been shown conclusively to be an independent prognostic indicator. A meta-analysis of 32 eligible studies involving 7642 patients noted that only about 15% of the colorectal cancer population had microsatellite instability reflecting inactivation of mismatch repair genes. In the remainder of the colorectal population (85%), colon cancer developed from the microsatellite stable pathway and included aneuploidy, allelic losses, amplifications, and translocations. In this study microsatellite instability was associated with a better prognosis.

**ANSWER:** A

41. A 54-year-old man underwent right hemicolectomy. Pathologic analysis showed invasion of tumor into muscularis propria, with 2 of 18 lymph nodes positive for tumor. What is his pathologic staging?

A. Dukes A

B. Astler-Coller A

C. T2N1 (stage IIIA)

D. T2N1 (stage IIB)

E. T3N2 (stage IIIA)

*Ref.:* 1, 3

**COMMENTS:** The **Dukes classification** (1932) was the original standardized method for **staging** colorectal cancer. In subsequent years, however, confusion had arisen because of numerous modifications. In 1954, V. B. Astler and F. A. Coller modified the classification as follows: an "A" lesion is confined to the mucosa and submucosa, "B$_1$" does not penetrate beyond the muscularis propria and nodes are negative, "B$_2$" is through the wall with negative nodes, and "C$_1$" and "C$_2$" parallel the above but nodes are positive.

The American Joint Committee on Cancer (AJCC) has proposed a **TNM** classification that is the most widely used classification of colorectal cancer presently used (Table 22-1). The TNM classification stages a tumor according to the extent of bowel wall involvement and the presence or absence of lymph node involvement and distant metastases. A T1 tumor penetrates only into the submucosa, whereas a T2 tumor demonstrates partial invasion of the muscularis. Transmural penetration imparts a T3 designation, and a T4 lesion invades adjacent structures. An N0 lesion has not metastasized to regional nodes, an N1 lesion involves three or fewer positive lymph nodes, and an N2 lesion has metastasized to four or more lymph nodes. The designations M0 and M1 indicate the absence and presence, respectively, of metastases. A minimum of 12 lymph nodes should be removed en bloc with the specimen for proper staging.

TNM stage 1 colon cancer patients have a 5-year survival rate of about 90%. Stage II patients that have had appropriate surgical resection have a 5-year survival of about 75%. Stage III cancer treated by surgery alone has a 5-year survival of about 50%. Stage

---

**TABLE 22-1   Definitions of TNM**

**Primary Tumor (T)**

| | |
|---|---|
| TX | Primary tumor cannot be assessed |
| T0 | No evidence of primary tumor |
| Tis | Carcinoma in situ: intraepithelial or invasion of lamina propria* |
| T1 | Tumor invades submucosa |
| T2 | Tumor invades muscularis propria |
| T3 | Tumor invades through the muscularis propria into pericolorectal tissues |
| T4a | Tumor penetrates to the surface of the visceral peritoneum** |
| T4b | Tumor directly invades or is adherent to other organs or structures**,*** |

*Note*: Tis includes cancer cells confined within the glandular basement membrane (intraepithelial) or mucosal lamina propria (intramucosal) with no extension through the muscularis mucosae into the submucosa.

**Note*: Direct invasion in T4 includes invasion of other organs or other segments of the colorectum as a result of direct extension through the serosa, as confirmed on microscopic examination (for example, invasion of the sigmoid colon by a carcinoma of the cecum) or, for cancers ina retroperitoneal or subperitoneal location, direct invasion of other organs or structures by virtue of extension beyond the muscularis propria (i.e., respectively, a tumor on the posterior wall of the descending colon invading the left kidney or lateral abdominal wall; or a mid or distal rectal cancer with invasion of prostate, seminal vesicles, cervix, or vagina).

***Note*: Tumor that is adherent to other organs or structures, grossly, is classified cT4b. However, if no tumor is present in the adhesion, microscopically, the classification should be pT1-4a depending on the anatomical depth of wall invasion. The V and L classifications should be used to identify the presence or absence of vascular or lymphatic invasion whereas the PN site-specific factor should be used for perineural invasion.

**Regional Lymph Nodes (N)**

| | |
|---|---|
| NX | Regional lymph nodes cannot be assessed |
| N0 | No regional lymph node metastasis |
| N1 | Metastasis in 1-3 regional lymph nodes |
| N1a | Metastasis in one regional lymph node |
| N1b | Metastasis in 2-3 regional lymph nodes |
| N1c | Tumor deposit(s) in the subserosa, mesentery, or nonperitonealized pericolic or perirectal tissues without regional nodal metastasis |
| N2 | Metastasis in four or more regional lymph nodes |
| N2a | Metastasis in 4-6 regional lymph nodes |
| N2b | Metastasis in seven or more regional lymph nodes |

*Note*: A satellite peritumoral nodule in the pericolorectal adipose tissue of a primary carcinoma without histologic evidence of residual lymph node in the nodule may represent discontinuous spread, venous invasion with extravascular spread (V1/2), or a totally replaced lymph node (N1/2). Replaced nodes should be counted separately as positive nodes in the N category, whereas discontinuous spread or venous invasion should be classified and counted in the Site-Specific Factor category Tumor Deposits (TD).

**Distant Metastasis (M)**

| | |
|---|---|
| M0 | No distant metastasis |
| M1 | Distant metastasis |
| M1a | Metastasis confined to one organ or site (e.g., liver, lung, ovary, nonregional node) |
| M1b | Metastases in more than one organ/site or the peritoneum |

*Continued*

**TABLE 22-1 Definitions of TNM—cont'd**

**Anatomic Stage/Prognostic Groups**

| STAGE | T | N | M | DUKES* | MAC* |
|---|---|---|---|---|---|
| 0 | Tis | N0 | M0 | — | — |
| I | T1 | N0 | M0 | A | A |
|  | T2 | N0 | M0 | A | B1 |
| IIA | T3 | N0 | M0 | B | B2 |
| IIB | T4a | N0 | M0 | B | B2 |
| IIC | T4b | N0 | M0 | B | B3 |
| IIIA | T1-T2 | N1/N1c | M0 | C | C1 |
|  | T1 | N2a | M0 | C | C1 |
| IIIB | T3-T4 | N1/N1c | M0 | C | C2 |
|  | T2-T3 | N2a | M0 | C | C1/C2 |
|  | T1-T2 | N2b | M0 | C | C1 |
| IIIC | T4a | N2a | M0 | C | C2 |
|  | T3-T4a | N2b | M0 | C | C2 |
|  | T4b | N1-N2 | M0 | C | C3 |
| IVA | Any T | Any N | M1a | — | — |
| IVB | Any T | Any N | M1b | — | — |

*Note*: cTNM is the clinical classification, pTNM is the pathologic classification. The y prefix is used for those cancers that are classified after neoadjuvant pretreatment (e.g., ypTNM). Patients who have a complete pathologic response are ypT0N0cM0 that may be similar to Stage Group 0 or I. The r prefix is to be used for those cancers that have recurred after a disease-free interval (rTNM).
*Dukes B is a composite of better (T3 N0 M0) and worse (T4 N0 M0) prognostic groups, as is Dukes C (Any TN1 M0 and Any T N2 M0). MAC is the modified Astler-Coller classification.

**Histologic Grade (G)**

| | |
|---|---|
| GX | Grade cannot be assessed |
| G1 | Well differentiated |
| G2 | Moderately differentiated |
| G3 | Poorly differentiated |
| G4 | Undifferentiated (corresponds to the histologic type "undifferentiated carcinoma" as below) |

It is recommended that the terms "low-grade" (G1-G2) and "high-grade" (G3-G4) be applied, because data indicate that low and high grade may be associated with outcome independently of TNM stage group for both colon and rectum adenocarcinoma. Some authors suggest that G4 lesions be identified separately because they may represent a small subgroup of carcinomas that are very aggressive. However, these tumors would be designated as "undifferentiated" carcinomas within the classification histologic types shown previously.
Used with the permission of the American Joint Committee on Cancer (AJCC), Chicago, Illinois. The original source for this material is the *AJCC Cancer Staging Manual, Seventh Edition (2010)* published by Springer Science and Business Media LLC, www.springer.com.

IV colon cancer carries a poor prognosis, with a 5-year survival rate of less than 5%.

**ANSWER:** C

42. Which of the following is the appropriate operation for a sigmoid cancer that has not metastasized distantly?

A. Segmental resection of the sigmoid

B. Resection of the entire sigmoid and distal descending colon, sparing the main left colic artery

C. Resection of the sigmoid and the descending colon, including the inferior mesenteric artery at its origin

D. Resection of the entire colon proximal to the lesion with ileorectostomy

E. Including routine concomitant oophorectomy at the time of colectomy

*Ref.: 3, 5, 9*

**COMMENTS:** The respective draining mesenteric lymph nodes and the vascular supply to an area of the colon determine the amount of resection necessary when one is operating with intent to cure. The inferior mesenteric artery arises from the aorta 3 to 4 cm above the aortic bifurcation. It bifurcates after 3 cm into the left colic artery, which ascends in the mesentery and into the sigmoidal branches. For a **sigmoid cancer** without evidence of distal spread, the resection should include, at a minimum, the entire sigmoid and distal descending colon and the accompanying mesentery to include the sigmoidal and superior hemorrhoidal vessels but sparing the left colic artery. A more extensive mesenteric resection, with ligation of the inferior mesenteric artery at its origin, is advocated by some, although there is no conclusive evidence that it improves survival rates. In fact, if there are positive nodes at the root of the inferior mesenteric artery, the patient may not be curable. Therefore, this is not considered the standard approach to the mesentery. Resection of the entire intra-abdominal colon can be considered for patients with an obstructing cancer because resection of a dilated stool-laden colon may safely permit an ileorectostomy rather than a colostomy. Other indications for total colectomy include synchronous cancers in separate segments of the colon or cancer in high-risk (younger) patients who require lifelong surveillance. Oophorectomy may be considered in postmenopausal women because approximately 6% of these patients have simultaneous drop metastases to the ovaries. It has not been established that routine prophylactic oophorectomy improves survival. Furthermore, only 1.4% of women with colorectal cancer subsequently require an operation for a recurrence in the ovary.

**ANSWER:** B

43. At the time of surgery for left colon obstruction, you find a thickened segment of colon with a narrow lumen and proximal bowel impacted with stool. There are no liver masses palpated. The following are appropriate initial operative strategies for this patient except:

A. Stricturoplasty

B. Resection and primary anastomosis following intraoperative colonic irrigation

C. Initial decompressive colostomy followed by resection within 7 to 10 days

D. Primary left colectomy, colostomy, and either a Hartmann pouch or a mucous fistula

E. Primary subtotal colectomy and ileocolic anastomosis

*Ref.:* 1, 3, 5

**COMMENTS:** Cancer is the leading cause of **colon obstruction**, and left-sided tumors in particular are susceptible to obstruction. For left-sided tumors producing obstruction, the traditional surgical approach has been an initial decompressive transverse colostomy, followed at a second stage by resection within 7 to 10 days, and possibly a third-stage operation for closure of the colostomy. Initial treatment by decompressive colostomy alone is still appropriate, particularly for poor-risk patients, but resection of the obstructing pathologic entity is more commonly performed today. Therefore, for many patients with obstructing left-sided tumors, the preferred operation is primary resection accompanied by a **Hartmann procedure** or creation of a mucous fistula. The reanastomosis is performed at a second stage. Some advocate primary subtotal colectomy with an ileocolic anastomosis as a one-stage procedure. Most right and transverse colon cancers with obstruction can be treated safely by primary resection and reanastomosis as a one-stage procedure. This is now becoming an acceptable surgical option for left-sided, nonperforated obstructing lesions as well.

In the absence of peritonitis or perforation, an alternative approach consists of resection followed by intraoperative colonic irrigation and then primary anastomosis. The irrigation is accomplished with several liters of saline solution administered through either a cecostomy or an appendicostomy. The effluent is discharged through large-caliber tubing inserted into the open end of the left colon. This operative approach has a clinical leakage rate of 5% to 7%. Recently, colon **stents** have been used to palliate poor surgical candidates with impending obstruction. Stents in the setting of acute obstruction allow temporary relief of the obstruction. Ultimately, a full bowel preparation can be performed with an improved chance for an elective resection with primary anastomosis. Stricturoplasty has no role in managing colon obstruction when cancer has not been excluded.

**ANSWER:**   A

---

44. A 54-year-old man is evaluated by his physician for rectal bleeding. On evaluation, he also reveals a history of constipation and rectal fullness. He underwent a colonoscopy that showed a 3-cm mass 2 cm above the dentate line. Pathologic anlaysis and immunohistochemical staining revealed a neuroendocrine cancer that contained a large amount of amine precursor (5-hydroxytryptophan). Which statement is correct regarding this tumor?

A. This tumor occurs at equal frequency in the colon and rectum.

B. The incidence of invasive malignancy and metastases correlates with the location of the tumor.

C. This tumor, when found in the rectum, frequently causes flushing, diarrhea, and heat intolerance.

D. This malignant tumor of the colon and rectum can be treated by enucleation.

E. Invasive rectal lesions larger than 2 cm are best treated by APR.

*Ref.:* 9

**COMMENTS:** This patient has a **carcinoid** tumor of the rectum. Carcinoid, a **neuroendocrine tumor** of the colon and rectum, represents a wide and diverse group of neoplasms that range from completely benign lesions to poorly differentiated cancers with an extremely dismal prognosis. These lesions share the capability of storing large amounts of an amine precursor (5-hydroxytryptophan), and through the amine precursor uptake and decarboxylation (APUD) system, these lesions produce several biologically active amines. The gastrointestinal tract is the most common site for carcinoid formation. In decreasing order of frequency, the most frequent locations are the appendix, ileum, rectum, stomach, and colon. Colon carcinoids account for only 2.5% of all gastrointestinal carcinoids, whereas rectal carcinoids account for 12% to 15%. The incidence of invasive malignancy and metastases to regional lymph nodes correlates well with the size of the carcinoid for both colonic and rectal lesions. For example, when rectal carcinoids are larger than 2 cm, only 5% to 10% are benign, whereas a lesion less than 2 cm is malignant only approximately 5% of the time.

Because rectal carcinoids smaller than 2 cm rarely demonstrate invasion of the muscularis or lymph node metastases, they may be excised transanally. Rectal lesions larger than 2 cm or those that have penetrated into the rectal muscularis are best treated by APR or low anterior resection (LAR) if possible. If malignant, colon carcinoids should be treated by formal segmental resection with the accompanying lymph node–bearing tissue. Up to two thirds of patients with neuroendocrine cancers of the colon are found to have either local spread or systemic metastases at the time of diagnosis. If disseminated disease is present, resection of the primary lesion is still recommended to alleviate symptoms and avoid bleeding and obstruction. Carcinoids of the colon and rectum infrequently produce carcinoid syndrome unless systemic metastases have occurred.

**ANSWER:**   E

---

45. In which of the following situations should LAR be performed?

A. A circumferential villous adenoma beginning at the dentate line and extending proximally 8 cm

B. Palliation of obstructing rectal cancer just above the dentate line with minimal liver metastases

C. A rectal cancer that produces anal pain and tenesmus

D. Anastomotic recurrence after LAR of a distal rectal cancer

E. An elderly patient with preexisting urinary incontinence and a rectal cancer 5 cm above the dentate line.

*Ref.:* 1, 3

**COMMENTS:** The Miles **abdominoperineal resection** is frequently required for cancers of the mid and distal parts of the rectum. It includes a permanent colostomy and is accompanied by complications such as impotence and bladder dysfunction. Therefore, it is indicated for malignant rather than benign lesions.

Large and even circumferential rectal adenomas can be removed with a variety of transanal techniques that preserve the sphincter muscle and fecal continence. Curative resection of cancers in the mid and even distal portions of the rectum can be performed by **low anterior resection** and colorectostomy or by coloanal anastomosis without the need for permanent colostomy, depending on the exact extent of the lesion, the size of the patient's pelvis, and the skill of the surgeon. A distal mural margin of 2 cm and adequate mesorectal excision must be achieved. The end-to-end surgical stapling devices introduced through the rectum have greatly facilitated anastomoses deep in the pelvis. Because stapling devices have increased our capability of performing deep pelvic anastomoses, there is concern that local recurrence rates will be higher as a result of compromising the distal margin. In fact, the distal margins are not compromised, and the ability to obtain an even greater margin is enhanced. Recurrence rates after stapled and hand-sewn anastomoses are the same.

APR is usually performed with curative intent, although it is justified for symptomatic patients with minimal metastatic disease who are expected to survive 6 months or longer. A cancer that produces anal pain and tenesmus usually involves the sphincter muscle. Recurrent cancer following low resection of a distal cancer usually mandates APR. Fecal incontinence will probably worsen following LAR and a deep pelvic anastomosis.

**ANSWER:** E

46. A patient undergoes EUS for staging of a recently diagnosed rectal cancer 5 cm from the dentate line. Ultrasound shows a tumor extending through the muscularis propria with three surrounding lymph nodes, each measuring 1 cm. Which of the following is the most appropriate initial treatment for this patient?

   A. APR

   B. LAR with total mesocolon excision

   C. Preoperative chemotherapy and radiation therapy

   D. Preoperative external beam radiation therapy

   E. Preoperative chemotherapy

*Ref.:* 9, 21, 23-25

**COMMENTS:** Adjuvant **chemotherapy** and **radiation therapy** have been studied in an attempt to determine their impact on survival and recurrence rates for rectal cancer. The Gastrointestinal Tumor Study Group (GITSG) and the National Surgical Adjuvant Breast and Bowel Protocol (NSABP) R-01 have shown that postoperative radiation therapy reduces local recurrence rates, but its impact on survival was not significant. A randomized Swedish trial showed that a short course of 2550 cGy in five fractions administered preoperatively reduced local failure and improved 5-year survival in comparison with surgery alone. Another Swedish study compared this preoperative regimen with 6000 cGy in 30 fractions administered postoperatively and showed significantly better locoregional control with the preoperative treatment. No chemotherapy was administered.

The GITSG and the North Central Cancer Treatment Group (NCCTG) investigated the combined use of 5-fluorouracil (5-FU) and methyl-*N*-(2-chloroethyl)-*N*'-cyclohexyl-*N*-nitrosourea (methyl-CCNU) and postoperative irradiation for Dukes stages B and C cancers of the rectum and found a reduction in recurrence rates and improvement in 5-year survival rates. This combined therapy, however, is accompanied by significant toxicity. Only approximately 65% of patients are able to complete treatment. Side effects included diarrhea, leukopenia, and enteritis. Postoperative regimens now generally omit methyl-CCNU, and tolerance is better.

An encouraging trend in the management of rectal cancer is the use of preoperative combined chemotherapy and radiation therapy for stage T3 tumors or any tumor that has evidence of nodal metastases seen on rectal ultrasound. This regimen acts to downstage tumors and improve resectability. Advocates of this protocol claim that sphincter preservation is likely to be enhanced, but this advantage remains to be seen. It is of note that up to 20% to 30% of patients have a complete response to treatment; that is, no residual tumor is found in the resected specimen. Preoperative combined therapy is becoming the standard for locally advanced neoplasms.

In summary, (1) postoperative radiation therapy alone reduces locoregional recurrence rates but has not been shown to have an effect on survival; (2) postoperative radiation therapy combined with chemotherapy reduces recurrence rates, improves survival, and is indicated for lesions that either have penetrated into fat or exhibit lymph node metastases; (3) preoperative radiation therapy alone reduces recurrence rates and may improve survival; and (4) preoperative radiation therapy combined with chemotherapy downstages tumors, improves resectability, and induces a complete response in some patients.

**ANSWER:** C

47. Which of the following is true regarding anorectal ultrasound imaging?

   A. Sedation is required.

   B. The bowel must be prepared as that for colonoscopy or colectomy.

   C. Scanning is best performed with a 3.0-MHz crystal.

   D. Imaging of lesions more than 10 cm from the anus is not possible.

   E. Image-guided needle biopsy of extraluminal nodules is safe.

*Ref.:* 23

**COMMENTS: Anorectal ultrasound** is generally performed as an office procedure without the need for sedation or formal bowel preparation. Frequently, a single enema is given 1 to 2 hours before the examination to remove any stool from the rectal vault. Because minimal penetration of the rectal wall and perirectal tissues is required, a high-frequency ultrasound crystal is used (i.e., 7 or 10 MHz) to obtain high resolution of the superficial structures (Figure 22-4). It is possible to image lesions in the mid and upper portions of the rectum, but to be certain that the ultrasound probe is in contact with neoplasms at this level, it is necessary to insert the probe under direct vision through a 2-cm-wide proctoscope. Endorectal ultrasound is used to stage rectal cancer. It is superior to CT for locoregional staging and has an overall accuracy for predicting tumor stage of up to 80% to 95% as compared with CT, which is 65% to 75% accurate. EUS also provides the benefit of guiding fine-needle aspiration biopsies to improve the accuracy of nodal staging. EUS demonstrates the depth of invasion of the cancer (T stage) and nodal involvement (N stage). For endoscopic ultrasound to be accurate on staging lymph nodes, the nodes must be at least 5 mm. Interobserver variability in performing EUS can be a limitation. In addition, EUS is limited in restaging patients treated with neoadjuvant chemotherapy and radiation therapy because of the treatment-induced fibrosis. Ultrasound staging is as follows:

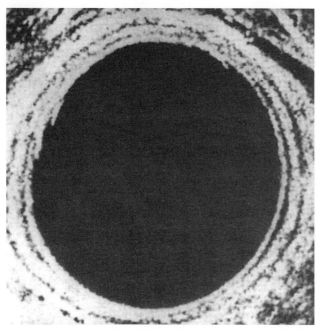

**Figure 22-4.** Sonographic layers of the rectal wall. Inner white, balloon interface; first dark, mucosa; middle white, submucosa; second dark, muscularis propria; outer white, interface with perirectal fat. *(From Saclarides TJ: Anorectal ultrasound. In Machi J, Staren ED, editors:* Ultrasound for surgeons, *ed 2, Philadelphia, 2005, Lippincott Williams & Wilkins, p 434.)*

uT1 is confined to the mucosa and submucosa, uT2 invades but does not penetrate through the muscularis propria, uT3 invades into the perirectal fat, uT4 invades into adjacent organs, uN0 has no lymph node enlargement, and uN1 has lymph node enlargement. Image-guided needle biopsy of extraluminal nodules is a safe procedure that can be performed under ultrasound guidance; suspicious perirectal nodules can also undergo biopsy in this fashion. Only if the biopsy specimen contains benign lymphoid tissue can it be assumed that the nodule in question is truly free of cancer.

**ANSWER:** E

48. A 62-year-old woman complains to her doctor of bright red blood per rectum, mixed with stool. On rectal examination she is found to have a palpable mass at the tip of the finger. Endoscopic examination of her rectum shows the presence of a 4-cm ulcerated mass at the dorsal aspect of her rectum that occupies 35% of its circumference. The tumor begins 4 cm from the dentate line. Which of the following is not indicated in the initial management of this patient?

A. Colonoscopy and tumor biopsy

B. Transrectal ultrasound

C. Transanal excision

D. CT of the abdomen and rectum

E. Rigid proctosigmoidoscopy

*Ref.:* 1, 26

**COMMENTS:** See Question 49

**ANSWER:** C

49. The patient from Question 48 undergoes a complete evaluation that shows a rectal adenocarcinoma and no evidence of distal metastasis or direct local tumor invasion. Her carcinoembryonic antigen (CEA) level is normal. The transrectal ultrasound is shown:

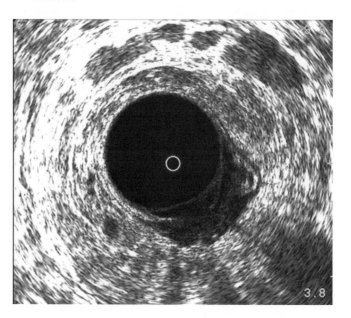

Select the most appropriate treatment for this patient:

A. Local excision

B. Transanal microscopic excision

C. APR

D. Preoperative chemotherapy and radiation therapy

E. Fulguration

*Ref.:* 1, 26

**COMMENTS:** The most common symptom of rectal cancer is hematochezia. Other symptoms include mucus discharge, tenesmus, and changes in bowel habits. The work-up for rectal cancer includes a complete colonoscopy to exclude synchronous colon tumors. Precise location is best determined by rigid proctosigmoidoscopy, which should be done even if the tumor has been diagnosed with colonoscopy to accurately and precisely assess the relationship of the tumor to the anal canal. EUS and magnetic resonance imaging can be used to assess the extent of tumor invasion through the bowel wall and to evaluate the adjacent lymph nodes. CT is useful in assessing the metastatic work-up. A baseline CEA level can be obtained and used to compare with subsequent CEA levels for monitoring of treatment or tumor recurrence. Transanal excision is not part of the initial management of rectal cancer and should be considered only after the evaluation is complete and the results assessed.

Tumors located in the distal 5 cm of the rectum can be difficult to treat. Ultrasound-staged T1 tumors can be treated via a transanal approach, which can be achieved with conventional instruments or transanal endoscopic microsurgery (TEM). TEM uses carbon dioxide insufflation through a 40-mm rectoscope to create better endoscopic visualization of the operative field. TEM is more likely to yield negative margins, an intact specimen, and lower recurrence than conventional instruments are. The pitfall with any transanal approach is an inability to assess lymph node status. In stage I cancers, the incidence of lymphatic metastases is less than 8%. Ultrasound-staged T2 rectal cancers should undergo radical surgery. The ultrasound image of this patient shows deep penetration of the muscularis propria and possibly the mesorectal fat. Suspicious lymph nodes (spherical, hypoechoic) are seen as well. Therefore, she should undergo chemoradiation therapy initially. In the United States, stages II and III rectal cancers are commonly treated with preoperative radiation therapy consisting of 4500 to 5040 cGy and 5-FU–based chemotherapy. Fulguration can be used in patients with lesions below the peritoneal reflection who are poor surgical candidates. This technique cannot provide a specimen to assess the pathologic stage. APR involves complete excision of the rectum and anus through a perineal and abdominal dissection. APR leaves the patient with a permanent colostomy. Thus, APR is indicated when the patient has poor preoperative sphincter control, the patient's body habitus is unfavorable, the tumor involves the anal sphincters, or part of the sphincter needs to be resected to obtain negative margins. LAR involves excision of the rectum and mesorectum through an abdominal approach. LAR may involve the use of a protective stoma (to protect the low colorectal anastomosis), which is often reversed at a later date.

**ANSWER:** D

50. With regard to radiation-induced enterocolitis, which of the following statements is true?

A. Histologically, subintimal foam cells are pathognomonic, and additional changes include progressive vasculitis of the submucosal arteries.

B. The splenic flexure is the most common site of injury.

C. Rectovaginal fistulas secondary to irradiation can be treated only by fecal diversion.

D. Long segments of strictured small bowel are best treated by resection.

E. The prevalence of rectal cancer in patients who have previously received pelvic radiation therapy is similar to that in patients without previous exposure to radiation.

*Ref.:* 3, 27

**COMMENTS:** The incidence of **radiation-induced enterocolitis** is dose dependent. Substantial bowel injury is uncommon with external doses of less than 4000 rad. In addition to the radiation dose, other factors that may predispose to injury include advanced age, hypertension, arteriosclerosis, diabetes, and adhesions that fix the bowel to a constant location. After cessation of radiation therapy, the denuded intestinal epithelium regenerates. In the vessels, however, a progressive vasculitis develops that may lead to thickening of the vessel wall and progressive diminution of the vessel lumen with occlusion or thrombosis (or both).

The rectum is the most common site of injury because of its proximity to the most frequently targeted organs (i.e., cervix, uterus, and prostate) and its fixed location within the pelvis. When rectal ulcers occur, they are located on the anterior wall about 4 to 6 cm from the dentate line. Rectal strictures usually occur at the 8 to 12 cm level. Hemorrhagic radiation-induced proctitis can occur as well. This disease usually arises 12 to 24 months after radiotherapy. Medical treatment, including hydrocortisone, sucralfate, fatty acid enemas, and 5-ASA, can have variable results. Four percent formalin per rectum is an alternative option that is generally well tolerated and safe. The argon plasma coagulator is a more invasive modality that is a popular option; however, it is associated with chronic rectal ulceration, strictures, rectovaginal fistulas, and bowel perforation.

In patients with a **rectovaginal fistula**, every attempt should be made to rule out recurrence of the cancer as the cause of the fistula. If cancer is present, fecal diversion usually palliates the symptoms. In the absence of recurrent cancer and in select patients, an attempt can be made to correct the fistula. Operative correction must interpose nonirradiated tissue between the rectum and the vagina after the fistulous openings have been closed. When possible, anterior resection or coloanal pull-through, with the nonirradiated intestine used for the proximal anastomotic limb, is preferred. The aforementioned precautions to ensure primary healing notwithstanding, proximal temporary fecal diversion in the form of a colostomy should be performed.

Previous pelvic irradiation does predispose to rectosigmoid cancer after a latent period of several years. For this reason, flexible sigmoidoscopy is advised on a periodic basis.

In summary, when treating radiation-induced enterocolitis, the following principles should be observed: (1) avoid an operation unless no other option exists, (2) resect short segments but bypass long segments of diseased small bowel, (3) avoid extensive adhesiolysis, and (4) safeguard against an anastomotic leak with a temporary proximal colostomy.

**ANSWER:** A

51. Which of the following pathology warrants APR?

A. Fixed circumferential adenocarcinoma just above the dentate line

B. Ulcerating adenocarcinoma whose lower edge is 7 cm from the dentate line, with infiltration and expansion of the second hypoechoic layer seen on ultrasound imaging

C. A 2-cm mobile adenocarcinoma arising in a villous adenoma 3 cm from the dentate line, with an intact second hypoechoic band seen on ultrasound imaging

D. Circumferential adenocarcinoma 12 cm from the anal verge

E. A 1.5-cm carcinoid 5 cm from the dentate line

*Ref.:* 9

**COMMENTS:** The most important determinant of which operation to perform for a **rectal cancer** is the location of the lesion within the rectum. Tumors located 0 to 5 cm from the anal verge, especially those that involve the sphincter muscle and are producing pain, are best treated by APR. Approximately 10% to 15% of tumors within this region, however, can be considered for local excision if they satisfy strict selection criteria. They should be no larger than 3 to 4 cm, exhibit minimal penetration of the rectal wall as seen on rectal ultrasound imaging, lack lymphovascular invasion, and be well differentiated. Occasionally, a coloanal anastomosis can be performed in thin patients, especially if there has been a significant reduction in the size of the tumor as a result of preoperative radiation therapy and chemotherapy.

Lesions in the upper part of the rectum (10 to 15 cm) are amenable to anterior resection with restoration of intestinal continuity by descending colorectostomy.

Lesions located in the midrectum (5 to 10 cm) are treated by a variety of operations, depending on the skill of the surgeon and the patient's body habitus. Most cancers in this region can be treated by LAR with colorectostomy (which has been facilitated by the use of surgical staplers) or coloanal anastomosis. In the latter case, a proximal temporary colostomy is constructed to divert stool away from the anastomosis. Impaired fecal continence has been noted in 10% to 35% of patients after coloanal anastomosis. However, construction of a colonic J pouch or performance of coloplasty may avoid frequent stools and incontinence. The decision with regard to the appropriateness of sphincter preservation must be individualized, and safety is a primary concern. If the patient is obese or the pelvis is narrow and a satisfactory anastomosis cannot be performed, APR or LAR with coloanal anastomosis is an option for midrectal cancers. In addition, if sphincter impairment is present preoperatively because of age or previous surgery, a low anastomosis should be avoided.

For low rectal carcinoids larger than 2 cm, transabdominal surgery with lymphadenectomy should be performed. APR would probably be indicated for the patient described in choice E if penetration into the muscularis propria were noted, but LAR with coloanal anastomosis could be considered as well.

**ANSWER:** A

---

**52.** A 58-year-old man is found to have biopsy-proved sigmoid colon cancer during colonoscopy. Staging abdominal CT does not reveal any evidence of metastatic disease. In consultation about laparoscopic versus open colectomy, you inform the patient that:

A. Open colectomy has lower a disease-free survival rate.

B. Laparoscopic colectomy has a higher recurrence rate.

C. Laparoscopic colectomy has higher complication rates.

D. There is no difference in parenteral narcotic use between postoperative laparoscopic and open colectomy.

E. There is no difference in reoperation rates between laparoscopic and open colectomy.

*Ref.:* 19

**COMMENTS: Laparoscopic colectomy** for cancer was first considered in 1990. At the time there was concern for dissemination of tumor and a question of proper oncologic resection for patients undergoing laparoscopic colectomy. The COST Study Group conducted a randomized controlled trial involving 872 patients between 1994 and 2001 to compare laparoscopic and open colectomy for curative resection of colon cancer. This trial concluded that there is no difference in disease-free survival, recurrence rates, complication rates, and reoperation rates between the laparoscopic and open groups when laparoscopy was performed by skilled and experienced surgeons. The laparoscopic group was found to have a shorter hospital stay and shorter use of parenteral narcotics. Patients with intraoperative evidence of locally advanced disease should undergo conversion to open resection to ensure proper tumor management. Thus, laparoscopy is an acceptable option for colon cancer without evidence of distal metastasis or locally advanced disease.

**ANSWER:** E

## REFERENCES

1. Fry RD, Mahmoud N, Maron DJ, et al: Colon and rectum. In Townsend CM, Beauchamp RD, Evers BM, et al, editors: *Sabiston textbook of surgery: the biological basis of modern surgical practice*, ed 18, Philadelphia, 2008, WB Saunders.
2. Pemberton JH, Phillips SF: Colonic absorption, *Perspect Colon Rectal Surg* 1:89–103, 1988.
3. Bullard KM, Rothenberger DA: Colon, rectum and anus. In Brunicardi FC, Andersen DK, Billiar TR, et al, editors: *Schwartz's principles of surgery*, ed 9, New York, 2010, McGraw-Hill.
4. Hookman P, Barkin JS: Clostridium difficile associated infection, diarrhea and colitis, *World J Gastroenterol* 15:1554–1580, 2009.
5. Corman ML: *Colon and rectal surgery*, ed 5, Philadelphia, 2005, JB Lippincott.
6. Mazier WP, Levien DH, Luchtefeld MA, et al: *Surgery of the colon, rectum and anus*. Philadelphia, 1995, WB Saunders.
7. Kaleya RN, Boley SJ: Colonic ischemia, *Perspect Colon Rectal Surg* 3:62–81, 1990.
8. Taylor I: Intestinal blood flow, *Perspect Colon Rectal Surg* 1:49–57, 1988.
9. Gordon PM, Nivatvongs S: *Principles and practice of surgery for the colon, rectum and anus*, ed 2, St. Louis, 1999, Quality Medical.
10. Saund M, Soybel DI: Ileus and bowel obstruction. In Mulholland MW, Maier RV, Lillemoe KD, et al, editors: *Greenfield's surgery scientific principles and practice*, ed 4, Philadelphia, 2006, Lippincott Williams & Wilkins.
11. Fischer JE, Bland KI, editors: *Mastery of surgery*, ed 5, Philadelphia, 2007, Lippincott Williams & Wilkins.
12. Boley SJ, Brandt LJ, Frank MS: Severe lower intestinal bleeding: diagnosis and treatment, *Clin Gastroenterol* 10:65–91, 1981.
13. Browder W, Cerise EJ, Litwin MS: Impact of emergency angiography in massive lower gastrointestinal bleeding, *Ann Surg* 204:530–536, 1986.
14. Wilhelm SM, McKenney KA, Rivait KN, et al: A review of infliximab use in ulcerative colitis, *Clin Ther* 30:223–230, 2008.
15. Sleisenger MH, Fordtran JS: *Gastrointestinal disease: pathophysiology, diagnosis and management*, ed 4, Philadelphia, 1989, WB Saunders.
16. Fazio VW, editor: *Current therapy in colon and rectal surgery*, St. Louis, 1990, BC Decker.
17. Howe JR, Guillem JG: The genetics of colorectal cancer, *Surg Clin North Am* 77:175–196, 1997.
18. Gordon MS, Cohen AM: Management of invasive carcinoma in pedunculated colorectal polyps, *Oncology* 3:99–105, 1989.
19. Nelson H, Sargent DJ, Wieand HS, et al: A comparison of laparoscopically assisted and open colectomy for colon cancer. The Clinical Outcomes of Surgical Therapy Study Group, *N Engl J Med* 350:2050–2059, 2004.
20. Popat S, Hubner R, Houlston RS: Systematic review of microsatellite instability and colorectal cancer prognosis, *J Clin Oncol* 23:609–618, 2005.
21. Ahuja N: Rectal cancer. In Cameron JL, editor: *Current surgical therapy*, ed 9, Philadelphia, 2008, CV Mosby.
22. Kukreja SS, Agusti EE, Velasco JM, et al: Increased lymph node evaluation with colrectal cancer resection: does it improve detection of stage III disease? *Arch Surg* 144:612–617, 2009.
23. Saclarides TJ: Anorectal ultrasound. In Machi J, Staren ED, editors: *Ultrasound for surgeons*, ed 2, Philadelphia, 2005, Lippincott Williams & Wilkins.
24. Diaz-Canton EA, Pazdur R: Adjuvant therapy for colorectal cancer, *Surg Clin North Am* 77:211–228, 1997.
25. Fleshman JW, Myerson RJ: Adjuvant radiation therapy for adenocarcinoma of the rectum, *Surg Clin North Am* 77:15–26, 1997.
26. Turner J, Saclarides T: Transanal endoscopic microsurgery, *Minerva Chir* 63:401–412, 2008.
27. Haas EM, Bailey R, Farragher I: Application of 10 percent formalin for the treatment of radiation-induced hemorrhagic proctitis, *Dis Colon Rectum* 50:213–217, 2006.

# B. Anus

*Kyle G. Cologne, M.D., and Theodore J. Saclarides, M.D.*

1. A 54-year-old woman comes to your office complaining of incontinence. She has a history of three vaginal deliveries, the last one occurring 20 years ago. Which of the following is true regarding her anal sphincteric mechanism?

   A. The longitudinal muscle of the rectal wall eventually forms the internal anal sphincter.

   B. The internal sphincter is made up of smooth muscle, and its lowest edge is above the lowest edge of the external sphincter.

   C. The puborectalis is a part of the levator ani muscle.

   D. The anorectal ring is composed entirely of the palpable deep portion of the external sphincter.

   E. The pudendal nerve is completely responsible for her condition.

   *Ref.:* 1, 2

**COMMENTS:** The taeniae of the sigmoid colon fuse at the upper aspect of the rectum to completely encircle it with longitudinal muscle, in addition to an inner circular muscle layer. In the anal canal, the longitudinal muscle forms the conjoined longitudinal muscle, which descends in the plane between the internal and external sphincters. The circular muscle of the rectum thickens to form the involuntary **internal anal sphincter**. It is smooth muscle and in a state of continuous contraction until relaxation is induced by a bolus of feces or gas. The lowest edge of the internal sphincter is 1.0 to 1.5 cm below the dentate line and is just cephalad to the lowest portion of the external sphincter. The **external sphincter** is formed from three parts—subcutaneous, superficial, and deep—which are striated muscles, under voluntary control, and are innervated by the pudendal nerve. Clinically, these components of the external sphincter are not distinguishable as separate layers. The **puborectalis muscle** is fused with the deep portion of the external sphincter and is also innervated by the pudendal nerve. It is not part of the levator muscle. The puborectalis originates from the posterior surface of the symphysis pubis and runs in a posterior direction to form a U-shaped loop around the rectum. Contraction of the puborectalis muscle pulls the rectum forward, thereby establishing a resting anorectal angle of 90 to 110 degrees. Unhindered defecation requires relaxation of the puborectalis. Inappropriate contraction during straining renders the anorectal angle more acute, which impairs defecation. The puborectalis muscle and the deep portion of the external sphincter, along with the upper portion of the internal sphincter, form the palpable anorectal ring.

**ANSWER: B**

2. All of the following are accepted applications of EUS except:

   A. Assessing sphincter integrity in patients complaining of fecal incontinence

   B. Determining whether a rectal cancer is suitable for local excision

   C. Ruling out recurrent cancer

   D. Evaluating anal fistulas

   E. Routine screening for rectal cancer

   *Ref.:* 3

**COMMENTS: Endorectal ultrasound** imaging has had a significant impact on the diagnosis and management of a variety of anorectal diseases. The initial use of ultrasound instrumentation was for staging of rectal cancers. The depth of penetration and the presence of abnormal lymph nodes were used to determine the stage of the cancer and its suitability for transanal, local excision. Generally, tumors that demonstrate deep penetration of the rectal wall have an increased likelihood of lymph node metastases and are not suitable candidates for transanal excision because of the unacceptably high recurrence rates associated with local excision of these advanced neoplasms. Recently, the use of ultrasound imaging for staging rectal cancers has been expanded to determine whether a lesion is advanced enough to warrant preoperative radiation therapy and chemotherapy. Ultrasound imaging can be used to assess the rectal wall and the extraluminal tissue for any sign of recurrent cancer following surgery. In this respect, it has distinct advantages over other imaging modalities, such as CT, in that the probe is placed in direct contact with the area of maximal interest, namely, the operative site. Resolution capabilities are much better with ultrasound than with CT.

Regarding benign diseases of the anus and rectum, the EUS device can also be used to image the sphincter mechanism in patients complaining of fecal incontinence (Figures 22-5 and 22-6). In fact, before a diagnosis of idiopathic or neurogenic incontinence is made, an ultrasound scan must be done to inspect the integrity of the sphincter. Although most anorectal abscesses and fistulas can be managed without elaborate imaging studies, ultrasound imaging has proved useful for determining the extent of abscess collections laterally and in a cephalad direction. Furthermore, the relation of the tract of the fistula to the sphincter muscle can be assessed with ultrasound imaging; the internal opening can be identified as a hypoechoic disruption of the internal sphincter muscle. In some instances, hydrogen peroxide has been injected into the fistula tract during ultrasound scanning to further delineate the fistula tract.

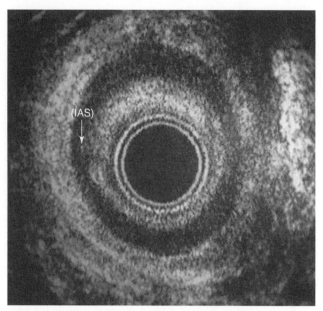

**Figure 22-5.**   The internal anal sphincter (*arrow*, IAS) is a dark hypoechoic band. *(From Saclarides TJ: Anorectal ultrasound. In Machi J, Staren ED, editors: Ultrasound for surgeons, ed 2, Philadelphia, 2005, Lippincott Williams & Wilkins, p 433.)*

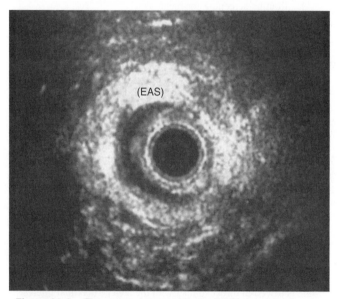

**Figure 22-6.**   The external anal sphincter (EAS) consists of loosely arranged hyperechoic bands. *(From Saclarides TJ: Anorectal ultrasound. In Machi J, Staren ED, editors: Ultrasound for surgeons, ed 2, Philadelphia, 2005, Lippincott Williams & Wilkins, p 433.)*

**A N S W E R :**   E

3.  A 35-year-old man with chronic constipation has noticed the passage of bright red blood per rectum. Anoscopy demonstrates hemorrhoids. Which of the following is true regarding the anatomy of the anal canal?

A.  The dentate line lies above the columns of Morgagni.

B.  Anal gland ducts are completely separate from the anal crypts.

C.  The columns of Morgagni overlie the internal hemorrhoidal plexus.

D.  The typical locations for internal hemorrhoids are right lateral and left anterior.

E.  Anal glands are frequently found in the ischiorectal space.

*Ref.:* 1, 2

**COMMENTS:**  The dentate line is at the level of the anal crypts. Above it are vertical mucosal folds, the columns of Morgagni, that overlie the internal hemorrhoidal plexus. The typical locations for hemorrhoids are left lateral, right anterior, and right posterior. The anal mucosa proximal to the dentate line is innervated by the autonomic nervous system and is **insensitive** to most painful stimuli. By contrast, the anoderm distal to the dentate line is supplied by somatic nerves and is quite sensitive. Anal glands, which number between 6 and 10, usually lie in the intersphincteric space, and their ducts open into the anal crypts.

**A N S W E R :**   C

4.  A 42-year-old man with no previous medical history has had a 4-day history of increasing rectal pain and difficulty sitting. Examination shows a 3-cm area of erythema and fluctance consistent with a perirectal abscess. Which of the following is true regarding the perirectal spaces where this might occur?

A.  The supralevator space is situated above the levator muscle and is connected with the contralateral side anteriorly.

B.  The retrorectal space lies between the rectum and the sacrum but below the rectosacral fascia.

C.  The deep postanal space lies between the levator ani and the superficial external sphincter posteriorly.

D.  The perianal space and the superficial postanal space lie deep to the superficial anal sphincter.

E.  The intersphincteric space lies just outside the conjoined longitudinal muscle.

*Ref.:* 2, 4

**COMMENTS:**  The **supralevator space** is located above the levator ani on both sides and communicates with the contralateral side *posteriorly*. The space is bounded superiorly by the peritoneum, laterally by the pelvic wall, medially by the rectum, and inferiorly by the levator ani. Infection in this space can arise from a pelvic source (e.g., diverticulitis or pelvic inflammatory disease) or as an upward extension from an anorectal source. The **retrorectal space** lies above the rectosacral fascia between the upper two thirds of the rectum and sacrum. The fascia runs downward and forward from the sacrum to the anorectal junction. The retrorectal space contains loose connective tissue and is a site for the formation of tumors arising from embryologic remnants (i.e., dermoids, teratomas, and chordomas). The retrorectal space is bounded anteriorly by the rectum, posteriorly by the presacral fascia, laterally by the pelvic side wall, superiorly by the peritoneal reflection, and inferiorly by the rectosacral fascia, below which is the supralevator space. The **ischiorectal space** lies below the levator muscle, above the transverse septum of the ischiorectal fossa, and between the external sphincter and the lateral pelvic wall. This space communicates posteriorly through the **deep postanal space**, which lies between the levator ani and the superficial external sphincter. The lower border of the deep postanal space is the anococcygeal ligament, which originates from the superficial portion of the external sphincter in the posterior midline. This communication allows an abscess in the deep postanal space to extend to both ischiorectal spaces (horseshoe abscess). The **perianal space** (the most common space involved in abscesses) lies superficial to the superficial external anal sphincter. The **intersphincteric space** lies within the conjoined longitudinal muscle, where the anal glands are also located. The perianal, ischiorectal, and supralevator spaces may connect posteriorly with their counterparts on the contralateral side to form a horseshoe connection in any of these spaces.

**ANSWER:** C

5. A 36-year-old woman has prolapsing rectal tissue and blood seen both in the toilet following forceful defecation and on toilet paper. On examination, she has several large vascular lesions that are reducible with direct pressure. Which of the following statements regarding her most likely condition is true?

A. Internal hemorrhoids are vascular cushions above the dentate line and are covered by anoderm.

B. Prolapsing hemorrhoids are external hemorrhoids covered by anoderm.

C. Bleeding internal hemorrhoids are best managed by surgical excision.

D. Thrombosed hemorrhoids are best treated by hemorrhoidectomy with the patient under general anesthesia.

E. Recurrence is uncommon after surgical hemorrhoidectomy.

*Ref.:* 1, 2, 5

**COMMENTS:** **Internal hemorrhoids** are submucosal cushions normally located above the dentate line and are therefore covered by the transitional mucosa of the anal canal and not by anoderm. **External hemorrhoids** are the dilated veins of the inferior hemorrhoidal plexus located below the dentate line and are covered by anoderm. Prolapsing hemorrhoids are internal hemorrhoids that prolapse beyond the dentate line. Bleeding is the main manifestation of smaller internal hemorrhoids and is managed initially by rubber banding, infrared coagulation, or injection sclerotherapy. Surgery is reserved for internal hemorrhoids that do not respond to these conservative measures. Surgery is the best initial therapy for prolapsing hemorrhoids that require manual reduction or for those that are incarcerated. Thrombosed hemorrhoids are best treated by incising the overlying anoderm with evacuation of the thrombus. Recurrence should be rare after surgical hemorrhoidectomy. When it does occur, it is usually related to inadequate removal of the rectal mucosa and hemorrhoidal tissue.

**ANSWER:** E

6. A 40-year-old woman is evaluated for pain with defecation. The pain started acutely after a large bowel movement, is exquisitely severe following the passage of any stool, and persists for several hours. She is barely able to tolerate examination, which demonstrates a small defect in the anoderm located at the posterior midline. Which of the following statements regarding her condition is true?

A. Most are located above the dentate line.

B. It is located at the posterior midline in all patients.

C. The operation of choice for a posterior midline lesion is excision and posterior internal sphincterotomy.

D. Lateral partial subcutaneous sphincterotomy for lesions not in the midline is considered definitive treatment.

E. Pharmacologic therapy with nitroglycerin, calcium channel blockers, or botulinum toxin (Botox) may prove beneficial.

*Ref.:* 1, 2, 6

**COMMENTS:** An **anal fissure**, a tear of the skin-lined part of the anal canal, is located at or below the dentate line. Gentle spreading of the buttocks is frequently all that is needed to reveal the fissure. About 90% of fissures (acute or chronic) are located in the posterior midline, an area where the anoderm is least supported by the sphincter and blood flow is the poorest. The anterior midline is the second most common location and is involved in 10% of women. Fissures located laterally should arouse suspicion for Crohn's disease, ulcerative colitis, syphilis, tuberculosis, leukemia, or other causes, and therapy is directed toward the underlying disease. The initial treatment of a midline fissure is conservative and involves lubricants and bulk laxatives. Topical nitroglycerin or calcium channel blockers may produce healing of the fissure in approximately 60% of patients; however, several weeks of treatment may be needed. Botox injected directly into the internal sphincter on either side of the fissure may also produce healing. Operative treatment consists of lateral subcutaneous partial internal sphincterotomy to relax the internal sphincter, with the sphincterotomy being carried up to the dentate line. Posterior fissurectomy and sphincterotomy can lead to a keyhole defect and constant soiling. It can be avoided by performing the sphincterotomy in the lateral location. External sphincterotomy should not be performed because it leads to higher rates of incontinence.

**ANSWER:** E

7. A 37-year-old man with suspected Crohn's disease has a recurrent perirectal abscess. The abscess was drained in the emergency department and he is now being seen for follow-up care. Which of the following is true about perirectal suppuration?

A. The pathophysiology of perirectal abscesses is related to infection of the perianal skin.

B. A horseshoe abscess is best drained at the bedside with the use of local anesthesia.

C. An intersphincteric abscess causes pain deep in the rectum, frequently without external manifestations.

D. Ischiorectal abscesses should be drained with the patient under general anesthesia, and the fistula must be identified and treated.

E. Because of Crohn's disease, this patient is at low risk for recurrent disease.

*Ref.:* 1, 2, 4

**COMMENTS:** A **perirectal abscess** starts in the anal glands lying in the intersphincteric space. Horseshoe abscesses include bilateral ischiorectal, supralevator, or perianal abscesses that communicate. Horseshoe abscesses usually arise from infection of the posterior midline glands. A **horseshoe ischiorectal abscess** starts in the deep postanal space and extends in a U-shaped manner into each ischiorectal space. The patient is treated in the operating room under regional or general anesthesia by incising the skin from the external sphincter to the coccyx. This step exposes the superficial external sphincter, which is split longitudinally but not transected. The incision provides access to the deep postanal space. A probe is inserted into the posterior midline crypt and then into the deep postanal space. A rubber seton is placed in this space and wrapped around the internal sphincter and superficial external sphincter. Small counterincisions are made laterally along extensions of the abscess. Sequential tightening of the seton should result in minimal, if any sphincter impairment. An **intersphincteric abscess** is usually accompanied by pain and bulging inside the rectum but no external swelling. Treatment consists of transanally laying open the internal sphincter, beginning at the lower edge of the abscess and extending cephalad to the top of the abscess cavity. Most perianal abscesses can be drained with the use of local anesthesia, but if the patient has a high fever, significant leukocytosis, or extreme pain, treatment in the operating room under general anesthesia is preferable. Identification of a fistula may be deferred until there are clinical signs that a fistula is present, namely, nonhealing of an abscess wound or recurrence of the abscess at the same location. Patients with anorectal Crohn's disease may experience recurrent abscesses despite maximal therapy. Anorectal abscesses may be the first manifestation of Crohn's disease in 5% to 30% of patients, whereas in 20% to 50% of patients with Crohn's disease, fistula in ano develops at some point in their disease process.

**ANSWER:** C

8. A 49-year-old man with Crohn's disease is found to have recurrent perianal abscesses. He is brought to the operating room and found to have a fistula in ano. Which of the following is true?

A. The internal openings of fistulas whose external opening is in the posterior quadrants are always in the posterior midline.

B. The most common type of fistula is intersphincteric.

C. Excision of the entire fistulous tract is necessary for cure.

D. Fistulas associated with Crohn's disease are usually lower and less complex than spontaneous ones.

E. Fibrin glue is the most effective means of treating most fistulas.

*Ref.:* 1, 2, 4

**COMMENTS: Anal fistulas** are classified as intersphincteric (most common), trans-sphincteric, suprasphincteric, and extra-sphincteric. **Goodsall's rule** states that if the external opening is anterior to an imaginary line drawn between the ischial tuberosities, the fistula usually runs directly into the anal canal, and if the external opening is posterior, the tract curves to the posterior midline. Anal fistulotomy and establishment of adequate drainage constitute sufficient therapy. Excision of the tract is unnecessary and prolongs healing. High trans-sphincteric fistulas can be managed by means of a **seton suture**. Alternatives include the use of fibrin glue, collagen plugs, or a rectal advancement flap to close the internal opening. Success rates with fibrin glue are variable, but typically 30% to 60% heal over time. Collagen plugs are inserted directly into the fistula tract and serve as a template for migrating fibroblasts. It is thought that deposition of collagen will obliterate the tract, but initial optimism has waned. With advancement flaps, the internal opening is excised, and a flap consisting of mucosa, submucosa, and circular muscle is raised, advanced, and sutured. Success rates are high even for patients with Crohn's disease, provided that the rectum is relatively healthy. A horseshoe fistula, which starts with infection at the posterior midline anal glands, is best treated by opening the deep postanal space and identifying and performing curettage of the lateral extensions. Laying open the fistula extensions could be done but would result in large,

gaping wounds that may require a long time to heal. The external opening in the posterior midline can be managed by placement of a seton suture. Fistulas associated with Crohn's disease are typically higher and more complex than spontaneously occurring ones. If there is mucinous drainage or an inflammatory tract that persists, biopsy should be done because there is increased risk for perianal carcinoma.

**ANSWER:** B

9. A 41-year-old patient with pruritus ani is seen for further treatment after having undergone a biopsy. Which of the following statements is correct regarding diseases of the anal margin?

A. Bowen disease progresses rapidly to invasive cancer and requires urgent wide local excision.

B. Paget disease of the perianal skin is often associated with an underlying breast malignancy.

C. Basal cell carcinomas of the anal margin have an excellent prognosis.

D. Buschke-Löwenstein tumors are primarily treated by chemotherapy.

E. Bowen disease and Paget disease both require 5-cm margins of resection.

*Ref.:* 1, 2, 7, 9

**COMMENTS:** Precursors to malignant disease are often found in the anal margin. Anal intraepithelial neoplasias, such as Bowen or Paget disease, can cause symptoms such as itching. Skin changes are usually present, and biopsy is indicated whenever the pruritus does not resolve with conservative measures. **Bowen disease** represents high-grade dysplasia or squamous cell carcinoma in situ of the perianal skin. It is associated with human papillomavirus (especially HPV types 16 and 18). It is usually indolent and less than 5% progress to invasive cancer. Treatment consists of wide local excision. **Paget disease** is an adenocarcinoma in situ of the perianal skin. It has a 50% to 70% association with an underlying lower gastrointestinal malignancy, and typically these are rectal or anal carcinomas. Treatment is wide local excision, and a search for underlying malignancy is indicated. Margins of resection for Bowen disease and Paget disease are often determined by mapping biopsies or frozen section. **Basal cell carcinoma** of the perianal skin is rare and has a 5-year survival rate of almost 100% following surgery. **Buschke-Löwenstein tumors** are also called giant condylomas and are verrucous tumors that resemble condylomas microscopically. They are rarely metastatic but may invade local structures around the anal canal or margin. Treatment consists of wide local excision or APR if the sphincter is compromised. Radiation therapy may be used preoperatively to shrink large cancers or for patients with recurrent tumors.

**ANSWER:** C

10. A 59-year-old woman complains of mucous discharge, fecal incontinence, and tenesmus. Digital rectal examination and anoscopy demonstrate a 2-cm lesion in the anal canal. Biopsy of the lesion demonstrates squamous cell cancer. When compared with similar tumors of the anal margin, which of the following is true?

A. They are more common in men.

B. They are more often associated with benign anal conditions.

C. They are more advanced when diagnosed.

D. They infrequently involve the anal sphincter.

E. They are effectively treated by local excision only.

*Ref.:* 1, 2, 7

**COMMENTS:** The anal canal is generally considered to be the region from the dentate line to the top of the anorectal ring (see Question 1). The anal margin is distal to the dentate line. **Squamous cell cancers of the anal canal** are more common in women. Because they are often mistaken for benign anal disorders, they are usually advanced at the time of diagnosis and therefore have a worse prognosis. **Basaloid and cloacogenic carcinomas** are a histologic variant of squamous cell cancer of the anal canal. Conversely, perianal (anal margin) squamous cell carcinoma is four times more common in men and is usually slow growing and late to metastasize. Basaloid features are uncommon. Wide local excision with a 2-cm margin may be adequate therapy for superficial squamous cell cancers of the anal margin, whereas squamous cell cancers of the anal canal generally necessitate multimodality treatment involving radiation therapy and chemotherapy. Up to 50% of patients exhibit local spread to the perianal tissues or anal sphincter at the time of diagnosis.

**ANSWER:**  C

11. Survival after treatment of squamous cell cancer of the anus is related to which of the following factors:

A. Tumor size, depth, and lymph node involvement

B. Tumor size, lymph node involvement, and histologic features

C. Tumor size, depth, and degree of differentiation

D. Basaloid versus squamous histologic features

E. HPV subtype detected

*Ref.:* 1, 2, 7, 9

**COMMENTS:** The prognosis of patients with **squamous cell carcinoma** of the anal canal is related to the delay in diagnosis, which can lead to large tumor size, deep invasion, and lymph node metastases. In basaloid cancers, there is good correlation between histologic differentiation and 5-year survival rates (90% for well-differentiated, 50% for moderately differentiated, and 0% for anaplastic lesions). The presence of basaloid histologic features versus squamous histologic features alone has not been conclusively shown to affect prognosis. Similarly, the degree of differentiation does not in itself appear to affect prognosis (except that less differentiated tumors are often initially seen later with larger tumor size). Although squamous cell cancer of the anus is frequently associated with HPV (most frequently HPV-16), there is no prognostic significance of different types. In addition to HPV infection, risk factors for the development of anal cancer include infection with multiple HPV types, infection with human immunodeficiency virus, receptive anal intercourse, smoking, and renal transplantation.

**ANSWER:**  A

12. A 27-year-old man who engages in anal intercourse has white, cauliflower-shaped masses throughout his perianal region and in the anal canal. Which of the following statements regarding his most likely condition is true?

A. The causative agent appears to be HPV.

B. Podophyllin, administered in a 25% solution, results in resolution of the warts in 80% of patients, and recurrence rates are less than 10%.

C. Immunotherapy with vaccination is used as the initial treatment of small lesions.

D. Carcinoma frequently develops if the lesions are left untreated.

E. Surgical treatment involves excision and is not associated with any risk of transmission to health care providers.

*Ref.:* 7, 10

**COMMENTS:** **Anal infection** with HPV is responsible for **condyloma acuminatum**, which appears as a group of cauliflower-shaped masses on the perianal skin and anal canal. The disease is transmitted by close contact and is seen in both genders regardless of whether anal intercourse is practiced. It is especially prevalent in anal-receptive men who have sex with men, and in this population it is seen more often than genital warts. Another high-risk population consists of those receiving immunosuppression after organ transplantation. Podophyllin, a cytotoxic agent available in 10% and 25% solutions, must be applied by a physician. However, the results have been disappointing. Clearance of the warts has been noted in 22% to 77% of patients, with recurrence rates being as high as 65%. Podophyllin may cause skin burns and cannot be used within the anal canal. Multiple treatments may be necessary. Failure to treat intra-anal lesions may cause higher recurrence rates. An autologous vaccine prepared from the condyloma can be injected weekly for 6 weeks. No adverse reactions have been seen, and resolution of lesions has been noted in up to 95% of patients. At present, such therapy is considered for extensive, persistent, or recurrent cases of condyloma. Although malignant transformation can occur, it rarely does so. Surgical treatment includes excision by one of three techniques (scissors, laser therapy, or electrocautery fulguration). Electrocautery is the preferred therapy and is associated with a recurrence rate of 10% to 25%. There is a risk of surgeon infection within the trachea from the inhalation of vaporized viral particles. This risk can be minimized by using smoke evacuators and special masks.

**ANSWER:**  A

13. A 24-year-old woman with frequent emergency room visits for gastrointestinal complaints is found to have a fistula in ano after recurrent perianal abscesses. A diagnosis of Crohn's disease is suspected. Which of the following regarding perianal involvement in Crohn's disease is true?

A. It is the first sign of disease in 50% of patients.

B. Anal involvement is more common in patients with small bowel than with colonic disease.

C. Multiple fistulas are the most common anal manifestation.

D. One third of low fistulas may demonstrate spontaneous healing.

E. Healing after fistulectomy has no correlation with Crohn's disease activity elsewhere in the gastrointestinal tract.

*Ref.:* 4, 10

**COMMENTS:** Anal or perianal disease is the first sign of **Crohn's disease** in approximately 10% of patients. Ultimately, up to 30% of patients with Crohn's disease present with anal disease. The anus is more likely to be involved with distal gastrointestinal involvement; it affects about 50% of patients with Crohn's colitis versus 25% of patients with Crohn's disease of the small intestine. The most common anal manifestation is edematous, thickened skin tags 1 to 2 cm in size. They can cause pain and difficulty achieving satisfactory local hygiene. Nonhealing of the wounds may occur after ill-advised tag excision. Fistula in ano is the second most common manifestation. Most fistulas are low and simple. Approximately one third demonstrate spontaneous healing. If a fistula is symptomatic and persistent, fistulotomy can be performed, but healing may not occur. Preoperatively, every attempt should be made to control proximal disease within the gastrointestinal tract. Failure to do so is associated with a higher incidence of nonhealing. The absence of rectal disease correlates with successful healing after fistulotomy. Surgery for perianal Crohn disease should be directed at relieving symptoms and should include such measures as draining of abscesses, gentle dilation of strictures, and promoting drainage of fistula tracts with curettage or placement of noncutting seton sutures.

**ANSWER:** D

14. A 60-year-old woman complains of air and stool coming from her vagina. Digital rectal examination reveals an area of induration on the rectovaginal septum, although contrast barium enema does not demonstrate any abnormality. Which of the following statements regarding her probable condition is true?

    A. Eighty-five percent of fistulas caused by obstetric trauma heal spontaneously.

    B. Low rectovaginal fistulas may be treated effectively by fistulotomy.

    C. Rectovaginal fistulas associated with Crohn's disease usually necessitate proctectomy.

    D. Radiation-induced fistulas generally necessitate a colostomy.

    E. High rectovaginal fistulas respond well to fibrin glue.

    *Ref.:* 8, 10

**COMMENTS: Rectovaginal fistulas** are classified according to location and cause, which influence the type of corrective surgery required. **High fistulas** require an abdominal approach, whereas **low or midline fistulas** can be repaired through a transanal, transperineal, or transvaginal approach. The causes of these fistulas include obstetric injuries, irradiation for pelvic cancers, recurrent cancer, inflammatory bowel disease, violent trauma, or infection (e.g., tuberculosis or lymphogranuloma venereum). Five percent of all vaginal deliveries are accompanied by third- or fourth-degree **perineal lacerations.** Approximately 10% of the repairs become disrupted and result in incontinence and, potentially, a rectovaginal fistula. Approximately 50% of these obstetric fistulas heal spontaneously (not 85%); therefore, if the patient's symptoms are not disabling, a 3- to 6-month waiting period is recommended. This waiting period also allows the tissue inflammation and edema to subside before surgical intervention. **Repair of a fistula** secondary to an obstetric injury can be performed transvaginally or transrectally. With the former, the tract is excised and the rectovaginal septum is inverted with serial purse-string sutures. With the latter, a flap consisting of mucosa, submucosa, and muscularis is advanced to cover the rectal side of the fistula. A diverting colostomy is not required unless multiple previous surgical attempts have failed. An **anovaginal fistula** may be treated by fistulotomy, but rectovaginal fistulas (even distal ones) should not be treated by this method. Partial or total incontinence may result if the fistula tract is divided.

High rectovaginal fistulas are best treated through a transabdominal approach so that coexisting pathologic conditions such as diverticulitis, cancer, or inflammatory bowel disease can be addressed. The rectovaginal septum is mobilized, the fistula is divided, the vagina is closed, and normal tissue (such as omentum or a muscle flap) is used to buttress the repair. Because the colon is not usually normal (inflammation or radiation injury), bowel resection is generally necessary.

Fistulas secondary to Crohn's disease do not necessitate proctectomy if the symptoms are minimal, the rectum is relatively healthy, and continence is normal. In such cases, an advancement flap can lead to healing. Refractory rectal Crohn's disease (especially the stricturing form) or incontinence usually necessitates proctectomy. **Radiation-induced fistulas** may necessitate a colostomy as sole therapy (e.g., poor-risk patient with recurrent, unresectable cancer) or to divert stool from an anastomosis after resection of diseased bowel.

**ANSWER:** D

15. A patient is referred to you from the emergency department with a posterior midline anal fissure. He brings extensive literature on possible treatments and has several questions regarding the most effective and appropriate nonsurgical therapy. Which of the following statements regarding the medical management of anal fissures is true?

    A. Glyceryl trinitrate (GTN) ointment relaxes the internal sphincter by acting as a nitric oxide donor.

    B. GTN heals fissures in approximately 65% of patients with a 2% ointment applied four times daily.

    C. The main side effect of GTN is orthostatic hypotension.

    D. Injectable calcium channel blockers reduce the resting anal pressure and heal fissures in up to 90% of patients.

    E. Botulinum toxin is an effective treatment and should be injected directly into the internal sphincter at monthly intervals.

    *Ref.:* 1, 2, 6, 9

**COMMENTS:** Internal sphincterotomy for **anal fissures,** although highly effective, may cause problems with fecal soilage or control of flatus. As a result, nonoperative forms of treatment have been pursued as initial management. GTN acts as a nitric oxide donor, which induces relaxation of the internal sphincter. It is applied topically to the anoderm at doses of 0.2% (not 2%) two to three times daily (not four times daily). Its main side effect is headache. Topical calcium channel blockers (such as nifedipine or diltiazem) are capable of healing fissures in up to 90% of patients. Oral calcium channel blocker therapy is much less effective and associated with increased side effects (because topical agents have limited systemic absorption). These medications are not injected into the sphincter. Botox is a powerful inhibitor of neuromuscular transmission. When injected directly into the anal sphincter on either side of the fissure, healing has been noted, although success rates are variable and range from 40% to 88%. Complications from the injection of botulinum toxin include incontinence (often temporary) and perianal thrombosis. Botox is usually effective after a single injection, although a second dose may be required.

**ANSWER:** A

16. A 38-year-old patient with Crohn's disease is being evaluated for significant perianal involvement and a rectovaginal fistula.

Which of the following statements regarding the use of infliximab (Remicade) for this patient is true?

A. Infliximab is a monoclonal antibody to TNF-α, which has been implicated in the pathogenesis of Crohn's disease.

B. Approximately 90% of patients will achieve significant remission of their disease.

C. Adverse side effects include opportunistic infections, pulmonary fibrosis, and bone marrow toxicity.

D. The endoscopic appearance of the bowel is not correlated with response to infliximab.

E. Before beginning therapy, all patients require screening for tuberculosis and varicella.

*Ref.:* 2, 4, 9

**COMMENTS:** TNF-α has been implicated in the pathogenesis of Crohn's disease. **Infliximab**, a monoclonal antibody to TNF-α, has been studied extensively and has shown great promise in treating active disease. Overall, approximately two thirds of patients respond and one third enter remission. The majority of patients maintain their response for several weeks. Infliximab is better suited to fistulizing Crohn's disease (30% to 60% of fistulas heal spontaneously with therapy, including rectovaginal fistulas). It is not as well suited for nonfistulizing Crohn's disease, in which the symptoms can actually worsen. The endoscopic appearance of the bowel improves after successful treatment with infliximab. Infliximab can cause serum sickness, sepsis, autoimmune phenomena, and opportunistic infections. Because it can reactivate tuberculosis, it is advised that patients be skin-tested and have a chest radiograph before beginning therapy. Varicella screening is not required. Infliximab is rarely required for mild to moderate disease, which is often controlled with aminosalicylates (5-ASA compounds, e.g., sulfasalazine), with or without steroids as needed. Severe disease may require 6-mercaptopurine, azathioprine, or monoclonal antibody to TNF-α.

**ANSWER:** A

**REFERENCES**

1. Bullard KM, Rothenberger DA: Colon, rectum and anus. In Brunicardi FC, Andersen DK, Billiar TR, et al, editors: *Schwartz's principles of surgery*, ed 9, New York, 2010, McGraw-Hill.
2. Nelson H, Cima RR: Anus. In Townsend CM, Beauchamp RD, Evers BM, et al, editors: *Sabiston textbook of surgery: the biological basis of modern surgical practice*, ed 18, Philadelphia, 2008, WB Saunders.
3. Saclarides TJ: Anorectal ultrasound. In Machi J, Staren ED, editors: *Ultrasound for surgeons*, ed 2, Philadelphia, 2005, Lippincott Williams & Wilkins.
4. Glasgow SC, Dietz DW: Anorectal abscess and fistula. In: Cameron JL, editor: *Current surgical therapy*, ed 9, Philadelphia, 2008, Mosby.
5. Gregorcyk SG, Huber PJ Jr: Hemorrhoids. In: Cameron JL, editor: *Current surgical therapy*, ed 9, Philadelphia, 2008, Mosby.
6. Costedio M, Cataldo PA: Anal fissures. In: Cameron JL, editor: *Current surgical therapy*, ed 9, Philadelphia, 2008, Mosby.
7. Ayscue JM, Smith LE: Tumors of the anal region. In: Cameron JL, editor: *Current surgical therapy*, ed 9, Philadelphia, 2008, Mosby.
8. Tran NA, Thorson AG: Rectovaginal fistula. In: Cameron JL, editor: *Current surgical therapy*, ed 9, Philadelphia, 2008, Mosby.
9. Corman ML: *Colon and rectal surgery*, Philadelphia, 2005, JB Lippincott.
10. Gordon PH, Nivatvongs S: Principles and practice of surgery for the colon, rectum and anus, St. Louis, 1999, Quality Medical.

# LIVER, BILIARY TRACT, PANCREAS, AND SPLEEN

# CHAPTER 23

# Liver and Portal Venous System

*Kiranjeet Gill, M.D., and Daniel J. Deziel, M.D.*

1. Which of the following statements about the anatomy of the liver is true?

   A. The right lobe extends to the umbilical fissure and falciform ligament.

   B. The left lobe end at the falciform ligament.

   C. The quadrate lobe is a portion of the medial segment of the right lobe.

   D. The left lobe contains the anterior and lateral segments.

   E. The lateral segment of the left lobe in the American system consists of segments II and III.

   *Ref.:* 1-3

**COMMENTS:** The **surgical anatomy of the liver** is based on the distribution of the hepatic veins and portal structures and has been modified several times. There are two main anatomic classification systems for the liver, the American system and the French system. In both these systems, the liver is divided into right and left lobes by the Cantilie line, a longitudinal plane that extends from the gallbladder fossa to the inferior vena cava. This plane, also called the portal fissure, contains the middle hepatic vein and the bifurcation of the portal vein. In the American system, the liver is further broken down into four segments, with each lobe containing two segments. The right lobe of the liver consists of posterior and anterior segments. The left lobe consists of a medial segment (quadrate lobe) and a lateral segment divided by the falciform ligament. The caudate lobe can be considered anatomically independent of the right and left lobes because it receives portal and arterial blood supply from both sides and has venous drainage directly into the inferior vena cava.

In the French system, developed by C. **Couinaud**, the two lobes of the liver are broken down into eight segments. These eight segments are formed by three vertical planes (scissurae) created by the right, middle, and left hepatic veins, which results in four sectors. These four sectors are further divided by a plane created by the branching portal system. Therefore, the left lobe, according to the French system, is divided into medial and lateral segments by the left hepatic vein. The lateral sector of the left lobe consists of a superior segment (II) and an inferior segment (III). The medial sector of the left lobe is segment IV. The right lobe consists of anteromedial and posterolateral sectors divided by a vertical plane containing the right hepatic vein. The anteromedial sector is made up of segment V (inferior) and segment VIII (superior), and the posterolateral sector is made up of segment VI (inferior) and segment VII (superior).

**ANSWER:** E

2. Which of the following statements is true about the hepatic arterial supply?

   A. Aberrant hepatic arterial anatomy is present in less than 5% of all patients.

   B. The cystic artery is usually a branch off the proper hepatic artery.

   C. A "replaced" right hepatic artery arises from the superior mesenteric artery.

   D. The hepatic artery provides 75% of blood flow to the liver.

   E. The hepatic artery lies dorsal to the portal vein within the hepatic hilum.

   *Ref.:* 1-3

**COMMENTS:** The **hepatic arterial supply** is normally derived from the celiac axis by way of the common hepatic artery, which becomes the proper hepatic artery after giving off the gastroduodenal branch and subsequently bifurcates into right and left hepatic branches. The hepatic artery lies ventral to the portal vein. The middle hepatic artery is usually a branch off the left hepatic artery, and the cystic artery is generally a branch off the right hepatic artery. There is, however, significant variability in hepatic arterial anatomy in up to 50% of patients. In approximately 15% of individuals, the right hepatic artery arises from the superior mesenteric artery (replaced right hepatic artery) and is found in the right dorsal border of the hepatoduodenal ligament. In roughly 10% of individuals, the left hepatic artery originates from the left gastric artery and is located in the gastrohepatic ligament. These commonly encountered variants can have important surgical implications during upper abdominal operations. The arterial blood supply accounts for only 25% of hepatic blood flow, with the remainder being supplied by the portal vein.

**ANSWER:** C

3. Which of the following statements about the anatomy of the hepatic veins is true?

   A. The left hepatic vein drains the entire left lobe.

   B. Veins from the caudate lobe enter the inferior vena cava directly.

   C. The middle hepatic vein usually drains into the right hepatic vein.

   D. There are valves in the hepatic venous system.

E. Hepatic veins have prominent hyperechoic walls on ultrasound imaging.

*Ref.:* 1-4

**COMMENTS:** The **hepatic veins** begin in the liver lobules as the central veins and coalesce to form the right, left, and middle hepatic veins, which drain into the inferior vena cava and are of considerable surgical importance because they define the three vertical scissurae of the liver. The right vein, which is generally the largest, drains most of the right lobe. The left vein drains the lateral segment of the left lobe and a portion of the medial segment as well. The middle vein drains the inferoanterior portion of the right lobe and the inferomedial segment of the left lobe. This vein joins the left hepatic vein in 80% of individuals and enters the inferior vena cava directly in the remainder. There are also smaller veins, particularly those draining the caudate lobe dorsally, that enter directly into the inferior vena cava. The human hepatic venous system has no valves. The portal veins and hepatic veins can readily be differentiated from each other on the basis of their distinctive sonographic features. The portal veins (not the hepatic veins) have prominent hyperechoic walls.

**ANSWER:** B

4. Which of the following statements is true about the portal vein?

   A. It is formed by the junction of the inferior mesenteric vein and splenic vein.

   B. It is the most dorsal structure in the hepatoduodenal ligament.

   C. It contains the valves of Mirizzi.

   D. The right portal vein typically branches later than the left portal vein.

   E. It carries deoxygenated blood and provides only 10% of the liver's oxygenation

*Ref.:* 1-3

**COMMENTS:** The **portal vein** is usually formed dorsal to the neck of the pancreas by the junction of the superior mesenteric vein and splenic veins. It ascends posterior to the common bile duct and hepatic artery in the hepatoduodenal ligament. These three structures make up the portal triad. There are no valves in the portal venous system (Pablo Mirizzi described valves in the common hepatic duct that do not exist). The portal vein bifurcates just outside the liver. The right portal vein has anterior and posterior branches that typically diverge only a short distance from the bifurcation and then quickly dive into the liver parenchyma. The left portal vein has a longer transverse portion (pars transversus) and then angulates anteriorly in the umbilical fissure (pars umbilicus), where it gives off medial branches to segment IV and lateral branches to segments II and III. The portal vein provides approximately 75% of hepatic blood flow, and although the blood is largely deoxygenated, it provides up to 50% to 70% of the liver's oxygenation secondary to the portal system's large volume flow rate.

**ANSWER:** B

5. Which of the following hepatic resections involves dissection in the plane of the falciform ligament or umbilical fissure?

   A. Right lobectomy

   B. Right trisegmentectomy

C. Left lobectomy

D. Left lateral segmentectomy

E. None of the above

*Ref.:* 1-3

**COMMENTS: Hepatic resections** can be broken down into (1) anatomic resections, (2) nonanatomic resections (wedge resections), and (3) enucleation procedures. Anatomic resections are based on either the American or the French segmental system. Right lobectomy includes segments V, VI, VII, and VIII. Right trisegmentectomy also includes segment IV. Left lobectomy includes segments II, III, and IV. Left lateral segmentectomy includes only segments II and III. The umbilical fissure is the segmental plane between the medial and lateral segments of the left lobe of the liver. A portion of the left branch of the portal vein, known as the pars umbilicus, runs in the inferior portion of the umbilical fissure. Dissection is therefore never carried out directly in the segmental fissure. During left lateral segmentectomy, the plane of the parenchymal dissection is to the left of the fissure, whereas with right trisegmentectomy, the parenchyma is divided to the right of the fissure. Both right and left lobectomies involve dissection well to the right of this plane.

**ANSWER:** E

6. Which of the following characteristics is typically seen on ultrasound imaging of the hepatic portal vein branches?

   A. Hyperechoic vessel walls

   B. Hepatofugal blood flow

   C. Diastolic reversal of blood flow

   D. Location between hepatic segments

   E. Vertical orientation

*Ref.:* 4

**COMMENTS:** The portal veins and hepatic veins can readily be differentiated from each other on the basis of their distinctive sonographic features. The portal vein and its branches have prominent hyperechoic walls. This appearance has been attributed to the accompanying intrahepatic branches of the hepatic artery and bile duct, which are not generally seen individually on external ultrasound imaging. In contrast, the hepatic veins appear to be essentially "wall-less." They are anechoic or hypoechoic tubular structures that are vertically oriented and increase in caliber as they course toward the inferior vena cava. The portal veins are more transversely oriented and of larger caliber centrally. The portal vein branches are located within the anatomic liver segments, and the hepatic veins are found between the segments. Doppler ultrasound permits characterization of flow patterns in the **hepatic vessels.** Under normal circumstances, portal vein flow is toward the liver (hepatopedal). Flow in the portal vein is usually of fairly low velocity, with minor undulations and continued forward flow during diastole. Flow in the hepatic veins is hepatofugal and varies according to the cardiorespiratory cycle. The portal veins are horizontally oriented, whereas the hepatic veins are vertically oriented.

**ANSWER:** A

7. A 40-year-old woman arrives at the emergency department complaining of right upper abdominal pain. Her vital signs and laboratory values are normal; however, ultrasound demonstrates a hyperechoic liver with a geographic hypoechoic area

adjacent to the gallbladder. What does this finding probably represent?

A. Duplication of the gallbladder

B. Reverberation artifact

C. Focal fatty sparing

D. Hepatic abscess

E. Bowel gas

*Ref.:* 4

**COMMENTS: Fatty infiltration of the liver** is a common finding that produces a hyperechoic parenchymal pattern on ultrasound. It is not unusual to have focal areas of fatty sparing within an otherwise steatotic liver. These areas typically appear as zonal hypoechoic regions and are usually found adjacent to the gallbladder or anterior to the porta hepatis. Duplication of the gallbladder is a rare occurrence. Reverberation artifacts are echoes within cystic structures. The sonographic appearance of hepatic abscesses is variable, depending on the cause and duration. Pyogenic abscesses are usually complex, with cystic characteristics and internal echoes caused by debris or septations. Bowel gas is highly reflective and impedes ultrasound imaging.

**ANSWER: C**

8. Which of the following is true regarding the hepatic functional unit?

A. The center of the hepatic lobule is the portal triad.

B. Blood flows from the hepatic vein to the portal triad.

C. Zone III is the most susceptible to hypoxic injury.

D. Hepatocytes in zone I have the lowest oxygen tension.

E. Bile flows toward the centrilobular hepatic venule.

*Ref.:* 1, 3

**COMMENTS:** The functional **histologic unit of the liver** is the acinus. At the center of the acinus is the portal triad, which consists of a terminal branch of the portal vein (portal venule) along with a hepatic arteriole and bile ductule. Blood from the terminal portal venule goes into the hepatic sinusoids, around which hepatocytes are located. Eventually, the blood returns to the central vein leading to the terminal hepatic venules at the periphery of the acinar unit. The hepatocytes of the acinus are divided into three zones, with zone I being closest to the afferent portal venule and zone III being nearest the efferent central hepatic venule. Zone II is between these two points. Within the acinus, there is a gradient of solute concentration and oxygen tension that is greatest near the portal venules at the center of the acinus. The hepatocytes in zone I are therefore exposed to more oxygen and are less subject to hypoxia than are the hepatocytes near the periphery of the acinus (zone III). This explains the histologic pattern of centrilobular necrosis that occurs following ischemia. The hepatic venule is at the center of the histologic hepatic lobule. Each hepatic lobule is thus surrounded by several peripheral acini. Bile is formed within the hepatocytes and empties into terminal canaliculi, which coalesce into bile ducts. The bile then flows toward the portal triad.

**ANSWER: C**

9. Alkaline phosphatase is primarily located in which portion of the hepatocyte plasma membrane?

A. Sinusoidal membrane

B. Basolateral membrane

C. Canalicular membrane

D. Basement membrane

E. None of the above

*Ref.:* 1, 3

**COMMENTS:** The plasma membrane of the **hepatocyte** has different regions, or domains, with ultrastructures designed for various functions. The sinusoidal membrane is the domain that borders the perisinusoidal space of Disse. It is covered with microvilli that project into the perisinusoidal space. These microvilli increase the absorptive area in contact with sinusoidal blood and allow proteins, solutes, and other substances to be transported across this border of the hepatocyte. The flat basolateral membrane connects the adjacent hepatocytes and is important for attachment and cellular interactions. The canalicular membrane is a specialized section of the hepatocyte membrane that is involved in bile formation and the transport of various substances into bile. The canalicular regions are separated from the pericellular space by tight junctions. The canalicular membrane contains enzymes such as alkaline phosphatase and 5′-nucleotidase. Thus, high levels of alkaline phosphatase are noted with extrahepatic bile duct obstruction.

**ANSWER: C**

10. During fasting, the liver provides energy substrates by all but which of the following mechanisms?

A. Glycogenolysis

B. Glycolysis

C. Gluconeogenesis from alanine

D. Gluconeogenesis from lactate

E. Formation of ketone bodies from fatty acids

*Ref.:* 1, 3, 5

**COMMENTS:** The **liver** plays a pivotal role in **energy metabolism**. In the fed state, glucose is converted to glycogen for storage. The liver itself obtains its energy primarily from ketoacids rather than glucose, although it can use glycolysis during periods of glucose excess (fed state). During fasting, the liver provides glucose by breakdown of the stored glycogen (glycogenolysis). Glucose is a critical energy source for red blood cells, the central nervous system, and the kidneys. Because glycogen stores are depleted after about 48 hours, the liver generates glucose from other sources. Alanine, other amino acids, lactate, and glycerol can serve as carbon sources for gluconeogenesis. Lipolysis occurs during prolonged fasting, and the fatty acids released from adipose stores are oxidized in hepatocytes to form ketone bodies. Ketone bodies are an important alternative fuel source for brain and muscle.

**ANSWER: B**

11. The reticuloendothelial function of the liver is primarily dependent on which of the following cells?

A. Hepatocytes

B. Kupffer cells

C. Histiocytes

D. Ito cells

E. All of the above

*Ref.: 1, 3, 5*

**COMMENTS:** The **reticuloendothelial system** (RES) functions to clear the circulation of particulate matter and microbes. The RES consists of fixed phagocytic cells located primarily in the liver, spleen, and lungs. Kupffer cells are responsible for the reticuloendothelial function of the liver. Located along the lining of the hepatic sinusoids (along with the sinusoidal endothelial cells), they are uniquely positioned to phagocytize and process gut antigens from the splanchnic and systemic circulation. Kupffer cells play an important role in the production and control of various cytokines and inflammatory regulators. Histiocytes are macrophages in connective tissue. Ito cells, also call hepatic stellate cells, are perisinusoidal cells involved in collagen and vitamin A metabolism.

**ANSWER:** B

12. Which of the following proteins is not primarily synthesized in the liver?

A. Albumin

B. Fibrinogen

C. von Willebrand factor

D. Transferrin

E. Factor VII

*Ref.: 1, 3, 5*

**COMMENTS:** The liver is the primary or sole source of numerous **plasma proteins**, including albumin, α-globulins, and an array of other transport proteins such as transferrin, hepatoglobulin, ferritin, and ceruloplasmin. Eleven proteins involved in hemostasis are synthesized in the liver, including fibrinogen (factor I); the vitamin K–dependent factors (II, VII, IX, and X); and all of the procoagulation factors except for von Willebrand factor, which is synthesized by vascular endothelial cells. Because factor VII has the shortest half-life, 5 to 7 hours, measurements of factor VII levels are useful for determining liver failure.

**ANSWER:** C

13. The cytochrome P-450 system transforms compounds by all of following mechanisms except?

A. Oxidation

B. Hydrolysis

C. Conjugation

D. Reduction

E. Both A and C

*Ref.: 1, 3, 5*

**COMMENTS:** The liver is responsible for **biotransformation** of many endogenous and exogenous substances. For the most part, this process detoxifies potentially injurious substances and facilitates their elimination. In some instances, however, hepatic biotransformation produces more toxic metabolites. There are two general mechanisms by which the liver accomplishes biotransformation: oxidation, reduction, and hydrolysis (phase I reactions) and conjugation (phase II reactions). The cytochrome P-450 enzyme system catalyzes phase I reaction. The second mechanism involves an array of enzymes that conjugate substances with other endogenous molecules. These reactions are referred to as phase II reactions, and their purpose is to convert hydrophobic compounds to hydrophilic ones that are water soluble and can thus be eliminated in bile or urine. The liver is also the principal site of conversion of ammonia to urea via the urea cycle, which is a separate process.

**ANSWER:** C

14. The liver is integral to which of the following steps in vitamin D metabolism?

A. Intestinal absorption

B. 1-Hydroxylation

C. 25-Hydroxylation

D. Formation of cholecalciferol

E. Both A and C

*Ref.: 1, 3*

**COMMENTS:** The liver is integral to **metabolism of the fat-soluble vitamins** A, D, E, and K. Each of these vitamins requires fatty acid micellization for adequate intestinal absorption, which requires the bile salts made in the liver. The liver is not only integral to the intestinal absorption of vitamin D but also plays an active role in one of its activation steps, 25-hydroxylation. Vitamin D is either produced in the skin when 7-dehydrocholestrol reacts with ultraviolet B light to form cholecalciferol or is ingested. As already mentioned, the liver aids in intestinal absorption via fatty acid micellization. Once in the liver, vitamin D undergoes 25-hydroxylation. It then undergoes 1-hydroxylation in the kidneys to arrive at its metabolically active form, which is important in the homeostasis of calcium and phosphorus.

**ANSWER:** E

15. In a patient with obstructive jaundice, which of the following enzymes is usually elevated?

A. Alkaline phosphatase

B. Leucine aminopeptidase

C. γ-Glutamyltransferase (GGT)

D. 5′-Nucleotidase

E. All of the above

*Ref.: 1*

**COMMENTS:** Aspartate transaminase (AST, formerly serum glutamic oxaloacetic transaminase [SGOT]), alanine transaminase (ALT, formerly serum glutamate pyruvate transaminase [SGPT]), and lactate dehydrogenase (LDH) are indicators of the integrity of the cell membrane, and elevated levels reflect hepatocyte injury with leakage. Levels of these **enzymes** are usually only mildly or moderately elevated in pure **obstructive jaundice**. Other enzymes, including alkaline phosphatase, 5′-nucleotidase, leucine aminopeptidase, and GGT, reflect the excretory capacity of the liver. Levels of these enzymes are typically elevated in the presence of extrahepatic bile duct obstruction or intrahepatic cholestasis. Elevations are also seen in patients with hepatic parenchymal disease or liver tumors. Transferrin and albumin levels decrease with liver disease because they reflect changes in liver function and nutritional status.

**ANSWER:** E

**16.** Which of the following operative techniques limits blood loss during major hepatic resection?

A. Portal triad clamping

B. Normothermic total hepatic vascular isolation

C. Total hepatic vascular isolation with venovenous bypass

D. Anesthesia with low central venous pressure

E. All of the above

*Ref.:* 6, 7

COMMENTS: **Hemorrhage** is one of the major hazards during **liver resection**. Troublesome bleeding is most likely to occur during division of the hepatic parenchyma, and life-threatening hemorrhage is most commonly from the hepatic veins and their branches. A variety of intraoperative techniques have been used in an effort to avoid this problem. A disadvantage of any vascular occlusion, however, is the potential for ischemic injury to the liver, particularly in patients with underlying hepatocellular disease. Occlusion of the portal triad (Pringle maneuver) can be useful for limiting bleeding from the hepatic artery and portal vein branches. It has generally been suggested that periods of occlusion should not exceed 20 minutes and perhaps should be shorter. Total hepatic vascular isolation requires occlusion of the inferior vena cava above and below the liver, in addition to the Pringle maneuver. Such management can be complex and is not well tolerated by some patients. Venovenous bypass, which has commonly been used during hepatic transplantation, has also been applied to major hepatic resections at some centers. Attempts to protect the liver during vascular occlusion via local hepatic hypothermia or systemic steroids have not been uniformly practiced or successful. Anesthesia with low central venous pressure minimizes hepatic venous bleeding by fluid restriction, head-down positioning, and the vasodilatory effects of standard anesthetics. Low–central venous pressure anesthesia during major hepatic resection decreases the need for perioperative blood transfusion. This technique has been accomplished with low rates of mortality and postoperative renal compromise.

ANSWER: E

**17.** Resection of hepatic metastases has most clearly benefited patients with which of the following cancers?

A. Colon

B. Breast

C. Stomach

D. Pancreas

E. Lung

*Ref.:* 1-3

COMMENTS: Resection of **hepatic metastases** from colorectal cancer provides a clear survival advantage over any other treatment and should be performed whenever possible. The 5-year survival rate is approximately 25% and is as high as 40% in favorable subgroups. Resection of metastatic neuroendocrine tumors (e.g., carcinoid, insulinoma, and gastrinoma) can be valuable for controlling the symptoms of excessive endocrine secretion. Experience with hepatic resection for metastases from other portal sites (e.g., stomach, pancreas, and biliary) or nonportal sites (e.g., lung, breast, melanoma, gynecologic, head and neck, and renal) has been more limited, and the results have not generally been as encouraging. Occasionally, a patient with a noncolorectal primary malignancy is cured when the isolated hepatic metastasis is resected. However, the natural history of noncolorectal primary malignancies is such that metastases isolated to the liver rarely develop. Hepatic resection for direct, contiguous growth of the primary tumor (e.g., stomach and biliary) into the liver sometimes produces long-term survivors.

ANSWER: A

**18.** A 50-year-old woman is incidentally found to have a 4-cm hepatic cyst with no internal echoes on ultrasound imaging. Which of the following would be the most appropriate management?

A. Observation of the cyst

B. Tamoxifen to prevent enlargement

C. Resection because of the risk for hemorrhage

D. Percutaneous aspiration for cytologic study

E. Magnetic resonance imaging (MRI) for further characterization of the cyst

*Ref.:* 1, 3, 5

COMMENTS: Simple, **nonparasitic hepatic cysts** are presumed to be congenital. They may be single or multiple, are more common in women, and are usually asymptomatic. The absence of internal echoes is diagnostic of a simple rather than a complex cyst, a cystic neoplasm, or a solid lesion. No further intervention is indicated for asymptomatic liver cysts when the diagnosis is secure, which can be ascertained by ultrasound, computed tomography (CT), or MRI. If the diagnosis of a simple cyst is made by ultrasound, there is no need to perform MRI. Complications such as hemorrhage or infection are rare, and these lesions are not premalignant. Exogenous hormones are not recognized to be harmful, nor is antihormonal therapy indicated. Occasionally, large cysts are symptomatic, primarily secondary to local pressure, which may cause biliary obstruction. Treatment of symptomatic cysts is operative resection or unroofing. This may be performed via an open or laparoscopic technique. Percutaneous drainage or injection of alcohol or other sclerosing agents does not suffice and is not recommended. If the cyst is found to communicate with the bile ducts, either excision or Roux-en-Y cystojejunostomy may be performed.

ANSWER: A

**19.** A 30-year-old Hispanic man visiting from Mexico comes to the emergency department with a history of 2 weeks of right upper quadrant pain and tenderness, fevers, chills, and diarrhea. He is febrile to 102.9° F. His heart rate and blood pressure are 120 beats/min and 100/75 mm Hg, respectively. Laboratory results include a white blood cell count of 16,000/mm³, AST of 50 IU/L, and ALT of 93 IU/L. Ultrasound of the abdomen shows a 4 × 7-cm round, hypoechoic, nonhomogenous lesion abutting the liver capsule without rim echoes. Subsequent CT also demonstrates a non–rim-enhancing hypoechoic lesion with a smaller adjacent lesion measuring 2 × 2 cm. Which of the following is the most appropriate course of action?

A. Observation

B. Open surgical drainage

C. Broad-spectrum antibiotics and percutaneous drainage

D. Serologic testing for *Entamoeba histolytica* and oral metronidazole

E. Therapeutic fine-needle aspiration

*Ref.:* 1, 2

**COMMENTS:** The clinical signs and symptoms of **pyogenic (bacterial) and amebic liver abscesses** may be similar and consist predominantly of fever and pain, but it is important to differentiate between the two for therapeutic purposes. *Escherichia coli* or other gram-negative bacteria are the organisms most commonly isolated from pyogenic abscesses. *Streptococcus* spp. and anaerobes such as *Bacteroides* are also common. Today, the most frequent source of pyogenic abscess is contiguous infection in the biliary tract, such as cholangitis. Other sources include infectious foci within the portal venous drainage system, direct extension from perihepatic sites, and hematogenous spread. The right lobe is the most commonly involved, which has been attributed to a streaming effect on the portal vein. Approximately 20% of pyogenic abscesses are cryptogenic. The diagnosis is based on the clinical findings and hepatic imaging and may be confirmed by fine-needle aspiration. Treatment of pyogenic abscess requires eradication of both the abscess and the source. Treatment of the abscess usually requires drainage by operative or percutaneous approaches. Antibiotic therapy alone may suffice for the treatment of multiple small abscesses.

Amebic abscesses are caused by the protozoan *E. histolytica*, which is spread through the fecal-oral route. Once ingested, the cysts pass into the intestines, where the trophozoite is released and transmitted to the colon. These trophozoites can then invade the colonic mucosa and subsequently reach the liver via the portal vein. In the liver, these trophozoites produce a liquefaction necrosis responsible for the classic "anchovy paste" appearance. Protozoa are not usually isolated from the abscess because they are located in the peripheral rim of tissue. Diagnosis requires hepatic imaging (usually ultrasound or CT) and serologic testing for the presence of *E. histolytica* antibodies, as well as a thorough history and physical examination. The patient in this question is a young man from an endemic region who has signs and symptoms similar to those of a pyogenic liver abscess; however, his classic history and the lack of rim enhancement on imaging suggest the diagnosis of amebic abscess rather than pyogenic abscess. Hepatic amebiasis is treated primarily by the administration of amebicidal drugs, with metronidazole being the drug of choice. Percutaneous aspiration may be indicated if the patient does not respond to medical management or the diagnosis is in question. Percutaneous or operative drainage is also indicated in the presence of secondary bacterial infection, which occurs in about 10% of amebic abscesses.

**ANSWER: D**

20. A 50-year-old woman complains of a 4-month history of right-sided abdominal pain and nausea. Her vital signs are stable and she is afebrile. Her physical examination is unremarkable except for hepatomegaly. Ultrasound of the abdomen shows an 8-cm well-circumscribed cyst with a rosette appearance. What is the preferred treatment of this patient?

A. Pericystectomy

B. Percutaneous catheter drainage

C. Transperitoneal surgical drainage

D. Metronidazole

E. Albendazole

*Ref.:* 1

**COMMENTS:** The helminth ***Echinococcus granulosus*** is responsible for most **hydatid diseases** of the liver. It is usually a unilocular process involving the right lobe, although it may be manifested as multiple cysts. Complications include intrabiliary, intraperitoneal, or intrapleural rupture; secondary infection; anaphylaxis; and mass replacement of the liver. These lesions often have a calcified wall and can be diagnosed serologically by indirect hemagglutination tests, complement fixation tests, serum immunoelectrophoresis, and formerly, the Casoni skin test. CT and ultrasound may demonstrate characteristic daughter cysts (hydatid sand) or granddaughter cysts (rosette appearance) within the cyst. Treatment is primarily surgical. Percutaneous aspiration or drainage is generally contraindicated because of the risk for intraperitoneal dissemination; however, since the advent of chemotherapeutic agents such as albendazole, some clinicians have proposed percutaneous drainage. The principles of surgical therapy are to avoid spillage and remove the entire germinal layer. The cyst consists of an inner germinal layer (endocyst) and an outer fibrous membrane layer (pericyst). Resection is usually accomplished by pericystectomy. Anatomic hepatic resection is not generally required but may be used. Surgery in addition to preoperative and postoperative benzimidazole compounds have been shown to be very effective. Metronidazole is used for the treatment of amebic liver abscesses. Because 20% of echinococcal cysts exhibit biliary communication, assessment by preoperative endoscopic retrograde cholangiopancreatography or intraoperative cholangiography is important in any patient with jaundice, cholangitis, elevated liver enzyme levels, or bile noted during resection. Scolicidal agents should be used with caution because of the risk of sclerosing the bile ducts in the event that the agent finds its way into the ductal system.

**ANSWER: A**

21. A 28-year-old asymptomatic, white woman is incidentally found to have a 3.5-cm hypervascular lesion with a central scar in the right lobe of her liver. On delayed images there is increased uptake of contrast material in the scar in comparison with the surrounding liver parenchyma. She is otherwise healthy and takes no medications. Liver enzyme and α-fetoprotein levels are within normal limits. Which of the following is the most appropriate management of this patient?

A. Open liver resection

B. Open surgical biopsy

C. Observation

D. Chemoembolization

E. Hepatic artery embolization

*Ref.:* 1-3, 5

**COMMENTS:** This patient has **focal nodular hyperplasia** (FNH), which is often found incidentally on imaging or during laparotomy. FNH is a benign liver tumor that predominantly occurs in women in the third to fifth decades of life. It is similar to hepatic adenoma (HA), but with important differentiating clinical and histologic features and therapeutic implications. Both occur most commonly in women of childbearing age; however, HA is associated with the use of oral contraceptives and anabolic steroids and is also seen in certain glycogen storage diseases. HA is usually symptomatic (80% of cases) and is associated with rupture and bleeding in a substantial proportion of patients, whereas FNH is usually asymptomatic and found incidentally. Furthermore, HA has potential for malignant transformation, whereas the risk for malignancy in FNH is unlikely but uncertain. Histologically, HA consists of hepatocytes without bile ducts or Kupffer cells. FNH contains Kupffer cells along with a central stellate scar surrounded by fibrous tissue. Scanning for Kupffer cell activity with technetium-99m ($^{99m}$Tc)-labeled sulfur colloid is thus useful in differentiating the lesions. Because of the asymptomatic nature of this patient, small size of the lesion, and negligible risk for malignant transformation, observation is appropriate. Surgical resection is reserved for symptomatic patients or when the diagnosis is uncertain.

**ANSWER:** C

22. Right upper quadrant abdominal pain develops in a 25-year-old woman taking oral contraceptives. CT demonstrates a hypodense, 6-cm mass in the right lobe of the liver. A $^{99m}$Tc-labeled scan reveals a defect in the area of the mass. Angiography reveals a hypervascular tumor with a peripheral blood supply. Which of the following is the appropriate management?

   A. Discontinuation of oral contraceptives and observation with serial CT

   B. Percutaneous needle biopsy

   C. Hepatic resection

   D. Arterial embolization

   E. Radiation therapy

*Ref.:* 1-3, 5

**COMMENTS:** The imaging characteristics described are typical of **hepatic adenoma**. Because HA does not contain Kupffer cells, it does not take up radioisotope. This point may be useful for differentiating HA from FNH but not necessarily from other mass lesions of the liver. Percutaneous biopsy of suspected HA is not advisable because of the risk for hemorrhage. HAs associated with oral contraceptives tend to be larger and have a higher risk for bleeding. Regression does not reliably occur with cessation of oral contraceptives. However, for lesions smaller than 4 cm, a trial of cessation of contraceptives or steroids with observation may be attempted. Resection is indicated for most suspected HAs, particularly for symptomatic lesions, for patients not taking oral contraceptives, and if the diagnosis is uncertain. Embolization may be useful for treating hemorrhage in a patient whose HA is inoperable. Radiation has no role in the management of HA.

**ANSWER:** C

23. An asymptomatic 45-year-old woman is found to have a 4-cm liver mass. CT demonstrates an initial hypodense lesion with peripheral-to-central enhancement by contrast material. MRI shows a dense T2-weighted phase. Which of the following is the appropriate management?

   A. Arteriography

   B. Observation

   C. Percutaneous needle biopsy

   D. Resection

   E. Radiation therapy

*Ref.:* 1-3, 5

**COMMENTS:** **Hemangiomas** are the most common benign liver tumors and occur in 7% of the population. They are characterized by collections of dilated blood vessels that can be diagnosed by their appearance on noninvasive imaging studies. Contrast-enhanced CT reveals a typical pattern of enhancement. A dense T2-weighted image on MRI is a sensitive (although not specific) finding. Radiolabeled red blood cell scans can also diagnose

hemangiomas. Angiography would likewise be diagnostic but is not necessary. These lesions are usually asymptomatic and can simply be observed. They do not have a high risk for spontaneous rupture. Percutaneous biopsy is contraindicated because of the risk for bleeding. Resection by enucleation is appropriate for symptomatic lesions, for enlarging lesions, or if the diagnosis is uncertain. There is no established role for such treatments as arterial ligation, embolization, or radiation therapy.

**ANSWER:** B

24. Hepatocellular carcinoma is epidemiologically associated with all of the following except:

   A. Hepatitis A virus (HAV) infection

   B. Hepatitis B virus (HBV) infection

   C. Hepatitis C virus (HCV) infection

   D. Wilson disease

   E. Alcoholic cirrhosis

*Ref.:* 1, 3

**COMMENTS:** **Primary hepatocellular cancer**, although less common in North America, is the most common malignant neoplasm worldwide. Endemic areas include sub-Saharan Africa, Southeast Asia, and Japan. The primary risk factors are chronic liver disease with cirrhosis (from essentially any cause), chronic infection with HBV or HCV, and various hepatotoxins. Hepatocellular carcinoma can develop in patients with liver disease related to alcohol abuse, hemochromatosis, $\alpha_1$-antitrypsin deficiency, Wilson disease, HA, and other conditions. Exogenous risk factors include dietary aflatoxins (found in grains, dairy products, and peanuts), oral contraceptives, anabolic steroids, vinyl chloride, and certain pesticides. HAV is not associated with hepatocellular cancer.

**ANSWER:** A

25. Which of the following statements is true regarding intrahepatic cholangiocarcinoma?

   A. Survival following resection is generally lower than that for distal bile duct cancer.

   B. Resection is contraindicated unless histologically negative margins can be obtained.

   C. The best survival is achieved with liver transplantation.

   D. Adjuvant chemotherapy improves survival following resection.

   E. None of the above

*Ref.:* 1, 7, 8

**COMMENTS:** **Cholangiocarcinoma** arises from the bile duct epithelium and can occur anywhere along the biliary tract. It constitutes 5% to 20% of primary liver cancers. Tumors arising from the extrahepatic bile ducts differ from those located intrahepatically in terms of their clinical findings, therapy, and prognosis. Tumors of the extrahepatic bile ducts are typically manifested as biliary obstruction. Intrahepatic tumors appear similar to hepatocellular cancer, a liver mass with absent or vague symptoms such as pain, weight loss, nausea, and anorexia. The treatment of choice is surgical excision, which is associated with a 15% to 20% 5-year survival rate. The prognosis is best for tumors of the distal bile ducts that can be resected by pancreaticoduodenectomy. Tumors involving the bifurcation of the bile duct (Klatskin tumor) are less often resectable. Tumor size and the presence of satellite nodules are correlated with outcome. Histologically negative margins are always desirable, but prolonged survival can be attained even with microscopically involved margins. If the tumor cannot be resected, improved survival has been noted with bypass or stenting procedures. **Liver transplantation for cholangiocarcinoma** has been associated with frequent recurrence and has not generally been encouraging. Adjuvant chemotherapy has not typically been useful for bile duct cancer.

**ANSWER: A**

26. A 60-year-old African-American man with a history of right hemicolectomy for colon cancer comes to the office for routine follow-up. His laboratory work-up is significant for a carcinoembryonic antigen level of 80 ng/mL. CT of the chest/abdomen/pelvis shows an isolated hepatic lesion in the right lobe of the liver suspicious for metastasis. Which of the following is the best management option?

    A. Chemotherapy alone

    B. Chemotherapy and radiation therapy

    C. Colonoscopy and hepatic resection

    D. Hepatic resection

    E. Chemoembolization

*Ref.: 1, 3, 7*

**COMMENTS:** Surgical resection remains the "gold standard" for select patients with **hepatic metastases from colorectal cancer**. Systemic chemotherapy alone is ineffective, with a 1-year survival rate of approximately 20% to 30%, whereas surgical resection has a cure rate of approximately 20% in appropriately selected patients. Over the last 2 decades, improvements in intraoperative techniques have afforded improved outcomes in liver surgery. Experienced centers demonstrate 5-year survival rates of 25% to 40% with mortality rates of less than 5%. Careful preoperative patient selection is paramount. Inadequate liver reserve, the presence of extrahepatic metastases (except limited pulmonary metastases or colonic anastomotic recurrence), total hepatic involvement, advanced cirrhosis, and vena cava or portal vein invasion are generally considered contraindications to curative resection. The goal is to resect all hepatic disease. Survival is adversely affected by margins that are positive for cancer or are less than 1 cm. As long as the resection margin is adequate, the specific type of liver resection (anatomic versus "wedge") does not influence survival. Synchronous lesions discovered at the initial operation for colorectal cancer may be removed at the original operation if the length of the original procedure, general condition of the patient, extent of hepatic resection, and experience of the surgeon allow such resection. Otherwise, resection can be performed at a later date. This patient should undergo surveillance colonoscopy to evaluate for local recurrence, as well as resection of the isolated metastatic lesion.

   **Hepatic arterial infusion** of chemotherapeutic agents has a higher response rate than does systemic administration, although adjuvant chemotherapy has not prolonged survival following hepatic resection in randomized studies. Radiation therapy is not useful for hepatic metastases. Ablative therapies, such as radiofrequency hyperthermia, may be useful for patients who cannot undergo resection.

**ANSWER: C**

27. Which of the following is the most accurate method for identifying hepatic metastases?

    A. Transabdominal ultrasound

    B. CT

    C. Laparoscopy

    D. Intraoperative palpation

    E. Intraoperative ultrasound imaging

*Ref.: 4*

**COMMENTS: Transabdominal ultrasound** is as accurate as CT for detecting **liver tumors** that are 2 cm in size or larger. For smaller lesions, **computed tomography** is more accurate, although it can miss the smallest lesions (<1 cm). **Laparoscopy** is useful for identifying small metastases on the liver or peritoneal surfaces that escape discovery by noninvasive preoperative imaging modalities. Laparoscopy has been incorporated into the staging work-up of a variety of intra-abdominal malignancies, including those of the liver. However, one of its limitations is its ability to assess the interior structure of solid organs. It is now well recognized that **intraoperative ultrasound** is the most accurate method for detecting and assessing hepatic tumors. Not only does intraoperative ultrasound discover more lesions than any other modality (including palpation), but it also clearly demonstrates the anatomic relationship of tumors to important vascular structures, which is a critical determinant of resectability and the extent of resection necessary. Intraoperative ultrasound can be performed with hand-held or laparoscopic transducers. Experience with intraoperative ultrasound for liver tumors has shown that the sonographic findings affect the surgical management of one third to one half of patients. Intraoperative ultrasound imaging has become an indispensable component of hepatic surgery.

**ANSWER: E**

28. A 56-year-old woman with cirrhosis of the liver secondary to alcohol abuse has had worsening mental status that has now progressed to hepatic coma. Which of the following can be used for initial treatment of a patient in hepatic coma?

    A. Reduction of dietary protein to 50 g/day or less

    B. Control of active bleeding

    C. Lactulose

    D. Neomycin

    E. All of the above

*Ref.: 1-3*

**COMMENTS:** Treatment of **hepatic encephalopathy** and coma is aimed at limiting the nitrogen that the liver must metabolize by eliminating nitrogenous material from the gastrointestinal tract and by inhibiting its absorption. At the same time, precipitating causes are sought and treated. Nutritional support is important and can be initiated with standard amino acids and restriction of dietary protein. Cessation of any gastrointestinal bleeding from varices is an important step in reducing the conversion of intraluminal blood to ammonia. Lactulose acts as a cathartic and also inhibits the absorption of ammonia by acidifying the colon. Nonabsorbable antibiotics, such as neomycin and kanamycin, reduce colonic flora and the production of ammonia. Systemic antibiotics may be useful for treating specific infections that precipitate encephalopathy but are not indicated empirically. Because the colon is the major site of ammonia absorption, colon resection or exclusion has been suggested to improve encephalopathy but is not a widely used therapeutic measure.

**ANSWER:** E

29. A 43-year-old man with alcoholic cirrhosis has had increasing abdominal distention over the last month. His vital signs are stable and he is afebrile. Physical examination reveals a distended abdomen with a fluid wave. The initial management of the patient's ascites should include all of the following except:

A. Transjugular intrahepatic portocaval shunt (TIPS)

B. Sodium restriction

C. Diuretic administration

D. Fluid restriction

E. Diagnostic paracentesis

*Ref.:* 9

**COMMENTS:** **Ascites** is the most common major complication of hepatic cirrhosis. It is associated with a 2-year survival rate of 50%, and its onset in a cirrhotic patient should prompt an evaluation for liver transplantation. Treatment of ascites depends on its cause, and therefore diagnostic paracentesis is required after a history and physical examination. Abdominal ultrasound can confirm the presence of ascites if it is not certain by examination. The serum-ascites albumin gradient is useful diagnostically. A high gradient (1.1 g/dL) indicates portal hypertension and suggests that the patient will be responsive to medical management consisting of sodium restriction (2000 mg/day) and oral diuretics. Usually, both spironolactone and furosemide are administered to produce fluid loss and natriuresis. Spironolactone alone may cause hyperkalemia, and furosemide alone is less effective. **Medical therapy** controls ascites in about 90% of patients. When the ascites is refractory, serial **therapeutic paracenteses** (with or without the administration of albumin or other plasma volume expanders) is indicated. **Liver transplantation** is the ultimate treatment. A **peritoneovenous shunt** is an option for patients with refractory ascites who are not transplantation candidates or who cannot undergo repeated paracenteses. These shunts are fraught with potential complications, however, and do not prolong survival in comparison with medical management. **Transjugular intrahepatic portosystemic shunts** or operative side-to-side–type portosystemic shunts may control the ascites in select patients.

**ANSWER:** A

30. Which of the following is an indication for TIPS?

A. Recurrent variceal bleeding

B. Ascites

C. Spontaneous bacterial peritonitis (SBP)

D. Hepatorenal syndrome

E. Portal gastropathy

*Ref.:* 1, 3

**COMMENTS:** **Portal hypertension** is responsible for the majority of the morbidity and mortality associated with cirrhosis, such as variceal bleeding, refractory ascites, and hepatic hydrothorax. First-line therapy for patients with primary variceal bleeding is endoscopic therapy with variceal band ligation or sclerotherapy. However, there is a high risk for rebleeding not amenable to

endoscopic techniques (refractory bleeding) or continuation of bleeding (recurrent bleeding). The **transjugular intrahepatic portosystematic shunt procedure** decompresses the portal system by creating a portosystemic shunt and has been effective in up to 90% of patients. The primary treatment of ascites is medical management, although in patients with refractory ascites that is unresponsive to sodium restriction, high-dose diuretics, and other medical therapies, TIPS does improve their ascites. However, there is no survival benefit in this population. Hepatorenal syndrome, SBP, and portal gastropathy are not indications for a TIPS procedure.

**ANSWER:** A

31. Which of the following statements is true regarding SBP?

A. The diagnosis can be made clinically without paracentesis.

B. Infection is most commonly polymicrobial.

C. Antibiotic therapy is reserved for patients with positive findings on ascitic fluid culture.

D. Gram-negative enteric bacteria are often present.

E. None of the above

*Ref.:* 3, 9

**COMMENTS:** **Spontaneous bacterial peritonitis** is a potentially lethal complication of ascites that affects about 10% of patients with cirrhotic ascites. Fever and abdominal pain are common manifestations, but the signs and symptoms may be subtle. Diagnosis requires paracentesis with demonstration of an elevated ascitic fluid polymorphonuclear neutrophil (PMN) count (>250 cells/mm$^3$) or, eventually, positive findings on culture. Antibiotic therapy should be instituted promptly based on an elevated ascitic fluid PMN count or on symptoms even if the PMN count is lower. Infection is usually from one organism, most commonly *E. coli*, *Klebsiella*, or pneumococcus. A third-generation cephalosporin is typically the preferred antibiotic. Differentiation from bacterial peritonitis secondary to a surgical condition is critical. Patients with SBP typically respond to appropriate antibiotics within 48 hours, and ascitic PMN counts decrease. Failure to improve, the presence of polymicrobial infection, or ascitic fluid with a total protein level greater than 1 g/dL, an LDH level greater than the serum level, or a glucose level less than 50 mg/dL suggests secondary peritonitis. Risk factors for SBP include previous SBP, variceal hemorrhage, and low-protein ascites (<1.0 g/dL). Short- or long-term prophylactic antibiotics may be appropriate for high-risk patients.

**ANSWER:** D

32. With regard to hernias in patients with ascites, which of the following statements is true?

A. Increased abdominal pressure is one cause of umbilical hernias in patients with ascites.

B. Umbilical hernia recurrence rates for patients with and without ascites are the same.

C. Patients with asymptomatic groin hernias should be treated surgically.

D. Preoperative paracentesis is not a helpful strategy for electively repairing these hernias.

E. All of the above.

*Ref.:* 10

**COMMENTS:** Umbilical and, less frequently, inguinal **hernias** occur in approximately 20% of patients with **ascites**. They develop as a result of increased intra-abdominal pressure, muscle wasting, fascial thinning, and nutritional deficits. The recurrence rate following repair of umbilical hernias in patients with ascites may be as high as 73%. Because of the high complication rate following hernia repair, it should not be entertained for asymptomatic hernias. Preoperative optimization with paracentesis helps decrease intra-abdominal pressure. Ascites leakage following a surgical procedure should be treated aggressively, and early wound exploration with repair of fascial dehiscence is necessary. Diuretic therapy alone is ineffective in this situation.

**ANSWER: A**

33. Which of the following is a contraindication to radiofrequency ablation (RFA) of liver tumors?

   A. Proximity of the tumor to major vascular structures

   B. Multiple lesions

   C. In conjunction with liver resection

   D. Metastatic colon cancer

   E. None of the above

*Ref.:* 11, 12

**COMMENTS: Radiofrequency ablation** is a technique in which a needle electrode is inserted into a malignant liver tumor. A radiofrequency generator is connected to the electrode, which produces localized tumor destruction with coagulative necrosis as the temperature of the tissue exceeds 50° C. Introduction of the electrode can be performed through a laparotomy incision, laparoscopically, or even percutaneously with the use of ultrasound guidance. This method has been used in patients with hepatocellular carcinoma, as well as in those with metastatic colon and rectal cancers. Some institutions combine the treatment with resection when multiple lesions are involved and resection alone would not leave enough viable hepatic parenchyma for survival. RFA works well when lesions are close to major vascular structures. The maximum size of lesion that can be ablated by RFA is unclear because multiple applications can be used, but it does appear to be more effective on smaller lesions (<5 to 6 cm).

**ANSWER: E**

34. Eight weeks after open heart surgery with transfusions, a 56-year-old man notes dark urine, fatigue, and anorexia. Physical examination discloses only mild, tender hepatomegaly. Laboratory investigations reveal a bilirubin level of 2 mg/dL; an AST level of 540 IU/L; an ALT level of 620 IU/L; an alkaline phosphatase level of 1120 IU/L; and negative assay results for hepatitis B surface antigen (HBsAg), hepatitis B core antibody (anti-HBc), immunoglobulin M anti-HAV antibody (IgM anti-HAV), and anti-HCV antibody (anti-HCV). Which of the following is the most likely explanation for the patient's clinical condition?

   A. Acute viral hepatitis A

   B. Acute viral hepatitis B

   C. Acute viral hepatitis C

   D. Acute viral hepatitis D

   E. Acute viral hepatitis E

*Ref.:* 1, 3

**COMMENTS: Post-transfusion non-A, non-B hepatitis** is mostly the result of HCV infection. The incubation period is usually 5 to 10 weeks, and the mean peak aminotransferase levels are 500 to 1000 IU/L. Anti-HCV antibody is commonly not detectable until 18 weeks after onset of the illness. Approximately 70% of patients with acute hepatitis C progress to chronic hepatitis and potentially cirrhosis. The negative serologic study results exclude acute infection with HAV and HBV. Hepatitis D (delta) virus (HDV) is capable of infecting only patients who also have HBsAg because HDV is an incomplete RNA virus. Hepatitis E (epidemic) virus is rare, except in association with water-borne epidemics in India, the Middle East, and South America.

**ANSWER: C**

35. Which of the following clinical conditions is indicated by the presence of serum antibodies against hepatitis B surface antigen (anti-HBs) and anti-HBc in the absence of HBsAg?

   A. Active, acute infection with HBV

   B. Normal response to vaccination with the hepatitis B vaccine

   C. Chronic active hepatitis secondary to HBV

   D. Recovery with subsequent immunity following acute hepatitis B

   E. Asymptomatic chronic carrier of HBV

*Ref.:* 1, 3

**COMMENTS:** The pattern of negative HBsAg, positive anti-HBs, and positive anti-HBc assays is seen during the recovery phase following acute hepatitis B and clearance of HBsAg from the liver. This antibody pattern may persist for years and is not associated with liver disease or infectivity. Vaccination with the hepatitis B vaccine (genetically manufactured HBsAg particles without HBcAg or HBV DNA) is associated with the development of anti-HBs antibody alone. Active, ongoing infection with HBV, whether acute hepatitis, chronic active hepatitis, or an asymptomatic chronic carrier state, is manifested by the presence of HBsAg and anti-HBc in serum.

**ANSWER: D**

## REFERENCES

1. D'Angelica M, Fong Y: The liver. In Townsend CM, Beauchamp RD, Evers BM, et al, editors: *Sabiston textbook of surgery: the biological basis of modern surgical practice*, ed 18, Philadelphia, 2008, WB Saunders.
2. Geller DA, Goss JA, Tsung A: Liver. In Brunicardi FC, Anderson DK, Billar TR, et al, editors: *Schwartz's principles of surgery*, ed 9, New York, 2010, McGraw-Hill.
3. Hepatobiliary and Portal Venous System Section. In Mulholland MW, Lillemoe KD, Doherty GM, et al, editors: *Greenfield's surgery: scientific principles and practice*, ed 4, Philadelphia, 2006, Lippincott Williams & Wilkins.
4. Deziel DJ: Hepatobiliary ultrasound, *Probl Gen Surg* 14:13–24, 1997.
5. Mulvihill SJ: Liver, biliary tract and pancreas. In O'Leary JP, Tabuenca A, editors: *The physiologic basis of surgery*, ed 4, Philadelphia, 2008, Lippincott Williams & Wilkins.
6. Melendez JA, Arslan V, Fischer ME, et al: Perioperative outcomes of major hepatic resections under low central venous pressure anesthesia: blood loss, blood transfusion and the risk of postoperative renal dysfunction, *J Am Coll Surg* 187:620–625, 1998.

7. Blumgart LH: *Surgery of the liver, biliary tract and pancreas*, ed 4, Edinburgh, 2006, Churchill-Livingstone.
8. Roayaie S, Guarrera JV, Ye MQ, et al: Aggressive surgical treatment of intrahepatic cholangiocarcinoma: predictors or outcome, *J Am Coll Surg* 187:365–372, 1998.
9. Runyon BA: Management of adult patients with ascites caused by cirrhosis, *Hepatology* 27:264–272, 1998.
10. Rosemurgy AS, Statman RC, Murphy CG, et al: Postoperative ascitic leaks: the ongoing challenge, *Surgery* 111:623–625, 1992.
11. Curley SA, Izzo F, Ellis LM, et al: Radiofrequency ablation of hepatocellular cancer in 110 patients with cirrhosis, *Ann Surg* 232:381–391, 2000.
12. Wong SL, Edwards NJ, Chao C, et al: Radiofrequency ablation for unresectable hepatic metastases, *Am J Surg* 182:552–557, 2001.

# CHAPTER 24

# Gallbladder and Biliary Tract

*Daniel J. Deziel, M.D.*

1. Which surgeon performed the world's first known cholecystectomy?

   A. Karl Langenbuch

   B. Justus Ohage

   C. Hans Kehr

   D. Lawson Tait

   E. Eric Mühe

   *Ref.:* 1

**COMMENTS:** Karl Langenbuch performed the first operation to remove the gallbladder on July 15, 1882. Before that and, in fact, even for years afterward, patients with symptomatic gallstone disease were treated only with ineffective medical remedies or, occasionally, by cholecystostomy to drain the gallbladder. The **first cholecystectomy** in the Western Hemisphere was performed 4 years later by Justus Ohage in St. Paul, Minnesota. Hans Kehr of Halberstadt and Berlin was an early pioneer in biliary surgery. In 1901, he published a remarkable book describing more than 500 operations for gallstones, including 96 common bile duct operations. Kehr died of sepsis caused by a hand infection incurred after digital exploration of the common bile duct. Lawson Tait was a famed nineteenth-century English surgeon who advocated cholecystostomy rather than cholecystectomy. Eric Mühe performed the first "**laparoscopic**" **cholecystectomy** in Germany in 1985. Although technically different from modern laparoscopic cholecystectomy, it was a landmark contribution. Mühe was severely criticized and, in fact, vilified by the surgical community at the time. Only years later was the significance of his accomplishment recognized.

**ANSWER:** A

2. During palpation of the hepatoduodenal ligament, a pulsation is felt dorsal and slightly to the right of the common bile duct. Which of the following does this pulsation most likely represent?

   A. A normal common hepatic artery

   B. A normal right hepatic artery

   C. A replaced right hepatic artery

   D. A gastroduodenal artery

   E. A right renal artery

   *Ref.:* 2, 3

**COMMENTS:** The most common variation in **hepatic arterial anatomy** is origination of the right hepatic artery from the superior mesenteric artery. This is a replaced hepatic artery and not simply an accessory vessel that can be sacrificed with impunity. When an operation is performed in the right upper part of the abdomen, the pulsations encountered in the porta hepatis and gastrohepatic ligaments should be assessed. If the hepatic artery is absent or small, the surgeon must be alert to the possibility of a replaced hepatic vessel. When the right hepatic artery originates from the superior mesenteric artery, it courses dorsal to the head of the pancreas and the portal vein and is usually identified dorsolateral to the common bile duct. This vessel and its origin can readily be identified with intraoperative ultrasonography. Only rarely does a replaced right hepatic artery course through the pancreas. A replaced left hepatic artery originates from the left gastric artery and is located in the gastrohepatic ligament, where it is frequently encountered during operations on the stomach and gastroesophageal junction.

**ANSWER:** C

3. Which of the following an anatomic features may contribute to stricture formation after injury to the common bile duct?

   A. The blood supply to the supraduodenal bile duct has a longitudinal pattern.

   B. The blood supply to the supraduodenal bile duct has a lateral pattern.

   C. The blood supply to the supraduodenal bile duct has a segmental end-artery arrangement.

   D. The blood supply to the common bile duct is derived primarily from the common hepatic artery.

   E. The blood supply to the common bile duct has a fragile anastomotic network.

   *Ref.:* 2-4

**COMMENTS: Ischemia** is an important contributing factor to the development of postoperative **bile duct stricture**. The blood supply to the area of the bile duct bifurcation and the distal retropancreatic duct is primarily lateral in arrangement, whereas the blood supply to the supraduodenal portion of the bile duct has a primarily axial or longitudinal pattern. The so-called 3- and 9-o'clock arteries and other small vessels arise from the right hepatic artery and the retroduodenal artery, which is a branch of the gastroduodenal artery, and form the skeleton of a pericholedochal plexus of vessels. An additional source of blood supply to the common bile duct can be the retroportal artery. This vessel arises from the celiac axis or the superior mesenteric artery and generally joins the retroduodenal artery; however, in approximately one third of individuals it ascends the back of the common bile duct to the right hepatic artery. The portion of the bile duct supplied by the longitudinal vessels receives most of its arterial blood supply from below, thus rendering the proximal portion of the duct subject to ischemia after injury or transection.

**ANSWER:** A

4. In this intraoperative cholangiogram, the arrow points to what duct?

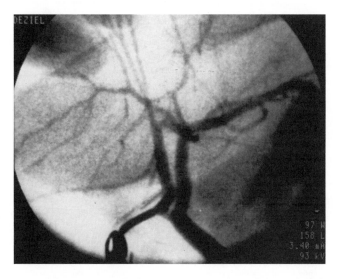

A. Common hepatic duct

B. Accessory right hepatic duct

C. Separately inserting right sectional duct

D. "Crossover" right hepatic duct

E. Cystic duct

*Ref.:* 2, 4, 5

**COMMENTS:** Variations in the **anatomy of the extrahepatic bile ducts** occur commonly. The surgeon must be cognizant of these variations and learn to recognize and identify them to prevent inadvertent injury to the bile ducts during cholecystectomy. Approximately two thirds of individuals have the "textbook" anatomy, with the anterior (segments V and VIII) and posterior (segments VI and VII) sectional ducts from the right joining to form the main right hepatic duct, which then joins the main left hepatic duct to form the common hepatic duct. In 15% to 25% of individuals, the anterior or posterior sectional duct from the right lobe inserts separately into the common hepatic duct. When the posterior duct inserts separately, it is usually at a greater distance caudally from the junction of the left duct and the other right duct than when the anterior duct inserts separately. This duct is therefore at risk for injury during cholecystectomy if the anatomy is not recognized.

One of the most common variations in cystic duct anatomy is direct insertion into one of these separately inserting right hepatic ducts, as the pictured cholangiogram demonstrates. The terms "crossover duct" and "accessory duct" are misnomers for this arrangement. True accessory ducts are rare and occur when there is embryologic duplication of the bud that forms the bile ducts and liver.

**ANSWER:** C

5. In this longitudinal laparoscopic ultrasound scan of the hepatoduodenal ligament, what structure is labeled B?

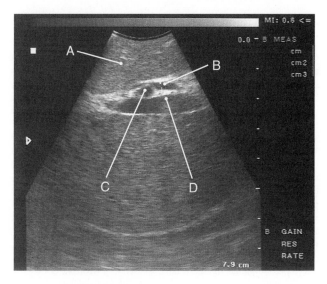

A. Portal vein

B. Common hepatic artery

C. Right hepatic artery

D. Common bile duct

E. Right hepatic duct

*Ref.:* 6

**COMMENTS:** See Question 6.

**ANSWER:** D

6. In this transverse laparoscopic ultrasound scan of the hepatoduodenal ligament, which structure is labeled B?

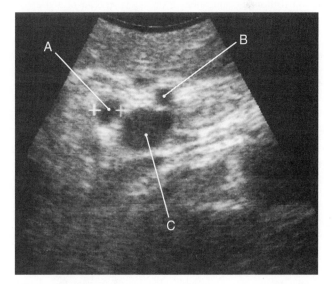

A. Portal vein

B. Common hepatic artery

C. Right hepatic artery

D. Common hepatic artery

E. Right hepatic duct

*Ref.: 6*

**COMMENTS:** A general principle of **ultrasonography** is that any structure visualized in one plane should also be examined in a second plane at a 90-degree angle to the first view to ascertain where and what the structure is. **Intraoperative ultrasound** imaging, whether laparoscopic or open, is an accurate method for identifying bile duct anatomy and assessing the bile duct for stones during cholecystectomy. The longitudinal and transverse scans of the hepatoduodenal ligament in Questions 5 and 6 depict typical anatomy. In the longitudinal plane, the common bile duct appears as a hypoechoic, tubular structure parallel and anterior to the portal vein. The normal upper-limit diameter of the duct at this location is 6 mm by ultrasound imaging criteria. In other words, a nondilated duct should not exceed one half the diameter of the neighboring portal vein. The right hepatic artery most commonly crosses behind the bile duct and is viewed in cross section on the longitudinal scan. In the transverse plane, the structures of the hepatoduodenal ligament have a "**Mickey Mouse**" configuration. The cross sections of the bile duct and common hepatic artery appear as smaller hypoechoic circles anterior to the larger portal vein. The structures labeled in the scan from Question 5 are as follows: A, liver; B, common bile duct; C, right hepatic artery; D, portal vein. The structures labeled in the scan from Question 6 are as follows: A, common bile duct; B, common hepatic artery, C, portal vein.

**ANSWER:** B

7. If a patient has complete bile duct obstruction, which of the following does not occur?

A. Triglyceride absorption

B. Vitamin K absorption

C. Cholesterol synthesis

D. Bilirubin conjugation

E. All of the above

*Ref.: 4*

**COMMENTS:** Bile has a number of critical functions related to the digestion and absorption of fats and the elimination of various endogenous and exogenous substances. Bile interacts with pancreatic lipase and colipase in the intraluminal hydrolysis of dietary triglycerides. It subsequently solubilizes the monoglycerides and fatty acids produced by triglyceride metabolism by forming mixed micelles. The micelles facilitate mucosal uptake of triglycerides by permitting transport across the water barrier adjacent to the enterocyte membrane. Although bile therefore plays an important role in triglyceride absorption, a substantial amount of triglycerides can be absorbed, even in the absence of bile, because of the long length of the intestine. The same is not true for the fat-soluble vitamins A, D, E, and K, which are minimally water soluble and are not absorbed in any substantial amount in the absence of micelles. Patients with long-standing **cholestasis** generally require supplementation of these fat-soluble vitamins to prevent the clinical effects of deficiency. Bile is the sole pathway for elimination of bilirubin and cholesterol from the body. Bilirubin is secreted into hepatic bile by an active transport mechanism following hepatic uptake and conjugation. Cholesterol is eliminated both by synthesis of bile acids from cholesterol and by solubilization of cholesterol in bile during secretion.

**ANSWER:** B

8. What change in bile flow would be expected in a patient with an external biliary fistula?

A. Increased total canalicular flow

B. Decreased bile acid–dependent canalicular flow

C. Increased bile acid–dependent canalicular flow

D. Decreased bile acid–independent canalicular flow

E. Increased bile acid–independent canalicular flow

*Ref.: 2, 4*

**COMMENTS:** Approximately 600 mL of **hepatic bile** are produced daily. Seventy-five percent of hepatic bile is formed by the bile canaliculi, and the remainder is secreted by the ducts. Canalicular bile can be divided into approximately equal bile acid–dependent and bile acid–independent fractions. The bile acid–dependent fraction results from active secretion of bile acids by the hepatocyte. This secretion depends on intestinal absorption and enterohepatic circulation of bile acids. Patients with external bile losses therefore have reduced bile acid–dependent canalicular flow and consequently reduced total canalicular flow. The bile acid–independent portion of canalicular flow is the result of secretion of inorganic electrolytes. Ductular secretion modifies canalicular bile flow by adding fluid and inorganic electrolytes.

**ANSWER:** B

9. Cholic acid is converted by bacteria to which of the following secondary bile acids?

A. Deoxycholic acid

B. Chenodeoxycholic acid

C. Lithocholic acid

D. Ursodeoxycholic acid

E. None of the above

*Ref.: 2-4, 7*

**COMMENTS:** The primary human **bile acids** cholic acid and chenodeoxycholic acid are synthesized from cholesterol in the liver. The secondary bile acids deoxycholic acid and lithocholic acid are formed in the intestine as the result of bacterial enzyme activity. 7-Ketolithocholic acid is also a secondary bile acid. It is converted to the tertiary bile acid ursodeoxycholic acid in the liver.

**ANSWER:** A

10. Conjugated bile acids are primarily absorbed in the intestine by which of the following mechanisms?

A. Active transport in the colon

B. Passive transport in the colon

C. Active transport in the ileum

D. Passive transport in the ileum

E. Bacterial translocation

*Ref.: 2-4, 7*

**COMMENTS: Enterohepatic cycling** of bile acids begins at the hepatocyte level. Bile acids are conjugated in the liver with glycine or taurine, secreted into the biliary system, concentrated and stored in the gallbladder, and then delivered to the duodenum after gallbladder contraction. Most bile acids are efficiently resorbed in the intestine. The site and mechanism of intestinal absorption differ according to the form of the bile acid and its corresponding lipid solubility. Conjugated bile acids are predominantly ionized in the intestinal pH range and are relatively lipid insoluble. Conjugated forms are therefore absorbed by an active transport mechanism in the terminal ileum. This mechanism accounts for approximately 70% to 80% of the enterohepatic circulation. Bacterial deconjugation of bile acids occurs in the colon and small intestine, as does conversion of primary bile acids to secondary forms. Deconjugation raises the $pK_a$ of bile acids and enables resorption by passive non-ionic diffusion, which occurs predominantly in the colon but to some extent in the small intestine as well. Both primary and secondary bile acids are resorbed and taken back to the liver. Unconjugated forms are then reconjugated and resecreted. Hepatic bile therefore contains both primary and secondary bile acids, with the primary bile acids normally constituting 60% to 90% of the total bile pool. Hepatic synthesis of new bile acids approximates fecal losses of 300 to 600 mg/day.

The bile acid pool cycles four to eight times per day, and hepatic secretion is dependent on enteral return. Disruption of this cycle therefore diminishes bile acid secretion. Clinical conditions that may be associated with bile acid malabsorption include ileal disease or resection, small bowel dysmotility or obstruction, and blind loop syndrome. Clinical consequences of this disordered physiology may include fat malabsorption, deficiencies of fat-soluble vitamins (A, D, E, and K), choleretic diarrhea caused by impaired colonic water absorption by bile acids, and formation of gallstones.

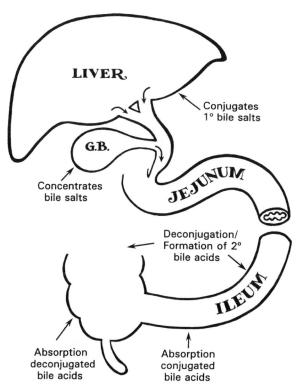

*G.B.*, Gallbladder; *1°*, primary; *2°*, secondary.

**ANSWER:** C

**11.** Normal functions of the gallbladder epithelium include all but which of the following?

A. Absorption of water

B. Absorption of sodium and chloride

C. Absorption of conjugated bile acids

D. Secretion of hydrogen ion

E. Secretion of glycoproteins

*Ref.:* 3, 7

**COMMENTS:** The primary **functions of the gallbladder** are to concentrate and store bile between feedings. The gallbladder epithelium absorbs solutes and water across concentration gradients by both active and passive mechanisms. The main concentrating force is active absorption of sodium (coupled to chloride transport), which leads to passive absorption of water. Abnormalities in gallbladder absorption are part of the pathophysiologic process of gallstone formation. Absorption of organic solutes is normally minimal and depends on their lipid solubility. Unconjugated bile acids are more lipid soluble than their conjugated forms. Absorption of unconjugated bile acids that form in the presence of bacteria or inflammation damages the mucosa, thereby promoting absorption of other solutes and destabilizing cholesterol in solution. The gallbladder epithelium is also secretory. Secretion of hydrogen ion lowers the pH of gallbladder bile in relation to hepatic bile. Mucin glycoproteins secreted by the mucosa may have both a protective function and a critical role as a nucleating factor during gallstone formation.

**ANSWER:** C

**12.** Which of the following usually produces gallbladder contraction?

A. Adrenergic stimulation

B. Vasoactive intestinal peptide (VIP)

C. Somatostatin

D. Cholecystokinin (CCK)

E. Secretin

*Ref.:* 3

**COMMENTS: Gallbladder function** is subject to many neurohormonal influences. Generally, stimulation of parasympathetic vagal nerves causes gallbladder contraction, and stimulation of sympathetic nerves from the celiac ganglion causes gallbladder relaxation. Regulation of gallbladder function is actually a complex process that involves the interaction of various neural, hormonal, and peptidergic stimuli on various receptors located on the gallbladder muscle, blood vessels, and nerves. Cholinergic stimuli (including vagal) and CCK cause contraction. CCK receptors can be found on both gallbladder smooth muscle cells and intrinsic cholinergic nerves. Adrenergic stimulation (sympathetic) usually causes relaxation, but selective stimulation of certain adrenergic receptors can cause contraction. VIP and somatostatin inhibit gallbladder contraction, which can account for clinical biliary manifestations in patients with tumors that secrete those substances or in patients being administered somatostatin agonists. Many other peptides, hormones, and neurotransmitters may also affect gallbladder function, although their clinical significance is not completely known.

**ANSWER: D**

13. Which of the following is true regarding gallbladder emptying in between meals?

   A. It does not occur.

   B. It is stimulated by CCK.

   C. It is inhibited by CCK.

   D. It depends on peristalsis of the common bile duct.

   E. It is stimulated by motilin.

*Ref.:* 3, 7

**COMMENTS: Bile flow** in the biliary tract varies according to the fasting or fed state of the individual. **Cholecystokinin**, which is released by the duodenum in response to the ingestion of food substances, facilitates delivery of bile to the intestine by stimulating contraction of the gallbladder and relaxation of the sphincter of Oddi. Normal contraction of the gallbladder in response to meals results in approximately 80% emptying in 2 hours. The common bile duct is for the most part a passive conduit in humans and does not play an active role in biliary motility. Filling of the gallbladder after it has emptied depends on neural and hormonal factors that relax the gallbladder and increase resistance of the sphincter of Oddi. During the interdigestive period, the gallbladder gradually fills, but this filling is interrupted by cyclic periods of emptying, during which time approximately one third of the gallbladder volume is dispensed. This cyclic pattern during fasting is correlated with the interdigestive myoelectric migratory complex of the intestine and is related to increased levels of plasma motilin. Motilin is a 21–amino acid peptide, and plasma motilin levels vary cyclically during the fasting period.

**ANSWER: E**

14. Which of the following levels of enzyme activity is most likely to be present in a nonobese individual with cholesterol gallstones?

   A. Increased 3-hydroxy-3-methylglutaryl coenzyme A (HMG-CoA) reductase activity

   B. Decreased HMG-CoA reductase activity

   C. Increased 7α-hydroxylase activity

   D. Decreased 7α-hydroxylase activity

   E. Decreased enterokinase activity

*Ref.:* 2

**COMMENTS: Cholesterol solubility** in bile depends on the concentration of cholesterol relative to bile acids and phospholipids. Although an increase in hepatocyte cholesterol synthesis and secretion has been implicated in obese patients with gallstones, a relative deficiency of bile acid secretion is thought to be responsible for gallstone formation in many nonobese patients. HMG-CoA reductase catalyzes the conversion of HMG-CoA to mevalonate and is the early rate-limiting enzyme in cholesterol synthesis. The primary bile acids are formed from cholesterol, and the rate-limiting enzyme in this process is 7α-hydroxylase. Relative imbalances in the activities of these enzymes therefore affect cholesterol solubility in bile.

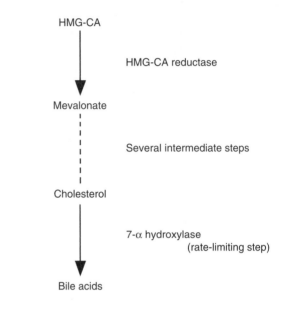

**ANSWER: D**

15. Which of the following is decreased after cholecystectomy?

   A. Size of the bile acid pool

   B. Rate of enterohepatic recycling

   C. Rate of bile acid secretion

   D. Cholesterol solubility in bile

   E. Rate of bilirubin conjugation

*Ref.:* 2

**COMMENTS:** The total size of the **bile acid pool** is diminished after **cholecystectomy** as a result of loss of the gallbladder reservoir. However, cholecystectomy produces a more continuous flow of bile into the intestine, which increases the frequency of enterohepatic cycling and stimulates bile acid secretion. For these reasons, even though the size of the bile acid pool is diminished, cholecystectomy improves cholesterol solubility in bile. The solubility of cholesterol in bile depends on the relative molar concentration of cholesterol in relation to the concentration of bile acids and the phospholipid lecithin. This relationship, described by W. Admirand and D. M. Small in 1969, is graphically depicted by the following familiar diagram:

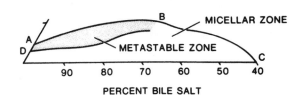

D. Aggregation of cholesterol monomers

E. Stone growth

*Ref.:* 2, 3, 7

**COMMENTS: Cholesterol gallstone formation** is a complex physicochemical process. The requisite steps in the genesis of cholesterol stones can be conceptually simplified as cholesterol saturation, nucleation, and stone growth. The cholesterol content of bile can exceed the capacity for bile to solubilize cholesterol in vesicles and micelles. Cholesterol supersaturation alone, however, is not sufficient to cause stones because this process can occur in normal individuals. Nucleation must also take place; that is, cholesterol monohydrate crystals must form and aggregate. Finally, the crystals must enlarge by fusion or continued solid deposition to produce a stone large enough to be clinically relevant. Bacterial infection is thought to be an important pathogenic factor in the development of some pigment stones but not generally cholesterol stones. Bacterial infection is associated with deconjugation of bilirubin and subsequent formation of insoluble calcium bilirubinate complexes. Bacterial infection can also result in the production of glycocalyx, an adhesive glycoprotein that plays a role in pigment stone formation.

**ANSWER:** B

---

**18.** Nucleation during cholesterol gallstone formation involves all but which of the following?

A. Mixed micelles

B. Biliary vesicles

C. Biliary calcium

D. Gallbladder stasis

E. Mucus secretion

*Ref.:* 3, 7

**COMMENTS:** Nucleation, or the formation and aggregation of solid cholesterol monohydrate crystals, is a necessary step in **gallstone formation**. There are factors that promote nucleation and some antinucleating factors that may protect against stone formation. Mucin glycoproteins secreted by the gallbladder epithelium are thought to be key nucleating factors. Increased mucus secretion occurs whenever there is gallbladder stasis, and this precedes the development of cholesterol crystals. Prostaglandins stimulate mucus production in animal models, and prostaglandin inhibitors can prevent stones. Nucleation is associated with the vesicular fraction of bile rather than with the mixed micelles. Biliary calcium also plays a role in the formation of both cholesterol and pigment stones. Calcium levels in gallbladder bile are increased during cholesterol stone formation. Calcium affects the absorptive function of the gallbladder epithelium and also promotes nucleation from vesicles. An understanding that the events of vesicle fusion, nucleation, and stone growth occur in the gallbladder is the basic foundation for cholecystectomy as the definitive treatment of cholesterol gallstone disease.

**ANSWER:** A

---

**19.** Cholesterol gallstones are associated with all except which of the following?

A. Obesity

B. Rapid weight loss

---

**ANSWER:** A

---

**16.** Which of the following is the primary form in which cholesterol is transported in bile?

A. Dissolved as free cholesterol

B. Dissolved as conjugated cholesterol

C. Attached to a protein carrier

D. Solubilized in mixed micelles

E. Solubilized in phospholipid vesicles

*Ref.:* 3, 7

**COMMENTS:** Cholesterol is insoluble in water, and bile is a solution composed of 90% water. The **solubility of cholesterol** in bile depends on the presence of bile acids and the phospholipid lecithin. These molecules aggregate into physicochemical structures that shelter cholesterol within a nonpolar, hydrophobic center and thus permit dissolution. For many years, the mixed micelle was recognized as the structure principally responsible for cholesterol solubility. Subsequently, it has been found that most cholesterol is usually solubilized in larger bilayered lipid structures known as vesicles. The balance between micelles and vesicles is a dynamic process. Recognition of these vesicles is particularly important because crystallization of cholesterol to form stones occurs from this phase.

**ANSWER:** E

---

**17.** Which of the following is not part of the process of cholesterol gallstone formation?

A. Supersaturation of bile with cholesterol

B. Bilirubin deconjugation

C. Crystal nucleation

C. Total parenteral nutrition (TPN)

D. Exogenous estrogen

E. High-calorie diet

*Ref.: 2, 3*

**COMMENTS:** Changes in bile composition that either increase the relative concentration of cholesterol or decrease the relative concentration of bile acids favor **cholesterol gallstone formation**. Situations that lead to increased hepatocyte cholesterol secretion include obesity, rapid weight loss, diets high in calories and polyunsaturated fats, and estrogen therapy. Drugs that inhibit HMG-CoA reductase are used to treat hypercholesterolemia and may prevent gallstone formation. Theoretically, a relative decrease in the size of the bile acid pool would predispose a person to cholesterol gallstone formation in situations in which there were excessive bile acid losses (e.g., ileal disease or resection) or decreased bile acid synthesis (e.g., reduced $7\alpha$-hydroxylase activity). Stones associated with ileal disease or resection are of the pigment type, however. TPN is also associated with pigment gallstones in a high proportion of patients, depending on the duration of therapy.

**ANSWER: C**

20. Which of the following is the main chemical component of pigment gallstones?

A. Cholesterol

B. Calcium bilirubinate

C. Calcium carbonate

D. Calcium phosphate

E. Calcium oxalate

*Ref.: 2, 7*

**COMMENTS: Pigment gallstones** are composed primarily of calcium precipitated with bilirubin, carbonate, phosphate, or palmitate anions. Two relatively distinct types of pigment gallstones are recognized: black pigment gallstones and brown pigment gallstones. There are differences between black and brown pigment gallstones in terms of gross appearance, chemical composition, pathogenesis, and clinical implications. Black pigment gallstones are small and spiculated. They contain calcium bilirubinate primarily in polymerized form, as well as calcium carbonate or phosphate. Brown pigment gallstones are soft and yellow-brown, are also composed primarily of calcium bilirubinate, but contain more calcium palmitate (fatty acid derived from lecithin) and cholesterol than do black stones. The oxalate salts of calcium play no role in gallstone disease.

**ANSWER: B**

21. Which of the following features is more characteristic of black pigment gallstones than brown pigment gallstones?

A. Association with hepatic cirrhosis

B. Association with bacterial infection

C. Location in the common bile duct

D. Treatment requiring bile duct drainage

E. Higher risk for cholangitis

*Ref.: 2, 3, 7*

**COMMENTS:** There are some important clinical differences between patients with **black pigment gallstones** and those with **brown pigment gallstones**. It is postulated that these stones form by different pathogenic mechanisms. Stasis and infection are critical factors in the formation of brown pigment gallstones. Bile culture results are positive in most patients with brown pigment gallstones, and scanning electron microscopy demonstrates bacterial colonies or casts within the stones. Brown pigment gallstones are found more frequently in the common bile duct than in the gallbladder. They occur in older patients with stasis and in postcholecystectomy patients.

Black pigment gallstones are thought to have a metabolic cause. They often occur in patients with cirrhosis or hemolysis. The precise role of stasis and infection in black stone formation remains unclear, however. Approximately 20% of patients with black pigment gallstones have positive bile culture results, and some investigators have demonstrated bacteria in black stones. A subset of patients with gallstones have combined features of both black and brown pigment gallstones. The important therapeutic implication in differentiating black from brown pigment gallstones is that patients with brown pigment gallstones may require a definitive biliary drainage procedure to prevent recurrence, whereas patients with black pigment gallstones may be treated successfully by cholecystectomy alone.

**ANSWER: A**

22. Which of the following sonographic findings is not a feature of gallstone disease?

A. Hyperechoic intraluminal structure

B. Mobility of the intraluminal structure

C. Shadowing posterior to the structure

D. Acoustic enhancement posterior to the structure

E. Sonographic Murphy sign in acute cholecystitis

*Ref.: 6*

**COMMENTS:** External ultrasound imaging has a sensitivity of about 95% for the diagnosis of gallstones. The three **sonographic criteria for gallstones** are (1) the presence of a hyperechoic intraluminal focus, (2) shadowing posterior to that focus, and (3) movement of the focus with changes in position of the patient. Problems in interpretation arise when all of these criteria are not fulfilled. For example, small stones may not shadow well, and impacted stones do not move. Ultrasound imaging may also fail to diagnose stones if the gallbladder cannot be visualized well because it is contracted or close to excessive bowel gas. For an optimal elective ultrasound scan, the gallbladder should be examined after the patient has fasted for about 6 hours. Posterior acoustic enhancement is a sonographic feature of hypodense structures such as cysts. The signals behind the structure are "whiter" because the sound wave energy is less attenuated as it passes through. The gallbladder itself is a cystic structure and demonstrates this phenomenon, whereas gallstones do the opposite. A sonographic Murphy sign refers to tenderness when the ultrasound transducer is placed over the gallbladder. This is a typical finding in a patient with gallstones and acute cholecystitis.

**ANSWER: D**

23. Ultrasound imaging reveals gallstones in an asymptomatic 50-year-old woman. Which of the following is the recommended treatment?

A. Observation

B. Laparoscopic cholecystectomy

C. Open cholecystectomy

D. Ursodeoxycholic acid

E. Extracorporeal shock wave lithotripsy (ESWL)

*Ref.:* 2, 3, 7

**COMMENTS:** The appropriate management of **asymptomatic cholelithiasis** is sometimes controversial. First, the physician must determine whether the patient is in fact asymptomatic, because gastrointestinal complaints other than pain may be attributable to biliary tract disease. It was formerly thought that symptoms would eventually develop in most patients with silent gallstones and that the risk for subsequent complications was high. Subsequent studies suggested that symptoms develop in about 1% to 2% of patients each year and that serious complications are relatively infrequent. The morbidity, mortality, and cost of intervention in these patients may exceed those of expectant therapy. The availability of laparoscopic cholecystectomy has not changed the basic indications for surgery, although it has probably altered the symptomatic threshold for surgical referral. Nonoperative pharmacologic dissolution and ESWL are neither definitive nor cost-effective.

Currently, therefore, the incidental finding of asymptomatic cholelithiasis is not an indication for therapy in most situations. Circumstances that may be exceptions and that merit consideration on an individual basis include (1) a transplant patient with anticipated immunosuppression because of the risk for sepsis, (2) anticipated long-term parenteral nutrition because of associated stasis and sludge formation, (3) anticipated pregnancy because of the possibility of becoming symptomatic as gallbladder emptying is impaired and because of the potential risk imposed on both the mother and fetus if complicated cholelithiasis occurs, (4) concurrent abdominal surgery for an unrelated problem because of the relative ease and safety of incidental cholecystectomy in most situations and in consideration of the potential for postoperative cholecystitis otherwise, and (5) bariatric operations because of the high incidence of gallstones associated with obesity and during rapid weight loss. In patients requiring massive intestinal resection, concomitant cholecystectomy has been recommended even when the gallbladder is normal because disease will probably develop during parenteral nutrition.

**ANSWER:** A

24. In patients with which of the following conditions is early elective cholecystectomy for symptomatic gallstones not indicated?

A. Elderly status

B. Diabetes mellitus

C. Child class C cirrhosis

D. TPN-induced gallstones

E. Chronic renal failure

*Ref.:* 3

**COMMENTS:** Patients with certain medical conditions are often considered to be at higher risk for morbidity and mortality from gallstone disease. Complications of cholelithiasis, such as sepsis, perforation, and choledocholithiasis, more frequently develop in elderly patients. They also have a higher mortality rate during emergency operations. Elective cholecystectomy can usually be performed safely in the elderly and is recommended for symptomatic patients. Although the supportive evidence has not always been conclusive, diabetic patients may also be at increased risk, particularly if emergency intervention is required, and should therefore be considered for early elective cholecystectomy. Gallstones develop in a high proportion of patients maintained on long-term TPN, and reports suggest that complications, emergency operations, and mortality are more frequent in this population as well. Early cholecystectomy is therefore indicated. **Cholecystectomy** is also indicated for patients with chronic renal failure, particularly if they are candidates for renal transplantation. Patients with hepatic cirrhosis, however, have high morbidity and mortality rates related to cholecystectomy, especially those with hepatocellular dysfunction and portal hypertension. Cholecystectomy should be approached with great caution in these circumstances and is usually reserved for patients with complications of cholelithiasis or for patients with substantial symptoms and less advanced hepatic disease (Child class A).

**ANSWER:** C

25. A patient with abdominal pain has a CCK-stimulated hepatobiliary iminodiacetic acid (HIDA) scan that demonstrates 25% gallbladder emptying. Ultrasound imaging of the gallbladder is normal. What is true regarding cholecystectomy in this situation?

A. Cholecystectomy is not indicated because persistent or recurrent symptoms are likely.

B. Cholecystectomy is indicated only if duodenal drainage yields cholesterol crystals or bilirubinate granules.

C. Cholecystectomy can alleviate symptoms in most patients if the pain is episodic and located in the right upper part of the abdomen.

D. Cholecystectomy improves symptoms in most patients regardless of the location or characteristics of the pain.

E. When compared with operations on patients with gallstones, there is a greater chance that laparoscopic cholecystectomy will need to be converted to an open procedure.

*Ref.:* 3, 8

**COMMENTS:** Surgeons are often confronted with the challenge of evaluating patients for abdominal pain that may or may not be of biliary origin. If the symptoms are typical of biliary "colic" and ultrasound imaging demonstrates gallstones, the situation is straightforward. However, when the symptoms are less typical (even the presence of gallstones) or when ultrasound imaging does not identify any abnormality, further evaluation is necessary to determine whether cholecystectomy is warranted. Other diagnoses must be excluded, and additional investigations may be appropriate, depending on the specific circumstances (e.g., esophagogastroduodenoscopy, computed tomography [CT], endoscopic retrograde cholangiopancreatography [ERCP], gastrointestinal contrast-enhanced studies, and colonoscopy).

**Cholecystokinin-stimulated cholescintigraphy** can be useful for identifying patients who may have symptoms as a result of motility disorders of the gallbladder. However, the test does not always reliably predict the long-term outcome of cholecystectomy. If the symptoms are more typical of biliary origin and findings on CCK scintigraphy are abnormal (<30% ejection), data suggest that most patients (>70%) can benefit from cholecystectomy. Histologic abnormalities of the gallbladder are found in a reasonable number of these patients. If the symptoms are less typical, the results of cholecystectomy cannot be expected to be as favorable, even though emptying is abnormal. Additional testing, such as repeated ultrasonography or duodenal drainage with CCK cholecystography, might sometimes be useful for evaluating these patients.

**ANSWER: C**

26. Laparoscopic cholecystectomy is most strongly contraindicated in which of the following situations?

    A. Pregnancy

    B. Previous upper abdominal surgery

    C. Known common bile duct stones

    D. Chronic obstructive pulmonary disease

    E. Gallbladder cancer

    *Ref.:* 3, 9

**COMMENTS:** When **laparoscopic cholecystectomy** was first introduced worldwide during the late 1980s, there were a number of circumstances in which it was more or less strongly contraindicated. Today, most contraindications are relative, and in fact the laparoscopic approach is preferred when possible in certain situations that were initially considered contraindications (e.g., acute cholecystitis, choledocholithiasis, and obesity). Basically, the surgeon must be adequately trained and the patient reasonably fit for an operation and give informed consent that includes the possibility of laparotomy. It must be recognized that there are patients for whom the potential physiologic consequences of $CO_2$ pneumoperitoneum are more important, and the presence of underlying disease itself does not prohibit a laparoscopic approach. In fact, laparoscopic cholecystectomy may be more beneficial to the postoperative course of a compromised patient. Pregnancy is not a contraindication with appropriate precautions, although the physiologic effects on the fetus are not completely known. Perhaps the strongest contraindication currently involves patients with suspected or known gallbladder cancer because of the risk for dissemination.

**ANSWER: E**

27. Most major bile duct injuries during laparoscopic cholecystectomy occur in patients under which of the following circumstances?

    A. Acute cholecystitis

    B. Gallstone pancreatitis

    C. Choledocholithiasis

    D. Elective cholecystectomy

    E. Conversion of a laparoscopic procedure to an open procedure

    *Ref.:* 10

**COMMENTS:** There are several **risk factors** for **bile duct injury** during **laparoscopic cholecystectomy**. Pathologic risk factors include severe acute or chronic inflammation. Several studies have found a statistical correlation between the rate of duct injury and the presence of acute cholecystitis. Bleeding has long been implicated as a factor predisposing to duct injury during open or laparoscopic cholecystectomy. Injuries are sometimes attributed to the "anomalous" anatomy of the bile ducts. More often than not, however, such "anomalies" are simply common anatomic variations that the surgeon must recognize to prevent injury (see Question 4). The surgeon's experience, or the "learning curve," is

clearly a risk factor, because higher rates of duct injury have been well documented in less experienced surgeons. It is interesting to note that there is no convincing evidence that duct injury is more frequent during cases involving laparoscopic management of common bile duct stones, possibly because these procedures are performed by more experienced surgeons. Unfortunately, most major bile duct injuries during laparoscopic cholecystectomy have occurred in elective and otherwise uncomplicated cases. Despite the presence or absence of risk factors, the primary problem resulting in duct injury is misidentification of the anatomy. The most frequent mechanism of injury is mistaking a major bile duct for the cystic duct and clipping and cutting it. This pitfall is best avoided by correct operative strategy, which means appropriate retraction and adequate dissection to obtain the "critical view of safety." The **critical view** is achieved by dissecting the base of the gallbladder off the liver for an adequate distance to visualize the cystic plate and to verify that the only structures entering the gallbladder are the true cystic duct and the cystic artery. Intraoperative bile duct imaging with cholangiography or laparoscopic ultrasonography can also aid in discerning the anatomy. If the cystic duct cannot be conclusively identified, the surgeon must resort to alternative approaches such as laparoscopic subtotal cholecystectomy, conversion to an open operation, or termination of the procedure.

**ANSWER: D**

28. A surgeon encounters difficulty during an elective laparoscopic cholecystectomy in a healthy 25-year-old woman and converts to an open procedure. The 4-mm common hepatic duct has been transected 1 cm below the bifurcation. Which of the following procedures is the most appropriate?

    A. Duct-to-duct repair over a T tube

    B. Duct-to-duct repair without a stent

    C. Roux-en-Y hepaticojejunostomy

    D. Hepaticoduodenostomy

    E. Ligation of the duct and placement of a drain

    *Ref.:* 11

**COMMENTS:** When a transection or resection **injury of the extrahepatic biliary tree** is discovered at the time of cholecystectomy, the surgeon must make some careful decisions. Repair at the time is preferable, provided that the surgeon is adequately experienced in performing such a repair so that a successful outcome is likely. Unfortunately, the weight of evidence indicates that most primary repairs by the initial operating surgeon have failed, thus necessitating repeated operations and other interventions. The initial repair of a major duct injury has the best chance for long-term success. A less experienced surgeon should not attempt anastomosis of a small bile duct but seek the help of an experienced colleague if available. Otherwise, drains should be placed and transfer to an experienced hepatobiliary surgeon arranged. If repair at the time is appropriate, the standard reconstruction for this type of injury is a Roux-en-Y hepaticojejunostomy. Duct-to-duct repairs usually fail in this situation. Hepaticoduodenostomy is not recommended for an injury at this level.

**ANSWER: C**

29. How would the bile duct injury described in Question 28 be classified?

    A. Bismuth type 1

    B. Bismuth type 2

C. Bismuth type 3

D. Bismuth type 4

E. Bismuth type 5

*Ref.:* 4

**COMMENTS:** The **Bismuth classification of bile duct injuries** and strictures describes the level of injury in relation to the bifurcation of the main right and left hepatic ducts. Higher injuries are more difficult. They require a greater degree of technical skill and expertise to reconstruct, and reconstructions may have a lower long-term success rate. Many of the injuries resulting from laparoscopic cholecystectomy have been higher than those seen with open cholecystectomy. Moreover, many injuries, initially lower, end up being higher when repaired because of the need to débride unhealthy ductal tissue as a result of ischemia or inflammation and infection caused by bile leakage. With a type 1 injury, 2 cm or more of the common hepatic duct is preserved below the bifurcation. With a type 2 injury, less than 2 cm remains. A type 3 injury reaches the bifurcation with preservation of continuity between the right and left ducts. A type 4 injury involves destruction of the hepatic duct confluence with separation of the right and left hepatic ducts. A type 5 injury involves a separate inserting right sectoral duct with or without injury to the common duct.

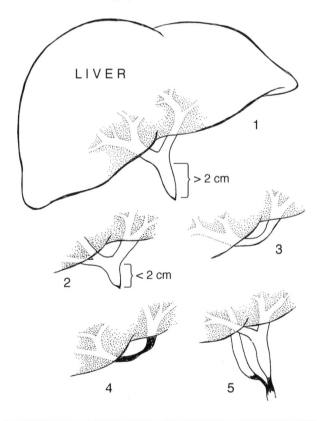

**A N S W E R :**   B

30. On the second postoperative day following elective laparoscopic cholecystectomy, a 40-year-old woman complains of nausea and abdominal pain. Examination shows a temperature of 100° F (37.8° C), a pulse of 100 beats/min, mild abdominal distention, and moderate right upper quadrant tenderness. Which of the following would next be appropriate?

A. Administration of intravenous antibiotics

B. Magnetic resonance cholangiopancreatography (MRCP)

C. HIDA scan

D. ERCP

E. Percutaneous transhepatic cholangiography (PTC)

*Ref.:* 11, 12

**COMMENTS:** Serious delays in the **postoperative diagnosis of bile duct injuries** can compound a patient's problems. A patient should be investigated promptly when the clinical course suggests anything other than the anticipated straightforward recovery that most patients experience. The primary concern is development of a bile leak, which occurs in 1% to 2% of patients. Other problems, such as retained bile duct stones or intestinal injury, can occur as well, although they are less frequent.

The various imaging studies can provide complementary information. An HIDA scan shows an ongoing bile leak and is often the most reasonable initial investigation after the patient is examined. Ultrasound or CT can demonstrate fluid collections or intrahepatic bile duct dilation. If a fluid collection is seen, percutaneous aspiration can determine whether the fluid is bile. If a bile leak is confirmed, cholangiography is necessary to establish the site of leakage and help determine further therapy. **Endoscopic cholangiography** is generally the first choice and may be all that is necessary for bile leaks that originate from lateral injuries, the cystic duct stump, or the gallbladder fossa. **Percutaneous transhepatic cholangiography** is necessary for complete anatomic definition in patients with transection or resection injuries or injuries to sectoral hepatic ducts that may not be in continuity with the rest of the extrahepatic bile ducts. MRCP is not an initial diagnostic examination but can be useful for delineation of bile duct anatomy in complex situations.

**A N S W E R :**   C

31. A stable patient underwent endoscopic cholangiography following laparoscopic cholecystectomy 2 days previously. What should be done next?

A. Endoscopic balloon dilation and stent placement

B. PTC

C. Reoperation for bile drainage

D. Reoperation for bile duct reconstruction

E. Percutaneous catheter drainage

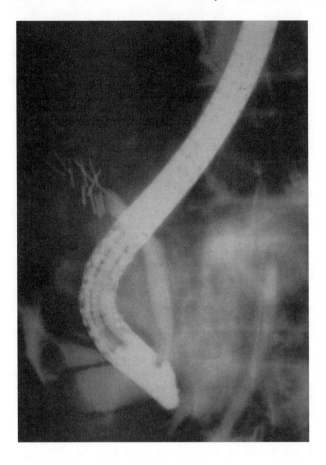

*Ref.:* 11, 13, 14

**COMMENTS:** The endoscopic cholangiogram demonstrates complete occlusion of the supraduodenal common bile duct without extravasation of dye. A classic mechanism of major **bile duct injury during laparoscopic cholecystectomy** involves clipping the distal common bile duct and resecting a portion of the extrahepatic ductal system. The proximal level of injury is variable but typically high. Bile leakage or obstruction occurs, depending on the status of the proximal ducts. The first priority when managing these injuries is to control sepsis and ensure adequate drainage of any bile leak. Generally, this can be accomplished by nonoperative percutaneous or endoscopic methods. Urgent reoperation for bile drainage is not typically necessary. Complete cholangiographic definition of the injury is recommended before definitive repair. For resection or transection injuries, as depicted above, PTC is used to assess the status of the proximal ducts. Endoscopic cholangiography alone may be adequate for lateral injuries when the continuity of the ducts is preserved. Occasionally, a "fistulogram" done through a percutaneous drainage catheter may visualize the proximal ducts. After complete cholangiography, long-term success is best achieved by an elective, expert reconstruction.

**ANSWER:** B

32. Which of the following is true regarding the use of intraoperative cholangiography (IOC) and bile duct injury during laparoscopic cholecystectomy?

    A. Selective use of IOC effectively prevents bile duct injury.

    B. Routine use of IOC effectively prevents bile duct injury.

    C. Selective use of IOC is associated with a higher rate of bile duct injury.

    D. The severity of bile duct injury is independent of the use of IOC.

    E. Use of IOC increases the intraoperative diagnosis of injury.

*Ref.:* 15

**COMMENTS:** As long as there are imaging studies to assess the bile ducts intraoperatively, the debate between proponents of routine versus selective use of such studies will continue. Proponents of IOC argue that its routine or liberal use can be advantageous in terms of bile duct injury and that there is an association between routine IOC and lower rates of duct injury. **Cholangiograms** can be incomplete or misinterpreted, however, and injuries can occur after IOC has been done. Properly performed IOC does not cause **duct injury**. There is a compelling argument that IOC may limit the severity of duct injury. For example, IOC may allow a surgeon to recognize that the cholangiogram catheter has been placed in the common duct and not the cystic duct before transection of the common duct. Some evidence suggests that the number of high duct injuries and anastomotic repairs required to remedy duct injuries has been lower when IOC was performed. The use of IOC increases the intraoperative recognition of any injury that has occurred. About 70% to 90% of injuries have been identified intraoperatively when IOC has been performed as compared with only 15% to 25% when IOC has not been done. Failure to interpret the results of IOC correctly can account for missed injuries. The two primary reasons for misinterpreting the results of IOC are failure to completely visualize the proximal ducts (including both the right anterior and posterior ducts) and extravasation of dye of uncertain origin.

**ANSWER:** E

33. Which of the following is an early event in the pathophysiology of acute calculous cholecystitis?

    A. Increased biliary lysolecithin

    B. Gallbladder ischemia

    C. Bacterial infection

    D. Prostaglandin depletion

    E. CCK receptor depletion

*Ref.:* 3, 7

**COMMENTS: Acute cholecystitis** is thought to be initiated by gallbladder obstruction and activation of various inflammatory mediators, which lead to mucosal damage, gallbladder distention, and eventually ischemia. Bacteria can be identified in the bile of about 50% (30% to 70%) of patients with acute cholecystitis, but bacterial infection is a secondary phenomenon. The primary **pathophysiology** depends on the biochemical events that take place. Some of the mediators that may be involved in the inflammatory process of acute cholecystitis are bile acids, lithogenic bile, pancreatic juice, prostaglandins, phospholipids, and lysolecithin. Lysolecithin is formed from lecithin by the enzyme phospholipase, and levels are elevated in patients with acute cholecystitis. The role of prostaglandins as mediators in this process has also received considerable attention.

**ANSWER:** A

**34.** Which of the following is most accurate in the diagnosis of acute cholecystitis?

A. Plain abdominal radiographs

B. Ultrasound imaging

C. Oral cholecystography

D. Technetium-99m pertechnetate and HIDA scans

E. Leukocytosis with elevated transaminases

*Ref.:* 2, 3

**COMMENTS: Radionuclide scanning** with $^{99m}$Tc-iminodiacetic acid agents normally allows visualization of the liver, gallbladder, and extrahepatic biliary tree. In the presence of **acute cholecystitis**, the gallbladder cannot be seen because of obstruction of the cystic duct. This finding is present in approximately 98% of patients with acute cholecystitis. Cholescintigraphy is not necessary in most patients with acute cholecystitis because the diagnosis is founded on clinical examination and demonstration of gallstones by ultrasound imaging. However, it can be quite useful in less typical situations and to exclude acute cholecystitis (by normal gallbladder uptake) in patients with other diagnoses. **Ultrasound** imaging of acute cholecystitis may demonstrate gallstones, pericholecystic fluid, thickening of the gallbladder, intramural edema, or a positive sonographic Murphy sign, but the morphologic findings are not specific. Although oral cholecystography fails to allow visualization of the gallbladder in patients with acute cholecystitis, this technique is not as diagnostically reliable as a radioisotope study because of the high frequency of gallbladders that cannot be visualized as a result of impaired dye absorption, hepatic uptake, or the presence of chronic cholecystitis. Plain abdominal radiographs reveal up to 15% of gallstones and demonstrate emphysematous cholecystitis but otherwise play no specific role in the diagnosis of acute cholecystitis. Elevations of the white cell count and transaminases are nonspecific.

**ANSWER: D**

**35.** A $^{99m}$Tc-iminodiacetic acid scan in a fasting patient demonstrates the following: normal liver activity, no gallbladder visualization at 60 minutes, intestinal activity present at 60 minutes, and gallbladder visualization at 120 minutes. These findings are most consistent with which of the following situations?

A. Normal study results

B. Acute calculous cholecystitis

C. Acute acalculous cholecystitis

D. Chronic cholecystitis

E. Partial bile duct obstruction

*Ref.:* 2, 3

**COMMENTS:** Since the mid-1970s, technetium-labeled derivatives of iminodiacetic acid (i.e., **HIDA**, PIPIDA, and DISIDA) have been important in the evaluation of **biliary tract disease**. After intravenous injection, these radioisotopes are taken up by the liver and excreted into the biliary tract. The characteristics of a normal study include visualization of the gallbladder within 60 minutes in fasting patients and the appearance of radioisotope in the duodenum by about the same time. In nonfasting patients, visualization of the gallbladder may be delayed. The hepatic phase of the study may demonstrate mass lesions or diminished uptake in patients with hepatic dysfunction. Such results are similar to those of a liver scan. With both calculous and acalculous acute cholecystitis, the gallbladder is not visualized because of cystic duct obstruction. No visualization or delayed visualization is common with chronic cholecystitis. The distinction between acute and chronic cholecystitis therefore depends on the clinical findings, not simply on abnormal scan results. Bile duct obstruction may cause delayed or absent clearance of isotope from the liver or delayed hepatic uptake. Radioisotope scans can be useful in the clinical assessment of disorders other than cholecystitis, including biliary motility, biliary enteric anastomosis, bile fistulas or leaks, and enterogastric reflux.

**ANSWER: D**

**36.** What is the preferred treatment of acute calculous cholecystitis?

A. Early laparoscopic cholecystectomy

B. Delayed laparoscopic cholecystectomy

C. Early open cholecystectomy

D. Delayed open cholecystectomy

E. Intravenous antibiotics

*Ref.:* 2, 3

**COMMENTS:** The former debate over early versus late **cholecystectomy** for **acute cholecystitis** has for the most part been put to rest. Prospective studies have demonstrated that early cholecystectomy within the first few days is not associated with higher morbidity or mortality and that delayed surgery requires longer hospitalization, is more expensive, and risks recurrent biliary problems before definitive therapy. Most patients are treated effectively by stabilization and prompt surgery. From a technical standpoint, cholecystectomy is often easier during the first day or two of the patient's illness, when the inflammation tends to be more edematous rather than necrotic and hyperemic, as it becomes when the process progresses. Laparoscopic cholecystectomy is the preferred treatment in most circumstances, although conversion to an open procedure is required more often than when the procedure is performed electively for nonacute symptoms.

**ANSWER: A**

**37.** With regard to acalculous cholecystitis, which of the following statements is true?

A. It most commonly affects elderly patients in an outpatient setting.

B. The primary pathophysiologic feature involves gallbladder stasis.

C. HIDA scan results are usually normal.

D. Ultrasound imaging of the gallbladder is usually normal.

E. Treatment requires cholecystectomy.

*Ref.:* 2, 3

**COMMENTS:** Approximately 5% to 10% of acute cholecystitis cases occur in patients without gallstones. The primary predisposing factor is gallbladder stasis with subsequent distention and ischemia. **Acalculous cholecystitis** typically develops in hospitalized patients, often after trauma, unrelated surgery, or other critical illnesses. Factors present in these patients that may contribute to biliary stasis include hypovolemia, intestinal ileus, absence of oral nutrition, multiple blood transfusions, narcotic use, and positive pressure ventilation. Because of the clinical situation in which acute acalculous cholecystitis occurs, the diagnosis may not be readily apparent. The patient may have fever or unexplained sepsis, and abdominal signs may not be initially appreciated. The results of imaging studies are generally abnormal. Because of stasis and functional obstruction of the cystic duct, HIDA scanning fails to allow visualization of the gallbladder, and ultrasonography may demonstrate sludge, thickening of the gallbladder wall, or pericholecystic fluid. None of these findings is specific for the presence of acute acalculous cholecystitis, however, and the diagnosis must rely on clinical suspicion.

Standard surgical treatment consists of cholecystectomy (or cholecystostomy for patients who are too infirm to withstand general anesthesia). Percutaneous cholecystostomy can be a valuable technique for establishing gallbladder decompression in these critically ill patients. Later cholecystectomy may not be required if stones are not present and subsequent cholangiography demonstrates a patent cystic duct. Cholecystectomy is the only effective treatment if the gallbladder is necrotic or gangrenous.

**ANSWER:  B**

38. The pertinent area of a plain x-ray film of the abdomen of a 78-year-old diabetic man with right upper quadrant pain is shown below. Which of the following is the appropriate next step?

   A. Ultrasound imaging of the gallbladder

   B. CT

   C. HIDA scan

   D. Cholecystectomy

   E. ERCP

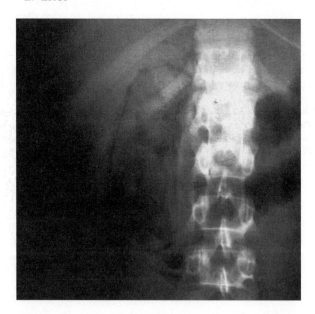

*Ref.:* 2, 3

**COMMENTS: Emphysematous cholecystitis** occurs most typically in elderly diabetic men. Curvilinear radiolucencies in the right upper quadrant have the configuration of the gallbladder, are in the location of the gallbladder, and are diagnostic of gas in the gallbladder wall. In their totality, they are pathognomonic of emphysematous cholecystitis. Gas may also be seen in the gallbladder lumen. This condition is associated with a high incidence of

gallbladder necrosis, perforation, and sepsis. Unnecessary diagnostic examinations would only delay prompt surgical therapy and possibly affect the outcome adversely. Urgent surgery is needed. An ultrasound study of an emphysematous gallbladder would show highly reflective shadows as a result of the gas. Differentiation from bowel gas may be difficult, although the diagnosis is usually evident. About one third of patients do not have stones. CT would show the abnormal gas in the gallbladder wall, lumen, or both. HIDA scans would fail to allow visualization of the gallbladder. ERCP is unnecessary.

**ANSWER:  D**

39. A 24-year-old woman who is 10 weeks pregnant is hospitalized with gallstone pancreatitis and recovers after 2 days of nonoperative management. Which of the following recommendations is the most appropriate?

   A. Laparoscopic cholecystectomy before discharge

   B. Open cholecystectomy before discharge

   C. Laparoscopic cholecystectomy in 4 weeks

   D. Open cholecystectomy in 4 weeks

   E. Nonoperative management until term and postpartum laparoscopic cholecystectomy

*Ref.:* 16

**COMMENTS:** Symptomatic **gallstone disease** is second to appendicitis as the most common nonobstetric surgical problem that affects **pregnant women**. The overwhelming majority of women who become symptomatic during the first trimester of pregnancy will have continuing or recurrent symptoms before delivery. Without definitive treatment, rehospitalizations are frequent and there is ongoing risk to both the mother and fetus. This has been particularly so when biliary pancreatitis has been the symptomatic manifestation. Cholecystectomy is therefore indicated and is preferably performed during the second trimester of pregnancy if the clinical situation will allow. **Laparoscopic cholecystectomy** has been performed successfully during all stages of pregnancy. In late term, however, the size of the gravid uterus interferes with trocar placement. For this reason, many surgeons prefer an open approach if surgery is necessary during the third trimester.

**ANSWER:  C**

40. During a difficult laparoscopic cholecystectomy for acute cholecystitis, you recognize that the patient has hepatic cirrhosis and portal hypertension. Which of the following is the best option?

   A. Conversion to open cholecystectomy

   B. Completion of the laparoscopic cholecystectomy

   C. Laparoscopic subtotal cholecystectomy

   D. Terminating the procedure and arranging for transjugular intrahepatic portosystemic shunt (TIPS) surgery

   E. Placement of drains and termination of the procedure

*Ref.:* 17

**COMMENTS:** See Question 41.

**ANSWER:  C**

41. A patient has undergone subtotal cholecystectomy with a portion of the gallbladder infundibulum left in situ. On the second postoperative day, bile is coming from a subhepatic drain placed at the time of surgery. Which of the following is the most appropriate step?

    A. Endoscopic retrograde cholangiography

    B. PTC

    C. Removal of the drain

    D. Leaving the drain in place and monitoring

    E. Returning to the operating room for completion of the cholecystectomy

    *Ref.:* 17

COMMENTS: Safe management of a patient with a difficult laparoscopic cholecystectomy requires technical skill, considerable judgment, and familiarity with a spectrum of operative options. Such options include open cholecystectomy, "fundus first" cholecystectomy, laparoscopic or open cholecystostomy, and laparoscopic or open subtotal cholecystectomy. Alternatives to total cholecystectomy can help avoid major bile duct or vascular injury under difficult circumstances. Cholecystostomy tube placement can be lifesaving; potential disadvantages include tube complications, the possible need for a reoperation later, and possible inability to place a tube if the gallbladder is necrotic or gangrenous. Subtotal cholecystectomy can help avoid injury and bleeding and reduce the need for cholecystostomy and reoperation. The ability to safely perform subtotal excision of the gallbladder laparoscopically can decrease the rate of conversion to an open operation and potential morbidity in critically ill patients. There are several variations of **subtotal cholecystectomy** that can be appropriate: leaving portions of the gallbladder infundibulum, posterior wall, or both, depending on the situation. Bile leakage is not uncommon following subtotal cholecystectomy, but most bile leaks are self-limited. Those that persist have often been associated with retained common bile duct stones and have been successfully treated endoscopically. Problems with retained stones in the gallbladder remnant have not been common in reports of subtotal cholecystectomy.

ANSWER: D

42. When compared with standard three- or four-port laparoscopic cholecystectomy, single-incision laparoscopic surgery (SILS) is associated with which of the following?

    A. Lower rate of trocar site hernias

    B. Increased rate of bile duct injury

    C. Increased rate of retained common bile duct stones

    D. Increased rate of gallbladder perforation

    E. None of the above

    *Ref.:* 18

COMMENTS: There has been substantial interest in the development of single-incision laparoscopic approaches for many operations, including cholecystectomy, colectomy, fundoplication, and gastric band placement. Proponents of **single-incision laparoscopic surgery** cite the potential advantages of decreased pain and improved cosmesis in comparison with laparoscopic operations using multiple trocar sites. However, these advantages have not yet been clearly validated. So far, for most surgeons, SILS has been more difficult and time-consuming than standard laparoscopic approaches. At the time of this writing, there are no results from randomized prospective trials to judge the outcomes of SILS cholecystectomy versus standard laparoscopic cholecystectomy with multiple trocar sites.

ANSWER: E

43. To date, cholecystectomy using natural-orifice transluminal endoscopic surgery (NOTES) has most commonly been performed by which of the following approaches?

    A. Hybrid transgastric

    B. Hybrid transvaginal

    C. Hybrid transcolonic

    D. Pure endoscopic transvaginal

    E. Pure endoscopic transgastric

    *Ref.:* 19

COMMENTS: The worldwide experience with NOTES is increasing and it has moved into human trials. To date, the majority of procedures have involved hybrid techniques using at least one laparoscopic port in addition to the endoscopic instrument placed via the transvaginal, transgastric, transcolonic, or transesophageal routes, depending on the operation. The largest current **natural-orifice transluminal endoscopic surgery** experience is with hybrid transvaginal cholecystectomy. Dedicated collaboration between teams of surgeons, endoscopists, scientists, and engineers is enabling the development of NOTES technology and investigation of relevant applications.

ANSWER: B

44. With regard to choledocholithiasis, which of the following statements is true?

    A. Common duct stones are present in one third of patients undergoing cholecystectomy.

    B. The incidence of common duct stones is highest in elderly patients.

    C. Most common duct stones are composed of calcium bilirubinate.

    D. Common duct stones are found more frequently when cholecystectomy is performed for chronic cholecystitis than for acute cholecystitis.

    E. Laparoscopic cholecystectomy is contraindicated if choledocholithiasis is suspected.

    *Ref.:* 2, 3

COMMENTS: About 8% to 18% of patients with symptomatic gallstones have **choledocholithiasis**, which has a spectrum of clinical manifestations. Approximately 6% of patients undergoing cholecystectomy have common bile duct stones that were completely unsuspected. Proper recognition of common duct stones is important because of the associated risk for biliary tract obstruction and cholangitis. The incidence of choledocholithiasis increases with each decade over the age of 60. Most common duct calculi originate in the gallbladder and are therefore of the cholesterol variety. Friable "earthy" stones (brown pigment gallstones) contain calcium complexed with bilirubinate and other anions and arise de novo in the common duct in association with biliary stasis and infection. Choledocholithiasis occurs as often with acute cholecystitis as with chronic cholecystitis. Therefore, appropriate evaluation of the patient for potential choledocholithiasis is mandatory. Laparoscopic cholecystectomy is the preferred approach for patients with choledocholithiasis. This can be accomplished in conjunction with preoperative ERCP for patients with a high likelihood of common duct stones. For those at intermediate or low risk for common duct stones, intraoperative duct imaging (cholangiography, laparoscopic ultrasound) is performed. If stones are found in the common duct, most can then be cleared with laparoscopic techniques.

**ANSWER: B**

45. Which of the following is the best indication for preoperative ERCP in a patient with gallstones?

   A. Obstructive jaundice

   B. Gallstone pancreatitis

   C. History of jaundice

   D. Alkaline phosphatase levels elevated to twice the normal

   E. A 10-mm common bile duct seen on ultrasonography

*Ref.:* 20

**COMMENTS:** The rationale for **preoperative endoscopic retrograde cholangiopancreatography** is to identify and remove common bile duct stones so that patients may subsequently undergo laparoscopic cholecystectomy and, it is hoped, avoid the potential need for an open operation or for operative treatment of the common bile duct. However, because endoscopic evaluation of the bile duct entails its own risks, it should be selected for patients at the highest risk for choledocholithiasis. Unfortunately, there are no absolute predictors of common bile duct stones. The yield of ERCP in identifying common bile duct stones is highest in patients with obstructive jaundice or clinical cholangitis or when a duct stone is actually seen on ultrasound. In all other circumstances, most patients have negative endoscopic cholangiograms, and the examination was not necessary for most of these patients. As the number of parameters suggestive of common bile duct stones increases, however, so does the likelihood of finding stones. There is no substitute for good clinical judgment in the use of preoperative ERCP. It is an unquestionably valuable tool for diagnosing and removing common bile duct stones, but its overuse is dangerous and must be discouraged. **Magnetic resonance cholangiopancreatography** can be a useful noninvasive screening tool for choledocholithiasis that allows ERCP to be reserved for those with positive studies.

**ANSWER: A**

46. An intraoperative cholangiogram obtained during laparoscopic cholecystectomy shows several 2- to 3-mm filling defects in the distal common duct. What should be done next?

   A. Complete the laparoscopic cholecystectomy and perform ERCP postoperatively.

   B. Perform open surgical common bile duct exploration.

   C. Administer glucagon and flush the common bile duct through the cystic duct.

   D. Laparoscopically dilate the cystic duct and perform transcystic choledochoscopy.

   E. Perform laparoscopic choledochotomy.

*Ref.:* 21

**COMMENTS: Choledocholithiasis** discovered **intraoperatively** can often be managed laparoscopically, depending on a number of considerations, such as the size, number, and location of the stones and the size and anatomy of the bile ducts. When approaching common bile stones laparoscopically, one should start with simple techniques and progress to more complex maneuvers

as necessary. Small stones can often be cleared by flushing the common duct through a transcystic catheter after glucagon has been administered to relax the choledochoduodenal sphincter. Other transcystic manipulations can be used if the cystic duct is dilated or dilatable (with hydrostatic balloons) and provided that there is a relatively direct course between the cystic duct and the common bile duct. Such techniques include retrieval with balloon catheters or stone baskets under fluoroscopic or choledochoscopic visualization. Experienced laparoscopic surgeons can perform choledochotomy when the common bile duct is sufficiently large and simpler efforts have failed. In general, the surgeon should not leave common duct stones untreated but may elect to terminate the procedure when (1) the stones are very small or questionable, (2) the common bile duct is narrow, (3) laparoscopic clearance is not feasible, and (4) the morbidity of an open common bile duct exploration is judged to be too high for a particular patient. Intraoperative endoscopic retrieval of common bile duct stones has been successful but may be logistically impractical. Relying on postoperative endoscopy for intentionally neglected stones carries the risk that endoscopic removal may fail. A traditional open common bile duct exploration is a safe, reliable fallback for most patients when laparoscopic methods are unsuccessful and the duct is not too small.

**ANSWER: C**

47. When compared with IOC, laparoscopic ultrasound for evaluation of the common bile duct during cholecystectomy is most associated with each of the following except:

   A. Better sensitivity for detecting common duct stones

   B. Less time requirement

   C. Increased risk for common bile duct injury

   D. Less accurate identification of the proximal bile ducts

   E. Better identification of vascular variations

*Ref.:* 22

**COMMENTS: Intraoperative cholangiography** and **intraoperative ultrasonography** are the most commonly used methods for evaluating the bile ducts during cholecystectomy. Some of the advantages of sonography are that it is relatively quick, it can be performed without the need for dissection of the cystic duct, and it can easily be repeated. Intraoperative ultrasound is more sensitive than IOC for the detection of small stones or sludge in the common bile duct, although these findings may not necessarily be clinically relevant. Sonography can also demonstrate the vascular anatomy of the hepatoduodenal region. Ultrasound is less reliable than cholangiography for delineation of the anatomy of the proximal bile ducts, such as the presence of separately inserting segmental hepatic ducts. Both imaging methods can be useful in the avoidance of bile duct injury.

**ANSWER: C**

48. Which of the following is the best treatment for a patient with choledocholithiasis 3 years after cholecystectomy?

   A. Administration of ursodeoxycholic acid

   B. Percutaneous transhepatic stone extraction

   C. Endoscopic sphincterotomy and stone extraction

   D. Common bile duct exploration and T-tube placement

   E. Common bile duct exploration and choledochoduodenostomy

*Ref.:* 2, 3

**COMMENTS:** Most **common bile duct stones** found in patients after cholecystectomy can be treated successfully by nonoperative methods. **Stone extraction** through a T tube or endoscopically after endoscopic sphincterotomy if the patient does not have a T tube in place results in successful duct clearance with a low complication rate in more than 90% of patients. By definition, bile duct stones occurring more than 2 years after cholecystectomy are considered primary common duct stones. These are pigment gallstones related to biliary stasis and infection rather than the typical cholesterol stones found in the gallbladder. In addition to stone removal, some type of ductal drainage procedure is therefore also indicated in most of these patients to prevent stone recurrence.

When performed by experienced clinicians, endoscopic sphincterotomy is successful in more than 90% of patients and, when combined with endoscopic extraction with the use of balloon catheters or baskets, results in stone clearance in 85% to 90% of patients. Duct stones have been removed successfully via the percutaneous transhepatic route when endoscopic approaches are not successful.

A number of situations may make endoscopic clearance of bile duct stones difficult or unsuccessful, including large impacted stones, the presence of a distal bile duct stricture, previous gastrectomy with gastroenterostomy or Roux-en-Y anastomosis, complications of endoscopic sphincterotomy before stone extraction, or the presence of a duodenal diverticulum. If access to the bile duct can be achieved endoscopically, adjuvant modalities, such as **intracorporeal fragmentation techniques** (i.e., mechanical, electrohydraulic, or laser lithotripsy) or ESWL, may allow successful removal of even difficult stones. Reoperation on the biliary tract for clearance of duct stones is reserved for physiologically fit patients in whom other extraction techniques are unsuccessful. Ursodeoxycholic acid does not dissolve pigment stones.

**ANSWER:** C

49. Which of the following is the most appropriate initial test for the evaluation of obstructive jaundice?

    A. HIDA scan

    B. Ultrasound imaging

    C. CT

    D. PTC

    E. ERCP

*Ref.:* 2, 3

**COMMENTS:** All of the aforementioned **imaging** modalities may be useful for evaluating a patient with **obstructive jaundice**. Overall, ultrasound is the most cost-effective initial examination. It permits identification or visualization of ductal dilation, suggests the level of obstruction, and provides information about the liver, the pancreas, and the presence or absence of calculous disease. CT or magnetic resonance imaging may best delineate the anatomy of mass lesions in the hepatobiliary and pancreatic region and assist in the preoperative assessment of resectability. **Magnetic resonance cholangiography** can provide precise delineation of ductal anatomy and is increasingly important in the evaluation of malignant disease. **Percutaneous transhepatic cholangiography** can demonstrate the proximal extent of obstruction and is useful for assessing the suitability of the proximal hepatic ducts for anastomosis. **Endoscopic retrograde cholangiopancreatography** is particularly useful in cases of distal biliary tract obstruction and allows evaluation of the ampullary region. Both PTC and ERCP allow cytologic or histologic sampling, and both can be used to place catheters for decompression of the obstructed biliary tract. Although [99mTc]-iminodiacetic acid scans can demonstrate ductal

obstruction, they do not provide sufficient anatomic definition to determine cause or assist in making therapeutic decisions.

**ANSWER:** B

50. Two weeks following hepaticojejunostomy for the treatment of a benign bile duct stricture, a patient has a serum bilirubin level of 6 mg/dL. The patient was jaundiced for 4 weeks before the operation and had a preoperative serum bilirubin level of 12 mg/dL. Which of the following is the most likely explanation for this current serum bilirubin level?

    A. Anastomotic stricture

    B. Persistent delta-bilirubinemia

    C. Postoperative hepatitis

    D. Normal expected decline after relief of any obstructive jaundice

    E. Renal failure

*Ref.:* 4

**COMMENTS:** After relief of biliary obstruction, there is a prompt increase in bile flow, and normal bile acid secretion resumes within several days. Serum bilirubin levels decline approximately 50% by 36 to 48 hours after surgery and 8% per day thereafter. This rate varies, depending on the duration of the jaundice. **Delta-bilirubin** is a form of bilirubin that is covalently bonded to albumin and is measured as part of the direct bilirubin fraction. As such, it is not filtered by the kidneys and has the same serum half-life as albumin, approximately 18 days, which accounts for the slow decline in serum bilirubin levels observed in patients following relief of longstanding jaundice. Although 90% of patients who had jaundice for 1 week or less have a normal serum bilirubin level 3 to 4 weeks postoperatively, only one third of patients who had jaundice for 4 weeks or longer obtain normal levels by the same time. Anastomotic stenosis does not usually develop early during the postoperative period. Postoperative hepatocellular dysfunction as a result of hepatitis or other causes can occur early in the postoperative period, but it is a less likely cause of hyperbilirubinemia in a patient whose serum bilirubin levels are gradually declining and who would be anticipated to have persistent delta-bilirubinemia.

**ANSWER:** B

51. Which of the following is the most likely explanation for a serum bilirubin level of 40 mg/dL in a patient with obstructive jaundice?

    A. The patient has complete biliary obstruction.

    B. The duration of obstruction has exceeded 2 weeks.

    C. The patient has associated renal dysfunction.

    D. The patient has malignant biliary obstruction.

    E. The patient also has Gilbert disease

*Ref.:* 4

**COMMENTS:** In the presence of **complete biliary obstruction**, **serum bilirubin** levels generally plateau at 25 to 30 mg/dL. At this point, the daily bilirubin load equals that excreted by the kidneys. Situations in which even higher bilirubin levels can be found include renal insufficiency, hemolysis, hepatocellular disease, and rarely, a bile duct–hepatic vein fistula. Hyperbilirubinemia tends to be more pronounced in patients with obstruction caused by malignant disease than with obstruction resulting from benign causes. However, malignant obstruction in the absence of the previously enumerated factors does not produce this degree of hyperbilirubinemia.

**ANSWER: C**

52. The pathophysiology of acute renal failure in a patient with biliary obstruction is related to which of the following conditions?

    A. Renal hypertension

    B. Hyperbilirubinemia

    C. Hepatorenal syndrome

    D. Bile acidemia

    E. Acute glomerulonephritis

    *Ref.:* 4

**COMMENTS: Acute renal failure** is a frequent and commonly fatal complication of **biliary sepsis**. A number of factors contribute to the development of this complication. Renal hypoperfusion occurs as a result of bacteremia, systemic hypotension, and hypovolemia. Circulating bacterial endotoxins are also nephrotoxic. Patients with biliary obstruction are at higher risk for renal failure than are patients with sepsis from other causes. Evidence suggests that circulating bile acids themselves may induce tubular damage and exacerbate the effects of renal ischemia. Therapy for patients with biliary sepsis must focus on adequate fluid and vasopressor support, antibiotic coverage, and biliary decompression to prevent renal failure. Additional treatment, such as the administration of bile acids to minimize gut absorption of bacterial endotoxins, has also been used. Little evidence exists to indicate that renal damage is caused by bilirubin, even though it may predispose the tubular cells to ischemia.

**ANSWER: D**

53. Which of the following conditions is usually associated with the highest incidence of positive bile culture results?

    A. Acute cholecystitis

    B. Chronic cholecystitis

    C. Choledocholithiasis

    D. Postoperative bile duct stricture

    E. Bile duct malignancy

    *Ref.:* 2, 4

**COMMENTS:** Recognition of clinical situations in which bacteria are likely to be present in bile is important because the presence of bacteria in bile is correlated with the risk for postoperative infectious complications. Prophylactic antibiotics have decreased infectious morbidity in patients older than 50 years and in those with jaundice, acute cholecystitis, or choledocholithiasis and **cholangitis**. Bile cultures are positive in approximately 5% to 40% of patients with chronic cholecystitis, 30% to 70% of patients with acute cholecystitis, 60% to 80% of patients with choledocholithiasis, and nearly all patients with bile duct stricture. Bacterial infection of bile occurs in 25% to 50% of patients with malignant obstruction. Bile culture results are expected to be positive in any patient with an indwelling biliary tube.

**ANSWER: D**

54. Which of the following organisms is most commonly isolated from bile?

    A. *Escherichia coli*

    B. *Clostridium* spp.

    C. *Bacteroides fragilis*

    D. *Pseudomonas* spp.

    E. *Enterococcus* spp.

    *Ref.:* 2, 4, 7

**COMMENTS:** All of the aforementioned organisms are found in the biliary tract, but gram-negative aerobic organisms, particularly *E. coli* and *Klebsiella*, are found most frequently. Other gram-negative aerobic bacteria that can be cultured are *Proteus*, *Pseudomonas*, and *Enterobacter* spp. Gram-positive organisms, especially *Enterococcus* spp. and *Streptococcus faecalis*, are also frequently observed. Anaerobes are now recognized in 25% to 30% of cases, most commonly *B. fragilis*, followed by *Clostridium* spp. Polymicrobial infection occurs in approximately 60% of cases. Prophylactic or therapeutic antibiotic therapy must be effective against the anticipated organisms. Severe **biliary sepsis** is usually treated with broad-spectrum or combination antibiotics that are effective against gram-negative organisms, anaerobes, and enterococci.

**ANSWER: A**

55. Which of the following is the most common mechanism leading to bacteria in bile?

    A. Ascending infection from the duodenum

    B. Hematogenous portal venous spread

    C. Hematogenous arterial spread

    D. Lymphatic spread

    E. Systemic immunosuppression

    *Ref.:* 2, 4

**COMMENTS:** Bile is usually sterile. There are various routes by which bacteria can reach the biliary tract, and although not proved, dissemination from the portal venous system via the liver is favored as the most common mechanism. Ascending infection from the duodenum does not occur to a significant extent. In addition, evidence suggests that the direction of lymphatic flow is from the liver downward rather than in the reverse direction. Hematogenous dissemination via hepatic arterial flow is a mechanism of hepatic abscess formation and may lead to bactibilia but is thought to be less common than portal venous spread.

**ANSWER: B**

56. Which of the following conditions is sufficient to cause cholangitis with bacteremia?

    A. Bacteria in bile

    B. Partial bile duct obstruction

    C. Complete bile duct obstruction

    D. Any of the above

    E. None of the above

    *Ref.:* 2, 7

**COMMENTS:** The pathophysiology of **cholangitis** requires both bacterial infection of bile and bile duct obstruction with elevated intraductal pressure. Neither the presence of bacteria in bile nor biliary obstruction alone is sufficient to produce bacteremia. When bacteria are present in bile and common duct pressures exceed 20 cm $H_2O$, cholangiovenous and cholangiolymphatic reflux occurs and results in systemic bacteremia. Partial or complete bile duct obstruction may produce cholangitis if bacteria are present. In fact, cholangitis occurs more commonly with partial obstruction because it is more frequently associated with stone disease, whereas complete obstruction is more often found with malignancy. Calculous disease is the most common cause of cholangitis, which is understandable because it is associated with both bile duct obstruction and bacterial infection.

**ANSWER:** E

57. If an antibiotic is effective against the bacteria present in bile, which of the following is the most important consideration for effective treatment of biliary tract infection?

A. Serum concentration of the antibiotic

B. Bile concentration of the antibiotic in an unobstructed biliary tract

C. Bile concentration of the antibiotic in an obstructed biliary tract

D. Potential renal toxicity of the antibiotic

E. Hospital Surgical Care Improvement Project (SCIP) guidelines

*Ref.:* 2, 4

**COMMENTS:** The most important pharmacologic considerations pertaining to selection of **antimicrobial agents** for the treatment of **biliary sepsis** are the spectrum of antibacterial activity of the agent and achievement of adequate serum levels of the drug. Therapy cannot be adequate if the agents selected are not effective against the anticipated organisms (i.e., gram-negative Enterobacteriaceae, enterococci, and anaerobes) or if dosing does not produce sufficient serum levels. The significance of biliary levels of antibiotics is often discussed, but they are of little clinical importance. High bile levels of an antibiotic are meaningless if the agent is not effective against the bacteria present. Moreover, agents that achieve high concentrations in the normal biliary tract may not reach such levels in the presence of biliary obstruction. The aminoglycoside gentamicin, for example, has traditionally been an effective agent against the gram-negative organisms that cause biliary sepsis, but it is not concentrated in bile. The potential nephrotoxicity of an antibiotic is an important consideration because the risk for renal compromise already exists in a patient with sepsis and biliary obstruction. This has encouraged the use of nonaminoglycoside drugs for gram-negative coverage, but this consideration is not as important as the activity spectrum and adequate serum levels of the drugs.

**ANSWER:** A

58. In addition to fluid resuscitation and intravenous antibiotics, most patients with acute cholangitis require urgent treatment with which of the following?

A. Laparoscopic cholecystectomy

B. Percutaneous transhepatic drainage

C. Endoscopic sphincterotomy and drainage

D. T-tube decompression of the common bile duct

E. None of the above

*Ref.:* 2, 7

**COMMENTS:** **Charcot's triad**, which consists of fever, jaundice, and upper abdominal pain, is the clinical hallmark of acute cholangitis. When accompanied by shock and changes in mental status, it is referred to as **Reynold's pentad**. Cholangitis varies widely in severity, and treatment must be individualized according to the patient's condition. Initial therapy consists of fluid resuscitation and antibiotics that are effective against gram-negative organisms, enterococci, and anaerobes. Approximately 5% to 10% of patients initially have severe toxic cholangitis and manifestations of the Reynold pentad. Patients who fail to improve or who deteriorate despite antibiotic and fluid support require urgent biliary decompression. This can generally be accomplished nonoperatively by percutaneous transhepatic or endoscopic approaches, depending on the suspected location of the obstruction based on ultrasonographic findings and on the availability of local expertise in these procedures. The ability to decompress the biliary tract nonoperatively in these cases has been advantageous because it not only allows stabilization of a high percentage of patients but also permits diagnostic cholangiography to be performed when the patient has stabilized. When initial operative decompression of the biliary tract was the only approach for these critically ill patients, the mortality rate was high, and there was a frequent need for subsequent reoperation on the biliary tract because of the inability to identify or deal with the underlying pathologic condition at the time of the initial operation. If effective nonoperative drainage of the biliary tract is not possible, surgery should not be delayed in these critically ill patients. T-tube decompression of the common bile duct is performed. Choledochoduodenostomy is not performed in critically ill patients, but it can be considered if the common bile duct is dilated to 15 mm or greater, the patient is physiologically stable, and other conditions permit safe performance of an anastomosis. The current mortality rate in patients with acute cholangitis is approximately 5%. Poor prognostic factors include renal failure, liver abscess, cirrhosis, and proximal malignant obstruction.

**ANSWER:** E

59. Ultrasound of the gallbladder demonstrates a 5-mm hyperechoic focus along the gallbladder wall that does not move or produce shadowing and that has a "comet tail" echo pattern behind it. What is the most likely diagnosis?

A. Adenomatous polyp

B. Cholesterol polyp

C. Gallstone

D. Adenomyomatosis

E. Xanthogranulomatous inflammation

*Ref.:* 6

**COMMENTS:** The term *hyperplastic cholecystosis* describes a group of benign proliferative conditions of the gallbladder, including cholesterolosis and adenomyomatosis, or adenomatous hyperplasia. These conditions can be symptomatic and are often diagnosed on the basis of their sonographic features. **Cholesterolosis** consists of deposits of cholesterol in foamy histiocytes in the gallbladder wall. A localized collection of such cholesterol-laden cells covered by a normal layer of epithelium and connected to the mucosa by a small pedicle is known as a cholesterol polyp. Ultrasound imaging shows hyperechoic foci with a "comet tail" artifact.

Unlike gallstones, the foci do not move or produce acoustic shadowing. **Adenomatous hyperplasia** is a proliferative lesion characterized by increased thickness of the mucosa and muscle along with mucosal diverticula known as Rokitansky-Aschoff sinuses. Segmental, diffuse, and localized forms of adenomyomatous hyperplasia have been described. Of these, a localized form involving the fundus of the gallbladder is most frequently encountered. Ultrasound demonstrates a mass lesion or "pseudotumor." **Adenomatous polyps** are true neoplasms derived from the glandular epithelium of the gallbladder. **Xanthogranulomatous inflammation** is a condition in which foamy histiocytes are found in conjunction with inflammatory cells and a fibroblastic vascular reaction, often with mucosal ulceration.

**ANSWER:  B**

60. With regard to adenomyomatosis of the gallbladder, which of the following statements is true?

    A. It is a premalignant lesion.

    B. It results from chronic inflammation.

    C. It may cause right upper quadrant pain in the absence of gallstones.

    D. It is rarely associated with cholelithiasis and cholecystitis.

    E. It is not an indication for cholecystectomy in asymptomatic patients.

    *Ref.:* 1, 2

**COMMENTS:** Adenomyomatosis is a hyperplastic abnormality of the gallbladder that is not related to inflammation or neoplasia. Approximately one half or more of patients with adenomyomatosis also have cholelithiasis and cholecystitis, but the relationship is not causal. Adenomyomatosis is not a premalignant lesion. The hyperplastic conditions of adenomyomatosis and cholesterolosis may be associated with functional abnormalities of the gallbladder, as evidenced by disturbances in motility or hyperconcentration during oral cholecystography. These abnormalities may be the cause of biliary tract symptoms in patients with hyperplastic cholecystosis in the absence of cholelithiasis. Cholecystectomy can relieve the symptoms in these patients.

**ANSWER:  C**

61. Which of the following is the most common type of biliary enteric fistula?

    A. Cholecystocolic

    B. Cholecystoduodenal

    C. Cholecystoduodenocolic

    D. Choledochoduodenal

    E. Choledochogastric

    *Ref.:* 2, 4

**COMMENTS:** Almost all **internal biliary fistulas** are acquired communications between the extrahepatic biliary tree and the intestinal tract. In rare instances, acquired or congenital bronchobiliary or acquired pleurobiliary fistulas occur. Biliary enteric fistulas most commonly involve the gallbladder and the duodenum (70% to 80% of cases) and are the result of chronic inflammation caused by gallstone disease. The second most common fistula occurs between the gallbladder and colon; infrequently, the stomach or multiple sites (cholecystoduodenocolic) are involved. Occasionally, the biliary site of the fistula is the common bile duct. Choledochoduodenal fistulas are most frequently caused by penetrating peptic ulcers, but they might occur in patients with choledocholithiasis and previous cholecystectomy. Other, less common causes of biliary enteric fistulas are malignancy and penetrating trauma.

**ANSWER:  B**

62. With regard to the management of a patient with gallstone ileus, which of the following statements is true?

    A. Initial tube decompression and nonoperative management allow spontaneous stone passage in one third of patients.

    B. Operative treatment attempts to displace the stone into the colon without enterotomy.

    C. Operative treatment involves enterotomy proximal to the site of obstruction.

    D. Cholecystectomy and fistula repair at the time of stone removal are contraindicated.

    E. Standard treatment is initial laparotomy for stone removal and reoperation for cholecystectomy when the patient is stable.

    *Ref.:* 2, 4

**COMMENTS: Gallstone ileus** is mechanical obstruction of the gastrointestinal tract caused by a gallstone that has entered the intestine via an acquired biliary enteric fistula. Although gallstone ileus accounts for only 1% to 3% of all small bowel obstructions, it is associated with a higher mortality rate than other nonmalignant causes of bowel obstruction because it tends to occur in the elderly population and typical cases are characterized by diagnostic delay as a result of waxing and waning of symptoms ("tumbling obstruction"). Pathognomonic radiologic features include a gas pattern of small bowel obstruction with pneumobilia and an opaque stone outside the expected location of the gallbladder. Not all of these radiologic features are usually present, however. The most common site of obstruction is the terminal ileum. Infrequently, sigmoid obstruction occurs in an area narrowed by intrinsic colonic disease.

Initial therapy is appropriate resuscitation followed by surgery. Spontaneous passage is a rare phenomenon, and nonoperative management is associated with a prohibitive mortality rate. Stone removal is best accomplished with an enterotomy placed proximal to the site of obstruction. Care must be taken to search for additional intestinal stones, which are present in 10% of patients. Attempts to crush the stone extraluminally or to milk it distally are contraindicated because they may cause bowel injury. In rare instances, small bowel resection is necessary if there is ischemic compromise or bleeding at the site of impaction.

The main controversy regarding surgical treatment of gallstone ileus is whether a definitive biliary tract operation with **cholecystectomy, fistula repair**, and possible common duct exploration should be performed at the time of stone removal. This decision must be based on sound surgical judgment and consideration of the underlying physiologic status of the patient and the anatomic status of the right upper quadrant. Up to one third of patients who do not undergo definitive biliary surgery experience recurrent biliary symptoms, including cholecystitis, cholangitis, and recurrent gallstone ileus. Furthermore, the rate of spontaneous fistula closure is open to question. For these reasons, a definitive one-stage procedure should be considered in physiologically fit patients if right upper quadrant dissection does not prove unduly hazardous from a technical standpoint, particularly if residual stones can be demonstrated in the right upper quadrant. In properly selected patients, a definitive one-stage procedure is not associated with higher operative morbidity or mortality rates. However, because most of these patients are elderly and have a high incidence of comorbid disease, surgical therapy has been limited to stone removal in most instances. **Interval cholecystectomy** should be considered for patients with postoperative biliary symptoms and for those with residual right upper quadrant stones, provided that they are physiologically fit. In reality, because of the compromised underlying status of many of these patients, interval elective procedures are not commonly performed.

**ANSWER:** C

63. Which of the following is the preferred management of a type I choledochal cyst?

   A. Cyst excision

   B. Cyst duodenostomy

   C. Cyst jejunostomy

   D. External drainage

   E. Endoscopic sphincterotomy

*Ref.:* 2

**COMMENTS: Cystic disease of the biliary tract** may involve the intrahepatic ducts, extrahepatic ducts, or both. The most common form of involvement is cystic dilation of the extrahepatic bile duct (type I). Combined intrahepatic and extrahepatic cysts (type IV) are next in frequency of occurrence. A diverticulum of the common bile duct (type II), a "choledochocele" extending from the distal duct into the duodenum (type III), and cystic disease confined to the intrahepatic ducts (type V) are less common. Bile duct cysts may be associated with jaundice, abdominal pain, and cholangitis in both adult and pediatric patients. Furthermore, their association with biliary tract malignancy and with anomalous relationships between the pancreatic duct and bile duct is well recognized. For these reasons, complete cyst excision with Roux-en-Y hepaticojejunostomy is the preferred treatment. Internal drainage procedures are followed by a high rate of recurrent jaundice, cholangitis, and stricture. In some instances, because of the intrahepatic or retroduodenal extent of disease or because of technical considerations, complete excision may not be feasible, and the surgeon may have to settle for partial excision. Endoscopic treatment by sphincterotomy or resection is occasionally appropriate for the rarely occurring choledochocele.

**ANSWER:** A

64. With regard to balloon dilation of benign biliary strictures, which of the following statements is true?

   A. Dilation can be performed via the transhepatic or endoscopic route.

   B. Repeated dilations are not often required.

   C. Perforation of the bile duct is the most frequent complication.

   D. Better success is obtained with anastomotic strictures than with primary duct strictures.

   E. The long-term success rate is better than that achieved with surgical repair.

*Ref.:* 2, 3

**COMMENTS:** Nonoperative **dilation of benign biliary strictures** via endoscopic or percutaneous transhepatic access is an alternative to surgery that may be appropriate for some patients. Repeated dilations are often required, but overall success rates of 70% to 80% at 2 to 3 years of follow-up have been reported. Success has generally been somewhat higher in patients with primary ductal strictures than in those with strictures of biliary enteric anastomoses. Bleeding and sepsis have been the most frequent complications and can be life-threatening. Data on long-term results are limited. Comparison between balloon dilation and surgery has demonstrated better long-term results (approximate mean follow-up at 5 years) with surgery, but no difference in overall morbidity, hospitalization, or cost between the two therapies. It cannot be ensured that the treatment groups are comparable, however. Nonoperative dilation of biliary strictures may be appropriate as initial treatment of a strictured biliary anastomosis or for patients in whom surgical repair is deemed excessively difficult or dangerous. The decision about how a biliary stricture is initially treated and when nonoperative maneuvers are abandoned in favor of surgery should be made in consultation with a skilled endoscopist, an interventional radiologist, and an experienced hepatobiliary surgeon.

**ANSWER:** A

65. A 40-year-old man is evaluated for fluctuating jaundice, pruritus, and fatigue. Liver enzyme levels demonstrate cholestasis. Ultrasound imaging does not show gallstones or bile duct dilation. What diagnostic test should be obtained next?

   A. Measurement of serum antimitochondrial antibodies

   B. CT

   C. HIDA scan

   D. ERCP

   E. Liver biopsy

*Ref.:* 2-4

**COMMENTS:** The findings described are fairly typical of **sclerosing cholangitis**, which can also be discovered in asymptomatic patients based on a cholestatic liver enzyme pattern. Sclerosing cholangitis is a disease of undetermined cause characterized by inflammatory fibrosis and stenosis of the bile ducts. The process can be considered primary when no specific etiologic factor is identified or secondary when associated with specific causes, such as bile duct stones, operative trauma, hepatic arterial infusion of chemotherapeutic agents, or intraductal instillation of various irritants for the treatment of echinococcal disease. Primary sclerosing cholangitis may be an isolated finding or may occur in conjunction with a variety of other disease processes, most commonly ulcerative colitis and pancreatitis. Although the cause of primary sclerosing cholangitis is unknown, most attention has focused on an autoimmune or infectious cause. Evidence of an autoimmune cause is largely inferential and based on the association of sclerosing cholangitis with a variety of autoimmune diseases. Abnormal immunologic parameters can be found in the serum of some patients with sclerosing cholangitis, but there are no specific serologic markers for the disease. Antimitochondrial antibodies are generally associated with primary biliary cirrhosis. The diagnosis is usually made following ERCP showing multiple strictures and dilations, which give a "beaded" appearance to the ducts. Magnetic resonance imaging of the bile ducts may also show abnormalities. Typically, sclerosing cholangitis is a diffuse process that affects both the intrahepatic and extrahepatic bile ducts. In some cases, more limited involvement of the distal bile duct, the intrahepatic ducts, or the area of the bifurcation can be seen. Liver biopsy may show fibro-obliterative cholangitis or cirrhosis as the disease progresses.

**ANSWER: D**

66. Definitive treatment of a patient with sclerosing cholangitis and biliary cirrhosis involves which of the following?

    A. Ursodeoxycholic acid

    B. Corticosteroids

    C. Endoscopic balloon dilation and stenting

    D. Extrahepatic bile duct resection and transhepatic stenting

    E. Hepatic transplantation

*Ref.:* 2-4

**COMMENTS:** Once **sclerosing cholangitis** has progressed to cirrhosis, the only definitive treatment is **hepatic transplantation**. The results of transplantation are generally similar to those obtained when it is performed for other indications. Before the development of cirrhosis, a number of medical and surgical therapies may be useful. Pharmacologic approaches have included the use of immunosuppressants, bile acid–binding agents, and antifibrotic and antimicrobial drugs. Unfortunately, there is little evidence that any medical therapy has been effective in slowing progression. Some hopeful results have been reported with ursodeoxycholic acid, which may improve liver enzyme test results and liver histologic study results. Dominant strictures can be treated operatively or by nonoperative dilation via endoscopic or percutaneous transhepatic approaches. The long-term efficacy of nonoperative approaches has often been limited, however. Select patients with predominantly extrahepatic or bifurcation strictures have been treated successfully with bile duct resection followed by Roux-en-Y reconstruction and long-term anastomotic stenting.

**ANSWER: E**

67. Following cholecystectomy, an adenocarcinoma of the gallbladder extending into the subserosa is discovered incidentally. The recommended treatment includes which of the following?

    A. Nothing further at this time

    B. External beam radiation therapy

    C. Radiation therapy and chemotherapy

    D. Reoperation for liver resection and lymphadenectomy

    E. Reoperation for performance of pancreaticoduodenectomy

*Ref.:* 22

**COMMENTS:** When **gallbladder cancer** is discovered postoperatively during pathologic examination of the specimen, the depth of tumor invasion is an important determinant of further therapy. Tumors limited to the mucosa (T1a) are usually cured by cholecystectomy alone. Patients with tumors extending into the muscle layer (T1b) or into the subserosal connective tissue layer (T2) are those most likely to benefit from resection of the adjacent liver segments (IV and V) and hepatoduodenal lymphadenectomy. A substantial proportion of patients with T2 lesions can be found to have lymph nodes positive for cancer or residual disease. Reoperation may increase the 5-year survival rate to 70% to 90% as compared with 40% for cholecystectomy alone. More extensive invasion through the serosa (T3) or more than 2 cm into the liver

(T4), with or without invasion of adjacent organs, may be recognized by the surgeon at the time of cholecystectomy, but such is not always the case. Cholecystectomy is inadequate for cure of these lesions. Radical resection of these cancers may certainly benefit some patients, but the morbidity and mortality may be high, and conclusive evidence of benefit to many patients is lacking. Other pathologic findings in the gallbladder specimen that favor reoperation are a cancer-positive cystic duct margin (in which case bile duct resection must be considered) or a cancer-positive cystic duct lymph node. Radiation therapy and chemotherapy have generally been ineffective for the treatment of gallbladder cancer.

**ANSWER: D**

68. Ultrasound imaging demonstrates a 15-mm polypoid lesion in the gallbladder of an asymptomatic 60-year-old patient. Which of the following best describes the recommended treatment?

    A. Observation with repeated ultrasound studies in 6 months

    B. Cholecystectomy

    C. Cholecystectomy if the patient is female

    D. Cholecystectomy only if symptoms develop

    E. Cholecystectomy only if the patient also has gallstones

*Ref.:* 23

**COMMENTS: Polypoid lesions** of the gallbladder may be benign, premalignant, or malignant. Inflammatory polyps and cholesterol polyps are benign, nonneoplastic lesions. Benign adenomas are neoplasms that have a malignant potential similar to that of adenomas arising in other areas of the gastrointestinal tract. Polypoid lesions are typically diagnosed by ultrasound imaging and occasionally by other imaging modalities, such as CT. The indications for cholecystectomy for the treatment of a polypoid lesion are (1) symptoms and (2) possible malignancy.

The **risk for malignancy** is related to the size of the lesion; it is higher for lesions that are 10 mm or larger and is quite substantial for lesions measuring 15 mm. Therefore, cholecystectomy is performed if the patient has biliary tract symptoms—regardless of polyp size or the presence or absence of gallstones—or if the lesion is larger than 10 mm. Polypoid lesions in patients 60 years or older are also more frequently malignant. The use of **laparoscopic cholecystectomy** for polypoid lesions is controversial. Proponents argue that the laparoscopic approach is appropriate, because most polyps are benign and even limited cancers may be cured by cholecystectomy alone. However, gallbladder leakage is not infrequent during laparoscopic cholecystectomy, and consequent dissemination of otherwise "curable" early cancers has been reported. It is generally advised that "**open cholecystectomy**" be performed for patients considered at risk for gallbladder cancer.

**ANSWER: B**

69. Which of the following is a contraindication to resection of an adenocarcinoma of the bile duct?

    A. Tumor location in the distal common bile duct

    B. Tumor location at the bifurcation of the bile duct

    C. Peritoneal metastases

    D. Invasion of the right portal vein and right hepatic artery

    E. None of the above

*Ref.:* 3, 4

**COMMENTS: Cancers of the extrahepatic bile ducts** usually carry a poor prognosis because these tumors are frequently beyond the confines of surgical resection at the time of diagnosis. Substantial palliation can often be achieved with therapy directed at the relief of biliary obstruction. The prognosis is related to tumor location, resectability, and histologic pattern. Proximal lesions at or near the hepatic bifurcation are most common but are also least often resectable and therefore have a less favorable prognosis. Aggressive resection of proximal lesions, usually including hepatic resection, can improve survival. Hilar cholangiocarcinoma (Klatskin tumor) is considered unresectable if there is metastatic disease, bilateral involvement of the portal vein or hepatic artery, or bilateral extension of the tumor to second-order biliary radicles. **Hepatic transplantation** for otherwise unresectable tumors has had poor results. Distal lesions resectable by pancreaticoduodenectomy have the best prognosis, with a 5-year survival rate of approximately 30%. Palliative decompression can be achieved by surgical anastomosis, surgical intubation, or endoscopic or percutaneous catheter placement. The most appropriate method of palliative decompression for a particular patient depends on tumor location and extent, the patient's underlying condition, the expertise of the surgeon, and the anticipated complications associated with each technique. Nonoperative decompression is preferred for patients who are demonstrated to have metastasis or otherwise unresectable disease before surgery.

**ANSWER: C**

70. How is a contusion of the gallbladder from blunt abdominal trauma best managed?

    A. Observation

    B. Placement of a percutaneous cholecystostomy tube

    C. Placement of an endoscopic biliary stent

    D. Suture imbrication of the contusion

    E. Cholecystectomy

*Ref.:* 2

**COMMENTS:** The **gallbladder** may be injured as a result of **blunt or penetrating trauma**. Penetrating injury is the most common. Most injuries of the gallbladder and extrahepatic biliary tree are associated with involvement of other organs, such as the liver, small bowel, and colon. Blunt injuries, including contusion, avulsion, and rupture, are treated by cholecystectomy. Penetrating injuries occasionally cause isolated injury to the gallbladder. Treatment in such instances is usually cholecystectomy, although cholecystostomy or simple closure plus drainage is conceivable. The prognosis following a nonoperative injury to the biliary tract is related to the significance of the associated injuries.

**ANSWER: E**

## REFERENCES

1. Deziel DJ: The journey of the surgeon-hero, *Surg Endosc* 22:1–7, 2008.

2. Chari RS, Shah SA: Biliary system. In Townsend CM, Beauchamp RD, Evers BM, et al, editors: *Sabiston textbook of surgery: the biological basis of modern surgical practice*, ed 18, Philadelphia, 2008, WB Saunders.

3. Mullholland MW, Lillemoe KD, Doherty GM, et al, editors: *Greenfield's surgery: scientific principles and practice*, Hepatobiliary and Portal Venous System Section, ed 4, Philadelphia, 2006, Lippincott Williams & Wilkins.

4. Blumgart LH: *Surgery of the liver, biliary tract and pancreas*, ed 4, Edinburgh, 2006, Churchill-Livingstone.

5. Yoshida J, Chijiwa K, Yamaguchi K, et al: Practical classification of the branching types of the biliary tree: an analysis of 1,094 consecutive direct cholangiograms, *J Am Coll Surg* 82:37–40, 1996.

6. Machi J, Staren ED: *Ultrasound for surgeons*, Philadelphia, 2005, Lippincott Williams & Wilkins.

7. Mulvihill SJ: Liver, biliary tract, and pancreas. In O'Leary JP, Tabuenca A, editors: *The physiologic basis of surgery*, ed 4, Philadelphia, 2008, Lippincott Williams & Wilkins.

8. Canfield AJ, Hetz SP, Schriver JP, et al: Biliary dyskinesia: a study of more than 200 patients and review of the literature, *J Gastrointest Surg* 2:443–448, 1998.

9. Fong Y, Brennan MF, Turnbulla A, et al: Gallbladder cancer discovered during laparoscopic surgery, *Arch Surg* 128:1050–1054, 1993.

10. Strasberg SM, Hertle M, Soper NJ: An analysis of the problem of biliary injury during laparoscopic cholecystectomy, *J Am Coll Surg* 180:101–125, 1995.

11. Lillemoe KD: Current management of bile duct injury, *Br J Surg* 95:403–405, 2008.

12. Deziel DJ: Complications of cholecystectomy, *Surg Clin North Am* 74:809–823, 1994.

13. Stewart L, Way LW: Bile duct injuries during laparoscopic cholecystectomy: factors that influence the results of treatment, *Arch Surg* 130:1123–1129, 1995.

14. Lillemoe KD, Martin SA, Cameron JL, et al: Major bile duct injuries during laparoscopic cholecystectomy, *Ann Surg* 225:459–471, 1997.

15. Woods MS, Traverso LW, Kozarek RA, et al: Biliary tract complications of laparoscopic cholecystectomy are detected more frequently with routine intraoperative cholangiography, *Surg Endosc* 9:1076–1080, 1995.

16. Date RS, Kaushal M, Ramesh A: A review of the management of gallstone disease and its complications during pregnancy, *Am J Surg* 196:599–608, 2008.

17. Palanivelu C, Rajan PS, Jani K, et al: Laparoscopic cholecystectomy in cirrhotic patients: the role of subtotal cholecystectomy and its variants, *J Am Coll Surg* 203:145–151, 2006.

18. Podolsky ER, Curcillo II PG: Single port access (SPA) surgery: a 24-month experience, *J Gastrointest Surg* 14:759–767, 2010.

19. Horgan S, Mintz Y, Jacobsen GR, et al: NOTES: transvaginal cholecystectomy with assisting articulating instruments, *Surg Endosc* 23:1900, 2009.

20. Barkun AN, Barkun JS, Fried GM, et al: Useful predictors of bile duct stones in patients undergoing laparoscopic cholecystectomy, *Ann Surg* 220:32–39, 1994.

21. Petelin J: Laparoscopic approach to common duct pathology, *Am J Surg* 165:487–491, 1993.

22. Perry KA, Myers JA, Deziel DJ: Laparoscopic ultrasound as the primary modality for bile duct imaging during cholecystectomy, *Surg Endosc* 22:208–213, 2008.

23. D'Angelica M, Dalal KM, DeMatteo RP, et al. Analysis of the extent of resection for adenocarcinoma of the gallbladder, *Ann Surg Oncol* 16:806–816, 2009.

# CHAPTER 25

# Pancreas

*Daniel J. Deziel, M.D.*

1. Which of the following vascular relationships is not an important consideration during resection of the head of the pancreas?

   A. Arterial supply of the pancreatic head from the splenic artery

   B. Confluence of the splenic vein and superior mesenteric vein dorsal to the pancreatic neck

   C. Absence of ventral portal vein branches dorsal to the pancreatic neck

   D. Origin of the right hepatic artery from the superior mesenteric artery

   E. Origin of the middle colic artery from the superior mesenteric artery

   *Ref.:* 1-4

COMMENTS: The relationship of the pancreas to neighboring organs and to critical vascular structures is of great surgical significance. The **arterial supply** to the head of the gland is derived from both the gastroduodenal and the superior mesenteric arteries via the anterior and posterior pancreaticoduodenal arcades. For the most part, the head of the pancreas and the duodenum have a shared blood supply, so they must generally be resected together. However, techniques for "duodenal-sparing" resection of the pancreatic head or "pancreatic-sparing" duodenectomy are appropriate in select circumstances.

   The body and tail of the **pancreas** receive their blood supply mainly from multiple branches of the splenic artery, which also connect with superior mesenteric sources. Variations in major arteries—such as the origin of the right hepatic artery from the superior mesenteric artery and the origin of the middle colic artery from the superior mesenteric artery or dorsal pancreatic artery—place these vessels in close proximity to the head and neck of the pancreas, where they are subject to injury during pancreatectomy. The junction of the splenic vein and superior mesenteric vein to form the portal vein lies behind the neck of the pancreas. Usually, these vessels do not have large anterior tributaries in this area, but appropriate caution must nonetheless be exercised when developing this plane during pancreatic operations.

ANSWER: A

2. Endoscopy demonstrates a 1-cm submucosal nodule with central umbilication in the second portion of the duodenum. This finding is usually associated with which of the following?

   A. Peptic ulceration

   B. Increased risk for pancreatic cancer

   C. Islet cell hyperplasia

   D. Absence of symptoms

   E. Intussusception

   *Ref.:* 1, 2, 4

COMMENTS: A **heterotopic pancreas** is pancreatic tissue located at sites other than the normal location of the gland. Ectopic pancreatic tissue has been described at many anatomic locations but is typically found in the stomach, the duodenum, or a Meckel diverticulum. Theories of origin include metaplasia (the favored theory) and transplantation. Histologic findings range from those of a rudimentary structure to a fully formed gland. Most heterotopic rests contain ducts, and both endocrine and exocrine elements may be present. This entity is not uncommon, being described in 1% to 2% of autopsies. It is usually asymptomatic. When symptoms occur, they are related to the location of the ectopic site and include obstruction (as a result of intussusception), ulceration, and bleeding. Although malignancy has been reported, there is no evidence that heterotopic pancreatic tissue is predisposed to cancer. The typical gross appearance is a submucosal nodule, often with central umbilication. Resection is indicated for symptomatic lesions and is appropriate diagnostically for incidental lesions discovered during operations for other reasons.

ANSWER: D

3. The embryologic ventral pancreas forms which area of the fully developed gland?

   A. Superior head

   B. Uncinate process

   C. Neck

   D. Body

   E. None of the above because it regresses

   *Ref.:* 1, 3, 4

COMMENTS: The pancreas is formed from two outpouchings of the primitive gut. The **dorsal pancreas** originates from the duodenum, and the **ventral pancreas** begins as a bud from the hepatic diverticulum, which itself is an outpouching of the duodenum. Other outgrowths from the hepatic diverticulum mature into the liver, gallbladder, and bile ducts. During normal fetal development, the ventral pancreas rotates along with the primitive gut and fuses with the dorsal component. The ventral pancreas constitutes the uncinate process and the inferior portion of the head of the gland in the fully developed state, and the dorsal pancreas forms the remainder of the gland. Abnormalities in this developmental process result in recognized congenital anomalies that can be clinically important. An understanding of this embryologic development is also important to recognizing the relationship of the pancreas to adjacent vascular structures during pancreatic operations.

**ANSWER:**  B

---

**4.** The uncinate process of the pancreas is adjacent and dorsal to which of the following?

A. Splenic vein

B. Inferior vena cava

C. Superior mesenteric artery

D. Left renal vein

E. Fourth portion of the duodenum

*Ref.:* 1-4

**COMMENTS:** The pancreas can be divided into various parts: head, uncinate, neck, body, and tail. The uncinate process is the portion of the gland that extends to the left, dorsal to the portal vein and superior mesenteric artery and ventral to the aorta and inferior vena cava. The uncinate process is located caudad and ventral to the left renal vein and cephalad to the distal duodenum. Understanding the extent and location of the uncinate is important during resection of the head of the pancreas. The blood supply of the uncinate is derived from numerous short branches of the superior mesenteric artery and portal vein. When performing pancreaticoduodenectomy, these branches must be carefully controlled to prevent bleeding and avoid injury to the superior mesenteric artery or portal vein.

**ANSWER:**  C

---

**5.** What is the recommended treatment of duodenal obstruction caused by an annular pancreas?

A. Endoscopic division of the associated duodenal web

B. Gastrojejunostomy

C. Duodenoduodenostomy

D. Surgical division of the annular tissue

E. Pancreaticoduodenectomy

*Ref.:* 1, 2, 4

**COMMENTS:** An **annular pancreas** is a congenital anomaly involving a band of pancreatic tissue encircling the second portion of the duodenum. The annular tissue appears to originate from the embryologic ventral pancreas. Causal theories include abnormal fixation of the ventral pancreatic primordium before gut rotation, failure of involution of part of the ventral pancreas, and the development of heterotopic pancreatic tissue in the duodenum. Approximately one half of these cases are diagnosed in infants and the remainder in adults, with a peak during the fourth decade of life. Most patients are asymptomatic. Clinical findings are obstruction in infants and children and obstruction, ulceration, or pancreatitis in adults. Associated anomalies include duodenal stenosis or atresia and Down syndrome. Treatment of symptomatic patients consists of surgical bypass by duodenoduodenostomy or duodenojejunostomy. Gastrojejunostomy can also alleviate obstruction but risks marginal ulceration. Resection or division of the annular band is

not advised because it risks the development of a pancreatic fistula and may fail to relieve the obstruction.

**ANSWER:**  C

---

**6.** Which of the following developmental anomalies best characterizes pancreas divisum?

A. Aplasia of the dorsal pancreatic anlage

B. Aplasia of the ventral pancreatic anlage

C. Incomplete rotation of the ventral pancreatic anlage

D. Failed fusion of the ventral and dorsal pancreatic parenchyma

E. Failed fusion of the ventral and dorsal pancreatic ducts

*Ref.:* 1, 4, 5

**COMMENTS:** See Question 7.

**ANSWER:**  E

---

**7.** The diagnosis of pancreas divisum is usually made by which of the following?

A. Laparoscopic exploration

B. Endoscopic ultrasound (EUS)

C. Computed tomography (CT)

D. Endoscopic retrograde cholangiopancreatography (ERCP)

E. Genetic testing

*Ref.:* 4

**COMMENTS: Pancreas divisum** currently refers to congenital variations of the pancreatic ducts that result from failed or incomplete fusion of the embryologic ventral and dorsal ductal systems. (Historically, the term may also refer to the rare failure of parenchymal fusion.) There may be complete separation of the ducts, an absent or minimal ventral duct, or only a few meager connections between the systems. As a consequence, most of the pancreatic duct drainage is through the dorsal duct joining the duodenum at the minor papilla. Any existing ventral ducts (Wirsung) drain only the uncinate process and the caudal head of the gland rather than the bulk of the gland at the major papilla, as when normally developed. Some variation of pancreas divisum is present in about 10% of the population. In some individuals, it is clinically significant if the relatively stenotic minor papilla imposes an obstruction to ductal flow. This can potentially result in recurrent abdominal pain, acute pancreatitis, or even chronic pancreatitis. The diagnosis is usually made by ERCP, and cannulation of the minor papilla may be required to image the dorsal duct. Magnetic resonance cholangiopancreatography (MRCP) might also demonstrate this ductal anatomy.

**ANSWER:**  D

---

**8.** Which of the following is appropriate treatment of a patient with pancreas divisum, chronic abdominal pain, a dilated dorsal pancreatic duct, and an enlarged, calcified pancreatic head?

A. Pancreaticoduodenectomy

B. Endoscopic dorsal sphincterotomy

C. Operative dorsal sphincterotomy

D. Endoscopic or operative ventral sphincterotomy

E. Splanchnic nerve ablation

*Ref.:* 1, 4

**COMMENTS:** The vast majority (95%) of individuals with **pancreas divisum** are asymptomatic. Whether there is a true relationship between the anatomic diagnosis of pancreas divisum and any clinical symptoms that may be present is often difficult to determine. Symptomatic patients with pancreas divisum require thorough evaluation of the nature of their symptoms and for any other causes of abdominal pain or pancreatitis. When it is reasonable to suspect that a stenotic lesser papilla is the cause of recurrent abdominal pain or recurrent acute pancreatitis, therapeutic considerations include endoscopic treatments (dilation, stenting, sphincterotomy) or operative sphincterotomy/sphincteroplasty, which may be combined with cholecystectomy and sphincteroplasty of the major papilla. Occasionally, there are patients (as described in this question) with established findings of chronic pancreatitis and pancreas divisum. Sphincter operations are not successful in this setting. Rather, surgical treatment involving resection or decompression of the pancreatic head may be indicated.

**ANSWER:** A

9. Which of the following is not characteristic of pancreatic acinar cells?

A. Zymogen granules

B. Carbonic anhydrase

C. Golgi apparatus

D. Rough endoplasmic reticulum

E. Contractile proteins

*Ref.:* 4, 5

**COMMENTS:** The twofold function of the **exocrine pancreas**—to secrete bicarbonate-rich fluid and to synthesize digestive enzymes—is accomplished by two cell types. Acinar cells, which elaborate and secrete digestive enzymes, are designed for protein synthesis. They contain abundant rough endoplasmic reticulum, Golgi apparatus, and secretory zymogen granules. Contractile proteins are also abundant near the apical membrane of the cell and facilitate exocytosis of the enzyme bundles into the ductal lumen. The centroacinar cells are part of the ductal system. They secrete bicarbonate and therefore contain carbonic anhydrase, which dissociates carbonic acid into bicarbonate and hydrogen ion:

$$H_2O + CO_2 \rightarrow H^+ + HCO_3^-$$

Some ductal cells also contain synthetic and secretory organelles for the production of mucoproteins.

**ANSWER:** B

10. The bicarbonate concentration of pancreatic secretions is:

A. Primarily increased by cholecystokinin (CCK)

B. Primarily decreased by secretin

C. Independent of acinar cell secretion

D. Reciprocally related to the chloride concentration

E. Reciprocally related to the sodium concentration

*Ref.:* 1, 3, 5

**COMMENTS:** The **centroacinar cells** secrete a bicarbonate-rich solution by an active transport mechanism, primarily in response to secretin. **Cholecystokinin** is the primary stimulant of enzyme secretion from the acinar cells. The bicarbonate and chloride contents of pancreatic juice are reciprocally related. As ductal flow rates increase, the bicarbonate concentration increases and the chloride concentration decreases. This is the result of two processes: (1) changes in passive exchange of intraductal bicarbonate for intracellular chloride and (2) changes in the relative contribution of acinar cell secretion. Acinar cells secrete fluid high in chloride in addition to digestive enzymes. In contradistinction to anion concentrations, the concentrations of sodium and potassium in pancreatic duct secretions remain relatively constant despite the flow rate and are similar to their concentrations in plasma.

**ANSWER:** D

11. Normally, activation of pancreatic trypsinogen involves which of the following?

A. Pancreatic amylase

B. pH greater than 7.0

C. Lysosomal hydrolase

D. Pancreatic enterokinase

E. Duodenal enterokinase

*Ref.:* 1-3, 5

**COMMENTS:** The **pancreatic acinar cells** secrete digestive enzymes for fats, carbohydrates, and proteins. Except amylase, these enzymes are secreted in inactive forms to protect the pancreas from autodigestion. Activation of the proenzyme trypsinogen to trypsin is the primary event that leads to activation of the other various proteases and phospholipases. It occurs in the duodenum via the action of enterokinase. Trypsinogen activation can also occur in acidic environments (pH <7.0). With acute pancreatitis, intraglandular activation can take place when the inactive enzymes are exposed to lysosomal hydrolases.

**ANSWER:** E

12. Which pancreatic islet cell type produces a hormonal peptide to stimulate glycogenolysis and gluconeogenesis?

A. Alpha cell

B. Beta cell

C. Delta cell

D. F cell

E. PP cell

*Ref.:* 1-3, 5

**COMMENTS:** See Question 13.

**ANSWER:** A

13. Pancreatic delta cells secrete which inhibitory peptide?

A. Bombesin

B. Glucagon

C. Somatostatin

D. Insulin

E. Pancreatic polypeptide

*Ref.:* 1-3, 5

**COMMENTS: The endocrine pancreas** is composed of various cells located in the islets of Langerhans, approximately 1 million of which are interspersed with the acinar and ductal elements throughout the gland. The hormonal peptides produced by the islets effect a wide range of metabolic and physiologic actions. The primary function of the endocrine pancreas is to regulate glucose homeostasis. Beta cells, which are the most numerous, produce insulin. Insulin promotes glucose transport, stimulates protein synthesis, and inhibits glycogenolysis and lipolysis. Alpha cells secrete glucagon, which counterbalances insulin by stimulating hepatic glycogenolysis, gluconeogenesis, ketogenesis, and lipolysis. Glucagon also inhibits intestinal motility and gastric acid and pancreatic exocrine secretion. Somatostatin, produced by delta cells, has a broad range of inhibitory effects on the gastrointestinal tract, including inhibition of secretion of other pancreatic peptides; inhibition of gastric, biliary, intestinal, and pancreatic exocrine secretions; and inhibition of gastrointestinal motility. PP cells are the source of pancreatic polypeptide. Pancreatic polypeptide inhibits pancreatic exocrine secretion and biliary and gut motility. Clinically, deficiency of pancreatic polypeptide has been linked to diabetes following resection of the pancreatic head or chronic pancreatitis. Because postprandial secretion of pancreatic polypeptide is dependent on vagal innervation, it has been used to assess the completeness of vagotomy.

**ANSWER:** C

---

**14.** Which is the principal cell type located at the center of the islets of Langerhans?

A. Alpha cell

B. Beta cell

C. Delta cell

D. F cell

E. Varies according to the location of the islet in the pancreas

*Ref.:* 1, 3

**COMMENTS:** Each **islet of Langerhans** is composed of an average of 3000 cells, with the major types as listed earlier and discussed in the preceding Comments. Beta cells are located at the core and make up about 70% of the islet. The other cell types are located at the periphery of the islet. This cellular anatomy has potential functional implications that are as yet not well understood. The distribution of cell types within the islet varies in different areas of the gland. Islets in the uncinate process derived from the embryologic ventral pancreas contain PP cells but few alpha cells. Islets in the body and tail of the gland have abundant alpha cells but no PP cells.

**ANSWER:** B

---

**15.** Which of the following statements is true regarding blood flow to the pancreas?

A. Islet cells receive a greater proportion of pancreatic blood flow than do the exocrine elements.

B. CCK and secretin regulate secretion by altering blood flow.

C. Fragile anastomotic networks predispose the gland to ischemia.

D. The blood supply to the islet cells is independent of the acinar supply.

E. Pancreatic blood flow is highly sensitive to changes in systemic blood pressure.

*Ref.:* 3-5

**COMMENTS:** The microcirculation of the pancreas is complex and has important correlations with the endocrine and exocrine functions of the gland. The rich anastomotic supply from various sources makes pancreatic ischemia unusual. The islets receive a disproportionately large amount of total **pancreatic blood flow** (10% to 25%) relative to their mass (1% to 2%). Both the islets and exocrine tissue have arteriolar blood supply. The acinar tissue is also perfused by blood that drains from the islets, a mechanism referred to as the islet-acinar or insuloacinar portal system. This system is the structural basis for endocrine regulation of exocrine function. Insulin receptors are present on acinar cells, and the density of receptors is higher on acini located near the islets. Because the islets themselves often have a central-to-peripheral pattern of perfusion, insulin from the centrally located beta cells can influence the other peripheral islet cell types. In addition, some islets are apparently perfused in a peripheral-to-central pattern. CCK and secretin have relatively little effect on blood flow and thus exert their stimulatory effects independently. Pancreatic blood flow is maintained relatively constant despite changes in arterial pressure.

**ANSWER:** A

---

**16.** Which of the following events occurs in acinar cells with acute pancreatitis?

A. Accelerated extrusion of zymogen granules

B. Impaired synthesis of zymogen granules

C. Fusion of lysosomes and zymogen granules

D. Fusion of mitochondria and zymogen granules

E. Impaired protein synthesis

*Ref.:* 3-5

**COMMENTS:** The **pathogenesis of pancreatitis** involves intrapancreatic activation of digestive enzymes that are normally secreted in inactive form. This results in "autodigestion" of the gland. Although the mechanisms by which the various causes of clinical pancreatitis lead to this state are incompletely understood, experimental observations have identified certain derangements in acinar cell biology that may be the underlying common pathway to pancreatic injury. The primary defects involve blocked extrusion of zymogen granules containing inactive digestive enzymes and alterations in intracellular transport that result in fusion of zymogen granules with lysosomes to form large cytoplasmic vacuoles. This sequence results in co-localization of digestive enzymes and lysosomal hydrolases. Lysosomal enzymes, such as cathepsin B, activate trypsinogen and initiate a cascade of intracellular digestive enzyme activation. Amino acid uptake and protein synthesis are not impaired during this process.

**ANSWER:** C

---

**17.** The mechanism of alcohol-induced acute pancreatitis is thought to involve all of the following except:

A. Pancreatic ductal obstruction

B. Pancreatic exocrine hypersecretion

C. Hypertriglyceridemia

D. Acetaldehyde toxicity

E. Genetic defect in lysosomal membranes

*Ref.:* 1, 3

**COMMENTS:** Ethanol is the prevalent etiologic factor in acute pancreatitis. There are several contributory mechanisms by which **alcohol-induced pancreatic injury** occurs. Ethanol causes pancreatic ductal hypertension by increasing ampullary resistance and by intraductal deposition of stone proteins. Concomitantly, ethanol stimulates gastric acid secretion and increases pancreatic exocrine secretion via release of secretin. The combination of ductal obstruction with stimulated secretion may result in enzyme extravasation. Acetaldehyde, the metabolic product of ethanol, injures acinar cells by increasing membrane permeability and disrupting the microtubule structure. The elevated levels of serum triglycerides induced by alcohol are a source of cytotoxic free fatty acids. Alcohol also impairs normal trypsin inhibition and reduces pancreatic blood flow. All of these effects may contribute to intraglandular enzyme activation and the development of acute alcoholic pancreatitis.

**ANSWER: E**

18. Hyperamylasemia is diagnostic of acute pancreatitis when associated with which of the following laboratory findings?

A. Hyperlipasemia

B. Increased urinary amylase levels

C. Amylase-creatinine clearance ratio (ACCR) greater than 5%

D. Hypocalcemia

E. None of the above

*Ref.:* 1-4

**COMMENTS:** The **diagnosis of acute pancreatitis** is based on signs and symptoms, supported by biochemical findings and morphologic abnormalities seen on imaging studies such as CT. No biochemical feature is pathognomonic of acute pancreatitis. Hyperamylasemia, hyperlipasemia, and elevations in urinary amylase levels and the ACCR are typical of acute pancreatitis but are not specific or sensitive, and they can occur with other abdominal and extra-abdominal disorders. Hypocalcemia may occur as a consequence of pancreatitis, but it is also nonspecific. There is no absolute level of serum amylase or lipase that is diagnostic of acute pancreatitis. Marked elevations are more indicative of pancreatitis but are not themselves diagnostic. Both amylase and lipase levels may be elevated in a number of conditions that can be confused with acute pancreatitis, such as acute cholecystitis, perforated peptic ulcer, and intestinal infarction. Moreover, severe pancreatitis can occur without substantial elevations in these serum enzymes.

**ANSWER: E**

19. A patient with abdominal pain is found to have a serum amylase level of 1200 IU/L, a normal urinary amylase level, and an ACCR of less than 2%. Based on these findings, the probable diagnosis is which of the following conditions?

A. Acute pancreatitis

B. Chronic pancreatitis

C. Renal failure

D. Choledocholithiasis without pancreatitis

E. Macroamylasemia

*Ref.:* 4

**COMMENTS:** Elevations in serum and urinary **amylase** levels and in the ACCR, as determined by the following equation, are typical of acute pancreatitis.

$$ACCR = U_{amy}/S_{amy} \times S_{cr}/U_{cr} \times 100$$

where U = urine, S = serum, amy = amylase, and cr = creatinine. Elevation of the **amylase-creatinine clearance ratio** above the normal 2% to 5% range is not specific for pancreatitis, but a normal ratio in the presence of hyperamylasemia suggests that the hyperamylasemia is the result of something other than pancreatitis. Serum and urinary amylase levels and the ACCR may be normal in patients with chronic pancreatitis or elevated during an acute exacerbation. Renal disease may be associated with low urinary amylase levels and an elevated ACCR. Common duct stones may produce hyperamylasemia without true pancreatitis. The urinary amylase level is elevated, although the ACCR may be normal. With macroamylasemia, amylase forms complexes with serum proteins too large for glomerular filtration. The serum amylase level is therefore elevated, but urinary amylase levels and the ACCR are low. The diagnosis can be confirmed by electrophoresis. Abdominal pain has been reported in more than one half of patients with macroamylasemia, although the biochemical abnormality is probably not etiologically related to the pain. Hyperamylasemia predominantly caused by salivary amylase may also be associated with a low urinary amylase level and ACCR because the salivary isoenzyme is cleared more slowly by the kidneys than the pancreatic isoenzyme.

**ANSWER: E**

20. Which of the following is an unfavorable prognostic factor in patients with acute alcoholic pancreatitis?

A. Initial white blood cell count higher than 16,000/mm$^3$

B. Elevated serum triglycerides during the initial 48 hours

C. Serum amylase level higher than 1200 IU/L on admission

D. Serum lipase level more than three times normal

E. Serum blood urea nitrogen (BUN) level elevated more than 2 mg/dL during the initial 48 hours

*Ref.:* 1, 3, 4

**COMMENTS:** Several systems have been devised to gauge the severity of acute pancreatitis. These systems involve multiple clinical, biochemical, and sometimes radiologic criteria. The most widely used system in the United States, developed by Ranson, was based on retrospective analysis and subsequent prospective verification. The **Ranson criteria** include 11 parameters determined at the time of admission or during the subsequent 48 hours. Patients with three or more criteria have more severe disease and are at increased risk for septic complications and death. The criteria reflect the patient's underlying status, the severity of the retroperitoneal inflammatory process, and the effects on renal and respiratory function. The Ranson criteria were originally developed for alcoholic pancreatitis and have been modified somewhat for gallstone pancreatitis. For example, a rise in the serum BUN level of more than 2 mg/dL is one of the 10 criteria for gallstone pancreatitis, but the rise must be more than 5 mg/dL to meet the criteria for alcoholic pancreatitis (a subtle point). Other physiologic scoring systems, such as the Acute Physiology, Age, and Chronic Health Evaluation II (APACHE II), are also useful prognostically, although they are not designed specifically for acute pancreatitis.

**ANSWER:** A

21. What is the leading cause of death from acute pancreatitis?

   A. Hemorrhage

   B. Pseudocyst rupture

   C. Secondary pancreatic infection

   D. Biliary sepsis

   E. Renal failure

*Ref.:* 6

**COMMENTS:** Formerly, death from acute pancreatitis often occurred early in the course of the disease as a result of the acute effects of hypovolemia and inadequate resuscitation. In the current era, about 80% of deaths are attributed to secondary pancreatic infection, which develops in approximately 10% of patients with acute pancreatitis. Fatal pancreatic sepsis typically progresses to multisystem organ failure, and deaths occur later in the course of the disease. To have an impact on this disease, therapeutic efforts have therefore focused on the prevention and early diagnosis of pancreatic infection and on more effective methods of surgical therapy.

**ANSWER:** C

22. Which of the following complications of acute pancreatitis is associated with the highest mortality rate?

   A. Peripancreatic abscess

   B. Infected pancreatic pseudocyst

   C. Infected pancreatic necrosis

   D. Sterile pancreatic necrosis

   E. Bile duct obstruction

*Ref.:* 4, 6

**COMMENTS: Retroperitoneal infection** is a serious, often fatal complication of **acute pancreatitis**. The early literature pertaining to the local infectious sequelae of pancreatitis may be confusing because of nonselective use of the term pancreatic abscess to describe infectious complications, which vary in severity. Pancreatic abscess best describes a localized collection of drainable pus in or around the pancreas. Pancreatic abscess and infected pseudocyst can be treated effectively by external drainage, and the anticipated mortality rate for each is about 5%. Pancreatic necrosis is a manifestation of severe pancreatitis. When accompanied by infection, it has been associated with a mortality rate that may exceed 40%, which is higher than that for noninfected necrosis. Infected pancreatic necrosis is treated by operative débridement and open or closed retroperitoneal drainage. Patients with sterile necrosis may require operative intervention as well but are generally treated nonoperatively with intensive support as long as their condition permits.

**ANSWER:** C

23. A 45-year-old man is admitted with severe alcoholic pancreatitis. Forty-percent pancreatic necrosis is estimated on CT. Which of the following statements best describes the current use of antibiotics for this patient?

   A. Systemic antibiotics are not indicated unless his condition deteriorates.

   B. Systemic antibiotics are indicated for coverage of gut-derived bacteria.

   C. Systemic antibiotics are indicated for coverage of gut-derived bacteria and fungal organisms.

   D. Nonabsorbable antibiotics are indicated for gut decontamination.

   E. Systemic antibiotics are not indicated if enteric feeding can be tolerated.

*Ref.:* 7

**COMMENTS:** The risk for **infected pancreatic necrosis** is related to the clinical severity and duration of disease and to the extent of necrosis. Strategies to decrease secondary pancreatic infection focus on patients at higher risk. Unfortunately, controlled trials of systemic antibiotics for prophylaxis against secondary infection have yielded conflicting results. These differences are probably because of numerous factors, including heterogeneity in the severity of disease, patient characteristics, and concomitant therapy among those studied, as well as to differences in study methodologies. Current practice favors systemic antibiotics for patients with severe disease and more extensive (>30%) necrosis based on studies demonstrating fewer septic complications and perhaps decreased mortality. However, not all studies have shown benefit, and the risk for subsequent infection with multiresistant bacterial or fungal organisms may be increased, particularly if prophylactic antibiotic use is prolonged. Because the gut is typically the source of the offending organisms, the use of nonabsorbable enteral antibiotics for selective gut decontamination has had some appeal. The effect of this measure remains unclear, and it is not typically used. Enteric feedings are beneficial to maintain the gut mucosal barrier to bacterial translocation. However, the efficacy of enteric feeding alone for prevention of secondary pancreatic infection has not been demonstrated.

**ANSWER:** B

24. Which of the following types of antibiotics does not achieve adequate levels in the pancreas?

   A. Imipenem

   B. Third-generation cephalosporins

   C. Metronidazole

   D. Aminoglycosides

   E. Fluoroquinolones

*Ref.:* 8

**COMMENTS:** Early studies of **antibiotic prophylaxis** in patients with **acute pancreatitis** showed no efficacy, in part because they involved individuals with mild pancreatitis and in part because they used antibiotics that did not achieve adequate therapeutic levels in the pancreas and retroperitoneum. Aminoglycosides, first-generation cephalosporins, and aminopenicillins do not adequately penetrate the pancreas. Drugs with penetration include the other choices listed, as well as piperacillin and mezlocillin.

**ANSWER:** D

25. An alcoholic patient has acute pancreatitis with five of the Ranson criteria. He gradually improves over a 14-day hospitalization, but then a pulse of 120 beats/min, a temperature of 39° C, and abdominal distention develop. CT is performed and the results are shown below. The next most appropriate therapy is which of the following measures?

A. Antibiotics

B. Percutaneous catheter drainage

C. Peritoneal lavage

D. Endoscopic cyst gastrostomy

E. Operative drainage

*Ref.:* 4, 6

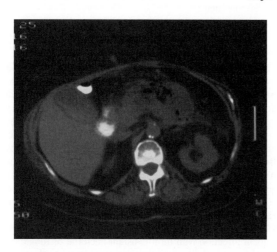

**COMMENTS: Pancreatic infection** complicating acute pancreatitis should be suspected in any patient who fails to improve following supportive medical therapy or improves but then demonstrates deterioration. Pancreatic infection occasionally occurs early during the chronologic course of the disease, but it typically occurs later, as in the patient described. CT is the best method for imaging the pancreas. The results of CT in this patient demonstrate air in the pancreas, which is characteristic of pancreatic infection. The technique of dynamic pancreatography can identify ischemic areas of pancreas and is useful for evaluating patients who may have pancreatic necrosis. **Dynamic pancreatography** is performed by serially imaging the pancreas after bolus injection of an intravenous contrast agent. Percutaneous needle aspiration of fluid collections or necrotic areas found on CT can be performed to identify the presence of infection and guide therapeutic decisions about the need for drainage. When pancreatic infection is present, operative drainage and débridement are indicated. Interest has focused on the selection of closed or open methods of operative drainage. Minimal-access operative approaches are also used to drain and débride pancreatic necrosis in the hope of lowering morbidity in these ill patients. Percutaneous catheters can drain thin fluid but are usually inadequate for the management of infected pancreatic necrosis. Peritoneal lavage has been used early in the course of patients with severe acute pancreatitis. Endoscopic cyst gastrostomy may be appropriate for some patients with pancreatic pseudocysts. These latter two modalities have no role in the management of infected pancreatic necrosis.

**A N S W E R :**  E

26. Acute gallstone pancreatitis is diagnosed in a 54-year-old man. Which of the following is considered standard treatment?

A. Urgent (within 24 hours) cholecystectomy and common bile duct exploration

B. Urgent ERCP and subsequent laparoscopic cholecystectomy

C. Initial supportive therapy with cholecystectomy performed during the same admission

D. Initial supportive therapy with cholecystectomy performed in 6 to 8 weeks

E. Initial supportive therapy with cholecystectomy performed only if symptoms recur

*Ref.:* 9

**COMMENTS: Gallstone pancreatitis** is related to the passage of stones through the ampulla of Vater. Patients with smaller gallstones have an increased risk for the development of this manifestation. **Cholecystectomy** is indicated because gallstone pancreatitis is a recurrent problem in 30% to 50% of patients if surgery is not performed. The traditional controversy has involved the timing of surgery. Proponents of immediate intervention have found a higher incidence of choledocholithiasis but have not demonstrated that this approach is safer than delayed surgery or that it is necessary for most patients. Most surgeons advise initial nonoperative therapy until the patient's signs and symptoms subside (most do within 2 to 3 days), followed by elective cholecystectomy with intraoperative imaging of the common bile duct by cholangiography or intraoperative ultrasonography during the same hospitalization.

The role of urgent **endoscopic retrograde cholangiopancreatography** and **endoscopic sphincterotomy** for the **management of biliary pancreatitis** has been controversial. The vast majority (97%) of patients with gallstone pancreatitis have mild pancreatitis that improves rapidly. ERCP finds common duct stones in only a small percentage of patients and is not indicated routinely. Some trials comparing urgent ERCP and sphincterotomy with traditional treatment have suggested benefit in patients with severe pancreatitis, but this has not been consistently observed. ERCP is indicated for patients with concomitant obstructive jaundice and biliary sepsis. Less invasive methods of duct imaging, such as **magnetic resonance cholangiopancreatography** or EUS, might be useful in patients with an intermediate risk for choledocholithiasis but is not necessary for most with biliary pancreatitis. For the small proportion of patients with severe biliary pancreatitis, early cholecystectomy should be avoided. Treatment in this group is directed at resolution of the pancreatitis and its complications. When the pancreatitis has subsided, delayed cholecystectomy is indicated.

**A N S W E R :**  C

27. Which of the following is the preferred nutritional support for a patient with severe pancreatitis?

A. Nasogastric feeding

B. Feeding via percutaneous endoscopic gastrostomy

C. Nasojejunal feeding

D. Parenteral amino acids and glucose

E. Parenteral amino acids, glucose, and lipids

*Ref.:* 10

**COMMENTS: Nutritional support** is a critical component of the successful management of patients with severe **pancreatitis**. Mortality is reduced by positive nitrogen balance. Direct delivery of nutrients into the jejunum is the preferred route. **Enteral jejunal feeding** does not stimulate pancreatic exocrine secretion and helps maintain the intestinal mucosal barrier. Jejunal feeding is associated with a lower risk for infection and shorter hospital stay than parenteral nutrition. Moreover, enteric feeding avoids catheter-related sepsis and other complications of central venous lines. Feeding into the stomach does stimulate the pancreas and is not usually tolerated because of retrogastric inflammation and delayed gastric emptying. Nasojejunal tubes may require radiologically guided or endoscopic placement.

If nutritional goals cannot be met within a few days of initiation, parenteral nutritional support may also be necessary. Intravenous lipids are not detrimental and prevent essential fatty acid deficiency.

**ANSWER:** C

28. In North America, chronic pancreatitis is most commonly related to chronic alcohol ingestion. Which of the following is the second most common cause?

A. Gallstones

B. Drugs

C. Infection

D. Malnutrition

E. Idiopathic

*Ref.:* 3

**COMMENTS:** In the Western world, **alcohol** use accounts for about 75% of cases of **chronic pancreatitis**. Approximately 20% of cases are considered idiopathic. In parts of Africa and Asia, protein malnutrition is an important etiologic factor. Other, less common causes of chronic pancreatitis include pancreatic duct obstruction (secondary to stenosis or pancreas divisum), hyperparathyroidism, trauma, cystic fibrosis, and hereditary causes. Unlike acute pancreatitis, calculous biliary disease is not a typical cause of chronic pancreatitis. Certain infections (particularly viral) and drugs are among the many factors that can produce acute, rather than chronic pancreatitis.

**ANSWER:** E

29. With regard to the histologic characteristics of chronic pancreatitis, all but which of the following is observed?

A. Increased interstitial connective tissue

B. Loss of acinar cells

C. Loss of islet cells

D. Neural hypertrophy

E. Damaged perineurium

*Ref.:* 4

**COMMENTS: Chronic pancreatitis** is characterized on histologic examination by the loss of exocrine acinar cells and a marked increase in interstitial fibrous connective tissue. The islets of Langerhans are preserved and constitute a relatively greater proportion of the pancreatic tissue. Hyperplasia of islet cells is also seen. The sizes and number of nerves are increased, but the protective perineural sheath is damaged, and nerves are found in proximity to inflammatory foci. There appear to be selective increases in certain peptidergic nerves. These histologic observations may be related to the cause of pain in chronic pancreatitis.

**ANSWER:** C

30. Pain is the predominant clinical manifestation of chronic alcoholic pancreatitis. Most patients also have which of the following associated manifestations?

A. Clinical diabetes mellitus

B. Hypoglycemia

C. Steatorrhea

D. Subclinical fat malabsorption

E. Hepatic cirrhosis

*Ref.:* 1-3

**COMMENTS:** Recurrent or persistent abdominal pain is the predominant symptom of **chronic pancreatitis**. Patients usually have varying degrees of nausea, anorexia, and weight loss. Mechanisms that may contribute to pain include ductal obstruction, parenchymal hypertension, acute inflammation, and perineural inflammation. About two thirds of patients have abnormal glucose tolerance test results and subclinical fat malabsorption, whereas overt diabetes is present in perhaps 30% to 50% and frank steatorrhea in only 10% to 15%. Endocrine and exocrine insufficiency progresses during the course of the disease. Diabetes mellitus may be related to impaired insulin release because the islet cells themselves are relatively preserved. Despite the common etiologic factor of ethanol, most patients with chronic pancreatitis do not have hepatic cirrhosis.

**ANSWER:** D

31. Which of the following would not be appropriate for the management of steatorrhea in a patient with chronic pancreatitis?

A. Restriction of fat to 75 g/day

B. Encapsulated pancreatic enzymes

C. Encapsulated pancreatic enzymes and a proton pump inhibitor

D. Nonencapsulated pancreatic enzymes

E. Nonencapsulated pancreatic enzymes and a proton pump inhibitor

*Ref.:* 3, 4

**COMMENTS:** Gross **steatorrhea** and diarrhea occur when pancreatic exocrine function is reduced to about 10% of normal. Therapy involves limitation of fat intake and administration of adequate amounts of exogenous pancreatic enzyme preparations to provide at least 10% of normal lipolytic activity in the duodenum at the time that the food substrate is present. Various commercial formulations of pancreatic enzymes are available. Nonencapsulated forms may improve the malabsorption but can be ineffective because of inactivation in the stomach when the pH falls below 4. The addition of $H_2$ blockers may then be useful. Enteric-coated preparations release their enzymes at a pH above 5. Therefore, they are useful for patients whose gastric pH remains low to ensure that the enzyme is not released until it reaches the duodenum. The use of encapsulated forms with $H_2$ blockers is counterproductive because the enzyme is released in the stomach and is then inactivated if the pH falls. In addition, enteric-coated preparations are microspheres of varying sizes, and the larger ones do not empty into the duodenum until after the food substrate does.

**ANSWER:** C

32. A 58-year-old woman with jaundice underwent ERCP (results shown below) as part of her diagnostic work-up. On the basis of this radiograph, what diagnosis is considered the most likely?

    A. Chronic pancreatitis

    B. Pancreatic cancer

    C. Cholangiocarcinoma

    D. Pancreas divisum

    E. Ectopic pancreas

*Ref.:* 1, 2

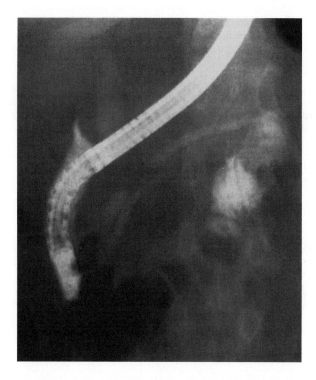

**COMMENTS:** This ERCP study shows the classic "double-duct sign:" dilation of the biliary system above an area of abrupt narrowing and abrupt termination of the main pancreatic duct. These findings place the primary abnormality in the geographic location of the pancreatic head, and it is not uncommon for a pancreatic neoplasm to involve both ducts. Chronic pancreatitis may cause biliary obstruction, but the obstruction in the biliary systems is usually more distal. Likewise, there are no coexistent changes in this patient, such as irregular beading of the pancreatic duct, to suggest that chronic pancreatitis is present. Cholangiocarcinoma may be responsible for the stenosis in the biliary system, but cholangiocarcinomas rarely become large enough to involve the pancreatic duct. With pancreas divisum, injection of the major papilla opacifies only a short, tapering ventral duct draining the caudal portion of the pancreatic head and uncinate process. Injection of the minor papilla demonstrates the dorsal duct draining the major portion of the gland.

**ANSWER:** B

33. A 45-year-old nondiabetic patient with chronic alcoholic pancreatitis and intractable abdominal pain has a 10-mm pancreatic duct. Which of the following choices constitutes the best treatment?

    A. Sphincteroplasty

    B. Lateral pancreaticojejunostomy

    C. Caudal (tail) pancreatectomy

    D. Total pancreatectomy

    E. Continued nonoperative therapy

*Ref.:* 1, 4, 11

**COMMENTS: Pain** is the primary indication for surgery in patients with **chronic pancreatitis**. Selection of the best **operation** for a particular patient must include consideration of the anatomy of the gland, preexisting endocrine or exocrine dysfunction, compliance and the rehabilitative capacity of the patient, postoperative endocrine or exocrine deficiency, and the likelihood of postoperative pain relief. Patients with a dilated duct (>6 mm) are candidates for ductal drainage, with lateral pancreaticojejunostomy being the best choice of these procedures. It is important to achieve adequate decompression of the enlarged pancreatic head and uncinate process during drainage procedures. Variations such as the **Frey or Beger procedure** are intended to accomplish this. Sphincteroplasty does not play a role in the management of patients with established chronic pancreatitis.

Patients with small ducts disease are treated by resection if surgery is necessary. Resection of the pancreatic head in properly selected patients has generally yielded better long-term results for pain relief than has tail resection. The head of the pancreas is often enlarged and bulky in chronic pancreatitis and has been considered to be the "pacemaker" of the disease. A number of operative techniques are available for resection of the pancreatic head. Total or nearly total (95%) resections have higher long-term morbidity and mortality rates related to postoperative endocrine insufficiency. Although endocrine and exocrine function tends to deteriorate over time in patients with chronic pancreatitis, some evidence suggests that pancreaticojejunostomy halts or delays this decline better than nonoperative therapy.

**ANSWER:** B

34. Ascites develops in a 60-year-old patient with acute pancreatitis. Paracentesis demonstrates that the ascitic fluid amylase level is higher than the serum amylase level and that the fluid protein level is higher than 3 g/dL. Which of the following best explains the ascites?

    A. Pancreatic duct leak

    B. Secondary bacterial peritonitis

    C. Portal vein thrombosis

    D. Underlying pancreatic cancer

    E. Resuscitative fluid overload

*Ref.:* 1, 2

**COMMENTS: Pancreatic ascites** can be differentiated from ascites of other causes by the characteristic high amylase and protein content of the peritoneal fluid. Pancreatic ascites and pleural effusion are the results of a disruption in the pancreatic duct, usually consequent to pancreatitis. The ascites may resolve with conservative management consisting of paracentesis (thoracentesis), total parenteral nutrition, and administration of a somatostatin analogue to inhibit pancreatic exocrine secretion. Otherwise, an operation may eventually be required for internal drainage of the pancreatic duct fistula or pseudocyst.

**ANSWER:** A

35. CT demonstrates a 5-cm peripancreatic fluid collection in a patient 3 weeks after an episode of acute pancreatitis. The patient is eating and does not have clinical signs of infection. What is the recommended treatment?

A. Expectant management without intervention

B. Nothing by mouth and total parenteral nutrition

C. Percutaneous catheter drainage of the fluid collection

D. Endoscopic drainage

E. Re-imaging in 3 to 6 weeks and surgery for internal drainage if the collection persists

*Ref.:* 1, 4, 12

**COMMENTS: Peripancreatic fluid collections** can be found in about 20% of patients with acute pancreatitis. Many of them resolve spontaneously and should not be mistaken for pancreatic pseudocysts. If the patient is stable, can eat, and does not have clinical evidence of infection or other complications, expectant management is indicated. The fluid collection can be monitored with ultrasonography or CT in 1 to 3 months. If the patient has persistent pain and is unable to eat, nutrition by postpyloric enteral feeding, or parenteral nutrition if necessary, may be instituted for several weeks to allow resolution or maturation of the collection into a pseudocyst. If the patient has a symptomatic or complicated fluid collection that requires early intervention, some method of external drainage must be used. If the fluid is thin, endoscopic or percutaneous catheter drainage may suffice. Operative drainage is preferred if there is substantial necrotic debris, as there often is, or if there is concern about infection. Operative drainage might be accomplished with minimal-access approaches.

**ANSWER:** A

36. Which of the following is the most important determinant of the need for drainage of a pancreatic pseudocyst?

A. Pseudocyst symptoms

B. Pseudocyst size

C. Pseudocyst duration

D. Associated chronic pancreatitis

E. Patient age

*Ref.:* 1, 4, 12

**COMMENTS:** Historically, **pancreatic pseudocysts** larger than 5 to 6 cm and present for longer than 6 weeks were thought to have a low rate of spontaneous resolution and a high rate of complications. They were therefore treated by operative drainage. Current understanding of the natural history of pseudocysts is that the rate of spontaneous resolution is higher and the rate of complications lower than previously thought. Pseudocyst size and duration are therefore no longer absolute criteria for intervention. Rather, pseudocyst-related symptoms are the primary indication for treatment. Large pseudocysts are more likely to be symptomatic and less likely to resolve spontaneously than are small pseudocysts. In addition, pseudocysts in patients with chronic pancreatitis are unlikely

to resolve but may not require intervention if they are stable, asymptomatic, and uncomplicated.

**ANSWER:** A

37. A patient with chronic pancreatitis is unable to eat because of persistent postprandial pain. CT is performed (shown below). What is the recommended treatment?

A. Nothing by mouth and total parenteral nutrition for 4 to 6 weeks

B. Percutaneous catheter drainage

C. Endoscopic drainage

D. Operative internal drainage

E. Operative external drainage

*Ref.:* 1, 4, 12

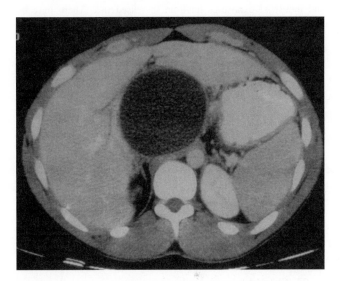

**COMMENTS: Pseudocysts** that develop in patients with **chronic pancreatitis** can be considered mature when they are discovered unless there has also been a recent episode of acute pancreatitis. The indications for treatment of a pancreatic pseudocyst are (1) persistent symptoms (pain, inability to eat, or biliary or gastrointestinal obstruction), (2) enlargement, or (3) the onset of a pseudocyst-related complication (infection, hemorrhage, or rupture). Operative internal pseudocyst drainage into the stomach, jejunum, or duodenum is generally the preferred treatment, depending on the location of the pseudocyst. For patients with chronic pancreatitis, it is critical to evaluate the pancreatic duct to determine whether a concomitant duct drainage procedure is necessary. **Pseudocyst drainage** can be accomplished laparoscopically in some situations. Pseudocysts in the tail of the gland are sometimes best treated by distal pancreatectomy. Percutaneous or endoscopic drainage of established pseudocysts is still being debated. These techniques can successfully treat pseudocysts in some circumstances but have definite limitations and potential complications.

**ANSWER:** D

38. Which of the following risk factors is most strongly associated with ductal adenocarcinoma of the pancreas?

A. Chronic pancreatitis

B. Diabetes mellitus

C. Cigarette smoking

D. Coffee consumption

E. Alcohol consumption

*Ref.:* 1, 3, 4

**COMMENTS: Epidemiologic studies** have identified various demographic, medical, environmental, and dietary factors that have some relationship to **pancreatic cancer**. The most firmly established risk factor is cigarette smoking. Experimentally, nitrosamines have been found to be carcinogenic. In addition, the carcinogens in cigarettes have been related to K-*ras* oncogene mutations, which are frequent in pancreatic cancer. Alcohol has not been demonstrated conclusively to be a risk factor independent of cigarettes. The previously reported association of pancreatic cancer with coffee consumption is questionable. Diets high in fats and meat may be associated with pancreatic cancer, whereas diets high in fruits and vegetables may be protective. Certain occupational and industrial exposures have an increased risk. There may be some association with diabetes mellitus and certain forms of chronic pancreatitis, but the relationship is not considered causal. Previous gastrectomy has been associated with increased risk, whereas tonsillectomy has been observed to be protective.

**ANSWER: C**

39. A jaundiced, otherwise healthy patient is noted to have a 3-cm mass in the head of the pancreas on CT. EUS-guided fine-needle aspiration shows cancer. The mass abuts the portal vein, but there is no clear evidence of vessel involvement or metastatic disease. Which of the following is the most appropriate next step?

A. MRCP to better assess vascular involvement

B. Direct angiography to better assess vascular involvement

C. Operative exploration and potential resection

D. Endoscopic placement of a biliary stent

E. Chemotherapy and radiation therapy

*Ref.:* 1, 2, 4

**COMMENTS:** When the clinical situation suggests a resectable **pancreatic neoplasm** in a good-risk patient with biliary obstruction, surgery for potential resection is generally indicated without additional tests. Routine **preoperative biliary decompression** is not advantageous in this setting because it does not improve operative outcomes and may increase the morbidity associated with resection. Endoscopic biliary decompression is invaluable, of course, for palliation of obstruction in patients deemed inoperable or if operation is to be delayed. Angiography was formerly popular for the preoperative staging of pancreatic cancer, but its accuracy in determining resectability has limitations, and it generally adds little to good-quality **Computed tomography** or **magnetic resonance imaging**. EUS is extremely useful for identifying small tumors that are inapparent on CT, for obtaining cytologic material, and somewhat for assessing vascular invasion. Neoadjuvant chemotherapy with radiation therapy is increasingly being used before surgery for patients whose imaging studies suggest "borderline" resectability. Imaging criteria for what constitutes a borderline case vary but would commonly include tumors that abut a substantial (half or greater) circumference of adjacent vessels (hepatic artery, superior mesenteric artery, portal vein) or that narrow the portal-splenic vein confluence.

**ANSWER: C**

40. In which of the following situations is resection of a ductal carcinoma of the pancreas contraindicated?

A. Age older than 80 years

B. Tumor located in the body of the pancreas

C. Inability to verify malignancy histologically before resection

D. Presence of small peritoneal metastases

E. Tumor invading the portal vein

*Ref.:* 1-4

**COMMENTS: Resection of a pancreatic malignancy** offers the only chance for cure. Most commonly, resection of ductal carcinomas involves pancreaticoduodenectomy, because most potentially resectable tumors are located in the head or uncinate process of the gland. Tumors originating in the body or tail of the pancreas are often not diagnosed until they are beyond the confines of surgical resection. However, location alone does not contraindicate resection because, stage for stage, tumors in the body have the same survival as tumors in the head of the pancreas. Resection is indicated for physiologically fit patients (age alone is not a contraindication) who do not have metastases beyond the field of resection. Histologic or cytologic confirmation of malignancy can often be obtained intraoperatively but is not necessary before resection if the clinical circumstances suggest cancer and the surgeon is appropriately experienced. For some tumors with local vascular invasion, en bloc resection with reconstruction of the involved vessels is appropriate if a tumor-free resection can be accomplished. **Positive lymph nodes** outside the resection field, peritoneal metastases, and liver metastases generally contraindicate resection for adenocarcinoma of the exocrine pancreas. However, tumor "debulking" and resection of liver metastases can be beneficial in patients with functioning tumors of the endocrine pancreas.

**ANSWER: D**

41. Which of the following operations could be appropriate for a 2-cm ductal adenocarcinoma in the head of the pancreas?

A. Pancreaticoduodenectomy (Whipple procedure) with preservation of the stomach and pylorus

B. Duodenum-sparing pancreatectomy

C. Total pancreaticoduodenectomy

D. Laparoscopic enucleation

E. All are potentially appropriate

*Ref.:* 1-4

**COMMENTS:** A standard **Whipple-type resection** with partial gastrectomy or with preservation of the stomach and pylorus is indicated for a resectable ductal cancer in the head of the pancreas. Each of these operations yields a 5-year survival rate of approximately 15% to 20%. There is a higher incidence of initially delayed gastric emptying with pyloric-preserving operations. However, long-term studies demonstrate normal emptying and good nutritional outcomes. Likewise, the postprandial gastrin and acid responses are normal despite the loss of duodenal inhibitory factors, and marginal ulcer has not been a prohibitive problem. Additional advantages of the pyloric-preserving technique are shorter operative time and lower operative blood loss. Of course, preservation of the stomach and most proximal portion of the duodenum is not appropriate for patients with tumors in close proximity if the margins would be compromised. Duodenum-sparing resection of the pancreatic head has been used in some centers for patients with chronic pancreatitis and has been reported to better maintain enteropancreatic hormonal relationships and glucose homeostasis. This operation is not indicated for cancer.

**Total pancreaticoduodenectomy** is not advocated for pancreatic cancers that can otherwise be resected. It has been used based on the grounds that it produces better clearance of the lymph nodes and possible multicentric disease and avoids a pancreatic anastomosis. However, long-term survival is not improved, and total pancreatectomy is associated with a higher rate of both early and late complications. Extended pancreaticoduodenectomy involves removal of more retroperitoneal soft tissue and regional lymph nodes. U.S. studies have not demonstrated improved survival with this approach, and the rate of operative complications may be higher. Pancreatic resections can be accomplished laparoscopically, but enucleation is never an appropriate method for removing a pancreatic ductal cancer.

**ANSWER:** A

---

42. At laparotomy, a jaundiced patient is found to have an unresectable pancreatic cancer obstructing the bile duct. Which of the following statements regarding biliary decompression is correct?

   A. The preferred management is to close the patient and place an endoscopic stent postoperatively.

   B. Cholecystectomy plus T-tube placement is the preferred management.

   C. Choledochoduodenostomy is contraindicated.

   D. Cholecystojejunostomy should not be performed if the patient has cholelithiasis.

   E. Roux-en-Y choledochojejunostomy is not appropriate because of limited life expectancy.

*Ref.:* 1-4

**COMMENTS:** Most patients with **pancreatic cancer** do not have resectable disease. **Palliative treatment** is directed to relieve obstruction of the bile duct and duodenum and to alleviate pain. For lesions demonstrated to be unresectable before laparotomy, nonoperative relief of biliary obstruction can be achieved by the endoscopic (preferred) or transhepatic route. Surgical bypass with some form of biliary enteric anastomosis generally provides more durable relief with less need for further intervention. It is preferred for patients when unresectability is determined at the time of laparotomy. Cholecystojejunostomy, choledocho- or hepatico jejunostomy, and choledochoduodenostomy are each appropriate for the management of distal bile duct obstruction.

**Choledochojejunostomy** usually provides the most durable relief. A Roux-en-Y configuration is preferred by many surgeons, although a simple loop (with or without distal enteroenterostomy) also suffices. Cholecystojejunostomy is relatively simple but should be avoided if the gallbladder is diseased or when cystic duct patency cannot be demonstrated or may be jeopardized by tumor proximity. It is sometimes taught that choledochoduodenostomy should be avoided with malignant obstruction because of possible tumor growth and eventual reobstruction. In reality, choledochoduodenostomy can be an effective solution provided that the common bile duct is sufficiently dilated and the duodenum is pliable and unobstructed.

**ANSWER:** D

---

43. When should gastrojejunostomy be performed at the time of biliary bypass in a patient with unresectable pancreatic cancer?

   A. Always

   B. Never

   C. If the tumor is locally unresectable and there are no peritoneal metastases

   D. Only if symptomatic duodenal obstruction is present at the time of surgery

   E. Only if endoscopic stent placement is not available

*Ref.:* 1-4

**COMMENTS:** In addition to biliary obstruction, **pancreatic cancers** can obstruct the duodenum or the proximal jejunum near the ligament of Treitz. Traditionally, many surgeons have favored routine "double bypass" (biliary and duodenal) for operated patients because the rate of duodenal obstruction that develops later in patients treated by biliary bypass alone has been cited to be 5% to 30%. However, duodenal obstruction does not develop in most patients, and gastrojejunostomy is sometimes associated with problems such as bleeding or delayed gastric emptying. The selective approach is therefore appropriate. Patients with obstructive symptoms or impending obstruction as a result of tumor location should undergo gastrojejunostomy. **Gastrojejunostomy** is also advisable for patients with an anticipated longer survival, such as those whose lesions are not resected because of local tumor invasion rather than because of hepatic or peritoneal metastases. Endoscopic placement of a **duodenal stent** is another option, but the results are not always satisfactory.

**ANSWER:** C

---

44. A 45-year-old woman who is not an alcoholic has a septated 10-cm cystic mass in the head of the pancreas. Which of the following statements constitutes appropriate advice?

   A. The lesion is benign and requires no intervention.

   B. The lesion is malignant and probably incurable.

   C. Pancreaticoduodenectomy is indicated.

   D. Percutaneous needle biopsy is indicated.

   E. Drainage by Roux-en-Y cyst jejunostomy is indicated.

*Ref.:* 1-4

**COMMENTS: Cystadenoma** and **cystadenocarcinoma** are **cystic neoplasms of the pancreas** that are most commonly manifested as mass lesions in middle-aged women. Serous and mucinous types are recognized, and the risk for malignancy is significant with the mucinous variety. Cystadenoma is more common than its malignant counterpart, but malignant transformation may occur. EUS with sampling for cytology, mucin, and carcinoembryonic antigen (CEA) can be useful for gauging the likelihood of cancer. Without resection, however, exclusion of malignancy can be difficult. Internal drainage of cystic neoplasms is not appropriate therapy. Complete excision should be carried out whenever possible. The 5-year survival rate after resection of cystadenocarcinoma is approximately 50%. Occasionally, islet cell tumors, ductal adenocarcinomas, or other unusual tumors (e.g., papillary and cystic pancreatic neoplasms) have cystic components.

**ANSWER:** C

45. A 64-year-old man is evaluated for abdominal pain. CT shows segmental dilation of the main pancreatic duct to greater than 10 mm in the head of the gland with mural nodules. Which of the following is the next most appropriate recommendation?

    A. EUS

    B. ERCP

    C. Serum CA 19-9

    D. Total pancreatectomy

    E. Abstinence from alcohol and CT repeated in 3 months

    *Ref.:* 13

COMMENTS: An **intraductal papillary mucinous neoplasm** (IPMN) of the pancreas is a premalignant condition characterized by papillary projections of mucin-secreting epithelial cells, excessive mucin production, and cystic dilation of the pancreatic duct. The patient may already have cancer when initially seen or may be at some other stage along the process of malignant transformation, which occurs relatively slowly. IPMNs are divided into a main duct type and a branch duct type, depending on the areas of the pancreatic ducts that are involved. The goals of evaluation are to identify factors associated with a higher risk for malignancy and to determine the anatomic extent of disease. EUS is usually the next step in evaluation when IPMN is suspected. EUS can identify diffuse or segmental dilation of the pancreatic duct and the size of cystic lesions or mural nodules and can guide fine-needle aspiration to assess cytology and molecular tumor markers. ERCP shows duct dilation without strictures, filling defects from mucus or nodules, and commonly a patulous papillary orifice with mucus. ERCP also permits sampling of mucus and therapeutic clearance if mucus obstruction is a problem. If available, direct pancreatoscopy and intraductal ultrasound can be adjuncts to ERCP for determining the extent of an IPMN.

ANSWER: A

46. Which of the following features of IPMN of the pancreas is associated with the lowest risk for cancer?

    A. Branch duct type with mural nodularity

    B. Branch duct type smaller than 3 cm

    C. Main duct type with diffuse dilation to greater than 10 mm

    D. Main duct type with segmental dilation

    E. Multifocal IPMN

    *Ref.:* 14, 15

COMMENTS: Progression of **intraductal papillary mucinous neoplasm** through the adenoma cancer sequence is considered a slow process that requires perhaps 10 to 20 years. Main duct–type tumors have a greater risk for malignancy than the branch duct type. The Sendai Consensus Guidelines identified the following features as risk factors for cancer and as general indicators for resection: main pancreatic duct dilation to greater than 10 mm, cyst size larger than 3 cm, presence of mural nodules, and atypical cytology. Additional risk factors include high-grade dysplasia, multifocal or synchronous tumors, and increasing cyst size during follow-up. In branch duct–type tumors, mural nodularity or atypical cytology may be more important determinants than size.

ANSWER: B

47. Which of the following would you recommend to a 60-year-old woman with an established diagnosis of IPMN?

    A. Mammography

    B. Transvaginal ultrasound

    C. Colonoscopy

    D. Genetic testing

    E. Screening CT for first-degree relatives

    *Ref.:* 16

COMMENTS: Extrapancreatic malignancies have been observed more commonly in patients with **intraductal papillary mucinous neoplasm** than in those with ductal cancer of the pancreas or other cystic pancreatic neoplasms. The reason for this is not known. No particular genetic predisposition for IPMN has been identified. Extrapancreatic cancer has been reported in approximately one third of patients with IPMN. Gastric cancer and colon cancer have been the most frequent. No specific guidelines exist, but based on these findings, screening upper gastrointestinal endoscopy and colonoscopy would be appropriate recommendations.

ANSWER: C

48. Which of the following is true regarding the diagnosis of insulinoma?

    A. The Whipple triad is pathognomonic.

    B. The serum insulin-to-glucose ratio is less than 0.3.

    C. An oral glucose tolerance test permits differentiation from reactive hypoglycemia.

    D. The tolbutamide test is useful for excluding factitious hyperinsulinemia.

    E. CT is the most accurate preoperative method for tumor localization.

    *Ref.:* 1-3

COMMENTS: The **Whipple triad** (fasting hypoglycemia, symptoms of hypoglycemia, relief of symptoms following the administration of glucose) clinically establishes hypoglycemia, the differential diagnosis of which requires further evaluation. The biochemical diagnosis of **insulinoma** is based on the findings of fasting hypoglycemia (<50 mg/dL) and hyperinsulinemia (>20 μU/mL) that yield an insulin-to-glucose ratio of greater than 0.3. The use of tolbutamide or leucine as a provocative test to release insulin may be dangerous and is not required. C peptide is cleaved from insulin before its release, and determination of C-peptide levels may be useful for excluding factitious hyperinsulinemia. In the case of organic hyperinsulinism, serial blood sampling results following oral glucose administration and subsequent fasting will demonstrate persistent hypoglycemia and hyperinsulinemia. When reactive hypoglycemia is present, insulin levels initially rise and glucose levels fall, but the levels become normal after several hours. Most insulinomas are small. Arteriography or selective venous sampling may provide useful preoperative localization. EUS and intraoperative ultrasonography can also aid in identification.

ANSWER: C

49. Which of the following statements is true regarding the treatment of insulinoma?

   A. Diazoxide is the preferred initial method of management.

   B. Enucleation is acceptable for localized pancreatic lesions.

   C. Because most lesions are multiple or diffuse, total or nearly total pancreatectomy is generally necessary.

   D. Because most lesions are malignant, adjuvant streptozocin is usually indicated.

   E. Parathyroid adenoma should be excluded or treated before pancreatic resection.

*Ref.:* 1-3

**COMMENTS: Insulinomas** are usually single and benign and are rarely ectopic. Localization of an insulinoma can be difficult, and preoperative imaging along with thorough mobilization and exploration of the pancreas are mandatory. Intraoperative ultrasonography is indispensable. For localized lesions, simple enucleation is the preferred treatment, but the integrity of the pancreatic duct must be ascertained. If the lesion cannot be identified and the biochemical basis of the diagnosis is firm, blind distal pancreatic resection with careful histologic examination of the specimen may be necessary. Intraoperative monitoring of serum glucose levels has also been used. Diazoxide inhibits insulin release from beta cells and is occasionally used for preoperative control or for patients with recurrent postoperative hypoglycemia. For patients with metastatic malignant insulinoma, tumor debulking may be beneficial, as is the use of streptozocin and 5-fluorouracil. Gastrinoma, not insulinoma, is the most common pancreatic adenoma associated with multiple endocrine adenomatosis type I syndrome. Parathyroid disease should be excluded or treated before surgical intervention for gastrinoma.

**ANSWER: B**

50. Which of the following features is characteristic of Zollinger-Ellison syndrome but not of Verner-Morrison syndrome?

   A. Diarrhea

   B. Hypercalcemia

   C. Hypocalcemia

   D. Increased gastric acid secretion

   E. Malignancy

*Ref.:* 1-3

**COMMENTS: Zollinger-Ellison syndrome** is caused by a gastrin-producing islet cell tumor. Verner-Morrison syndrome is caused by an islet cell tumor that produces vasoactive intestinal peptide. Zollinger-Ellison syndrome is associated with a marked increase in gastric acid secretion and with diarrhea. Hypercalcemia may occur because of associated parathyroid abnormalities. Verner-Morrison syndrome is characterized by watery diarrhea, hypokalemia, and achlorhydria. Hypercalcemia may occur, but the parathyroids are usually normal. Both syndromes are frequently the result of malignant islet cell tumors.

**ANSWER: D**

51. Which of the following is not a feature of the clinical syndrome associated with a glucagon-producing islet cell tumor?

   A. Rash

   B. Diabetes

   C. Seizures

   D. Glossitis

   E. Anemia

*Ref.:* 1-3

**COMMENTS:** Patients with **glucagon-secreting tumors** have diabetes, anemia, weight loss, venous thrombosis, glossitis, and a characteristic cutaneous lesion known as necrolytic migratory erythema. The lesion is rare and often metastatic at the time of diagnosis. Treatment is directed at achieving as complete a resection as possible. Postoperatively, chemotherapy with dacarbazine or streptozocin may be useful for residual or recurrent disease.

**ANSWER: C**

52. Which of the following statements is true about pancreatic trauma?

   A. Blunt trauma is the most common mechanism of injury.

   B. Trauma is the most common cause of pancreatic pseudocyst.

   C. Hyperamylasemia following penetrating abdominal injury is pathognomonic.

   D. Negative peritoneal lavage findings following blunt trauma usually exclude pancreatic injury.

   E. Central retroperitoneal hematomas should be explored to exclude pancreatic injury.

*Ref.:* 1-3

**COMMENTS:** Most **pancreatic injuries** are the result of penetrating trauma, although the gland is vulnerable to blunt trauma because of its fixed position anteriorly over the vertebral column. The presence of significant pancreatic injury following blunt trauma is often not initially apparent. Hyperamylasemia in serum or peritoneal fluid suggests the diagnosis, but a negative peritoneal tap or lavage does not exclude retroperitoneal injury. Retroperitoneal hematomas in the upper part of the abdomen should be explored to exclude pancreatic ductal injury. Pancreatitis is the most common cause of pseudocyst, although about 25% occur as a result of trauma.

**ANSWER: E**

53. At operative exploration following blunt abdominal trauma, complete transection of the pancreatic neck is identified. There are no associated organ injuries. Which of the following treatments is most appropriate?

   A. Placement of drains and closure of the abdomen

   B. Distal pancreatectomy with ligation of the proximal duct

   C. Roux-en-Y pancreaticojejunostomy to the distal pancreas with ligation of the proximal duct

   D. Roux-en-Y pancreaticojejunostomy to both the proximal and distal segments of the pancreas

   E. Pancreaticoduodenectomy with Roux-en-Y pancreaticojejunostomy to the distal duct

*Ref.:* 1-3

**COMMENTS: Pancreatic contusions or lacerations** without ductal disruption are managed by drainage alone. The pancreatic neck is a frequent site of pancreatic injury when it occurs with blunt trauma. Distal pancreatectomy with identification and closure of the proximal duct and drainage is safe, and resections involving up to 80% of an otherwise normal gland can be accomplished without subsequent endocrine insufficiency. In theory, Roux-en-Y pancreaticojejunostomy may be desirable to preserve pancreatic tissue, but it is not recommended for the management of acute injuries because of the risk associated with a pancreatic anastomosis and the need to open the gut. Pancreaticoduodenectomy is indicated for patients with severe combined duodenal, pancreatic, and bile duct injuries.

**ANSWER: B**

## REFERENCES

1. Steer ML: Exocrine pancreas. In Townsend CM, Beauchamp RD, Evers BM, et al, editors: *Sabiston textbook of surgery: the biological basis of modern surgical practice*, ed 18, Philadelphia, 2008, WB Saunders.
2. Fisher WE, Andersen DK, Bell RH, et al: Pancreas. In Brunicardi FC, Andersen DK, Billar TR, et al, editors: *Schwartz's principles of surgery*, ed 9, New York, 2010, McGraw-Hill.
3. Mulholland MW, Lilleomoe KD, Doherty GM, et al, editors: *Greenfield's surgery: scientific principles and practice*, ed 4, Philadelphia, 2006, JB Lippincott.
4. Howard J, Idezuki Y, Ihse I, et al, editors: *Surgical diseases of the pancreas*, ed 3, Baltimore, 1998, Williams & Wilkins.
5. Mulvihill SJ: Liver, biliary tract, and pancreas. In O'Leary JP, Tabuenca A, editors: *The physiologic basis of surgery*, ed 4, Philadelphia, 2008, JB Lippincott.
6. Deziel DJ, Prinz RA: Bacteriology of necrotizing pancreatitis, *Probl Gen Surg* 13:22–28, 1996.
7. Villatoro E, Bassi C, Larvin M: Antibiotic therapy for prophylaxis against infection of pancreatic necrosis in acute pancreatitis, *Cochrane Database Syst Rev* 4:CD002941, 2006.
8. Buchler M, Malfertheiner P, Freiss H, et al: Human pancreatic tissue concentration of bactericidal antibiotics, *Gastroenterology* 103:1902–1908, 1992.
9. Sharma VK, Howden CW: Meta-analysis of randomized controlled trials of endoscopic retrograde cholangiography and endoscopic sphincterotomy for the treatment of acute biliary pancreatitis, *Am J Gastroenterol* 94:3211–3214, 1999.
10. McClave SA, Chang WK, Dhaliwal R, et al: Nutrition support in acute pancreatitis: a systematic review of the literature, *J Parenter Enteral Nutr* 30:143–156, 2006.
11. Prinz RA, Deziel DJ, editors: Chronic pancreatitis, *Probl Gen Surg* 15, 1998.
12. Deziel DJ, Prinz RA: Drainage of pancreatic pseudocysts: indications and long term results. *Dig Surg* 13:101–108, 1996.
13. Pais SA, Attasaranya S, Leblanc JK, et al: Role of endoscopic ultrasound in the diagnosis of intraductal papillary mucinous neoplasms: correlation with surgical histopathology, *Clin Gastroenterol Hepatol* 5:489–495, 2007.
14. Tanaka M, Chari S, Adsay V, et al: International consensus guidelines for management of intraductal papillary mucinous neoplasms and mucinous cystic neoplasms of the pancreas, *Pancreatology* 6:17–32, 2006.
15. Schmidt CM, White PB, Waters JA, et al: Intraductal papillary mucinous neoplasms: predictors of malignant and invasive pathology, *Ann Surg* 246:644–651, 2007.
16. Yoon WJ, Ryu JK, Lee JK, et al: Extrapancreatic malignancies in patients with intraductal papillary mucinous neoplasm of the pancreas: prevalence, associated factors, and comparison with patients with other pancreatic cystic neoplasms, *Ann Surg Oncol* 15:3193–3198, 2008.

# CHAPTER 26

# Spleen and Lymphatic System

*Kyle Cologne, M.D., and Tina J. Hieken, M.D.*

1. Which of the following statements regarding splenic anatomy is true?

   A. The splenic ligaments are all avascular.

   B. The tail of the pancreas is often contained in the splenorenal ligament.

   C. The average weight of the adult spleen is 300 g.

   D. The first branches of the splenic artery are the short gastric arteries.

   E. Accessory spleens are most commonly found in the greater omentum.

   *Ref.:* 1-3

COMMENTS: Although the majority of the **splenic ligaments** are in fact avascular, the gastrosplenic ligament contains the short gastric vessels. Additionally, in the case of portal hypertension, other splenic ligaments may become vascularized. The tail of the pancreas may be injured during splenectomy because it often lies within the splenorenal ligament. The average weight of the adult spleen is 150 g (range, 75 to 300 g). The first branches of the **splenic artery** are the pancreatic branches and then the short gastric, the left gastroepiploic (which may also give rise to the short gastric arteries), and the terminal splenic branches. The splenic artery divides into segmental branches that enter the trabeculae of the spleen. There are two types of anatomy of the splenic artery: the distributive and magistral types. The distributive subtype is much more common (70% of individuals) and is characterized by a short splenic artery trunk and multiple long branches entering the spleen. Conversely, the magistral type has a long main trunk that divides relatively near the hilum. **Accessory spleens** are common, especially in patients with hematologic disorders, and are found in 15% to 35% of patients. In decreasing order of frequency, they are found in the splenic hilum, the gastrosplenic ligament, the splenocolic ligament, the splenorenal ligament, the greater omentum and mesentery, and the left pelvis along the left ureter or by the left testis or ovary, but they have been identified anywhere within the peritoneal cavity.

ANSWER: B

2. Which statement regarding the segments and function of the spleen is true?

   A. The white pulp consists of lymphatic sheaths surrounding vessels and is where B-lymphocyte precursors mature before migrating to the red pulp.

   B. The white pulp usually constitutes 50% of the normal spleen.

   C. The major function of the red pulp is to store old or defective erythrocytes for future use.

   D. The marginal zone is the zone usually absent except in the presence of lymphoma.

   E. The spleen can act as a large reservoir of platelets, erythrocytes, and other lymphatic cells.

   *Ref.:* 1, 4

COMMENTS: The **white pulp** of the spleen consists of lymphatic sheaths that usually surround splenic blood vessels. The white pulp contains plasma cells and lymphocytes and functions as the immune center of the spleen. The lymphatic sheaths contain mostly T cells, as well as some B-cell follicles that can be either primary or secondary (after stimulation by antigen). The white pulp makes up approximately 25% of a normal spleen. The **red pulp** is the largest component of the spleen and represents a network of sinuses that filter the blood. Here, red cells are removed from the circulation and destroyed. The junction between the red pulp and white pulp is the **marginal zone**, which allows additional antigen presentation and contributes further to the lymphatic functions of the spleen. The spleen serves as a large reservoir. As much as 30% of an individual's platelets reside in the normal spleen. In disease states such as portal hypertension, splenic sequestration can trap an even larger proportion of the body's circulating cells, including as much as 90% of the total number of platelets.

ANSWER: E

3. A 49-year-old woman with Felty's syndrome undergoes successful splenectomy. Several years after surgery, examination of her peripheral blood smear would reveal which one of the following to be true?

   A. Howell-Jolly bodies, which are suggestive of the presence of an accessory spleen

   B. Stippling, spur cells, and target cells because of the lack of filtration

   C. High levels of properdin and tuftsin

   D. No change in the level of antibodies needed to clear organisms as in the presplenectomy state

   E. Red blood cells undergoing maturation more quickly

   *Ref.:* 1, 2

COMMENTS: Howell-Jolly bodies are abnormal cytoplasmic inclusions within red blood cells. They are seen in individuals who have undergone **splenectomy** because normally they are removed by a functioning spleen, and thus their absence would suggest the presence of an **accessory spleen**. Stippling, spur cells, and target cells are all functionally altered erythrocytes that are normally cleared from the circulation by the spleen and thus are commonly seen following splenectomy. Properdin and tuftsin are important opsonins manufactured in the spleen. Properdin helps initiate the alternative pathway of complement activation, which is particularly useful for fighting encapsulated organisms. Tuftsin enhances the phagocytic activity of granulocytes. Asplenic individuals lack the ability to produce these substances. The spleen is the initial site of IgM synthesis in response to bacteria. Without this primary defense mechanism, asplenic individuals require increased levels of antibodies to clear organisms relative to the presplenectomy state. Erythrocytes do not undergo maturation more quickly after splenectomy. As part of its "pitting" function, the spleen removes cytoplasmic inclusions (particles such as nuclear remnants [Howell-Jolly bodies], insoluble globin precipitates [Heinz bodies], and endocytic vacuoles) from within circulating red blood cells. **Felty's syndrome** is an uncommon disorder marked by splenomegaly, neutropenia, and rheumatoid arthritis. Patients may have thrombocytopenia and anemia, with a predisposition to infections. Splenectomy in patients with Felty syndrome is beneficial in correcting the anemia and neutropenia associated with this syndrome.

**ANSWER:  B**

4. A 55-year-old individual has a history of a splenectomy following a motor vehicle accident as a child. The patient now comes to the physician about other complaints. This patient:

   A. Has decreased susceptibility to infection with malarial parasites and *Bartonella* species.

   B. Is likely to require vaccination against *Haemophilus influenzae*, *Streptococcus pneumoniae*, and meningococci.

   C. Is subject to an increased risk for infection and should have been vaccinated at least 1 month before splenectomy.

   D. Requires revaccination every 10 years.

   E. Should be vaccinated with the newest 14-valent vaccine against *S. pneumoniae*.

   *Ref.:* 1, 2, 5

**COMMENTS:** The spleen has the ability to clear unopsonized bacteria and microorganisms for which the body has no antibodies. It can clear organisms contained within erythrocytes (such as malaria and *Bartonella* species); thus, an asplenic individual is more susceptible to these infections. Individuals who have undergone **splenectomy** are more susceptible to infection with encapsulated organisms, especially *H. influenzae*, *S. pneumoniae*, and meningococci. If preoperative **vaccination** is possible, administration should be undertaken at least 2 weeks before splenectomy for optimal antibody response. For patients undergoing emergency splenectomy, vaccines should be given 2 weeks postoperatively or at the time of hospital discharge if the patient is deemed unlikely to comply with follow-up care. The recommended reimmunization interval for pneumococcal and meningococcal vaccines is 5 years, not 10 years. The benefit of revaccination for *H. influenzae* is unclear. A 23-valent pneumococcal vaccine is now used for immunization.

**ANSWER:  B**

5. A 5-year-old child with sickle cell anemia who underwent splenectomy several months earlier following a sequestration crisis is now being evaluated because of several days of fever

and fatigue after exposure to a sick contact at school. When he arrives at the emergency department, he is hypotensive, tachycardic, and lethargic. Which of the following is true about his current condition?

   A. The incidence is lower when splenectomy is performed for hematologic disease.

   B. The incidence is highest within 6 months of splenectomy.

   C. Patients require lifelong antibiotic prophylaxis, usually with penicillin, especially those older than 5 years.

   D. Mortality rate approaches 90%.

   E. Complications include peripheral gangrene, deafness, and endocarditis.

   *Ref.:* 1, 2, 5

**COMMENTS: Overwhelming post-splenectomy infection** (OPSI) is a life-threatening disorder that must be recognized promptly and treated appropriately. Typically, it manifests as a prodromal phase of 1 to 2 days of nonspecific symptoms such as sore throat, malaise, myalgias, diarrhea, vomiting, fevers, and chills. This situation can progress rapidly to hypotension, disseminated intravascular coagulation, respiratory distress, and death. Mortality rates may exceed 50%, and it is often complicated by severe sequelae such as those in choice E. The incidence of OPSI is higher following splenectomy performed for hematologic disorders and in younger patients. OPSI may occur at any time following splenectomy, although the incidence is highest within the first 2 years after splenectomy. Daily prophylactic penicillin therapy for asplenic patients remains controversial. The main reason for prophylaxis is to decrease the incidence of OPSI. The duration of and need for therapy have been contested, although many advocate prophylaxis for 3 to 5 years, especially in younger children undergoing splenectomy.

**ANSWER:  E**

6. A 43-year-old man has thrombocytopenia, ecchymoses, and a history of melena. His primary doctor suspects that he might have idiopathic thrombocytopenia purpura (ITP). Which of the following is true about this condition?

   A. It is characterized by a low platelet count, mucosal hemorrhage, normal bone marrow, and an enlarged spleen.

   B. It is caused by splenic overproduction of IgM, which attacks the platelet membrane and causes platelet destruction.

   C. The bone marrow often hypertrophies to counteract the increased platelet destruction.

   D. It affects young men more commonly than women.

   E. Diagnosis requires exclusion of other causes of thrombocytopenia.

   *Ref.:* 1, 2

**COMMENTS: Idiopathic thrombocytopenia purpura** is a disorder of increased platelet destruction caused by autoantibodies to platelet membrane components. This results in platelet phagocytosis in the spleen, and the bone marrow does not adequately compensate for this increased destruction. Although ITP is characterized by a low platelet count, mucosal hemorrhage, and relatively normal bone marrow (not hyperactive), the spleen is not enlarged. The autoantibodies are IgG antibodies, not IgM, directed against the platelet fibrinogen receptor. The mechanism underlying the use of intravenous IgG for the treatment of ITP is that IgG saturates the fibrinogen receptors so that they will not bind and thus destroy platelets. This autoimmune disorder affects women more commonly than men. A diagnosis of ITP requires exclusion of other potential causes of thrombocytopenia such as drugs, myelodysplasia, thrombotic thrombocytopenia purpura (TTP), systemic lupus erythematosus, lymphoma, and chronic disseminated intravascular coagulation.

**ANSWER:** E

7. The patient described in Question 6 undergoes a complete work-up and ITP is diagnosed. Which of the following about the treatment of ITP is true?

    A. Platelet transfusions are best given before ligation of the splenic artery.

    B. Initial medical therapy includes steroid therapy with the possible addition of intravenous IgG.

    C. Initial response rates to medical therapy in adults are as high as 75%, with permanent cure from medical therapy being achieved in greater than 50%.

    D. Spontaneous resolution is rare in children.

    E. Splenectomy is indicated if ITP does not improve after 1 year of steroid therapy or if thrombocytopenia recurs following steroid taper.

*Ref.:* 1, 2

**COMMENTS:** Initial therapy for **idiopathic thrombocytopenia purpura** is medical and consists of high-dose corticosteroids, usually prednisone, 1 mg/kg/day. The goal of therapy is to induce remission and achieve platelet counts higher than 100,000/mm³. This is effective initially in approximately 75% of patients, usually within 1 week, but up to 3 weeks of therapy may be required. Treatment is generally initiated when platelet counts fall to less than 20,000 to 30,000/mm³ or for individuals with platelet counts of less than 50,000/mm³ and mucous membrane bleeding or significant risk factors for bleeding. Although the initial response to treatment is good, only 15% to 25% of patients achieve a lasting response. If platelet counts remain low despite steroid therapy, intravenous IgG is indicated at doses of 1 g/kg for 2 days. In most cases, this increases platelet counts within 3 days. In contrast to adults, 70% to 80% of children will experience spontaneous permanent remission. **Splenectomy** is considered if platelet counts remain below 10,000/mm³ after 8 weeks of therapy, regardless of whether bleeding is present. Splenectomy is also recommended for those who experience a relapse after initial success with glucocorticoid treatment or who have significant morbidity from continued high-dose steroids. Intracranial bleeding in patients with ITP is usually managed by prompt administration of intravenous IgG followed by splenectomy. Finally, women in their second trimester of pregnancy are offered splenectomy if they have platelet counts of less than 10,000/mm³ or bleeding with counts of less than 30,000/mm³ despite appropriate medical therapy. Platelet transfusion during splenectomy should be withheld until after ligation of the splenic artery, if possible, to prevent platelet consumption.

**ANSWER:** B

8. A 17-year-old girl is evaluated for fever, purpura, hemolytic anemia, and hematuria with renal insufficiency. Focal neurologic defects soon develop, and head computed tomography (CT) demonstrates an intracranial hemorrhage. Which of the following is true regarding this condition?

    A. Splenectomy is curative in most patients and should be considered after a trial of steroids.

    B. It is caused by hyaline membranes that form within arterioles and capillaries and resultant platelet aggregation.

    C. Plasmapheresis is considered as a last resort when other therapy fails.

    D. Administration of platelets can result in clinical improvement, thereby allowing splenectomy to be delayed.

    E. Even with rapid progression, the prognosis is generally good because of the high success of medical therapy with splenectomy for salvage.

*Ref.:* 1, 2

**COMMENTS:** This patient has **thrombotic thrombocytopenic purpura**. The disease is characterized by occlusion of arterioles and capillaries by hyaline deposits of aggregated platelets and fibrin. First-line therapy is **plasmapheresis**. Fresh frozen plasma and high-dose corticosteroids may be used to control bleeding. Splenectomy is not curative and is considered only for salvage therapy. Mortality rates in patients with TTP can approach 50%, mostly from intracranial hemorrhage or renal failure. The disease can have a rapidly fulminant course. Most long-term survivors of TTP have undergone splenectomy. Platelet transfusion does not control the bleeding; therapy should be focused on high-volume plasmapheresis.

**ANSWER:** B

9. A 10-year-old boy is found to have an abnormal complete blood count notable for an elevated mean cell hemoglobin concentration, an elevated red cell distribution width, and reticulocytosis. On examination of his peripheral smear, the red blood cells exhibit a lack of central pallor and loss of the usual biconcave shape, and the cells are fairly uniform in size and shape. Which of the following is true regarding this condition?

    A. It is usually transmitted as an autosomal recessive disorder and causes a membrane abnormality that results in decreased osmotic fragility.

    B. Splenectomy can decrease the incidence of secondary complications such as jaundice, pigmented gallstones, and anemia.

    C. Surgery should be delayed until after the age of 10 because of the risk for overwhelming post-splenectomy sepsis in younger patients.

    D. It is less severe than other heredity membrane disorders, including pyruvate kinase deficiency, sickle cell anemia, thalassemia, and elliptocytosis, and less likely to require splenectomy than these conditions.

    E. It is associated with a small spleen.

*Ref.:* 1, 2, 6

**COMMENTS: Hereditary spherocytosis** (HS) is generally inherited as an autosomal dominant disease, although up to 25% of cases in the United States are inherited in an autosomal recessive manner. It is the most common hereditary hemolytic disorder in persons of northern European descent, with an incidence of approximately 1 in 5000 or less. HS results from deficiency of an erythrocyte cytoskeletal membrane protein, most commonly spectrin. Lack of spectrin produces spherical erythrocytes that are small and rigid with increased osmotic fragility and results in increased destruction of erythrocytes as they pass through the trabeculae of the spleen. The clinical manifestations are variable. Anemia may develop, as well as jaundice, splenomegaly, and pigmented gallstones from hemolysis. **Splenectomy** can decrease these secondary complications but should be delayed until after 6 years of age, if possible, to preserve immunologic function in young children (who are at greatest risk for **overwhelming post-splenectomy infection**). Cholecystectomy may be required in patients with symptomatic cholelithiasis but otherwise mild HS. Splenectomy is clearly indicated for patients with severe anemia. The hereditary disorders listed in choice D are often less severe than those in HS and much less likely to require splenectomy. **Splenomegaly** is a prominent feature of HS.

**ANSWER:** B

10. A 47-year-old woman with a history of a radical mastectomy 20 years previously has had long-standing lymphedema of her upper extremity on the treated side. She is now complaining of a reddish blue nodule on her arm and dyspnea on exertion. Which one of the following is not true regarding her condition?

   A. The lymphatic system is a collection of small lymphatic vessels that parallel the major blood vessels and may contain red blood cells, bacteria, and proteins.

   B. The lymphatic system has valves.

   C. Her reddish blue nodule probably represents a benign condition related to long-standing lymphedema.

   D. Extrinsic factors such as muscle contraction, arterial pulsation, and respiratory movement aid in the movement of lymph flow.

   E. Measurement of the protein content of edema fluid can be used to assess the lymphatic function of her arm.

*Ref.:* 7-9

**COMMENTS:** This patient has a **lymphangiosarcoma** following mastectomy complicated by untreated chronic **lymphedema**, or **Stewart-Treves syndrome**. This malignant tumor is rare and typically occurs in patients with long-standing lymphedema. It is characterized by a rapid and aggressive course and a tendency to metastasize to the lungs early, as suggested by her history of dyspnea. Treatment often involves multimodality therapy, and amputation of the limb may be necessary. The **lymphatic system** begins as a network of valveless capillaries in the superficial dermis that drain into a secondary system of valved vessels in the deep or subdermal layer, which then drain into major lymphatic channels that parallel the major blood vessels. Intradermal lymphatics can be evaluated by the intradermal injection of blue dye. Lymphangiography is rarely done as a mapping technique for patients with lymphedema because it may worsen the symptoms. Proteins, red blood cells, and lymphocytes that make their way into the extracellular fluid readily enter the lymphatic vessels. Measurement of the protein content of edema fluid in an extremity can be used to assess the status of lymphatic function. The protein content should be less than 1.5 mg/dL; higher values suggest declining lymphatic return.

**ANSWER:** C

11. A 23-year-old woman is seen with left supraclavicular adenopathy. She has no history of fever, chills, night sweats, or weight loss. CT of the chest and abdomen shows no other findings. Bone marrow biopsy is negative. Biopsy of the lymph node

discloses nodular sclerosing Hodgkin's disease. Which of the following statements regarding further surgical intervention for this patient is not true?

   A. Staging laparotomy (or laparoscopy) for Hodgkin's disease, when indicated, includes thorough abdominal exploration, splenectomy with splenic hilar lymphadenectomy, bilateral wedge and core needle liver biopsies, bilateral retroperitoneal lymph node sampling, bone marrow biopsy, and oophoropexy for female patients.

   B. Staging laparotomy (or laparoscopy) has largely been supplanted by CT and positron emission tomography (PET) for assessing the extent of disease.

   C. Eighty percent of patients undergoing splenectomy will have evidence of Hodgkin's involvement of the spleen.

   D. The spleen is the only site of intra-abdominal disease in approximately one half of patients with Hodgkin's disease found to have splenic involvement.

   E. Except for patients with early-stage Hodgkin disease, who may be treated with radiation therapy alone, most patients receive systemic chemotherapy.

*Ref.:* 1, 2

**COMMENTS: Staging laparotomy (or laparoscopy)** for **Hodgkin lymphoma** is now largely of historical interest because PET and CT have all but replaced the need for operative staging. The components of a staging laparotomy (laparoscopy) are listed in choice A. When splenectomy is performed, approximately 40% of patients will be found to have splenic involvement. In one half of these patients with splenic involvement, there will be no other site of disease in the abdominal cavity or pelvis.

**ANSWER:** C

12. Which of the following descriptions of the extent of Hodgkin's disease is paired with the correct clinical stage?

   A. Bilateral involvement of the axillary lymph nodes with no subdiaphragmatic disease is considered stage I.

   B. Epigastric lymph node and liver hilar lymph node involvement is stage III if there is no disease above the diaphragm.

   C. The presence of positive left cervical and right mediastinal nodes denotes stage IV disease because of involvement of the contralateral side.

   D. Splenic involvement in the presence of mediastinal lymph node involvement represents stage III disease.

   E. Bone marrow involvement represents stage II disease but carries a poor prognosis.

*Ref.:* 1, 2

**COMMENTS:** According to the **Ann Arbor classification**, **Hodgkin's disease** is staged as follows: stage I—one or two contiguous areas of lymph node involvement on the same side of the diaphragm; stage II—two noncontiguous areas on the same side of the diaphragm; stage III—involvement of lymph node groups on both sides of the diaphragm (the spleen is considered a lymph node for this classification); and stage IV—involvement of the liver, bone marrow, lungs, or any other non–lymph node tissue, exclusive of the spleen. A superscript E signifies extranodal involvement adjacent to the involved lymph nodes. In addition, patients are subcategorized as being asymptomatic (A) or having constitutional symptoms (B) if they have had fever (>38° C), night sweats, or 10% weight loss within 6 months.

**ANSWER:** D

13. Hairy cell leukemia is diagnosed in a 58-year-old man with pancytopenia and palpable splenomegaly. He is referred to your office for a second opinion after another surgeon did not offer him a splenectomy. Which of the following is true regarding his condition?

    A. It is a B-cell lymphoma characterized by cytoplasmic protrusions that first invade the thymus and then the spleen secondarily.

    B. The mainstay of treatment is methotrexate chemotherapy.

    C. It is associated with a two- to threefold risk for the development of a second malignancy, including prostate, skin, and lung cancers.

    D. Splenectomy may be palliative but is infrequently done because of the lack of sustained response.

    E. The 5-year survival rate is less than 20%.

*Ref.:* 1, 2

**COMMENTS: Hairy cell leukemia** is a clonal disorder of B lymphocytes that involve the blood and bone marrow (not the thymus). It usually affects elderly men and is characterized by filamentous cytoplasmic projections on lymphocytes and splenomegaly. Pancytopenia is common because of bone marrow replacement by leukemic cells. It is associated with a two- to threefold risk for a second solid tumor, most commonly prostate, skin, lung, or gastrointestinal tract adenocarcinoma. As many as 10% of affected patients have an indolent course requiring no specific therapy. Survival after medical treatment with purine analogues (cladribine) is generally good (80% at 5 years). **Splenectomy** is now reserved for patients who fail medical management or have bleeding complications from thrombocytopenia. Splenectomy results in improvement of the pancytopenia in 40% or more of patients and may be sustained for many years.

**ANSWER:** C

14. A 32-year-old woman comes to the emergency department complaining of pain in her foot and calf. She reports that her left leg has been swollen for the last 15 years. She has a temperature of 101.5° F and reports that she had a splinter removed from her leg 1 week earlier. Her left lower extremity is swollen from the foot to the inguinal ligament, and she has erythema of the foot and calf. In addition to cellulitis, what is the most likely underlying diagnosis?

    A. Chronic venous insufficiency

    B. Deep venous thrombosis

    C. Lymphedema praecox

    D. Meige's disease

    E. Milroy's disease

*Ref.:* 7, 8, 10

**COMMENTS:** Chronic venous insufficiency is usually bilateral and marked by signs of venous stasis such as hemosiderin deposits and possibly ulceration. Deep venous thrombosis would be manifested acutely and would be unlikely to have such a long-standing

history. Swelling of an extremity from a pathologic condition of the lymphatic system is classified as primary or secondary **lymphedema**. Primary lymphedema is an uncommon condition and is not related to any extrinsic process. Primary lymphedema is divided into three groups, depending on age at diagnosis. With onset before completion of the first year of life it is called congenital lymphedema (or Milroy's disease if associated with a family history). **Lymphedema praecox** refers to the onset of primary lymphedema before the age of 35. It is the most common form of primary lymphedema and affects women four times more commonly than men. Onset is usually in puberty, and 70% of cases are unilateral, with the left side more commonly affected than the right. **Lymphedema tarda** (or Meige's disease) refers to swelling of the legs that occurs after the age of 35. It is the least common form of primary lymphedema. Secondary lymphedema can be the result of multiple disease processes, including but not limited to infection, trauma, filariasis, lymph node dissection, and exposure to radiation. The mainstay of **lymphedema treatment** is conservative and nonoperative. The goals of therapy are prevention of infection and reduction of subcutaneous fluid volume with the use of decongestive massage therapy, pneumatic compression devices, and fitted elastic stockings. Diuretics are not used routinely but may be useful in women with premenstrual fluid retention. Recurrent lymphangitis is common following injury, and streptococci are the usual offending organisms. Penicillin is appropriate therapy. Rarely, a protein-losing enteropathy attributed to lymphatic obstruction of the small bowel develops in patients with lymphedema. Various surgical procedures have been described for the treatment of lymphedema, including removal of skin, subcutaneous tissue, and fascia, followed by split-thickness skin graft reconstruction (the Charles operation); excision of strips of skin and subcutaneous tissue, followed by primary closure; and creation of buried dermal flaps. All these procedures are associated with significant failure rates.

**ANSWER:** C

15. A 56-year-old African-American man with a history of lung disease is referred to your office for evaluation of an abnormality seen in his spleen on abdominal CT. He also has a history of sarcoidosis. Which of the following is not true about splenic involvement in his case?

    A. One fourth of patients have splenomegaly from granulomatous involvement of the spleen.

    B. Not all patients who have splenomegaly experience thrombocytopenia.

    C. Splenic rupture can occur as a result of granulomatous involvement of the spleen.

    D. Caseating granulomas are the hallmark of sarcoidosis.

    E. Patients with active sarcoidosis may have elevated levels of angiotensin-converting enzyme, which may be secreted by cells within the granuloma.

*Ref.:* 2

**COMMENTS: Sarcoidosis** is a disease that is characterized by noncaseating granulomas. One quarter of patients will have granulomatous involvement of the spleen, although bilateral lung involvement is even more common. Granulomas may also be found in the liver. Splenic involvement can lead to splenomegaly, but of those affected, only 20% have hypersplenism (increased hemolytic function of the spleen resulting in a deficiency of one or more peripheral blood elements, hypercellularity of the bone marrow, and splenomegaly). Thrombocytopenia usually resolves following splenectomy. Complications of granulomatous involvement of the spleen include splenic rupture, anemia, and neutropenia. Epithelial cells within the sarcoid granulomas may produce angiotensin-converting enzyme, thereby resulting in elevated serum levels of this enzyme.

**ANSWER:** D

16. A 61-year-old heavy smoker undergoes CT of the abdomen after a motor vehicle accident. The scan reveals a 4-cm irregular hypodensity in the spleen without other associated lymphadenopathy or masses. Which of the following statements is true regarding primary and metastatic tumors of the spleen?

   A. Vascular neoplasms, including hemangiomas and angiosarcomas, are the most common primary tumors of the spleen.

   B. With the exception of lymphomas, the spleen is rarely a site of metastatic involvement from primary tumors.

   C. Splenectomy is often curative for primary tumors of the spleen.

   D. A laparoscopic approach to splenectomy for malignancy is associated with inferior outcomes.

   E. Most splenic metastases are symptomatic.

   *Ref.:* 1, 11

**COMMENTS:** Not infrequently, lung cancer metastasizes to the spleen. Other common primary tumors that may metastasize to the spleen include breast cancer and melanoma, as well as ovarian, gastric, and colon cancers. The most common **primary splenic tumors** are vascular in origin and include hemangiomas (benign) and angiosarcomas (malignant). The latter may be associated with environmental exposure to vinyl chloride or thorium dioxide. Most **splenic metastases** are asymptomatic and are found at autopsy in about 7% of cancer patients. Occasionally, secondary tumors in the spleen may cause symptomatic splenomegaly or splenic rupture. By the time that metastases are detected, splenectomy is rarely curative, but it may be palliative in appropriately selected symptomatic patients or be reasonable therapy for isolated splenic metastases. The laparoscopic approach to splenectomy is appropriate for most splenic tumors.

**ANSWER:** A

17. A 41-year-old man is referred to you with chronic abdominal pain after abdominal CT demonstrates a 7-cm solitary splenic cyst. This is proposed as the source of his symptoms. Which of the following is true about splenic cysts?

   A. A large majority of splenic "cysts" are actually pseudocysts that are mostly post-traumatic in origin.

   B. Echinococcal parasitic cysts should be suspected when a solitary simple cyst has a calcified wall.

   C. Treatment should be considered for cysts larger than 10 cm or for those producing symptoms.

   D. True congenital splenic cysts may have an epithelial lining that secretes carcinoembryonic antigen (CEA) and CA 19-9. These cysts should be removed to prevent malignant transformation.

   E. All can be treated effectively by percutaneous aspiration under image guidance.

   *Ref.:* 1, 11

**COMMENTS:** The most commonly diagnosed **splenic cysts** are actually pseudocysts and are usually post-traumatic in origin. **Echinococcal parasitic cysts** are calcified but have internal daughter cells, which gives them a complex appearance on imaging studies. The diagnosis of echinococcal or hydatid cysts can be confirmed by serologic testing. When excising these cysts, just as for echinococcal cysts of the liver, care must be taken to avoid spillage into the abdominal cavity because of the possibility of anaphylactic shock or dissemination of parasites. Cysts can be sterilized by the injection of 3% sodium chloride, alcohol, or 0.5% silver nitrate. Treatment should be considered for symptomatic cysts or those larger than 5 cm (not 10 cm). True congenital splenic cysts may in fact secrete tumor markers such as CEA or CA 19-9. They are, however, benign and have no malignant potential. Splenic pseudocysts or simple cysts may be aspirated percutaneously, but not all cysts can be treated effectively in this way; the success rate for elimination and resolution of symptoms is higher with splenic cystectomy or partial or total splenectomy.

**ANSWER:** A

18. A 23-year-old sustains blunt force trauma in a high-speed motor vehicle accident. Abdominal CT demonstrates a subcapsular hematoma involving 60% of the surface area of the spleen without obvious injury to the hilum. The patient has a heart rate of 110 beats/min and blood pressure of 105/60 mm Hg. Correct statements regarding the management of this patient include which of the following?

   A. A Kehr's sign is a contraindication to nonoperative management given the high associated severity of injury.

   B. Diagnostic peritoneal lavage is not sensitive for the detection of splenic injury.

   C. For patients with moderate to severe splenic injuries managed nonoperatively, follow-up abdominal CT is indicated in 2 to 3 days.

   D. Angiography is required in all patients with splenic injury to exclude unsuspected areas of active hemorrhage not seen on CT.

   E. Nonoperative management may be pursued, provided that the patient is hemodynamically stable, the injury can be clearly classified by imaging, and transfusion requirements remain less than 6 units of packed red blood cells.

   *Ref.:* 1, 12

**COMMENTS:** This patient has a grade III splenic injury (see Table 26-1 online at www.expertconsult.com). Kehr's sign (pain referred to the left shoulder) does correlate highly with **splenic injury** but does not mandate operative management. Diagnostic peritoneal lavage is perhaps too sensitive in detecting significant splenic injury and has largely been replaced by ultrasound. Follow-up scans are recommended to exclude any **vascular blush** not seen on initial imaging because of sampling error with larger cuts or subsequent lysis of clot. Angiography, with possible angioembolization, should be pursued if a vascular blush appears on CT in patients with grade III and higher injuries or in patients with any grade of injury if frank hemorrhage from the splenic artery is seen. It is not required for all patients. Criteria for nonoperative management include hemodynamic stability, documented CT classification of injury, absence of additional injuries necessitating surgery, and transfusion of 2 or fewer units of red blood cells (not 6 units). The success of nonoperative management is reported to be 70% to 90% for children and 40% to 50% for adults treated in trauma centers. The differing success rates may be related to both anatomic considerations and mechanisms of injury.

**ANSWER:** C

**19.** A 14-year-old girl is involved in a high-speed car accident and has a mildly distended abdomen, a seat belt sign, and a positive focused abdominal sonography for trauma (FAST) examination. She is tachycardic and found on CT to have a splenic injury; she fails nonoperative management over the next day because of transfusion requirements. At the time of exploration, which of the following is most correct?

A. Eighty percent of the spleen can be sacrificed at splenorrhaphy before total splenectomy should be performed.

B. Although available techniques for splenorrhaphy include argon beam coagulation, fibrin glue, and mattress suturing with pledgets, mesh wrap should not be done because of the increased risk for infection.

C. Splenorrhaphy is especially advantageous in the setting of pancreatic or hollow viscus injury because it decreases the occurrence of subphrenic abscess.

D. Splenorrhaphy may be attempted safely in patients with severe head injuries.

E. Splenorrhaphy is best used only for grades I and II injuries.

*Ref.: 1, 12*

**COMMENTS: Splenorrhaphy** is a useful tool to allow preservation of the spleen. Only one third of the spleen is required for retention of its immunologic benefit; injuries requiring sacrifice of more than two thirds of the spleen are best treated by splenectomy. Available tools for splenorrhaphy include all those listed in choice B. The use of a mesh wrap has not contributed to an increased incidence of infection following splenorrhaphy, even in the setting of associated hollow viscus injury. It is true that splenorrhaphy decreases the incidence of abscess formation following pancreatic or hollow viscus injury. In unstable patients or those with severe head injuries, expeditious splenectomy should be performed if needed instead of partial splenectomy or splenorrhaphy because the latter tends to be more time-consuming. There is no grade restriction for performing splenorrhaphy after injury, and it may be done as long as one third of the spleen remains viable for continued immunologic function.

**ANSWER: C**

**20.** After failing medical therapy, a 46-year-old woman with ITP is referred to you for splenectomy. She is very interested in a laparoscopic procedure and was told by her hematologist that she is a good candidate. Review of her CT scan shows a normal-sized spleen and normal splenic vascular anatomy. Which of the following is true about laparoscopic splenectomy?

A. Operative mortality rates are the same regardless of the underlying disease type.

B. Laparoscopic splenectomy has similar success rates as open splenectomy, except when performed for ITP.

C. The rate of conversion from laparoscopic to open splenectomy is 0% to 20%.

D. Laparoscopic splenectomy can be considered for spleen sizes up to 35 cm.

E. Laparoscopic splenectomy results in a higher incidence of splenosis than does the open approach.

*Ref.: 1, 2*

**COMMENTS: Laparoscopic splenectomy** is increasingly being selected as the technique when elective splenectomy is indicated. The operative morbidity and mortality rates after splenectomy are higher for patients with malignant hematologic disease than for those with benign disease. The risk for postoperative **portal venous thrombosis** is greatest for patients with myeloproliferative disorders. For **idiopathic thrombocytopenic purpura**, laparoscopic splenectomy has success rates similar to those of open splenectomy. Regardless of the surgical approach, when splenectomy is performed for hematologic disease, a careful search for **accessory spleens** must be performed. Their appearance may mimic that of a lymph node, and they may more easily be palpated than visualized, thus giving rise to concern that the laparoscopic approach may overlook some accessory spleens. The conversion rate to an open procedure is reported to range from 0% to 20%. Conversion is usually secondary to bleeding, but extensive adhesions, obesity, and splenomegaly may also be factors. Spleens up to 20 to 25 cm in size are amenable to laparoscopic splenectomy. A splenic size of 35 cm is generally too large for a laparoscopic approach. The laparoscopic approach does not result in a higher incidence of **splenosis** (autotransplantation and subsequent growth of splenic fragments from an injured spleen that may remain functional and occasionally cause pain or symptoms related to a mass effect).

**ANSWER: C**

**21.** A 41-year-old with chronic myelogenous leukemia and massive splenomegaly underwent splenectomy after successful bone marrow transplantation. Which of the following is true?

A. The most common site of postoperative bleeding is the splenic hilum.

B. Nasogastric tube decompression is recommended for 1 to 2 days postoperatively in all patients to prevent gastric expansion and disruption of the ligated short gastric vessels.

C. There is a higher risk for thromboembolism and pulmonary embolism following splenectomy than with other types of intra-abdominal surgery.

D. Injury to the tail of the pancreas occurs in 5% to 10% of patients undergoing splenectomy.

E. Seventy-five percent of postoperative infections after splenectomy are respiratory in nature.

*Ref.: 1-3*

**COMMENTS:** For **chronic myelogenous leukemia, splenectomy** has not been shown to improve survival when done before bone marrow transplantation. Thrombosis and thromboembolic events are reported in 2% to 4% of patients after splenectomy. There is an increased incidence of deep venous thrombosis, pulmonary embolism, and splenic venous thrombosis in postsplenectomy patients, particularly those with myeloproliferative disorders. The mesenteric, portal, and renal veins are particularly at risk. The most common site of bleeding following splenectomy is from the diaphragmatic portion of the splenic bed, not the splenic hilum. Nasogastric tube decompression, although theoretically of benefit to prevent gastric distention and disruption of short gastric vessels, is no longer done routinely. Injury to the tail of the pancreas is reported in 2% of patients after splenectomy and may be secondary to either devascularization or direct injury (such as when pancreatic tissue is included with ligation of the splenic vessels). Respiratory infections account for approximately one half of postoperative infections in patients after splenectomy.

**ANSWER: C**

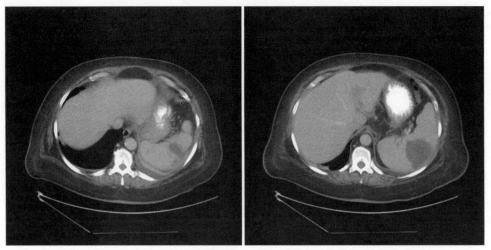

**Figure 26-1.** Abdominal computed tomographic scans of a morbidly obese female.

**22.** A 66-year-old morbidly obese woman has fever, tachycardia, abdominal pain, and bacteremia after an infected lap band was removed 4 weeks earlier. CT of the abdomen demonstrates a splenic fluid collection with rim enhancement (Figure 26-1). All of the following may be part of the appropriate treatment of this patient except:

A. Broad-spectrum antibiotics

B. Splenectomy

C. Percutaneous drainage of the splenic fluid collection

D. Open or laparoscopic splenotomy

E. Echocardiography

*Ref.:* 1, 11

**COMMENTS:** The images show a hypodense fluid collection with rim enhancement within the spleen. **Splenic abscesses** are rare but are associated with high mortality and complication rates because of delayed detection and treatment. Patients often have vague symptoms and signs such as fever and nonspecific abdominal or chest pain. Less than one half of patients complain of left upper quadrant pain. One half of patients will have positive blood cultures. The majority of splenic abscesses arise from hematogenous spread from a distant focus such as endocarditis, pyelonephritis, or direct inoculation from intravenous drug use, but spread from a contiguous infected organ or adjacent intra-abdominal infection or secondary infection of a post-traumatic hematoma can occur as well. The most commonly cultured organisms are gram-positive aerobes, but gram-negative or polymicrobial infections can also occur, as can infection with mycobacteria and fungi. Broad-spectrum antibiotics are begun empirically until culture data are available. Splenectomy is effective treatment. However, in the interest of splenic preservation, image-guided percutaneous drainage has gained popularity over the past decade. The success rate for treatment of unilocular abscesses in this fashion exceeds 75%. Thus, splenectomy may be reserved for failure of nonoperative management or for patients with multiple abscesses in whom percutaneous drainage is not feasible. Splenotomy would not be beneficial for this patient. Echocardiography to evaluate for valvular vegetations is prudent in patients with positive blood cultures and splenic abscess.

**ANSWER:** D

**REFERENCES**

1. Beauchamp RD, Holzman MD, Fabian TC, et al: The spleen. In Townsend CM, Beauchamp RD, Evers M, et al, editors: *Sabiston textbook of surgery: the biological basis of modern surgical practice,* ed 18, Philadelphia, 2008, WB Saunders.
2. Sebastian ML, Marohn MR: Splenectomy for hematologic disorders. In Cameron JL: *Current surgical therapy,* ed 9, Philadelphia, 2008, CV Mosby.
3. Hoyt DB, Coimbra R: Splenectomy and splenorrhaphy. In Fisher JE, Bland KE, editors: *Mastery of surgery,* ed 5, Philadelphia, 2007, Lippincott Williams & Wilkins.
4. Griffin J, Arif S, Mufti A, editors: *Crash course immunology and haematology,* ed 2, Toronto, 2003, CV Mosby.
5. Mourtzoukou EG, Pappas G, Peppas, et al: Vaccination of asplenic or hyposplenic adults, *Br J Surg* 95:273–280, 2008.
6. Gonzalez G, Eichner R: Spherocytosis, hereditary: treatment & medication. In Besa E, editor: *eMedicine Clinical Knowledge Base, Hematology.* Available at www.emedicine.medscape.com/article/206107-overview. Accessed July 19, 2009.
7. Pipinos I, Baxter T: The lymphatics. In Townsend CM, Beauchamp RD, Evers M, et al, editors: *Sabiston textbook of surgery: the biological basis of modern surgical practice,* ed 18, Philadelphia, 2008, WB Saunders.
8. Park JE, Manson PN, Deune EG: Lymphedema. In Cameron JL: *Current surgical therapy,* ed 9, Philadelphia, 2008, CV Mosby.
9. Liem TK, Moneta GL: Venous and lymphatic disease. In Brunicardi FC, Andersen DK, Billiar TR, et al, editors: *Schwartz's principles of surgery,* ed 9, New York 2010, McGraw-Hill.
10. Rutherford RB, editor: *Vascular surgery,* ed 6, Philadelphia, 2005, WB Saunders.
11. McIntyre T, Zenilman ME: Cysts, tumors, and abscesses of the spleen. In Cameron JL: *Current surgical therapy,* ed 9, Philadelphia, 2008, CV Mosby.
12. Haider AH, Cornwell EE III: Splenic salvage procedures: therapeutic options. In Cameron JL: *Current surgical therapy,* ed 9, Philadelphia, 2008, CV Mosby.

# CARDIOVASCULAR AND THORACIC

# CHAPTER 27

# Cardiac Surgery

## A. Congenital Defects

*Anastasios C. Polimenakos, M.D., F.A.C.S., F.A.C.C.; Eric J. Okum, M.D.;*
*R. Anthony Perez-Tamayo, M.D., Ph.D.;*
*and Robert S. D. Higgins, M.D., M.S.H.A.*

1. Which of the following statements is true regarding the fetal circulation?

   A. Blood flows through the ductus arteriosus from the pulmonary artery to the aorta.

   B. Less than 25% of cardiac output flows through the lungs.

   C. The blood in the ductus venosus is unoxygenated.

   D. The atrial septum is intact.

   E. The right side of the heart pumps against lower resistance than the left side.

   *Ref.:* 1-3

COMMENTS: The circulation in utero differs markedly from postnatal circulation. Gas exchange occurs in the placenta, which receives blood from the umbilical arteries. Oxygenated blood then returns through the ductus venosus, which joins the inferior vena cava at the level of the hepatic veins. This blood is mixed with the venous return from the superior vena cava in the right atrium. Blood in the right atrium may be shunted across the foramen ovale to the left atrium, where it goes to the left ventricle and is pumped into the circulation. Blood in the right atrium may also go to the right ventricle and be pumped into the pulmonary artery. Pulmonary vascular resistance is very high in utero, and much of the blood pumped into the pulmonary artery goes through the ductus arteriosus and into the descending aorta. Because the ductus arteriosus is large and communicates with the aorta, pressure in the pulmonary artery is the same as that in the aorta (systemic). After birth the umbilical cord is ligated, thereby decreasing ductus venosus return to zero and causing the ductus venosus to constrict and obliterate. Pulmonary vascular resistance drops with expansion of the lungs, which causes pulmonary blood flow to increase. Because return to the left atrium is increased, left atrial pressure causes the foramen ovale to close. Increased oxygen tension causes the ductus arteriosus to constrict and close. The pulmonary and systemic circulations at this point become separate.

ANSWER: A

2. Which of the following choices best characterizes right-to-left shunts?

   A. Obstructive lesions

   B. Decreased pulmonary blood flow

   C. Increased pulmonary blood flow

   D. Increased ventricular work

   E. No change in pulmonary blood flow

   *Ref.:* 1-3

COMMENTS: **Congenital heart defects** can be divided into four categories, each associated with distinct physiologic abnormalities. Obstructive lesions (e.g., aortic stenosis, coarctation of the aorta) restrict the flow of blood and increase the workload of the obstructed ventricle. Without an associated lesion, there is no shunting or mixing of blood between the pulmonary and systemic circulations. Left-to-right shunts occur in the setting of a communication between the pulmonary and systemic circulations at the levels of the atria (e.g., atrial septal defect [ASD]), ventricles (e.g., ventricular septal defect [VSD]), or great vessels (e.g., patent ductus arteriosus [PDA]). When there is no obstruction to pulmonary blood flow, these communications usually result in flow of blood across the defect from the systemic to the pulmonary circuit. The amount of pulmonary blood flow per minute may be as much as four or five times as great as the amount that flows in the systemic circulation. Clinically significant shunts occur when pulmonary blood flow is greater than 1.5 to 2 times systemic flow. Right-to-left shunts occur in the setting of a similar communication but when there is obstruction to pulmonary blood flow (e.g., tetralogy of Fallot, subaortic or doubly committed double-outlet right ventricle). Obstruction of pulmonary blood flow causes blood to flow from the right to left side without having passed through the lungs. If a sufficient amount of desaturated blood enters the systemic circuit without passing through the lungs, the patient becomes cyanotic. Complex lesions include defects such as transposition of the great arteries and hypoplastic left heart syndrome, in which the pathophysiologic features cannot be so easily described. A child with a complex lesion may suffer from cyanosis, pulmonary overcirculation, and obstructive lesions simultaneously.

ANSWER: B

3. With regard to increased pulmonary blood flow (left-to-right shunts), which of the following statements is true?

   A. A shunt becomes physiologically important when pulmonary blood flow is five times as great as systemic flow.

   B. High pulmonary artery pressures preclude surgical correction of the defect.

C. Delivery of 100% oxygen to the patient during transesophageal echocardiography may provide crucial information for determining whether the patient is an operative candidate.

D. The rapidity with which pulmonary vascular disease develops depends on the magnitude of the shunt regardless of the anatomic location of the defect.

E. Increased fixed pulmonary vascular resistance precludes surgical correction of the defect.

*Ref.:* 1-3

**COMMENTS:** Large **left-to-right shunts** have, by definition, an increased amount of pulmonary blood flow. Frequently, pulmonary artery pressure and left atrial pressure are elevated. The combination of these factors causes increased extravascular fluid in the pulmonary parenchyma and thus congestive heart failure. A shunt in which pulmonary blood flow is less than 1.5 times systemic flow is unlikely to produce symptoms and does not usually represent an indication for surgical repair. If a patient has a large communication at the level of the ventricles or the great vessels, pulmonary artery pressure is equal to systemic pressure because there is free communication between systemic pressure and the pulmonary artery. This does not necessarily imply that the patient has pulmonary vascular disease. High pulmonary artery pressure with a large pulmonary flow (Qp)–to–systemic flow (Qs) ratio (e.g., Qp/Qs = 3) implies low pulmonary vascular resistance, thus making the child an appropriate candidate for repair. If a child has high pulmonary artery pressure at cardiac catheterization and relatively low pulmonary blood flow (Qp/Qs < 2), pulmonary vascular resistance is high and the child may not tolerate surgical correction. One hundred percent oxygen is a potent pulmonary vasodilator. If during cardiac catheterization the shunt significantly increases with the administration of 100% oxygen or iNOS, it implies that the pulmonary vascular disease is reversible and the child may yet be a candidate for surgical correction. Because the development of pulmonary vascular disease depends on pressure, as well as flow, severe pulmonary vascular obstructive disease uncommonly develops in patients with large atrial-level shunts, whereas it usually does in patients with large ventricular- or arterial-level shunts.

**ANSWER:** E

4. Resolution of congestive heart failure without surgical correction in a patient who has had a large left-to-right shunt:

A. Indicates increased pulmonary vascular resistance

B. Is a sign of increased left-to-right shunting

C. Is a sign of unchanged left-to-right shunting

D. Indicates reversible pulmonary vascular resistance

E. Is a harbinger for early death in the fourth decade of life

*Ref.:* 1-3

**COMMENTS:** The natural history of a large **left-to-right shunt** (especially at the ventricular or atrial level) is progressive pulmonary vascular obstructive disease. There are considerable variations in the progression of pulmonary vascular disease. In a child with a large **ventricular septal defect**, pulmonary vascular disease usually develops at 2 to 4 years of age. A child with a large left-to-right shunt may have considerable congestive heart failure during the first year of life. However, as the pulmonary vascular obstructive disease progresses, the left-to-right shunt decreases as pulmonary vascular resistance approaches systemic vascular resistance. During this period, the child's symptoms may improve, and chest radiographic findings of cardiomegaly and pulmonary plethora may also improve. However, this finding is grave because the pulmonary vascular disease is usually progressive at this point despite surgical correction or any other currently available therapies. Pulmonary vascular disease progresses until pulmonary vascular resistance exceeds systemic vascular resistance. Shunting ceases to be left to right and becomes right to left, thereby resulting in the patient becoming cyanotic. This condition is referred to as Eisenmenger syndrome. This process usually continues until it results in the patient's death. Most patients who succumb from Eisenmenger syndrome die during their teens or twenties.

**ANSWER:** A

5. With regard to left obstructive congenital heart lesions, which of the following statements is true?

A. The most common obstructive lesions are pulmonary valve stenosis, aortic valve stenosis, and coarctation of the aorta.

B. Obstructive congenital heart lesions produce systolic pressure overloading and concentric hypertrophy.

C. Concentric hypertrophy produces marked cardiac enlargement, which can be detected by physical examination and routine chest radiography.

D. Myocardial oxygen demand will be unchanged if cardiac catheterization demonstrates normal-appearing coronary arteries ("clean coronaries").

E. A and B

*Ref.:* 1-3

**COMMENTS:** The concentric hypertrophy of obstructive congenital heart lesions is not easily detected by chest radiography. Auscultation may give some indication of the severity of aortic or **pulmonary stenosis**. Coarctation of the aorta may be indicated by differences in the pulses and blood pressure between the arms and legs. The electrocardiogram (ECG) and echocardiogram with Doppler examination are additional noninvasive modalities useful for assessing chamber size, degree of obstruction, and function. Although often not necessary, cardiac catheterization is the definitive modality for assessing the gradient across obstructive lesions. **Aortic stenosis** causes increased myocardial oxygen demand while reducing supply, especially to the subendocardium. This may lead to myocardial ischemia with all its sequelae, including angina pectoris, arrhythmia, a predisposition to sudden death, and end-stage cardiac failure.

**ANSWER:** E

6. Lesions that produce large left-to-right shunts during the newborn period are:

A. Multiple muscular VSDs: "Swiss cheese"

B. Primum ASD

C. Dextro-transposition of the great arteries

D. Secundum ASD

E. Tetralogy of Fallot

*Ref.:* 1-3

**COMMENTS:** Large **left-to-right shunting** occurs because of a communication between the pulmonary and systemic circuits, combined with lower resistance in the pulmonary circuit. Blood is directed toward the lower resistance. The pulmonary vascular resistance of newborns is at systemic levels and then falls during the first few weeks of life. As pulmonary vascular resistance falls, the shunt becomes greater in magnitude, and signs and symptoms of left-to-right shunting appear.

**A N S W E R :**  A

7. With regard to right-to-left shunts, which of the following statements is true?

    A. Polycythemia may lead to venous thrombosis and, in patients with a long-standing right-to-left shunt, to systemic emboli.

    B. The degree of cyanosis depends on both oxygen saturation and hemoglobin concentration.

    C. Cardiac catheterization is mandatory to determine the degree of pulmonary stenosis and the suitability of the patient for surgery.

    D. A $Po_2$ of 45 mm Hg is life-threatening and requires immediate surgical treatment if it cannot be increased.

    E. An oxygen saturation of 75% is life-threatening and requires immediate surgical treatment if it cannot be increased.

*Ref.:* 1-3

**COMMENTS: Cyanosis** is present when the amount of desaturated hemoglobin present in the systemic circulation exceeds 5 g/dL. Thus, cyanosis is dependent on both oxygen saturation and hemoglobin level. A patient with severe hypoxia who also has a relatively low hemoglobin concentration may be minimally cyanotic. Conversely, patients with a similar oxygen saturation may appear profoundly cyanotic if they are polycythemic. Polycythemia is a physiologic response to cyanosis that can lead to a hematocrit of greater than 60%. A high hematocrit increases blood viscosity and predisposes individuals to venous thrombosis. Systemic emboli, particularly cerebral emboli, may be life-threatening. In particular, children with long-standing right-to-left shunts are at risk for cerebral abscesses. Most children who have right-to-left shunts can be well evaluated with echocardiography alone. Cardiac catheterization is reserved for those who require better delineation of small branch pulmonary arteries. Children tolerate saturations down to around 75%, which corresponds to a $Po_2$ of 40 mm Hg. A child who chronically has a $Po_2$ of around 45 mm Hg usually does well while waiting for an elective operation.

**A N S W E R :**  E

8. Which of the following best characterizes the tetralogy of Fallot?

    A. Egg-shaped heart

    B. Left atrial and ventricular enlargement

    C. Figure-of-eight abnormality of the pulmonary venous ("snowman") drainage

    D. Boot-shaped heart (coeur en sabot)

    E. Right atrial and ventricular enlargement

*Ref.:* 1-3

**COMMENTS:** The chest radiograph plays an important role in the evaluation of congenital heart disease. The right ventricular hypertrophy characteristic of the **tetralogy of Fallot** tends to produce a boot-shaped heart with an upturned apex. With transposition of the great arteries, the great arteries usually overlie each other, with a resultant narrow mediastinum. The heart looks like an egg on a string. Supracardiac total anomalous pulmonary venous return (TAPVR) has a large vertical vein and a large innominate vein, which results in a wide mediastinum and a figure-of-eight contour, or a "snowman." ASDs cause right-sided enlargement because of the atrial-level shunt. VSDs cause left-sided heart enlargement (blood goes through the VSD to the pulmonary artery, left atrium, left ventricle, and then back through the VSD; hence, the left atrial and ventricular enlargement). Atrioventricular (AV) valve regurgitation also causes enlargement on its respective side (Ebstein anomaly of the tricuspid valve on the right and the mitral valve on the left) secondary to the volume overload.

**A N S W E R :**  D

9. With regard to the tetralogy of Fallot, which of the following statements is true?

    A. Cyanosis occurs because of the septal defect associated with the right ventricular hypertrophy.

    B. A right-to-left shunt occurs because of the septal defect associated with obstruction of the right ventricular outflow tract.

    C. Patients often become anemic.

    D. Patients learn to squat because it lowers their pulmonary artery pressure.

    E. The aorta is overriding, which exacerbates the right-to-left shunt.

*Ref.:* 1-3

**COMMENTS:** The classic congenital abnormality producing a right-to-left shunt is the **tetralogy of Fallot**, a combination of a VSD, pulmonary stenosis, overriding of the aorta, and right ventricular hypertrophy. The amount of shunting across the VSD is related to the amount of pulmonary stenosis. In patients with little pulmonary stenosis, the shunting may be left to right, as with an uncomplicated VSD. Most patients with the tetralogy of Fallot have enough pulmonary stenosis that some of the desaturated blood in the right ventricle goes through the VSD to the systemic circulation. Because of the chronic cyanosis, polycythemia with hemoglobin values exceeding 20 mg/dL may develop. Patients will learn to squat if the problem remains uncorrected past a few years of age. Squatting increases systemic vascular resistance, thereby forcing more blood to go to the lungs. Squatting does nothing directly to the pulmonary vasculature.

**A N S W E R :**  B

10. Treatment strategies for repair of the tetralogy of Fallot during infancy are:

    A. Always a complete repair

    B. Staged approach with palliative surgery first followed by complete repair

    C. Selective use of palliative surgery in early cyanosis and when small pulmonary arteries are present

    D. Staged approach with balloon valvuloplasty first followed by complete repair

    E. All of the above

*Ref.:* 1-3

**COMMENTS:** Repair of the tetralogy of Fallot involves closure of the VSD and relief of the right ventricular outflow tract obstruction. About 15 to 20 years ago, most patients with the **tetralogy of Fallot** underwent palliation with a **Blalock-Taussig shunt** followed by complete repair at 3 to 6 years of age. At that time, complete repair during infancy carried significant morbidity and mortality. Since then, improvements in surgical, anesthetic, and perfusion techniques have allowed single-stage correction during infancy for most patients with the tetralogy of Fallot. Elective repair is usually performed at approximately 6 months of age. Earlier repair may be done if a child is too cyanotic to wait until 6 months. A staged approach may still be performed. One such circumstance involves patients with very small pulmonary arteries. VSD closure may cause right ventricular pressure to become supra-systemic in an attempt to pump blood through the small pulmonary arteries. A staged approach may allow time for growth of the pulmonary artery and definitive repair at a later date.

**ANSWER: C**

11. Which of the following statements is true regarding systemic-to-pulmonary artery shunts?

   A. They join one of the great vessels with the pulmonary vein, either directly or by means of a prosthetic graft.

   B. They are used to decrease pulmonary blood flow in patients with the tetralogy of Fallot.

   C. Based on shunt size, a systemic-to-pulmonary shunt may widen the pulse pressure (after shunt construction), and an increase in diastolic runoff will promote coronary flow insufficiency.

   D. A successful shunt may make definitive surgery unnecessary.

   E. A shunt is commonly used in a cyanotic infant to delay definitive surgery until the patient is older.

*Ref.:* 1-3

**COMMENTS: Blalock-Taussig shunts** are part of the broader classification of systemic-pulmonary artery shunts. Although other kinds of shunt connections were made in the past, most shunts today consist of Gore-Tex grafts between the aorta or one of the great vessels (e.g., innominate artery) and the pulmonary artery. Pulmonary blood flow may be increased to relieve severe hypoxia. A shunt may delay the need for definitive surgery in young patients with complex heart disease. Shunt physiology is inherently inefficient, because the blood going through the lungs via the shunt is already partly oxygenated. Thus, a shunt is never considered the final repair, except in complex cases in which definitive repair is not possible. Because there is runoff through the shunt into the low-resistance pulmonary circuit during diastole, systemic diastolic pressure tends to be low, thus making pulse pressures wide.

**ANSWER: C**

12. Which of the following auscultatory findings is associated with an ASD.

   A. "Innocent" systolic murmur

   B. A significantly increased second heart sound ($S_2$)

   C. Diastolic murmurs

   D. Widely split and "fixed" $S_2$

   E. Continuous murmur

*Ref.:* 1-3

**COMMENTS:** Proper auscultation of the heart often leads to the correct diagnosis of a **congenital cardiac abnormality**. $S_2$ is heard best at the left upper sternal border and should be evaluated in terms of its degree of splitting and relative intensity. The degree of splitting of $S_2$ normally varies with respirations (increases with inspiration and decreases or becomes single with expiration). An abnormal $S_2$ may be in the form of (1) wide splitting, (2) narrow splitting, (3) single $S_2$, (4) abnormal increase or decrease in the pulmonary component of the second sound ($P_2$), or (5) paradoxical splitting of $S_2$. **Systolic murmurs** occur between $S_1$ and $S_2$ and may be (1) ejection (through stenotic semilunar valves or secondary to increased flow through normal semilunar valves) or (2) regurgitant (pansystolic or holosystolic). The latter are associated with a VSD, mitral regurgitation, or tricuspid regurgitation. Diastolic murmurs may occur because of an incompetent semilunar valve or increased flow through an AV valve. Diastolic murmurs are virtually always pathologic. **Continuous murmurs** begin during systole and continue through $S_2$ into all or part of diastole. They are caused by an aortopulmonary or arteriovenous connection (e.g., PDA, arteriovenous fistula, or after a systemic-pulmonary shunt) or a flow disturbance in veins (e.g., venous hum) or arteries (e.g., coarctation or peripheral pulmonary artery stenosis).

**ANSWER: D**

13. With regard to echocardiography for the evaluation of congenital heart disease, which of the following statements is true?

   A. It is the most accurate method by which to delineate intracardiac anatomy.

   B. It may indicate the gradient across a valve.

   C. It may indicate whether right ventricular pressure is at or well below systemic pressure.

   D. It may precisely define pulmonary artery anatomy.

   E. A, B, and C

*Ref.:* 1-3

**COMMENTS: Echocardiography** has become the dominant imaging modality for **congenital heart disease**. It is the most accurate method by which to delineate intracardiac anatomy, and nearly all diagnoses are determined by echocardiography. Doppler echocardiography measures velocities across valves and outflow tracts, and these velocities may be translated into gradients with the formula $\Delta P = 4V^2$ (V is velocity). The velocity of a small amount of tricuspid regurgitation may be translated into the right ventricular–right atrial (RV/RA) gradient and be a good estimate of right ventricular pressure. Pulmonary artery distortion may be difficult to assess by echocardiography, and better delineation is often needed by cardiac catheterization. Coronary arteries may be assessed with a good deal of accuracy, although the images obtained do not always yield definitive information.

**ANSWER: E**

14. With regard to pulmonic stenosis, which of the following statements is true?

   A. The most common morphologic feature is hypoplasia of the pulmonic valve annulus.

   B. The physiologic abnormality is obstruction of flow from the right ventricle with hypoplasia.

   C. The intervention of choice is surgical commissurotomy.

*Ref.:* 1-3

D. The most common symptom is dyspnea at rest.

E. Echocardiography best delineates the anatomy and severity of obstruction.

*Ref.:* 1-3

**COMMENTS: Pulmonic stenosis** accounts for 10% of congenital abnormalities. It most commonly involves fusion of the cusps of the pulmonary valve, post-stenotic dilation of the main pulmonary artery, and concentric hypertrophy of the right ventricle. Less common morphologic conditions include hypoplasia of the pulmonary valve annulus, supravalvar stenosis, and subvalvular obstruction from hypertrophied muscle (infundibular stenosis). The condition is usually asymptomatic, but when symptoms are present, the most common is dyspnea on exertion. Echocardiography accurately delineates the nature and severity of the obstruction by visualizing the anatomy and measuring the velocity of the jet across the obstruction. The current treatment of choice is **balloon valvotomy**, which works in most patients who do not have hypoplasia of the valve annulus. Surgical therapy is reserved for patients with annular hypoplasia, infundibular obstruction, or failed balloon valvuloplasty.

**ANSWER: E**

15. With regard to coarctation of the aorta, which of the following statements is correct?

A. The lesion involves narrowing of the descending aorta just distal to the left subclavian artery and is surgically correctable.

B. Early left ventricular failure requiring surgical correction is common when coarctation is present in a neonate.

C. Late recurrence of the coarctation does not occur provided that the appropriate repair technique is used.

D. Arm hypertension, decreased or absent leg pulses, and a systolic murmur over the left hemithorax are the typical physical findings early in infancy.

E. A and B

*Ref.:* 1-3

**COMMENTS: Coarctation of the aorta** accounts for 10% to 15% of congenital heart defects and occurs twice as frequently in males. Associated anomalies include a bicuspid aortic valve, VSD, PDA, and mitral valve disorders. Coarctation of the aorta usually occurs distal to the left subclavian artery in association with the ligamentum arteriosum. When severe, coarctation is manifested in neonates as severe left ventricular failure, which requires immediate surgical correction. Patients who are initially seen later in childhood often do not have symptoms but exhibit severe arm hypertension. The presence of differential pulses or blood pressure between the arms and legs strongly suggests the diagnosis. Because collateral flow via the intercostal arteries is sufficient, ischemic symptoms in the lower part of the body are uncommon when the patient is initially seen after the neonatal period. Findings on physical examination and an ECG showing left ventricular hypertrophy establish the diagnosis. Echocardiography is the diagnostic method of choice. Coarctation is one of the classic causes of surgically correctable hypertension (others include pheochromocytoma, aldosterone-secreting tumor, and renal artery stenosis). Postoperative hypertension may continue to exist even after adequate surgical repair. Repair may be accomplished by several means, including predominantly resection with extended end-to-end anastomosis or, alternatively, a left subclavian flap. Both are associated with a small but definite percentage of late recoarctation. Patch aortoplasty is now seldom used because of a high rate of late pseudoaneurysm formation.

**ANSWER: C**

16. With regard to valvular aortic stenosis, which of the following statements is true?

A. Aortic stenosis predisposes to sudden death only in children.

B. Valve replacement is the treatment of choice.

C. A gradient alone is not an indication for intervention, even without symptoms.

D. Surgical or balloon valvotomy for aortic stenosis has a high likelihood of causing aortic regurgitation.

E. A bicuspid aortic valve is virtually always stenotic.

*Ref.:* 1-3

**COMMENTS: Valvular aortic stenosis** may develop from a bicuspid or tricuspid aortic valve. Newborns may be affected with critical aortic stenosis, or the stenosis may progress with time and be manifested at any time in the patient's life. Newborns with critical aortic stenosis have severe cardiomegaly and heart failure. The symptoms and indications for surgery in older children are similar to those in adults. Symptoms of congestive heart failure, angina, and syncope may develop. A gradient of greater than 50 mm Hg on exertion or greater than 30 mm Hg at rest is thought to be a risk factor for sudden death. The presence of symptoms or an asymptomatic gradient higher than 50 mm Hg is thought to be an indication for intervention. Unlike the situation in adults, aortic stenosis in children does not usually involve calcified leaflets. Therefore, **valvuloplasty** (surgical or balloon) is an option. Valvuloplasty has produced good results in terms of relieving stenosis as long as the annulus is adequate, but a high rate of postvalvuloplasty aortic regurgitation (20%) is encountered, which often results in valve replacement at a future date. Both balloon valvuloplasty and surgical valvuloplasty are associated with a 50% reintervention rate at 5 years. An increasingly common valve replacement option is a pulmonary autograft (Ross procedure). In addition to not requiring anticoagulation, a pulmonary autograft has growth potential. A bicuspid valve constitutes a common underlying morphologic condition for aortic valve stenosis. However, most people who have a bicuspid aortic valve do not suffer from clinically significant aortic stenosis.

**ANSWER: D**

17. Which of the following statements is true regarding subaortic stenosis?

A. It is usually caused by diffuse narrowing of the subaortic area.

B. A turbulent bloodstream may hit the aortic valve and cause inflammation and valvar aortic stenosis.

C. The indications for surgery are the same as those for valvular aortic stenosis.

D. Subvalvular aortic stenosis is amenable to balloon valvuloplasty.

E. The area of resection of subaortic stenosis is adjacent to the conduction tissue.

*Ref.:* 1-3

**COMMENTS: Subaortic stenosis** can occur as a discrete membrane or as a diffuse tunnel-like narrowing, but it is more commonly discrete. Surgery involves removal of the membrane with or without septal myotomy to further widen the outflow tract. Because valve replacement is rarely necessary and the jet from the subaortic stenosis may precipitate aortic regurgitation, the threshold for surgical treatment of subaortic stenosis is far less than for valvar aortic stenosis. Because the membrane requires resection in patients with subaortic stenosis, transcatheter interventions have little role. Despite the fact that the membrane directly overlies the conduction tissue, careful resection of a subaortic membrane rarely leads to heart block.

**ANSWER: D**

18. Which of the following statements is not true regarding aortic regurgitation?

   A. Discrete subaortic stenosis or VSD may be responsible for producing aortic regurgitation.

   B. The symptoms are those of congestive heart failure.

   C. Echocardiography accurately estimates the degree of regurgitation and chamber size.

   D. Because effective cardiac output is reduced, the pulses are weak and the pulse pressure is narrowed.

   E. Surgery is indicated when symptoms develop.

   *Ref.:* 1-3

**COMMENTS: Aortic regurgitation** causes volume overload on the left ventricle, which eventually results in left ventricular dilation and failure. Stroke volume is increased because of the regurgitant fraction, and bounding pulses and wide pulse pressure result. The symptoms are those of congestive heart failure. Angina may occur as a late finding. Syncope is not generally associated with aortic regurgitation, as it is with aortic stenosis. Echocardiography facilitates accurate diagnosis of aortic regurgitation and monitoring of the patient's condition. Indications for surgery include an onset of symptoms or increased left ventricular dimensions even before symptoms occur. Aortic regurgitation may occur as the primary valve pathology, be secondary to valvuloplasty for aortic stenosis, or develop after damage to a normal aortic valve caused by discrete subaortic stenosis or a VSD. The possibility of creating aortic insufficiency is one of the indications for repair of subaortic stenosis and VSDs.

**ANSWER: D**

19. With regard to ASDs, which of the following statements is true?

   A. The magnitude of the shunt is determined by the difference in compliance between the ventricles.

   B. The left ventricle frequently becomes pressure-overloaded.

   C. Increased pulmonary vascular resistance may develop in approximately 40% of patients.

   D. An ASD should be surgically corrected before the patient is 1 year of age to avoid pulmonary hypertension.

   E. Surgical closure with cardiopulmonary bypass (CPB) is the only option for closure.

   *Ref.:* 1-3

**COMMENTS:** Atrial septal defects may produce **large left-to-right shunts** without high pulmonary artery pressure. The magnitude of the shunt is determined by the difference in compliance

between the two ventricles. The shunt occurs during diastole, when blood goes from the atria to the ventricles. Because of the defect, the atria have equal pressure, so the filling pressure for the two ventricles is similar. The amount of blood that goes to each side depends on the amount that each ventricle distends given that filling pressure. Because the right ventricle is more compliant, blood from the left atrium has a tendency to cross the defect and enter the right ventricle, thereby creating the left-to-right shunt. Pulmonary artery pressure may be normal or nearly normal because there is no communication between the two sides during systole. Congestive heart failure eventually develops in about 25% of individuals with ASDs, usually during the third to fourth decade of life if the ASD is left untreated. Pulmonary vascular obstructive disease occurs in about 10% if the ASD is left untreated. Because symptoms rarely occur during the first decade of life, repair is entirely elective. Repair is usually done when the child is at a preschool age (3 to 4 years), a time when the child is large enough for easy closure but has few psychological effects from undergoing the surgery. During the current era, many defects are now closed with transcatheter devices by interventional cardiologists. The majority of **atrial septal defects** are now closed percutaneously. The published literature shows a success rate of 90% to 95% for percutaneous closure and greater than 98% for surgical closure.

**ANSWER: A**

20. Which of the following statements is true regarding TAPVR?

   A. TAPVR is categorized as supracardiac, cardiac, infracardiac, or mixed.

   B. The pathologic condition occurs when the pulmonary veins fail to empty into the right atrium and, instead, connect directly to the left atrium.

   C. The connection between the pulmonary veins and the systemic veins may be obstructed with equal frequency, regardless of whether the connection is supracardiac, cardiac, or infracardiac.

   D. When a patient has obstructed TAPVR, there is reduced pulmonary blood flow, which leaves the lungs relatively dark on a chest radiograph.

   E. A VSD must be present for survival.

   *Ref.:* 1-3

**COMMENTS:** During embryologic development, the four pulmonary veins form a confluence that merges with the back of the left atrium. **Total anomalous pulmonary venous return** is an anomaly in which this connection fails to occur. The pulmonary venous flow then goes through an anomalous vessel that most commonly connects to the innominate vein (supracardiac), the coronary sinus (cardiac), or the portal vein (infracardiac). Supracardiac TAPVR occurs in approximately 50% of cases, cardiac TAPVR in 25%, and infracardiac TAPVR in 20%, with 5% of cases being mixed. Because both systemic and pulmonary venous return goes to the right side of the heart, an ASD must be present to allow blood to go into the left side of the heart and the systemic circulation. The blood returning to the atrium distributes itself between the right and left ventricles according to their relative compliance, as with any large ASD. Because the right ventricle has greater compliance than the left ventricle, there is more pulmonary flow than systemic flow. This is equivalent to a large left-to-right shunt. A serious complication of TAPVR occurs when the connection between the pulmonary venous confluence and the systemic veins is obstructed. With infracardiac TAPVR, obstruction is the rule because pulmonary venous return must go through the hepatic capillary bed. With supracardiac TAPVR, obstruction occurs in only a few patients, and with cardiac TAPVR, obstruction is rare. When obstruction occurs, pulmonary venous pressure is high, which causes severe pulmonary edema.

**ANSWER:** A

21. Which of the following statements is true for ASDs?

    A. Secundum ASDs rarely cause symptoms during infancy.

    B. Secundum ASDs rarely cause residual problems after closure.

    C. Secundum ASDs are part of the spectrum of AV canal defects.

    D. Left ventricular outflow tract obstruction typically develops with secundum ASDs.

    E. Secundum ASDs are typically associated with left axis deviation.

*Ref.:* 1-3

**COMMENTS:** Secundum ASDs and primum **atrial septal defects** have in common left-to-right shunting at the atrial level but are different malformations. Because of their similar atrial-level shunting, they rarely cause symptoms during infancy and generally require elective repair at 1 to 4 years of age. Secundum ASDs seldom cause any residual problems after closure. However, primum ASDs are truly part of the spectrum of AV canal defects (endocardial cushion defects). Therefore, the AV valves are abnormal, and frequently the left AV valve (mitral valve) becomes insufficient with time. Long-term insufficiency requiring valve repair or replacement is a well-known complication. Left ventricular outflow tract obstruction may also develop in patients with primum ASDs. Patients with primum ASDs have left axis deviation on their ECGs, which also distinguishes them from secundum ASDs. Children with Down syndrome have a high incidence of endocardial cushion defects, although secundum ASDs and typical VSDs may be found as well.

**ANSWER:** B

22. With regard to VSDs, which of the following statements is true?

    A. Multiple muscular VSDs ("Swiss cheese") with a large left-to-right shunt may become symptomatic within 1 year of age.

    B. Defects less than 2 cm in diameter are generally well tolerated.

    C. Irreversible pulmonary vascular obstructive disease is relatively common before 1 year of age.

    D. Banding of the pulmonary artery is the operation of choice in infants younger than 2 years.

    E. Subaortic VSDs will close spontaneously.

*Ref.:* 1-3

**COMMENTS: Ventricular septal defects** account for 20% to 30% of congenital heart defects. Associated anomalies are common (e.g., PDA, coarctation, ASD, aortic insufficiency). Defects smaller than 4 to 5 mm in diameter are associated with pulmonary blood flow less than two times systemic flow, with few adverse physiologic consequences. Larger defects can produce cardiac failure, pulmonary hypertension, and death. VSDs are usually asymptomatic during the newborn period. Pulmonary vascular resistance is high, which keeps the left-to-right shunting and pulmonary overcirculation minimized. At 1 to 2 months of age, pulmonary vascular resistance decreases and allows a large left-to-right shunt, which produces symptoms of congestive heart failure. In symptomatic infants with large lesions, surgical correction is indicated. If such infants are left untreated, the increased pulmonary vascular resistance may become irreversible by the age of 2 years. It is rare for irreversible pulmonary vascular resistance to occur before 1 year of age. Up to 40% of VSDs close spontaneously by 2 years of age. Pulmonary artery banding, once widely used in infants with significant VSDs, is now rarely used with the increasing success of definitive closure in younger patients. It may be reserved for patients with multiple muscular VSDs ("Swiss cheese"), a large left-to-right shunt, and early symptomatology within 1 year of age. Repair of a VSD was traditionally performed via ventriculotomy. Advances in operative technique now allow most defects to be closed through the right atrium, with retraction of the tricuspid valve. This procedure avoids disruption of the ventricular wall and potential coronary artery damage. Some defects, particularly muscular defects, may still require ventriculotomy.

**ANSWER:** A

23. Eisenmenger syndrome represents:

    A. A classic conduction defect resulting from inappropriate repair of a VSD

    B. A condition that can occur with VSD, PDA, AV canal defects, transposition of the great arteries, and truncus arteriosus and rarely in association with a large ASD

    C. A condition in which the increased pulmonary vascular resistance from the left-to-right shunt eventually exceeds systemic vascular resistance and causes reversal to a right-to-left shunt and cyanosis

    D. B and C

    E. A and B

*Ref.:* 1-3

**COMMENTS: Eisenmenger syndrome** is the end stage that results from a large left-to-right shunt with fixed pulmonary hypertension secondary to irreversible pulmonary vascular resistance. It can occur with VSD, PDA, AV canal defects, transposition of the great arteries, and truncus arteriosus and rarely in association with a large ASD. The increased pulmonary vascular resistance from the left-to-right shunt eventually exceeds systemic vascular resistance and causes reversal to a right-to-left shunt and cyanosis.

**ANSWER:** D

24. With regard to PDA, which of the following statements is true?

    A. It produces a right-to-left shunt at the level of the great arteries.

    B. Irreversible, increased pulmonary vascular disease generally occurs only in association with another defect.

    C. Because of low cardiac output, children with PDA tend to have narrow pulse pressure.

    D. Indomethacin can be used to close PDAs in term infants but not in premature babies.

    E. The presence of cyanosis is a contraindication to closure.

*Ref.:* 1-3

**COMMENTS: Patent ductus arteriosus** is an abnormal communication between the descending aorta and the pulmonary artery. The ductus arteriosus ordinarily closes after birth in response to rising oxygen tension and numerous other hormonal factors. PDA in premature babies usually involves a structurally normal ductus that fails to close because of the low oxygen tension and surrounding mediators (e.g., increased prostaglandins) that maintain patency of the ductus. By changing the hormonal environment with indomethacin (which blocks prostaglandin production), a PDA in a premature infant may be closed. In a term baby, a PDA is caused by a structurally abnormal ductal wall. Indomethacin therefore has little effect on term infants. If a PDA is large, there is a large left-to-right shunt, with the pulmonary artery being exposed to systemic pressure. These children experience the same course of congestive heart failure followed by increased pulmonary vascular resistance as do children with a large VSD. Like children with a large VSD, Eisenmenger syndrome may develop in children with a large PDA. Cyanosis from Eisenmenger syndrome is a contraindication to closure of a PDA. Because of runoff from the aorta into the low-resistance pulmonary artery during diastole, diastolic pressure in children with a PDA tends to be low, with large pulse pressure.

**ANSWER: E**

25. Prostaglandins may be indicated to maintain ductal patency in which of the following lesions?

    A. Pulmonary atresia with an intact ventricular septum

    B. VSD

    C. Interrupted aortic arch

    D. A and C

    E. All of the above

*Ref.:* 1-3

**COMMENTS: Prostaglandins** (prostacyclin [PGE$_1$]) are useful for maintaining ductal patency in newborns. The indications may be for either right- or left-sided obstructive lesions. If a patient has a right-sided obstructive lesion (e.g., **pulmonary atresia**), pulmonary blood flow may be duct dependent. Prostaglandins may be used to keep the ductus patent until a surgically created systemic-pulmonary artery shunt or definitive repair can be accomplished. With left-sided lesions, such as an **interrupted aortic arch**, blood flow to parts of the systemic circulation may be duct dependent; that is, before repair can be undertaken, the ductus is the only means by which part of the systemic circulation can receive blood flow. Closure of the ductus is lethal in the setting of a severe left-sided obstruction, such as an interrupted aortic arch. In this situation, blood through the ductus flows from the pulmonary artery to the aorta.

**ANSWER: D**

26. Which of the following statements is true regarding complete AV canal defects?

    A. They are associated with cystic fibrosis.

    B. There is one AV orifice with clearly defined mitral and tricuspid valves.

    C. Because most of the shunting occurs at the ventricular level, the natural history of the disease is similar to that of a VSD.

D. The decompression through the atrial part of the defect protects against pulmonary vascular disease.

E. Recurrent ventricular-level shunting is the most common long-term complication of repair.

*Ref.:* 1-3

**COMMENTS:** Common **atrioventricular canal defects** involve abnormal development of the endocardial cushion. The atrial septum, ventricular septum, and AV valves should join at a central point but fail to do so. The patient is usually left with a large defect in the inferior atrial septum and inlet ventricular septum. Instead of the usual mitral and tricuspid valves, there is one large AV valve that separates both atria from both ventricles. Most patients with complete AV canal defects also have Down syndrome. The pathophysiology is that of a large left-to-right shunt, as with a VSD. Pulmonary vascular disease develops somewhat faster with an AV canal than with a VSD, partly because the shunt is both atrial and ventricular and partly because children with Down syndrome have a tendency for the development of early vascular disease. Significant postoperative AV valve regurgitation, usually of the left-sided AV (mitral) valve, may develop. The incidence of reoperation for left-sided AV valve regurgitation is approximately 10% to 15% at 10 years.

**ANSWER: C**

27. Which of the following statements regarding extracorporeal membrane oxygenation (ECMO) is true?

    A. The survival rate is less than 50% when used for neonatal respiratory support.

    B. Survival is equal in adults and children.

    C. Survival with cardiac ECMO is greater than that with respiratory ECMO.

    D. The overall survival rate is 40%.

    E. The lowest survival rate occurs in neonates with meconium aspiration syndrome.

*Ref.:* 1-3

**COMMENTS: Extracorporeal membrane oxygenation** can be used in infants, children, or adults for acute cardiac or respiratory support. Common indications in the pediatric population include meconium aspiration, congenital diaphragmatic hernia, sepsis, and primary pulmonary hypertension, as well as after repair of intracardiac defects. The survival rate in neonates is higher with respiratory than with cardiac causes (77% versus 38%). Adults have much lower survival rates than children. Overall, the survival rate when extracorporeal life support is used is approximately 40%. The highest survival rate is for meconium aspiration syndrome (94%).

**ANSWER: D**

28. With regard to transposition of the great vessels, which of the following statements is not true?

    A. The aorta arises from the right ventricle and carries unoxygenated blood to the body.

    B. The pulmonary artery arises from the left ventricle and carries unoxygenated blood to the lungs.

    C. PDA, VSD, or ASD is necessary for survival (before definitive correction).

D. Pulmonary stenosis occurs in approximately 10% of patients.

E. VSD occurs in approximately 25% of patients.

*Ref.:* 1-3

**COMMENTS: Transposition of the great arteries** is a common form of complex cyanotic heart disease. The aorta arises from the right ventricle and carries unoxygenated blood to the body. The pulmonary artery arises from the left ventricle and carries oxygenated blood to the lungs. For any oxygen to be delivered to the body, there must be mixing between the systemic and pulmonary circuits. This mixing is necessary for survival. The common points of mixing are an ASD, a VSD, and a PDA. If the patient has an intact ventricular septum and a small ASD, it may be necessary to use a large balloon-tipped catheter to enlarge the atrial septum to stabilize the child preoperatively. Transposition of the great arteries has many associated defects, the most common being VSDs and pulmonary stenosis (i.e., left ventricular outflow tract obstruction). Other associations include interrupted aortic arches, coarctation of the aorta, and hypoplastic ventricles. The associated lesions may greatly affect prognosis and treatment. The usual surgical treatment of transposition of the great arteries is the **arterial switch operation**. This operation involves transecting the great vessels just above the semilunar valves and "switching" their positions such that the aorta would come off the left ventricle and the pulmonary artery off the right ventricle. The difficulty of the arterial switch operation involves switching the coronary arteries.

**ANSWER:** B

29. Which of the following statements is true of vascular rings?

A. They may cause decreased perfusion to the lower extremities.

B. The most common associated anomaly is a Kommerell diverticulum.

C. A vascular ring may be manifested as recurrent respiratory infections.

D. Repair of a vascular ring requires a bypass graft.

E. Dysphagia is the most common sign of a vascular ring.

*Ref.:* 1-3

**COMMENTS: A vascular ring** is an encirclement of the trachea and esophagus by an abnormal formation of the arch and great vessels. The most common form is a **double aortic arch**. During early development all fetuses have two aortic arches: a right (posterior) arch and a left (anterior) arch. These arches encircle the forming trachea and esophagus. Ordinarily, the right arch regresses. If both arches persist, the trachea and esophagus become encircled. A double aortic arch may be asymptomatic, but it often causes symptoms related to compression. The trachea is more often

affected, and there may be recurrent respiratory infections. Esophageal compression may be present with or without tracheal symptoms. Although they may occur at any age, symptoms usually develop during infancy or early childhood. Repair consists of dividing the smaller of the two arches, as determined by ultrasound imaging, by magnetic resonance imaging, or at the time of surgery. Repair is generally performed through a left thoracotomy and does not involve CPB. A bypass graft is not necessary for repair. There are other vascular rings in addition to the double aortic arch, and their clinical manifestations, natural history, and principles of repair are similar. A pulmonary artery sling is a vascular congenital anomaly in which the left pulmonary artery originates from the right pulmonary artery and courses posterior to the trachea. Patients are seen in infancy with stridor or recurrent pulmonary infections. One third to one half of patients have associated tracheal stenosis or complete rings, thus giving rise to the term *ring-sling complex*.

**ANSWER:** B, C

30. Which of the following statements regarding pulmonary artery banding is definitely not true?

A. May result in pulmonary artery distortion

B. May result in pulmonary valve damage

C. May result in the development of outflow tract narrowing by muscle band hypertrophy

D. Results in volume loading of the ventricle

E. May not result in adequate protection of the pulmonary vascular bed

*Ref.:* 1-3

**COMMENTS: Pulmonary artery banding** remains a useful palliative maneuver in selected patients with increased pulmonary blood flow. It may result in pulmonary artery distortion, pulmonary damage, or outflow tract narrowing via muscle band hypertrophy. It always results in pressure loading of the ventricle. A loose pulmonary artery band may not adequately protect the pulmonary vascular bed. However, some patients may "grow into" a loose pulmonary artery band.

**ANSWER:** D

## REFERENCES

1. Baue AE, Geha AS, Hammond GL, et al, editors: *Glenn's thoracic and cardiovascular surgery*, Stamford, Conn., 1996, Appleton & Lange.
2. Kirklin JW, Barratt-Boyes BG, editors: *Cardiac surgery*, New York, 1993. Churchill Livingstone,
3. Sellke FW, del Nido PJ, Swanson SJ, editors: *Sabiston and Spencer: surgery of the chest*, ed 8, Philadelphia, 2010, WB Saunders.

# B. Acquired Diseases

*R. Anthony Perez-Tamayo, M.D., Ph.D.; Edward B. Savage, M.D.;
Eric J. Okum, M.D.; and Robert S. D. Higgins, M.D., M.S.H.A.*

1. A 60-year-old man is successfully resuscitated after an episode of sudden cardiac death. Appropriate evaluation and treatment may include all of the following except:

   A. Cardiac catheterization and coronary angiography

   B. If significant coronary stenosis or a left ventricular aneurysm is identified, surgical intervention directed at these targets to achieve satisfactory control of the arrhythmia

   C. Automatic implantable cardioverter-defibrillator (AICD) in patients whose ventricular tachycardia cannot be mapped or medically/surgically controlled

   D. Electrophysiologic studies (EPSs) to determine the mechanism, origin, inducibility, and suppressibility of the arrhythmia

   E. EPS-directed resection

   *Ref.:* 1-3

**COMMENTS: Sudden cardiac death** is a major cause of morbidity and mortality in the United States. Most cases are thought to be of arrhythmogenic origin. The number of survivors is increasing as a result of the rising number of laypeople trained in cardiopulmonary resuscitation, as well as improved prehospital and emergency medical care. Survivors, however, have a 60% chance of recurrence resulting in sudden death during the first 2 years after hospitalization. When evaluating these patients, one must include the following: EPSs to determine the mechanism of the arrhythmia (automatic versus reentrant), to identify the origin of the arrhythmia, and to identify the inducibility and assess the suppressibility of induced arrhythmias by various pharmacologic agents. Cardiac catheterization and coronary angiography should be performed to identify significant coronary stenosis and the presence of a ventricular aneurysm, which may be the arrhythmogenic focus. However, coronary revascularization alone fails to control the arrhythmia, and blind aneurysmectomy (non–EPS directed) often fails because the endocardial origin of the arrhythmia may be distant from the border of the aneurysm. EPS-directed endocardial resection plus encircling endocardial ventriculotomy with or without adjunctive cryoablation has success rates in the range of 90%.

   For inpatients whose arrhythmia cannot be mapped or controlled medically and surgically, an AICD is a last alternative. An AICD is a device that senses ventricular tachycardia/fibrillation through an epicardial or endocardial lead and delivers a defibrillating pulse, originally between two epicardial patches. Currently, the most common form delivers the pulse through a transvenous coil in the right ventricle. An AICD terminates more than 98% of episodes of ventricular fibrillation or ventricular tachycardia and provides the greatest benefit for patients with reduced left ventricular systolic function. A coronary arteriogram should precede the implantation or testing procedure, which has a mortality rate of about 0.5%.

**ANSWER:** B

2. Which of the following is the maximum amount of time that extracorporeal circulation can be tolerated before significant risk for physiologic injury and metabolic defects occurs?

   A. 2 to 4 hours

   B. 6 to 8 hours

   C. 10 to 12 hours

   D. 14 to 16 hours

   E. 18 to 20 hours

   *Ref.:* 1, 2

**COMMENTS:** Tolerance of **extracorporeal circulation (CPB)** is variable. Six to 8 hours is an acceptable range, although physiologic injury may occur earlier. Occasionally, patients undergo longer perfusion with relatively few consequences. With proper myocardial preservation, the heart can be arrested safely for up to 4 hours. Physiologic defects observed with extracorporeal circulation include progressive sludging of blood elements in the capillary microcirculation, red blood cell hemolysis, coagulation defects, denaturation of plasma proteins, fibrinolysis, and activation of inflammatory cascades. The primary culprit within the CPB circuit for these derangements is the oxygenator and its vast surface area for blood–foreign body exposure. **Extracorporeal membrane oxygenation** circuits are increasingly being used in adult patients for circulatory and respiratory support and can be used for weeks at a time. There are several distinctions between CPB and ECMO. Blood–foreign body exposure is limited by shortening the length of the circuit tubing and minimizing priming volume in ECMO. ECMO is used for partial support, and therefore some measure of the circulating volume remains in the patient's native cardiopulmonary system. Advances in technology have produced hollow-fiber oxygenators with a tight and very biocompatible gas-blood interface. This tight interface prevents leakage of plasma, thereby extending the durability of the oxygenator, and keeps the formation of gaseous microbubbles in blood to a minimum, thereby preventing hemolysis and organ damage from gaseous emboli.

**ANSWER:** B

3. All of the following are complications of prolonged extracorporeal circulation except:

   A. Postoperative bleeding

   B. Pancreatitis

   C. Hypertension

   D. Psychosis

   E. Hepatic insufficiency

   *Ref.:* 1, 2

**COMMENTS:** The physiologic and metabolic injuries resulting from **prolonged extracorporeal circulation** are exhibited in several ways. Postoperative bleeding may occur as a result of dilution of clotting factors, destruction of platelets, impairment of platelet function, and improper titration of protamine to reverse systemic heparinization. The coagulation defect may be transient and usually resolves within the first 12 hours following perfusion. The importance of meticulous surgical hemostasis is apparent. Renal and respiratory insufficiency is usually transient and often requires only supportive treatment. Hepatic injury can occur with prolonged support, partly from low cardiac output but potentially from derangements in splanchnic and portal flow. A variety of central nervous system changes may occur. These changes have both metabolic and organic causes and may be manifested as localized or generalized deficits of variable severity and duration. With prolonged nonpulsatile CPB and hypothermia, some patients have elevated serum amylase levels, which fortunately is less frequently associated with the signs and symptoms of pancreatitis.

**ANSWER: C**

4. After aortic valve replacement for calcific aortic stenosis, a patient experiences seizures. All of the following are the most likely causes except:

   A. Air embolism

   B. Calcium emboli

   C. Emboli from a left atrial thrombus

   D. Emboli from aortic atherosclerosis

   E. Extracorporeal circulation

   *Ref.:* 1, 2

**COMMENTS: Seizures** may occur as a manifestation of focal injury to the central nervous system. Air embolism is a result of incomplete evacuation of air from the cardiac chambers following open heart surgery. Evacuation may be facilitated by the use of a left ventricle vent, an aortic vent, or both. The vents are left in place until after the heart is beating. During this time, CPB is gradually reduced, the patient is rotated, and the heart is manipulated to assist in removing air from within the cardiac chambers. Calcium fragments may embolize after the removal of calcific debris from a diseased aortic valve. Cannulation or clamping of a diseased aorta may result in dislodgement of arteriosclerotic debris. Left atrial thrombi are another potential source of cerebral emboli, although these usually occur in patients with mitral stenosis. The usual neurologic deficit observed following prolonged extracorporeal circulation is a transient generalized depression of cerebral function related to sludging of blood elements in the cerebral capillaries, which results in focal areas of stasis and hypoperfusion of the microcirculation.

**ANSWER: E**

5. Indications for coronary artery bypass graft (CABG) surgery include all of the following except:

   A. Severe triple-vessel occlusive disease

   B. Stenosis of the left main coronary artery

   C. Persistent angina and changes on the ECG following percutaneous coronary stenting

   D. Acute myocardial infarction

   E. Development of complications during percutaneous transluminal coronary angioplasty (PTCA)

   *Ref.:* 1, 4

**COMMENTS: Surgical revascularization** provides relief of angina in more than 90% of patients and improves survival in select groups. Patients are referred to as having single-, double-, or triple-vessel disease if significant stenoses are present in one, two, or all three of the major coronary arteries. Numerous studies have concluded that patients with significant triple-vessel disease, especially impaired left ventricular function, are best treated with surgery. Left main artery disease is also a well-accepted indication. Most surgeons and cardiologists agree that double-vessel disease is not always an indication for surgery unless the left anterior descending artery has a severe (>50%) proximal stenosis. Acute myocardial infarction is not an unequivocal indication for surgery. In less than 1% of patients undergoing PTCA do complications requiring surgery develop. Most authorities consider congestive heart failure with pulmonary hypertension (in the absence of mechanical defects such as left ventricular aneurysm, mitral regurgitation, or VSD) the only cardiac contraindication to bypass grafting. Improvements in anesthetic and surgical techniques and methods of myocardial protection have reduced the mortality rate associated with elective coronary artery bypass to approximately 2%. The risk is somewhat higher in certain groups of patients, but even in higher-risk categories, in situations of emergency coronary artery bypass surgery or during revision of failed surgery, the risk rarely exceeds 3% to 5%.

**ANSWER: D**

6. With regard to the surgical treatment of atrial fibrillation with the maze procedure, which of the following is true?

   A. More than 90% of cases of paroxysmal atrial fibrillation arise from an ectopic focus in the sinoatrial node.

   B. The need for mitral valve repair represents a contraindication.

   C. The maze procedure results in a greater than 90% long-term cure rate of atrial fibrillation without antiarrhythmic medications.

   D. The majority of patients will require permanent pacemaker implantation within 1 year of the procedure.

   E. Pulmonary artery ablation alone will reduce the incidence of atrial fibrillation by 50%.

   *Ref.:* 2

**COMMENTS: The Cox maze procedure** is designed to cure atrial fibrillation by creating a series of lesions in the left and right atria that insulate against conduction and propagation of fibrillatory impulses. The lesions, created in the earliest forms of the procedure by incision and anastomosis and currently using different forms of ablative energy, subdivide the atria into a maze of channels, with no channel large enough to allow the formation of macro-reentrant loops. The set of lesions isolating the pulmonary veins is especially important in patients with paroxysmal atrial fibrillation, which originates from ectopic foci in these structures in 95% of cases. The maze procedure can be performed alone or in combination with various other cardiac surgery procedures and is ideally applied in patients with pathologic conditions of the mitral valve, because these disease states are often complicated by atrial fibrillation and exposure of the left atrium is already necessary. The greater than 90% long-term cure rate for atrial fibrillation without antiarrhythmic medication resulting from the maze procedure will often unmask a dysfunctional AV node that requires permanent pacemaker implantation in 20% of patients.

**ANSWER: C**

**7.** After a documented acute myocardial infarction, surgery is indicated in all but which of the following situations?

   A. Postinfarction angina with anatomic lesions not amenable to PTCA

   B. VSDs

   C. Acute mitral regurgitation

   D. Free wall rupture

   E. Atrial tachyarrhythmia

*Ref.: 2, 4*

**COMMENTS: Postinfarction angina** occurs in 10% to 15% of patients, with the incidence increasing to 30% if a thrombolytic agent was used. It generally indicates residual myocardial tissue at risk for subsequent cell death and extension of the infarct. In this setting, cardiac angiography is indicated, with PTCA or surgery performed, depending on the anatomy. **Ventricular septal defects** occur in about 2% of patients following myocardial infarction, generally 3 to 5 days later. Advocates of delayed repair point to better intraoperative demarcation of necrotic and living tissue and a lower incidence of recurrent VSD because of suture line dehiscence. Nevertheless, early surgical intervention is indicated because natural history studies indicate a 25% mortality rate in the untreated at 24 hours and 80% at 4 weeks, respectively. Acute mitral regurgitation resulting from papillary muscle infarction and rupture occurs in less than 2% of patients. Surgery results in a better survival rate than does medical therapy. **Ventricular free wall rupture** occurs 3 to 6 days following transmural myocardial infarction. Although the incidence is not precisely known, medical therapy almost certainly leads to death, thus leaving surgical repair as the only therapeutic option. Postinfarct ventricular tachyarrhythmias can drive a decision for early revascularization, following the dictum that the best antiarrhythmic is oxygenated blood.

**ANSWER: E**

**8.** Refractory angina develops in a 70-year-old woman in the coronary care unit 2 days after being hospitalized for acute myocardial infarction. With regard to coronary artery bypass in this situation, which of the following statements is true?

   A. It should be performed only if left main coronary disease is present.

   B. Operative mortality and long-term survival rates are poor in comparison with those in patients who have unstable angina not precipitated by myocardial infarction.

   C. It should be preceded by thrombolytic therapy if multivessel disease is also present.

   D. The operative mortality rate is less than 5%.

   E. The preoperative work-up should include dobutamine stress echocardiography to assess viability.

*Ref.: 1, 2, 4*

**COMMENTS: Unstable angina** is preceded by myocardial infarction in approximately 50% of patients. The initial treatment of patients with unstable angina involves intensive medical therapy with β-blockers, nitrates, and calcium channel blockers. Patients with refractory angina should undergo emergency PTCA with stenting or CABG surgery. PTCA with stenting may be tried for one- and two-vessel disease, but significant left main artery disease should be approached surgically. Most trials have demonstrated reduced in-hospital and 1-year mortality rates when thrombolytic therapy has been effective in reestablishing flow to ischemic tissue within 4 hours. PTCA with stenting has been used alone and in conjunction with thrombolytic therapy and is associated with a 90% successful reperfusion rate, 10% in-house mortality rate, and 10% to 30% reocclusion rate within 6 months. These modalities have been less effective for multivessel disease and in older patients, those in cardiogenic shock, women, and those with poor left ventricular function. CABG surgery is associated with a 4% mortality rate in patients with unstable angina, with approximately 80% of patients surviving 10 years and 80% experiencing long-term relief of angina. The observation of angina during a hospitalization has no bearing on the benefits of the use of CPB during myocardial revascularization. Persistence of the angina is a strong enough suggestion that viable tissue is at risk and the stress of dobutamine echocardiography would not be justified.

**ANSWER: D**

**9.** Angina develops in a patient 5 years after CABG surgery. Angiography most likely reveals which of the following?

   A. Vein graft thrombosis

   B. Progressive atherosclerosis in the vein graft

   C. Progressive atherosclerosis in the coronary arteries

   D. A dominant right coronary system

   E. Occlusion of the left internal mammary arterial graft

*Ref.: 1, 2, 4*

**COMMENTS:** The rate of **recurrence of angina** following CABG surgery is approximately 5% to 7% per year. Surgery, unfortunately, does not slow the progression of atherosclerosis, which is the primary cause of recurrent symptoms. Graft occlusion may also occur as a result of thrombosis, intimal fibrosis, or fibrous endarteritis. Vein grafts may also be involved with atherosclerosis, which usually occurs later during the postoperative course. Overall, the rate of vein graft patency is approximately 70% to 80% after 5 years. Internal mammary artery grafts have significantly higher long-term patency and improved event-free survival rates in comparison with vein grafts.

**ANSWER: C**

**10.** Indications for surgical resection of a left ventricular aneurysm include all of the following except:

   A. Angina

   B. Congestive heart failure

   C. Systemic arterial emboli

   D. Presence of paradoxical motion with systole

   E. Ventricular tachyarrhythmias refractory to drug therapy

*Ref.: 2, 4*

**COMMENTS:** See Question 11.

**ANSWER: D**

**11.** With regard to surgical treatment of ventricular aneurysm, which of the following statements is true?

   A. Preservation of the left anterior descending artery is mandatory.

   B. All aneurysms should be excised because of the progressive nature of this lesion and the poor prognosis if it is untreated.

C. Complete aneurysmectomy is preferred.

D. Concomitant coronary bypass is generally performed.

E. Repair must be undertaken before a probable rupture.

*Ref.:* 1, 2, 5

COMMENTS: Most **ventricular aneurysms** result from transmural infarction. They frequently involve the anterior left ventricle in the distribution of the left anterior descending artery. The most common complication is congestive heart failure, followed by arrhythmias and angina. Peripheral emboli may occur but are infrequent. Death from rupture of a ventricular aneurysm is an unusual event. Ventricular aneurysms may also be totally asymptomatic, in which case observation rather than resection is usually indicated. Preservation of the left anterior descending artery is preferred, if possible, to provide blood flow to the septum, but preservation is not mandatory. Small aneurysms are generally asymptomatic and can be observed. During surgical resection, total scar removal is not generally performed, but rather, a rim of scar tissue is left by the surgeon to facilitate closure of the defect. Because of the high incidence of concomitant multivessel coronary occlusive disease, approximately 75% of patients considered for aneurysm resection also undergo coronary bypass. The indications for surgical ventricular restoration (SVR) in patients with coronary artery disease and left ventricular aneurysms are a subject of controversy as a result of the **Surgical Treatments for Ischemic Heart Failure** (STICH) trial, reported in 2009. This prospective randomized controlled trial did not demonstrate any difference in mortality or readmission for heart failure in patients who underwent bypass grafting and SVR versus bypass grafting alone a median of 48 months after surgery. Critics of this trial believe that determination of aneurysm size and left ventricular volume did not identify patients most likely to benefit from SVR and that the 19% reduction in end-systolic volume index reported for patients in the SVR plus CABG group falls short of the 30% reduction that they believe is necessary for clinical improvement after this type of surgery. Subgroup analysis and comparison of medical and surgical therapies are still pending from this trial. Actual rupture of a true ventricular aneurysm is rare.

ANSWER: D

12. Treatment of acute pyogenic pericarditis may require which of the following?

A. Parenteral antibiotics active against *Streptococcus* and *Mycobacterium*

B. Initial pericardial aspiration followed by pericardial stripping if there is a recurrence

C. Subxiphoid pericardiotomy

D. Radical pericardiectomy

E. Anterior (phrenic-to-phrenic) pericardiectomy

*Ref.:* 1, 5

COMMENTS: **Pyogenic pericarditis** is rare. Today, it is usually seen in infants or young children, in whom it is associated with a high mortality rate. *Staphylococcus* and gram-negative species are the most common organisms in adults, whereas *Staphylococcus* and *Haemophilus influenzae* predominate in infants and children. Parenteral administration of antibiotics combined with serial pericardial aspiration and occasional intrapericardial instillation of antibiotics is usually adequate treatment. Surgical drainage may be necessary, but radical pericardiectomy is not indicated.

ANSWER: C

13. With regard to chronic constrictive pericarditis, which of the following statements is true?

A. It is usually caused by a previous streptococcal infection.

B. It is characterized by equalization of right- and left-sided pressure.

C. It is best treated with a combination of diuretics and β-blocking agents.

D. Pericardiectomy is successful in 50% of patients.

E. The "RSR sign" on pulmonary artery catheterization during systole is pathognomonic.

*Ref.:* 1, 2, 5

COMMENTS: **Chronic constrictive pericarditis** often occurs secondary to a viral infection, although in most cases the true cause is unknown. Tuberculosis was once thought to be the most frequent cause. The disease is marked by progressive edema, ascites, hepatic enlargement, and dyspnea on exertion. Hemodynamic findings include elevation of right ventricular end-diastolic, right atrial, and central venous pressure to levels equal to those of pulmonary artery wedge and left ventricular end-diastolic pressure. Pericardiectomy is the treatment of choice and is successful in 90% of cases if adequate resection is performed. The "square root sign" is the appearance of the right ventricular waveform during cardiac catheterization in the presence of constrictive pericarditis. It is attributed to rapid filling of the ventricle in early diastole. Initially, filling pressure is normal but becomes substantially increased because of the constrictive pathophysiology. The relatively sudden rise in filling pressure appears as a dip and plateau, or the "square root sign," on the ventricular pressure tracing.

ANSWER: B

14. Following open heart surgery, a patient experiences chest pain, fever, tachycardia, and a pericardial friction rub. Which of the following statements is true?

A. The most likely diagnosis is postoperative mediastinitis.

B. Primary treatment should include surgical exploration.

C. The patient most likely responds well to antibiotics.

D. There is usually an associated leukocytosis or lymphocytosis.

E. This syndrome is generally accompanied by pleural effusion and shortness of breath.

*Ref.:* 1, 5

COMMENTS: Following procedures in which the pericardium is entered, transient pericardial inflammation, known as the **postpericardiotomy syndrome** or **Dressler syndrome**, may occur. Clinical manifestations include fever, pericarditis, pleuritis, and sometimes a pericardial friction rub. The syndrome usually appears 2 to 4 weeks postoperatively, and the erythrocyte sedimentation rate is elevated. There is also leukocytosis with an increase in lymphocytic cells. Patients generally respond well to a short course of an anti-inflammatory agent, although sometimes a corticosteroid is required.

ANSWER: D

15. Three hours after aortic valve replacement, a patient suddenly becomes hypotensive. The cardiac index has decreased from 2.5 to 1.6 L/min. Central venous pressure is 19 mm Hg with a pulmonary artery wedge pressure of 20 mm Hg. Mediastinal drainage over the last hour has been minimal. Immediate treatment should include which of the following?

A. Echocardiogram to assess prosthetic valve function

B. Volume resuscitation to increase cardiac output

C. Afterload reduction with nitroprusside

D. Preload reduction with nitroglycerin

E. Mediastinal exploration

*Ref.:* 1, 2, 4

COMMENTS: Hypotension and low cardiac output following open heart surgery necessitate prompt, careful evaluation. Specific causes include inadequate blood volume, occult bleeding, cardiac tamponade, arrhythmias, myocardial insufficiency, and acidosis. The finding of elevated filling pressure with equalization of right- and left-sided pressures suggests the diagnosis of cardiac tamponade, in which case immediate reoperation is mandatory. Substantial elevation of filling pressure in association with low cardiac output may also be indicative of cardiac failure, which may be treated with inotropic agents, digitalis, and intra-aortic balloon counterpulsation. Chest radiography is of variable diagnostic value but occasionally allows detection of occult accumulation of blood in a pleural space.

ANSWER: E

16. Aortic stenosis in an adult may result from all of the following except:

A. Ehlers-Danlos syndrome

B. Marfan syndrome

C. Rheumatic fever

D. Syphilis

E. Bacterial endocarditis

*Ref.:* 1, 5

COMMENTS: Aortic stenosis in an adult may result from rheumatic fever or from a congenital valve deformity. A congenital bicuspid valve may remain asymptomatic for many years, but the deformed valve is susceptible to endocarditis, and calcification and symptomatic stenosis eventually develop. Aortic insufficiency commonly follows bacterial endocarditis. Aortic insufficiency may also result from dilation of the aortic annulus because of an ascending aortic aneurysm, as seen with Marfan syndrome, Ehlers-Danlos syndrome, or more rarely, syphilis.

ANSWER: C

17. Clinical manifestations of severe aortic valve stenosis include all of the following except:

A. Syncope

B. Holosystolic murmur

C. Angina pectoris

D. Dyspnea on exertion

E. Atrial fibrillation

*Ref.:* 1, 5

COMMENTS: Characteristically, patients with **aortic stenosis** remain asymptomatic for many years but deteriorate rapidly once symptoms begin. Angina pectoris develops in about two thirds of patients. Left ventricular hypertrophy, increased left ventricular diastolic volume, and prolongation of the isometric contraction phase and systolic ejection time are compensatory mechanisms to allow a longer period of ventricular emptying. However, the duration of diastolic coronary perfusion to the hypertrophied ventricle is decreased, which gives rise to angina pectoris, even in the absence of primary coronary artery disease. Syncope, present in one third of patients, also reflects impaired cardiac output. Signs of left ventricular failure and atrial fibrillation resulting in elevated left atrial pressure are evidence of more advanced disease. A crescendo-decrescendo murmur that radiates to the neck and is accompanied by a thrill is typical of severe aortic stenosis.

ANSWER: B

18. Indications for surgery in patients with aortic stenosis include all of the following except:

A. All symptomatic patients

B. Systolic pressure gradient greater than 50 mm Hg in asymptomatic patients

C. Associated pericardial effusion

D. Valvular cross-sectional area smaller than 1 cm$^2$

E. Serial radiographic evidence of rapid cardiac enlargement

*Ref.:* 1, 5

COMMENTS: Once symptoms develop in patients with **aortic stenosis**, the prognosis is poor. With angina or syncope, the average life expectancy of untreated patients is 2 to 3 years. Death occurs 1 to 2 years after left ventricular failure. Sudden death occurs more frequently with aortic stenosis than with any other valvular lesion. It accounts for approximately 20% of deaths from aortic stenosis and is always a risk, but it occurs more frequently in symptomatic patients. The loudness of the classic systolic diamond-shaped ejection murmur heard over the aortic area and the apex does not have prognostic significance. All symptomatic patients require prompt **valve replacement** because of the high risk for sudden death and deterioration. Peak systolic gradients across the valve of greater than 50 mm Hg and cross-sectional areas of 0.8 to 1.0 cm$^2$ are generally found with moderate to severe aortic stenosis and are indications for valve replacement, even if symptoms are absent. Serial radiographic evidence of rapid cardiac enlargement is an ominous sign in patients with aortic stenosis and is an urgent indication for surgery. Severe stenosis (based on the cross-sectional area) but a low transvalvular gradient may result from compromised ventricular function, which increases the risk associated with valve replacement. The 5-year survival rate following aortic valve replacement is approximately 80%.

ANSWER: C

19. With regard to the selection of prosthetic heart valves, all of the following statements are true except:

A. Free aortic homograft valves have a lower incidence of infective endocarditis than do porcine valves.

B. Bioprosthetic valves should be avoided in patients with chronic renal failure.

C. Mechanical valves should be avoided in children.

D. Current bioprosthetic valves now have durability equivalent to that of mechanical valves.

E. Reconstructed mitral valves have limited durability and offer no advantage over valve replacement.

*Ref.:* 1, 2, 4, 5

**COMMENTS:** The ideal **prosthetic heart valve** has yet to be developed. Selection is based on the patient's characteristics, the operative findings, and the surgeon's preference. **Bioprosthetic valves** (glutaraldehyde-fixed porcine heterografts or bovine pericardium) have a low rate of associated thromboembolism, and therefore these patients do not require long-term anticoagulation. The problem with bioprosthetic valves, however, is long-term durability. Although the latest-generation valves are more durable, the reoperation rate at 10 years is less than 5% in patients older than 65. These valves are contraindicated in children and in patients younger than 20 to 30 years because structural deterioration begins to develop at 8 to 10 years. In the past, they were not recommended for renal failure patients because of calcification, but recent series show no survival advantage over mechanical valves in this population.

Mechanical heart valves are more durable, but their usefulness is limited by the need for permanent anticoagulation, which is contraindicated in certain clinical states (e.g., pregnancy, coagulopathy, ulcer disease). Thromboembolic complications occur at an annual rate of 1% to 2%, even in patients with adequate anticoagulation. Patients with mechanical valves require permanent anticoagulation therapy, which carries a risk for major hemorrhage of approximately 1% per year. The risk for prosthetic valve endocarditis is about 1% to 2% per year for both bioprosthetic and mechanical valves. Because of the low recurrence rate of endocarditis, free aortic homograft valves are advantageous in the setting of active endocarditis. Even with small valves, there is virtually no gradient across the homograft valve and a markedly decreased incidence of valve cusp calcification in young patients.

Mitral valve reconstruction is preferable to replacement whenever possible because of the freedom from prosthetic valve complications. Chronic anticoagulant therapy is not needed, and endocarditis is rare. Durability has been satisfactory, with approximately 90% of patients remaining free of the need for late valve replacement at 5 years after surgery.

**ANSWER:** D

20. Cardiac catheterization of a 50-year-old man with a recent history of dyspnea on exertion, hemoptysis, and paroxysmal nocturnal dyspnea demonstrates a left atrial pressure of 28 mm Hg. One of the primary determinants of this pressure includes which of the following?

A. Pulmonary artery pressure

B. Cross-sectional area of the mitral opening

C. Temperature of the blood

D. Plasma viscosity

E. Mean systemic arterial pressure

*Ref.:* 1, 2

**COMMENTS:** The primary physiologic consequences of **mitral stenosis** are increased left atrial pressure, decreased cardiac output, and increased pulmonary vascular resistance. The clinical manifestations of these changes include the typical symptoms of congestive heart failure, pulmonary edema, and right-sided heart failure,

as well as atrial fibrillation and arterial embolism. Left atrial pressure is determined by the size of the mitral orifice, cardiac output, and heart rate. The severity of disease is best classified by calculating the cross-sectional area of the valve, which takes into consideration both the pressure gradient and cardiac output. A mitral valve area of approximately 1 cm$^2$ or less is indicative of significant stenosis, although low flow rates and the presence of mitral regurgitation may influence calculations. When left atrial pressure exceeds plasma oncotic pressure (24 to 30 mm Hg), pulmonary edema develops.

**ANSWER:** B

21. Indications for valve replacement in patients with significant mitral stenosis include all of the following except:

A. Congestive heart failure

B. Pulmonary hypertension

C. Atrial fibrillation

D. Asymptomatic status

E. Systemic embolization

*Ref.:* 1

**COMMENTS:** See Question 22.

**ANSWER:** D

22. With regard to the results of surgical treatment of symptomatic mitral stenosis, which of the following statements is false?

A. The survival rate is higher than that after medical therapy.

B. Commissurotomy decreases the risk for systemic embolization and endocarditis.

C. Pulmonary vascular resistance usually diminishes following valve replacement or commissurotomy.

D. The 10-year survival rate exceeds 90%.

E. Recurrent valvular dysfunction is best treated by mitral valve repair.

*Ref.:* 1

**COMMENTS:** The natural history of **mitral stenosis** is one of progressive manifestation of symptoms. Treatment of mitral stenosis is a judicious combination of medical and surgical therapies. Most asymptomatic patients are treated medically and observed. Symptomatic patients who receive only medical treatment eventually die of their cardiac disease. Indications for operative intervention include congestive heart failure (with New York Heart Association class III or IV symptoms), onset of atrial fibrillation with significant mitral stenosis, pulmonary hypertension, systemic embolization, and infective endocarditis. Surgical therapy is also recommended for patients who have mild symptoms and a severe reduction in valvular area. In this situation, mitral commissurotomy can be performed if leaflet flexibility and the subvalvular apparatus are preserved. This operation produces physiologic and clinical improvements, but these benefits tend to deteriorate. Recurrent valvular dysfunction that necessitates treatment is almost always best treated by valve replacement.

**ANSWER:** E

23. Which of the following is the most common cause of mitral insufficiency in Western countries?

A. Bacterial endocarditis

B. Degenerative mitral valve disease

C. Marfan syndrome

D. Silent myocardial infarction

E. Rupture of the chordae tendineae

*Ref.:* 1, 2, 5

COMMENTS: See Question 24.

ANSWER: B

24. With regard to patients with mitral regurgitation versus those with mitral stenosis, which of the following statements is true?

A. Left ventricular failure is more common.

B. Atrial fibrillation rarely develops.

C. Systemic emboli are frequent.

D. The postoperative prognosis is better with replacement than with repair.

E. Pulmonary hypertension usually fails to resolve following valve replacement.

*Ref.:* 1, 4

COMMENTS: **Degenerative mitral valve disease** (e.g., **Barlow disease**) is the most common cause of mitral regurgitation. Worldwide, rheumatic heart disease is a major cause, and it produces both stenosis and regurgitation. Although mitral stenosis almost exclusively results from rheumatic fever, mitral regurgitation may have other causes, including mitral valve prolapse, idiopathic calcification, bacterial endocarditis, chordae rupture, and ischemic heart disease. A cause other than rheumatic fever is often suspected on the basis of the history and clinical findings. The physical signs of pulmonary hypertension and right heart failure produced by mitral regurgitation are similar to those seen with mitral stenosis. Unlike patients with mitral stenosis, however, moderate to severe mitral regurgitation can be tolerated for many years with minor symptoms until left ventricular failure ultimately develops as a result of chronic overload. Atrial fibrillation is a common manifestation of mitral regurgitation. Embolization does occur, but it is less common than with mitral stenosis. The natural history of mitral regurgitation and the results of operative correction are somewhat more variable than those of mitral stenosis because of the different etiologic factors that may produce mitral incompetence. Clinical severity depends on the degree of regurgitation, the status of left ventricular function, and the course of valve disease.

In patients with infective endocarditis, trauma, or chordae rupture, emergency surgery is required and can be lifesaving. The long-term prognosis with surgery is poor in patients with ischemic mitral regurgitation and poor ventricular function and in elderly patients with severe associated conditions. Pulmonary hypertension usually resolves after successful valve repair or replacement. Repair is associated with better survival rates than replacement. Some measure of this advantage may be attributed to preservation of the subvalvular apparatus and its relationship to the ventricular walls.

ANSWER: A

25. A 75-year-old man with a history of dyspnea on exertion, palpitations, and episodes of severe diaphoresis has a high-pitched diastolic murmur along the left sternal border and a blood pressure of 140/60 mm Hg. Expected findings include which of the following?

A. Systolic ejection murmur

B. Enlargement of the left ventricle on chest radiographs

C. Atrial fibrillation

D. History of syphilis

E. Weak peripheral pulses

*Ref.:* 1

COMMENTS: Common symptoms of **aortic insufficiency** include angina, progressive dyspnea, palpitations, and peripheral vasomotor changes. Signs of pulmonary congestion occur later as left ventricular failure develops. Findings on physical examination include a normal cardiac rhythm and bounding peripheral pulses because of the widened pulse pressure. The classic diastolic murmur is present and is accentuated when the patient leans forward. A systolic ejection murmur may also be heard but usually represents aortic stenosis. Enlargement of the left ventricle is seen on chest radiographs or echocardiography and represents the ventricular response to the mixed pressure and volume overload of aortic insufficiency.

ANSWER: B

26. Indications for operative intervention to correct aortic insufficiency include which of the following?

A. The finding of aortic insufficiency alone, which warrants correction even in asymptomatic patients

B. Loudness and length of the diastolic murmur

C. Left ventricular end-diastolic volume of 40 mL/m$^2$

D. Magnitude of the regurgitation

E. Age of the patient

*Ref.:* 1, 4

COMMENTS: Patients with **aortic insufficiency** generally remain asymptomatic for many years, although there is substantial variability. Progressive symptoms of heart failure or ischemia and increasing left ventricular size on chest radiography or echocardiography are considered indications for surgery. The loudness of the diastolic murmur is not correlated with the severity of the disease. The length of the murmur to some extent reflects the patient's physiologic status in that a longer murmur indicates a greater degree of regurgitation. Short murmurs may be heard, however, in patients with early disease and minimal regurgitation and in those with end-stage disease and elevated left ventricular end-diastolic pressure. A left ventricular end-diastolic volume of 55 mL/m$^2$ is generally accepted as an indication for aortic valve surgery. Severe ("wide-open") aortic insufficiency is poorly tolerated and indicates the need for replacement.

ANSWER: D

27. All of the following statements commonly apply to tricuspid valvular disease except:

A. Replacement carries a significant risk for heart block.

B. Intravenous drug abuse is a common cause of tricuspid valvular endocarditis.

C. Total valve excision is well tolerated because of the passive nature of the right atrium.

D. Permanent epicardial pacing leads may be necessary with mechanical valves.

E. The lower-pressure right-sided valve lends itself well to repair.

*Ref.:* 1, 5

**COMMENTS:** The location of the AV node along the base of the septal leaflet (triangle of Koch) exposes this structure to injury. Because transvenous pacing leads are not practical with a mechanical valve replacement, epicardial leads are often left in place in anticipation of treatment of complete heart block. Isolated organic disease of the **tricuspid valve** is most commonly seen as a result of endocarditis secondary to intravenous drug abuse. Total valve excision without replacement has occasionally been an alternative in this difficult situation but is not well tolerated long term. The lower pressures of the right ventricle and right atrium and the size of the tricuspid annulus allow the opportunity for a variety of repair techniques, including bicuspidization, wherein one third of the circumference of the valve can be sewn shut.

**ANSWER: C**

28. A 30-year-old man arrives at the emergency department following a high-impact automobile accident. The initial chest radiograph demonstrates a widened mediastinum. Which of the following statements is true?

A. Despite normal blood pressure, the patient should be explored to drain the hemopericardium before impending tamponade occurs.

B. The finding of normally palpable femoral pulses makes aortic rupture unlikely, and the patient should be managed medically with β-blocking agents.

C. Aortography is the "gold standard" diagnostic evaluation.

D. The most common site of aortic disruption is the proximal arch, which should be approached through a left thoracotomy.

E. Surgical repair of traumatic aortic rupture carries a 15% to 20% incidence of paraplegia, but it is the only effective therapy.

*Ref.:* 1, 4

**COMMENTS: Traumatic rupture of the aorta** requires urgent diagnosis and therapy. Most patients with this lesion do not reach the hospital alive. The history of a sudden deceleration injury along with chest radiographic findings of a widened mediastinum and loss of the aortic knob contour is strongly suggestive of the diagnosis. Aortography demonstrates the site of injury. Ninety-five percent of traumatic disruptions occur in the proximal descending aorta, just distal to the left subclavian artery, and are best approached through a left thoracotomy. Open surgical repair is the traditional treatment option and is associated with paraplegia in approximately 5% of patients. In the past, simple cross-clamping during repair was often used, but techniques that provide distal perfusion during clamping, such as left atriofemoral bypass, femorofemoral partial bypass, and the Gott shunt, have become the standards of care. Endovascular approaches using stent grafts to exclude the transection are being used with increasing frequency, particularly in patients with complex multisystem trauma, who might not tolerate the anticoagulation necessary during CPB. These grafts can be deployed with or without exclusion of the left subclavian artery as required by the pathology, with subsequent bypass of this vessel performed if needed. Although stent grafts appear to be safe and effective for this application, the long-term results are still being studied.

**ANSWER: C**

29. Which cardiac chamber is most frequently injured by penetrating trauma?

A. Left ventricle

B. Right ventricle

C. Left atrium

D. Right atrium

E. Equivalent incidence in all four chambers

*Ref.:* 1, 2

**COMMENTS:** The right ventricle is the most anterior chamber of the heart and consequently is the area most susceptible to penetrating injury. **Cardiac injury** may produce exsanguination, cardiac tamponade, and rarely, cardiac failure secondary to damage to a major coronary artery, a valve, or the conduction system. The key to saving patients who arrive at the emergency department with cardiac injury is prompt recognition and treatment of tamponade while other resuscitative measures are instituted. Pericardiocentesis can be lifesaving as well as diagnostic while the operating room is being made ready. Most penetrating injuries can be treated without the need to resort to pump support. Nonpenetrating cardiac trauma usually produces diffuse contusion, which warrants cardiac monitoring.

**ANSWER: B**

30. Which of the following is the most common primary cardiac neoplasm?

A. Myxoma

B. Rhabdomyoma

C. Sarcoma

D. Lymphoma

E. Metastatic sarcoma

*Ref.:* 1, 2

**COMMENTS:** The most common **cardiac neoplasms** are metastatic. Primary cardiac tumors are rare, with an incidence of 0.33% noted on postmortem studies. Most primary cardiac neoplasms are benign, and of them, myxoma is the most common, followed by rhabdomyoma. Approximately 20% of primary tumors are malignant. They are almost always rhabdomyosarcomas and angiosarcomas, and they generally have systemic metastases at the time of diagnosis. The clinical manifestations of cardiac tumors are the result of local invasion, mass effect, embolization, or systemic constitutional signs such as fever, malaise, weight loss, and autoimmune phenomena, particularly associated with atrial myxomas. Echocardiography is the initial diagnostic technique of choice, followed by computed tomography, magnetic resonance imaging, and transesophageal echocardiography. Myxomas constitute 50% of benign primary cardiac tumors. They are most frequently found in women and are usually located in the left atrium.

**ANSWER: A**

**31.** The physiologic effects of the intra-aortic balloon pump (IABP) include which of the following?

A. Decreased cardiac afterload

B. Decreased coronary blood flow

C. Increased left ventricular end-diastolic pressure

D. Decreased cerebral perfusion

E. Increased left ventricular preload

*Ref.:* 1, 2

**COMMENTS:** An electronically synchronized **intra-aortic balloon pump** that inflates during diastole and deflates at the onset of systole has physiologic effects that both decrease myocardial oxygen consumption and increase coronary blood flow. The IABP decreases systolic blood pressure, decreases time during systole, and improves emptying of the heart (decreased radius). Deflation of the IABP reduces impedance to aortic flow, thereby reducing afterload and improving cardiac output. Left ventricular end-diastolic volume and pressure are reduced, and diastolic coronary blood flow is enhanced, particularly in failing hearts. Pulmonary artery diastolic pressure is decreased, thereby reducing left ventricular preload.

**ANSWER:** A

**32.** Which of the following statements describes the clinical effects of the IABP?

A. Use of an IABP in patients with myocardial infarction and cardiogenic shock decreases infarct size.

B. Most patients using an IABP for cardiogenic shock after myocardial infarction can be weaned from this device.

C. An IABP effectively relieves pain in patients with unstable angina.

D. An IABP is not indicated for support of cardiac failure following CBP because of the availability of ventricular assist devices.

E. An IABP is indicated in patients with severe aortic insufficiency to decrease peripheral resistance.

*Ref.:* 1

**COMMENTS:** Indications for use of the **intra-aortic balloon pump** include the following: cardiac failure after CPB, refractory unstable angina, preoperative treatment of septal defects, mitral regurgitation, arrhythmias, ventricular aneurysms, and occasionally, cardiogenic shock. The IABP is used to treat cardiogenic shock associated with myocardial infarction, but only 15% to 20% of patients can be weaned successfully from this device, and there is no conclusive evidence that an IABP decreases infarct size. The IABP is particularly effective in controlling pain in patients with angina refractory to pharmacologic manipulation. The device has also been successful in the support of patients with cardiac failure following CPB. Most such patients can be weaned successfully, with excellent long-term survival. Severe aortic insufficiency is a contraindication to use of the IABP because regurgitation and cardiac failure are exacerbated with its use.

**ANSWER:** C

**33.** Which of the following is not an indication for placement of a permanent cardiac pacemaker?

A. Sick sinus syndrome

B. Complete AV block

C. Mobitz type I AV block

D. Mobitz type II AV block

E. Stokes-Adams attacks

*Ref.:* 1, 3

**COMMENTS:** There is some disagreement regarding the indications for temporary or permanent **cardiac pacing**. Most agree that the indications for permanent pacing include the following: severe or symptomatic sick sinus syndrome, Mobitz type II AV block (because it frequently leads to complete AV block), complete AV block, symptomatic bilateral bundle branch block, and bifascicular or incomplete trifascicular block with an intermittent complete AV block following myocardial infarction. Stokes-Adams attacks, which consist of intermittent syncopal episodes and sometimes convulsions, are manifestations of complete heart block. Mobitz type I AV block (Wenckebach block) rarely necessitates pacing.

**ANSWER:** C

**34.** Open cardiac massage may be indicated in patients with which of the following?

A. Blunt thoracic trauma

B. Penetrating thoracic trauma

C. Barrel chest

D. Spinal deformities

E. Postoperative CABG patient with cardiac arrest

*Ref.:* 1

**COMMENTS:** **External cardiac massage** transmits pressure and flow energy to the cardiovascular system by direct cardiac compression. The stroke work is generated through forceful displacement of the chest wall, which compresses the ventricles, closes the mitral valve, opens the aortic valve, and produces unidirectional pressure and flow. Intrathoracic pressure, once considered a more plausible explanation for the beneficial effect of closed cardiac massage, accounts for less than 25% of cavitary cardiac pressure. Stroke volume is optimized by compressions of high velocity, moderate force, and brief duration. Coronary artery flow occurs during diastole and is optimized at a compression rate of 100 to 120/min. Open methods are used when arrest occurs after cardiac surgery and in cases of thoracic injury when cardiac tamponade, massive intrathoracic hemorrhage, penetrating cardiac injury, or an open pericardium is suspected. It may be necessary in patients with a barrel chest, emphysema, or spinal deformities because closed chest resuscitation is sometimes unsuccessful in such settings. Most patients with cardiac arrest in the field following blunt thoracic trauma cannot be successfully resuscitated even by open cardiac massage. Those who survive the initial episode may have a dismal outcome.

**ANSWER:** A

**35.** With regard to blood conservation during cardiac surgery, which of the following statements is true?

A. Transfusion of blood components during or after cardiac surgery is largely unavoidable.

B. The risks associated with transfusions are primarily related to red blood cells, not plasma.

C. Cardiotomy suction can reclaim blood while not increasing the incidence of microembolization.

D. Antifibrinolytics, such as ε-aminocaproic acid, can reduce bleeding.

E. Aprotinin has both antifibrinolytic and renal-protective effects.

*Ref.:* 5

**COMMENTS:** Strict **blood conservation** should be practiced by meticulous hemostasis during surgery and the use of blood reclamation systems such as the Cell Saver suction. During routine procedures, transfusions can usually be avoided. The risks associated with the transfusion of blood components such as platelets and plasma are similar to those associated with the transfusion of red blood cells. Cardiotomy suction returns blood shed from the mediastinum to the CPB circuit but in so doing draws up lipid globules and pericardial debris that can escape the filters. ε-Aminocaproic acid (Amicar) and tranexamic acid (Cyklokapron) are antifibrinolytic agents that have been shown to reduce postoperative blood loss. Aprotinin (Trasylol) is also an effective antifibrinolytic, but large retrospective series suggested an increased incidence of renal dysfunction and mortality, and the drug was withdrawn from use in 2008.

**ANSWER:** D

**36.** Which of the following statements regarding adult cardiac transplantation is true?

A. Despite improved immunosuppression, the 5-year survival rate following cardiac transplantation is approximately 50%.

B. The number of cardiac transplants performed annually in the United States is limited by the number of donors rather than by the number of suitable recipients.

C. Patients with ventricular assist devices who survive to transplantation have significantly greater 1-year mortality rates than do those who receive transplants primarily.

D. Coronary occlusive disease, otherwise known as "graft vasculopathy," is relatively rare and has the same pathophysiology and morphology as atherosclerosis.

E. With improved medical therapy available, the number of patients awaiting a heart transplant has remained relatively constant.

*Ref.:* 1, 2, 4

**COMMENTS:** Results following **cardiac transplantation** have continued to improve, largely because of improved immunosuppression. Currently, the 1-year survival rate is approximately 80%, and the 5-year survival rate is 65% to 70%. The number of transplants performed annually is limited almost solely by the number of available donors. The development of coronary occlusive disease in the transplanted heart, or "graft vasculopathy," remains a major determinant of long-term survival. Many researchers believe that it is a manifestation of a low-intensity, chronic form of rejection. The number of cardiac transplants performed annually has remained relatively constant, whereas the number of patients waiting continues to increase. Although patients requiring ventricular assist devices as a bridge to transplantation are clearly sicker, those who survive to transplantation have comparable posttransplant survival rates at 1 year.

**ANSWER:** B

**REFERENCES**

1. Sellke FW, del Nido PJ, Swanson SJ, editors: *Sabiston and Spencer: surgery of the chest,* ed 8, Philadelphia, 2010,WB Saunders.
2. Cohn LH, Edmunds LH, editors: *Cardiac surgery in the adult,* ed 3, New York, 2009, McGraw-Hill.
3. American Heart Association, American College of Cardiology, North American Society of Pacing and Electrophysiology: 2002 Guidelines, *J Am Coll Cardiol* 51:1–62, 2008.
4. Yang SC, Cameron DE, editors: *Current therapy in thoracic and cardiovascular surgery,* Philadelphia, 2004, CV Mosby.
5. Kaiser LF, Kron IL, Spray TL, editors: *Mastery of cardiothoracic surgery,* ed 2, Philadelphia, 2007, Lippincott-Raven.

# CHAPTER 28

# Vascular Surgery

*Chad E. Jacobs, M.D., and Walter J. McCarthy, M.D.*

## A. Vascular Surgery Principles

*Ferenc P. Nagy, M.D.*

1. Which of the following is not an independent risk factor for the development of coronary and peripheral atherosclerosis?

   A. Cigarette smoking

   B. Hypercholesterolemia

   C. Diabetes mellitus

   D. Hypertension

   E. Hypercoagulable conditions

   *Ref.:* 1-3

**COMMENTS:** Hypercoagulable conditions are associated with an increased risk for thrombosis, but they have not been shown to be an independent **risk factor for atherosclerosis**. Smoking is a risk factor because of the release of oxidative free radicals, which damage the vascular endothelium. Hypercholesterolemia with total serum levels greater than 200 mg/dL and elevated low-density lipoprotein fractions is also associated with increased risk. Diabetes mellitus and hypertension are independent risk factors in proportion to their severity.

**ANSWER:** E

2. Which of the following statements regarding claudication is true?

   A. The term *claudication* originated from the Latin root word meaning "to shuffle."

   B. Without intervention, the risk for limb loss approaches 15% at 5 years.

   C. It is not alleviated significantly with cilostazol.

   D. It can be managed successfully without arteriography, balloon angioplasty, or surgery in most cases.

   E. The optimal treatment is limited exercise and minimal walking per day.

   *Ref.:* 1-5

**COMMENTS: Claudication** is derived from the Latin verb meaning "to limp." The risk for loss of limb in all claudicant patients is 5% over a 5-year period. The risk for limb loss drops substantially, from 12% to 2%, if a patient successfully stops smoking. Claudication can usually be treated safely with medication. Several medications, including pentoxifylline and cilostazol, have been shown to improve walking distance. "Stop smoking and keep walking" are five words that sum up the treatment strategy for most patients. A regular, organized walking program generally doubles walking distance.

**ANSWER:** D

3. Which of the following describes chronic leg ulcers?

   A. The cause of ulcers often cannot be determined by their locations on the leg.

   B. Venous ulcers are seldom located on the foot.

   C. Arterial ulcers are seldom located on the leg.

   D. Leg ulcers affect diabetic patients less often than other patient groups.

   E. Ulcer healing is improved more significantly with balloon angioplasty than with arterial bypass.

   *Ref.:* 1, 4, 5

**COMMENTS:** Chronic venous insufficiency causes characteristic dermal changes, including hyperpigmentation, thickened skin, and ulceration in the gaiter region, named for an item of clothing that covers the leg from the ankle to the knee. **Venous ulcers** usually occur at the medial malleoli but seldom extend below the ankles. **Arterial ulcers** form at the distal aspect of the region that has compromised arterial circulation. They usually result in ulcers of the toes or foot, but islands of ischemia can occur more proximally on the leg, especially the anterior aspect. Diabetic patients can form neurotrophic ulcers. The neuropathy that afflicts patients with long-standing diabetes causes wasting of the muscles of the foot and collapse of the standard architecture of the foot, which leads to pressure points between the toes and at the metatarsal heads. Strict avoidance of weight bearing is essential for these pressure ulcers to heal when the arterial circulation is adequate. If the arterial circulation is compromised, these patients usually need arterial leg bypass operations, although balloon angioplasty can also heal these ulcers.

**ANSWER:** B

4. Which of the following is characteristic of ischemic extremity rest pain?

   A. Initially occurs mostly in the morning

   B. Can be relieved by placing the involved extremity in the supine position

   C. Usually located at the toes

   D. Can be relieved by intravenous heparin

   E. Can be relieved with cilostazol (Pletal)

   *Ref.:* 1-4

**COMMENTS:** Extremity angina occurs most commonly at night because when patients with severe lower extremity arterial insufficiency lie supine, they lose the added benefit of gravity for perfusing the lower extremity. Patients with nocturnal **ischemic rest pain** quickly discover that walking, standing, or sleeping in a chair relieves this pain, which is centered over the metatarsal heads, not the toes. Pain in the toes suggests gout or an infection. Intravenous heparin causes vasodilation by promoting the release of nitric oxide, thereby improving extremity arterial circulation. Intravenous heparin can reduce rest pain until the arterial circulation can be improved with a bypass operation or angioplasty. Cilostazol improves claudication-impaired distance walking but has not been shown to be effective in treating ischemic rest pain.

**ANSWER:** D

5. Which of the following characteristics of leg swelling from venous insufficiency or lymphedema is true?

   A. Edema forms when hydrostatic pressure in the interstitium is higher than that in the lymphatics or venules.

   B. Venous insufficiency causes pigmentation and hypertrophic changes in the skin over the ankle and results in late lymphedema with fibrosis.

   C. Lymphedema can be diagnosed by ultrasound imaging.

   D. Operative intervention can treat venous insufficiency and is commonly used for lymphedema.

   E. Lymphedema may be pitting in form.

   *Ref.:* 1-3

**COMMENTS: Edema formation** is governed by the balance between hydrostatic and oncotic pressure in the interstitium versus the lymphatics and venules. Hyperpigmentation with cicatrix formation in the gaiter region (legs from the ankles to the knees) is pathognomonic of venous insufficiency and is caused by the breakdown of extravascular red blood cells and subcutaneous scar tissue (liposclerosis). With severe cases of untreated chronic venous insufficiency, such scar tissue formation can cause local destruction of the leg lymphatics and secondary formation of lymphedema. Any severe hypoproteinemia can cause lymphedema. Lymphedema may appear early as a pitting form, but after subsequent protein deposition in the extremity and damage to the lymphatics, the adipose tissue fibroses and the skin thickens. **Venous insufficiency** can be recognized clinically by filling of varices, as well as on color Doppler imaging. Because of the size of the lymphatics, they are not visible on ultrasound imaging, and only nonspecific subcutaneous edema may be visible. Operations for lymphedema are not generally performed. Operations for venous insufficiency include perforator vein ligation, varicose vein ligation

and stripping, deep vein valvoplasty, and laser and radiofrequency ablation of the greater and lesser saphenous veins.

**ANSWER:** B

6. A patient with severe peripheral vascular disease underwent aortobi-iliac bypass grafting 9 months earlier and now has hematochezia and suffered a syncopal episode. Along with the administration of intravenous antibiotics, appropriate treatment or diagnostic modalities include which of the following?

   A. Upper endoscopy (esophagogastroduodenoscopy) and magnetic resonance imaging (MRI)

   B. Angiography and tagged red blood cell scanning

   C. Bilateral axillofemoral bypass and delayed removal of the graft

   D. Unilateral axillofemoral and femorofemoral bypass followed by removal of the graft

   E. Colonoscopy

   *Ref.:* 1, 3

**COMMENTS:** The general approach to the treatment of **aortoenteric fistulas** and infections involves prompt diagnosis, administration of antibiotics, removal of the entire prosthesis, and re-establishment of vascular continuity through noncontaminated fields. MRI has the highest sensitivity for diagnosing graft infections but is ill suited to unstable patients, whereas computed tomography (CT) is fast and shows abnormal findings 91% of the time in patients with aortoenteric fistulas. Abnormal findings on CT include perigraft fluid, gas, and tissue inflammation. It actually demonstrates aortoenteric fistulas in only 33% of cases. Although arteriography may help in planning the site of distal anastomosis, it rarely demonstrates the fistula and can take considerably longer. Colonic ischemia is more common in the immediate postoperative period.

In hemodynamically unstable patients, esophagogastroduodenoscopy of the third and fourth portions of the duodenum should be performed first, with aggressive resuscitation and rapid transfer to the operating room. Extra-anatomic routes of axillofemoral or femorofemoral grafts permit revascularization through a clean field distal to the original site. In situations requiring revascularization through a contaminated area, autologous tissue such as superficial femoral vein can be used. Bilateral axillofemoral grafts should be used as a secondary option because of their diminished outflow in comparison with unilateral axillofemoral and femorofemoral grafts. Delayed excision of the graft is recommended only in patients who are hemodynamically stable and do not have a false aneurysm at the site of the fistula.

**ANSWER:** D

7. Fasciotomy should be performed in patients with which of the following signs or symptoms?

   A. Tense fullness of the compartment in an otherwise asymptomatic patient

   B. Extremity ischemia for longer than 4 hours

   C. Progressively worsening neurologic signs after revascularization

   D. Traumatic injuries to the popliteal artery

   E. Compartmental pressure higher than 15 mm Hg and unreliable findings on physical examination

   *Ref.:* 1-3

COMMENTS: **Compartment syndromes** occur whenever tissue pressure within a confined anatomic space becomes sufficiently elevated to impair venous return. It can be caused by bleeding within a compartment or by reperfusion edema. Successful treatment is based on early, accurate diagnosis. There is no absolute pressure above which the syndrome invariably occurs, but nutrient blood flow in the muscle ceases between 30 and 40 mm Hg. However, isolated measurement of compartment pressure is neither sensetive nor specific for determining the degree of muscle ischemia. The important variable is the gradient between diastolic blood pressure and the compartment pressure. At minimum, such elevated pressures mandate close follow-up neurovascular examinations in reliable patients. Fasciotomy is indicated when measured compartment pressure is within 20 to 30 mm Hg of diastolic blood pressure. Prolonged ischemia is associated with compartment syndrome because of the reperfusion injury and release of free radicals. Diminished or absent pulses is a late finding, after which irreversible neurologic damage may have occurred. Compartment syndromes are best diagnosed by having a high index of suspicion. A tense compartment alone in the absence of elevated pressures or physical findings is not an absolute indication for fasciotomy. Traumatic injury to the popliteal artery is not an absolute indication for fasciotomy unless the repair/revascularization occurred more than 4 hours after the time of injury.

**ANSWER: C**

8. In a low-resistance arterial vascular system, at which percent reduction in diameter does a stenosis become flow limiting?

    A. 10%

    B. 20%

    C. 40%

    D. 50%

    E. 80%

*Ref.:* 4, 6

COMMENTS: In low-resistance arterial systems, such as the internal carotid artery, total blood flow across a stenosis does not decrease until the diameter is reduced by approximately 50%. This corresponds to a 75% reduction in cross-sectional area. Total blood flow is maintained by increasing the velocity. Shear stress (drag along the wall) and viscosity limit further increases in velocity once the reduction in diameter exceeds 50%. This hemodynamic fact is the reason for not repairing short stenoses of less than 50% because total blood flow is not altered. A longer stenosis increases shear stress and causes a lesser degree of stenosis over a long enough length to be flow limiting.

**ANSWER: D**

9. Which of the following characterizes duplex ultrasound imaging?

    A. It is a combination of Doppler and D-mode ultrasound imaging.

    B. Lower frequencies (e.g., 3 MHz) are better suited for deep abdominal imaging, and higher frequencies (e.g., 7 MHz) are better for more superficial structures, such as in situ vein grafts.

    C. High-frequency ultrasound waves have higher energy than low-frequency ultrasound waves.

    D. The diagnosis of deep venous thrombosis (DVT) is made with the use of color flow imaging alone.

    E. Calcification within a diseased artery is usually severe enough to prevent an adequate vascular ultrasound examination.

*Ref.:* 4-6

COMMENTS: **Duplex ultrasound imaging** consists of the B-mode image (picture) and Doppler shift, which measures the velocity of flowing blood. High-frequency transducers (7 to 10 MHz) are used for superficial structures, with applications such as saphenous vein mapping and in situ vein bypasses or pedal bypasses. These higher-frequency transducers have greater resolution but lower energy and cannot penetrate deeper tissues, as can lower-frequency, higher-energy transducers (3 or 5 MHz). Because venous flow velocity is slower than arterial flow velocity, artifacts can more easily be introduced by transducer movement when performing a venous examination, especially to rule out DVT. For these reasons, a more accurate venous examination to look for DVT is one without color that demonstrates a dilated uncompressible vein. The black-and-white image allows better assessment of vein compressibility and is not confused by an artifact introduced by transducer movement. Absence of flow in the segment of vein with augmentation and lack of respiratory variation confirm the diagnosis. Arterial wall calcium occasionally interferes with vascular ultrasound scans by blocking transmission of the ultrasound wave, but it is unusual that one cannot perform an adequate vascular examination of the carotid artery or other structure because of severe calcification.

**ANSWER: B**

10. The advantages of lower extremity arterial Doppler examinations performed with waveform analysis versus the ankle-brachial index (ABI) alone include which of the following?

    A. Calcification of the artery by diseases such as diabetes mellitus and chronic renal failure makes the arterial wall incompressible, thereby causing the ABI to be artificially decreased and unreliable.

    B. Inflow disease can be recognized by the delay in the downstroke of the waveform.

    C. Loss of reversal of flow when the arterial waveform transforms from triphasic to biphasic is observed with exercise or with moderate atherosclerosis.

    D. The ABI can be used to diagnose an arteriovenous fistula (AVF).

    E. The ABI can be used to diagnose DVT.

*Ref.:* 4-6

COMMENTS: The **ankle-brachial index** is a measurement for quantifying ischemia in an extremity based on the assumption that flow in the limb is proportional to blood pressure in the limb. The ABI is obtained with a blood pressure cuff and a handheld Doppler instrument. The cuff is applied at the point at which the pressure measurement is desired. The Doppler device is placed over any vessel distal to the cuff, but routinely it is the radial artery in the upper extremity or the posterior tibial or dorsal pedal artery in the lower extremity. The cuff is inflated to a pressure greater than systolic pressure. The pressure at which the arterial Doppler signal returns as the cuff is deflated is the pressure used to calculate the ABI. Diabetes and renal failure cause calcification of the axial extremity arteries, which makes the arteries noncompressible. The ABI is artificially elevated with these conditions.

When the ABI is unreliable (ABI >1.2), the Doppler waveform is used to assess the degree of ischemia in the extremity. Waveforms become monophasic in diseased arteries regardless of whether the vessels are compressible. The degree of arterial inflow disease (above the inguinal ligament) can be assessed by examining the femoral artery waveform. An arterial upstroke prolonged to more than 180 ms is consistent with significant iliac disease. Digital artery pressures are useful for quantifying ischemia in patients with diabetes and renal failure because these vessels are usually compressible even under such conditions. Toe pressures lower than 30 mm Hg are consistent with severe ischemia in non-diabetic patients, and those lower than 50 mm Hg are consistent with severe ischemia in diabetic patients.

Reversal of the direction of blood flow is caused by vascular resistance. Exercise causes vasodilation in the muscular beds and decreases resistance. The first change in waveform morphology that one observes in patients with mild atherosclerotic disease is loss of flow reversal when the waveform goes from triphasic to biphasic. Duplex imaging is required to diagnose AVFs and DVTs. The ABI alone is inadequate for diagnosing these conditions.

**A N S W E R :   C**

11. When performing duplex ultrasound imaging of the carotid arteries, what factors help distinguish the external carotid artery from the internal carotid artery?

    A. The internal carotid artery has continuous forward flow, and the external carotid artery exhibits reversal of flow during diastole.

    B. The external carotid artery is larger.

    C. The internal carotid artery is generally seen first.

    D. The superior thyroid artery is the first branch of the internal carotid artery and aids in identifying the internal carotid artery.

    E. The internal carotid artery has triphasic flow with flow reversal.

*Ref.:* 4, 5

**COMMENTS:** The external **carotid artery** is usually found anteromedially on a **duplex examination**, whereas the internal carotid artery is usually found posterolaterally. The external carotid artery is generally the first artery seen. It has triphasic flow, not continuous flow, as found in the internal carotid artery. The first branch of the external carotid artery is the superior thyroid artery. The internal carotid artery has biphasic continuous flow because it feeds the brain, a low-resistance system. The external carotid artery has triphasic flow with flow reversal because it feeds the face and its musculature, all high-resistance systems. Both arteries are approximately the same size in their proximal aspects. The internal carotid artery has no branches in the neck, in contrast to the external carotid artery.

**A N S W E R :   A**

12. Which of the following statements regarding percutaneous transluminal balloon angioplasty (PTA) for the treatment of occlusive atherosclerotic arterial blockage or stenosis is not true?
    A. Rates of intimal hyperplasia following PTA in a small artery (<5 mm) exceed those observed following operative repair of arteries of a similar size.

    B. The short- and long-term results of balloon angioplasty for lesions longer than 10 cm are better than those for operative intervention.

    C. Balloon angioplasty has demonstrated excellent results for stenotic lesions of the common iliac artery, but the results are not as good for occlusive lesions of the external iliac artery.

    D. Complications of PTA include dissection, thrombosis, and atheroembolization.

    E. The patency rate following PTA of the renal artery is only 60% at 2 years.

*Ref.:* 4-6

**COMMENTS:** **PTA** is performed via the percutaneous intravascular passage of balloon-tipped catheters. During **balloon dilation**, the atherosclerotic intima is ruptured and compressed, thereby allowing the media to become overstretched. PTA works best for short stenoses or occlusions in large arteries, such as may be found in the common iliac artery. Success rates for PTA of the common iliac artery are 80% at 1 year. The results of PTA of the external iliac artery fall to approximately 55% at 2 years.

Myointimal hyperplasia affects all blood vessels that have undergone intervention, but this process exerts its greatest influence on small arteries with diameters of less than 5 mm. Stents have been introduced to combat this problem, but they have not eliminated this complication of PTA. Myointimal hyperplasia can lead to failure rates of up to 40% at 6 months for small arteries that have undergone PTA, with the outcome being recurrent stenosis or thrombosis. PTA of long superficial femoral artery lesions has a success rate of only 22% at 1 year, whereas femoropopliteal bypass has a patency rate of 90% at 1 year. PTA of the renal artery works well for fibromuscular dysplasia but not as effectively for atherosclerotic lesions. The patency rate following PTA of the renal artery is only 60% at 2 years. Atheroembolization, dissection, and thrombosis can complicate any attempted percutaneous intervention and lead to loss of the limb.

**A N S W E R :   B**

13. What is the most common cause of a congenital hypercoagulable disorder?

    A. Protein S deficiency

    B. Protein C deficiency

    C. Antithrombin III deficiency

    D. Activated protein C resistance (APC-R; factor V Leiden mutation)

    E. Homocysteinemia

*Ref.:* 4-6

**COMMENTS:** Hemostasis is a finely tuned balance between coagulation and fibrinolysis. The existence of a congenital defect in procoagulant or anticoagulant proteins can shift this balance and cause increased bleeding or increased thrombotic tendencies, respectively. **Hypercoagulable states** are the most common cause of early bypass graft failure in young adults who require vascular interventions for limb salvage. More than 50% of patients younger than 50 years who require a lower extremity bypass and experience early graft thrombosis have a hypercoagulable state.

**Protein C**, **protein S**, and **antithrombin III deficiencies** have been known to exist for years, but until recently a specific inherited hypercoagulable state could not be identified in as many as 80% of patients.

It is now known that APC-R is the most common inherited hypercoagulable state; it is found in more than 50% of patients with inherited thrombotic tendencies. The cause of APC-R is an amino acid substitution in factor V of glutamine for arginine 506. Patients with APC-R have a poor anticoagulant response to APC, a vitamin K–dependent anticoagulant protein. When protein C is activated, it normally degrades activated clotting factors Va and VIIa. The altered factor V, or Leiden mutation (named for the Dutch city where it was first found), is resistant to the degrading action of APC. The altered, activated factor V retains its procoagulant activity, and the hemostatic balance is shifted toward thrombosis.

**Antithrombin III** is the major plasma inhibitor of thrombin. Heparin performs its anticoagulant function by forming a trivalent molecule of heparin–antithrombin III–thrombin to inactivate thrombin. This deficiency is rare, with an incidence of only 1 in 5000. Thrombotic events are usually triggered by trauma, surgery, or pregnancy.

**Proteins C and S** are both vitamin K–dependent anticoagulant proteins synthesized by the liver. The incidence of congenital protein C deficiency is 1 in 200. Proteins C and S deficiencies are found in 20% of patients younger than 50 years with arterial thrombosis, but the combined incidence is much less than the incidence of APC-R.

Treatment of antithrombin III, protein C, and protein S deficiencies is lifelong warfarin anticoagulation. Heparin must be given before initiating warfarin anticoagulation in these patients to protect against warfarin-induced skin necrosis. All patients with thrombosis who are to receive warfarin therapy should be administered heparin during the first 3 to 4 days of warfarin therapy because the half-life of the anticoagulant protein C is much less because it is degraded much faster than the procoagulant vitamin K–dependent factors II, IX, and X.

Mild homocysteinemia exists in 5% to 7% of the population. Elevated levels of homocysteine occur because of a defect in the pathway that metabolizes methionine. Treatment of homocysteinemia is with the B vitamin folate, 1 to 5 mg/day.

**A N S W E R :  D**

---

14. What is the most common cause of an acquired hypercoagulable state?

    A. Smoking

    B. Heparin-induced thrombocytopenia (HIT)

    C. Antiphospholipid antibody (e.g., lupus anticoagulant)

    D. Warfarin

    E. Oral contraceptives

*Ref.:* 4-6

**COMMENTS:** Smoking is the most common cause of **acquired hypercoagulability**. It is the most important factor that determines the short- and long-term results of any vascular intervention. The mechanisms of action of smoking are multiple and include both vasoconstriction and a measurable elevation in plasma fibrinogen levels, which itself is a risk factor for thrombosis.

The next most common cause of acquired hypercoagulability is HIT. This condition affects 2% to 3% of all patients who receive heparin. Antibodies form to heparin because it is obtained from bovine or porcine sources. The clinical manifestations are a falling platelet count, increasing resistance to anticoagulation with heparin, and new paradoxical thrombotic events while undergoing heparin treatment. Although low-molecular-weight heparin is responsible for a lower incidence of HIT than standard heparin, 25% of patients with HIT who receive low-molecular-weight heparin present with heparin allergy. Treatment of HIT is cessation of all heparin. Warfarin-induced skin necrosis is unusual as long as heparin is administered for the first 3 days that warfarin is given.

**Antiphospholipid syndrome** (APS) is common and affects 1% to 5% of the population. Specific types are lupus anticoagulant and anticardiolipin antibodies. Because the incidence of APS increases with age, 50% of patients older than 80 years have APS. This syndrome is recognized by prolongation of the baseline partial thromboplastin time (PTT). Brain thromboplastin is the reagent used for triggering the intrinsic clotting system when the PTT is measured. Patients with APS have serum antibodies that consume this reagent, thereby resulting in a prolonged PTT. This is an unforgiving hypercoagulable state, with an incidence of thrombotic complications approaching 50%.

Warfarin and oral contraceptives are less common causes of hypercoagulability.

**A N S W E R :  A**

---

15. A 70-year-old man who had undergone repair of an endovascular abdominal aneurysm 1 year earlier collapses and complains of back and abdominal pain. His blood pressure is 90/40 mm Hg. The patient denies a history of peptic ulcer or alcohol abuse. What is the most likely diagnosis?

    A. Aortoenteric fistula

    B. Bleeding duodenal ulcer

    C. Ruptured abdominal aortic aneurysm (AAA)

    D. Pancreatitis

    E. Diverticulitis

*Ref.:* 7

**COMMENTS:** The diagnosis of a **ruptured abdominal aortic aneurysm** must be considered in a patient with abdominal pain, back pain, and hypotension. After **endovascular repair**, an **endoleak** (persistent flow within an aneurysm sac despite an excluded aneurysm) develops in up to 50% of patients. Type 1 endoleak occurs when a persistent channel of blood flow develops as a result of an inadequate or ineffective seal at the graft ends. Type 2 endoleak occurs when there is persistent collateral blood flow retrograde into the aneurysm sac from patent lumbar arteries or the inferior mesenteric artery. Type 3 is a graft defect endoleak, such as when the sections pull apart. Type 4 is a graft fabric porosity endoleak. However, only about 1% of patients with stent graft repair of AAAs have a late rupture.

**A N S W E R :  C**

---

16. Which of the following statements concerning fibromuscular dysplasia of the carotid arteries is true?

    A. The incidence in males and females is approximately equal.

    B. Atherosclerosis is common when fibromuscular dysplasia is present.

C. Patient should undergo operative dilation before transient ischemic attacks (TIAs) or stroke occurs.

D. The process can also occur in the subclavian, internal iliac, and mesenteric vessels.

E. Approximately 25% of patients have associated intracranial aneurysms.

*Ref.:* 7

**COMMENTS: Fibromuscular dysplasia** occurs predominantly in females and can also involve the renal, external iliac, carotid, and vertebral arteries. The subclavian and mesenteric vessels are not involved. Symptomatic patients may undergo graded intraluminal dilation via arteriotomy in the common carotid artery or percutaneous treatment with balloon angioplasty. Asymptomatic patients may be monitored.

Approximately 13% to 35% of patients have atherosclerosis of the carotid bifurcation. The incidence of intracranial aneurysm is 23%.

**ANSWER:** E

**REFERENCES**

1. Vascular Section. In Townsend CM Jr, Beauchamp RD, Evers BM, et al, editors: *Sabiston textbook of surgery: the biological basis of modern surgical practice*, ed 18, Philadelphia, 2008, WB Saunders.
2. Lin PH, Kougias P, Bechara C, et al: Arterial Disease. In Brunicardi FC, Andersen DK, Billiar TR, et al, editors: *Schwartz's principles of surgery*, ed 9, New York, 2010, McGraw-Hill.
3. Ernst CB, Stanley JC: *Current therapy in vascular surgery*, ed 4, St. Louis, 2001, CV Mosby.
4. Moore WS: *Vascular and endovascular surgery*, ed 7, Philadelphia, 2006, WB Saunders.
5. Yao STJ, Pearce WH: *Practical vascular surgery*, Stamford, CT, 1999, Appleton & Lange.
6. Porter JM, Taylor LM Jr: *Basic data underlying clinical decision making in vascular surgery*, St. Louis, 1994, Quality Medical Publishing.
7. Cronenwett J, Johnston W, editors: *Rutherford's vascular surgery*, ed 7, Philadelphia, 2010, WB Saunders.

# B. Cerebrovascular Disease
*Muhammad Asad Khan, M.D.*

1. The most common cause of cerebral ischemia involves which of the following?

   A. Extracranial arterial stenosis

   B. Intracranial arterial thrombosis

   C. Arterioarterial embolization (atheroembolization)

   D. Cardioarterial embolization

   E. Traumatic arterial thrombosis

   *Ref.:* 1, 2

COMMENTS: **Atherosclerosis** is the most common cause of **ischemic stroke**. Arterioarterial embolization of plaque fragments from degenerative plaque or platelet-fibrin aggregates from a thrombogenic plaque surface is believed to be responsible for the neurologic injury. A small proportion of ischemic strokes may be caused by processes other than atherosclerosis, such as emboli from cardiac sources, fibromuscular hyperplasia, occlusive arteritis of the aortic arch vessels (Takayasu arteritis), dissecting thoracic aortic aneurysms, and trauma.

ANSWER: C

2. What percentage of patients with cerebral ischemia have a surgically accessible lesion?

   A. 95%

   B. 75%

   C. 50%

   D. 25%

   E. 5%

   *Ref.:* 2

COMMENTS: Of the patients with **cerebrovascular ischemia** who are studied by four-vessel angiography (common carotid and vertebral arteries), 75% are found to have significant extracranial disease that is surgically accessible. In the carotid vessels, lesions characteristically involve the carotid bifurcation and the proximal 1 to 2 cm of the internal carotid artery. In patients with vertebral basilar insufficiency, plaques or stenotic lesions characteristically occur near the origin of the vertebral arteries from the subclavian vessels. Because stroke is the third leading cause of death in the United States and the lesions responsible are often surgically accessible, endarterectomy benefits a significant proportion of patients with symptoms of cerebral ischemia.

ANSWER: B

3. In which patients is carotid endarterectomy not indicated?

   A. Acute stroke, 70% carotid stenosis, rapid recovery, and negative findings on head CT

   B. Forty-five percent carotid stenosis with continued or worsening TIAs while the patient was treated with aspirin and clopidogrel (Plavix)

   C. Transient neurologic deficit (<24 hours) and 70% stenosis

   D. Completed stroke and totally occluded internal carotid artery

   E. Eighty-five percent stenosis, completed stroke, mild deficit, and ulcerated carotid plaque

   *Ref.:* 1-3

COMMENTS: In patients with symptoms of **cerebrovascular ischemia** and greater than 50% stenosis, those with TIAs are optimal candidates for **carotid endarterectomy** because their risk for subsequent stroke is decreased significantly by operative intervention. Endarterectomy may also benefit patients with a completed stroke if the neurologic deficit is not severe and there is no evidence of a stroke on CT. A large stroke evident on CT means that the patient should wait 4 to 6 weeks for endarterectomy. Endarterectomy of the internal carotid artery has no benefit for a patient who has had a completed stroke with total occlusion of the artery. The role of carotid endarterectomy in an acute or evolving stroke is controversial. Restoration of flow is not usually indicated in patients with acute, fixed deficits and may in fact worsen symptoms and produce death by causing hemorrhage in the area of infarction. In patients with an evolving stroke (so-called crescendo TIAs) and fluctuating neurologic deficits, emergency endarterectomy may be of benefit. Symptomatic stenosis in carotid arteries with ulcerated plaques should be treated by endarterectomy because of the propensity of such plaques to activate platelets and form emboli.

ANSWER: D

4. Which of the following is characteristic of a TIA?

   A. Symptoms lasting longer than 24 hours

   B. Weakness, paralysis, or dysarthria in one side of the face or extremity

   C. Unilateral eye pain lasting 1 second

   D. Bilateral paresthesias, numbness, or aphasia

   E. Incontinence of bowel and bladder

   *Ref.:* 1-3

COMMENTS: **Transient ischemic attacks** are defined as completely resolving within 24 hours. They commonly last 2 to 15 minutes and resolve completely afterward. Attacks lasting longer than 24 hours but less than 3 weeks are referred to as reversible ischemic neurologic deficits. After 3 weeks, the attack is completed and referred to as a completed stroke. TIAs typically involve unilateral motor or sensory deficits of the extremities or face. Pain is not an associated feature, and episodes lasting only a few seconds are unlikely to be TIAs. Isolated symptoms of unconsciousness without other symptoms, dizziness alone, dysarthria alone, diplopia alone, incontinence of bowel or bladder, focal symptoms associated with migraines, confusion alone, and amnesia alone are also unlikely to be TIAs.

**ANSWER: B**

5. Which of the following is the best screening test for significant carotid stenosis in a patient with an asymptomatic bruit?

   A. Magnetic resonance angiography

   B. Four-vessel cerebral angiography

   C. Digital subtraction angiography

   D. CT of the brain with infusion

   E. Duplex ultrasound scanning

   *Ref.:* 1, 2

COMMENTS: Because of their sensitivity, safety, and repeatability, **noninvasive cerebrovascular studies** provide the best means of screening patients with asymptomatic bruits to detect significant stenotic lesions. Duplex scanning (real-time B-mode ultrasound imaging), which combines ultrasound and frequency spectrum analysis, provides a noninvasive method of quantifying the degree of stenosis and assessing morphologic characteristics. Accordingly, it is the single best screening test for evaluating carotid disease. Angiography is the definitive method for evaluating carotid anatomy in most centers, but it is not advocated as a screening procedure because it carries a 0.5% to 1.0% combined risk for mortality and major neurologic injury. Digital subtraction angiography has been evaluated as a screening tool in asymptomatic patients but has been found to have limited usefulness. CT of the brain and electroencephalography are rarely indicated for screening. CT angiography is a valuable tool but is not the first-line screening modality.

**ANSWER: E**

6. With regard to the Asymptomatic Carotid Atherosclerosis Study (ACAS), which of the following patients could be recommended for carotid endarterectomy?

   A. A 65-year-old woman with 30% stenosis and complaints of lower extremity claudication

   B. A 70-year-old man with a carotid bruit and a 60% stenosis revealed on an angiogram

   C. An 80-year-old woman with atrial fibrillation, complete left hemiplegia, and a 30% stenosis on duplex ultrasound imaging

   D. A 70-year-old man with hyperlipidemia, a recent myocardial infarction, and a 50% carotid stenosis

   E. An 80-year-old man with obstructive pulmonary disease and 90% stenosis of the left internal carotid artery

   *Ref.:* 1-3

COMMENTS: The value of **prophylactic carotid endarterectomy** for patients with asymptomatic stenosis is predicated on a progressive natural history of the disease process and the ability to perform endarterectomy with morbidity and mortality rates of less than 2%. Several studies have shown that in asymptomatic patients with hemodynamically significant carotid stenosis (exceeding 60%), the percentage of cerebral ischemic events is higher than in patients without stenosis and that carotid endarterectomy in a prophylactic setting decreases the expected risk for cerebral ischemic events. No data to date, however, support the use of endarterectomy for patients with less than 60% asymptomatic stenosis. Duplex ultrasound imaging as a diagnostic modality may also underestimate or overestimate the degree of stenosis and lead to an erroneous conclusion from the study data. The ACAS and North American Symptomatic Carotid Endarterectomy Trial (NASCET) studies were predicated on angiographic stenosis or reduction in diameter, which underestimates the reduction in area. Carotid endarterectomy can be recommended only for asymptomatic patients with otherwise low operative risk and few comorbid conditions.

**ANSWER: B**

7. Of the following factors that contribute to flow through a stenotic artery, which is the most important?

   A. Diameter of the stenosis

   B. Length of the stenosis

   C. Blood viscosity

   D. Blood pressure

   E. All of the above

   *Ref.:* 1

COMMENTS: **Stenosis** is usually considered hemodynamically significant if the diameter of the lumen is reduced by 50% or more, which corresponds to a 75% decrease in cross-sectional area. Blood flow is best described by Poiseuille's law, written as $Q = \pi(P_1 - P_2)r^4/8\,L\eta$, where Q is flow, P is pressure, r is radius, L is length, and $\eta$ is viscosity. Flow is proportional to pressure and inversely proportional to the length of the stenosis and to blood viscosity, but flow is directly related to the fourth power of the radius. The radius is thus the most important factor when determining total blood flow.

**ANSWER: A**

8. A patient with symptomatic 85% carotid stenosis is found to have 50% stenosis of the contralateral carotid artery that is asymptomatic. Appropriate initial treatment includes which of the following?

   A. Simultaneous bilateral carotid endarterectomy

   B. Staged bilateral carotid endarterectomy with a 1-week interval between stages

   C. Carotid endarterectomy on the symptomatic side only

   D. Carotid endarterectomy on the side with the greatest stenosis, regardless of symptoms

   E. Antiplatelet therapy and follow-up with duplex scans

   *Ref.:* 3

COMMENTS: The long-term risk for **asymptomatic carotid stenosis** is not fully defined. The Toronto Asymptomatic Bruit Trial observed an 18% annual incidence of neurologic events in patients with 75% stenosis. Evaluation of patients with symptomatic disease who are found to have asymptomatic stenosis on the contralateral side suggests that TIAs related to the asymptomatic lesion may develop in 10% to 15% of patients and that approximately 1% of patients suffer stroke. The latter rate occurs in patients whose lesions have 50% to 75% stenosis. The risk in patients with more significant narrowing is not known and may be higher. It therefore appears that patients with asymptomatic contralateral disease can be managed expectantly and that cerebral ischemic symptoms, when they do develop, are predominantly in the form of TIAs, which can be treated when they occur.

**ANSWER:** C

9. After elective carotid endarterectomy, a patient is noted to have a new severe neurologic deficit while in the recovery room. Appropriate management of this perioperative neurologic deficit includes which of the following?

A. Immediate return of the patient to the operating room for neck exploration

B. CT of the head with intravenous contrast enhancement to evaluate for ischemia

C. Cerebral angiography

D. Observation overnight

E. Immediate heparinization

*Ref.:* 3

**COMMENTS:** The overriding concern for this patient is to be certain that no technical causes are responsible for this patient's **postoperative, deteriorating neurologic condition**—the most common technical error is creation of an intimal flap. This possibility can be determined most effectively by immediately returning the patient to the operating room for neck exploration. The patient should be heparinized once the neck is opened and the artery checked for a pulse, a thrill, or intracarotid thrombosis. If the pulse is diminished or there is evidence of thrombosis, the artery is reopened to examine it for thrombosis or flap elevation. If there are no signs of a carotid problem when the neck is opened, an intraoperative duplex scan should be considered to identify intraluminal debris. Intraoperative angiography may also be a useful maneuver in this desperate situation.

**ANSWER:** A

10. With regard to the long-term results of carotid endarterectomy, which of the following statements is true?

A. The rate of restenosis is 10% to 15%.

B. Restenosis is most commonly manifested as stroke.

C. Ischemic cerebral events are the main cause of late death.

D. Restenosis rates are higher when endarterectomy is performed for symptomatic disease than for asymptomatic disease.

E. The combined operative morbidity and mortality rate for carotid endarterectomy is 7%.

*Ref.:* 2

**COMMENTS:** The combined operative morbidity and mortality rate for **carotid endarterectomy** should be less than 5%. Coronary

artery disease is the main cause of both immediate and late postoperative death. There is a significant rate of restenosis (10% to 15%) after carotid endarterectomy, although most of these lesions are asymptomatic, not hemodynamically significant, and do not require intervention. It is therefore recommended that patients undergo annual B-mode duplex scanning to look for restenosis after having scans two or three times the first year.

**ANSWER:** A

11. With regard to symptoms of ischemia secondary to vertebral basilar insufficiency, which of the following statements is correct?

A. They include diplopia, ataxia, vertigo, and tinnitus.

B. They are usually indistinguishable from those of carotid insufficiency.

C. They usually reflect unilateral vertebral disease.

D. They are most commonly caused by emboli.

E. They are caused by diffuse, ulcerated stenosis of the artery

*Ref.:* 2

**COMMENTS: Stenosis of the vertebral artery** usually involves a localized segment near its origin from the subclavian artery. Unlike carotid plaques, the stenotic lesions are usually smooth and nonulcerated, and the ischemia is generally attributed to decreased flow rather than an embolic phenomenon. Although one vertebral artery is usually dominant, unilateral vertebral stenosis rarely produces symptoms. Symptoms generally reflect bilateral disease. Associated atherosclerotic involvement of the basilar artery is also common. Symptoms of ischemia caused by vertebral basilar insufficiency are the same as those of brainstem ischemia and produce a characteristic clinical syndrome (diplopia, dysarthria, vertigo, and tinnitus) quite distinct from the cerebral hemispheric ischemia produced by carotid disease.

**ANSWER:** A

12. Most patients with "subclavian steal" syndrome have which of the following conditions?

A. Reversal of flow in the ipsilateral vertebral artery

B. Disabling neurologic symptoms

C. Upper extremity claudication

D. Equal systolic blood pressure in both arms

E. Require operative intervention

*Ref.:* 1, 2

**COMMENTS: "Subclavian steal" syndrome** results from occlusion of a subclavian artery, rarely the innominate, with decreased systolic pressure distal to the obstruction. This causes blood to flow up the contralateral vertebral artery and across the basilar artery (from which more blood is "stolen") as it courses down (in a retrograde manner) the ipsilateral vertebral artery to help supply the affected subclavian artery. Most patients with this phenomenon are asymptomatic and do not require intervention, although limb weakness and paresthesias or symptoms of vertebral artery insufficiency may occur, in which case intervention is appropriate.

**ANSWER:** A

**13.** Amaurosis fugax is brought about by occlusion of which of the following arteries?

   A. Facial artery

   B. Occipital artery

   C. Retinal artery

   D. Posterior auricular artery

   E. Ophthalmic artery

*Ref.:* 1, 2

**COMMENTS:** About 75% of patients who suffer a stroke have had a previous TIA. **Amaurosis fugax**, one type of TIA (lasting minutes to hours), is manifested as ipsilateral blindness, described by the patient as being like a window shade pulled across the eye. It is caused by emboli traveling via the ophthalmic artery—the first intracerebral branch of the internal carotid artery—and lodging in the retinal artery. These emboli may be seen on funduscopic examination and are called Hollenhorst plaques. The other arteries listed are branches of the external carotid artery. There are eight branches of the external carotid artery: superior thyroid, lingual, facial, ascending pharyngeal, occipital, posterior auricular, superficial temporal, and maxillary.

**ANSWER:** C

**14.** Carotid body tumors are most commonly manifested by which of the following?

   A. Hypertension

   B. Painless neck mass

   C. Cranial nerve deficit

   D. Horner syndrome

   E. Cerebral ischemia

*Ref.:* 1, 2

**COMMENTS:** The carotid body is 3 to 4 mm in size and located within the adventitial tissue of the carotid bifurcation. It arises from paraganglionic cells of neural crest origin. **Carotid body tumors (chemodectomas)** are uncommon, slow growing (they may even remain stationary for long periods), and usually manifested as a painless mass. There are two types of carotid body tumors: sporadic (5% of which are bilateral) and autosomal dominant familial (32% of which are bilateral). The criteria for malignancy are controversial and influenced by the tumor's location, its biologic behavior, or evidence of local invasion or distal spread. Most are benign. Definitive treatment is excision.

**ANSWER:** B

**15.** Regarding carotid artery stenting (CAS), which of the following statements is true?

   A. CAS is the new "gold standard" of care for cerebrovascular occlusive disease.

   B. It is especially beneficial for people older than 80 years.

   C. CAS has no role in patients who have previously undergone carotid endarterectomy and restenosis develops.

   D. Cerebral embolic protection devices have improved the results of CAS.

   E. All of the above.

*Ref.:* 1, 2

**COMMENTS:** The precise role of **carotid artery stenting** is still undefined. Currently available data have shown CAS to be suitable for postendarterectomy restenosis, surgically difficult neck dissections secondary to radiation treatment, and other indications. The interim results from the Carotid Revascularization Endarterectomy vs Stent Trial (CREST) have shown increased stroke and death rates in patients older than 80 years in the stenting group. Cerebral protection devices, or temporary filters placed above the stent during deployment, have been a major advance in stent technology, and their use has now become standard practice. Carotid endarterectomy continues to be the gold standard treatment for carotid occlusive disease.

**ANSWER:** D

**REFERENCES**

1. Riles TS, Rockman CB: Cerebrovascular disease. In Townsend CM Jr, Beauchamp RD, Evers BM, et al, editors: *Sabiston textbook of surgery: the biological basis of modern surgical practice*, ed 18, Philadelphia, 2008, WB Saunders.
2. Lin PH, Kougias P, Bechara C, et al: Arterial disease. In Brunicardi FC, Andersen DK, Billiar TR, et al, editors: *Schwartz's principles of surgery*, ed 9, New York, 2010, McGraw-Hill.
3. Ernst CB, Stanley JC: *Current therapy in vascular surgery*, ed 4, St. Louis, 2001, CV Mosby.

# C. Thoracic Aorta

*Muhammad Asad Khan, M.D.*

1. With regard to ascending aortic aneurysms, which of the following statements is true?

   A. They are most often caused by connective tissue abnormalities.

   B. They are not related to earlier venereal disease.

   C. Primary tumors of the aorta are common.

   D. They are usually associated with aortic insufficiency.

   E. Death is generally caused by rupture with resulting hemothorax.

   *Ref.:* 1, 2

**COMMENTS:** Etiologic factors involved in **aortic aneurysms** vary according to the location of the aneurysm. In the ascending aorta, a connective tissue abnormality recognized histologically as cystic medial necrosis is the most common underlying abnormality and is the defect seen in aneurysms associated with **Marfan syndrome**. Other known causes, such as syphilitic aneurysms, are steadily decreasing in frequency, and atherosclerotic aneurysms of the ascending aorta are relatively uncommon. Primary tumors originating from the aorta are extremely rare. The most common primary tumors are sarcomas. Aortic insufficiency occurs only when there is associated annular dilation or when one or more aortic cusps are sheared off by an acute dissection. Death from an ascending aortic aneurysm is usually caused by cardiac failure secondary to chronic untreated aortic insufficiency or rupture into the pericardium with pericardial tamponade.

**ANSWER:** A

2. With regard to the clinical characteristics and management of ascending aortic aneurysms, which of the following statements is true?

   A. Most ascending aortic aneurysms are symptomatic.

   B. Valvar murmurs are rare.

   C. Aortography is contraindicated because of the risk of causing dissection of the aneurysm with the catheter.

   D. Operative management with placement of a composite graft of aortic conduit and aortic valve is the treatment of choice for all ascending aortic aneurysms.

   E. CT with contrast enhancement is a good noninvasive modality with which to delineate the size and extent of an aortic aneurysm.

   *Ref.:* 1, 2

**COMMENTS:** Although relatively uncommon, an **ascending aortic aneurysm** may be manifested as a mass in the anterior aspect of the chest. Patients are usually asymptomatic, in which case the aneurysm is likely to be detected on routine chest radiographs. Aneurysms can be localized (saccular) or more generalized (fusiform). When symptoms are present, they are commonly related to congestive heart failure caused by dilation of the aortic annulus, which results in aortic insufficiency and its characteristic murmur (an early diastolic murmur at the second interspace along the right sternal border). This murmur is often present even in asymptomatic patients.

Aortography confirms the diagnosis and is important for defining the dimensional extent of the aneurysm and its relationship to the rest of the aorta, its major branches, and the coronary ostia.

Surgical correction is clearly the treatment of choice, and treatment depends on the presence of valve pathology. Valve-sparing operations are carried out in patients with preserved valve function. If aneurysms are associated with massive dilation of the aortic root, aortic annulus, and aortic leaflets, a composite graft is used (**Bentall operation**).

CT with intravenous contrast enhancement and MRI are excellent noninvasive modalities that can delineate the extent and size of an aneurysmal aorta.

**ANSWER:** E

3. Superior vena cava (SVC) syndrome is characterized by which of the following?

   A. Bronchogenic carcinoma with invasion into the mediastinum is the leading cause of SVC syndrome.

   B. Venous pressure in the SVC rarely exceeds 15 mm Hg.

   C. Acute obstruction of the SVC is seldom clinically significant because of the large number of collateral vessels available.

   D. Occlusion of the SVC between the azygos vein and the right atrium is more symptomatic than an occlusion above the azygos vein.

   E. Surgical correction is usually indicated.

   *Ref.:* 1, 2

**COMMENTS:** More than 90% of **superior vena cava obstructions** are caused by malignant tumors, most often mediastinal invasion by bronchogenic carcinoma. When obstruction occurs, venous pressures rise to 20 to 50 mm Hg.

Acute complete obstruction allows little time for the formation of collateral vessels and can therefore produce significant edematous laryngeal obstruction and even fatal cerebral edema. A more gradual onset of obstruction results in the characteristic clinical picture of facial swelling and dilation of the collateral veins of the head and neck, arms, and upper thoracic areas. Obstruction between the azygos vein and the right atrium is less disabling because the azygos vein provides a large collateral venous channel for drainage of the SVC system into the inferior vena cava (IVC) system. Obstruction above the azygos vein eliminates this collateral channel and is not as well tolerated.

The treatment of choice for obstruction caused by associated malignancy is prompt radiation therapy, often in association with diuretics and chemotherapy. An operation is rarely indicated for management of SVC obstruction because of the technical difficulties associated with vena cava grafts, the underlying poor prognosis in patients with malignant conditions, and the usual adequacy of collateral venous circulation in the rare instances of slowly developing obstruction caused by benign conditions. The only indication for surgery is the unusual instance of a benign problem in which the collateral circulation does not relieve the symptoms. Surgical management consists of either a replacement graft or a bypass. In general, autologous grafts have performed better than prosthetic grafts. Balloon angioplasty and stenting can be useful.

**A N S W E R :** A

4. Regarding thoracic aortic aneurysms in patients with Marfan syndrome, which of the following statements is true?

   A. Less than 50% of patients with Marfan syndrome survive past the age of 45 years.

   B. The descending aorta is always affected.

   C. All aneurysmal dilations greater than 4 cm should be treated with prophylactic replacement of the aortic root.

   D. Surgical repair of an ascending aortic aneurysm usually requires aortic repair only.

   E. The perioperative mortality rate exceeds 15%.

*Ref.:* 3

**COMMENTS:** The severely diminished longevity of patients with **Marfan syndrome** has been well documented. Less than 50% of all male and female patients with the syndrome survive past the age of 45 years. Cardiac deaths account for more than 90% of early deaths of known cause, and 75% of these deaths are secondary to aortic root dilation or aortic dissections and their complications. Prophylactic aortic root replacement is recommended for all aneurysms larger than 6 cm in diameter. In contrast to atherosclerotic aneurysmal disease, aneurysmal dilations in patients with Marfan syndrome involve not only the entire aorta, including the coronary sinuses, but also the cardiac valvular tissues. Therefore, replacement of the entire aortic root, including the aortic valve, with a composite valve graft is required in the majority of patients. Improved techniques of myocardial protection have resulted in perioperative mortality rates of less than 5% in most recent series.

**A N S W E R :** A

5. With regard to thoracic aortic trauma, which of the following is true?

   A. CT angiography should be performed in most stable patients if injury is suspected.

   B. Cardiac tamponade is a major cause of death in patients with blunt trauma to the chest.

   C. Fatal hemorrhage is sometimes prevented by the aortic adventitia in penetrating trauma.

   D. Immediate surgical intervention is rarely indicated.

   E. Widening of the mediastinum to greater than 12.0 cm remains the key to diagnosis.

*Ref.:* 1, 2

**COMMENTS:** Both penetrating and deceleration **injuries of the thoracic aorta** are commonly fatal. When the patient is in extremis from exsanguination, thoracotomy in the emergency department to control hemorrhage may be indicated, even though success is unlikely. In clinically stable patients, CT angiography is indicated for both types of injury to define the anatomy of the injury because it may influence the choice of surgical approach. With penetrating injuries, pericardial tamponade, in addition to exsanguination, is a major cause of death. With deceleration injuries, complete disruption of the aorta is nearly always fatal. In some instances, however, the adventitia remains intact, thus confining the hemorrhage and allowing time for surgical correction. With severe blunt trauma to the chest, the possibility of aortic injury must be suspected, and CT angiography should be used liberally. Mediastinal widening (>8.0 cm) with loss of the aortic window contour remains the key to diagnosis.

**A N S W E R :** A

6. With regard to aortic dissection and the DeBakey classification:

   A. Type I dissections are limited to the descending aorta.

   B. Type II dissections are primarily treated nonoperatively.

   C. Death from cardiac tamponade and acute aortic insufficiency is common with ascending aortic dissections.

   D. Aneurysm development is rare in the acute or chronic phase of dissection.

   E. Type III dissections are primarily treated surgically.

*Ref.:* 1, 2

**COMMENTS: Aortic dissections** have been classified by Michael DeBakey according to their site of origin and extent of aortic involvement. **Type I** originates in the ascending aorta and dissects throughout the entire thoracic and abdominal aorta. **Type II** originates in the ascending aorta but is confined to that segment of the aorta and is the type commonly seen in patients with Marfan syndrome. **Type III-A** originates distal to the left subclavian artery but remains confined to the descending thoracic aorta. It is readily accessible to surgical repair. **Type III-B** originates distal to the left subclavian artery but dissects down into the abdominal aorta, which complicates its surgical repair. Definition of the origin and extent of aortic dissection is of paramount importance because these considerations dictate therapy. Most dissections occur in the inner one third or one half of the aortic wall. The underlying defect is destruction of the media from an unknown cause. Hypertension is present in 80% to 90% of patients and in well in excess of 95% of those with dissection of the descending aorta. Dissections originating in the ascending aorta most commonly occur throughout the entire length, whereas those originating distal to the subclavian artery occur distal to that point. Multiple entry and reentry points are seen in type I dissections.

After initial evaluation and diagnosis, antihypertensive therapy (nitroprusside) and β-blockade should be instituted. Nearly all patients with ascending aortic dissection (types I and II) should undergo surgery immediately. Early causes of death in patients with types I and II dissections are coronary artery occlusion, rupture with cardiac tamponade, and acute aortic valve insufficiency. The goal of surgery is to correct the aortic insufficiency and graft the ascending aorta, with obliteration of the false lumen. Dissections of the descending aorta require prompt surgery if signs of visceral ischemia are present or if rupture has occurred. In the absence of the aforementioned indications, surgery can be postponed. Thirty percent of such patients ultimately require an operation because of an enlarging aneurysm. The **Stanford classification** includes dissections starting in the ascending aorta as type A and those starting in the descending aorta as type B. The principles of management are the same as those for the **DeBakey classification**.

**ANSWER: C**

7. Regarding treatment of acute Stanford type B aortic dissections, which of the following statements is true?

   A. The most important initial treatment is control of hypertension to prevent proximal extension of the dissection.

   B. Surgical treatment is required for all patients with limb, renal, or mesenteric ischemia.

   C. Surgical treatment always requires a left thoracotomy.

   D. Cardiopulmonary bypass has no role in reducing complications during replacement of the descending thoracic aorta.

   E. Endovascular techniques have no role in these patients.

*Ref.:* 1, 2

**COMMENTS:** For patients with acute **Stanford type B dissection**, hemodynamic stabilization with control of hypertension to levels adequate for maintenance of cerebral, myocardial, and renal perfusion is the immediate goal of medical therapy. Although sodium nitroprusside is the traditional pharmacologic therapy of choice, intravenous esmolol more effectively reduces the aortic and left ventricular hyperdynamic state and helps prevent proximal extension of the dissection. Patients with renal, mesenteric, or limb ischemia can be treated nonoperatively with stents, stent grafts, or balloon septostomy. Placement of a thoracic aortic stent graft in the proximal descending thoracic aorta results in obliteration of the false lumen and redirection of flow into the true lumen and has been associated with significantly lower perioperative mortality. If endovascular techniques fail or are not available, patients with ischemic symptoms require surgical revascularization. This can be accomplished through a left posterolateral thoracotomy, with placement of an interpositional graft in the proximal descending aorta and obliteration of the false lumen. Distal aortic perfusion with the use of left atriofemoral or femorofemoral cardiopulmonary bypass reduces renal, visceral, and spinal cord ischemia time during this procedure and thereby the incidence of perioperative complications. An alternative approach is infrarenal aortic graft placement with surgical septotomy and obliteration of the distal false lumen to restore lower extremity blood flow. If only the leg is ischemic, femorofemoral or axillobifemoral bypass is a less invasive procedure if leg ischemia cannot be treated with endovascular techniques.

**ANSWER: A**

8. With regard to blunt traumatic rupture of the aorta, which of the following statements is correct?

   A. The most common site of rupture is distal to the left subclavian artery at the point of insertion of the ligamentum arteriosum.

   B. Patients rarely die at the scene of the accident.

   C. The intima provides nearly 60% of the strength of the thoracic aorta and must remain intact for the patient to survive.

   D. There is still a high risk for free aortic rupture, even in patients who survive the first 6 weeks after injury.

   E. Bypass support is mandatory for its correction.

*Ref.:* 1, 2

**COMMENTS:** About 85% to 90% of patients who sustain an **aortic rupture** die at the scene of the accident. Patients who sustain rupture of the ascending aorta rarely reach the hospital alive. In most patients who survive, the rupture is located at the aortic isthmus (immediately distal to the origin of the left subclavian artery). The aortic adventitia provides 60% of the tensile strength of the thoracic aorta. For someone to survive blunt trauma to the aorta, this layer must remain intact to prevent a free rupture and exsanguinating hemorrhage. Of the patients who initially survive and are merely observed because the pathologic process is not recognized or for some other reason, 20% die within 6 hours and 72% within 1 week. If a patient survives 6 to 8 weeks after the injury, the risk of free aortic rupture is low. There is evidence that if an operation is performed expeditiously with appropriate monitoring of somatosensory potentials to prevent paraplegia, adequate physiologic support, and control of blood pressure with nitroprusside, simple aortic clamping without bypass is equally safe, and the operative time and blood loss are significantly less. Cardiopulmonary bypass is, however, commonly used for these operations.

**ANSWER: A**

9. With regard to thoracoabdominal aneurysms, which of the following statements is true?

   A. Symptoms of compression of adjacent structures are rare.

   B. Paraplegia and renal failure are the most common complications of elective repair.

   C. Type IV aneurysms are associated with the highest incidence of paraplegia.

   D. Endovascular repair is not feasible for these aneurysms.

   E. Sixty percent of patients are asymptomatic.

*Ref.:* 1, 2

**COMMENTS: Thoracoabdominal aneurysms** occur primarily in older patients with extensive atherosclerosis and are infrequent in comparison with infrarenal aortic aneurysms. The cephalad location of the abdominal component frequently precludes palpation because of the overlying pancreas and stomach. Thirty percent of patients in a large series were asymptomatic, and the condition was first diagnosed on routine chest radiographs, which revealed dilation of the aorta at the diaphragm. A major advance in the treatment of these aneurysms was made by E. Stanley Crawford, who developed the intraluminal graft technique. This procedure has significantly reduced the rates of morbidity and mortality associated with surgical repair. Technical difficulties during surgical repair, including the need to reimplant the celiac, superior mesenteric, and renal arteries, increase the risk associated with this operation sufficiently that repair is usually warranted only for symptomatic or significantly enlarging aneurysms. **Paraplegia** as a result of temporary or permanent loss of spinal cord blood flow can occur in 7% to 12% of patients. Its frequency can be reduced by draining spinal fluid with a lumbar drain. Distal aortic pressure higher than 60 mm Hg, rather than flow rate, is the key to perfusion of the spinal cord. Reattachment of large lumbar vessels has helped lower the incidence of paraplegia.

Thoracoabdominal aneurysms can compress the mainstem bronchus, pulmonary tissue, and esophagus. Type IV aneurysms—from the diaphragm distally—have the lowest risk for paraplegia with repair. Endovascular repair of thoracoabdominal aneurysms is possible, and the limitation of anatomic landing zones can be overcome by debranching with the so-called hybrid procedure.

**ANSWER: B**

10. With regard to transverse aortic arch aneurysms, which of the following statements is true?

    A. Cystic medial necrosis is a major cause.

    B. Repair is associated with the highest operative mortality rate of any of the aortic aneurysms.

    C. Differentiation from mediastinal tumors is usually possible on standard chest radiographs.

    D. Deep hypothermia with circulatory arrest and cardiopulmonary bypass is rarely used.

    E. All of the above.

    *Ref.:* 1, 2

**COMMENTS: Transverse aortic arch aneurysms** are almost always the result of atherosclerosis. In asymptomatic individuals, they are most often detected on routine chest radiographs. Aortography and CT, however, are required to differentiate them from mediastinal tumors and to define the vascular anatomy before repair. Concomitant association with coronary and cerebrovascular disease, together with the need to disrupt flow to the brain temporarily during repair, has resulted in an operative mortality rate exceeding that for repair of other aortic aneurysms. The introduction of cardiopulmonary bypass and hypothermic circulatory arrest has significantly reduced this operative mortality rate. Spiral CT is used rather than aortography in some centers.

**ANSWER: B**

11. Radiographic signs of aortic injury secondary to blunt chest trauma include all of the following except

    A. Widening of the mediastinum

    B. Blunting of the aortic knob

    C. Right apical capping

    D. Depression of the left main bronchus

    E. Deviation of the trachea to the right

    *Ref.:* 1, 2

**COMMENTS: Blunt injury to the thoracic aorta** may occur without clinical signs or symptoms that such an injury is present. Frequently, the mechanism of injury (sudden deceleration from

vehicular accidents or falls) and a high index of suspicion obligate the examining physician to rule out aortic trauma by aortography or CT angiography. Radiographic signs of aortic injury, when present, include blunting of the aortic knob, widening of the mediastinum (to 7.0 cm), deviation of the trachea to the right, left apical blunting, and depression of the left main bronchus. Even when these radiographic signs are present, aortography is required to precisely define the anatomy and the extent of the vascular injury. Spiral CT is used rather than aortography in many centers.

**ANSWER: C**

12. With regard to diagnosis and treatment of aortic dissection, which of the following statements is true?

    A. Aortography and coronary angiography are essential before surgery for type A acute aortic dissection.

    B. Transesophageal echocardiography is not useful for diagnosing acute aortic dissection.

    C. Type B acute aortic dissection is treated primarily by surgery.

    D. Surgical treatment of acute type A dissection is similar in patients with or without Marfan syndrome.

    E. With chronic type B dissection, the indications for surgery are related to the size of the aneurysm, symptoms of pain, and development of visceral, renal, and neurologic ischemia.

    *Ref.:* 1, 2, 4, 5

**COMMENTS:** Coronary angiography before emergency repair of **acute proximal aortic dissection** is not recommended. Even in the presence of moderate coronary artery disease, early repair of the dissection has precedence over other procedures. Since its introduction in 1984, the use of transesophageal echocardiography to diagnose aortic dissection has gained acceptance by many surgeons. It has a sensitivity and specificity of 99% and 98%, respectively. Because it can be performed in the emergency department or the operating room, it does not require transferring the patient to a separate area, as does angiography. It can also be used to assess the function of the left ventricle, the aortic valve, and the mitral valve.

Type B aortic dissection is primarily treated medically by instituting strict control of hypertension. Indications for surgery for acute type B dissection are limited to prevention or relief of life-threatening complications (i.e., aortic rupture, ischemia of limbs and organ systems, persistent pain, or uncontrolled hypertension).

Patients with Marfan syndrome have more extensive pathologic involvement of the tissue, which necessitates a more extensive dissection process. There is general agreement that a composite root replacement with an aortic valve and aortic graft, rather than an interposition graft alone, is the surgical treatment of choice for patients with Marfan syndrome.

**ANSWER: E**

13. A 50-year-old man involved in a deceleration-type motor vehicle accident is brought to the emergency department. He has a systolic blood pressure of 90 mm Hg. Chest radiographs reveal a widened mediastinum. He has a bilateral pelvic fracture and a tender abdomen. Which of the following statements is true about this patient?

    A. Management should begin with aortography to evaluate the widened mediastinum.

B. The most common site of traumatic aortic rupture is the ascending aortic arch.

C. Repair of this type of injury virtually always requires cardiopulmonary bypass.

D. Rarely, this type of injury is manifested 10 years after the accident.

E. The risk for paraplegia following repair of the thoracic aorta can be avoided if certain precautions are taken.

*Ref.:* 1, 2, 5

**COMMENTS:** Patients with multiple injuries and a suspected **aortic tear** should have certain associated injuries addressed first (e.g., extensive pelvic fractures or intra-abdominal injuries). In this patient, diagnostic peritoneal lavage or immediate abdominal CT should be performed along with evaluation of the widened mediastinum. The most common site for an aortic tear is just distal to the left subclavian artery. Although cardiopulmonary bypass may be required in certain patients with an extensive aortic tear, tears can be treated by placement of a covered stent in some cases. Even though patients with a thoracic aortic tear can live to undergo successful repair, many patients with this injury die at the scene of the accident. Some arrive at the hospital and die during initial resuscitation. Rarely, such patients are found to have a chronic pseudoaneurysm up to 15 years after the accident.

    **Paraplegia** following repair of the thoracic aorta remains one of the most distressing complications associated with the operation. Aortic cross-clamp time, distal aortic pressure monitoring, and cerebrospinal fluid drainage by spinal tap have been used. However, none of these steps has proved reliable in eliminating the risk for postoperative paraplegia, which is 3% to 10%.

**ANSWER: D**

14. Regarding endovascular repair of thoracic aortic aneurysms (TEVAR), which of the following statements is true?

A. Neck diameter is rarely considered in preoperative planning for TEVAR.

B. Thoracic stents have no role in a trauma situation.

C. Small iliac vessels are an absolute contraindication to TEVAR.

D. Benefits include improved mortality and paraplegia rates.

E. No surveillance is required after TEVAR.

*Ref.:* 1

**COMMENTS:** Neck diameter at the proximal and distal landing zones is an important consideration in preoperative planning for **endovascular repair of thoracic aortic aneurysms**. Debranching of the arch and visceral vessels has been helpful in certain situations to increase landing zones. In patients with small iliac vessels, an iliac conduit can be placed to accommodate a large-profile delivery system. When comparing open repair with TEVAR, prospective randomized trials have shown improvements in mortality (11.7% to 2.1%) and paraplegia rates (14% to 3%) with TEVAR. Lifelong surveillance is required after TEVAR: CT scans at 1, 6, and 12 months and then yearly afterward. Endovascular repair of blunt thoracic aortic trauma is gaining popularity and has shown improved morbidity and paraplegia rates. Long-term results are not available yet.

**ANSWER: D**

**REFERENCES**

1. Safi HJ, Estrera AL, Miller CC, et al: Thoracic vasculature with emphasis on the thoracic aorta. In Townsend CM Jr, Beauchamp RD, Evers BM, et al, editors: *Sabiston textbook of surgery: the biological basis of modern surgical practice*, ed 18, Philadelphia, 2008, WB Saunders.
2. LeMaire SA, Sharma K, Coselli JS: Thoracic aneurysms and aortic dissection. In Brunicardi FC, Andersen DK, Billiar TR, et al, editors: *Schwartz's principles of surgery*, ed 9, New York, 2010, McGraw-Hill.
3. Moffatt-Bruce SD, Mitchell RS: Thoracic aortic aneurysms. In Mullholland MW, Lillemoe KD, Doherty GM, et al, editors: *Greenfield's surgery: scientific principles and practice*, ed 4, Philadelphia, 2006, Lippincott Williams & Wilkins.
4. Cohn LH, editor: *Cardiac surgery in the adult*, ed 3, New York, 2008, McGraw-Hill.
5. Crawford ES, Crawford JL, Safi HJ, et al: Thoracoabdominal aortic aneurysms: preoperative and intraoperative factors determining immediate and long-term results of operations in 605 patients, *J Vasc Surg* 3:389–404, 1986.

# D. Abdominal Aorta

*Muhammad Asad Khan, M.D.*

**1.** The following may be acceptable treatments of occlusive aortoiliac disease except for:

A. Thromboendarterectomy (TEA)

B. Aortofemoral bypass

C. Axillofemoral bypass

D. Percutaneous balloon angioplasty

E. Percutaneous atherectomy

*Ref.:* 1-3

**COMMENTS:** The basic goal of arterial revascularization for **occlusive arterial disease** is to reestablish adequate blood flow to the tissue being supplied. In patients with occlusive aortoiliac disease who require surgery, a variety of techniques are applicable, depending on the site and extent of obstruction, the presence or absence of aneurysmal disease, and the patient's underlying medical condition. **Thromboendarterectomy** is appropriate for rare patients with disease confined to the distal aorta and common iliac arteries. The results of TEA are similar to those with aortofemoral bypass grafting. TEA is contraindicated in patients with aneurysmal disease and disease that extends to the external iliac arteries and is gradually being abandoned with the development of percutaneous endovascular techniques. **Aortofemoral bypass grafts** produce excellent results in terms of immediate and long-term patency and relief of claudication. The long-term patency rates are reported to be as high as 90% at 10 years. Axillofemoral and thoracofemoral bypass grafts have been successful in patients in whom an abdominal operation may pose excessive risk, including those with infected aortic prosthetic grafts, those with previously occluded aortofemoral grafts, and patients with a "hostile" abdomen. **Femorofemoral and ileofemoral bypass grafts** are used when only one iliac artery is diseased. Percutaneous balloon angioplasty is successful for isolated short-segment lesions of the iliac arteries in patients with good distal runoff. This may yield 5-year patency rates as high as 80%. **Angioplasty** can also be used to dilate an iliac stenosis before a more distal bypass. The addition of intraluminal stents has broadened the number and location of lesions amenable to balloon angioplasty and has increased the technical success rates of these procedures. Disadvantages of percutaneous angioplasty include a lower rate of overall success in patients with poor distal runoff or limb-threatening ischemia and the potential complications of intimal dissection, vascular occlusion or rupture, and distal embolization.

**ANSWER:** E

**2.** Which of the following is the most common graft-related late complication of aortic bypass grafts?

A. Graft occlusion caused by progressive atherosclerosis

B. Suture line pseudoaneurysm

C. Aortoenteric fistula

D. Distal embolization

E. Infection caused by transient bacteremia

*Ref.:* 2

**COMMENTS:** The long-term **patency rates** of **aortofemoral bypass grafts** are reported to range from approximately 65% to 90%. The most common graft-related late complication is graft occlusion, which develops in 10% to 35% of patients. The most frequent cause of graft occlusion is progressive atherosclerosis, which usually occurs at or just beyond the distal anastomosis. Other late complications include anastomotic pseudoaneurysm (1% to 5%) and graft infection (1%), both of which occur more often when a femoral anastomosis is involved. An aortoenteric fistula is rare but carries a high mortality rate (50%). Therefore, it should be a primary consideration in any patient with a previous abdominal aortic graft who has gastrointestinal bleeding. Most frequently, there is bleeding into the third portion of the duodenum from the proximal aortic suture line.

**ANSWER:** A

**3.** What is the most common cause of death after recovery from a successful aortic bypass graft operation?

A. Pseudoaneurysm rupture

B. Acute graft thrombosis

C. Cerebrovascular accident

D. Coronary artery disease

E. Renal failure

*Ref.:* 1, 3

**COMMENTS:** Associated **coronary artery disease** is the leading cause of death after **aortic reconstruction**. Risk factors predictive of postoperative cardiac events include age older than 70 years, previous myocardial infarction, history of ventricular arrhythmias, diabetes mellitus, and angina pectoris. The dipyridamole thallium stress test has an excellent negative predictive value for postoperative cardiac complications. Combining clinical markers with dipyridamole thallium stress testing increases the specificity of dipyridamole thallium alone. Aggressive preoperative cardiac evaluation is justified to define a patient's operative risk and to identify patients who would benefit from further invasive cardiac evaluation and therapy.

**ANSWER:** D

**4.** Which of the following is the most common manifestation of an AAA?

A. Incidental finding on physical examination or CT performed for unrelated disease

B. Back or abdominal pain

C. Acute rupture

D. Spontaneous thrombosis with peripheral ischemia

E. Peripheral embolization

*Ref.:* 1, 2, 4

COMMENTS: Approximately three fourths of all **abdominal aortic aneurysms** are discovered incidentally and are asymptomatic. The most common complaint in patients with symptoms is vague abdominal pain. Patients may also note back or flank pain. AAAs may expand without symptoms, erode into the adjacent vertebral bodies, partially obstruct the duodenum or ureters (inflammatory aneurysms), embolize, thrombose, or rupture. Rare manifestations include aortoenteric fistula and aortocaval fistula. The latter are accompanied by an abdominal bruit, venous hypertension, and high-output cardiac failure. Rupture may mimic other acute intra-abdominal emergencies, such as diverticulitis and renal colic, and may be manifested as acute abdominal pain followed by transient hypotension and eventually vascular collapse. Signs and symptoms of acute ischemia in the lower extremities may follow thrombosis or embolization from an abdominal aneurysm.

ANSWER: A

5. With regard to preoperative imaging of AAAs, which of the following statements is true?

A. High-quality CT without intravenous contrast enhancement provides adequate information for surgical planning in the majority of AAAs.

B. Arteriography provides more accurate measurements of the size of the aneurysm than CT.

C. Arteriography is not helpful when there is clinical suspicion of occlusive disease of the renal, mesenteric, or iliofemoral arteries.

D. Arteriography is the test of choice for identifying candidates for endovascular repair.

E. The presence of a horseshoe kidney or an ectopic kidney on CT is an indication for arteriography before elective AAA repair.

*Ref.:* 1, 3, 4

COMMENTS: **Computed tomography** with intravenous contrast enhancement is the most commonly used preoperative study to obtain the anatomic information necessary to plan surgical repair of **abdominal aortic aneurysms**. CT provides the most accurate measurement of aneurysm size and important anatomic information regarding the proximal and distal extent of the aneurysm, the degree of calcification of the aortic wall, and anatomic variants that could complicate surgery. The current spiral CT scanners offer three-dimensional reconstructions that are particularly helpful in identifying candidates for endovascular repair. Therefore, CT has largely replaced arteriography for the evaluation of patients with AAAs. **Arteriography** is still helpful for patients with occlusive disease of the renal, mesenteric, or iliofemoral arteries who might benefit from a simultaneous repair. It is also indicated in patients with an ectopic or horseshoe kidney for accurate delineation of aberrant renal arteries. CT without contrast enhancement is useful

to define the outside diameters of aneurysms and can be used to monitor them chronically.

ANSWER: E

6. The following are acceptable indications for repair of an AAA except:

A. Any AAA regardless of size

B. Symptomatic aneurysm of any size

C. Symptomatic aneurysm larger than 5 cm in diameter

D. Asymptomatic aneurysm larger than 6 cm in diameter

E. Asymptomatic 4.5-cm aneurysm that was 3.5 cm 1 year earlier

*Ref.:* 2, 4

COMMENTS: The **natural history of most abdominal aortic aneurysms** is progressive enlargement. The risk for rupture is directly related to the size of the aneurysm. This relates to the law of Laplace, according to which the mean tension (T) in the wall of a vessel is directly proportional to the product of the radius (R) and intraluminal pressure (P). Therefore, an increase in radius (expansion) or pressure (hypertension) results in an increase in wall tension: $T = P \times R$. Approximately one half of the deaths in patients with untreated AAAs are caused by rupture. The risk for rupture of an aneurysm 5 to 5.9 cm in diameter is approximately 3.4% per year. Two recent independent studies in the United States and the United Kingdom have shown no survival benefit for elective repair of asymptomatic aneurysms measuring up to 5.5 cm in diameter. Because the risk for rupture increases dramatically with diameters larger than 5.5 cm, elective repair is indicated for all aneurysms above that size. **Ruptured aneurysms** carry a 50% mortality rate in patients who reach the hospital alive. Any patients with symptoms suggestive of impending rupture or with a proved contained rupture should be operated on immediately. Ultrasound imaging provides a reliable noninvasive method for observing patients with small asymptomatic aneurysms. The anticipated growth rate is 0.4 cm/yr. When the growth rate exceeds 0.6 cm/yr, the risk for rupture is high, and elective repair is a reasonable approach for aneurysms measuring at least 4.5 cm in diameter, provided that the patient is a good surgical candidate. Diastolic hypertension and severe chronic obstructive pulmonary disease are believed to be predictors of expansion and rupture, especially for large aneurysms. The decision to operate must therefore be based on considerations of size, shape (saccular is more ominous than fusiform), presence of symptoms, cardiac risk, and the presence of cerebrovascular or chronic obstructive pulmonary disease. The mortality rate with elective repair is approximately 3% to 5%.

ANSWER: A

7. With regard to the operative approach for open repair of AAAs, which of the following statements is true?

A. There is no true indication for a retroperitoneal approach.

B. Extension of the aneurysm to the right common iliac artery is a contraindication to a retroperitoneal approach.

C. The retroperitoneal approach is associated with a higher incidence of paralytic ileus.

D. The midline transperitoneal approach is associated with a higher incidence of pulmonary complications.

E. The retroperitoneal approach can be used for repair of ruptured AAAs.

*Ref.:* 3

**COMMENTS:** There are many reported indications for the retroperitoneal approach to the **infrarenal aorta**. A "hostile abdomen," usually resulting from multiple transabdominal procedures, irradiation, or the presence of enteric or urinary stomas, is the most common. The **retroperitoneal approach** is also useful for patients with ascites, peritoneal dialysis catheters, morbid obesity, inflammatory aneurysms, and a horseshoe kidney. Relative contraindications to use of the retroperitoneal approach include the presence of right renal artery stenosis, ruptured AAA, and an AAA with a left-sided IVC. The presence of a right common iliac artery aneurysm is not an absolute contraindication to the retroperitoneal approach. In these cases, the right iliac aneurysm is excluded by oversewing the ostium of the right common iliac artery through the open aorta, making a right lower quadrant transplant incision, ligating the distal neck of the iliac aneurysm, and extending the right limb of the bifurcated aortic graft to the right external iliac or right common femoral artery. Alternatively, the distal neck of the aneurysm is not ligated, but the distal right external iliac or the proximal right common femoral artery is ligated, followed by extension of the right limb of the graft to the right common femoral artery. The latter approach has the disadvantage of allowing backflow to the iliac aneurysm via the right internal iliac artery, which may result (on rare occasion) in enlargement and rupture of the iliac aneurysm. Although most surgeons avoid the retroperitoneal approach for ruptured AAAs, several centers with extensive experience have reported successful use of this approach in select cases of ruptured AAAs.

At least four prospective randomized studies have confirmed that the retroperitoneal approach is associated with a decreased incidence of postoperative ileus and a shorter hospital stay. There was no significant difference in the incidence of pulmonary complications, perhaps because of the increasing use of epidural analgesia in the postoperative period for patients undergoing AAA repair.

**ANSWER:** E

8. With regard to the operative technique of AAA repair, which of the following statements is true?

A. Bifurcation grafts are preferable to straight grafts, even if the iliac vessels are not involved.

B. An endoaneurysmal approach is most commonly used today.

C. Bleeding lumbar vessels are routinely ligated from outside the aneurysm sac.

D. The inferior mesenteric artery (IMA) is routinely reimplanted in elderly patients to prevent ischemia of the left colon.

E. Flow should first be restored to the external iliac vessels when the cross-clamps are removed.

*Ref.:* 1, 2, 4

**COMMENTS:** Details of the operative technique for **repair of abdominal aortic aneurysms** vary somewhat, depending on individual circumstances, but several general principles should be emphasized. Proximal control is established distal to the renal vessels after identifying the left renal vein. Manipulation of the aorta is kept to a minimum to prevent embolization of the contents of the aneurysm. After the proximal and distal clamps are applied, the aneurysm is opened and the thrombus evacuated. The lumbar vessels are ligated from within the aneurysm sac. The **inferior mesenteric artery** can usually be safely ligated precisely at its origin, thereby avoiding damage to collateral vessels within the mesentery of the left colon. If backflow from the IMA is poor, consideration should be given to reimplanting the artery to the side of the prosthesis. Some surgeons evaluate backflow by viewing the IMA orifice from inside the opened aneurysm. Others measure IMA stump pressure and find that a pressure lower than 40 mm Hg is a reason for reimplantation.

Flow to at least one hypogastric artery should be preserved to maintain collateral flow to the colon via the middle hemorrhoidal arteries. If ischemic injury to the left colon is suspected, a second-look laparotomy should be performed 24 hours later.

Because most of the aneurysm sac is preserved, the posterior suture lines consist of a double thickness of aorta. This provides more suture line strength and hemostasis because the graft is sutured to the aorta from within the aneurysm sac in an end-to-end manner.

A tube graft is preferable to a bifurcation graft when the common iliac arteries are uninvolved. Tube grafts obviate the need for an additional anastomosis, obviate an increased risk for dissection, and obviate the increased incidence of infection associated with anastomosis performed in the groin.

In some instances in which the aneurysm is extensive, the celiac, superior mesenteric, and renal arteries are involved. These aneurysms require more complex revascularization procedures, including reimplantation of the vessels previously mentioned.

After graft placement, proper techniques of aortic flushing and sequential unclamping are important to minimize the risk for hypotension, declamping shock, and distal embolization. The latter is accomplished by adequate flushing before completing the distal anastomosis and opening the circulation first into the internal iliacs and then into the external iliac arteries.

The surgeon should control systemic arterial pressure with finger pressure on the graft until appropriate volume replacement has been accomplished.

Hypotension after removal of the aortic cross-clamp is believed to occur as a result of washout of acidic metabolites and vasoactive substances from the ischemic lower extremities, third-space loss into permeable distal tissues, and sudden flow into vasodilated beds, as well as vascular steal secondary to reactive hyperemia in the lower extremities.

The aneurysm sac is not extensively resected and is closed over the prosthetic graft to isolate the graft from the duodenum and to minimize the risk for erosion and fistulization.

**ANSWER:** B

9. Two days after uncomplicated open repair of an AAA, bloody diarrhea develops. The most likely diagnosis is which of the following?

A. Coagulopathy

B. Ischemic colitis

C. Aortoenteric fistula

D. Acute hepatic failure

E. Diverticulitis

*Ref.:* 1-3

**COMMENTS:** The main concern in this situation is that **ischemic colitis** may have developed as a result of interruption of flow to the IMA without adequate collateral blood supply from the superior mesenteric or hypogastric artery (or both) to the sigmoid colon. It is important to realize that diarrhea, whether Hemoccult positive or negative, is one of the first signs of ischemic colitis. Less commonly, ischemic colitis can also develop as a result of embolization of atheromatous debris into the mesenteric circulation during aneurysm repair. The reported incidence of clinically significant ischemia is 1% to 2%. Additional risk factors related to ischemia include the duration and placement of cross-clamping, hypotension, and cardiac arrhythmias. Ischemia occurs more commonly in patients with previous colon resection and those undergoing a total aortic graft reoperation or operation for a ruptured aortic aneurysm. Immediate proctosigmoidoscopy is important during the initial evaluation of such a patient to assess colonic viability. The rectum is usually spared, and ischemic changes, seen through the sigmoidoscope as pale, patchy areas with membranes, can be visualized 10 to 20 cm from the anal verge. Ischemic colitis may be limited to the mucosa or may be transmural. Management must be individualized. The presence of associated increasing abdominal tenderness, peritoneal signs, fever, and an elevated white blood cell count point to a transmural process that necessitates surgery. Resection of the descending and sigmoid colon with the Hartmann pouch and end-colostomy are required for transmural necrosis to prevent gross spillage and contamination of the graft. Aortoenteric fistula is a late complication of aortic aneurysm repair that results from erosion of a false aneurysm at the proximal aortic suture line into the duodenum or, on occasion, the sigmoid colon. It is not a likely diagnosis in this clinical scenario. Coagulopathy is not usually manifested as bloody diarrhea, but hepatic function and the coagulation profile should be assessed promptly if a bleeding diathesis is suspected.

**ANSWER:** B

10. With regard to rupture of an AAA, which of the following statements is true?

   A. It is the most common cause of death in patients with an untreated AAA.

   B. The operative mortality rate of patients with a ruptured AAA is 5%.

   C. Control of the proximal aorta cannot be accomplished endoluminally.

   D. The lowest mortality rates occur in patients with preexisting coronary artery disease.

   E. Female patients with ruptured AAAs have a better chance of survival than males.

*Ref.:* 1-4

**COMMENTS:** **Rupture of an abdominal aortic aneurysm** is a catastrophic complication that may be heralded by abdominal, back, or flank pain followed by vascular collapse. It is the most common cause of death in patients with untreated abdominal aneurysms, with a mortality rate of 30% to 50%, although nearly that many patients die of associated atherosclerotic problems, including cardiac, cerebral, or renal disease. The mortality rate associated with elective, nonruptured repair is 5% or less.

Immediate surgery plus control of the proximal aorta is mandatory if patients are to survive. These procedures are best accomplished transabdominally at a level just below the diaphragm.

Although there are proponents of retroperitoneal exposure for surgical management of a ruptured AAA, most surgeons believe that a midline incision allows better exposure and control of the ruptured abdominal aorta. With free abdominal rupture or retroperitoneal rupture above the renal vein, manual compression of the aorta can be used at the level of the crus of the diaphragm for control. Infrarenal control can then be achieved in the same manner as during elective aneurysm repair. A large Foley or Fogarty catheter can be placed in the aneurysm and inflated to achieve immediate control.

The most significant predictors of mortality are the presence of preoperative hypotension and a low hematocrit. Other factors include age, intraperitoneal rupture, transfusion requirements, and gender (females have a higher mortality rate). The presence of preexisting coronary disease is not the most significant preoperative factor in the mortality from a ruptured AAA.

**ANSWER:** A

11. Which one of the following complications occurs most commonly after successful repair of an AAA in a 58-year-old man?

   A. Sexual dysfunction

   B. Ischemic colitis

   C. Renal failure

   D. Peripheral embolization

   E. Leg paralysis

*Ref.:* 1, 2, 4

**COMMENTS:** All of these complications may occur after **repair of an abdominal aortic aneurysm**, but with appropriate operative technique, most of them are uncommon, except for changes in sexual function. Retrograde ejaculation has been reported in as many as two thirds and loss of potency in as many as one third of such patients. These changes may result from injury to the autonomic nerve fibers overlying the anterior aorta near the origin of the IMA or from injury to fibers overlying the proximal left common iliac artery and aortic bifurcation. Avoiding excessive aortic dissection in this region can help minimize this complication. Documentation that sexual dysfunction existed preoperatively is of obvious importance in aortoiliac surgery because the incidence of impotence in men of this age with no aortoiliac occlusive disease is considerable. Unilateral, isolated iliac artery obstruction in men is often best treated by femorofemoral bypass to avoid the potential for postoperative impotence. Revascularization of the internal iliacs at the time of aortoiliac reconstruction for occlusive disease can reverse vasculogenic impotence in patients with distal obstructive disease.

**ANSWER:** A

12. With regard to inflammatory AAA, which of the following statements is true?

   A. Less than 1% of AAAs are considered inflammatory.

   B. There is a characteristic gross appearance consisting of a thick, white fibrotic retroperitoneal process with adherence of the aneurysm to the duodenum and IVC.

   C. An infectious cause is responsible for the inflammatory process.

D. The operative approach is the same as for the usual atherosclerotic aneurysm.

E. Most inflammatory AAAs occur in a suprarenal location.

*Ref.:* 2-4

**COMMENTS: Inflammatory abdominal aortic aneurysms** represent 2.5% to 15.0% of all AAAs. There is a male preponderance. This type of aneurysm is infrarenal and characterized by an intense adventitial fibroplastic reaction, with adherence of the aneurysm to the third and fourth portions of the duodenum and IVC. Ureteral entrapment is present in 25% of patients. No infectious cause has been found, and the inflammatory process is believed to be autoimmune. Abdominal and back pain, weight loss, and an elevated erythrocyte sedimentation rate (ESR) in a patient with an AAA suggest this diagnosis. Abdominal CT with contrast enhancement is the most definitive examination for securing a preoperative diagnosis. This scan demonstrates aortic wall thickening outside the rim of aortic calcification. In contrast to a leaking AAA, the inflammatory process is enhanced with contrast material and demonstrates less attenuation than blood. The operative strategy includes proximal aortic control above the left renal vein and the use of ureteral catheters if the inflammatory process extends to the iliac vessels. Dissecting off adherent structures (e.g., duodenum) should be avoided. Ureterolysis is rarely necessary. The risk for rupture is lower than with the usual atherosclerotic aneurysm. After aneurysmorrhaphy with graft placement, the inflammatory process gradually resolves, and the ESR returns to normal.

**A N S W E R :**  B

13. A patient who had an AAA repaired 5 years earlier is evaluated for fever and positive blood cultures. Which of the following statements is true?

A. Angiography is the preferred initial imaging technique for suspected graft infection.

B. Published mortality rates following surgery for infected aortic grafts range between 5% and 10%.

C. Graft infections identified within 4 months of AAA repair are associated with a more virulent course than later infections are.

D. *Pseudomonas* is the most common infecting pathogen.

E. Upper gastrointestinal bleeding is the most common initial manifestation of an infected abdominal aortic graft.

*Ref.:* 4

**COMMENTS:** Diagnosis of an **infected aortic graft** is often a difficult task. Clinical symptoms can be as subtle as prolonged ileus, abdominal pain or tenderness, or unexplained sepsis. The patient should be examined closely for anastomotic pseudoaneurysms or signs of septic embolization. CT with intravenous contrast enhancement is the preferred initial imaging technique for patients with suspected aortic graft infection. Fluid or gas around the graft, obliteration of the normal retroperitoneal tissue planes, and pseudoaneurysm formation suggest a graft infection. Published mortality rates range between 10% and 50%, with subsequent amputation rates ranging from 15% to 60%. The reasons for the high mortality rates are aortic stump blowout and persistent sepsis. Graft infections diagnosed within 4 months are more virulent than those diagnosed later. *Staphylococcus aureus* and gram-negative bacteria are the pathogens mainly implicated in early graft infection. Gram-negative bacteria are particularly virulent because the endotoxins (elastase and alkaline protease) that they produce can lead to compromise of the structural integrity of the anastomosis. *S. aureus* is the most prevalent pathogen in infected aortic grafts, although the incidence of *Staphylococcus epidermidis* infection is on the rise. *S. epidermidis* infection is more chronic and insidious in nature and is usually diagnosed more than 4 months postoperatively.

**A N S W E R :**  C

14. Which of the following statements is correct regarding endovascular repair of infrarenal AAA?

A. The most common complication with this technique is graft thrombosis.

B. Tube grafts are preferable to bifurcated grafts for endovascular repair of infrarenal AAAs.

C. Anatomic limitations prohibiting endovascular repair include a short neck and large angulation of the aneurysm.

D. Iliac stenosis is an absolute contraindication to endoluminal repair.

E. Use of this technique is more likely to be feasible for large aneurysms.

*Ref.:* 4, 5

**COMMENTS: Complications** following **endovascular repair of abdominal aortic aneurysms** include endoleaks, microembolization, improper or incomplete placement of the stent, graft migration, graft thrombosis, and delayed aneurysm rupture. An endoleak is defined as persistent arterial supply of the aneurysmal sac following deployment of the endograft. The incidence of this complication has been reported to be as high as 40%. Treatment of endoleaks varies. Some leaks can be managed conservatively, but others require treatment with further endovascular stenting or conversion to an open technique. Placement of tube endografts in the infrarenal aorta has been associated with a very high degree of complications (distal endoleaks) and has therefore been abandoned. Favorable anatomic characteristics for endovascular repair include a proximal neck at least 15 mm in length and a distal neck at least 10 mm in length. The aneurysmal aorta tends to have a significant degree of angulation. When the angulation exceeds 60 degrees, the incidence of graft migration and stent fracture increases significantly. Patients with iliac stenosis can undergo iliac artery angioplasty with or without stent placement preceding endovascular repair of the aneurysm, thus not making it an absolute contraindication to repair. The smaller the aneurysm, the more likely it is to have a proximal and distal neck and the less likely it is to exhibit mural thrombus formation.

**A N S W E R :**  C

15. Regarding endovascular repair of AAAs, which of the following statements is false?

A. Aneurysm rupture may occur in patients with successful repair in the absence of endoleaks.

B. Type II endoleaks are caused by patent lumbar, inferior mesenteric, or hypogastric arteries.

C. Types I and III endoleaks do not need any intervention.

D. Endoleaks may develop at any time after endograft placement.

E. Endotension is defined as aneurysm pressure in the absence of an endoleak.

*Ref.: 5*

**COMMENTS:** Continued perfusion plus pressurization of the aortic aneurysmal sac is called endoleak and is the most common **complication of endovascular repair of abdominal aortic aneurysms. Endoleaks** have been classified into five different types. Type I results from inadequate seal at the proximal or distal ends of the endograft. Type II is caused by branch flow through a patent IMA, lumbar artery, or hypogastric artery. Type III is a midgraft endoleak originating from holes in the fabric or an inadequate seal between endograft components. Type IV is caused by endograft porosity. Type V, or endotension, is aneurysm pressure and enlargement in the absence of identifiable perigraft flow. Endoleaks may develop at any time. Therefore, following successful endograft deployment, patients are monitored with various imaging modalities (commonly spiral CT) at 6-month intervals for the possible development of a new endoleak. Although aneurysm rupture in the absence of endoleak has been reported following endovascular repair, several studies have shown that the presence of an endoleak increases the risk for rupture. This risk is higher with type I and type III endoleaks. Therefore, once they are identified, these endoleaks require prompt repair. The risk for rupture from a type II endoleak is significantly smaller, and the need for secondary interventions to address such an endoleak is still a subject of debate. Usually, if the endoleak is associated with growth of the aneurysm, most experts recommend repair.

**ANSWER:** C

16. With regard to infected (mycotic) AAAs, which of the following statements is true?

A. Infected aneurysms account for 5% of all AAAs.

B. Most infected aneurysms develop when they are caused by an aortoenteric fistula.

C. *Salmonella* is the most commonly isolated bacterial pathogen.

D. Negative results of intraoperative Gram staining exclude the diagnosis of an infected AAA.

E. Most patients are treated by excision of the aneurysm and in situ aortic reconstruction.

*Ref.: 1, 3, 4*

**COMMENTS: Infected (mycotic) aneurysms** are a rare subset of AAAs that constitute only 0.1% to 1.5% of cases. Most infected aneurysms are caused by the spread of hematogenous bacteria that infect nonaneurysmal but atherosclerotic arteries, with subsequent aneurysmal degeneration. Other causes include arterial trauma leading to false aneurysm formation with concomitant bacterial contamination, septic emboli of cardiac origin, or infection of a preexisting aneurysm. *Salmonella* has been identified in almost 40% of patients with infected AAAs. Infections with gram-negative organisms are less common but are associated with a higher incidence of aneurysm rupture. The most common symptoms in patients with infected aneurysms are fever and abdominal or back pain. Laboratory data lack sensitivity and specificity when considered alone. Blood culture results are positive in approximately 35% to 50% of patients. CT is the preferred diagnostic study and may reveal an enhancing and eccentric periaortic mass, an aneurysm at an atypical location, periaortic fluid or gas, retroperitoneal soft tissue edema, prominent periaortic lymphadenopathy, and evidence of aneurysm rupture. When the diagnosis of an infected AAA is entertained, broad-spectrum antibiotics and prompt surgical intervention are mandatory. Excision of the aneurysm with débridement of all involved tissues, secure aortic stump closure, and extra-anatomic reconstruction, such as axillofemoral bypass, is recommended in most cases. Following surgery, patients are prescribed parenteral antibiotics for 4 to 6 weeks, depending on the virulence of the organism, the extent of infection, and the method of arterial reconstruction. Aneurysm excision with in situ aortic reconstruction may be performed in patients with minimal infection and low-virulence organisms, such as *S. epidermidis*. After in situ aortic graft reconstruction, lifelong oral antibiotics are advised.

**ANSWER:** C

17. With regard to prosthetic aortic graft infections, which of the following statements is true?

A. Infected prosthetic aortic grafts occur more commonly after aortofemoral bypass than after aortoiliac bypass.

B. *Salmonella* is the pathogen most commonly isolated from infected prosthetic aortic grafts.

C. Ultrasound is the preferred diagnostic modality for confirming prosthetic aortic graft infection.

D. Most prosthetic aortic graft infections are diagnosed within 1 year after implantation.

E. Graft excision, secure aortic stump closure, and extraanatomic reconstruction are required for all infected prosthetic aortic grafts.

*Ref.: 1, 3, 4*

**COMMENTS: Infected prosthetic aortic bypass grafts** have an incidence of approximately 1% following aortoiliac bypass and 1.5% to 2.0% following aortofemoral bypass. Mortality from infected grafts is as high as 50% in reported series. The most common pathogens isolated from infected prosthetic aortic grafts are *S. epidermidis* and *S. aureus*. Factors that contribute to graft infection include contact between the graft and skin during insertion, break in sterile technique, extension of contaminated wounds, contaminated lymphatics, arterial wall infection, and early transient bacteremia. CT has proved to be the most sensitive tool for diagnosing infected prosthetic grafts. Changes on CT suggestive of infected grafts include perigraft fluid or gas, soft tissue swelling, focal bowel wall thickening, increased soft tissue between the graft and the wrap, and false aneurysm formation. Radionuclide techniques have similar sensitivity but high false-positive rates because of labeling techniques, especially after graft implantation. Ultrasound provides limited information. MRI is limited by its inability to differentiate between infected and sterile fluid, especially during the early postoperative period. Most prosthetic graft infections are diagnosed more than 1 year after implantation. Early infection (<4 months) is associated with emergency operations for ruptured AAA, states of impaired immunocompetence, concomitant remote infection, and postoperative colonic ischemia. Most infected prosthetic aortic grafts are treated by graft excision, wide débridement of infected tissues, secure aortic stump closure, and extra-anatomic reconstruction. Patients with late graft infections of low virulence (*S. epidermidis*) and no gross contamination may be treated by segmental graft excision and in situ graft replacement. Regardless of the technique of reconstruction, patients are placed on a long-term antibiotic regimen and are subjected to close follow-up.

**ANSWER:** A

18. Which of the following is not an acceptable treatment option for a patient with late aortic graft limb occlusion?

A. Percutaneous atherectomy

B. Thrombolytic therapy

C. Graft limb thrombectomy

D. Femorofemoral bypass

E. Aortofemoral bypass reoperation

*Ref.:* 1, 3

**COMMENTS:** The most common **graft-related complication** following **aortofemoral bypass** is thrombosis of one limb. Graft limb occlusion occurs in 10% to 20% of patients, depending on the duration of follow-up. Late graft limb occlusion is most commonly caused by progressive atherosclerotic disease at or just beyond the distal anastomosis. Other causes include worsening disease of the outflow vessels, commonly the proximal profunda femoris artery; thrombosis of an anastomotic aneurysm; arterial embolism from a cardiac source; low-output states; hypercoagulable states; and iatrogenic injury to the graft or native vessels following cardiac catheterization or diagnostic angiography. Except in those with profound limb ischemia, preoperative angiography should be performed in all patients. In high-risk or inactive patients without evidence of limb-threatening ischemia, a nonoperative approach may be the most prudent course. Thrombolytic therapy has been used in patients with acute graft thrombosis. Its use is limited in patients with severe limb-threatening ischemia. Significant complications such as bleeding, distal embolization, and worsening ischemia may occur. Furthermore, surgical revision of the graft is usually required in most patients. Therefore, its use is limited to patients with acute occlusion and non–limb-threatening ischemia, particularly high-risk patients. Most patients with graft limb occlusion are treated via an operative approach. In patients with graft limb occlusion of short duration, absence of proximal aortic disease, and unilateral occlusion, graft limb thrombectomy has been shown to be 90% successful. To prevent further thrombosis, repair of the distal anastomosis may be required if a defect is present. Advantages of this approach include the use of a unilateral groin incision and the fact that the procedure may be performed with the patient under local or regional anesthesia. A common procedure for those with unilateral limb occlusion is a femorofemoral bypass. This procedure is not usually excessively time-consuming, may be done with the patient under local or regional anesthesia, and is technically easier than aortic reoperation. In patients with proximal aortic disease, anastomotic complications, or significant degeneration or dilation of the original prosthesis, aortofemoral bypass graft reoperation is the preferred approach. In patients with multiple occluded grafts or "hostile" abdomens in whom the other, less formidable options are contraindicated, extraanatomic reconstructions, such as axillofemoral or descending thoracic aortofemoral bypass, may be used. Regardless of the technique, revision of the outflow tract must be accomplished if necessary. It may require profundaplasty, graft limb extension, and bypass to the popliteal or tibial level. Distal grafts are required in 25% to 50% of all procedures for graft limb occlusion.

**ANSWER:** A

**REFERENCES**

1. Reddy DJ, Shepard AD: Aortoiliac disease. In Mullholland MW, Lillemoe KD, Doherty GM, et al, editors: *Greenfield's surgery: scientific principles and practice*, ed 4, Philadelphia, 2006, Lippincott Williams & Wilkins.
2. Lin PH, Kougias P, Bechara C, et al: Arterial disease. In Brunicardi FC, Andersen DK, Billiar TR, et al, editors: *Schwartz's principles of surgery*, ed 9, New York, 2010, McGraw-Hill.
3. Ernst CB, Stanley JC: *Current therapy in vascular surgery*, ed 4, St. Louis, 2001, CV Mosby.
4. Cronenwett J, Johnston W, editors: *Rutherford's vascular surgery*, ed 7, Philadelphia, 2010, WB Saunders.
5. Ouriel K: Endovascular aneurysm repair: an update, *Semin Vasc Surg* 16:87–175, 2003.

# E. Peripheral: Lower Extremity

*Ferenc P. Nagy, M.D.*

1. Which of the following statements is true regarding arterial occlusive disease of the lower extremities?

   A. Intermittent claudication is a symptom of acute arterial occlusion.

   B. Rest pain usually occurs in the same muscle groups affected by claudication and is often relieved by dependent positioning of the affected extremity.

   C. Changes such as hair loss, brittle nails, and muscle atrophy generally precede symptoms of claudication.

   D. Tissue necrosis is more likely in the presence of multilevel distal arterial disease.

   E. Arterial ulcerations, such as those of venous insufficiency, characteristically begin near the malleoli.

   *Ref.:* 1, 2

**COMMENTS:** **Chronic arterial occlusion of the lower extremities** is a result of atherosclerotic disease of the aorta and its branches and can be diagnosed by the presence of characteristic signs and symptoms. The classic symptom, intermittent claudication, is cramping pain in specific muscle groups that occurs when blood flow is inadequate for meeting the demands of exercise. The pain usually occurs below the level of occlusion. Hence, claudication of the buttock and thigh muscles is suggestive of aortoiliac obstruction, and calf claudication is suggestive of femoral artery obstruction. As the chronic ischemia progresses, trophic changes such as hair loss, nail brittleness, and muscular atrophy occur. Ischemic pain during rest is a manifestation of end-stage disease and characteristically involves the more distal aspects of the arterial circulation, such as the toes and feet. Pain is typically felt across the metatarsal heads. Associated physical findings include exacerbation of pain with elevation of the extremity, relief of pain by dependent positioning of the extremity, and dependent rubor (redness of the feet) caused by reactive hyperemia. Tissue necrosis usually signifies multilevel disease of the distal arterial tree inasmuch as chronic proximal occlusion alone is associated with the development of collateral circulation, which is normally adequate for preventing necrosis and gangrene. Most ulcers resulting from arterial insufficiency involve the toes or plantar surface of the foot and are painful, whereas venous ulcers are less painful and typically occur near the malleoli.

**ANSWER: D**

2. Which of the following is the most common site of atherosclerotic occlusion in the lower extremities?

   A. Aortic bifurcation

   B. Common femoral artery

   C. Profunda femoris artery

   D. Proximal superficial femoral artery

   E. Distal superficial femoral artery

   *Ref.:* 2

**COMMENTS:** Although atherosclerotic disease frequently involves the area of arterial bifurcations, such as the aortic, iliac, and common femoral bifurcations, the most common site of occlusion in the lower extremities is the distal superficial femoral artery. The occlusion occurs in the adductor canal proximal to the popliteal fossa and is related to the anatomic relationship of the artery to the adductor magnus tendon at this site. Affected patients frequently have disease at several levels, however, which emphasizes the need for accurate angiographic assessment before revascularization procedures. Involvement of the superficial femoral artery alone is generally associated with intermittent claudication but not generally with tissue loss or pain during rest. The profunda femoris artery is not usually occluded in this situation and serves as an important source of collateral blood flow.

**ANSWER: E**

3. With regard to aortoiliac atherosclerotic occlusive disease, which of the following statements is correct?

   A. Impotence is a common finding that results from decreased blood flow through the external iliac vessels.

   B. Thigh or buttock claudication (or both) is typical, and toe ulceration or gangrene secondary to atherosclerotic emboli is occasionally present.

   C. Lower extremity hair loss and nail brittleness occur in 60% of patients.

   D. Hemorrhage and sepsis are the principal causes of death after aortoiliac reconstruction.

   E. Percutaneous angioplasty with stenting of iliac lesions only occasionally relieves symptoms.

   *Ref.:* 1-3

**COMMENTS:** An accurate history and physical examination can help establish the diagnosis of **aortoiliac atherosclerotic occlusive disease**. Three common clinical manifestations, often referred to as the Leriche syndrome, include intermittent claudication of the thighs or buttocks, impotence, and diminished or absent femoral pulses. Impotence is caused by hypogastric (internal iliac) arterial occlusion, which reduces blood flow through the internal pudendal artery and the corpora cavernosa. With aortoiliac involvement alone, however, trophic changes are rarely present because collateral flow originating from the lumbar and epigastric arteries is preserved. Nutritional changes, such as hair loss and nail brittleness, when present, signify additional distal disease. Although distal tissue necrosis is often suggestive of more distal occlusive disease, the possibility of emboli from atherosclerotic plaque in the aortoiliac vessels must always be considered. This has been referred to as the "blue toe syndrome" and can occur even in the absence of occluding lesions. The principal cause of death in this group of patients is coronary artery disease. Iliac angioplasty with stenting is particularly successful in treating short-segment iliac disease. When multilevel disease necessitates conventional distal bypass techniques, adequate inflow may be established with balloon angioplasty of the iliac arteries.

**ANSWER:** B

**4.** Any patient with intermittent calf claudication should be advised of which of the following?

A. Angiography should be performed early to determine the extent of the arterial disease.

B. Surgical reconstruction should be performed to prevent progression of disease and the development of pain at rest with gangrene.

C. Nonoperative treatment is sufficient for 50% of patients.

D. There are no indications for arterial revascularization in patients with claudication.

E. Claudication progresses to gangrene in 2% to 3% of patients per year.

*Ref.:* 1-3

**COMMENTS:** The goals of **therapy for occlusive arterial disease** of the lower extremities are to relieve pain, prevent limb loss, and maintain bipedal gait. Most patients with intermittent claudication alone remain stable or even improve with appropriate conservative management. Such management includes a formal exercise program, smoking cessation, and risk reduction and may include medications such as cilostazol (Pletal). Daily aspirin ingestion has been shown to be beneficial for such patients by reducing the risk for morbidity from concomitant atherosclerotic disease, such as stroke and myocardial infarction. Prophylactic surgical intervention is not indicated. Patients with claudication have a low rate of progression to gangrene. In fact, more than 75% of these patients remain stable, and the amputation rate is less than 7% in patients treated nonoperatively and observed for up to 8 years. In patients with severe claudication and marked involvement of the tibial vessels, the disease progresses to gangrene in 2% to 3% of patients annually. This is in contrast to patients with pain at rest, ulceration, or gangrene, who are at risk for limb loss and should be evaluated for revascularization. Surgical intervention may be indicated for patients with claudication whose lifestyle or livelihood is impaired by their symptoms and who do not otherwise have limiting cardiac disease. Arteriography is indicated for patients who are considered candidates for surgery or angioplasty, but it should be preceded by less invasive testing, such as arterial blood flow studies.

**ANSWER:** E

**5.** With regard to nonoperative treatment of occlusive atherosclerotic disease of the lower extremities, which of the following statements is true?

A. Exercising to the point of claudication leads to improved muscle performance because of more efficient oxygen extraction.

B. Cessation of cigarette smoking reduces claudication but does not affect the risk for gangrene.

C. Aggressive foot care, including aggressive nail trimming and foot soaking, is recommended.

D. Anticoagulant therapy with warfarin (Coumadin) or heparin promotes healing of arterial ulcers.

E. All of the above.

*Ref.:* 1, 2

**COMMENTS:** Most patients in whom **intermittent claudication** is the only manifestation of peripheral vascular disease respond to conservative measures consisting of abstinence from tobacco and a graduated exercise program. Continued tobacco use has been associated with an increased risk for gangrene and a higher rate of premature graft failure after reconstructive procedures. For patients with more advanced ischemia, protection of the lower extremity is critical. Patients should avoid temperature extremes, improper footwear, or overly aggressive trimming of nails and calluses. It is not uncommon for relatively minor trauma to result in gangrene and eventual amputation of an already compromised foot. There is evidence that regular low-dose therapy with acetylsalicylic acid may be of benefit in preventing thrombosis in patients with atherosclerotic disease, but therapy with heparin or warfarin sodium has not proved beneficial.

**ANSWER:** A

**6.** Occlusive tibioperoneal disease does not occur commonly in patients with which of the following entities?

A. Buerger disease

B. Raynaud phenomenon

C. Diabetes mellitus

D. Arterial emboli

E. Tobacco use

*Ref.:* 2, 3

**COMMENTS:** Although the common pattern of **atherosclerotic occlusive disease** involves the femoral artery or the more proximal aortoiliac system, **diabetic patients** characteristically acquire a pattern of distal occlusive disease involving the distal popliteal artery and the tibial and metatarsal vessels. Buerger disease, or thromboangiitis obliterans, is associated with tobacco use and results in inflammatory thrombosis of the small and medium-sized vessels of the upper and lower extremities. This type of distal involvement may also be seen in patients with arterial embolism. Patients with tibioperoneal involvement are often initially found to have advanced ischemia rather than simple claudication, and arterial reconstruction may necessitate bypass grafting to target vessels at the ankle or proximal part of the foot. Raynaud syndrome is characterized by vasospasm of the small arteries and arterioles of the most distal portions of the extremities (i.e., the hands, fingers, feet, and toes).

**ANSWER:** B

**7.** With regard to the diabetic foot, which of the following statements is true?

A. Foot pain resulting from diabetic neuropathy is usually relieved by dependent positioning.

B. Trophic ulcers rarely occur if pedal pulses are palpable.

C. Débridement of infected tissue should be avoided until revascularization is accomplished because of the risk of nonhealing.

D. Surgical revascularization distal to the popliteal artery may be required to control infection and allow healing if arterial occlusion is present.

E. The ABI in a diabetic with an ischemic foot is most often lower than 1.0 because of calcified vessels.

*Ref.:* 1, 2

COMMENTS: **Diabetic patients** are at risk for foot disorders caused by diabetic neuropathy, occlusive arterial disease, and infection. **Diabetic neuropathy** generally has adverse consequences. Sensory neuropathy renders the foot susceptible to trauma because of analgesia, motor neuropathy causes imbalances in the intrinsic musculature of the foot that lead to ventral subluxation of the metatarsal heads and pressure necrosis of the plantar tissue, and autonomic neuropathy may alter the microcirculation, thereby further exacerbating the tissue ischemia. Ischemic pain during rest, unlike pain secondary to neuropathy, may be relieved by dependent positioning. Trophic ulcers, which are painless, often occur on the plantar surface over the metatarsal heads as a result of pressure necrosis and are seen frequently in patients with palpable pedal pulses. Such lesions provide sites of entry for infection, to which the diabetic foot is markedly susceptible. Control of infection requires aggressive initial débridement of all necrotic tissue, systemic antibiotics, and subsequent arterial revascularization if associated occlusive disease is present. Arterial reconstruction in diabetic patients by bypass or endovascular technique usually involves the tibioperoneal vessels and plays an important role in limb salvage. The ABI in diabetic patients is typically higher than 1.0 because of lower extremity arterial calcification and does not accurately reflect the degree of occlusive disease. Doppler waveforms obtained from noninvasive blood flow studies are a better guide to the degree of ischemia in this setting and are often markedly attenuated in diabetics with peripheral ischemia.

ANSWER: D

8. With regard to femoropopliteal bypass, which of the following statements is true?

A. The patency rates of prosthetic grafts are nearly equal to those of autologous vein grafts in both above- and below-knee bypasses.

B. Patency rates are higher when bypass is performed for claudication than when done for limb salvage.

C. Coronary artery disease adversely affects graft patency.

D. Diabetes adversely affects graft patency.

E. Patency rates are unaffected by vein size.

*Ref.:* 1, 2

COMMENTS: The **reversed saphenous vein autograft** has been the most successful arterial bypass graft below the inguinal ligament and is the standard against which the success of prosthetic grafts is measured. Some controversy exists with regard to the primary use of polytetrafluoroethylene or Dacron for above-knee popliteal bypasses, but the recent literature supports the preferential use of autologous vein graft even in the above-knee position. Therefore, autologous vein should be the first choice for all infrainguinal revascularizations. Patency rates for above-knee saphenous vein grafts are approximately 80% to 90% at 1 year and approximately 75% at 5 years.

**Patency rates** are generally higher when bypass is performed for claudication than for salvage of the limb because of the extent of the underlying pathologic process.

Patency is adversely affected by grafts performed below the knee, continued tobacco use, poor distal runoff, and small vein size (<4 mm). Small vein size and size mismatch can be corrected with the in situ technique.

Associated risk factors, such as diabetes, hypertension, and coronary artery disease, have not been shown to exert a detrimental effect on long-term graft patency. Limb salvage rates generally exceed graft patency rates. If healing is complete after distal bypass and the bypass subsequently becomes occluded, limb salvage can be achieved in more than 50% of patients.

ANSWER: B

9. Which of the following statements is not true regarding endovascular management of lower extremity ischemia?

A. Iliac stenoses may be treated with endovascular techniques, but occlusions must be addressed surgically.

B. Superficial femoral artery stenoses greater than 10 cm in length have much reduced patency when subjected to endovascular treatment.

C. Long-term patency rates for occlusion and stenosis are similar.

D. Endovascular stents can be placed primarily to treat long, complex arterial lesions, recurrent lesions, or obstructions or be placed secondarily to correct a dissection or residual stenosis after initial balloon angioplasty.

E. Infrapopliteal angioplasty results in a 2-year limb salvage rate of 50% to 80% despite much lower patency rates.

*Ref.:* 3

COMMENTS: **Endovascular approaches** play an integral role in the management of **atherosclerotic occlusive disease**. Long-term patency following angioplasty depends largely on the site being treated. Proximal, larger-caliber arteries have the best initial and long-term results, whereas distal sites have decreasing patency rates. Better results are obtained when treating short, focal stenoses rather than long, diffusely diseased arteries. Stenoses less than 2 cm are considered ideal lesions for percutaneous treatment, whereas those longer than 10 cm have poor patency with endovascular repair. Iliac stenoses and occlusions may both be treated with percutaneous endovascular technique. Although initial success rates in treating occlusions are somewhat lower, some series have shown similar long-term patency rates for both stenoses and occlusions of the iliac artery. This may be due partly to increased use of intravascular stents when treating occlusions. Although stents certainly have a role in treating postangioplasty dissections or residual stenoses, primary stent placement may be considered for treating longer, more complex lesions, recurrent lesions, lesions likely to embolize (ulcerated plaque), and occlusions. In poor operative candidates with limb-threatening ischemia, infrapopliteal angioplasty may be considered. Even though the 2-year limb salvage rate for such procedures has been reported to be 50% to 80%, patency rates are significantly lower, 30% to 40%.

ANSWER: A

**10.** Which of the following statements is true regarding infrainguinal revascularization in patients with end-stage renal disease (ESRD)?

A. Symptomatic lower extremity arterial occlusive disease will develop in more than one half of patients with ESRD.

B. Patients with ESRD have morbidity and mortality rates equal to those of the normal population when undergoing infrainguinal revascularization.

C. At 3 and 5 years, patency rates for infrainguinal revascularization are worse for patients with ESRD than for those with normal renal function.

D. Factors such as length of time on dialysis, availability of autogenous conduit, and size or location of ulceration may be prognostic indicators of successful revascularization for patients with ESRD.

E. Bypass to the tibial vessels should not be offered to patients with ESRD.

*Ref.:* 3, 4

**COMMENTS:** The frequency of **infrainguinal revascularization** in patients with **end-stage renal disease** has increased over the past decade. In addition, symptoms from arterial occlusive disease will develop in approximately 20% of patients with ESRD. Several studies have examined the efficacy of revascularization in this patient population. Although patients with ESRD do have higher rates of morbidity and mortality than the population with normal renal function, 3- to 5-year graft patency rates are quite similar. Many prognostic factors have been proposed to help predict success or failure in this tenuous patient population, including length of time maintained on hemodialysis, location of gangrene (heel or forefoot), size of ulceration (>2 to 4 cm), availability of autogenous conduit, and the presence of suitable target vessels. A global assessment of such patients that takes into account comorbid conditions, ambulatory status, and the prognostic factors just listed must be made. When this is performed, tibial bypass can often be undertaken successfully in the renal failure population.

**ANSWER:** D

**11.** Long-term patency of bypass grafts to the tibioperoneal vessels is influenced by which of the following?

A. Diabetes

B. Previous attempts at revascularization

C. Presence of a patent pedal arch

D. Level of distal anastomosis

E. All of the above

*Ref.:* 1-3

**COMMENTS: Bypass graft procedures to the tibial vessels** are typically performed for limb salvage (i.e., rest pain or ischemic tissue loss/gangrene) and in patients with significant multilevel occlusive arterial disease. Accordingly, they are less successful than bypasses performed for claudication, in which case the atherosclerotic burden is typically much lower. Patency is better when the pedal arch is angiographically intact, but absence of a pedal arch is not a contraindication to surgery. Grafts to the anterior or posterior tibial arteries are therefore preferred, but grafts to the peroneal artery are also useful. Concomitant endarterectomy of the

tibial vessels is more likely to result in dissection and is consequently rarely undertaken. The presence of diabetes does not significantly adversely affect patency on bypasses to the popliteal or tibial levels. Diabetes is, however, a significant risk factor for the development of tibioperoneal occlusive disease. Previously performed operative procedures have not adversely affected early or long-term patency rates or limb salvage. The role of distal vein patches for prosthetic grafts, the addition of an AVF to a bypass graft, and the use of postoperative antiplatelet drugs or anticoagulants have all been proposed as adjuncts to improve infrageniculate bypass graft patency. The level of the distal anastomosis does not influence graft patency. However, the quality of the distal runoff is a primary factor.

**ANSWER:** C

**12.** Sudden pain and weakness in the left leg develop in a patient with a history of coronary artery disease and atrial fibrillation. Examination reveals a cool, pale extremity with an absence of pulses below the groin and a normal contralateral leg. Which of the following is the most likely diagnosis?

A. Cerebrovascular accident

B. Arterial thrombosis

C. Arterial embolism

D. Acute thrombophlebitis

E. Aortic dissection

*Ref.:* 1, 2

**COMMENTS:** See Question 14.

**ANSWER:** C

**13.** For the initial evaluation of the patient described in Question 12, which of the following tests is mandatory?

A. Electrocardiography

B. Venography

C. Arteriography

D. Abdominal ultrasound studies

E. CT angiography of the affected extremity

*Ref.:* 1, 2

**COMMENTS:** See Question 14.

**ANSWER:** A

**14.** If the patient described in Question 12 had a history of intermittent left calf claudication and if examination showed, in addition, diminished pulses in the contralateral leg and trophic skin changes bilaterally, which of the following would be true?

A. Arteriographic findings are unlikely to help plan the appropriate surgical approach.

B. Venography is mandatory for ruling out phlegmasia alba dolens.

C. Indications for surgical intervention are unchanged.

D. The anticipated surgical procedure is unchanged.

E. Irreversible muscular necrosis may occur after 24 to 48 hours.

*Ref.:* 1, 2

**COMMENTS:** The classic signs of **acute arterial occlusion** are pain, pallor, absence of pulse, paralysis, and paresthesia (the five P's). The common causes of acute arterial occlusion are embolism, thrombosis, and trauma. In the patient described in Question 12, the history of atrial fibrillation, coupled with the classic findings of acute arterial occlusion, make arterial embolism the most likely diagnosis.

Clinical findings that suggest arterial thrombosis rather than embolism as the cause include an absence of cardiac disease commonly associated with embolization phenomena, symptoms of underlying occlusive atherosclerotic disease, and physical findings suggestive of chronic ischemia. It can be difficult, however, to differentiate embolism from thrombosis on clinical grounds alone. Embolism can certainly occur in patients with underlying peripheral vascular disease.

Prompt operative intervention is indicated, regardless of cause, when there is acute limb-threatening ischemia. It is important, however, to distinguish arterial embolism from arterial thrombosis superimposed on atherosclerotic plaque because the extent of surgery may vary considerably. Although embolism may be treated successfully by simple embolectomy and extraction of the thrombus that forms distal to the embolism, effective treatment of arterial thrombosis can be much more difficult, with arterial reconstruction sometimes being required. Arteriography may be helpful for differentiating between embolic and thrombotic occlusions. A careful history and physical examination permit a diagnosis of embolic occlusion in most cases. Arteriography is not always necessary and should not be performed if it will delay operative reestablishment of blood flow. Patients with arterial embolism should undergo electrocardiography and radiography of the chest because of the high association with intrinsic cardiac disease and its potential for myocardial infarction.

Acute arterial occlusion can be differentiated from acute venous thrombosis in that venous thrombosis is usually associated with edema and preservation of peripheral pulses. Severe venous obstruction produces phlegmasia cerulea dolens. When this is associated with arterial thrombosis and spasm, phlegmasia alba dolens may occur. Untreated, this process may progress to venous gangrene.

In rare instances, an aortic dissection mimics acute embolism by producing loss of peripheral pulses, but the diagnosis may be suspected because of the presence of back or chest pain and hypertension.

Acute arterial occlusion that rapidly produces paralysis and paresthesia may be mistaken for a stroke. However, the physical examination should direct attention toward the compromised extremity and eliminate stroke from the differential diagnosis.

Prompt diagnosis of arterial occlusion is critical because irreversible muscular necrosis necessitating amputation may occur within 4 to 6 hours.

**ANSWER:** C

15. For an acute arterial embolus to the lower extremity with limb-threatening ischemia, appropriate initial treatment includes which of the following?

A. Intravenous 5000-unit heparin bolus followed by continuous-drip administration

B. Delay in heparinization until anesthesia is administered because heparinization precludes spinal anesthesia

C. Routine preoperative trial of vasodilators

D. Attempt at thrombolytic therapy with drugs such as tissue plasminogen activator

E. Immediate angiography before an operation

*Ref.:* 1, 2

**COMMENTS:** Treatment of **arterial embolism** must be initiated promptly to prevent irreversible ischemic damage. Intravenous heparin should be administered to prevent the formation and propagation of thrombosis distal to the embolus and is the most important first step. Heparinization should not be delayed, particularly because most embolectomies can be performed with the use of local anesthesia. Furthermore, the degree of distal thrombosis is an important determinant of surgical success and limb salvage. Although arterial spasm accompanies acute arterial occlusion, the routine use of vasodilators is not advocated. Fibrinolytic agents have an important role in the treatment of patients with acute thrombosis superimposed on chronic ischemia. Their routine use to treat acute arterial embolism with limb-threatening ischemia is not advocated, however, because timely intervention is of utmost importance. Because patients with arterial embolism often have associated cardiac disease and may be compromised further by the metabolic effects of ischemic tissue, preoperative attention must be given to careful physiologic monitoring and to the fluid balance, electrolyte balance, and arterial blood gas status of the patient.

**ANSWER:** A

16. With regard to the operative management of lower extremity arterial embolism, which of the following statements is true?

A. Embolectomy can be performed in most cases via arteriotomy distal to the site of obstruction.

B. Suspected aortoiliac emboli should be removed through an abdominal approach.

C. Brisk backbleeding is a reliable indicator of successful complete distal embolectomy.

D. Wide fasciotomy should be avoided in heparinized patients because of the risk for hemorrhage.

E. Palpable pulses or audible Doppler signals are reliable indicators of complete embolectomy.

*Ref.:* 1, 2

**COMMENTS:** In most cases, **embolectomy** can be performed with the use of balloon catheters introduced through arteriotomies proximal to the embolic lodging site. Aortoiliac emboli can be removed successfully via bilateral femoral arteriotomies. Backbleeding does not necessarily indicate adequate removal of the embolus distally because it may originate from an arterial branch proximal to the thrombus that remains. For this reason, restoration of distal pulses or Doppler signals and intraoperative arteriography, when necessary, constitute the gold standard used to assess the completeness of thromboembolectomy. Fasciotomy is an important concomitant procedure if the limb has been subjected to ischemia for 4 to 6 hours or longer. Fasciotomy should be performed, even in heparinized patients. Compartment syndrome can develop after reperfusion of an ischemic limb, and close postoperative attention is thus required.

**ANSWER:** E

**17.** While a patient is in the recovery room after femoral embolectomy, a palpable pedal pulse disappears. The patient's leg is pale and swollen. Appropriate treatment includes which of the following?

A. Venography

B. Fibrinolytic therapy

C. Arteriography

D. Immediate reexploration and fasciotomy

E. Duplex ultrasound of the arterial repair.

*Ref.:* 1, 2

**COMMENTS:** During the immediate postoperative period, therapy focuses on maintenance of peripheral perfusion, treatment of the patient's underlying cardiac disease, and treatment of the potential metabolic complications after resumption of perfusion of an ischemic limb. Frequent evaluation of peripheral pulses by palpation and Doppler ultrasound studies and of limb temperature and color is mandatory. Any change that indicates **postoperative ischemia** warrants immediate reexploration. If swelling threatens the viability of peripheral musculature, fasciotomy is indicated. Fibrinolytic therapy has been used for arterial thrombosis but is contraindicated in patients who have undergone a recent operation because of the risk for hemorrhage at the operative site.

**ANSWER:** D

**18.** After undergoing femoral embolectomy and fasciotomy, a patient becomes oliguric, and the urine is brownish red. Immediate treatment includes which of the following?

A. Cessation of intravenous administration of heparin

B. Restoration of the serum potassium level

C. Intravenous administration of sodium bicarbonate and mannitol

D. Renal arteriography

E. Intra-arterial vasodilators

*Ref.:* 1

**COMMENTS:** When an extremity has been subjected to **ischemia** and **muscular necrosis** occurs, reperfusion can result in metabolic acidosis and profound hyperkalemia. Rhabdomyolysis releases myoglobulin, which precipitates in acidic urine and produces brownish red urine that is free of red blood cells. Treatment of patients in this situation requires prompt reversal of hyperkalemia to prevent cardiac arrest (intravenous insulin and glucose), administration of sodium bicarbonate to alkalinize the urine and to treat the systemic metabolic acidosis, and osmotic diuresis with mannitol to prevent renal tubular obstruction. Fasciotomy is indicated if it has not already been performed. Continuation of anticoagulation therapy is critical because the patient remains at significant risk for recurrent embolism from the underlying cardiac disease. Less than 10% of arterial emboli involve the renal vessels, and renal arteriography is not indicated in this case.

**ANSWER:** C

**19.** Most arterial emboli originate from which one of the following sites?

A. Cardiac valves

B. Left atrium

C. Left ventricle

D. Thoracic aorta

E. Abdominal aorta

*Ref.:* 1, 2

**COMMENTS:** By far, most **arterial emboli** originate in the heart. Less than 10% arise from ulcerated plaques in the aorta, carotid arteries, or subclavian arteries. The most common intracardiac site is the left atrium, in which thrombi form as a result of stasis in patients with atrial fibrillation, mitral valvular disease, or both. A rare source of left atrial emboli is a left atrial myxoma. Left ventricular thrombi are a potential source of embolism in patients with myocardial infarction, left ventricular aneurysm, congestive heart failure, or cardiomyopathy. Valvular sources of emboli include vegetative endocarditis and thrombi formed on mechanical prosthetic heart valves. Paradoxical emboli arising from the venous system may reach the arterial circulation through a patent foramen ovale.

**ANSWER:** B

**20.** Arterial emboli of cardiac origin most frequently produce occlusion of which of the following?

A. Cerebral vessels

B. Distal aorta

C. Common femoral artery

D. Superficial femoral artery

E. Popliteal artery

*Ref.:* 1, 2

**COMMENTS:** **Arterial emboli** usually lodge proximal to arterial bifurcations and most commonly involve the lower extremities. One third to one half of arterial emboli occlude the common femoral artery at the bifurcation of the superficial femoral and profunda femoris. Because the embolus lodges proximal to major bifurcations, there is significant and abrupt interruption of potential collateral flow, which results in severe ischemia.

**ANSWER:** C

**21.** After undergoing brachial artery catheterization for coronary angiography, a patient complains of hand numbness, and the previously present radial pulse is noted to be absent. Which of the following is the appropriate treatment?

A. Administration of systemic vasodilators

B. Surgical exploration and topical application of papaverine

C. Percutaneous balloon dilation of the brachial artery

D. Brachial artery exposure with direct repair of the injured segment

E. Arteriography to determine the presence of thrombus at the catheterization site

*Ref.:* 1

**COMMENTS:** **Iatrogenic arterial injuries** may result from the placement of needles and catheters for radiographic studies or monitoring purposes. Arterial occlusion usually occurs as a result of thrombosis in association with intimal injury. Treatment consists of prompt exploration with arteriotomy and thrombectomy. Intimal damage may be treated by segmental excision with direct anastomosis or by placing a short vein patch. Surgery should not be delayed by attributing the ischemia associated with arterial injury to arterial "spasm." Arteriography to confirm what is already clinically apparent delays the required surgical exploration and is not usually indicated.

**A N S W E R :**  D

22. Which of the following is the most common symptom of thoracic outlet syndrome?

    A. Raynaud phenomenon

    B. Pain or paresthesia in the C8-T1 nerve distribution

    C. Pain or paresthesia in the radial nerve distribution

    D. Ischemia or pain caused by arterial compression

    E. Arm edema caused by venous obstruction

    *Ref.:* 1, 2

**COMMENTS:** Anatomic compression of the brachial plexus, subclavian-axillary vessels, or both may occur at the **thoracic outlet** by a variety of mechanisms at several specific sites. The primary symptoms depend on which anatomic structures are compressed. Most patients have pain or paresthesias as a result of compression of the brachial plexus. Pain and paresthesias may affect any part of the shoulder or upper extremity but are most commonly noted in the C8-T1 area, or ulnar nerve distribution. Symptoms of arterial compression, such as ischemic pain, fatigue, and decreased temperature, are less common. Embolic events may produce digital gangrene. Symptoms of venous compression occur even less frequently than those of arterial compromise and may include edema, venous distention, and discoloration. In some instances, "**effort thrombosis**" of the subclavian vein (Paget-von Schroetter syndrome) may occur. Nerve conduction studies, arteriography, and dynamic CT may aid in the diagnosis of thoracic outlet syndrome. Physicians' maneuvers aimed at detecting a pulse deficit have low specificity. Resection of a cervical rib or a first rib with anterior scalenectomy is performed to decompress the thoracic outlet. Associated subclavian-axillary arterial lesions are corrected. A transaxillary or supraclavicular approach may be used.

**A N S W E R :**  B

23. With regard to Buerger disease, which of the following statements is correct?

    A. It is most frequently found in African-American men 20 to 40 years of age.

    B. Recurrent migratory superficial phlebitis often follows arterial involvement.

    C. Sympathectomy is effective in 50% of patients, but arterial reconstruction offers better long-term results.

    D. Cessation of cigarette smoking is the primary therapy.

    E. It can be treated successfully with anticoagulants, vasodilators, and steroids.

    *Ref.:* 1, 2

**COMMENTS: Buerger disease** (thromboangiitis obliterans) is an inflammatory process of uncertain etiology that produces thrombosis of medium-sized and small arteries and veins. The disease typically affects young men who are heavy smokers. It is rare in African Americans. Recurrent migratory superficial thrombophlebitis involving the pedal veins often predates arterial involvement by several years. Both the upper and lower extremities can be affected, and ischemic gangrene frequently results. Complete cessation of tobacco use is the most important aspect of treatment and may produce remission. Simply decreasing the frequency of tobacco use is ineffective. Arterial reconstruction is not usually possible because distal small vessels are frequently involved. Cervical or lumbar sympathectomy is useful in 50% of patients. No pharmacologic treatment has proved widely successful.

**A N S W E R :**  D

24. With regard to the appropriate management of popliteal aneurysms, which of the following statements is true?

    A. Popliteal artery aneurysms should be managed conservatively if less than 3 cm in diameter, asymptomatic, and stable.

    B. Popliteal aneurysms are bilateral in up to 25% of patients.

    C. Excision with end-to-end anastomosis is the procedure of choice for popliteal artery aneurysms.

    D. The presence of a popliteal aneurysm should heighten suspicion for arterial aneurysms in the abdomen and thorax.

    E. Rupture is the most common complication of a popliteal aneurysm.

    *Ref.:* 2

**COMMENTS: Peripheral aneurysms** are primarily atherosclerotic in origin, associated with hypertension, and frequently multiple. **Popliteal artery aneurysms** are the most common, they are bilateral in 50% to 70% of patients, and approximately 50% are associated with femoral or aortic aneurysms. Patients with bilateral popliteal artery aneurysms have a 70% chance of having an AAA. Patients with popliteal aneurysms therefore require thorough assessment to rule out other associated aneurysms. Popliteal aneurysms present a high risk for limb loss as a result of thrombosis or embolism, and rupture is very rare. Popliteal aneurysms should be operated on even when small, with diameters of 1.5 to 2.0 cm being a useful guideline. Proximal and distal ligation with bypass grafting is the procedure of choice. On occasion, if the aneurysm is small and the artery is tortuous, excision with end-to-end anastomosis is possible.

**A N S W E R :**  D

25. With regard to Raynaud disease or phenomenon, which of the following statements is correct?

    A. It is characterized by sequential phases of pallor, cyanosis, and rubor in the upper extremities that are initiated by exposure to heat or emotional stress.

    B. It is seen most frequently in elderly women.

    C. It is characterized by a pathologic mechanism that involves vasospasm with a reduction in dermal circulation.

    D. β-Blockers often yield symptomatic control.

    E. Cervical sympathectomy is usually the primary therapy.

    *Ref.:* 2

**COMMENTS: Raynaud disease** or phenomenon is the most common vasospastic disorder and most frequently affects young women (90% of patients are younger than 40 years). It may exist as a primary disorder (Raynaud disease), or it may be a secondary manifestation (Raynaud phenomenon) of disorders such as scleroderma, Buerger disease, or thoracic outlet syndrome. The classic pattern of pallor, cyanosis, and rubor occurs after exposure to cold or stress. Vasospasm with a decrease in dermal circulation results in pallor. Cyanosis occurs as a result of sluggish flow of blood. Reactive hyperemia then develops as the vasospasm subsides. Avoidance of initiating factors is often adequate. Calcium channel blockers are the initial drug of choice.

**ANSWER: C**

26. Appropriate management of frostbite includes which of the following?

    A. Rapid rewarming with dry heat rather than rapid rewarming with warm water

    B. Rapid rewarming with warm water

    C. Slow rewarming at room temperature if heparin or dextran is administered

    D. Thorough débridement of blisters and devitalized tissue

    E. Sympathectomy in the presence of tissue necrosis to minimize the extent of necrosis and prevent late vasomotor sequelae

    *Ref.:* 2

**COMMENTS: A cold-injured extremity** is best treated by rapid rewarming in warm water (40° C to 42° C). This results in less tissue damage than treatment by slow rewarming (i.e., at room temperature). Dry heat or water at higher temperature risks additional thermal injury because of decreased sensation of the injured part. The extremity should be elevated and exposed. Antibiotics are given if there is an open wound, and tetanus prophylaxis is administered as indicated. Opening of blisters and débridement of apparently devitalized tissue are contraindicated. True demarcation of nonviable tissue requires many weeks and should be allowed to develop spontaneously. The initial use of vasodilating drugs or antithrombotic agents such as heparin and dextran has not been shown to be effective. Sympathectomy may be useful for the treatment of the chronic sequelae of frostbite, such as paresthesia, hyperhidrosis, and coldness, but it does not minimize the amount of tissue necrosis.

**ANSWER: B**

27. With regard to popliteal entrapment syndrome, which of the following is true?

    A. The syndrome commonly affects men before the age of 40.

    B. Limb-threatening ischemia is the most common manifestation.

    C. Fibrous bands of the popliteus muscle most commonly cause arterial impingement.

    D. CT is the diagnostic procedure of choice.

    E. Symptoms are usually treated by exercise and antiplatelet medications.

    *Ref.:* 3, 4

**COMMENTS:** The **popliteal artery entrapment syndrome** most commonly affects men before the age of 40. The most common finding is mild, intermittent claudication. Arterial thrombosis or occlusion is rare. Other, less common causes of claudication in young adults include premature atherosclerosis caused by malignant hyperlipidemia, adventitial cystic degenerative disease, chronic exertional compartment syndrome, and vasculitis secondary to collagen vascular disorders. Physical examination typically reveals a loss of tibial pulses with active plantar flexion or passive dorsiflexion to tighten the gastrocnemius muscle. Noninvasive blood flow studies and duplex scanning may also reveal the abnormality when done in conjunction with these flexion maneuvers. The most sensitive diagnostic study is MRI, which can delineate the musculotendinous structures of the popliteal fossa and document their dynamic relationship with the popliteal vessels. The most common abnormality encountered is medial deviation of the popliteal artery around the medial head of the gastrocnemius muscle. Five other anatomic variants have been described. Surgical repair is the only effective treatment for symptomatic patients. Resection or release of the variant musculotendinous structures is performed. Arterial reconstruction is necessary when stenotic or aneurysmal lesions are present. Surgical repair is also recommended for asymptomatic patients who are noted to have anatomic variants on the opposite side to prevent the development of secondary vascular complications.

**ANSWER: A**

28. With regard to atheroembolic disease of the lower extremities, which of the following is true?

    A. Atheroemboli commonly cause acute occlusion of the common femoral bifurcation.

    B. Normal pedal pulses are commonly found in patients with atheroembolic disease.

    C. The most common source of atheroemboli is superficial femoral artery atherosclerotic disease.

    D. Medical therapy is associated with a low rate of recurrence.

    E. Aortofemoral bypass, femoropopliteal bypass, extra-anatomic bypass with aortic exclusion, and localized endarterectomy are not indicated for the management of atheroembolic disease.

    *Ref.:* 1-4

**COMMENTS:** The term *atheroemboli* describes cholesterol or atherothrombotic microemboli. Both aneurysms and atherosclerotic plaque may be the sources of microemboli. Aortoiliac atherosclerotic disease is the most common source of lower extremity microemboli. Although macroemboli from cardiac sources tend to lodge at the bifurcations of large vessels, microemboli commonly lodge in the distal small vessels, such as the digital arteries of the toes. Cholesterol debris is often found on pathologic review of patients with atheroemboli. Patients typically have the sudden appearance of painful, mottled areas on their toes. Microemboli may lodge in the capillaries of the skin and lead to livedo reticularis of the knees, thighs, and buttocks. Typically, patients have palpable pedal pulses. If the superficial femoral artery is the source, a bruit or thrill may be present. Duplex scans may help define atherosclerotic lesions, but biplane angiography is the most sensitive diagnostic method for determining the source of emboli.

Medical management with antiplatelet agents, steroids, aspirin, or warfarin is associated with a high rate of recurrence.

Warfarin may lead to exacerbation of the condition because of plaque destabilization. Surgical intervention is indicated to remove the embolic source and reconstruct the arterial tree if necessary. Aortofemoral bypass, femoropopliteal bypass, extra-anatomic bypass with aortic exclusion, and localized endarterectomy may all be indicated, depending on the location and extent of disease. Covered stents and in some cases bare stents are also used.

**A N S W E R :** B

29. True statements regarding anterior tibial compartmental syndrome include which of the following?

   A. It may be caused by severe exertion.

   B. Pain is the dominant symptom and is elicited on palpation of the calf.

   C. The dorsalis pedis pulse is always absent.

   D. Unlike the treatment of other compartment syndromes, fasciotomy is rarely needed.

   E. The presence of pulses does negate the diagnosis.

*Ref.:* 2

**COMMENTS: Anterior tibial compartmental syndrome** is related to pressure from tissue fluid within the closed compartment. The syndrome may be secondary to arterial trauma or arterial embolism and may be seen as a complication of cardiopulmonary bypass or femoropopliteal bypass. It may also be caused by severe exertion with no proven anatomic lesion. Pain is characteristically the first and dominant symptom and is located over the anterior compartment. As with other compartment syndromes, the presence of pulses does not negate the diagnosis. Early fasciotomy before neuromuscular necrosis is the treatment in the acute setting. Chronic recurrent pain is occasionally seen in athletes and is also sometimes treated with fasciotomy after careful work-up to exclude other causes of pain.

**A N S W E R :** A

**R E F E R E N C E S**

1. Belkin M, Owens CD, Whittemore AD, et al: Peripheral arterial occlusive disease. In Townsend CM Jr, Beauchamp RD, Evers BM, et al, editors: *Sabiston textbook of surgery: the biological basis of modern surgical practice,* ed 18, Philadelphia, 2008, WB Saunders.
2. Lin PH, Kougias P, Bechara C, et al: Arterial disease. In Brunicardi FC, Andersen DK, Billiar TR, et al, editors: *Schwartz's principles of surgery,* ed 9, New York, 2010, McGraw-Hill.
3. Cronenwett J, Johnston W, editors: *Rutherford's vascular surgery,* ed 7, Philadelphia, 2010, WB Saunders.
4. Ernst EB, Stanley JE: *Current therapy in vascular surgery,* ed 4, St. Louis, 2001, CV Mosby.

# F. Peripheral Venous and Lymphatic Disease

*Benjamin Lind, M.D.*

1. A 28-year-old overweight woman comes to the emergency department with a slightly reddened, painful "knot" 8 cm above the medial malleolus. Examination in the standing position demonstrates a palpable vein above and below a tender nonfluctuant 2-cm mass. The patient is afebrile and has no other abnormalities on physical examination. Which of the following is the most likely diagnosis?

   A. Early DVT

   B. Superficial venous thrombosis

   C. Suppurative thrombophlebitis

   D. Cellulitis

   E. Insect bite

   *Ref.:* 1-3

**COMMENTS: Superficial venous thrombi** may be associated with thrombophlebitis, which is an acute, nonbacterial inflammation that produces pain, redness, and swelling. Thrombi, however, may form without producing any signs or symptoms. Superficial thrombophlebitis usually appears as a localized process over the known course of a superficial vein. It occurs in association with intravenous catheters in the upper extremity and is generally seen at the sites of varicose veins in the lower extremity. The presence of distended varicosities above and below the lesion aids in the diagnosis. The diagnosis is usually readily made from the history and findings on physical examination. Lack of blood flow through the vein can be confirmed with Doppler ultrasound imaging, but this test is usually unnecessary unless there is concern about DVT or a question regarding the diagnosis. Venography is not indicated and may even exacerbate the condition.

The diagnoses of cellulitis, insect bite, subcutaneous hematoma, and traumatic ecchymosis must be considered when evaluating these lesions. An insect bite is frequently associated with itching. The presence of hematoma or ecchymosis may indicate trauma as the cause. Suppurative thrombophlebitis must also be considered, especially in patients with fever and leukocytosis. Suppurative thrombophlebitis is characterized by purulence within the vein and is generally a complication of intravenous cannulation. The presence of increased redness, pain, fluctuance, fever, and leukocytosis is more typical of bacterial infection than of superficial thrombophlebitis.

**ANSWER: B**

2. In a patient with superficial thrombophlebitis associated with varicose veins, the treatment plan may include which of the following measures?

   A. Excision of the entire vein and administration of intravenous antibiotics

   B. Iodine-125 ($^{125}$I)-labeled fibrinogen scan, hospitalization, and heparinization

   C. Ligation of the vein proximal and distal to the mass, bed rest, and intravenous antibiotics

   D. Bed rest, elastic support hose, leg elevation, and antibiotics

   E. Warm packs, elastic support hose, nonsteroidal antiinflammatory drugs, and ambulation with limited sitting or standing

   *Ref.:* 1, 2

**COMMENTS:** The usual aim when treating **superficial thrombophlebitis** is to relieve the symptoms. The inflammation is nonbacterial, and antibiotics are not necessary unless there is evidence of secondary infection. These thrombi almost never embolize to the lungs unless they have propagated to the deep venous system. Fortunately, superficial venous thrombosis does not usually progress to DVT. Anticoagulation is therefore not necessary. Ligation is reserved for superficial lesions in the greater saphenous system near its junction with the femoral vein and for lesions of the lesser saphenous system near the popliteal fossa, locations from which a thrombus may more easily extend to the deep venous system.

Superficial phlebitis in these locations is best evaluated with duplex ultrasound scanning. Unlike the recommendations made for DVT, with superficial thrombosis the risk for propagation of the thrombus is lessened by preventing venous stasis. This is accomplished by frequent walking, use of elastic stocking support, and keeping the leg elevated above the level of the heart when in the supine position. In other words, the patient should either walk or lie down with the leg elevated. Sitting and standing still for extended periods should be avoided whenever possible. Superficial thrombophlebitis is an acute problem, and symptoms from it usually resolve in 6 to 8 weeks. Anti-inflammatory drugs are of variable effectiveness. Aspirin usually suffices. Recurrent superficial thrombophlebitis may respond to proximal ligation followed by vein stripping.

**ANSWER: E**

3. Which of the following is true regarding ileofemoral venous thrombosis?

   A. Edema is rarely present.

   B. The left side is more frequently involved.

   C. It commonly results from an indwelling catheter.

D. It is the most common site of lower extremity DVT.

E. It rarely results in elevated venous pressure.

*Ref.:* 1, 2

**COMMENTS:** The signs and symptoms of **deep venous thrombosis** vary according to the vein involved. The most frequent site of thrombosis is the calf, with the lesion generally arising in the sinuses of the soleus muscle. Calf vein thrombi usually produce pain and localized tenderness. Little swelling occurs (typically less than a 1.5-cm difference in diameter between the calves, although it is entirely absent in 30% of patients), and venous pressure is normal. **Femoral vein thrombi** produce pain in the calf, popliteal region, or adductor canal. Swelling is generally present up to the midcalf, and venous pressure is elevated. Ileofemoral thrombi are often localized but may extend to the calf. The left leg is involved twice as often as the right, probably because of the longer course of the left iliac vein and its compression by the right iliac artery. As venous pressure becomes elevated, the leg becomes painful, edematous, swollen, and pale (phlegmasia alba dolens). In this condition, the blanched appearance of the limb is the result of edema and not arterial spasm, as previously thought. More extensive ileofemoral venous thrombosis, in which clot is propagated distally and into the ileofemoral venous tributaries, can obstruct all venous drainage, impair arterial inflow, and produce ischemia and threatened loss of the limb. This condition, phlegmasia cerulea dolens, is a surgical emergency. Pelvic vein thrombus can occur in women with pelvic inflammatory disease or in men with prostatic infections. The condition is detected by pelvic examination, and there are few leg signs. Venous thrombosis is less frequent in the upper than the lower extremities, and most commonly it is the result of subclavian vein thrombosis from an indwelling catheter. Upper extremity DVT may occur in patients with heart failure or cancer. In otherwise normal patients it has been termed **Paget-von Schroetter syndrome or "effort thrombosis"** and is a subclavian axillary vein thrombosis resulting from chronic repeated injury to the vein at the thoracic outlet. It is manifested as arm swelling and heaviness, with discomfort made worse by activity.

**ANSWER: B**

4. Which of the following factors is the least important independent risk factor associated with increased risk for DVT?

A. Obesity

B. Central venous catheters

C. Hospitalization with recent surgery

D. Trauma

E. Previous DVT

*Ref.:* 3

**COMMENTS: Venostasis of the lower extremities** is associated with prolonged bed rest, standing, or sitting. It is also caused by the immobilization and muscular paralysis associated with trauma and general and spinal anesthesia. The most significant risk factors include previous DVT and hospitalization with recent surgery. Additional risk factors include advanced age, diabetes mellitus, and the presence of malignancy. Obesity in conjunction with other risk factors leads to increased risk for DVT, but it may not be an independent risk factor. Patients with blood group type O are at lower risk for DVT, whereas patients with group A blood are at higher risk. In both instances the reason is unknown.

Oral contraceptives and pregnancy are associated with increased levels of fibrinogen and factors VII, VIII, IX, and X, and both are associated with increased risk for DVT.

The incidence of DVT in surgical patients is 20% to 50%. The incidence in patients with hip fractures or in those undergoing knee or hip replacement may exceed 50%.

**ANSWER: A**

5. Regarding the work-up of patients with DVT, which of the following statements is true?

A. Ascending venography has high specificity for the diagnosis of DVT.

B. MRI can detect central but not iliac venous thrombi.

C. Doppler ultrasound imaging and impedance plethysmography are equally useful in diagnosing femoral, popliteal, and major calf vein thromboses.

D. Doppler ultrasound and impedance plethysmography are equally sensitive in diagnosing ileofemoral venous occlusion.

E. Isotope scanning differentiates between active thrombosis and inflammatory fibrous exudate.

*Ref.:* 1-3

**COMMENTS: Isotope scans** with [125]I-labeled human fibrinogen are used to detect clot formation or thrombus propagation. Studies of even the sickest patient are possible with portable instrumentation. Isotope scanning is not useful in patients with superficial **thrombophlebitis**, overlying recent incisions, traumatic injuries, hematomas, cellulitis, active arthritis, or primary lymphedema because it cannot differentiate between active inflammatory fibrous exudate and thrombus formation. Upper thigh and pelvic lesions are often confounded by high background counts of the isotope within the pelvic organs. An isotope scan can be 90% accurate in detecting the onset of thrombosis when performed serially (daily) in high-risk patients. Isotope scanning is now almost never used for routine clinical diagnosis and is reserved for serial studies of patients in research studies. **Doppler ultrasound imaging** is useful for detecting occlusions of major venous channels. It can also detect incompetence of the deep and perforator veins, but it cannot differentiate between old and new thrombi, nor can it help diagnose small, nonobstructing thrombi. Duplex scanning with B-mode ultrasound imaging is the best noninvasive study for DVT. This test can reliably differentiate extrinsic venous compression from DVT and new thrombi from old, and it can determine valvular competence. Superficial and deep veins of the calf and thigh, as well as the iliac veins and IVC, can also be visualized. These tests are viewed as the preferred initial tests for DVT. Impedance plethysmography is more accurate than Doppler ultrasound for diagnosing femoral, popliteal, and major calf vein thrombosis but less accurate than duplex scanning. Venography is still considered the definitive test for the diagnosis of DVT and is used to resolve equivocal results obtained by the noninvasive techniques. It is rarely used, however.

**ANSWER: A**

6. Which of the following is true?

A. The calf muscle pump has minimal importance in regard to the venous flow rate.

B. Post-thrombotic syndrome may occur in more than one half of patients after an episode of DVT.

C. Veins are less stiff than arteries per unit of cross-sectional area.

D. Valvular incompetence contributes to the development of varicose veins but not to the development of venous stasis ulcers.

E. Venous pressure at the foot is greatly increased while walking.

*Ref.:* 3

**COMMENTS:** The **calf muscle pump** is the most important mechanism for preventing the accumulation of interstitial fluid. While standing, **venous pressure** may exceed 100 mm Hg. This pressure is greatly reduced while walking. Post-thrombotic syndrome occurs in up to 60% of patients following DVT. It is caused by valvular incompetence in deep veins below the knee and perforating veins. Venous hypertension results in brawny discoloration and venous stasis disease. Varicose veins result when incompetent valves allow reflux of blood proximally to distally. Veins have less elastic tissue than arteries and are stiffer per unit of cross-sectional area.

**ANSWER:** B

7. Regarding the medical treatment of DVT, which of the following statements is true?

A. Bed rest increases the risk for embolism.

B. Heparin is given to prevent attachment of thrombi to the venous wall.

C. Platelet counts lower than 75,000/mm$^3$ imply active clot formation and inadequate levels of heparin.

D. Anticoagulation should be continued for 12 months after the acute event, regardless of the site of involvement.

E. Tissue plasminogen activator and urokinase are contraindicated within 4 weeks of major operations or trauma.

*Ref.:* 1, 2

**COMMENTS:** Prevention of embolization from existing thrombi and inhibition of new thrombus formation are the goals of **medical therapy for deep venous thrombosis**. Bed rest with leg elevation decreases venous pressure and prevents fluctuations of pressure in the deep venous system. This allows the thrombus already present to become firmly attached to the vessel wall, minimizes venous distention, and reduces edema and pain. Elastic support is not needed if there is adequate elevation, but it should be used when ambulation is started.

**Heparin** prevents propagation of the thrombus. It inhibits thrombin by inactivating thrombin in the presence of antithrombin III (now called antithrombin). A PTT that is two times normal indicates adequate heparinization. Giving heparin by continuous intravenous infusion is the preferred method, but intravenous or subcutaneous administration as a bolus can be used. In some patients receiving heparin therapy, platelet clots develop in the arterial and venous system (HIT), which can be a catastrophic complication. Therefore, a platelet count that falls to less than 75,000/mm$^3$ is believed by some to be a reason to consider discontinuing heparin treatment. Antiplatelet antibody levels should be evaluated in these patients. Alternative anticoagulation medications such as lepirudin and argatroban should be used. **Warfarin** (Coumadin) derivatives are begun before stopping the heparin to allow anticoagulant therapy to be continued on an outpatient basis. Treatment is usually continued for 3 to 6 months until the risk for

recurrence diminishes. In patients with ileofemoral thrombosis, anticoagulation is continued for 6 months to allow time for the development of adequate collateral circulation, which decreases the risk for recurrence.

**Tissue plasminogen activator** and **urokinase** are capable of lysing thrombi via activation of plasminogen to plasmin. Both agents are most effective when given to patients with DVT of less than 5 to 7 days' duration, and the best results are obtained in patients who have had symptoms for less than 48 hours. Pyrogenic, allergic, and bleeding complications occur with both agents, and their use is contraindicated within 4 weeks of major operations or injury. Bleeding complications occur two to five times more frequently in patients treated with heparin alone, and intracranial bleeding may occur in 1% of patients. Thus, thrombolytic treatment of lower extremity DVT is limited to severe cases.

**ANSWER:** E

8. Which of the following statements is true?

A. The major indication for deep venous thrombectomy is recurrent pulmonary embolism (PE).

B. Thrombectomy for ileofemoral DVT rarely results in less swelling, pain, and venous stasis than conservative therapy does.

C. Thrombectomy is contraindicated in patients with phlegmasia cerulea dolens.

D. Ileofemoral thrombosis from a pelvic infection is best treated by thrombectomy.

E. Caval interruption should always precede ileofemoral thrombectomy.

*Ref.:* 1, 2

**COMMENTS:** The role of surgery in the treatment of **acute deep venous thrombosis** is limited because of the effectiveness of medical management, the high incidence of residual or recurrent venous obstruction, and the valvular incompetence that occurs after operative correction. Surgery is usually reserved for major obstruction of the subclavian, iliac, or femoral vein and when the immediate- or long-term function of the limb is in jeopardy. Clinical studies have not demonstrated that thrombectomy leads to less swelling, pain, and venostasis than nonoperative therapy. Progression of ileofemoral thrombosis to the stage of nearly total occlusion, with tenderness, massive edema, and cyanosis (phlegmasia cerulea dolens), may lead to venous gangrene. When it occurs, failure of the patient to respond promptly to treatment consisting of leg elevation and heparinization or thrombolytic therapy (or both) is an indication for thrombectomy.

Although there is a theoretical advantage to caval interruption before thrombectomy, ileofemoral thrombectomy can be performed safely without caval interruption.

Septic ileofemoral thrombi (usually as a result of pelvic infection) are a contraindication to thrombectomy.

Operations for subclavian vein thrombosis should include resection of the first rib or cervical rib (or both) because most thrombi originate at the point where the clavicle crosses the first rib. Failure to resect these structures is associated with a high rate of postoperative recurrence.

The success of venous thrombectomy depends on early surgery, good technique, and complete removal of the thrombus. Surgery is not as useful after 7 to 10 days, and the best results occur when thrombectomy is performed within 48 hours of the appearance of symptoms.

PE that recurs despite proper medical therapy is best treated with a caval filter.

**ANSWER:** B

9. Which of the following statements regarding the evaluation of patients with suspected PE is true?

   A. The triad of dyspnea, pain, and hemoptysis is present in more than 60% of patients.

   B. Normal aspartate transaminase (AST; also called serum glutamic-oxaloacetic transaminase [SGOT]) levels in the presence of elevated serum bilirubin and lactate dehydrogenase (LDH) levels are seen in more than 50% of patients.

   C. Pulmonary arteriography requires cardiac catheterization.

   D. Arterial blood gas analysis demonstrates hypoxemia and increased $P_{CO_2}$.

   E. Ventilation-perfusion scans must be compared with a recent chest radiograph to be of value.

*Ref.: 1, 2*

**COMMENTS:** Surgeons must have a low threshold for suspecting **pulmonary embolism** in postoperative patients. About 85% of cases of PE arise from the lower extremity, 10% from the right atrium, and 5% from the pelvic veins, vena cava, or arms. Up to 30% of patients with PE are free of symptoms, and only one third of patients with PE have physical evidence of DVT at the time of diagnosis. Emboli produce symptoms either by the direct effects of pulmonary artery obstruction or by secondary bronchospasm and vasoconstriction. The most common symptoms are dyspnea and pleuritic chest pain, and the most common signs are tachypnea, tachycardia, and rales. The classic triad of dyspnea, pain, and hemoptysis is present in less than 25% of patients. In fact, hemoptysis is indicative of frank pulmonary infarction and is uncommon. The classic biochemical triad of a normal AST level with elevated LDH and bilirubin levels is now considered unreliable. Few patients show diagnostic electrocardiographic changes other than tachycardia. Wedge-shaped defects on chest radiographs are seen only if infarction occurs. Decreased vascularity, pulmonary artery distention, and pleural fluid may be detected. Pulmonary arteriography is the most specific test for diagnosis and is performed by infusion of contrast agent through a right atrial or main pulmonary artery catheter. On ventilation-perfusion scans, areas of the lungs that are normally ventilated but not perfused and that appear normal on chest radiographs should be considered to have PE. These scans are safe, convenient, and reliable if the findings are strongly positive or normal. Arterial blood gas analysis typically demonstrates hypoxemia and decreased $P_{CO_2}$. This is the opposite of what is expected with "dead space" disease (i.e., normal ventilation with decreased perfusion), wherein $P_{O_2}$ is normal and $P_{CO_2}$ is usually elevated. This paradox is explained by a (presumably) chemically mediated right-to-left shunt induced by PE and tachypnea and leading to a normal or slightly decreased $P_{CO_2}$. **Spiral computed tomography** is a rapid and excellent means of diagnosing PE and is the initial test of choice in many medical centers but does require a bolus of contrast material.

**ANSWER:** E

10. Which of the following is true regarding DVT?

    A. Antithrombotic therapy following DVT minimizes postthrombotic sequelae such as phlegmasia cerulea dolens.

    B. The likelihood of thrombosed vein segment recanalization is lower with more distal location.

    C. Surgical thrombectomy is associated with a high rate of intraoperative PE.

    D. Early thrombus removal in patients with phlegmasia cerulea dolens can prevent progression to venous gangrene.

    E. Venous valve damage is common following catheter-based thrombolytic therapy for DVT.

*Ref.: 3*

**COMMENTS: Antithrombotic therapy** following **deep venous thrombosis** prevents extension of the DVT and lowers the risk for PE. Damage to distal valves can result in venous reflux and subsequent postthrombotic sequelae. The thrombosed vein segment is more likely to recanalize the more distally it is located. Approximately 95% of popliteal and tibial thromboses will recanalize. Most series show low rates of perioperative PE secondary to surgical thrombectomy. Early thrombus removal is indicated in active, healthy young patients to prevent late sequelae. It is also indicated in patients with phlegmasia cerulea dolens to prevent progression to venous gangrene. Catheter-based clot manipulation combined with thrombolysis is effective in removing acute thrombus and results in preservation of venous competence and minimization of postthrombotic sequelae.

**ANSWER:** D

11. Which of the following statements is true regarding the prevention of venous thrombosis?

    A. Mechanical prophylaxis has been shown to reduce the risk for death from venous thrombosis but not PE.

    B. Aspirin may be used for prevention of DVT in low-risk patients.

    C. Most thromboembolic events occur in medical patients.

    D. The incidence of DVT in cancer patients is not influenced by the type of cancer.

    E. Screening duplex ultrasound is an effective method of preventing complications secondary to DVT in certain high-risk groups, such as patients who have undergone major orthopedic surgery.

*Ref.: 4*

**COMMENTS: Prevention of venous thrombosis and pulmonary embolism** remains a critical quality-of-care issue. No **mechanical device** has been shown to reduce the risk for either PE or death, although they do reduce the incidence of DVT. They are an acceptable option in patients at high risk for bleeding. A large number of studies have shown that aspirin is ineffective in preventing DVT and should not be used in any patient group for prevention of DVT. Most cases of DVT and PE occur in medical patients; this population represents a significant opportunity for prevention. Risk factors for DVT in medical patients include advanced age, immobility, New York Heart Association classes III and IV heart failure, sepsis, and cancer. The risk for DVT varies by cancer type and is highest in patients with brain tumors and adenocarcinomas of the ovaries, pancreas, colon, stomach, lungs, prostate, and kidneys. Predischarge duplex ultrasound screening has never been found to decrease the risk for thromboembolic complication of DVT. It is costly and mainly identifies asymptomatic, small thrombi for which treatment may not be necessary.

**ANSWER:** C

**12.** A 56-year-old man has had heaviness, tiredness, and aching of the lower part of his left leg for the past several months. The symptoms are relieved by leg elevation. He mentions that he is awakened from sleep because of calf and foot cramping but that it is relieved by walking or massage. On physical examination, he has thick, darkly pigmented skin, nonpitting edema bilaterally, and a superficial ulcer 2 cm in diameter, 5 cm above and behind the medial malleolus, that is slightly painful. The most likely diagnosis is which of the following?

A. Arterial insufficiency with ulceration

B. Isolated symptomatic varicose veins

C. Diabetic neuropathy with ulceration

D. Deep venous insufficiency with incompetent perforator veins

E. Diabetic ulcer

*Ref.:* 1, 2

**COMMENTS:** The most common symptoms associated with **venous insufficiency** are aching, swelling, and night cramps of the involved leg. The symptoms often occur after periods of sitting or inactive standing. Elevation of the leg frequently provides relief. Although the edema of venous insufficiency can occur with varicose veins alone, it is usually associated with deep venous abnormalities and incompetent perforating veins. Night cramps are the result of sustained contractions of the calf and foot muscles and are relieved by massage, ambulation, and proper management of the underlying venous insufficiency. Brawny, nonpitting edema is the result of increased connective tissue in the subcutaneous tissue. Brown discoloration is the result of hemosiderin deposition. **Ulceration** is most common in patients with deep venous abnormalities and incompetent perforators. In such cases, the ulcers are usually located above and posterior to the malleoli (medial more than lateral), thus reinforcing their relationship with perforator abnormalities. When patients with a history of DVT are monitored beyond 10 years, ulcers ultimately develop in up to 20%.

In contrast to arterial ulcers, **venous ulcers** are superficial and rarely penetrate the fascia. The pain of arterial insufficiency is often increased with leg elevation. Ulcers associated with arterial insufficiency may occur anywhere on the lower part of the leg but usually occur distally, with the toe often being involved first. Arterial ulcers have an associated blue erythematous border and are more painful than venous ulcers. Shallow ulcers of the ankle that closely resemble venous stasis ulcers may develop in patients with diabetes mellitus. Treating them as venous stasis ulcers (i.e., with leg elevation, an Unna boot, and other measures) may be disastrous because of the associated arterial insufficiency. Diabetic ulcers frequently occur on the calf or ankle but are not associated with the edema and other skin changes seen with venous stasis ulcers. These ulcers result from arterial insufficiency and often begin with minor trauma to the affected area.

**ANSWER:** D

**13.** A surgeon has performed a Trendelenburg test on the patient described in Question 12 and has determined that he has incompetent varicose veins associated with incompetent perforating veins. How should this be interpreted?

A. Negative/negative Trendelenburg test

B. Negative/positive Trendelenburg test

C. Positive/negative Trendelenburg test

D. Positive/positive Trendelenburg test

E. None of the above

*Ref.:* 1, 2

**COMMENTS:** There are several **tests for diagnosing venous insufficiency**. The **Trendelenburg test** is a two-part test used to delineate the competence of the superficial and perforating veins. While in the supine position, the patient elevates the legs until the superficial veins empty.

In part I, the saphenofemoral junction is occluded digitally, and the patient is asked to stand. The superficial veins are observed for 30 seconds. This action allows assessment of the competence of the perforator veins. Slow, ascending, incomplete filling of the superficial veins during compression is a negative (normal) result, whereas rapid filling is a positive result indicative of incompetence of the deep and perforating veins.

In part II, the saphenofemoral occlusion is released while the veins are kept under observation. This action allows assessment of the competence of the superficial veins. Continued slow ascending filling after saphenofemoral release is a negative (normal) result. Rapid retrograde filling is a positive result indicating incompetence of the valves of the superficial system.

The percussion test is performed by tapping the superficial veins near the saphenofemoral junction while palpating over the knee for transmitted pulses. It can also be used to examine the lesser saphenous system. Transmission of a pulse suggests incompetent valves. Venous pressure studies help delineate abnormalities in the normal venous pressure relationships during exercise. Functional phlebography is performed in patients before and after a standard active exercise and can demonstrate important pathologic and physiologic abnormalities. The Perthes test involves the application of elastic wraps to a leg with varicosities (to occlude the superficial venous system) before the patient is asked to exercise. Pain during exercise suggests obstruction of the deep venous system. Although these tests based on physical examination yield useful information, Duplex scanning with direct observation of venous flow is now widely used in clinical practice to determine venous insufficiency.

**ANSWER:** D

**14.** The therapeutic plan for the patient in Question 12 should include which of the following measures?

A. Varicose vein ligation and stripping as soon as possible

B. Ligation of the medial perforating veins as soon as possible

C. Initial treatment consisting of appropriate leg wraps, leg elevation, and ambulation with avoidance of prolonged sitting or standing

D. Ulcer débridement, vein stripping, and skin grafting

E. Laser ablation

*Ref.:* 1, 2

**COMMENTS: Operative treatment of venous insufficiency** in most instances is an adjunct to aggressive conservative management. Leg elevation, active exercise, and elastic compression form the cornerstone of nonoperative management. The goals of compression are to relieve symptoms and reduce swelling. When ulcers are present, local medications should be avoided unless evidence of infection exists. Ulcers smaller than 3 cm in diameter often heal with the treatment just described.

The indications for superficial vein ligation, endovenous ablation, and stripping are moderate to severe symptoms without other signs of venous insufficiency, venous insufficiency with recurrent ulceration despite aggressive medical management, and occasionally, severe varicosities without symptoms. **Ligation of incompetent perforating veins** can be an important addition to the treatment of venous insufficiency, particularly if done before ulceration develops. Ligation was once often performed through a longitudinal incision placed posterior and superior to the malleoli, as first described by Robert Linton. Subfascial endoscopic techniques have recently reduced the morbidity associated with this technique. When present, incompetent superficial veins should be stripped as part of the procedure. Postoperatively, conservative measures must be continued aggressively. Obstructions of the ileofemoral or femoropopliteal veins have been bypassed with use of the ipsilateral (femoropopliteal occlusions) or contralateral (ileofemoral occlusions) saphenous veins.

**ANSWER: C**

15. Which is true regarding lymphatic anatomy?

    A. The limb lymphatic vessels are valveless.

    B. The lymphatic system begins just below the dermis as a network of fine capillaries.

    C. Red blood cells and bacteria do not enter lymphatic capillaries.

    D. Extrinsic factors (e.g., muscle contraction, arterial pulsations, respiratory movement, and massage) aid in the movement of lymph flow.

    E. All of the above.

*Ref.: 1, 2, 5*

**COMMENTS:** The **lymphatic system** begins as a network of valveless capillaries in the superficial dermis. There is a second valved plexus in the deep or subdermal layer that joins with the first to form the lymphatic vessels, and their course parallels that of the major blood vessels. Lymph flow toward the heart is aided by massage, arterial pulsations, respiratory movement, and muscle contraction. Intradermal lymphatics can be evaluated by the intradermal injection of patent blue dye. The capillaries normally become visible as a fine network 30 to 60 seconds after injection. Lymphangiography is rarely used to visualize the lymphatic vessels because it may make the lymphedema worse. Unlike veins, these vessels appear to be of uniform caliber throughout their course.

Lymphatic vessels are readily entered by the proteins present in extracellular fluid. Red blood cells and lymphocytes enter lymphatic vessels by separating the endothelial cells at their junctions.

Lymphedema occurs when the lymphatics are obstructed, too few in number, or nonfunctional, which results in the retention of interstitial fluid with a high protein concentration. Tissue oncotic pressure increases, and fluid is drawn into the interstitium. Measurement of the protein content of edema fluid (normally <1.5 mg/dL) can be used to assess the status of lymphatic function in the edematous extremity.

**ANSWER: D**

16. A 45-year-old woman comes to the emergency department complaining of pain in her left foot and calf. She reports that her left leg has been swollen for the last 5 years. She is febrile with a temperature of 101.5° F (38.6° C). The left leg is swollen from the inguinal ligament down, and she has erythema of the foot and calf. Besides the obvious cellulitis, what is the most likely underlying diagnosis?

    A. Chronic venous insufficiency

    B. DVT

    C. Lymphedema tarda

    D. Meige disease

    E. Milroy disease

*Ref.: 3, 5*

**COMMENTS:** Swelling of the extremity secondary to a pathologic condition of the lymphatic system is classified as primary or secondary. Primary **lymphedema** is an uncommon condition and is not related to any extrinsic process. Primary lymphedema is classified into three subtypes based on the age at onset of symptoms. The first group is congenital lymphedema, with onset before 1 year of age. The lower extremities are more commonly affected, but an upper extremity may also be involved. No specific therapy is needed. If associated with a family history, it is referred to as **Milroy disease**. The second group—the most common form—is **lymphedema praecox**, with the onset of symptoms before 35 years of age. If associated with a family history, it is referred to as **Meige disease**. **Lymphedema tarda** represents a minority of the cases. Patients have leg swelling after the age of 35. **Secondary lymphedema** can be the result of multiple processes, including infection, trauma, filariasis, lymph node dissection, and radiation, among others.

**ANSWER: C**

17. Which statement is true regarding the cause and complications of lymphedema?

    A. Primary lymphedema appears at birth, is more common in females, and occurs in the right leg more often than the left.

    B. Milroy disease is a form of primary lymphedema that is gender linked.

    C. A lymphangiogram usually demonstrates a point of obstruction of the lymphatics in primary lymphedema.

    D. Primary lymphedema almost always progresses to involve both lower extremities.

    E. The major complication of lymphedema is the later development of lymphangiosarcoma.

*Ref.: 1, 2, 5*

**COMMENTS: Primary lymphedema** is caused by abnormal development resulting in aplasia, hypoplasia, or varicosities of the lymphatic vessels. Congenital lymphedema (Milroy disease) is present at birth and is a familial, gender-linked condition, but a family history is present in less than 5% of patients. Primary lymphedema usually appears in individuals during their teens, more commonly in females, and it often develops insidiously. The left limb is more frequently involved than the right (3:1), and often only one limb is involved.

**Secondary lymphedema** is the result of obstruction or destruction of normal lymphatic channels and can be caused by tumor, repeated infection, or parasitic infection (particularly filariasis), or it can occur following radiation treatment or lymph node dissection. Lymphangiography often demonstrates a discrete obstruction. Recurrent infections of venous stasis ulcers can destroy lymphatic vessels and lead to lymphedema.

The inability to clear proteins leads to edema formation, which gradually increases over time and becomes woody because of the presence of fibrous tissue in the subcutaneous region. Repeated infection hastens the accumulation of this fibrous tissue. In some patients blisters develop that contain edema fluid, or chyle. The major complication of lymphedema is recurrent attacks of cellulitis or lymphangitis, often following minor injury. β-Hemolytic streptococci are the organisms responsible, and the infection spreads rapidly because the protein-containing edema fluid is an excellent culture medium.

Lymphangiosarcoma is a rare complication of long-standing lymphedema that is most frequently described in patients following radical mastectomy (Stewart-Treves syndrome). It appears as a blue or purple nodule with a satellite lesion. Metastases develop early, primarily to the lungs.

Rarely, a protein-losing enteropathy that has been attributed to lymphatic obstruction of the small bowel develops in patients with lymphedema.

**ANSWER:** B

18. Regarding the treatment of lymphedema, which of the following statements is true?

    A. More than 50% of patients ultimately require an operation.

    B. Diuretics have a crucial role in the conservative management of early lymphedema.

    C. Pneumatic compression devices can damage the remaining lymphatics and should not be used.

    D. Microsurgically constructed lymphovenous shunts are far more effective than excisional procedures.

    E. All surgical procedures for lymphedema have significant failure rates.

*Ref.:* 1, 2, 5

**COMMENTS:** The mainstay of **management of lymphedema** is conservative and nonoperative. Less than 5% of patients require an operation. The goals of therapy are prevention of infection and reduction of subcutaneous fluid volume. Fluid volume is reduced by elevating the extremity during sleep, the use of pneumatic compression devices, and carefully fitted elastic support stockings. Diuretics are not used routinely but may be useful in women who retain fluid during the premenstrual period. Patients prone to recurrent lymphangitis require intermittent long-term antibiotic therapy at the first sign of infection. The drug of choice is penicillin because streptococci are the usual infecting organisms. Secondary lymphedema requires treatment of the underlying cause, such as giving diethylcarbamazine for filariasis and appropriate antibiotics for tuberculosis or lymphogranuloma venereum.

Edema that is excessive and interferes with normal activity and the presence of severe recurrent cellulitis are indications for surgery. Patients with minimal edema, gross obesity, and progressing disease are not candidates for surgery. Excisional procedures include removal of skin, subcutaneous tissue, and fascia, followed by split-thickness skin graft reconstruction (the Charles operation); excision of strips of skin and subcutaneous tissue, followed by primary closure; and creation of buried dermal flaps. Physiologic procedures to restore or enhance lymphatic drainage include insertion of silk, Teflon, or polystyrene threads into the subcutaneous

tissue; construction of pedicle grafts from the involved limb to the trunk; and microsurgical lymphovenous shunts using dilated lymphatics or the capsule and efferent channels of isolated lymph nodes anastomosed to neighboring veins. All procedures are associated with significant failure rates.

**ANSWER:** E

19. Which of the following is least likely to occur with acquired peripheral AVFs?

    A. Bacterial endocarditis

    B. Distal embolization

    C. Peripheral arterial insufficiency

    D. Congestive heart failure

    E. Venous aneurysm formation

*Ref.:* 2, 3, 6

**COMMENTS: Acquired peripheral arteriovenous fistulas** are most commonly the result of penetrating trauma, which causes injury to an adjacent artery and vein. The upper and lower extremities are the most frequent sites. Other causes include suture ligation of adjacent vessels, vessel catheterization for diagnostic or therapeutic study, erosion of an adjacent vein by an atherosclerotic aneurysm, periarterial abscess, or neoplasm. Another cause is a remnant fistula following in situ peripheral artery bypass. Small fistulas may close spontaneously. Fistulas that persist lead to dilation and ectasia of the proximal artery, and the adjacent vein becomes thick walled, dilated, and aneurysmal. The intimal damage that occurs leads to increased risks for infection and bacterial endocarditis. Depending on the size and location of the fistula, significant flow may lead to arterial insufficiency distal to the fistula ("steal phenomenon"). Venous congestion, chronic venous stasis changes, edema, and venous varicosities may also occur. In young children, a peripheral fistula may lead to limb length inequality if it is present before closure of the epiphyseal plate. If the fistula is large, signs and symptoms of high-output congestive heart failure may develop. Temporary compression of the fistula may elicit a Branham-Nicoladoni sign with a rise in diastolic blood pressure and decreased heart rate. Peripheral AVFs do not cause thrombosis or distal embolization.

**ANSWER:** B

20. With regard to the diagnosis and treatment of peripheral acquired AVFs, which of the following is true?

    A. Acquired AVFs are rarely diagnosed by physical examination.

    B. Angiography is the initial preferred diagnostic study.

    C. Most AVFs can be observed without surgical intervention.

    D. Proximal arterial ligation is the surgical procedure required for repair of most AVFs.

    E. Percutaneous techniques, such as detachable balloons and embolization, are used to treat AVFs.

*Ref.:* 1, 3, 6

**COMMENTS:** Most **peripheral acquired arteriovenous fistulas** are easily detected with a careful history and physical examination. A history of penetrating trauma is usually elicited. Physical findings may include a continuous ("machinery") murmur heard over the site; a palpable thrill; distended, tortuous, or varicose veins; chronic venous stasis changes; elevated skin temperature; and the changes seen with congestive heart failure. Duplex scanning is useful for establishing an initial diagnosis. Arteriography is the preferred diagnostic study to document an AVF. The fistula is identified by the presence of a dilated afferent artery with early venous filling and simultaneous visualization of both arteries and veins. There is also diminished contrast enhancement distally. Duplex scanning is useful for diagnosing AVF formation in the groin after catheterization injury. In this instance, it may be the only test required before surgical repair.

Most acquired AVFs should be repaired soon after diagnosis because of the low rate of spontaneous closure and the long-term sequelae. The goals of surgical repair include complete closure of the arteriovenous connection and restoration of normal arterial and venous flow. Placement of an interposition arterial graft may be required. Autogenous vein is preferred when the repair is in the extremity. Most often, the venous defect is repaired with a lateral suture. Repair with proximal arterial ligation leads to early distal ischemia and long-term persistence of the fistula because of collateral circulation. In certain instances, surgical repair is not possible as a result of its location or technical difficulties. Percutaneous embolization with thrombogenic material or detachable balloons is useful in these situations. Both surgical repair and percutaneous embolization can lead to distal ischemia, infarction, and closure of an undesired artery. After repair of a long-standing AVF, long-term surveillance is required because of the risk for arterial aneurysmal degeneration.

**ANSWER:** E

21. With regard to axillary-subclavian vein thrombosis (Paget-von Schroetter syndrome), which of the following is true?

A. It is rarely associated with thoracic outlet compression syndrome.

B. Severe pain in the affected extremity is usually the initial symptom.

C. Venography is the gold standard for making the diagnosis.

D. Surgical thrombectomy is the treatment of choice for the management of acute disease.

E. Patients treated with thrombolytic and anticoagulant therapy alone have a low rate of recurrence.

*Ref.:* 3, 6

**COMMENTS:** Spontaneous thrombosis of the axillary-subclavian vein is termed **effort thrombosis or Paget-von Schroetter syndrome**. There is a strong male preponderance. Thrombosis typically follows upper extremity exertion. Swelling invariably develops and patients complain of heaviness and discomfort in the arm that are exacerbated with activity and relieved with rest. Severe pain is a rare complaint. As many as 80% of patients with effort thrombosis have an associated thoracic outlet compression syndrome. Symptoms of disabling venous hypertension develop in as many as 25% to 75% of patients if not treated appropriately. Venography remains the gold standard for diagnosis. CT, MRI, and arteriography are often required when planning surgical decompression of the thoracic outlet. Treatment with thrombolytic agents and anticoagulation is highly successful for short-term management of this disease. Diagnosis and staged treatment of thoracic

outlet compression are mandatory because of the high rate of rethrombosis in those treated with thrombolytic and anticoagulant therapy alone. Treatment involves removing the first rib.

**ANSWER:** C

22. Left lower extremity pain and swelling developed in a 53-year-old woman who underwent resection of a brain tumor 4 days earlier. A venous duplex scan was performed, and DVT of the femoral and popliteal vein on the left was diagnosed. Which treatment is most appropriate?

A. Begin ambulation and discontinue bed rest.

B. Order emergency venography, and if the results are abnormal, begin intravenous heparin administration.

C. Order spiral CT to rule out PE.

D. Use intermittent leg compression and graduated compression stockings.

E. Place an IVC filter.

*Ref.:* 3

**COMMENTS:** Well-known indications for **inferior vena cava filter placement** are DVT or PE in patients with contraindications to anticoagulation and recurrent PE or DVT despite anticoagulation. It is also performed after pulmonary embolectomy and failure of a previously placed filter. Among relative indications are the presence of large or free-floating thrombi in the iliofemoral system or vena cava, septic PE, chronic PE in a patient who has significant cardiac or respiratory impairment, trauma patients at high risk, spinal cord injury with paraplegia or quadriplegia, complex pelvic fracture with associated long-bone fractures, pregnancy with DVT, and patients with seizures or gait difficulties who are at high risk with warfarin (Coumadin) therapy. IVC filters are also used for patients with contraindications to anticoagulation. The list of absolute contraindications to anticoagulation therapy includes recent spinal or brain surgery, eye surgery, major trauma, hemorrhagic stroke, malignant hypertension, and active gastrointestinal hemorrhage. Relative contraindications to anticoagulation therapy are hemorrhagic diathesis, malignant hypertension, and severe renal or hepatic insufficiency.

**ANSWER:** E

23. A 17-year-old boy comes to the emergency department complaining of swelling of his left arm and cyanosis 1 hour after a strenuous workout involving weight lifting. Venography demonstrates subclavian-axillary vein thrombosis. Which treatment is most appropriate?

A. All patients can expect asymptomatic recovery if treated promptly with anticoagulants only.

B. The patient may be treated effectively with acetylsalicylic acid only.

C. The patient will need lifelong anticoagulation with Coumadin.

D. The patient requires catheter-directed thrombolysis and resection of the first rib if patency is restored and venous narrowing is demonstrated.

E. The patient requires first rib resection only.

*Ref.:* 3

**COMMENTS: Primary deep venous thrombosis of the upper extremity** is a rare entity that accounts for 2% to 3% of all patients with thoracic outlet syndrome. A young healthy athlete is a typical patient. Males are affected twice as often as females. Almost all have a history of strenuous or repetitive physical activity 24 to 48 hours earlier. During hyperabduction of the arm, the subclavian vein is compressed at the costoclavicular space, which is the most medial aspect of the thoracic outlet. Trauma at this location causes intimal injury, followed by thrombus formation in the axillary and subclavian veins. All patients complain of swelling and cyanosis of the affected extremity when initially seen, and pain develops in the majority of patients.

    **Catheter-directed thrombolysis** is the first line of treatment. If resolution of the thrombus is documented after thrombolysis and extrinsic compression is identified at the level of the costoclavicular space, resection of the first rib is recommended. It is performed through the axillary or supraclavicular approach during the same hospitalization or at a later date. If the lesion is inside the vein itself, there are several treatment options, including anticoagulation and delayed outlet decompression, outlet decompression with external venolysis, outlet decompression followed by angioplasty, and outlet decompression with venous reconstruction. The decision regarding which option to use is based on the level of the patient's discomfort and findings on venography.

**ANSWER:** D

---

24. A 67-year-old man is in the hospital for the treatment of bilateral PE and DVT. Heparin was continued for the last 2 days. On day 3, the patient's platelet count was 75,000/mm³, a decrease from an original level of 250,000/mm³. On physical examination, the patient was noted to have ischemic changes in the right upper extremity and right lower extremity. Which of the following statements is true?

    A. Low-molecular-weight heparin can be used safely as a substitute for unfractionated heparin.

    B. Venous thrombosis is the most likely cause of this patient's problem.

    C. Subcutaneous administration of heparin is not associated with this problem.

    D. Direct thrombin inhibitors are used as the first line of treatment.

    E. Antiplatelet agents are not necessary as additional treatment.

*Ref.:* 3

**COMMENTS: Heparin-induced thrombocytopenia** is an immune-mediated adverse drug reaction that can occur in up to 5% of patients undergoing treatment with unfractionated heparin. The initial diagnosis of this condition is clinical. The occurrence of HIT is independent of the route of administration. Two forms of acute HIT have been reported. Mild (type 1) thrombocytopenia occurs 2 to 7 days after the initiation of full-dose heparin therapy. It is nonimmune in nature. Platelet counts usually remain above 100,000/mm³, and treatment can be continued without any risk for complications. Severe (type 2) thrombocytopenia occurs much less frequently, 5 to 10 days after the initiation of full-dose or low-dose heparin therapy. It is an immune-mediated syndrome. Platelet counts drop below 100,000/mm³, or there is a more than 50% drop from baseline. Laboratory confirmation of the presence of heparin-induced antibodies is available, but not always in a timely fashion for decision making. Platelet-associated immunoglobulin G (IgG)

levels are almost always elevated, but testing for them is not very specific. The C-serotonin platelet release assay, heparin-induced platelet aggregation assay, and flow cytometric studies are very sensitive and specific. Paradoxically, severe HIT is associated with thrombotic complications, including arterial thrombosis with a platelet-fibrin clot (so-called white clot), which may cause myocardial infarction or stroke or necessitate amputation of a limb. Arterial or venous thrombosis may develop in up to 75% of patients, and the mortality rate is 25% to 30%. Direct thrombin inhibitors such as lepirudin and argatroban are the first line of treatment, with the choice of agent depending on the patient's comorbid conditions (lepirudin depends on renal clearance, and argatroban depends on hepatic functional status). Each agent has a relatively short half-life. Antiplatelet medications (e.g., aspirin and clopidogrel [Plavix]) should be used for all patients with HIT.

**ANSWER:** D

---

25. A 55-year-old woman comes to her physician's office with bilateral lower extremity swelling that she has had for the last 3 months. The list of differential diagnoses includes all but which of the following?

    A. DVT

    B. Congestive heart failure

    C. Lymphedema

    D. Retroperitoneal sarcoma

    E. Arterial occlusive disease

*Ref.:* 3

**COMMENTS: Leg swelling** may be secondary to a systemic disorder, acute or chronic obstruction of the venous system, or an abnormality of the lymphatic system. Physical examination and the patient's history are usually sufficient to find the cause of the limb swelling. Systemic disorders should be ruled out first. The list of differential diagnoses includes renal failure, liver disease, constrictive pericarditis, tricuspid regurgitation, congestive heart failure, malnutrition, and other causes of hypoproteinuria. Rare systemic causes of edema include endocrine disorders such as myxedema, type 1 allergic reactions, hereditary angioedema, and idiopathic cyclic edema. Among medications that can cause generalized swelling are angiotensin-converting enzyme inhibitors, which most frequently affect the extremities and the face; corticosteroids; antihypertensive drugs; and anti-inflammatory agents. Local or regional causes of leg swelling include chronic venous insufficiency, lipedema, congenital vascular malformation, AVF, trauma, snake bite, infection, hematoma, soft tissue tumor, and dependency.

**ANSWER:** E

---

26. A 45-year-old woman reports a recent onset of bilateral edema of the lower extremities. Which of the following statements is true about the appropriate work-up?

    A. Aspiration of tissue fluid to measure protein content is appropriate.

    B. CT is an unnecessary modality in the presence of bilateral disease.

    C. The diagnosis can be confirmed by means of lymphoscintigraphy.

D. Physical findings are not reliable.

E. Laboratory tests and urinalysis are not very useful for diagnosis.

*Ref.:* 3

**COMMENTS:** Although the physical examination and patient's history are usually sufficient to find the cause of **limb swelling**, several diagnostic modalities are available. Laboratory examinations should include a complete blood count, liver function tests, creatinine clearance testing, and urinalysis. One of the first diagnostic tests is **computed tomography**, which is used to differentiate inflammatory or infectious processes, enlargement of regional lymph nodes, and underlying local or abdominal malignancy. **Venous Doppler study** or strain-gauge plethysmography is sufficient to exclude venous thrombosis. Duplex scanning is used to detect venous insufficiency. MRI provides the most accurate information in patients with clinical signs of congenital vascular malformation, soft tissue tumor, or retroperitoneal fibrosis. **Direct contrast-enhanced lymphangiography** is a classic method for the diagnosis of lymphedema. Because it requires cutdown and has a risk of oil embolism and lymphangitis, however, this test is no longer used except in very unusual circumstances. Normal findings on lymphoscintigraphy essentially exclude the diagnosis of lymphedema. Subcutaneous injection of technetium-labeled colloid and a serial gamma camera are used.

**ANSWER:** C

27. A 35-year-old woman with three children has a large, painful varicose vein in her left extremity. Diagnosis and treatment should include all but which of the following?

A. Duplex scanning for venous insufficiency and evaluation of the deep venous system

B. Stripping of the left great saphenous vein (GSV) from the groin to the ankle

C. Stripping of the left GSV from the groin to the knee and excision of the calf varicose vein

D. Treatment of the left GSV with a radiofrequency or laser catheter and excision of the calf varicose vein

E. Treatment of the left GSV with a radiofrequency or laser catheter alone

*Ref.:* 3

**COMMENTS: Duplex scanning** is a combination of gray-scale ultrasound and Doppler examination—hence the name duplex. Preoperative examination with duplex scanning defines where the reflux is in the superficial and deep venous systems and ensures that the deep system is present and patent. If the deep system is occluded, stripping or excision of the superficial system is contraindicated. If the GSV refluxes significantly, interruption will help alleviate the symptoms. Treatment of the thigh-level portion of the GSV is usually sufficient to relieve venous hypertension. Excision of the GSV below the knee risks damage to the saphenous nerve. Stripping of the GSV is an established technique, but catheter ablation with radiofrequency or laser energy is very effective and less invasive. After treatment of the incompetent GSV, the residual calf and thigh varicose veins can be observed, excised with small incisions, or injected with a sclerotherapy technique. Fitted elastic stockings are useful for reducing symptoms in patients who do not desire intervention.

**ANSWER:** B

28. Which of the following regarding treatment of DVT is true?

A. Thrombus removal is associated with high morbidity and is rarely indicated.

B. Catheter-based thrombolysis has complication rates equivalent to those of systemic thrombolysis

C. Low-molecular-weight heparin and unfractionated heparin are associated with equivalent rates of HIT.

D. Intracranial bleeding, reported in 5% of patients, is the most common major complication of catheter-based thrombolysis.

E. Early thrombus resolution is associated with improved long-term outcomes.

*Ref.:* 3

**COMMENTS: Post-thrombotic syndrome** results in venous valvular incompetence and subsequent venous hypertension. Clinically, this is manifested as lower extremity edema, cutaneous stasis changes, venous varicosities, and venous stasis ulceration. These sequelae are termed *post-thrombotic syndrome*. Early clot resolution is associated with a reduced incidence of post-thrombotic syndrome. Substantial evidence suggests that patients with extensive clot burden (i.e., iliac vein clot) have improved outcomes with thrombus removal versus anticoagulation alone. Data regarding thrombus removal for infrainguinal DVT are lacking. Thrombolytics may be used to accelerate clot resolution. Catheter-based delivery of thrombolytic agents is associated with fewer complications than systemic thrombolytic delivery is. The most common complication is major bleeding, seen in 5% to 10% of patients; it is usually located at the puncture site. Intracranial bleeding was reported in less than 1% of patients in multiple studies.

**ANSWER:** E

## REFERENCES

1. Freischlag JA, Heller JA: Venous disease. In Townsend CM Jr, Beauchamp RD, Evers BM, et al, editors: *Sabiston Textbook of surgery: the biological basis of modern surgical practice*, ed 18, Philadelphia, 2008, WB Saunders.
2. Liem TK, Moneta GL: Venous and lymphatic disease. In Brunicardi FC, Andersen DK, Billiar TR, et al, editors: *Schwartz's principles of surgery*, ed 9, New York, 2010, McGraw-Hill.
3. Cronenwett J, Johnston W, editors: *Rutherford's vascular surgery*, ed 7, Philadelphia, 2010, WB Saunders.
4. Geerts WH, Pineo GF, Heit JA, et al: Prevention of venous thromboembolism. The Seventh ACCP Conference on Antithrombotic and Thrombolytic Therapy, *Chest* 126:338S–400S, 2004.
5. Pipinos II, Baxter BT: The lymphatics. In Townsend CM Jr, Beauchamp RD, Evers BM, et al, editors: *Sabiston textbook of surgery: the biological basis of modern surgical practice*, ed 18, Philadelphia, 2008, WB Saunders.
6. Ernst EB, Stanley JE, editors: *Current therapy in vascular surgery*, ed 3, St. Louis, 1995, CV Mosby.

# G. Amputations

*Ferenc P. Nagy, M.D.*

1. Which of the following describes a myodesis amputation?

    A. Antagonist muscles are sutured across the end of the bone.

    B. Skin, fascia, and muscle are transected at the level of the amputation and then closed over the bone.

    C. Transected muscles are attached to bone by suturing through drill holes placed in the distal end of the bone.

    D. Tissues are cut circularly and allowed to retract initially, and the wound may be closed secondarily or approximated with skin traction.

    E. It is used when the extremity is grossly infected and the patient is septic.

    *Ref.:* 1

**COMMENTS:** The conventional **amputation** uses curved skin and fascial flaps based at the level of amputation. When care is taken to ensure proper approximation of soft tissue over the bone stump, it lends itself to the potential for good rehabilitation. Fitting for a prosthesis is delayed until healing has occurred. An osteomyoplastic amputation (suturing antagonistic muscles across the end of the bone) and a myodesis amputation (attaching muscles directly to the bone) are typically used for special situations (e.g., young patients with trauma). They provide improved function and allow the immediate application of postsurgical prosthetic devices. An open, or "guillotine," amputation is reserved for emergency situations, unstable patients, or the presence of severe sepsis. The wound is left completely open, and the bone usually protrudes after soft tissue contraction occurs, thus requiring revision. This situation can be obviated by using appropriately elongated skin flaps or even by countering this tendency with postoperative skin traction. The stump is not usually amenable to easy rehabilitation.

**ANSWER:** C

2. The principles of postoperative management after amputation include which of the following?

    A. Splinting of the stump dressing to avoid shift in position

    B. Compression dressing over the stump to avoid postoperative edema and hematoma formation

    C. Exercise and positioning to avoid contracture

    D. Early evaluation and care by a qualified physical therapist and prosthetist

    E. All of the above

    *Ref.:* 1, 2

**COMMENTS:** Conventional postoperative care begins with the application of a light compression dressing in the operating room, followed by repeated application of elastic dressings to avoid stump edema. Damage to the skin can result from excessively compressive dressings applied over bony prominences (e.g., the anterior tibial area in a below-knee stump). Stump exercises and stretching prevent contracture after primary wound healing has taken place. Progressive training after suture removal allows the eventual application of a permanent prosthesis. Alternatively, application of a rigid dressing in the operating room allows the immediate use of a prosthetic device, but a rigid dressing may also be used without immediate prosthetic fitting. Rigid dressings offer the advantage of immediate use of the extremity. Wound healing may be enhanced by maximum control of edema and hematoma and by better tissue immobilization. When treatment is successful, resumption of full activity can be expected to occur within 4 to 6 weeks. All of the listed choices are important for proper **amputation management**.

**ANSWER:** E

3. Useful preoperative methods of evaluating the adequacy of blood flow in patients with peripheral vascular disease undergoing amputation include which of the following?

    A. Clinical assessment of cutaneous blood flow and assessment of the status of peripheral pulses

    B. Determination of transcutaneous $P_{O_2}$ and $P_{CO_2}$

    C. Segmental Doppler systolic blood pressure determinations

    D. Laser Doppler velocimetric studies

    E. All of the above

    *Ref.:* 1-3

**COMMENTS:** The healing ability of an amputation stump is determined by the adequacy of nutritional blood flow to the skin. Clinical assessment is successful in determining the level of amputation in approximately 80% of below-knee amputations and 90% of above-knee amputations. For **amputations** below the ankle, clinical judgment alone has been shown to be less effective, with a healing rate of only 40%. Physical examination findings such as the extent of tissue necrosis, skin temperature, capillary refill, and pulse evaluation help determine the clinical assessment. The presence of pulses immediately above the proposed amputation site is a good prognostic indicator, but the absence of such a pulse does not necessarily preclude adequate wound healing.

Several other methods have been used to preoperatively select amputation levels, including Doppler segmental blood pressure measurements, transcutaneous oxygen and carbon dioxide measurements, fluorescein dye measurements, laser Doppler velocimetric studies, isotope measurement of skin perfusion, conventional or magnetic resonance angiography, and others. Segmental Doppler blood pressure measurement is probably the most commonly used first test to assist in determining the level of amputation. An absolute pressure of at least 50 to 70 mm Hg at the calf and 80 mm Hg at the thigh is highly predictive of successful healing of a below-knee amputation. However, a major caveat of this test modality is the falsely elevated pressures that result from calcification of the arterial wall, particularly in the tibial vessels of diabetic patients. Transcutaneous $Po_2$ levels can also be measured and may help determine whether a particular level of amputation will heal. A transcutaneous $Po_2$ value greater than 40 mm Hg is associated with successful healing, and a value below 20 mm Hg is associated with failure.

**ANSWERS:** E

4. Which of the following statements regarding proper selection of the level of amputation is true?

   A. The extent of resection for malignant tumors must be compromised for functional considerations.

   B. The use of skin grafts and flaps to conserve bone length is appropriate in healthy, stable trauma patients.

   C. Unless 4 inches or more of tibia can be preserved, the knee joint should be sacrificed.

   D. The presence of contracture should not influence the level of amputation.

   E. None of the above.

*Ref.:* 1-3

**COMMENTS:** As a general principle, the longer the **amputation stump**, the more functional the limb. However, when performing amputations for malignancy, adequate tumor excision, not preservation of stump length, is the primary concern. The irregular damage to skin caused by trauma can be treated by skin grafts and flaps to preserve bone length. Full-thickness skin should be maintained for weight-bearing surfaces. Amputations in patients with peripheral vascular disease succeed best when performed at levels that have adequate nutritional blood flow to the skin. Below-knee stumps as short as 2 inches can be successfully fitted with prostheses, but function is much better if at least 4 inches of stump is maintained. Preservation of the knee joint allows a bent-knee, end-weight-bearing prosthesis to be used and is generally preferable to a long above-knee stump. Amputations above the knee should remove at least 4 inches of femur to facilitate fitting a prosthetic knee joint. Relative contraindications to below-knee amputation include the presence of a hip or knee contracture, which negates its functional advantage.

**ANSWER:** B

5. Which of the following statements regarding toe amputation is true?

   A. Empirical selection and clinical judgment are associated with a 95% healing rate regardless of the presence of pedal pulses.

   B. When the entire toe must be removed, disarticulation is preferred over transmetatarsal amputation.

   C. Toe amputations should not be attempted in patients who do not have pedal pulses.

   D. Rehabilitation after transmetatarsal amputation of all five toes is improved by a shoe filler prosthesis.

   E. None of the above.

*Ref.:* 1-3

**COMMENTS:** Empirical selection for **toe amputation** is associated with a 75% healing rate in the absence of palpable pedal pulses and a 98% healing rate in the presence of palpable pulses. Patients with palpable popliteal and pedal pulses who undergo toe or transmetatarsal amputations do better than those without, but the absence of these pulses is not considered an absolute contraindication. Therefore, if pedal pulses are not palpable, other measures should be used, such as Doppler toe and ankle pressure measurements. Toe pressures greater than 35 mm Hg are associated with a higher rate of successful healing. When the entire toe is to be amputated, a transmetatarsal procedure rather than a simple joint disarticulation is performed. The former prevents exposure of the avascular cartilage of the proximal joint capsule. Ambulation may be started after the incision has healed. No special shoe is required, but a shoe filler improves gait. A shoe modification that incorporates a steel shank in the sole allows normal toe push-off and prevents excessive dorsiflexion.

**ANSWER:** D

6. A Syme amputation is best suited for which of the following?

   A. An elderly patient with limited physical reserve

   B. Gangrene involving the heel pad

   C. A proximal ankle and foot destroyed by trauma

   D. A patient with a patent anterior tibial artery but a chronically occluded posterior tibial artery

   E. Isolated toe gangrene

*Ref.:* 1-3

**COMMENTS:** The **Syme amputation** is created at a bone level just distal to the tibial flare, with preservation of the heel pad. Therefore, any gangrene, infection, or open lesions of the heel create a contraindication to this amputation. It maintains the length of the lower extremity and allows the creation of an end-weight-bearing stump. It is usually performed when most of the forefoot has been destroyed by trauma or tissue necrosis. Because the heel flap for this amputation derives its entire blood supply from the posterior tibial artery, the patency of this vessel must be ascertained. A patient with a well-healed Syme amputation and a properly constructed prosthesis has only a 10% increase in ambulatory energy consumption in comparison with nonamputees.

**ANSWER:** A

7. Knee disarticulation has which of the following advantages?

   A. For adults, it is used to preserve bone length when severe ischemia contraindicates a below-knee amputation.

   B. For children, it is useful for maintaining the epiphysis for bone growth.

   C. It provides maximal length but poor end-weight-bearing characteristics.

   D. It is easily fitted with a simple prosthesis.

   E. None of the above.

*Ref.:* 1, 2

**COMMENTS: Knee disarticulation** is most often used for children because it allows maintenance of the epiphysis for bone growth. It is rarely used in situations in which there is impaired circulation and is rarely performed in adults. The procedure preserves maximum length, provides a good end-weight-bearing stump, and lends itself to a good fit between the stump and socket. However, because the femoral condyles are preserved, the stump is bulky, which can make prosthesis fitting difficult. The anterior flap is left longer than the posterior flap, and the patella is preserved if it is not involved by disease.

**ANSWER:** B

8. Which of the following statements regarding below-knee amputation is true?

   A. It may be performed on patients with significant knee contracture.

   B. When compared with above-knee amputation, below-knee amputation provides decreased potential for prosthetic ambulation.

   C. A below-knee prosthesis does not significantly increase the energy expenditure required for ambulation.

   D. The commonly used posterior myocutaneous flap involves the soleus and gastrocnemius muscles.

   E. The level of tibial transaction should be 20 cm (two hand-breadths) below the tibial tuberosity.

*Ref.:* 3

**COMMENTS: Below-knee amputation** is performed on patients who have gangrene, infection, or ischemic ulcers that preclude a more distal amputation and are not amenable to vascular reconstruction. A patient with a fixed contracture of the knee is not a candidate for a below-knee amputation. In such cases, fitting a prosthesis is not possible, use of the joint for ambulation is unlikely, and the stump is vulnerable to decubitus ulceration. However, in patients with a normal knee joint and distal disease, a below-knee amputation provides far superior rehabilitation potential than an above-knee amputation. Nonetheless, ambulation with a below-knee prosthesis increases the energy expenditure of ambulation by 10% to 40%.

Although several skin flap techniques have been used for below-knee amputation, the most commonly used is the posterior flap technique. The posterior myocutaneous flap is based on the underlying soleus and gastrocnemius muscles. The level of transection of the tibia should be approximately 10 to 12 cm below the tibial tuberosity. However, the absolute minimal length for a functional result is just below the tibial tuberosity. This preserves the insertion of the patellar tendon, which is critical for knee extension and successful ambulation.

**ANSWER:** D

9. Indications for an above-knee amputation do not include which of the following?

   A. Absent popliteal pulses

   B. Gangrene at the tibial tuberosity

   C. Calf muscle rigor

   D. Knee or hip contractures

   E. Patient with minimal potential for rehabilitation and ambulation

*Ref.:* 1, 2

**COMMENTS:** Assessment of vascular status at the **level of amputation** is important, but the absence of popliteal pulses or the presence of diabetes is not in itself an absolute indication for an above-knee amputation. The rigor of the calf muscles and the presence of gangrene of the skin at the level where the flaps would be constructed for a below-knee amputation are sufficient indications for an above-knee amputation. Because knee and hip contractures make rehabilitation after below-knee amputation unlikely and because an above-knee amputation has the highest healing rate and the lowest reamputation rate in patients with severe peripheral vascular disease, patients so afflicted do best with an above-knee amputation.

**ANSWER:** A

10. Which of the following statements regarding hip disarticulation and hemipelvectomy is true?

   A. Prostheses are unavailable for ambulation.

   B. The usual indications are bone tumors, soft tissue tumors, and occasionally, extensive trauma.

   C. Flaps are brought together posteriorly after hip disarticulation.

   D. The entire ilium must be removed during hemipelvectomy.

   E. None of the above.

*Ref.:* 1, 2

**COMMENTS:** The most common indications for **hip disarticulation** include tumors of bone or soft tissue and, in some cases, extensive trauma. **Hemipelvectomy** is indicated when an upper thigh tumor cannot be excised by disarticulation alone. The posterior flap after hip disarticulation is closed anteriorly so that the patient can sit comfortably on the socket of the prosthesis. Whenever possible, leaves of ilium and the pelvic rami are preserved during the hemipelvectomy to act as support points for the prosthesis. Both amputations can be fitted with a prosthesis that allows ambulation.

**ANSWER:** B

11. Which of the following statements regarding lower limb prostheses is true?

   A. They require more energy to use than crutch walking does.

   B. The shorter the stump, the greater the stump tip pressure.

   C. The main pressure point in a below-knee prosthesis is the stump end.

   D. A suspension belt is used for all above-knee prostheses.

   E. None of the above.

*Ref.:* 1, 2

**COMMENTS: Prostheses** are designed to restore function, mobility, and appearance. Properly fitted prostheses have lower energy requirements than crutch walking. Socket design has as its goals patient comfort and even distribution of forces on the stump. The longer the stump, the greater the surface area over which these forces can be distributed. Above-knee sockets are usually of the quadrilateral total-contact design and are suspended by stump suction or pelvic belts. The below-knee prostheses most commonly used are the patellar tendon–bearing type and the patellar tendon supracondylar type.

**ANSWER: B**

12. Which of the following statements regarding amputations distal to the elbow is true?

   A. Digital tourniquets should be used when possible to prevent excessive blood loss.

   B. The length of forearm preserved has little bearing on functional status.

   C. After suprametacarpal amputation, opposing tendons should be fixed to preserve muscle tone and strength.

   D. The precise nature of the operation requires a general anesthetic.

   E. None of the above.

*Ref.:* 1-3

COMMENTS: Most patients undergoing **lower extremity amputations** have peripheral vascular disease, and the use of tourniquets is not necessary. For the upper extremity, however, tourniquets are frequently used to provide a blood-free field so that critical nerve and tendon structures can be identified. Because of the risk for thrombosis, digital tourniquets such as rubber bands should be avoided. To best preserve muscle strength, tone, and hence function, opposing tendons should be fixed anatomically. The goal of amputation of the proximal part of the arm is preservation of as much viable tissue as possible. For distal arm amputations, the goal is to preserve the grasping function of the hand. Leaving as much forearm length as possible results in higher functionality of the residual limb and easier prosthetic fitting. Adequate anesthesia can often be accomplished by regional blockade. This is preferred in trauma patients, who may have a full stomach, because it avoids the risk of aspiration.

**ANSWER: C**

13. Which of the following statements regarding amputation of upper extremity digits is true?

   A. A shorter volar flap and a longer dorsal flap are desired.

   B. The root of the nail should always be preserved.

   C. During removal of the distal phalanx, the distal middle phalangeal cartilage should be preserved.

   D. Amputation at the metacarpophalangeal joint is preferable to amputation through the proximal phalanx.

   E. Even the smallest stump of the thumb is preferable to complete amputation with a prosthesis.

*Ref.:* 1, 2

COMMENTS: **Closure of the stump following amputation of an upper extremity digit** is best accomplished with a longer volar flap so that the scar can be positioned away from pressure-bearing surfaces. However, bone and viable tissue should never be sacrificed to achieve ideal scar placement. Unless more than one half of the nail bed can be preserved, the nail root should be removed. If the distal phalanx must be removed, the exposed middle phalangeal cartilage should be resected. Given a choice, resection through

the proximal phalanx is preferred over a metacarpophalangeal amputation. As is the case with the thumb, any stump, no matter how short, has function. When a digit must be removed in its entirety, preservation of function of the hand as a unit is the goal and may require a variety of secondary procedures.

**ANSWER: E**

14. Which of the following statements regarding wrist disarticulation is true?

   A. The stump is stronger than that left when the amputation is through the carpal bones.

   B. It provides better prosthesis control than does a long forearm amputation.

   C. The severed tendons and ligaments of the hand must be shortened to allow retraction of them.

   D. Preservation of the styloid processes is necessary for prosthetic fitting.

   E. None of the above.

*Ref.:* 1, 2

COMMENTS: **Wrist disarticulation** has several advantages over more proximal amputations. It preserves length and provides better control of the prosthesis. Although it is weaker than when the carpal bones remain, it accommodates a less conspicuous prosthesis. The styloid processes are removed to permit a smoother fit. The tendons of the hand are transected with the muscles at rest and fixed to the periosteum to prevent retraction and atrophy.

**ANSWER: B**

15. Which of the following statements is not true regarding forearm amputations?

   A. Unless significant forearm muscle mass and length can be preserved, an above-elbow amputation is preferred to enhance prosthetic function.

   B. Skin mobility is preserved by avoiding excessive dissection between the skin and fascia.

   C. A short stump of the ulna or radius can be lengthened secondarily.

   D. Cineplastic operations using the biceps or pectoralis muscles can provide function to artificial limbs when the amputation stump is extremely short.

   E. None of the above.

*Ref.:* 1, 2

COMMENTS: In cases of **forearm amputation**, dissection is kept to a minimum to avoid immobilization of skin by subsequent scar formation. Pronation and supination are preserved by striving for a longer stump. In addition, the procedure is conducted as atraumatically as possible to avoid fibrosis. Even an extremely short forearm stump is preferable to an above-elbow amputation. Functional control of a prosthesis fitted over a short stump can be provided by a cineplastic operation using the ipsilateral biceps or pectoralis muscle after the initial stump has healed. Other secondary procedures include the use of bone flaps or grafts to lengthen short stumps of the ulna or radius.

**ANSWER: A**

**16.** Which of the following statements regarding infection of a diabetic patient's foot is true?

    A. The infection within the foot is usually less severe than it appears on clinical evaluation.

    B. The pain expressed by the patient is generally greater than one would expect in relation to the degree of infection.

    C. The infection rarely has a bony or tendinous element at its base.

    D. Factors contributing to ulceration and infection in the foot of a diabetic patient are neuropathy, peripheral arterial occlusive disease, and impaired leukocyte phagocytic function.

    E. Conservative measures rarely succeed, with amputation often being necessary.

*Ref.:* 1, 2

**COMMENTS:** A **foot ulcer in a diabetic patient** may be caused by pressure on a dysesthetic extremity that may or may not be associated with peripheral vascular arterial insufficiency. There is often a bony or tendinous element at the base of the ulcer. The infection is usually more extensive in the foot than appears clinically. After adequate débridement, many extremities are salvageable. Aggressive open débridement is essential. Unless the need for amputation is urgent, an evaluation for arterial reconstruction should be made first.

**ANSWER:** D

**REFERENCES**

1. Frymoyer JW, editor: *Orthopaedic basic science*, Rosemont, IL, 1993, American Academy of Orthopaedic Surgeons.
2. Kasser JR, editor: *Orthopaedic knowledge update 5*, Rosemont, IL, 1996, American Academy of Orthopaedic Surgeons.
3. Nehler MR: Extremity amputation for vascular disease. In Rutherford RB, editor: *Vascular surgery*, ed 6, Philadelphia, 2005, WB Saunders.

# CHAPTER 29

# Thoracic Surgery

*Matthew J. Graczyk, M.D., and Anthony W. Kim, M.D.*

1. A patient who has remained intubated endotracheally for a prolonged period (>4 weeks) is at risk for the development of tracheal injury. All of the following are true of postintubation tracheal injury except:

   A. Symptoms usually appear many months after extubation.

   B. Dyspnea on exertion is the primary symptom.

   C. It is often misdiagnosed as asthma or bronchitis

   D. Bronchoscopy is the best mode of evaluation.

   E. Treatment options include tracheal dilation, laser resection, internal stent placement, and staged reconstruction.

   *Ref.:* 1, 2

**COMMENTS: Tracheal injury** after endotracheal intubation can occur at the cuff level, as a result of stomal injury, or at the glottic and subglottic areas. It is typically caused by scarring at the site of compression of the tracheal mucosa by the balloon from the endotracheal tube. Symptoms usually appear within 1 to 6 weeks after intubation. Dyspnea on exertion is the primary symptom. The severity usually correlates with the degree of tracheal stenosis. Dilation, laser treatment, and stent placement are most often used as temporizing measures to allow inflammation or the patient's overall condition to improve. Most functionally significant strictures are best treated by segmental resection and primary anastomosis.

**ANSWER: A**

2. Approximately 2 weeks after placement of a tracheostomy, copious bleeding from within and around the tracheostomy develops in a 65-year-old man. Which of the following choices is the best management for this problem?

   A. Removal of the tracheostomy tube at the bedside

   B. Replacement of the tracheostomy tube with an endotracheal tube

   C. Tracheal stent placement

   D. Resection of the innominate artery

   E. Arterial wall repair of the innominate artery

   *Ref.:* 1, 2

**COMMENTS: A tracheoinnominate artery fistula** is a rare, but often fatal complication of intubation or tracheostomy. It has a reported mortality rate of 86%. The most common cause is placement of the tracheostomy too low with subsequent erosion of the anterior tracheal wall into the innominate artery. Massive hemoptysis and episodic hemoptysis are the most common symptoms. Management includes hyperinflation of the tracheal tube cuff, finger compression of the innominate artery, and emergency return to the operating room for control of the airway and operative repair. Following orotracheal intubation, exposure is initially achieved via a collar incision at the stoma with extension into the midline for a sternotomy. The tracheal defect may be closed primarily and covered with soft tissue or be left open to heal by secondary intention if grossly infected. Repair of the innominate artery is associated with a high incidence of failure. Once the vascular defect is identified, the artery is divided proximal and distal to the defect and the divided edges are oversewn. The stumps are then buried under healthy tissue.

**ANSWER: D**

3. Hoarseness has developed in a 55-year-old woman following transhiatal esophagectomy. Which of the following is true about her complication?

   A. It is the result of injury to the superior laryngeal nerve.

   B. It is the result of injury to the recurrent laryngeal nerve.

   C. The nerve on the right side is more susceptible to injury.

   D. Seventy percent of bilateral nerve injuries are related to tracheal surgery.

   E. The most common mechanism of injury to the nerve is thermal from cautery burn.

   *Ref.:* 1, 2

**COMMENTS: Vocal cord paralysis** after thoracic surgery procedures has been reported to occur in 4% to 45% of patients. The nerve on the left side is more likely to be injured because of its course around the aortic arch. Seventy percent of bilateral injuries are associated with thyroid surgery. The most common mechanisms of injury to the recurrent laryngeal nerve are traction and division. Treatment is primarily surgical and includes injection, augmentation, and laryngeal framework surgery. Injury can result primarily in hoarseness, but it also can lead to incoordination of swallowing with a predisposition to aspiration.

**ANSWER: B**

4. A 53-year-old woman is evaluated for worsening stridor. She also complains of worsening dyspnea. Imaging studies demonstrate no lung pathology but are suggestive of an endotracheal lesion. Bronchoscopy confirms the presence of a primary tracheal tumor. Which of the following statements is true?

A. It occurs more frequently in women.

B. A tracheal tumor is best treated with radiation therapy to provide the optimal chance for long-term survival.

C. The most commonly histology is adenoid cystic and squamous cell.

D. It is usually found incidentally.

E. Imaging studies allow adequate characterization of tracheal tumors.

*Ref.:* 1, 2

**COMMENTS: Primary tumors of the trachea** are rare and account for less than 0.2% of all respiratory tract malignancies in the United States. A male-to-female ratio of 7:3 is reported. Patients typically have progressive respiratory symptoms, including cough and hemoptysis. Hoarseness and dysphagia are less common. Although endoscopic resection, radiotherapy, and tracheal resection are all available treatment modalities, surgical resection with airway reconstruction provides the best chance for long-term survival in appropriately select patients. Despite imaging studies visualizing these tumors, bronchoscopic evaluation is extremely important in planning resection.

**ANSWER: C**

5. All of the following are true of congenital malformations of the aortic arch system (also known as vascular rings) except:

A. Children typically have noisy breathing and varying degrees of respiratory distress.

B. Symptoms are usually caused by compression of the trachea or esophagus by the vascular abnormality.

C. Symptomatic patients rarely require surgical repair.

D. Late complications of unrepaired vascular rings include aortic dissection and aneurysm.

E. Contrast-enhanced computed tomography (CT) is the best diagnostic modality.

*Ref.:* 1, 2

**COMMENTS: Congenital malformations of the aortic arch** often cause symptomatic compression of the trachea and esophagus. Age at diagnosis and the severity of symptoms depend on the degree of compression. A newborn may exhibit dramatic airway compromise, whereas an adolescent may have subtle swallowing problems. The term *dysphagia lusoria* is used to describe the symptom occurring as a result of esophageal compression by an anomalous right subclavian artery arising from the thoracic aorta and passing behind the esophagus. Early surgical repair is recommended for symptomatic patients to avoid the complications of severe or recurrent respiratory infections, aortic dissection, and aneurysm formation. CT and magnetic resonance imaging are accurate imaging modalities, but they require sedation, which further jeopardizes the patient's tenuous respiratory status.

**ANSWER: C**

6. A 75-year-old woman is found to have bilious output from her tracheostomy that is associated with subcutaneous air, as well as pneumomediastinum. What is true about her problem?

A. Repair can be performed at anytime regardless of the need for ventilator dependence.

B. Acquired causes are more common than congenital forms.

C. It is best repaired by primary reapproximation of the esophagus and trachea.

D. The acquired form is most commonly caused by postintubation injury from endotracheal tube cuff pressure.

E. Muscle flap repair should be reserved for defects larger than 6 cm.

*Ref.:* 1, 2

**COMMENTS: A tracheoesophageal fistula** (TEF) can occur in two forms: from congenital abnormalities or acquired. Congenital TEF is more common than the acquired forms. There are several different types of congenital TEF, with the most common type being esophageal atresia with a distal TEF. The associated fistula in this type is typically small and is found in the midline of the membranous portion of the trachea proximal to the carina. Acquired TEFs result from destruction of the posterior membranous portion of the trachea. They can be secondary to erosion by malignant tumor or, more commonly, endotracheal tube cuff injury. Repair of an acquired TEF is best performed by segmental tracheal resection, primary closure of the esophagus, and interposition of soft tissue between the trachea and esophagus. The best results are obtained if the patient can be weaned from the ventilator before surgical repair. Endoscopic stents may be used to palliate or treat complications associated with esophageal malignancies causing fistulas.

**ANSWER: D**

7. A 32-year-old woman complains of a chronic and recurrent pulmonary infection. Closer evaluation of the CT scan demonstrates an abnormal vessel at the level of the diaphragm that appears to be perfusing a portion of the left lung. Which of the following statements is false regarding her process?

A. Intralobar sequestrations have their own pleural covering.

B. There are two forms of pulmonary sequestrations: intralobar and extralobar.

C. There is no communication between pulmonary sequestrations and the tracheobronchial tree.

D. The blood supply to the pulmonary sequestration is from a systemic arterial source.

E. Extralobar sequestration is frequently associated with congenital diaphragmatic hernias (CDHs).

*Ref.:* 1, 2

**COMMENTS: Pulmonary sequestration** is a congenital abnormality of the lungs. Both intralobar and extralobar types have in common the absence of communication with the tracheobronchial tree, blood supply to the lesion from a systemic source, and venous drainage into either the pulmonary or systemic circulation. The arterial supply is usually derived from the descending thoracic aorta (intralobar) or the abdominal aorta (extralobar). The intercostal arteries are rarely the arterial source. **Extralobar sequestration** is marked by having its own pleural covering separate from the surrounding normal lung, whereas the intralobar type does not. These lesions are most often located in the lower lung fields. Patients often have recurrent infections in the lungs. **Intralobar**

sequestrations constitute approximately 75% of all the sequestrations. Repeated pulmonary infections and hemoptysis are the most common symptoms. Extralobar sequestrations, in contrast to intralobar sequestrations, are associated with other congenital anomalies, particularly CDH.

**ANSWER: A**

8. Indications for an operation in patients with lung abscess include:

    A. Persistence of an abscess despite adequate therapy

    B. Empyema associated with a bronchopleural fistula (BPF)

    C. Inability to exclude a cavitating carcinoma

    D. Hemoptysis

    E. All of the above

    *Ref.:* 1, 2

**COMMENTS:** A **lung abscess** is a collection of pus contained in a cavity that is formed by the destruction of lung parenchyma. The bacteria responsible are numerous and include many gram positives, gram negatives, and anaerobes that cause pneumonia. The initial symptoms may include cough, fever, chills, fatigue, malaise, weight loss, pleuritic chest pain, dyspnea, and hemoptysis. Initial management consists of antibiotic therapy. Intervention for the aforementioned reasons is best achieved by percutaneous catheter drainage under CT or ultrasound guidance. Bedside tube thoracostomy is indicated for acutely ill patients with rupture of an abscess into the pleural space. Lung abscesses occur on the right side more than on the left side in most instances. Internal drainage with postural techniques and chest physiotherapy is usually sufficient for the management of this problem.

**ANSWER: E**

9. Regarding fungal infections of the lungs:

    A. Histoplasmosis is rarely found in an immunocompetent patient.

    B. No single staining technique demonstrates all the organisms.

    C. Coccidioidomycosis is endemic to the Mississippi River Valley.

    D. Blastomycosis is the most common cause of fibrosing mediastinitis.

    E. Untreated invasive *Aspergillus* infections gradually lead to the formation of an aspergilloma.

    *Ref.:* 1, 2

**COMMENTS: Mycotic lung infection** can be caused by many different organisms. The clinical manifestations vary widely from an asymptomatic patient with subclinical infection to an immunocompromised host with life-threatening opportunistic illness. The overall incidence of histoplasmin sensitivity (indicative of previous infection) in the United States is 20%. The incidence rises to 80% to 90% in the Midwest and Mississippi River Valley, where *Histoplasma capsulatum* is endemic. Fibrosing mediastinitis is a late complication of the mediastinal granuloma caused by **histoplasmosis**. **Coccidioidomycosis** is endemic to the southwestern region

of the United States. Immunocompetent patients with no or minimal symptoms and histoplasmosis, coccidioidomycosis, or **blastomycosis** can be monitored safely without antifungal treatment unless progression of the disease occurs. No single stain demonstrates all of the fungal organisms, but the two best stains to visualize fungal organisms are periodic acid–Schiff and methenamine silver. Aspergillomas are caused by noninvasive *Aspergillus* infections. They are characterized by a mass of fungal mycelia, sulfur granules, inflammatory cells, mucus, and tissue debris within a preformed lung cavity.

**ANSWER: B**

10. A 45-year-old man is admitted to the intensive care unit with septic syndrome and diffuse pulmonary infiltrates. Broad-spectrum antibiotics are initiated after collecting endobronchial specimens for culture and sensitivity. One week later, the patient remains intubated, cultures are negative, but he continues to exhibit a septic picture with negative findings on CT except for diffuse lung infiltrates. Select the most correct statement regarding surgical lung biopsy:

    A. Is indicated for patients with functional impairment and unexplained lung pathology

    B. Requires sampling only grossly abnormal lung tissue

    C. Is indicated to confirm the diagnosis of bacterial pneumonia

    D. Has diagnostic accuracy similar to that of transbronchial lung biopsy

    E. Should be placed in formalin and sent to the pathology laboratory for routine processing

    *Ref.:* 1, 2

**COMMENTS: Surgical lung biopsy** is a helpful diagnostic modality in a patient with unexplained lung pathology. It may be performed to obtain a suspected diagnosis or to assist in excluding other diagnoses that can be made only by histologic evaluation. Lung biopsy should not be used when the clinical diagnosis can be made by less invasive means, such as in the case of bacterial pneumonia. Lung biopsy can be performed by video-assisted thoracoscopic surgery (VATS) or by open thoracotomy. Surgical biopsy has much greater diagnostic accuracy than transbronchial techniques do. Obtaining tissue samples from multiple lobes, even if not grossly abnormal, is critical during diagnostic evaluation for such conditions as idiopathic interstitial pneumonia. Lung specimens should be sent fresh and in a variety of fixatives to maximize the diagnostic yield.

**ANSWER: A**

11. A 48-year-old man has a very round 2.5-cm nodule in the lower lobe of his right lung. It has a heterogeneous appearance on CT consistent with some fat within the mass itself. There are no other abnormal findings on CT, and no metabolic activity is seen on positron emission tomography. A benign diagnosis is entertained, and therefore which of the following choices is most accurate about this general category of tumors?

    A. Are usually symptomatic

    B. May be diagnosed from the radiographic appearance

    C. Often double in size within a 2-year period

D. Include the histologic subtype bronchoalveolar carcinoma

E. Frequently progress to malignant tumors

*Ref.:* 1, 2

**COMMENTS: Benign lung tumors** are usually asymptomatic and identified incidentally on imaging performed for other reasons. The radiographic appearance is unreliable in determining whether a lung nodule or mass is benign or malignant. Only specific patterns of calcification or the presence of fat density is considered to be an indicator of benign disease. Lung lesions are often monitored for changes in size over a specific interval to help determine benign versus malignant disease. A lesion that has not increased in size over a 2-year period is generally considered benign. An exception is bronchoalveolar carcinoma, which is a slow-growing malignant lesion with a characteristic ground glass opacity on CT. Malignant degeneration of a benign lung lesion is rare. Hamartomas are the most common benign lung lesions and account for more than 70% of all nonmalignant tumors. The majority of these lesions occur in the periphery.

**ANSWER:**    B

12. A 3-cm right upper lobe parenchymal mass and ipsilateral positive mediastinal lymph nodes (N2 disease) place a patient in which stage according to the new 7th edition of the American Joint Committee on Cancer (AJCC) staging system?

A. IB

B. IIA

C. IIB

D. IIIA

E. IIIB

*Ref.:* 1-3

**COMMENTS: Staging of lung tumors** is based on individual descriptors and their grouping. Stage IIIA disease in the new (seventh edition) staging system of the AJCC encompasses a range of disease from T1-3N2 to T4N0-1. Tables 29-1 and 29-2 delineate the individual T, N, and M descriptors and show the grouping of T, N, and M into their stages. The T designation typically refers to the status of the primary tumor in terms of size, location, visceral pleural involvement, and other factors. The N designation refers to

## TABLE 29-1    Definitions of TNM

**Primary Tumor (T)**

| | |
|---|---|
| TX | Primary tumor cannot be assessed, or tumor proven by the presence of malignant cells in sputum or bronchial washings but no visualized by imaging or bronchoscopy |
| T0 | No evidence of primary tumor |
| Tis | Carcinoma in situ |
| T1 | Tumor 3 cm or less in greatest dimension, surrounded by lung or visceral pleura, without bronchoscopic evidence of invasion more proximal than the lobar bronchus (i.e., not in the main bronchus)[a] |
| T1a | Tumor 2 cm or less in greatest dimension |
| T1b | Tumor more than 2 cm but 3 cm or less in greates dimension |
| T2 | Tumor more than 3 cm but 7 cm or less or tumor with any of the following features (T2 tumors with these features are classified T2a if 5 cm or less); Involves main bronchus, 2 cm or more distal to the carina; Invades visceral pleura (PL1 or PL2); Associated with atelectasis or obstructive pneumonitis that extends to the hilar region but does not involve the entire lung |
| T2a | Tumor more than 3 cm but 5 cm or less in greatest dimension |
| T2b | Tumor more than 5 cm but 7 cm or less in greatest dimension |
| T3 | Tumor more than 7 cm or one that directly invades any of the following: parietal pleural (PL3) chest wall (including superior sulcus tumors), diaphragm, phrenic nerve, mediastinal pleura, parietal pericardium; or tumor in the main bronchus (less than 2 cm distal to the carina[a] but without involvement of the carina; or associated atelectasis or obstructive pneumonitis of the entire lung or separate tumor nodule(s) in the same lobe |
| T4 | Tumor of any size that invades any of the following: mediastinum, heart, great vessels, trachea, recurrent laryngeal nerve, esophagus, vertebral body, carina, separate tumor nodule(s) in a different ipsilateral lobe |

**Regional Lymph Nodes (N)**

| | |
|---|---|
| NX | Regional lymph nodes cannot be assessed |
| N0 | No regional lymph node metastases |
| N1 | Metastasis in ipsilateral peribronchial and/or ipsilateral hilar lymph nodes and intrapulmonary nodes, including involvement by direct extension |
| N2 | Metastasis in ipsilateral mediastinal and/or subcarinal lymph node(s) |
| N3 | Metastasis in contralateral mediastinal, contralateral hilar, ipsilateral or contralateral scalene, or supraclavicular lymph node(s) |

**Distant Metastasis (M)**

| | |
|---|---|
| MX | Distant metastasis cannot be assessed |
| M0 | No distant metastasis |
| M1 | Distant metastasis |
| M1a | Separate tumor nodule(s) in a contralateral lobe; tumor with pleural nodules or malignant pleural (or pericardial) effusion[b] |
| M1b | Distant metastasis (in extrathoracic organs) |

[a]The uncommon superficial spreading tumor of any size with its invasive component limited to the bronchial wall, which may extend proximally to the main bronchus, is also classified as T1.
[b]Most pleural (and pericardial) effusions with lung cancer are due to tumor. In a few patients, however, multiple cytopathologic examinations of pleural (pericardial) fluid are negative for tumor, and the fluid is nonbloody and is not an exudate. Where these elements and clinical judgment dictate that the effusion is not related to the tumor, the effusion should be excluded as a staging element and the patient should be classified as T1, T2, T3, or T4.
Used with the permission of the American Joint Committee on Cancer (AJCC), Chicago, Illinois. The original source for this material is the *AJCC Cancer Staging Manual, Seventh Edition (2010)* published by Springer Science and Business Media LLC, www.springer.com.

**TABLE 29-2   Stage Grouping Comparisons: 6<sup>th</sup> Edition vs. 7<sup>th</sup> Edition Descriptors, T and M Categories, and Stage Groupings**

| 6<sup>th</sup> Edition T/M descriptor | 7<sup>th</sup> Edition T/M | N0 | N1 | N2 | N3 |
|---|---|---|---|---|---|
| T1 (≤2 cm) | T1a | IA | IIA | IIIA | IIIB |
| T1 (>2-3 cm) | T1b | IA | IIA | IIIA | IIIB |
| T2 (≤5 cm) | T2a | IB | **IIA** | IIIA | IIIB |
| T2 (>5-7 cm) | T2b | **IIA** | IIB | IIIA | IIIB |
| T2 (>7 cm) | T3 | **IIB** | **IIIA** | IIIA | IIIB |
| T3 invasion | T3 | IIB | IIIA | IIIA | IIIB |
| T4 (same lobe nodules) | T3 | **IIB** | **IIIA** | **IIIA** | IIIB |
| T4 (extension) | T4 | **IIIA** | **IIIA** | IIIB | IIIB |
| M1 (ipsilateral lung) | T4 | **IIIA** | **IIIA** | **IIIB** | **IIIB** |
| T4 (pleural effusion) | M1a | **IV** | **IV** | **IV** | **IV** |
| M1 (contralateral lung) | M1a | IV | IV | IV | IV |
| M1 (distant) | M1b | IV | IV | IV | IV |

Cells in **bold** indicate a change from the 6<sup>th</sup> edition for a particular TNM category. Used with the permission of the American Joint Committee on Cancer (AJCC), Chicago, Illinois. The original source for this material is the *AJCC Cancer Staging Manual, Seventh Edition (2010)* published by Springer Science and Business Media LLC, www.springer.com.

the level of lymph node involvement. The M descriptor refers to the presence of metastasis.

**ANSWER:   D**

13. A 56-year-old man has what appears to be early-stage non–small cell lung cancer and therefore resection is planned. Which of the following statements is most accurate in the treatment of this patient's problem?

   A. Cannot be performed with VATS

   B. Does not need to include mediastinal lymph node sampling or dissection

   C. Includes lobectomy and pneumonectomy only

   D. Should not be performed in conjunction with chemotherapy or radiation therapy given either preoperatively or postoperatively

   E. Is possible only in a minority of patients initially seen with lung cancer

*Ref.:* 1, 2

**COMMENTS:** Although most patients in whom **non–small cell lung cancer** is diagnosed eventually die of their disease, surgical resection is the most effective means of controlling the primary tumor and provides the best chance for cure. Because patients are often initially seen with advanced disease, only 20% to 35% of patients with non–small cell lung cancer are candidates for surgery. Presuming that the appropriate stage is assigned, the majority of this group typically represents those with stages I and II disease. Resection can include the removal of an entire lung, a lobe, or a portion/segment of a lobe of the lung. Surgery can be performed by **video-assisted thoracoscopic surgery** or thoracotomy with good results. Sampling or removal of mediastinal lymph nodes (or both) is paramount for complete pathologic staging. Complete and accurate staging determines whether a patient may receive adjuvant therapy in addition to surgical resection, such as chemotherapy, radiation therapy, or both. These adjuncts can be given before or after surgical resection, depending on tumor stage.

**ANSWER:   E**

14. Which of the following is not a criterion for resection of pulmonary metastases?

   A. The primary tumor is not controllable.

   B. More than one other extrapulmonary site of tumor exists.

   C. No better method or proven treatment is available.

   D. Complete resection of the metastatic focus is possible.

   E. Nonanatomic resection may be required.

*Ref.:* 1, 2

**COMMENTS:** Many patients with **lung metastases** from sarcomas and germ cell tumors may be candidates for metastasectomy, but with most cancers of epithelial origin, only 1% to 2% of patients may be treated in this manner because these patients often have concurrent distant metastases in other organs. The general criteria for pulmonary metastasectomy are outlined in the answers. In general, patients being considered should satisfy all these criteria. In very general terms, the survival rate with complete metastasectomy is 36% at 5 years, 26% at 10 years, and 22% at 15 years. These figures can obviously vary depending on the site of origin. The median survival after lung resection for metastatic disease is 35 months. It is not uncommon for anatomic resections (segmentectomy, lobectomy, and pneumonectomy) to be performed in the appropriate circumstances.

**ANSWER:   B**

15. A 20-year-old tall, thin man experiences spontaneous pneumothorax. On further questioning and examination, it is revealed that approximately 1 year earlier he was hospitalized and had a right chest tube placed for a similar problem. What is the optimal treatment option for this patient at this time?

   A. Observation and discharge

   B. Repeated tube thoracostomy maintained until resolution

   C. Needle aspiration and discharge

   D. Lobectomy and hospitalization

   E. Thoracoscopic resection

*Ref.:* 1, 2

**COMMENTS: Primary spontaneous pneumothorax** occurs in young patients without significant lung disease, whereas secondary spontaneous pneumothorax occurs in patients with chronic obstructive pulmonary disease. The most common cause of primary spontaneous pneumothorax is rupture of small apical blebs. In the United States, tube thoracostomy with water seal drainage is the usual first-line treatment of a moderate to large pneumothorax in a patient with a first-time occurrence. Needle aspiration of air from the pleural space is more commonly done in Europe. Patients with small first-time pneumothoraces can be safely observed. Approximately 20% to 30% of patients will have a recurrence within 2 years of the first episode. After three or more episodes of spontaneous pneumothorax, the rate of recurrence rises to 50% to 70% within the following 2 years. It is for this reason that surgery is indicated if there is a recurrence. Operative intervention may be considered after a first episode of spontaneous pneumothorax in patients with previous pneumonectomy, a history of untreated bilateral pneumothorax, or an occupation that poses an elevated risk for the development of pneumothorax, such as an airline pilot or underwater diver.

**ANSWER:   E**

16. The location of the thoracic duct at the level of the diaphragm is best described as:

A. Extrapleural along the right anterior surface of the vertebral bodies, posterior to the esophagus, between the aorta and azygous vein

B. Extrapleural along the left anterior surface of the vertebral bodies, posterior to the esophagus, between the aorta and azygous vein

C. Intrapleural along the right anterior surface of the vertebral bodies, posterior to the esophagus, between the aorta and azygous vein

D. Intrapleural along the left anterior surface of the vertebral bodies, posterior to the esophagus, between the aorta and azygous vein

E. Extrapleural along the right anterior surface of the vertebral bodies, anterior to the esophagus, between the aorta and azygous vein

*Ref.:* 1, 2

**COMMENTS:** See Question 17.

**A N S W E R :** A

17. Management of chylothorax includes all of the following except:

A. Drainage of the pleural space

B. Fluid, electrolyte, and nutritional support

C. External beam radiation therapy

D. Surgical ligation of the thoracic duct

E. Reduction of chyle production

*Ref.:* 1, 2

**COMMENTS: Chylothorax** is the accumulation of excess lymphatic fluid in the pleural space. It is usually a result of injury to the **thoracic duct** or one of its major branches and occasionally results from obstruction of the duct. The thoracic duct at the level of the diaphragm runs extrapleurally along the left anterior surface of the vertebral bodies, posterior to the esophagus, between the aorta and azygous vein. A triglyceride level of 110 mg/dL has a 99% likelihood of being chylous versus 5% when the drainage is 50 mg/dL. The most common causes are trauma, neoplasms, tuberculosis, and venous thrombosis. Treatment options are divided into operative and nonoperative categories. Drainage of the pleural space is the basic treatment of any significant accumulation of fluid. Prevention of dehydration and malnutrition and correction of electrolyte imbalance are important for higher-output chyle leaks. The most effective means of reducing chyle production is limitation or elimination of oral intake and institution of total parenteral nutrition. Somatostatin, octreotide, etilefrine, mechanical ventilation with positive end-expiratory pressure, and embolization of the thoracic duct have been used with variable success. In general, 25% to 50% of chyle leaks will close spontaneously within 2 weeks of nonoperative treatment. Surgical treatment is recommended for persistent leaks and can be performed with a variety of described techniques. Successful operative management relies on anatomic understanding of the course of the thoracic duct. Prolonged drainage only results in dehydration, malnutrition, and immunologic compromise secondary to the loss of fluid, fats, proteins, and T lymphocytes.

**A N S W E R :** C

18. A 60-year-old former smoker and plumber is being evaluated for progressive dyspnea and is found to have a large left-sided effusion. Work-up reveals that his effusion is secondary to a malignant pleural mesothelioma of sarcomatoid histology. Which of the following is true regarding his diagnosis?

A. Only approximately 20% of malignant pleural mesotheliomas are not asbestos related.

B. It is related to infection with *Histoplasma*.

C. Its incidence is decreasing.

D. Malignant pleural mesothelioma cannot be treated with surgery.

E. It has a 5- to 10-year latency period after exposure to asbestos.

*Ref.:* 1, 2

**COMMENTS: Malignant mesothelioma** is a rare tumor of the pleura. It is classified histologically into three subtypes: epithelioid, sarcomatoid, and mixed. The incidence is believed to be related to the industrial use of asbestos, particularly in occupations that expose individuals to the amphibole fibers of asbestos. Approximately 80% of malignant pleural mesotheliomas are secondary to asbestos exposure. Other factors that may contribute to the development of malignant pleural mesothelioma include radiation, non–asbestos-containing mineral fibers, organic chemicals, viruses, genetic predisposition, pleural scarring, and chronic inflammation. Despite governmental regulations on asbestos exposure in the second half of the 20th century, the incidence of malignant pleural mesothelioma has been rising in the United States since 1980. The latency period between exposure to asbestos and disease is 20 to 50 years. Twenty percent of cases are not related to **asbestos exposure**. Overall survival is grim. The best overall survival appears to be achieved with multimodality therapy consisting of combinations of surgery, chemotherapy, and radiation therapy. In appropriately selected patients, surgical treatment options include pleurectomy with decortication and extrapleural pneumonectomy. Controversy exists regarding which procedure is best.

**A N S W E R :** A

19. A 64-year-old woman has recurrent malignant pleural effusion that is not responding to repeated thoracentesis. She underwent mastectomy for stage II carcinoma of the breast 10 years earlier. In managing this malignant pleural effusion, the most effective agent for chemical pleurodesis is which one of the following?

A. Tetracycline

B. Talc

C. Bleomycin

D. Doxycycline

E. Erythromycin

*Ref.:* 1, 2

**COMMENTS: Malignant pleural effusion** is a common clinical problem that can lead to significant morbidity and reduction in quality of life in patients with advanced cancer. Lung cancer and breast cancer are the most common underlying primary malignancies. Relief of shortness of breath and improvement in quality of life are the mainstays of treatment. The diagnosis is usually made by cytologic evaluation of pleural fluid obtained via thoracentesis or thoracoscopy. Treatment options include repeated thoracentesis, tube thoracostomy with bedside pleurodesis, and placement of an indwelling pleural catheter. The most effective agent for achieving pleurodesis is talc. Talc can be instilled via closed tube thoracostomy as a "slurry" in solution or as an aerosol "poudrage" delivered at the time of thoracoscopy. Talc has been shown to control malignant pleural effusions in more than 90% of patients, generally with a success rate of between 85% and 96%. Although other series have reported high success rates with other agents, on average, the success rates are not as consistent as with talc **pleurodesis**. The other sclerosing agents listed are associated with success rates of 50% to 75%. It is important to point out that pleurodesis can be achieved only if the lung is not trapped and can re-expand to allow apposition of the visceral and parietal pleural surfaces. For patients with trapped lung associated with a malignant pleural effusion, an indwelling pleural catheter is a good option for ongoing drainage of the pleural space and control of symptoms. Erythromycin has no current role in pleurodesis.

**ANSWER: B**

20. Two months following right-sided pneumonectomy, empyema develops in a 60-year-old man. Conservative measures followed by lesser invasive measures to address this problem are not successful. Therefore, the patient is scheduled for open drainage of his empyema. Which of the following is true?

A. Is typically used in any patient able to tolerate general anesthesia

B. Is best suited if the underlying lung will re-expand after drainage and is not well adherent to the surrounding chest wall

C. Particularly useful if a BPF is present

D. Cannot be used in the setting of a BPF

E. Can be considered as an alternative first-line therapy in lieu of a chest tube

*Ref.:* 1, 2

**COMMENTS: Empyema** is defined as a purulent pleural effusion. The most common source of infection is the lung, but bacteria may enter the pleural space through the chest wall, from below the diaphragm, or through the mediastinum. The mainstays of treatment are antibiotics and drainage of the pleural space. Diagnostic thoracentesis is often performed, but definitive pleural drainage must be undertaken to control the infection. This can be performed by closed tube thoracostomy, pigtail catheter, VATS, or open thoracotomy. Open drainage of an empyema is best suited for chronic empyema with fixed underlying lung parenchyma that will not reexpand. Open drainage is particularly useful if a **bronchopleural fistula** is present. The drainage technique of open-window thoracostomy is credited to Dr. Leo Eloesser. In 1935 he described an open thoracic window for tuberculous empyemas in which a U-shaped flap of skin and subcutaneous tissue was created and sewn to the most dependent portion of the empyema cavity after removing two to three underlying ribs and intercostal muscles. The **Eloesser flap** is performed with a thoracotomy incision over the empyema, rib resection, and marsupialization of the skin edges to the parietal pleura to prevent closure of the incision. The **Clagett procedure** can be used if a BPF is not present and consists of open pleural drainage, serial operative débridement, and eventual chest closure after filling the chest cavity with antibiotic solution. It is most often used for an infected pneumonectomy space.

**ANSWER: C**

21. A 14-year-old boy has an anterior chest wall deformity that includes a depression in the body of the sternum, as well as in the lower costal cartilage. Which of the following statements regarding his chest wall deformity is accurate?

A. There is a 4:1 male-to-female preponderance.

B. Occurrence on the left side is more common than on the right side.

C. There is a high incidence of spontaneous resolution.

D. There is an association with Marfan syndrome in more than 10% of patients.

E. It is frequently associated with syndactyly.

*Ref.:* 1, 2

**COMMENTS: Pectus excavatum** and **carinatum** are the most common chest wall deformities. Carinatum is anterior angulation of the sternum, whereas excavatum is posterior angulation. Asymmetry of the depression can occur, such as the right side being more involved than the left side. It is usually present at birth but may worsen significantly during adolescence because of rapid growth of the individual. Pectus excavatum occurs four times more commonly in males than in females and is rarely seen in the African-American or Hispanic population. Although rare cases of spontaneous resolution occur, the majority of children have deformities that persist or worsen with time, especially during rapid growth periods. Approximately 65% of patients with Marfan syndrome have chest wall deformities, with pectus excavatum being the most common. However, only 2% of all patients with pectus excavatum have Marfan syndrome. **Poland syndrome** is a congenital anomaly characterized by absence of the sternal head of the pectoralis major and minor muscles. It is associated with anomalies, including hypoplasia of the breast/nipple complex, rib aplasia, lung hernia, small and elevated scapula (Sprengel deformity), cervical vertebral fusion (Klippel-Feil syndrome), syndactyly, and renal anomalies. Malignancies such as leukemia, lymphoma, cervical cancer, and lung cancer have also been associated.

**ANSWER: A**

22. A 45-year-old man is being evaluated for a painful right chest wall mass emanating from the ribs. Work-up suggests that this is a primary lesion of the chest wall. What is the most common primary malignant chest wall neoplasm in an adult?

A. Osteosarcoma

B. Soft tissue sarcoma

C. Ewing sarcoma

D. Chondrosarcoma

E. Plasmacytoma

*Ref.:* 1, 2

**COMMENTS:** Most **primary chest wall tumors** are benign, whereas most malignant chest wall neoplasms are metastatic. The most common primary malignant chest wall mass in adults is **chondrosarcoma**. It accounts for 50% of malignant chest wall tumors and 25% of all primary chest wall masses. Eighty percent of chondrosarcomas occur in the ribs and 20% in the sternum. Surgical resection is the best treatment of chondrosarcoma because these tumors are extremely resistant to radiation therapy and chemotherapy. Wide resection is typically curative. If left untreated, metastases typically occur late. Ewing sarcoma and primitive neuroectodermal tumors are the most common primary chest mall malignancies in children. These tumors are best treated by resection and radiation therapy. Chemotherapy can be used to control distant disease. Plasmacytoma is a local manifestation of multiple myeloma that is often manifested as a rib lesion in older men. Osteosarcomas have a bimodal distribution; they occur between the ages of 10 and 25 then again after the age of 40, often in association with many other diseases. Primary soft tissue sarcomas of the chest wall are uncommon.

**ANSWER:   D**

23. A 49-year-old woman after bilateral mastectomies for advanced cancer of the breast has a soft tissue skin metastasis in the midsternal region. After radiation therapy, a 5-cm, indolent, extremely painful necrotic ulcer develops. Following appropriate work-up, the patient is offered full-thickness resection of the chest wall. Which of the following is the most common soft tissue pedicled flap used for chest wall reconstruction?

   A. Transverse rectus abdominis muscle (TRAM)

   B. Serratus anterior

   C. Omentum

   D. Latissimus dorsi

   E. Trapezius

*Ref.:* 1, 2

**COMMENTS: Chest wall reconstruction** is often necessary after chest wall resection. Soft tissue reconstruction of the chest wall can be done with any of the flaps listed. They can be used either as free tissue flaps with microvascular anastomoses or, more commonly, as pedicled flaps using the native blood supply. The choice of flap is dictated by the location and size of the defect to be covered. The latissimus dorsi muscle is the most versatile and most common choice for chest wall reconstruction. However, the thoracodorsal vessels may have been compromised by the previous therapy, in which case a **transverse rectus abdominis muscle flap** can be used. It may be used as an isolated muscular flap or taken with the overlying paddle of skin and used as a myocutaneous flap. It the most commonly used flap because it has an extensive arc of rotation when the pedicle is based on the thoracodorsal neurovascular bundle. When used in such a manner, the latissimus dorsi flap can cover defects on the anterior, posterior, and lateral chest wall.

**ANSWER:   D**

24. Regarding the diagnosis and management of thoracic outlet syndrome:

   A. An operation is the primary treatment.

   B. It is recognized in approximately 2% of the population.

   C. Neurogenic symptoms primarily result from compression of the phrenic nerve between the anterior and middle scalene muscles.

   D. Patients may have primarily neurogenic symptoms, vascular symptoms, or a combination of both.

   E. Decreased nerve conduction velocity of the median nerve at the elbow is strongly suggestive.

*Ref.:* 1, 2

**COMMENTS: Thoracic outlet syndrome** is compression of the subclavian vessels or the brachial plexus (or both) as these structures exit the chest at the junction of the scalene muscles and the bony thorax. Most of the compression occurs at the first rib. It is present in approximately 8% of the population. Patients may have neurologic symptoms, signs of vascular compression, or a combination of both. Although the phrenic nerve lies on the anterior scalene muscle, neurogenic symptoms occur from compression of the brachial plexus between the scalene triangle and the bony thorax. Pain and paresthesia symptoms predominate, particularly in the ulnar nerve distribution. The initial treatment of most patients with thoracic outlet syndrome is nonoperative and consists of patient education on positioning, behavior modification, and physical therapy. Surgery is usually reserved for the 5% of patients with persistent symptoms despite nonoperative treatment. **Delayed nerve conduction velocity** across the thoracic outlet is consistent with thoracic outlet syndrome, and decreased velocity around the elbow is indicative of ulnar nerve entrapment or neuropathy.

**ANSWER:   D**

25. A minor league pitcher arrives at the hospital with complaints of edema, discoloration, and distention of the superficial veins in his throwing arm the day after he pitched for an extended period. What is true about his current condition?

   A. Is the result of a hypercoagulable state

   B. Is best treated with catheter-directed thrombolytic agents followed by surgical decompression of the thoracic outlet

   C. Is best treated with rest, elevation, and long-term warfarin therapy

   D. Is best treated with balloon angioplasty and intravascular stent placement

   E. Is not associated with occupational risk factors

*Ref.:* 1, 2

**COMMENTS: Effort thrombosis** of the axillary subclavian vein is known as **Paget-Schroetter syndrome**. It is usually caused by unusual or excessive use of the arm in association with some element of anatomic compression as described in thoracic outlet syndrome. Repetitive muscular activity such as that observed in professional athletes, painters, and beauticians can predispose the individual to this condition. It is not a direct result of a hypercoagulable state, although increased thrombogenicity can increase the incidence and exacerbate the symptoms. Treatment consisting of rest, elevation, and anticoagulation therapy was once the mainstay of management but has been shown to be associated with significant morbidity, including deep venous thrombosis, pulmonary embolism, and subsequent need for thrombectomy. The best treatment is catheter-directed lytic therapy combined with prompt surgical decompression of the thoracic outlet.

**ANSWER:   B**

26. Risk factors for poststernotomy mediastinitis include all of the following except:

   A. Male gender

   B. Advanced age (>75)

   C. Obesity (body mass index >30 kg/m²)

D. Diabetes with glucose levels higher than 200 mg/dL

E. Smoking

*Ref.:* 1, 2, 4

**COMMENTS:** The incidence of **post-sternotomy mediastinitis** is reported be between 0.7% and 1.5%. The mortality rate can be significant but averages between 4% and 10%. A number of risk factors are associated with this problem and are classified as modifiable versus unmodifiable or as preexisting, intraoperative, and postoperative. All of the risk factors listed are associated with an increased incidence of post-sternotomy mediastinitis except male gender. Female gender is an associated risk factor. The duration of cardiopulmonary bypass has also been shown to be a strong predictor of post-sternotomy mediastinitis. The principles of management for sternal wound infections are to (1) gain control the infectious process in the shortest amount of time and (2) ensure sternal stability.

**ANSWER:** A

27. During the performance of trisegmentectomy in a patient with colorectal metastasis to the right lobe of the liver, a brisk venous-like type of bleeding arises posterior to the liver. The surgeon decides to extend the incision through a median sternotomy. The best location to take down and repair the diaphragm so that the phrenic nerve is not injured is:

A. Centrally along the middle of the diaphragm, beginning medially at the central tendon and moving laterally toward the chest wall

B. Along the posterior third between the aorta and esophagus

C. Circumferentially at the periphery of the diaphragm

D. Centrally along the middle of the diaphragm in a vertical line from anterior to posterior

E. Medially in linear fashion at the junction of the diaphragm and mediastinal pleura

*Ref.:* 1, 2

**COMMENTS:** The **diaphragm** is innervated by the **phrenic nerves**. Arising from cervical roots C3, C4, and C5, the nerves originate at the superior border of the thyroid cartilage, pass along the anterior scalene muscles bilaterally, and descend through the mediastinum along the middle of the pericardium anterior to the hilum of the lungs. The right phrenic nerve reaches the diaphragm just lateral to the inferior vena cava. The left phrenic nerve enters the diaphragm lateral to the left border of the heart. Both nerves divide at the level of the diaphragm or just above it into several branches. There are three main muscular branches on the surface of the diaphragm. One is directed anteromedially toward the sternum, another is directed anterolaterally toward the central tendon, and the third is directed posteriorly. When taking down the diaphragm for surgical exposure it is of paramount importance to avoid injury to these branches. The best approach to divide the diaphragm is along the peripheral circumference with just enough muscle left on the chest wall for sturdy reapproximation. Generally, it is advised that one stay at least 5 cm lateral to the edge of the central tendon to avoid the posterolateral and anterolateral branches of the phrenic nerve.

**ANSWER:** C

28. Bochdalek CDH:

A. Is right sided 90% of the time

B. Is located anterior at the sternocostal junction

C. Usually has a hernia sac with associated abdominal contents

D. Is related to failure of development or fusion of the pleuroperitoneal membranes

E. Is associated with other congenital anomalies in less than 10% of patients

*Ref.:* 1, 2

**COMMENTS:** **Congenital diaphragmatic hernias** are divided into two subtypes, Bochdalek and Morgagni. Both types occur as a result of abnormalities during embryogenesis, specifically failure of development or fusion of the pleuroperitoneal membranes that usually make up the diaphragm between the fourth and eighth weeks of gestation. In **Morgagni hernias**, the defect occurs at the sternocostal hiatus through which the superior epigastric vessels pass from the abdomen to the retrosternal area. **Bochdalek hernias** occur in the posterolateral portion of the diaphragm and are left sided in 90% of cases. Most are found incidentally or are recognized after organ incarceration or volvulus. All Morgagni hernias have a sac that usually contains omentum and may also contain stomach, small bowel, or colon. Most (90%) Bochdalek hernias do not have a sac. CDH is associated with other congenital abnormalities in 45% to 50% of live births.

**ANSWER:** D

29. A newborn infant begins to experience respiratory distress approximately 4 hours after delivery. On examination, the newborn is tachypneic, with sternal, subcostal, and supraclavicular retractions. Decreased breath sounds are noted, and bowel sounds are present in the left side of the chest. The abdomen is scaphoid. Which of the following is not part of the management of this newborn?

A. Immediate operative repair

B. Extracorporeal membrane oxygenation (ECMO)

C. High-frequency oscillatory ventilation

D. Inhaled nitric oxide

E. Inotropic and vasopressor support

*Ref.:* 1, 2

**COMMENTS:** Treatment of **congenital diaphragm hernias** often begins with a prenatal diagnosis via ultrasound. If a prenatal diagnosis is made, delivery should take place in a center capable of delivering advanced neonatal and pediatric surgical care with reasonable experience in dealing with CDH. Stabilization of the patient and delayed surgical repair are the standard of care for newborns with CDH. Stabilization begins with respiratory support, including immediate intubation. Additional measures of support, including ECMO, oscillatory ventilation, inhaled nitric oxide, and hemodynamic support, can be used as the clinical condition warrants. Immediate surgical repair before stabilization and support is associated with significant morbidity and mortality. Tube thoracostomy is not routinely described as an adjunct in the preoperative care of patients with CDH, presumably because of the presence of herniated abdominal contents in the ipsilateral side of the chest and the absence of a true pneumothorax. The respiratory distress and hypoxia that are present are usually secondary to pulmonary hypoplasia. Finally, a tube thoracostomy is not typically used after repair because of concern for negative intrapleural pressure causing barotrauma and alveolocapillary membrane damage.

**ANSWER:** A

30. A 40-year-old man is evaluated for unremitting fevers and chills following a recent history of having a dental abscess. He neck is tender, and flexion and extension of the neck result in pain. What best characterizes this process?

    A. Arises commonly from a postoperative surgical site infection

    B. Is best treated by percutaneous drainage

    C. Can usually be treated in a single-stage operation

    D. Is a chronic, indolent disease process

    E. Is best diagnosed by CT of the neck and chest

    *Ref.:* 1, 2

**COMMENTS:** Acute descending **necrotizing mediastinitis** is a destructive, life-threatening condition similar to necrotizing fasciitis and acute necrotizing pancreatitis. Infection usually stems from an oropharyngeal source, with cultures yielding a polymicrobial mix of aerobic and anaerobic bacteria. The bacteria progress to the mediastinum via the pretracheal and retrovisceral spaces or along the carotid sheath. Although the diagnosis is often delayed, it is best made by early contrast-enhanced CT of the neck and chest. The principles of treatment are immediate parenteral broad-spectrum antibiotics and aggressive surgical treatment of both the neck and mediastinum. In most cases a cervical approach is sufficient, but a thoracic approach may need to be performed on occasion. Serial operations are often required. The best results are achieved with a multidisciplinary approach that includes thoracic surgeons, otolaryngologists, and oral maxillofacial surgeons when appropriate.

**ANSWER:** E

31. A stage I thymoma has been diagnosed in a 41-year-old woman. Through which of the following surgical approaches should a thymectomy not be performed?

    A. Transcervical collar incision

    B. Median sternotomy

    C. Partial sternal split

    D. VATS

    E. Posterolateral thoracotomy through the sixth intercostal space

    *Ref.:* 1, 2

**COMMENTS:** **Thymectomy** is performed most commonly for patients with myasthenia gravis. Indications for thymectomy include the presence of **thymoma** and a diagnosis of myasthenia without thymoma in patients whose disease is refractory to medical therapy or who cannot tolerate or are noncompliant with medical treatment. Thymectomy is also indicated for patients with other less common thymic neoplasms such as thymic carcinoma and

thymic carcinoid tumors. Various surgical techniques for thymectomy have been advocated and include all of the approaches listed. The debate regarding which technique has the best results has not been resolved. A posterolateral thoracotomy through the sixth intercostal space would be too low and provide suboptimal exposure.

**ANSWER:** E

32. All of the following mediastinal tumors are found in the anterior mediastinum except:

    A. Thymoma

    B. Thyroid mass

    C. Lymphoma

    D. Teratoma

    E. Ganglioneuroma

    *Ref.:* 1, 2

**COMMENTS:** **Mediastinal masses** are characterized by their location in the three compartments of the mediastinum: anterior, middle, and posterior. The **anterior mediastinum** extends vertically from the thoracic inlet to the diaphragm and is bounded anteriorly by the sternum and posteriorly by the brachiocephalic vessels, aorta, and pericardium. The **middle mediastinum** is defined as the space that contains the heart and pericardium. The posterior mediastinal compartment is defined anteriorly by the heart and trachea, laterally by the mediastinal pleura, and posteriorly by the vertebrae. The differential diagnosis of an anterior mediastinal mass includes thymoma, thyroid, lymphoma, and teratoma as the most common tumors. Neurogenic tumors, of which ganglioneuromas are one, are most often located in the **posterior mediastinum**.

**ANSWER:** E

33. A 58-year-old former heavily smoking man with a history of ethanol abuse recently ceased drinking and experienced a severe episode of ethanol withdrawal while hospitalized. Shortly after this episode he was noted to have pneumomediastinum on a chest radiograph. Which of the following is most likely the result of pneumomediastinum in the patient presented?

    A. Esophageal perforation

    B. Tracheobronchial injury

    C. Rupture of terminal alveoli from pressure generated by coughing or straining against a closed glottis

    D. Extension of a pneumothorax

    E. Penetrating trauma

    *Ref.:* 1, 2

**COMMENTS:** **Pneumomediastinum** refers to the presence of air in the mediastinal space. The most common source is rupture of terminal alveoli generated by coughing or straining against a closed glottis. The air escapes the distal lung tissue, but the visceral pleura remains intact. The air then courses along the perivascular or peribronchial space into the mediastinum. This process is rarely clinically significant and almost always requires no intervention except reassurance and a brief period of observation.

Pneumomediastinum may also arise from more significant injury to the tracheobronchial tree or from esophageal perforation. Tracheobronchial injuries should be evaluated with bronchoscopy. An esophagogram with or without esophagoscopy can be performed to evaluate for esophageal injury. Rarely, gas extension from the neck, usually secondary to trauma or surgical procedures, or from the abdominal cavity, usually after perforation of retroperitoneal hollow viscera, may result in pneumomediastinum.

**ANSWER: A**

34. A 23-year-old man is taken to the trauma department following a snowmobile accident in which his neck was injured in a "clothesline" fashion. In the field, he exhibited respiratory distress and was intubated. What is true about the laryngeal trauma that this patient experienced?

 A. It is graded on a four-point descriptive scale according to the severity of injury.

 B. Management begins with stabilizing the neck because of associated injuries.

 C. Minor injuries can be evaluated with endoscopy and managed nonoperatively.

 D. Early-stage blunt trauma classically causes symptoms.

 E. CT is not a sensitive diagnostic test for identifying traumatic laryngeal injury.

*Ref.:* 1, 2

**COMMENTS:** Because of the protected position of the larynx in the neck, external **laryngeal trauma** is rare. However, the mortality rates associated with these injuries can as high as 40% from blunt injury and 20% from penetrating injury. Death most often results from asphyxia secondary to laryngospasm, hemorrhage from an associated vascular injury, or laryngeal concussion. The signs and symptoms may be overt, with findings of subcutaneous emphysema, an expanding neck hematoma, hemoptysis, hematemesis, or a neurologic deficit. Alternatively, the clinical findings may be more subtle and consist of changes in voice, dyspnea, neck pain, dysphagia, coughing, or aspiration suggesting possible injury. CT is a sensitive diagnostic test for traumatic laryngeal injury and may be indicated despite normal findings on flexible laryngoscopy or bronchoscopy. Laryngeal injuries are graded on a five-point descriptive scale according to the severity of injury. Management, as with all trauma victims, begins with obtaining a stable airway. Minor injuries may be managed nonoperatively after careful and thorough endoscopic evaluation. Major injuries to the larynx require surgical exploration, with repair and reconstruction dictated by the extent of the injury.

**ANSWER: C**

35. A 24-year-old woman is a passenger in motor vehicle collision. On arrival to the trauma bay, a chest radiograph is suggestive of a left hemothorax. A tube thoracostomy is performed and a copious amount of bloody effusion is evacuated. Blood continues to be drained from her chest. In blunt chest trauma with hemothorax, what is an indication for surgical exploration that is listed among the following choices?

 A. Initial chest tube output exceeding 1500 mL

 B. Hourly chest tube output of up to 100 mL for 3 consecutive hours

 C. Declining hemoglobin or hematocrit

 D. Increasing opacities on chest radiography

 E. Presence of pneumothorax

*Ref.:* 1, 2

**COMMENTS: Blunt injury to the thorax** often results in varying degrees of hemothorax, pneumothorax, or both. Tube thoracostomy is the initial management of all injuries, both blunt and penetrating, to the thoracic cavity that result in **hemothorax** or **pneumothorax**. Many such injuries can be managed with tube thoracostomy alone. With regard to hemothorax, two metrics are generally accepted as indications for thoracotomy: (1) volume of initial drainage after tube thoracostomy of 1500 mL or more or (2) ongoing bloody chest tube output of greater than 200 mL/h. A drop in hemoglobin or hematocrit is often associated with a multiply injured trauma victim and is not by itself an indication for thoracotomy. Opacities on a chest radiograph in trauma patients are relatively nonspecific and may represent lung contusion, atelectasis, pneumonia, pleural effusion, or retained hemothorax. Their presence, although important to ongoing care of the patient, is not an indication for surgical exploration. Most pneumothoraces from trauma will resolve with tube thoracostomy.

**ANSWER: A**

36. A 26-year-old man was the driver in a high-speed motor vehicle collision in which the side of his car was hit in a lateral fashion ("T-boned"), and he sustained left-sided blunt chest wall injury. On evaluation, his primary survey is intact. He does have some left lateral rib fractures on the lower aspect of the left side of his chest. His chest radiograph shows an elevation in the costophrenic angle with air-fluid levels in the chest. Before undergoing chest CT, a nasogastric tube is placed, and during confirmatory radiographs, diagnosis of the injury is made. Which of the following is true regarding this patient's injury?

 A. Must be repaired with a patch

 B. Can be readily identified on radiographs or CT

 C. Heals spontaneously

 D. Is best identified and repaired via laparotomy

 E. Requires full excision of the diaphragm with prosthetic repair

*Ref.:* 1, 2

**COMMENTS:** Injury to the diaphragm accounts for only 3% of all trauma-related injuries, with the majority occurring on the left side rather than the right side. Blunt injuries usually occur secondary to high-speed motor vehicle crashes. A lateral impact is more likely to cause the injury than a frontal impact. Initial chest radiographic findings are normal in 50% of patients, and pneumothorax or hemothorax is seen in the remaining 50% of patients with **diaphragmatic injury**. CT, though helpful in the evaluation for other injuries to the thorax and abdomen, will aid in the diagnosis of a diaphragm injury only if abdominal viscera herniate into the pleural space. This is less common in the acute setting. The diagnosis of a diaphragm injury is best made with a high index of clinical suspicion based on the mechanism of injury and an injury pattern that is confirmed by thorough exploration via laparotomy. Recently, **laparoscopic exploration** of the abdomen has been used in the diagnosis of diaphragmatic injuries. Almost all trauma-related diaphragm injuries in the acute setting can be repaired primarily with a continuous monofilament suture 1-0 or larger in size. In general, in the acute setting a transabdominal approach is preferred, although some have advocated a right thoracic approach for right-sided injuries regardless of the time from injury. Classically, a thoracic approach is reserved for injuries seen in delayed fashion.

**ANSWER:** D

37. A 29-year-old man sustains a stab wound to the right side of his chest in approximately the sixth intercostal space in the anterior axillary line. He is found to have hemopneumothorax. In the management of penetrating injury to the lung, all of the following are appropriate except:

A. Tube thoracostomy

B. Oversewing of small lung lacerations

C. Wedge resection

D. Anatomic lung resection

E. Placement on continuous ECMO within hours of evaluation

*Ref.:* 1, 2

**COMMENTS: Penetrating injury to the lungs** results in varying degrees of hemothorax, pneumothorax, or both. Tube thoracostomy is the initial management of all injuries, both blunt and penetrating, to the thoracic cavity that result in hemothorax or pneumothorax. Most injuries can be managed by tube thoracostomy alone. Drainage of the pleural space with reestablishment of pleural apposition is usually sufficient to tapenade the low-pressure venous bleeding and serves to seal the air leak. Indications for early thoracotomy are massive hemothorax and massive air leak (only after the level of tracheobronchial injury, if present, has been identified by bronchoscopy). With regard to hemothorax, two metrics are generally accepted as indications for thoracotomy: (1) volume of initial drainage after tube thoracostomy of 1500 mL or greater or (2) ongoing bloody chest tube output greater than 200 to 250 mL/h for 3 to 4 consecutive hours after tube thoracostomy. All of the methods listed can be used to definitively control injury, depending on the extent of involved lung and associated blood vessels. Surgical exploration in a trauma patient should be expeditious and focused. Because anatomic lung resection may be time-consuming, other measures of controlling injury to the lung should be well known to the surgeon exploring the thorax in the setting of trauma. If surgical exploration is performed, some bronchial stump coverage is important because of contamination of the pleural space. Lung injury alone is not an indication for ECMO.

**ANSWER:** E

38. A 31-year-old man is brought to the trauma department 10 minutes after a gunshot wound to the left side of his chest. On arrival, he loses his vitals signs. He is already intubated with endotracheal tube placement confirmed, and an ongoing resuscitation effort is maintained. In preparing for emergency thoracotomy, which of the following best characterizes the necessary incision and position of the patient?

A. Posterolateral incision through the fourth intercostal space and the patient in the lateral decubitus position

B. Anterior incision through the second intercostal space and the patient supine

C. Anterolateral incision through the fourth or fifth intercostal space and the patient supine

D. Vertical incision along the anterior axillary line through the sixth intercostal space and the patient supine

E. Anterolateral incision through the sixth intercostal space and patient in the lateral decubitus position

*Ref.:* 1, 2

**COMMENTS:** The most common **emergency thoracotomy incision** is an anterolateral incision. It allows quick access to the thoracic cavity for control of life-threatening hemorrhage. This is performed with the patient supine and begins along the inframammary fold. The incision is turned superiorly along the medial aspect after crossing the midclavicular line so that if extension across the sternum is required, the incision will not be too low. The pericardium, lungs, pulmonary hilum, and descending thoracic aorta from the left side are readily accessible through this incision. If on entering the chest, high apical bleeding is encountered consistent with injury to a great vessel, the apex of the chest should be packed and the appropriate counterincision made. All of the other incisions listed are used in thoracic surgery for various exposures but are not generally indicated for trauma.

**ANSWER:** C

## REFERENCES

1. Patterson GA, Cooper JD, Deslauriers J, et al, editors: *Pearson's thoracic and esophageal surgery*, ed 3, Philadelphia, 2008, Churchill Livingstone.
2. Sellke FW, del Nido PJ, Swanson SJ, editors: *Sabiston and Spencer surgery of the chest*, ed 7, Philadelphia, 2005, WB Saunders.
3. Detterbeck FC, Boffa DJ, Tanoue LT: The new lung cancer staging system, *Chest* 136:260–271, 2009.
4. Shields TW, Locicero J, Reed CE, et al, editors: *General thoracic surgery*, ed 7, Philadelphia, 2009, Lippincott Williams & Wilkins.

# Subspecialties for the General Surgeon

# Metabolic and Bariatric Surgery

*Minh B. Luu, M.D., F.A.C.S., and Jonathan A. Myers, M.D.*

1. Which of the following statements regarding the prevalence of morbid obesity is true?

   A. Less than 50% of the U.S. population is considered overweight.

   B. The annual number of deaths from obesity in the United States exceeds that of breast and colon cancers combined.

   C. Approximately 10% of the U.S. adult population is morbidly obese.

   D. The rate of adolescent obesity has been stable in the last 10 years.

   E. All of the above.

   *Ref.: 1*

**COMMENTS:** Two thirds of the population in the United States is considered **overweight**, whereas 5% of the U.S. population is either **morbidly obese** or **clinically severely obese**. It is estimated that 280,000 Americans die annually of obesity-related causes whereas the total number of deaths from breast and colon cancers combined is roughly 90,000. The incidence of obesity in adolescents (40% above ideal body weight) is growing at an alarming rate and is estimated to be in the 20% range in most European countries and 35% in the United States. Obesity is the second leading cause of preventable death after tobacco use.

**ANSWER:** B

2. Which of the following definitions regarding body mass index (BMI) and obesity is not correct?

   A. BMI is calculated as weight in kilograms divided by the square of height in meters.

   B. Obese individuals have a BMI of 30 or higher.

   C. Normal weight is a BMI of 25 to 30.

   D. Morbid obesity is a BMI of 40 or greater.

   E. Morbid obesity is defined as being either 100 lb above ideal body weight or twice ideal body weight.

   *Ref.: 1*

**COMMENTS:** **Body mass index** is calculated by the equation $BMI = weight (kg)/height (m)^2$. Overweight individuals have a BMI of 25 to 29.9 kg/m². Obesity is defined as a BMI of 30 or higher. Morbid or "clinically severe obesity" is defined as being

either 100 lb above ideal body weight, twice ideal body weight, or a BMI of 40 kg/m² or greater.

**ANSWER:** C

3. Which of the following statements concerning the hormone ghrelin is true?

   A. It is produced mainly by the arcuate nucleus of the hypothalamus.

   B. Plasma levels increase after meals.

   C. Plasma levels are increased after gastric bypass.

   D. Plasma levels are increased in individuals following a low-calorie diet.

   E. Plasma levels are unchanged after sleeve gastrectomy.

   *Ref.: 1, 2*

**COMMENTS:** **Ghrelin** is a 28–amino acid peptide predominantly secreted by the oxyntic glands of the proximal part of the stomach with lesser amounts produced by the bowel, pancreas, and hypothalamus. Ghrelin is a potent orexigenic circulating hormone that causes release of growth hormone and influences the insulin signaling mechanism. Ghrelin secretion is increased by weight loss and by caloric restriction. Ghrelin levels are decreased after gastric bypass and sleeve gastrectomy.

**ANSWER:** D

4. Which of the following is not associated with morbid obesity?

   A. Metabolic syndrome

   B. Asthma

   C. Uterine cancer

   D. Hypoglycemia

   E. Hypercholesterolemia

   *Ref.: 1, 3, 4*

**COMMENTS:** Medical problems associated with obesity affect nearly every organ system. Most commonly, **arthritis** and degenerative **joint disease** affect more than 50% of patients seeking treatment. The **metabolic syndrome** is a constellation of medical conditions consisting of type 2 diabetes, impaired glucose tolerance, dyslipidemia, and hypertension. Other common comorbid conditions include obstructive sleep apnea, asthma, hypertension, diabetes, and gastroesophageal reflux disease. Additionally, accumulating evidence suggests an association between obesity and **multiple cancers**, including an increased risk for breast, colon, endometrial, renal, and esophageal cancers. The International Agency for Research on Cancer Working Group noted a similar association with gallbladder, liver, and pancreatic cancers. Furthermore, a linear relationship seems to exist between increasing BMI and higher mortality in patients with colon, renal, and esophageal cancers.

**ANSWER: D**

5. Concerning the medical treatment of obesity, which of the following is true?

   A. Very-low-calorie diets primarily restrict either fat intake or carbohydrate intake.

   B. Sibutramine is a medication that inhibits pancreatic lipase and thereby reduces the absorption of up to 30% of ingested dietary fat.

   C. Orlistat is a medication that blocks the presynaptic uptake of both norepinephrine and serotonin, thereby potentiating their anorexic effect in the central nervous system.

   D. Severely obese patients have a 10% chance of losing enough weight by dietary measures alone to achieve a BMI of less than 35 $kg/m^2$.

   E. For severely obese patients, medications have shown promising long-term weight loss.

*Ref.:* 1, 3

**COMMENTS:** Numerous programs exist to promote weight loss. However, all are encumbered by difficulty in helping patients sustain long-term weight loss. The National Institutes of Health (NIH) consensus conference recognized that **medical therapy** alone had been uniformly unsuccessful in treating the severely obese population. In fact, severely obese patients have a 3% or less chance of losing enough weight by dietary measures alone to achieve a BMI of less than 35 $kg/m^2$. **Surgical treatment** of obesity allows a loss of at least 50% of excess body weight in 80% to 90% of eligible individuals with concurrent improvement in comorbid conditions. Nonetheless, it is agreed that patients considering **bariatric surgery** need to be on a medically supervised diet program before being eligible for an operation. Diet options include **very-low-calorie diets**, which primarily restrict either fat intake or carbohydrate intake. Recent pharmacologic therapy focuses on two medications. **Sibutramine** blocks the presynaptic uptake of norepinephrine and serotonin, thereby potentiating their anorexic effect in the central nervous system. **Orlistat** inhibits pancreatic lipase and thereby reduces the absorption of up to 30% of ingested dietary fat. For severely obese patients, neither medication has shown promising long-term weight loss.

**ANSWER: A**

6. A 30-year-old woman who weighs 245 lb is seen in the office for a consultation regarding bariatric surgery. Which of the following is not a criterion for eligibility?

   A. BMI of 40 $kg/m^2$ or greater

   B. BMI between 30 and 34.9 $kg/m^2$ with significant obesity-related comorbidity

   C. Failure to lose weight in a supervised dietary program

   D. Demonstration of psychiatric stability to undergo the proposed procedure

   E. Medically fit for surgery

*Ref.:* 1, 3

**COMMENTS:** Approved guidelines (NIH, 1991) regarding eligibility for **weight reduction surgery** include a BMI greater than 40 $kg/m^2$ without associated comorbid medical conditions or a BMI of 35 $kg/m^2$ or greater with associated comorbidity. Additionally, patients must have failed dietary or other nonoperative weight loss attempts, be psychiatrically stable without substance abuse problems, have knowledge about the operation and its sequelae, and be medically able to safely undergo a surgical procedure. Furthermore, most institutions stress the importance of a **multidisciplinary team** that includes a dietitian, psychologist, and members of the cardiac, pulmonary, gastrointestinal, and endocrine specialties, among others. Appropriate preoperative evaluation of comorbid conditions is necessary to ensure safe patient care. Weight loss surgery offers resolution or improvement of most comorbid conditions, except for patients suffering from Prader-Willi syndrome. Certification of institutions as centers of excellence by the American College of Surgeons or the American Society for Metabolic and Bariatric Surgery is desirable, but not mandatory. There is no absolute age limit for weight loss surgery other than the patient's physiologic age and potential for longevity. Finally, it is essential for patients to have a strong family and social support network.

**ANSWER: B**

7. Which of the following statements regarding bariatric operations is not correct?

   A. Laparoscopic adjustable gastric banding (LAGB) is a restrictive procedure.

   B. Biliopancreatic diversion (BPD) is mainly a malabsorptive procedure.

   C. The Roux-en-Y gastric bypass is mainly a restrictive procedure with a malabsorptive component.

   D. Vertical sleeve gastrectomy is a malabsorptive procedure.

   E. Vertical banded gastroplasty is a restrictive procedure.

*Ref.:* 1, 3

**COMMENTS:** Bariatric operations are categorized according to their mechanism of action: restriction of oral intake and malabsorption of ingested food. Examples of restrictive procedures include the **adjustable gastric band**, **vertical sleeve gastrectomy**, and **vertical banded gastroplasty**. Malabsorptive procedures function by creating a long intestinal channel that extends from the stomach or gastric pouch to a distal anastomosis between the small intestine and the biliopancreatic limb. This results in the malabsorption of ingested food proximal to the common channel where bile and pancreatic enzymes digest the nutrients for absorption. An example of a malabsorptive procedure with a mild restrictive component is **biliopancreatic diversion**. The **Roux-en-Y gastric bypass** is a combined procedure that functions by creating a small restrictive pouch in addition to a malabsorptive Roux limb. The length of the Roux limb used varies from 75 to 150 cm depending on the severity of obesity. All of the aforementioned procedures can be performed through a laparoscopic or open approach. Advantages of the laparoscopic approach include a reduced rate of incisional hernias and shorter hospitalization.

**ANSWER:** D

8. Which operation was first used extensively for the treatment of morbid obesity during the 1960s?

A. Roux-en-Y gastric bypass

B. BPD

C. Jejunoileal bypass

D. Vertical banded gastroplasty

E. Adjustable gastric banding

*Ref.:* 1

**COMMENTS:** The surgical treatment of morbid obesity is referred to as **bariatric surgery**. Malabsorptive procedures were first developed in the 1950s for the treatment of severe hyperlipidemia. This prompted development of the **jejunoileal bypass** in the 1960s, which resulted in significant weight loss but was later abandoned because of unacceptable metabolic complications. **Gastric bypass** and **gastroplasty** were later developed to avoid the significant complications associated with jejunoileal bypass.

**ANSWER:** C

9. Laparoscopic placement of an adjustable gastric band requires completion of all of the following steps except:

A. Division of the peritoneum at the angle of His

B. Dissection around the upper part of the stomach via the perigastric technique

C. Placement of the band around the upper part of the stomach by buckling it in place

D. Suturing the fundus to the proximal part of the stomach to imbricate the anterior gastric wall over the band

E. Securing the port to the abdominal wall fascia

*Ref.:* 1, 5

**COMMENTS:** The surgical technique for the correct **laparoscopic placement of an adjustable band** requires careful retraction of the left lateral lobe of the liver followed by division of the peritoneum overlying the angle of His and the pars flaccida of the gastrohepatic omentum. After identifying the base of the right crus, a small defect is made to create an avascular tunnel from the lesser curvature to the angle of His (pars flaccida technique) (E-Figure 30-1; E-figures throughout this chapter can be found online at www.expertconsult.com). An articulating dissector or grasper is placed through this defect to grasp the band, pull it around the upper part of the stomach, and buckle it in place. The fundus of the stomach is then imbricated over the band with sutures to the proximal portion of the stomach superior to the band. The **perigastric technique** involves dissecting the neurovascular bundle off the lesser curve of the stomach and placing the posterior portion of the band free within the lesser sac. This resulted in a high incidence of slippage, and thus the **pars flaccida technique** has become the preferred approach. The tubing is attached to the port, which is secured to the abdominal wall fascia (E-Figure 30-2).

The port can be accessed starting several weeks postoperatively with a noncoring needle to adjust the band.

**ANSWER:** B

10. Which of the following outcomes regarding the use of LAGB is false?

A. Deficiencies of calcium and vitamin $B_{12}$ are common.

B. Excess weight loss after surgery averages nearly 50% at 2 years.

C. Resolution of type 2 diabetes occurs in nearly 50% of patients.

D. Resolution of hypertension occurs in more than 40% of patients.

E. Maximal weight loss is usually achieved by the third year.

*Ref.:* 1, 5

**COMMENTS:** Most studies have reported a mean excess weight loss of 47.5% after **laparoscopic adjustable gastric banding**. Additionally, its use was shown to resolve type 2 diabetes in 47.9% of patients and to improve the condition in 80.8% of patients. Hypertension was resolved in 42% of patients and improved in 70.8% of patients. Dyslipidemia, obstructive sleep apnea, gastroesophageal reflux disease, and venous stasis improved or resolved after weight loss occurred with adjustable gastric banding. Other advantages of the procedure include the fact that it is adjustable and reversible, carries a low risk for death, and has no malabsorptive effect leading to metabolic problems or vitamin deficiency after surgery.

**ANSWER:** A

11. A 37-year-old woman is seen in your office 2 years after placement of an LAGB. She has lost 80 lb and her BMI is down to 28 kg/m². She states that her port site is tender and red. Her last adjustment took place 3 months earlier. The most likely diagnosis is:

A. Trocar site hernia

B. Wound infection from poor sterile technique during her last band adjustment

C. Band erosion

D. Leakage of the access port tubing

E. Band slippage

*Ref.:* 1

**COMMENTS:** The mortality associated with **laparoscopic adjustable gastric banding** ranges from 0.02% to 0.1%, which is significantly lower than that associated with bypass (0.3% to 0.5%) or the malabsorptive operations (0.9% to 1.1%). The rate of perioperative complications with LAGB is 1.5%, with late complications occurring in up to 15% of patients: band slippage or prolapse (13.9%), erosion (3%), and port access problems (5.4%). Band slippage occurs when the fundus of the stomach herniates up through the band and causes obstruction; preferential use of the **pars flaccida technique** over the perigastric technique has resulted in a decrease in band slippage rates from 15% in early studies to 4% in recent studies. **Port access site problems** are the most common complication after LAGB and include leakage of the access tubing, kinking of the tubing as it passes through the fascia, or port flip. Most port site problems can be repaired with the patient under local anesthesia. **Port site infection** is rare (<1%) but should be evaluated with upper endoscopy because it may be indicative of band erosion. This phenomenon involves erosion of the band into the lumen of the stomach and may increase with the passage of time. The incidence remains low at 1%, and it may be manifested as abdominal pain or port access site infection. It may be caused by placement of a band that is too tight or be caused by imbrication sutures placed too close to the buckle of the band. Treatment involves removal of the band and repair of the stomach.

**ANSWER: C**

---

**12-15.** A 42-year-old woman with a 20-year history of morbid obesity wants to have a "gastric bypass" because her neighbor has undergone the procedure. She stands 5 feet 5 inches tall and weighs 280 lb with a BMI of 46.6 kg/m$^2$. She has a history of medication-controlled hypertension and hyperlipidemia. The patient has undergone several commercial and physician-directed diet and exercise programs with weight fluctuations from 260 to 295 lb.

**12.** Which of the following is true regarding gastric bypass?

A. The incidence of postoperative gallstone or sludge formation is about 5%.

B. The greater curvature of the stomach is removed.

C. The gastric pouch is completely divided from the distal part of the stomach.

D. Three anastomoses are required in the Roux-en-Y reconstruction.

E. A common channel of 100 cm is created by measuring proximal to the ileocecal valve.

*Ref.:* 1, 5

**COMMENTS:** The essential components of **gastric bypass** include creating a 10- to 15-mL proximal gastric pouch based on the upper lesser curvature of the stomach to prevent dilation and minimize acid production, complete division of the gastric pouch from the distal end of the stomach by creating a Roux limb at least 75 cm in length and constructing an enteroenterostomy that avoids stenosis or obstruction, and closure of all potential spaces for internal hernias. A gastrojejunostomy is created in an antecolic or retrocolic fashion, depending on surgeon preference. Incomplete division of the gastric pouch from the distal part of the stomach remnant has been associated with gastrogastric fistula formation and weight loss failure. A **gastrojejunostomy** and a **jejunojejunostomy** are the two anastomoses in the **Roux-en-Y reconstruction** after gastric bypass (E-Figure 30-3). The incidence of gallstone or sludge formation after gastric bypass is approximately 30%. Answer B refers to sleeve gastrectomy. Answer E describes BPD/duodenal switch (DS) and accounts for the malabsorptive component of the procedure.

**ANSWER: C**

---

**13.** The patient undergoes a laparoscopic Roux-en-Y gastric bypass. On postoperative day 5, she is tachycardic with a pulse of 130 beats/min, tachypneic, and oliguric. What clinical scenario are you most concerned about?

A. Hypovolemia

B. Postoperative bleeding

C. Pulmonary embolism

D. Anastomotic leak

E. Inadequate pain control

*Ref.:* 1, 3

**COMMENTS: Complications after gastric bypass** can be classified as early (<30 days) or late (>30 days) and vary depending on reporting. The most feared early complication specific to gastric bypass is a **leak at the gastrojejunostomy**. It is generally manifested as tachycardia, along with tachypnea and oliguria. Fever or signs of peritonitis may be absent. The leak rate has been reported to be approximately 2% to 3%, and leaks are a significant contributor to mortality. Imaging will show free fluid, air, or extravasation of contrast material. **Pulmonary embolism** is another leading cause of death in the early postoperative period. It may be manifested as tachycardia, tachypnea, and hypoxia. There are no data to support a superior prophylaxis regimen, but many centers use a combination of early ambulation, the use of sequential compression devices, and subcutaneous administration of fractionated or unfractionated heparin.

**ANSWER: D**

---

**14.** At her 3-month postoperative clinic visit, which of the following observations would require further investigation?

A. After an initial weight loss of 50 lb, she has not lost any weight in a week.

B. She is tolerating a general diet but because of the operation has vomited three times after eating steak.

C. She reports two to three loose bowel movements per day.

D. Her neck and trunk appear thinner but her lower extremities are unchanged.

E. She complains of fatigue.

*Ref.:* 1

**COMMENTS: Weight loss after gastric bypass** is nonlinear, and short periods without weight loss are expected. Change in appearance of the head, neck, and upper part of the body as a result of weight loss are more pronounced than of the lower extremities. Nausea and vomiting are not unusual in isolated circumstances after gastric bypass, especially in relation to the patient's adaptation to food restrictions. Persistent vomiting may lead to **Wernicke encephalopathy**. This neurologic deficit may be preventable with parenteral thiamine. **Loose bowel movements** are common after all malabsorptive procedures and vary in severity. Iron is preferentially absorbed in the duodenum and proximal jejunum. The incidence of **iron deficiency anemia** after gastric bypass is approximately 20%, and it will often be manifested clinically as fatigue.

**ANSWER: E**

---

**15.** The patient comes to the emergency department 6 months after surgery complaining of a 2-day history of epigastric abdominal pain and emesis without relief. In the emergency department her temperature is 98.9° F with a pulse of 99 beats/min and blood pressure of 140/70 mm Hg. Her abdomen is soft with mild distention, normal bowel sounds, and vague discomfort on palpation. Computed tomography of the abdomen reveals passage of oral contrast to the colon without evidence of free fluid, extravasation of contrast, or pneumoperitoneum. The excluded stomach and the entire length of the biliopancreatic limb are dilated. The biliopancreatic limb appears to be in its normal location. The patient will most likely require which one of the following?

A. Revision of the jejunojejunostomy

B. Revision of the gastrojejunostomy

C. Excision of the marginal ulcer

D. Hernia repair with mesh

E. Reversal of the gastric bypass

*Ref.:* 1, 3

**COMMENTS: Late complications** include marginal ulcers, stomal stenosis, and internal and incisional hernias. **Marginal ulcers** occur in 2% to 10% of gastric bypass patients and can vary in time of appearance. The majority resolve by treatment with proton pump inhibitors but, if untreated, can result in stenosis or perforation. This patient has a late complication manifested as **obstruction of the biliopancreatic limb** because of stenosis of the jejunojejunostomy and will probably require revision of the anastomosis. Contrast material is excluded from the biliopancreatic limb and will not aid in diagnosis. Other late complications include **gastrojejunostomy stricture** or **internal hernias**. Internal hernias can be difficult to diagnose but are repaired by reduction and primary closure. Many surgeons advocate closure of all mesenteric defects at the time of the original operation to reduce the risk for internal hernia formation.

**ANSWER: A**

**16-17.** A 35-year-old man with long-standing morbid obesity is evaluated for bariatric surgery. He is 5 feet 8 inches tall, weighs 475 lb with a BMI of 72.2 kg/m², and has limited mobility requiring the assistance of a walker. His medical history is significant for hypertension, type 2 diabetes, sleep apnea, and gastroesophageal reflux disease.

**16.** Which of the following is true when discussing BPD as an option for this patient?

A. Malabsorption of fat-soluble vitamins is rare.

B. Protein malnutrition is the most significant long-term complication seen after BPD.

C. Postoperative diarrhea is uncommon.

D. Long-term weight loss results are not as good as with gastric bypass.

E. A portion of the stomach is divided but not removed from the patient.

*Ref.:* 1, 3

**COMMENTS:** See Question 17.

**ANSWER: B**

**17.** Which of the following is not a benefit of the DS modification of BPD?

A. Decreased marginal ulcers

B. Decreased protein malnutrition

C. Decreased dumping syndrome

D. Decreased iron deficiency

E. A two-stage operation is an option

*Ref.:* 1, 3

**COMMENTS: Biliopancreatic diversion** involves performing a hemigastrectomy that is drained by a Roux limb anastomosed to the biliopancreatic limb 50 to 150 cm proximal to the ileocecal valve (Figure 30-1). Malabsorption is the essential weight loss mechanism with this approach. **Duodenal switch** is an American adaptation of the BPD that involves tubularizing the stomach with a vertical sleeve gastrectomy and preserving the pylorus (rather than performing a hemigastrectomy) in an effort to decrease the incidence of marginal ulcers after BPD. This provides a restrictive component to the operation. The pylorus is then connected to the Roux limb with downstream construction similar to the original BPD (Figure 30-2). In addition to decreased marginal ulcers, preservation of the pylorus results in reduced dumping syndrome and improved iron homeostasis. At a BMI of greater than 60 kg/m², some surgeons recommend a two-stage procedure in which sleeve gastrectomy only is performed during the first operation to decrease operative risk. The remainder of the operation is performed in a delayed time frame after initial weight loss from the sleeve gastrectomy. The most significant long-term complication following BPD/DS is **protein malnutrition**, which occurs in up to 12% of patients. **Malabsorption of fat-soluble vitamins** is another major

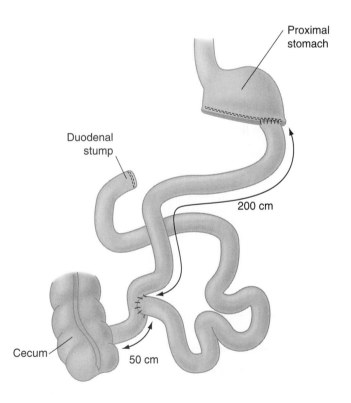

Alimentary channel = 250 (± 50) cm
Common channel = 50 cm

**Figure 30-1.** Anatomic configuration of biliopancreatic diversion.

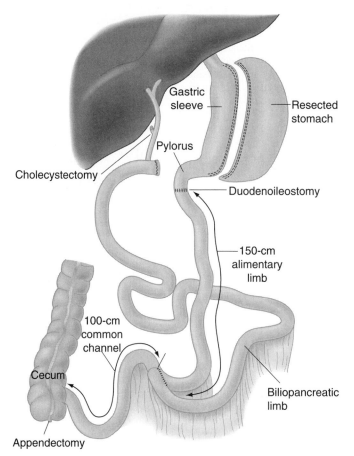

**Figure 30-2.** Configuration of the duodenal switch.

problem following surgery, with depressed levels of vitamins A, D, and K occurring in 63% to 69% of patients. Mortality rates have been reported at 1.1%, along with a 5.9% wound complication rate, 1.8% leak rate, and 4.2% reoperation rate. Following BPD/DS, three to four loose bowel movements a day, excessive flatulence, and foul-smelling stool may be normal and are results of the malabsorptive nature of the procedure. Difficulty in managing the protein and vitamin deficiencies coupled with the technical difficulty in performing BPD/DS has prevented its wide acceptance in the United States. Nonetheless, the procedure does result in significant weight loss, with studies demonstrating 70% to 78% loss of excess body weight up to 12 years after surgery.

**A N S W E R :** B

18. Advantages of laparoscopic gastric bypass with Roux-en-Y reconstruction over the open approach include all of the following except:

A. Shorter patient hospital stay

B. Lower wound infection rate

C. Lower internal hernia rate

D. Decreased rate of respiratory complications

E. Lower incisional hernia rate

*Ref.:* 1

**COMMENTS:** When compared with the open technique, laparoscopic gastric bypass results in a shorter hospital stay, lower rate of wound infections, and lower rate of incisional hernias. The short-term weight loss and leak rates are similar for the two techniques. Furthermore, a recent meta-analysis showed similar findings of decreased rates of incisional hernias and respiratory and wound complications. The rate of development of internal hernias was higher in the laparoscopic group, most likely because of decreased intraabdominal adhesion formation.

**A N S W E R :** C

19. Which of the following statements is true concerning sleeve gastrectomy?

A. Long-term data show 50% to 70% loss of excess body weight.

B. It works by restrictive and malabsorptive mechanisms.

C. Postoperative gastric emptying is delayed.

D. Postoperative plasma ghrelin levels are elevated.

E. It is a component of DS.

*Ref.:* 1, 3

**COMMENTS:** Sleeve gastrectomy is a component of the **duodenal switch modification of biliopancreatic diversion** and may be performed as a first stage to decrease operative risk in patients with a BMI of greater than 60 kg/m². Because of its short-term success in weight loss, sleeve gastrectomy has been applied as a primary operation, but its long-term outcomes, comparative results, and precise indications remain to be determined. Long-term data are not currently available. Aside from its restrictive component, the mechanism of weight loss is unknown. Ghrelin levels are decreased and gastric emptying is increased following sleeve gastrectomy. Other investigational procedures that are showing modest short-term weight loss include **gastric pacing** and **endoluminal sleeves**.

**ANSWER:** E

20. The most common indication for revision surgery after gastric bypass is:

    A. Perforation

    B. Protein deficiency

    C. Failure to lose weight

    D. Dumping syndrome

    E. Anastomotic bleeding

*Ref.:* 1

**COMMENTS:** Approximately 10% of gastric bypass patients fail to lose or maintain adequate weight loss and often seek **revision surgery**. When assessing these patients, it is important to determine whether there is an anatomic defect (dilated gastric pouch, enlarged gastrojejunostomy, gastrogastric fistula) that might be the cause of the failure. Reoperation on a patient who fails to lose weight with an anatomically intact and well-constructed gastric bypass is likely to be unsuccessful. Revision surgery is associated with an increased rate of infection, organ injury, and leakage.

**ANSWER:** C

21. The current procedure of choice for the surgical management of weight loss that combines optimal weight loss with acceptable morbidity is:

    A. Adjustable gastric banding

    B. Roux-en Y-gastric bypass

    C. BPD with DS

    D. Sleeve gastrectomy

    E. None of the above

*Ref.:* 1, 3

**COMMENTS:** Mortality after **adjustable gastric banding** (0.02% to 0.1%) is lower than that after **gastric bypass** (0.3% to 0.5%) or **biliopancreatic diversion/duodenal switch** (1.1%). However, mean excess weight loss for the procedures is 48%, 62%, and 70%, respectively. Advantages of the adjustable gastric band include low risk for death, reversibility, and no malabsorption. Disadvantages include pouch enlargement, slippage, erosion, port malfunction, esophageal dilation, and lower average excess weight loss. Advantages of gastric bypass include proved weight loss for more than 5 years and greater weight loss than that achieved with restrictive-only procedures. Disadvantages include malabsorption, risk for marginal ulcer formation, stomal stenosis, inability to access the distal end of the stomach, internal hernia, and vitamin deficiencies. Advantages of BPD/DS include excellent weight loss, ability to increase food intake, preserved pylorus with less dumping, and less risk for marginal ulcers. Disadvantages include increased risk for protein malabsorption, vitamin deficiencies, diarrhea and flatulence, internal hernia, and a high complication rate. Based on these data, the procedure of choice for the surgical management of weight loss must be tailored to each patient based on the history and physical examination, weight loss goals, and surgical risk tolerance.

**ANSWER:** E

**REFERENCES**

1. Richards WO, Schirmer BD: Morbid obesity. In Townsend CM, Beauchamp RD, Evers BM, et al, editors: *Sabiston textbook of surgery: the biological basis of modern surgical practice*, ed 18, Philadelphia, 2008, WB Saunders.
2. Mercer DW, Robinson EK: Stomach. In Townsend CM, Beauchamp RD, Evers BM, et al, editors: *Sabiston textbook of surgery: the biological basis of modern surgical practice*, ed 18, Philadelphia, 2008, WB Saunders.
3. McCarty TM, Lamont J: Morbid obesity. In Cameron JL, editor: *Current surgical therapy*, ed 9, Philadelphia, 2008, CV Mosby.
4. International Agency for Research on Cancer Working Group on Evaluation of Cancer-Preventive Strategies. *Weight control and physical activity*, Lyon, France, 2002, IARC Press.
5. Schweitzer M, Magnuson T: Laparoscopic surgery for morbid obesity. In: Cameron JL, editor: *Current surgical therapy*, ed 9, Philadelphia, 2008, CV Mosby.

# CHAPTER 31

# Gynecology, Neurosurgery, and Urology

## A. Gynecology

*Alfred S. Guirguis, D.O., M.P.H.*

1. A 53-year-old G3P3 (three pregnancies [gravida] with three births [para]) postmenopausal woman was found to have a right adnexal mass during a routine examination. The patient denies any pain, nausea, vomiting, or postmenopausal bleeding. Her past medical history is significant for borderline diabetes and hypertension. Her family history is significant for a first-degree relative with ovarian cancer diagnosed at the age of 39 years. Her initial work-up should include all of the following except:

   A. Transvaginal ultrasound

   B. Blood tumor markers, including CA 125

   C. Magnetic resonance imaging (MRI) of the pelvis and abdomen

   D. Genetic counseling and possible testing of the patient for *BRCA1* and *BRCA2* mutations

   E. National Comprehensive Cancer Network (NCCN) guidelines

   *Ref.:* 1-10

**COMMENTS:** Common **ovarian masses** include functional cysts, hemorrhagic cysts, paraovarian or paratubal wolffian remnants, endometrioma, and benign or malignant tumors (epithelial, germ cell, stromal). The single most effective and efficient modality for assessing pelvic anatomy and pathology is real-time ultrasonography, especially with a transvaginal transducer. In addition, the tumor marker CA 125 is a glycoprotein that is produced by certain tumors, however, it is not specific for ovarian cancer. In postmenopausal women with a pelvic mass and elevated CA 125 (normal, <35 U/mL), ovarian cancer is diagnosed in 80% of these patients. MRI rarely provides additional information in patients with benign pelvic pathology. First-degree relative (i.e., mothers, sisters, and daughters) of patients with breast and ovarian cancers have a two- to threefold excess risk for the disease. Women should be considered for genetic testing only if their chance of having a deleterious *BRCA* mutation is at least 10%. The U.S. Preventive Services Task Force currently recommends that genetic testing be considered for women who have a family history that suggests

inherited *BRCA1* and *BRCA2* mutations. Criteria for identifying individuals with at least a 10% risk of having a genetic mutation for referral to a genetic counselor and possible testing were also developed by the Kaiser Permanente Health Plan, NCCN, Family History Risk Assessment Tool, and the American College of Medical Genetics.

**ANSWER:** C

2. For the patient in Question 1, what ultrasound finding is not associated with higher risk for malignancy?

   A. Simple cyst and increased resistive index of ovarian vessels on Doppler ultrasound

   B. Cystic and solid components

   C. Low resistive indices of ovarian vessels

   D. Thickened septations

   E. Hyperechoic solid component

   *Ref.:* 1-10

**COMMENTS: High-risk ultrasonographic features** include (1) a solid component that is not hyperechoic and is often nodular or papillary; (2) septations or papillae, if present, that are thick (>2 mm); (3) color or power Doppler demonstration of flow in the solid component; (4) decreased resistive index of ovarian vessels, probably occurring as a result of neovascularization; (5) bilaterality; and (6) presence of ascites.

**ANSWER:** A

3. The patient in Question 1 was found to have a 3-cm simple cyst on transvaginal ultrasound and a CA 125 level of 15 U/mL. What is the most appropriate next step in her management?

   A. Exploratory laparotomy and a right salpingo-oophorectomy

   B. Computed tomography (CT) of the abdomen and pelvis

C. Oral contraceptive prescription

D. Repeated CA 125 determination and pelvic ultrasound in 2 to 3 months

E. MRI of the pelvis

*Ref.:* 1, 8

**COMMENTS:** Follow-up with serial **ultrasound examinations** and CA 125 measurements is appropriate for women who meet all the following criteria: simple unilateral ovarian cyst on ultrasound and Doppler imaging, asymptomatic pelvic examination not suggestive of malignancy, and normal cervical cytology and CA 125 concentration.

**ANSWER: D**

4. If the patient in Question 1 was considered to be at high risk for ovarian and breast cancers, what type of close surveillance should be recommended?

A. Annual mammograms and pelvic ultrasound starting at 20 years of age

B. Monthly breast self-examination (BSE) beginning at 25 years of age and annual mammography beginning at age 35

C. Annual MRI for *BRCA* mutation carriers and other high-risk women

D. Monthly BSE beginning at 18 years of age, annual mammography and MRI beginning at age 25, and ovarian cancer screening with ultrasound and serum CA 125 levels beginning age 35

E. None of the above

*Ref.:* 5, 6

**COMMENTS:** Unfortunately, the efficacy of early and increased surveillance for **breast and ovarian cancer** mortality is not known for women with genetic mutations. Although most guidelines recommend conventional annual mammography, there is no consensus regarding the optimal frequency of breast imaging screening for asymptomatic *BRCA* carriers. More frequent mammography (e.g., every 6 months) is sometimes considered because of the frequent development of interval malignancies. Nevertheless, the following screening strategies are typically recommended for women with *BRCA1* or *BRCA2* mutations who have not undergone risk-reducing surgery: monthly BSE beginning at age 18; clinical breast examination two to four times annually; annual mammography; and twice-yearly ovarian cancer screening with ultrasound and serum CA 125 levels beginning at age 35. In addition to a malignancy, benign findings such as leiomyomas, endometriosis, menstruation, pregnancy, pelvic inflammatory disease (PID), and liver cirrhosis may elevate CA 125 levels.

**ANSWER: D**

5. A 65-year-old woman was undergoing a routine abdominal hysterectomy and bilateral salpingo-oophorectomy for uterine prolapse. Intraoperatively, the gynecologist noted ascites, a 3-cm adnexal mass, and lesions on her omentum. Initially, a gynecologic oncologist was not available to assist on this surgery. Her past medical history was significant for an unintentional 20-lb weight loss, night sweats, abdominal bloating,

early satiety, and pelvic pain over the last 2 months. Of note, the patient emigrated from Asia approximately 2 years earlier. What is the differential diagnosis for this patient?

A. Ovarian cancer

B. Meigs syndrome

C. Uterine cancer

D. Tuberculosis

E. All except B

*Ref.:* 8, 11-15

**COMMENTS:** Seventy-five percent of women with **epithelial ovarian cancer** are initially found to have tumor that has spread throughout the peritoneal cavity or involves the para-aortic or inguinal lymph nodes (stage III) or tumor that has spread to more distant sites (stage IV). The association of ovarian fibroma with ascites or pleural effusion (or both) is termed *Meigs syndrome*. Papillary serous adenocarcinoma of the endometrium behaves more like an ovarian carcinoma than an endometrial cancer. Most cases of tuberculous peritonitis result from reactivation of latent peritoneal disease. The illness often develops insidiously, with patients having had symptoms for several weeks to months at the time of initial evaluation. Abdominal swelling secondary to ascites formation is the most common symptom, with most patients complaining of a nonlocalized, vague abdominal pain. Constitutional symptoms such as low-grade fever and night sweats, weight loss, anorexia, and malaise are reported in about 60% of patients. CT can demonstrate the thickened and nodular mesentery with mesenteric lymphadenopathy and omental thickening.

**ANSWER: E**

6. Upon exploration of the patient in Question 5, a biopsy of an accessible lesion is submitted for frozen section and reads as adenocarcinoma, most likely of gynecologic origin. What is not the most appropriate surgical strategy?

A. Operable resection of all visible disease, including possible splenectomy and bowel resections if necessary, with no disease greater than 1 cm in diameter remaining

B. Total abdominal hysterectomy, bilateral salpingo-oophorectomy, pelvic and paraaortic lymph node dissection, omentectomy, and optimal cytoreduction

C. Recommendation for ending the surgery given her advanced disease status and arranging follow-up with a medical oncologist for possible chemotherapy

D. Consultation with a gynecologic oncologist

E. None of the above

*Ref.:* 1, 3, 13-15

**COMMENTS:** Treatment of invasive epithelial **ovarian cancer** includes hysterectomy; bilateral salpingo-oophorectomy; omentectomy; peritoneal biopsy of the diaphragm, bilateral paracolic gutters, bilateral pelvis, and cul-de-sac; and lymph node sampling. If the cell type is mucinous, an appendectomy is also performed to rule out a metastasis from the appendix. Optimal debulking/cytoreduction is defined as residual disease no greater than 1 cm in diameter. Studies have consistently shown that surgical treatment by non-gynecologic oncologists and low-volume providers contributes to suboptimal surgical management and shorter median survival.

**ANSWER: C**

**7.** For the patient in Question 5, what would have been the appropriate work-up preoperatively if a pelvic mass and ascites were noted on pelvic examination and ultrasound?

A. CT of the chest, abdomen, and pelvis

B. Tumor markers such as CA 125, carcinoembryonic antigen (CEA), CA 19-9, and HE4

C. Colonoscopy

D. PPD and chest radiograph

E. All of the above

*Ref.:* 8, 11-13

**COMMENTS:** The single most effective and efficient modality for assessing pelvic anatomy and pathology is real-time ultrasound, especially with a transvaginal transducer. In addition, the tumor marker CA 125 is a glycoprotein that is produced by certain tumors. It is unfortunately not specific for ovarian cancer. In postmenopausal women with a pelvic mass and elevated **CA 125** (normal, <35 U/mL), ovarian cancer is diagnosed in 80% of these patients. CEA is probably the most studied cancer tumor marker and is predominantly used clinically in patients with cancers of the colon and rectum. Carbohydrate antigen 19-9 (CA 19-9) is widely used as a serum marker for pancreatic cancer, but it can also be elevated in women with colon and ovarian cancers. Recommendations for screening include annual fecal occult blood testing and flexible sigmoidoscopy every 5 years (with full colonoscopy for patients with positive occult blood or adenomatous polyps on flexible sigmoidoscopy) or colonoscopy every 5 to 10 years. Peritoneal tuberculosis often develops insidiously, with patients having had symptoms for several weeks to months at initial evaluation. Abdominal swelling secondary to ascites formation is the most common symptom and occurs in more than 80% of instances. Similarly, most patients complain of a nonlocalized, vague abdominal pain. Constitutional symptoms such as low-grade fever and night sweats, weight loss, anorexia, and malaise are reported in about 60% of patients. CT will demonstrate the thickened and nodular mesentery with mesenteric lymphadenopathy and omental thickening.

**ANSWER:** E

**8.** What is the most common histologic subtype of ovarian cancer?

A. Epithelial tumors

B. Papillary serous carcinoma

C. Germ cell carcinoma

D. Endometrioid adenocarcinoma

E. Transitional cell carcinoma

*Ref.:* 8, 16, 17

**COMMENTS:** Of all **ovarian epithelial tumors**, papillary serous carcinoma accounts for 30.7% to 52.7%, mucinous for 23.7% to 31.1%, endometrioid for 6.1%, clear cell for 2.6%, and transitional cell for 3.2%.

**ANSWER:** B

**9.** What is one of the most common causes of death in patients with ovarian cancer?

A. Uremia

B. Anemia

C. Liver failure

D. Bowel obstruction

E. Respiratory failure

*Ref.:* 8, 17-19

**COMMENTS:** One of the most common problems faced by women with recurrent **advanced ovarian cancer** is **bowel obstruction**. Rectosigmoid resection was the most common bowel operation overall, particularly in the primary surgery group (65%). Colostomy was performed at primary surgery in 30% of patients who underwent rectosigmoid resection. Small bowel resection was most common in the women treated surgically for recurrence or palliation.

**ANSWER:** D

**10.** A 49-year-old G0P0 perimenopausal woman was undergoing total abdominal hysterectomy and bilateral salpingo-oophorectomy for abnormal uterine bleeding lasting more than 1 year. Intraoperatively, on frozen section the uterus was found to have a deeply invasive adenocarcinoma. Of note, her past medical history is significant for diabetes and hypertension. What is the most appropriate surgical staging for endometrial cancer?

A. Total abdominal hysterectomy and bilateral salpingo-oophorectomy

B. Pelvic washings, total abdominal hysterectomy, bilateral salpingo-oophorectomy, and pelvic and para-aortic lymph node sampling or dissection

C. Pelvic washings, total abdominal hysterectomy, bilateral salpingo-oophorectomy, omentectomy, and pelvic lymph node dissection

D. Total abdominal hysterectomy, bilateral salpingo-oophorectomy, omentectomy, and pelvic and para-aortic lymph node dissection

E. Pelvic washings, total abdominal hysterectomy, bilateral salpingo-oophorectomy, omentectomy

*Ref.:* 8

**COMMENTS:** According to the International Federation of Gynecologists and Oncologists (FIGO) **Surgical Staging**, optimal staging for endometrial cancer requires the steps outlined in answer B. All other options are incomplete.

**ANSWER:** B

**11.** What is the most common histologic subtype of endometrial cancer?

A. Squamous cell carcinoma

B. Papillary serous carcinoma

C. Germ cell carcinoma

D. Endometrioid adenocarcinoma

E. Clear cell carcinoma

*Ref.:* 8, 17, 20

**COMMENTS:** The most common type of **endometrial cancer** is epithelial endometrioid adenocarcinoma. However, there are other types of epithelial carcinoma, including papillary serous, squamous, clear cell, mucinous, and neuroendocrine. Papillary serous, clear cell, and neuroendocrine tumors behave aggressively with a high risk for recurrence of disease.

**ANSWER:** D

12. Which of the following is not a risk factor for endometrial cancer?

A. Obesity

B. Smoking

C. Unopposed estrogen use

D. Nulliparity

E. Diabetes

*Ref.:* 17, 20

**COMMENTS:** Patients who have complex hyperplasia with atypia have a 20% to 30% chance for the development or presence of a coexisting adenocarcinoma. Risk factors for hyperplasia include obesity, hypertension, diabetes, anovulation, and unopposed estrogen use.

**ANSWER:** B

13. What is the single most important prognostic indicator for endometrial cancer?

A. Stage

B. Depth of invasion

C. Uterine size

D. Lymphovascular invasion

E. Histologic subtype

*Ref.:* 16, 17, 20

**COMMENTS:** Stage and histology are the most important **prognostic factors for endometrial cancer**, especially the presence of extrauterine disease, particularly pelvic and para-aortic lymphadenopathy.

**ANSWER:** A

14. For the patient in Question 10 with endometrial cancer, what preoperative work-up should have been done initially?

A. CT of the chest, abdomen, and pelvis

B. Endometrial biopsy or dilation and curettage

C. Pelvic transvaginal ultrasound

D. All of the above

E. Only B and C

*Ref.:* 8, 15, 16, 19

**COMMENTS:** Ultrasound measurement of the thickness of the endometrial stripe can assist in avoiding unnecessary biopsies. A postmenopausal woman with an endometrial stripe of less than 5 mm and no an irregularity in the cavity is very unlikely to have

a carcinoma. Endometrial biopsy or dilation plus curettage is the procedure for the evaluation and possible therapeutic treatment of menorrhagia, menometrorrhagia, and abnormal uterine bleeding.

**ANSWER:** E

15. A 63-year-old woman was undergoing a hysterectomy and debulking for a uterine sarcoma that appeared to be extending into the pelvic side walls. You were called in to assist with the intraoperative hemorrhage that occurred after the hysterectomy was performed. The estimated blood loss at this time was approximately 2 L, she was normothermic, and her total operative time was 3 hours. Her hemoglobin level dropped from 10 to 7 g/dL. However, her platelet count is still $175,000/mm^3$. Intraoperatively, brisk bleeding appeared to be coming from near the uterine vessels that were coated with tumor. As the surgeon, what options would appear to decrease the bleeding?

A. Administration of platelets

B. Bilateral ligation of the anterior division of the hypogastric artery

C. Ligation of the internal iliac vein

D. Use of fibrin sealant

E. Bilateral ligation of the anterior and posterior branches of the hypogastric artery

*Ref.:* 8, 16, 17

**COMMENTS:** Bilateral hypogastric artery ligation can reduce pulse pressure by 85% and blood flow by 50%. It is important to ligate only the anterior division of the hypogastric artery and not the posterior division. In addition, fibrin sealant can be used to stop bleeding from small and inaccessible blood vessels. These sealants mimic the last step of the coagulation cascade.

**ANSWER:** B

16. For the patient in Question 15, after the aforementioned was done and on further investigation, she has already received 8 units of packed red blood cells and a large volume of crystalloid and continues to have small but diffuse venous bleeding. What is the best next step in the management of this hemorrhage?

A. Continuation of the operation and finishing the surgery

B. Replacement of coagulation factors

C. Pelvic packing and reoperation in 24 to 48 hours

D. Only B and C

E. None of the above

*Ref.:* 8, 16, 17

**COMMENTS:** By now the patient most probably has a dilutional coagulopathy, and therefore replacement of clotting factors and pelvic pressure should be the next step. Application of pelvic pressure with tight packing plus reoperation when the patient is fully resuscitated in 24 to 48 hours has also been shown to help in multiple case series.

**ANSWER:** D

17. A 40-year-old G4P3 woman comes to the emergency department complaining of vaginal bleeding, pelvic pain, flank pain,

foul-smelling discharge, and disorientation. Her past medical history is significant for three normal vaginal deliveries and one miscarriage. In addition, she did have a history of abnormal Papanicolaou smears approximately 3 years earlier. What initial laboratory work-up must be done?

A. Complete metabolic panel

B. Complete blood count

C. β-Human chorionic gonadotropin (β-hCG)

D. Urine analysis

E. All of the above

*Ref.:* 16, 17, 20

**COMMENTS:** A good history and physical examination, including a pelvic examination, is an absolute in any patient with **abnormal vaginal bleeding** and can usually determine the origin of this bleeding. This patient's differential diagnosis includes PID, miscarriage, dysfunctional uterine bleeding, cervical lesions including cervical cancer, and urinary tract infections leading to pyelonephritis. A complete metabolic panel and a complete blood count are important in this patient because she is disoriented, which could be caused by electrolyte abnormalities or severe anemia. In addition, all patients younger than 50 years should have urine hCG determined to rule out a miscarriage. Finally, urine analysis and culture will determine whether this patient has a urinary tract infection and possibly pyelonephritis, as well as hematuria.

**ANSWER:** E

18. Assuming that the patient in Question 17 is not pregnant and was found to have cervical cancer extending to the side wall on pelvic examination, what is the most likely minimal stage of her cervical cancer?

A. Stage IB2

B. Stage IIB

C. Stage IIIA

D. Stage IIIB

E. Stage IV

*Ref.:* 5, 8, 16

**COMMENTS: Cervical cancer stage IIIB** includes T3b or T1-3, any N or N1, and M0, extension onto the pelvic side wall and/or causes hydronephrosis and/or a nonfunctional kidney (Figure 31-1).

**ANSWER:** D

19. Which of the following risk factors have the strongest association with cervical cancer?

A. Multiple sexual partners

B. Early onset of intercourse

C. Human papillomavirus (HPV)

D. Human immunodeficiency virus (HIV)

E. Smoking

*Ref.:* 8, 21

**COMMENTS:** Squamous cell **carcinoma of the cervix** is a disease of sexually active women. Infection with specific high-risk strains of HPV is central to the pathogenesis of cervical cancer. Risk factors that predispose to infection with HPV include early onset of intercourse, multiple sexual partners over time, and sexual partners who themselves have had multiple sexual partners. Cigarette smoking increases the risk for cervical cancer up to fourfold. Immunosuppression also significantly increases risk for the development of cervical cancer. Squamous cell carcinoma accounts for approximately 80% of cervical cancers, adenocarcinoma for 15%, and adenosquamous carcinoma for 3% to 5%.

**ANSWER:** C

20. Which is the most appropriate next step after an abnormal Papanicolaou smear?

A. Simple hysterectomy

B. Cold knife cone

C. Loop electrosurgical excision procedure

D. Colposcopy and possibly biopsy

E. Radical hysterectomy

*Ref.:* 8, 17, 20

**COMMENTS:** Pap smears are a screening test for dysplasia and malignancy. Abnormal Pap smears require further evaluation with colposcopy to exclude glandular lesions and atypical cells from low- and high-grade squamous intraepithelial lesions. Biopsy at the time of colposcopy can confirm the histologic diagnosis of mild, moderate, or severe dysplasia.

**ANSWER:** D

21. A patient in whom cervical cancer was diagnosed underwent CT that showed disease confined to her pelvis. Which of the following treatment modalities would be most appropriate?

A. Simple hysterectomy

B. Radical hysterectomy

C. Pelvic exenteration

D. Pelvic irradiation as well as brachytherapy

E. Chemoradiation therapy directed to the pelvis with brachytherapy

*Ref.:* 8, 16, 17, 19, 20

**COMMENTS:** For stages IIB to IVA tumors, treatment is a combination of extended field radiation therapy with cisplatin-based chemotherapy. Radical hysterectomy involves removal of the uterus, resection of parametrial tissue lateral to the ureter, ligation of the uterine arteries at their origin on the hypogastric arteries, transection of the uterosacral ligaments near the rectum, and removal of the upper third of the vagina. Pelvic lymphadenectomy is commonly done at the time of radical hysterectomy. The ovaries are preserved if they appear normal. This is usually done in conjunction with pelvic lymph node dissection for early cervical cancer stages IA2 to IB2. Extrafascial hysterectomy can be performed for stage IA1 cervical cancer; it involves removal of the uterus, preservation of the parametrium, ligation of the uterine vessels at the level of the cervical os, transection of the uterosacral

American Joint Committee on Cancer

# Cervix Uteri Cancer Staging

7th EDITION

## Definitions

### Primary Tumor (T)

| TNM CATEGORIES | FIGO STAGES | |
|---|---|---|
| TX | | Primary tumor cannot be assessed |
| T0 | | No evidence of primary tumor |
| Tis* | | Carcinoma in situ (preinvasive carcinoma) |
| T1 | I | Cervical carcinoma confined to uterus (extension to corpus should be disregarded) |
| T1a** | IA | Invasive carcinoma diagnosed only by microscopy. Stromal invasion with a maximum depth of 5.0 mm measured from the base of the epithelium and a horizontal spread of 7.0 mm or less. Vascular space involvement, venous or lymphatic, does not affect classification |
| T1a1 | IA1 | Measured stromal invasion 3.0 mm or less in depth and 7.0 mm or less in horizontal spread |
| T1a2 | IA2 | Measured stromal invasion more than 3.0 mm and not more than 5.0 mm with a horizontal spread 7.0 mm or less |
| T1b | IB | Clinically visible lesion confined to the cervix or microscopic lesion greater than T1a/IA2 |
| T1b1 | IB1 | Clinically visible lesion 4.0 cm or less in greatest dimension |
| T1b2 | IB2 | Clinically visible lesion more than 4.0 cm in greatest dimension |
| T2 | II | Cervical carcinoma invades beyond uterus but not to pelvic wall or to lower third of vagina |
| T2a | IIA | Tumor without parametrial invasion |
| T2a1 | IIA1 | Clinically visible lesion 4.0 cm or less in greatest dimension |
| T2a2 | IIA2 | Clinically visible lesion more than 4.0 cm in greatest dimension |
| T2b | IIB | Tumor with parametrial invasion |
| T3 | III | Tumor extends to pelvic wall and/or involves lower third of vagina, and/or causes hydronephrosis or nonfunctioning kidney |
| T3a | IIIA | Tumor involves lower third of vagina, no extension to pelvic wall |
| T3b | IIIB | Tumor extends to pelvic wall and/or causes hydronephrosis or nonfunctioning kidney |
| T4 | IVA | Tumor invades mucosa of bladder or rectum, and/or extends beyond true pelvis (bullous edema is not sufficient to classify a tumor as T4) |

### Regional Lymph Nodes (N)

| TNM CATEGORIES | FIGO STAGES | |
|---|---|---|
| NX | | Regional lymph nodes cannot be assessed |
| N0 | | No regional lymph node metastasis |
| N1 | IIIB | Regional lymph node metastasis |

### Distant Metastasis (M)

| TNM CATEGORIES | FIGO STAGES | |
|---|---|---|
| M0 | | No distant metastasis |
| M1 | IVB | Distant metastasis (including peritoneal spread, involvement of supraclavicular, mediastinal, or paraaortic lymph nodes, lung, liver, or bone) |

### ANATOMIC STAGE/PROGNOSTIC GROUPS (FIGO 2008)

| Stage | T | N | M |
|---|---|---|---|
| Stage 0* | Tis | N0 | M0 |
| Stage I | T1 | N0 | M0 |
| Stage IA | T1a | N0 | M0 |
| Stage IA1 | T1a1 | N0 | M0 |
| Stage IA2 | T1a2 | N0 | M0 |
| Stage IB | T1b | N0 | M0 |
| Stage IB1 | T1b1 | N0 | M0 |
| Stage IB2 | T1b2 | N0 | M0 |
| Stage II | T2 | N0 | M0 |
| Stage IIA | T2a | N0 | M0 |
| Stage IIA1 | T2a1 | N0 | M0 |
| Stage IIA2 | T2a2 | N0 | M0 |
| Stage IIB | T2b | N0 | M0 |
| Stage III | T3 | N0 | M0 |
| Stage IIIA | T3a | N0 | M0 |
| Stage IIIB | T3b | Any N | M0 |
| | T1–3 | N1 | M0 |
| Stage IVA | T4 | Any N | M0 |
| Stage IVB | Any T | Any N | M1 |

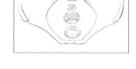

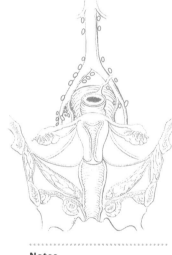

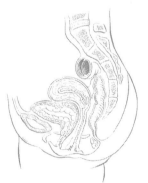

### Notes

\* FIGO no longer includes Stage 0 (Tis).

\*\* All macroscopically visible lesions—even with superficial invasion—are T1b/IB.

**American Cancer Society®**

Financial support for AJCC 7th Edition Staging Posters provided by the American Cancer Society

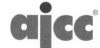

**Figure 31-1. AJCC Cervix Uteri Cancer Staging Poster.** (Used with the permission of the American Joint Committee on Cancer (AJCC), Chicago, Illinois. The original source for this material is the *AJCC Cancer Staging Manual, Seventh Edition (2010)* published by Springer Science and Business Media LLC, www.springer.com.)

ligaments at the uterus, and preservation of the vaginal cuff. Because of the more extensive and lateral dissection done during radical hysterectomy, there is a higher incidence of ureteral and bladder complications than with extrafascial hysterectomy.

ANSWER: E

22. The patient from Question 21 had initially been treated non-surgically and is now seen 2 years later with a pelvic recurrence of her cervical cancer. All of the following are acceptable criteria for surgical intervention except:

A. Central recurrence

B. Disease extending to the side wall

C. Disease invading the bladder and causing a vesicovaginal fistula

D. Disease invading the rectum and causing a rectovaginal fistula

E. Both B and C

Ref.: 8, 16, 17, 20

COMMENTS: Once there is evidence of local recurrence on pelvic examination, distant disease must be ruled out by imaging studies. After this has been completed, side wall involvement must be ruled out by examining the patient under anesthesia. Patients with central recurrence of cervical cancer who have previously undergone radiation therapy can be cured with pelvic exenteration.

ANSWER: B

23. One year after the patient underwent pelvic radiation therapy, she began having symptoms of bowel obstruction. Which segment of bowel is most commonly affected?

A. Terminal ileum

B. Cecum

C. Sigmoid colon

D. Rectum

E. None of the above

Ref.: 8, 17

COMMENTS: Patients treated by external radiation therapy, brachytherapy, and possibly extended field irradiation are at risk for bowel complications, particularly when the terminal ileum and other segments of bowel are fixed in place either physiologically or from previous surgery.

ANSWER: A

24. Two years after completing pelvic radiation therapy she started having rectal bleeding. All of the following are acceptable treatment options for hemorrhagic proctitis except:

A. Transfusions if necessary

B. Colonoscopy, biopsy to rule out recurrence, and focal cautery

C. Colonoscopy and focal cautery

D. Cortisone enemas

E. Colostomy with resection of the affected bowel

Ref.: 8, 16, 17

COMMENTS: Hemorrhagic proctitis can be managed with cortisone enemas and transfusion. Colonoscopy with focal cautery can also be performed. However, biopsies are avoided because of the risk for fistula formation. In some cases, colostomy with resection of the affected bowel may be indicated.

ANSWER: B

25. Regarding endometriosis, which of the following is not true?

A. Total abdominal hysterectomy with bilateral salpingo-oophorectomy is considered definitive surgical therapy.

B. Adenomyosis is a clinical variant of the disease.

C. Laparoscopy is considered the "gold standard" for diagnosis.

D. Minimal and mild stages of the disease can be associated with infertility.

E. Symptoms include pelvic pain and dysmenorrhea.

Ref.: 20, 22

COMMENTS: Endometriosis is defined as endometrial tissue outside the uterus. Symptoms can include pelvic pain, dysmenorrhea, and infertility. Minimal and mild stages of the disease have been associated with infertility. The diagnosis can be made empirically if the patient's symptoms are ameliorated after a short (3-month) trial of a gonadotropin-releasing hormone agonist and after all other causes have been ruled out. Laparoscopy, however, is considered the gold standard for diagnosis. Definitive surgery for endometriosis consists of total abdominal hysterectomy with bilateral salpingo-oophorectomy. Bilateral salpingo-oophorectomy is the key component because it results in surgical menopause. Adenomyosis, which refers to endometrial tissue within the myometrium, is not considered a variant of the disease. Symptoms of adenomyosis include abnormal uterine bleeding and dysmenorrhea. Medical therapy for adenomyosis is usually ineffective, and surgery (hysterectomy) is generally required for persistent symptoms.

ANSWER: B

26. Which ovarian tumor is correctly matched with the most appropriate characteristic?

A. Masculinizing—Endodermal sinus tumor (yolk sac)

B. α-Fetoprotein (AFP)—Sertoli-Leydig cell tumor

C. hCG—Choriocarcinoma

D. Elaborates estrogen—Granulosa-theca cell tumor

E. None of the above

Ref.: 16, 23, 24

COMMENTS: Ovarian tumors are frequently characterized by their ability to produce hormones or biologic markers. Sertoli-Leydig cell tumors produce androgens and frequently cause masculinization. Granulosa-theca cell tumors frequently produce estrogen and have been associated with precocious puberty in young patients and endometrial cancer in older patients. Endodermal sinus tumor (yolk sac tumor), which is the second most common germ cell ovarian tumor, secretes AFP. Choriocarcinoma produces hCG, which can be used as a marker to gauge response to treatment.

**ANSWER:** C

27. All of the following statements are true except:

    A. Clear cell carcinoma—Seen in adolescents or young adult females

    B. Sarcoma botryoides—Seen in infants

    C. Squamous cell carcinoma—Most common primary vaginal cancer

    D. Vaginal cancer—Most are secondary to direct spread from other organs

    E. Primary upper-third vaginal cancer—Should be treated as vulvar cancer

    *Ref.:* 16, 17, 23

**COMMENTS:** Squamous cell carcinoma is the most common primary vaginal malignancy. Most vaginal cancers are direct extensions from cancers arising in adjacent organs. Sarcoma botryoides is a bulky polypoid sarcoma commonly found in infants or young children. Clear cell carcinoma can develop in adolescent or adult children of mothers who took diethylstilbestrol during pregnancy.

**ANSWER:** E

28. Regarding vaginal cancer, which of the following is not true?

    A. It is rare.

    B. Tumor extending to the pelvic side wall is considered stage II disease.

    C. Primary vaginal cancer involving the upper third of the vagina should be treated as though it were cervical cancer.

    D. It is predominantly a disease of older women.

    E. All of the above are true.

    *Ref.:* 8, 16, 17

**COMMENTS:** Primary vaginal cancer is predominantly a disease of older women but is rare overall. Primary vaginal cancers involving the upper third of the vagina generally behave as cervical cancer and are treated as such. Similarly, tumors involving the lower third of the vagina are treated as vulvar cancer. Management of tumors involving the middle third of the vagina is challenging. Vaginal carcinoma is staged clinically. The tumor may be limited to the vaginal wall (stage I), extend to subvaginal tissue (stage II), extend to the pelvic side wall (stage III), spread to adjacent organs or to areas outside the true pelvis (stage IVA), or spread to distant organs (stage IVB).

**ANSWER:** B

29. Which of the following vulvar abnormalities is not considered a risk factor for invasive malignancy?

    A. Vulvar intraepithelial neoplasia (VIN) type III

    B. Paget disease

    C. Lichen sclerosis

    D. Hypertrophic dystrophy without atypia

    E. All of the above are risk factors

    *Ref.:* 17, 20

**COMMENTS:** Suspicious vulvar lesions should undergo biopsy to rule out malignancy. There are numerous risk factors for vulvar cancer, including a history of vulvar dysplasia, smoking, hypertension, diabetes, and chronic steroid use. Vulvar lichen sclerosis has an approximately 5% risk of progressing to invasive squamous cell carcinoma. Hypertrophic dystrophy without atypia of the vulva is a nonneoplastic epithelial disorder that is not considered a risk factor for malignancy. Paget disease is an intraepithelial lesion of the vulva associated with vulvar adenocarcinoma. Untreated VIN can progress to vulvar cancer in 5% of cases. VIN is commonly multifocal, and multiple biopsies are needed to determine the extent of the disease. Acetic acid can be used to help identify dysplastic vulvar lesions. Treatment of VIN consists of observation, wide local excision, skinning vulvectomy, laser ablation, or topical 5-fluorouracil (5-FU). Most lesions that undergo spontaneous regression do so within 6 months. Wide local excision requires removal of a full thickness of skin with a 2- to 3-cm cancer-free margin. Laser treatment to a depth of 1 mm in non–hair-bearing areas and 3 mm in hair-bearing areas is required for effective treatment. Topical 5-FU can be very effective but requires good compliance on the part of the patient and is associated with significant skin reactions.

**ANSWER:** D

30. Regarding vulvar carcinoma, which of the following is false?

    A. Squamos cell cancer is the most common type.

    B. There is an association with HPV infection in young patients.

    C. Pruritus is one of the most common symptoms.

    D. The disease is staged clinically.

    E. Ulceration lesion is one of the common initial complaints.

    *Ref.:* 17, 20

**COMMENTS:** Squamous cell cancer is the most common vulvar malignancy. Pruritus and the presence of an abnormal or ulcerating lesion are common initial complaints. High-risk subtypes of HPV have been associated with vulvar cancer in younger patients. Patients often have a history of cervical or vulvar dysplasia. Vulvar cancer, unlike cervical cancer, is staged surgically. Staging assists in guiding treatment and determining prognosis.

**ANSWER:** D

31. Which is the correct match for clinical pelvic organ prolapse with the appropriate description?

    A. Rectocele—Uterosacral ligament defect

    B. Cystocele—Defect in the pubocervical fascia

C. Enterocele—Defect in the rectovaginal septum

D. Uterovaginal prolapse—Herniation of the pouch of Douglas between the uterosacral ligaments

E. All of the above are matched correctly

*Ref.:* 20, 22

**COMMENTS:** Damage to endopelvic fascial support structures can lead to prolapse of pelvic organs. The pubocervical fascia provides major support to the urethra and bladder. Damage to this support structure can lead to a cystocele, which causes protrusion of the bladder through the anterior vaginal wall. The rectovaginal septum lies between the posterior vagina wall and the anterior part of the rectum. Damage to this septum results in a rectocele, which is a herniation of the rectum anteriorly. In addition to distressing symptoms from the bulge itself, rectoceles can cause a sensation of obstructed defecation from trapping of stool. The uterosacral ligaments, along with the cardinal ligaments, provide major support to the cervix and upper part of the vagina. Weakened or damaged uterosacral ligaments can lead to uterovaginal prolapse. The uterosacral ligaments also prevent the development of an enterocele, or herniation of small bowel into the pouch of Douglas.

**ANSWER:** B

32. Potential sites for ureteral injury during abdominal hysterectomy with bilateral salpingo-oophorectomy include all of the following except:

A. Transection of the round ligaments

B. Transection of the uterine arteries

C. Transection of the cardinal ligaments

D. Transection of the infundibulopelvic ligaments

E. All are potential sites of injury

*Ref.:* 19, 20

**COMMENTS:** Anatomic knowledge of the course of the ureters in the pelvis is essential for preventing ureteral injury. The ureters travel in the retroperitoneal space in the abdominal and pelvic segments. In the abdomen, they run downward and medially along the anterior surface of the psoas muscle. The iliopectineal line serves as the marker for the pelvic segment of the ureter. The ureters cross the iliac vessels as they enter the pelvis and travel in the medial leaf of the parietal peritoneum. They course near the ovarian and uterine vessels. Thus, they are susceptible to injury during transection of the infundibulopelvic ligaments and uterine arteries. The ureters travel through the cardinal ligaments about 1 to 2 cm lateral to the cervix.

Removal of the cervix during hysterectomy places the ureter at risk for injury. In general, the ureters do not travel near the round ligaments. In a pelvis with normal anatomy, this is not regarded as a common site for ureteral injury.

**ANSWER:** A

33. Regarding menopause, which of the following is false?

A. The average age at onset in the United States is 51.4 years.

B. It occurs as result of gradual depletion of functional ovarian follicles.

C. Unopposed estrogen is acceptable therapy for women with a uterus and vasomotor symptoms.

D. Vaginal atrophy, vasomotor symptoms, and osteoporosis are sequelae.

E. All of the above are true.

*Ref.:* 20

**COMMENTS:** The average age at menopause in the United States is 51.4 years. A gradual decrease in the number of ovarian follicles usually precedes its onset. The result is diminished estrogen production. This hypoestrogenic state may lead to vasomotor symptoms, vaginal atrophy, and osteoporosis. Menopausal hormone therapy is usually highly effective in ameliorating all of these symptoms. For patients who have contraindications to menopausal hormone therapy, alternative therapies exist for each of these symptoms. If menopausal hormone therapy is prescribed, it should never be given as an unopposed oral estrogen formulation in women with a uterus. Unopposed estrogen has been associated with an increased incidence of endometrial hyperplasia with atypia, the precursor to endometrial cancer. Combination oral menopausal hormonal therapy has been reported in a recent randomized controlled trial to be associated with increased risk for breast cancer, coronary heart disease, dementia, and venous thromboembolic events.

**ANSWER:** C

34. Regarding pelvic inflammatory disease (PID), which of the following is true?

A. *Neisseria gonorrhoeae* is the most common causative organism.

B. Physical examination is considered the gold standard for diagnosis.

C. Chronic pelvic pain and ectopic pregnancy are common sequelae.

D. It should initially be treated with parenteral antibiotics.

E. CT scan of the pelvis should be done routinely.

*Ref.:* 25

**COMMENTS:** Treatment of **pelvic inflammatory disease** is the most common reason for gynecologic hospital admissions in the United States. PID is a spectrum of inflammatory disorders of the upper genital tract in women that include salpingitis, endometritis, and tubo-ovarian abscess (TOA). Bacterial organisms involved include *N. gonorrhoeae*, *Chlamydia trachomatis*, endogenous aerobic and anaerobic bacteria, and *Mycoplasma*. *C. trachomatis* is the causative organism more often than *N. gonorrhoeae*. Although physical examination is frequently used to diagnose PID, laparoscopy is considered the gold standard for diagnosis. Patients who meet the diagnostic criteria can be treated as outpatients with broad-spectrum antibiotics, but a follow-up evaluation should be scheduled for 48 hours later. Patients who fail outpatient therapy should be admitted and treated with intravenous broad-spectrum antibiotics. Imaging studies are required if one suspects TOA. All patients with PID should be counseled about the common sequelae of the disease, which include chronic pelvic pain, infertility, and increased risk for ectopic pregnancies.

**ANSWER:** C

35. Regarding TOAs, which of the following is false?

A. Initial outpatient oral antibiotic therapy is currently considered suboptimal treatment.

B. Initial therapy should be nonsurgical.

C. TOAs are present in approximately 50% of patients with PID.

D. Unilateral removal can be used as conservative therapy for women desiring fertility.

E. None of the above.

***Ref.:* 19, 20**

**COMMENTS: Tubo-ovarian abscesses** are present in 10% of women with PID. They are more common in women with concurrent bacterial vaginosis or HIV infection. TOAs contain a mixture of anaerobic and facultative or aerobic organisms. Therefore, antibiotic therapy should cover a wide range of organisms, including *N. gonorrhoeae* and *C. trachomatis*. Initial therapy with oral antibiotics does not appear to provide sufficient serum antibiotic levels to treat TOAs. In general, broad-spectrum intravenous antibiotics should be used as initial therapy. If the patient's symptoms do not improve over a 24- to 48-hour period, alternative interventions such as surgery should be considered. TOAs can be drained laparoscopically or under radiologic guidance. There appears to be no difference in outcome between these approaches. Midline pelvic TOAs may be drained through a posterior colpotomy. Frequently, a temporary intraperitoneal catheter is left in place for drainage. For patients who are not candidates for conservative procedures, resection of TOAs via laparotomy is commonly done. TOAs involving both ovaries or the uterus are treated with hysterectomy and bilateral salpingo-oophorectomy. Unilateral TOAs can be treated with unilateral adnexectomy for patients desiring fertility. The abdominopelvic cavity should be irrigated extensively. Ideally, the vaginal cuff should be left open or an intraperitoneal catheter placed for postoperative drainage. Ruptured TOAs are surgical emergencies. Patients should undergo prompt surgical treatment via laparotomy after they are hemodynamically stabilized. These patients usually have acute and progressive pelvic pain, and they may be hemodynamically unstable. The mortality rate associated with a ruptured TOA is 5% to 10%. Delay in diagnosis and treatment results in higher mortality rates. Most patients undergo hysterectomy with bilateral salpingo-oophorectomy. Conservative surgeries for ruptured TOAs have not been well studied. Broad-spectrum intravenous antibiotics are continued until the patient is able to tolerate oral intake, and oral antibiotics are continued until the patient is afebrile.

**ANSWER:** C

**REFERENCES**

1. ACOG Committee Opinion: number 280, December 2002. The role of the generalist obstetrician-gynecologist in the early detection of ovarian cancer, *Obstet Gynecol* 100:1413–1416, 2002.
2. American Society of Clinical Oncology policy statement update: genetic testing for cancer susceptibility, *J Clin Oncol* 21:2397–2406, 2003.
3. Kaiser Permanente Guideline. *BRCA1* genetic screening, 1998.
4. Myers ER, Bastian LA, Havrilesky LJ, et al: Management of adnexal mass, *Evid Rep Technol Assessment* 130:1–145, 2006.
5. National Comprehensive Cancer Network (NCCN) Guidelines for Hereditary Breast and/or Ovarian Cancer, available online at www.nccn.com/physician_gls/index.html.
6. Scheuer L, Kauff N, Robson M, et al: Outcome of preventive surgery and screening for breast and ovarian cancer in BRCA mutation carriers, *J Clin Oncol* 20:1260–1268, 2002.
7. Statement of the American Society of Clinical Oncology: genetic testing for cancer susceptibility, Adopted on February 20, 1996, *J Clin Oncol* 14:1730–1736, 1996; discussion 1737–1740.
8. Townsend CM Jr, Beauchamp RD, Evers BM, et al, editors: *Sabiston textbook of surgery: the biological basis of modern surgical practice,* ed 18, Philadelphia, 2004, WB Saunders.
9. Genetic risk assessment and *BRCA* mutation testing for breast and ovarian cancer susceptibility: recommendation statement, *Ann Intern Med* 143:355–361, 2005 6.
10. Hampel H, Sweet K, Westman JA, et al: Referral for cancer genetics consultation: a review and compilation of risk assessment criteria, *J Med Genet* 41:81–91, 2004.
11. Sanai FM, Bzeizi KI: Systematic review. Tuberculous peritonitis: presenting features, diagnostic strategies and treatment, *Aliment Pharmacol Ther* 22:685–700, 2005.
12. Shakil AO, Korula J, Kanel GC, et al: Diagnostic features of tuberculous peritonitis in the absence and presence of chronic liver disease: a case control study, *Am J Med* 100:179–185, 1996.
13. Mullholland MW, Lillemoe KD, Doherty GM, et al, editors: *Greenfield's surgery: scientific principles and practice,* ed 4, Philadelphia, 2006, Lippincott Williams & Wilkins.
14. Petignat P, Vajda D, Joris F, et al: Surgical management of epithelial ovarian cancer at community hospitals: a population-based study, *J Surg Oncol* 75:19–23, 2000.
15. Schrag D, Earle C, Xu F, et al: Associations between hospital and surgeon procedure volumes and patient outcomes after ovarian cancer resection, *J Natl Cancer Inst* 98:163–171, 2006.
16. DiSaia PJ: *Clinical gynecologic oncology,* ed 6, St. Louis, 2002, CV Mosby.
17. Hoskins WJ: *Principles and practice of gynecologic oncology,* ed 3, Philadelphia, 2000, Lippincott Williams & Wilkins.
18. Tamussino KF, Lim PC, Webb MJ, et al: Gastrointestinal surgery in patients with ovarian cancer, *Gynecol Oncol* 80:79–84, 2001.
19. Thompson JD, Rock AR: *Te Linde's operative gynecology,* ed 9, Philadelphia, 2003, Lippincott Williams & Wilkins.
20. Herbst AL, Mishell DR, Stenchever MA, et al: *Comprehensive gynecology,* ed 4, St. Louis, 2001, Mosby–Year Book.
21. Walboomers JM, Jacobs MV, Manos MM, et al. Human papillomavirus is a necessary cause of invasive cervical cancer worldwide, *J Pathol* 189:12–19, 1999.
22. Bent AE: *Ostergard's urogynecology and pelvic floor dysfunction,* ed 5, Philadelphia, 2003, Lippincott Williams & Wilkins.
23. Berek JS: *Practical gynecologic oncology,* ed 3, Philadelphia, 2000, Lippincott Williams & Wilkins.
24. Briasoulis E, Karavasilis V, Pavlidis N. Megestrol activity in recurrent adult type granulosa cell tumour of the ovary, *Ann Oncol* 8:811–812, 1997.
25. Available online at www.cdc.gov/STD/treatment/2006/updated-regimens.htm.

# B. Neurosurgery

*Adam P. Smith, M.D., and Richard W. Byrne, M.D.*

1. Which of the following statements regarding diagnostic procedures used to evaluate the central nervous system (CNS) is false?

   A. MRI is the most useful initial test for the evaluation of spinal cord compression.

   B. Magnetic resonance angiography eliminates some of the risk associated with cerebral angiography.

   C. Water-soluble contrast material has decreased the incidence of arachnoiditis following myelography.

   D. CT is the best available radiographic test for soft tissue evaluation.

   E. MRI does not expose the patient to radiation.

   *Ref.:* 1-5

**COMMENTS:** In evaluating intracranial processes, **magnetic resonance imaging** is superior to **computed tomography** in many cases. MRI is associated with minimal bone artifact, yields high-grade differentiation of gray-white matter, can directly scan multiple planes (although CT reconstructions can be useful), and does not expose the patient to radiation. In the case of spinal cord compression, MRI will identify the degree of soft tissue or bone impingement on the spinal cord, hematoma within or around the spinal cord, and any changes in signal within the cord itself. CT identifies bone structures well, along with some indications of canal or foraminal stenosis, but it provides poor delineation of soft tissues or the degree of actual neural tissue compression. **Angiography** is the main method for identifying and evaluating vascular lesions, for preoperative evaluation and possible treatment of tumors, and for identifying vascular involvement in trauma to the brain and spinal cord. The risks involved in angiography are predominately vessel rupture, embolus formation, and vessel spasm, all of which could lead to stroke. Adverse reactions to contrast material may also occur. These risks may be obviated by the use of **magnetic resonance angiography**, but the images obtained are of slightly inferior quality. With the advent of higher-power MRI (i.e., 3-T or greater MRI), angiography is still believed to be superior. The use of water-soluble contrast media during **myelography** has decreased the incidence of postprocedure arachnoiditis. Most institutions use CT scanning in conjunction with myelography. **Computed tomographic myelography** is most commonly used to evaluate intervertebral disk disease, but it is also useful for patients with contraindications to MRI. Following trauma, CT myelography may identify nerve root avulsion. CT is at present the most useful diagnostic tool for identifying acute hemorrhage or fracture intracranially and for identifying spine fractures or subluxations. Modern units perform axial cuts of approximately 5 mm and provide resolution in the range of 1 mm. The major disadvantage of CT is the artifact created by bone and the poor resolution of neural tissue.

**ANSWER:** D

2. Which of the following statements regarding scalp injuries is true?

   A. The blood supply to the scalp lies between the periosteum and the galea.

   B. Most scalp laceration hemorrhages can be controlled by applying direct pressure.

   C. Subgaleal hematomas must be drained to avoid abscess formation and extensive scalp elevation.

   D. If a scalp laceration extends below the zygoma, facial weakness may result from damage to the ipsilateral trigeminal nerve.

   E. The scalp consists of two layers: the skin and the subcutaneous tissue.

   *Ref.:* 2, 3

**COMMENTS:** The **scalp** consists of five layers: skin, subcutaneous tissue, galea aponeurotica, loose areolar tissue, and periosteum (SCALP). The skin and galea are the layers of surgical importance, with the blood supply lying between the skin above and the galea below. Because the blood supply to the scalp is rich, lacerations can be accompanied by significant blood loss. When the underlying skull is intact, this blood loss can be controlled by simple pressure. If the skull is fractured, however, direct pressure may be hazardous to the underlying brain tissue. Pulling the retracted galea back over the wound edge with forceps often controls such hemorrhage. Contusions causing **subgaleal hemorrhage** can lead to the formation of large **subgaleal hematomas** that can elevate extensive portions of the scalp off the skull. In this instance, compression dressings can reduce the extent of hematoma formation. If the overlying scalp is viable and there is no evidence of infection, subgaleal hematomas may be left alone to resolve naturally over a period of several weeks. If the hematoma is infected, it is necessary to evacuate it. The occipitalis and frontalis muscles insert on the galea, and contraction of these muscles tends to separate areas of galeal disruptions. Therefore, even small lacerations of the galea should be closed. Regarding nonoperative treatment of subgaleal hematomas, large lacerations with significant loss of galeal or subgaleal tissue may be treated with compression dressings after appropriate débridement and closure to minimize the chance of residual subgaleal hematoma, infection, or both. The largest arteries supplying the scalp originate from the external carotid arteries and are the superficial temporal and occipital arteries. The **facial nerve** (cranial nerve VII) runs below the zygoma and may be injured if a laceration extends into the face. This may result in facial weakness, depending on which branch or branches are injured. As the facial nerve exits the cranium through the stylomastoid foramen, it penetrates the parotid gland and lies in a plane that separates the deep and superficial lobes of the parotid. It then divides into five main branches as it leaves the gland to innervate the muscles of facial expression. The temporal branch of the facial nerve lies within the deep temporal fascia, between the superficial layer of the deep temporal fascia and the superficial temporal fat pad. The superficial temporal fat pad splits the superficial and deep layers of the deep temporal fascia. Lacerations through this area may also damage the nerve. The **trigeminal nerve** supplies sensation to the face, and although **scalp** lacerations may also damage this nerve, such lacerations would not result in weakness of the muscles of facial expression.

**ANSWER:** B

3. Which of the following statements regarding hydrocephalus is the most accurate?

   A. It represents a primary process in up to two thirds of patients.

   B. It is classified as communicating or noncommunicating, depending on where the obstruction to cerebrospinal fluid (CSF) flow occurs.

   C. With proper, timely shunting, patients with hydrocephalus usually have intelligence equal to that of matched control groups without hydrocephalus.

   D. Hydrocephalus ex vacuo is more common in the young.

   E. Clinical signs of hydrocephalus are manifested the same ways in all age groups.

*Ref.:* 2, 3, 5

**COMMENTS: Hydrocephalus** is a secondary, not a primary problem. Causes of hydrocephalus include aqueductal stenosis, dysfunction of arachnoid granulations, subarachnoid scarring, blockage of **cerebrospinal fluid** by blood clot or tumor, or rarely excess production by some choroid plexus tumors. These causes may be classified as communicating or noncommunicating. With communicating hydrocephalus, obstruction to flow is outside the ventricular system, most commonly at the arachnoid granulations. Noncommunicating, or obstructive, hydrocephalus is caused by obstruction of CSF flow at any point within the ventricular system. The most common cause of congenital hydrocephalus is aqueductal stenosis. The clinical features of infantile hydrocephalus include diastasis of the cranial sutures, enlarging head circumference, bulging anterior fontanelle, and weakness of upward gaze (the "setting sun" sign). Clinical features of hydrocephalus past 1 year of age (when the cranial sutures are closed) include headache, nausea, vomiting, visual loss, and lethargy. In some cases, this progresses to coma and death without proper treatment of the increased intracranial pressure (ICP). Most cases of hydrocephalus are treated with pressure-activated shunts, the most common being a **ventriculoperitoneal shunt**. Other common distal catheter targets are the pleura, cardiac atrium, and gallbladder. Although treated patients usually attain acceptable levels of intelligence overall, patients with shunts do not commonly do as well intellectually as nonhydrocephalic matched control groups. The outcome largely depends on the cause of the hydrocephalus and how quickly and successful the hydrocephalus is treated. Hydrocephalus ex

vacuo refers to enlarged ventricles secondary to loss of cerebral tissue, commonly following a cerebral insult or atrophy. It occurs most commonly in the elderly.

**ANSWER:** B

4. Which of the following statements regarding ICP monitoring is false?

   A. Ventricular pressure catheters are the reference standard for ICP monitoring.

   B. ICP monitoring should be performed in salvageable patients with a Glasgow Coma Scale (GCS) score of 3 to 8 after resuscitation and an abnormal findings on head CT.

   C. Risk factors for elevated ICP after head injury include age younger than 40 years, open basal cisterns on CT, and systolic blood pressure higher than 90 mm Hg.

   D. Normal ICP is 0 to 15 mm Hg or 0 to 20 cm $H_2O$.

   E. ICP can be measured with either an intraparenchymal or ventriculostomy monitor.

*Ref.:* 5-9

**COMMENTS:** Because of the approximate 1% risk for hemorrhage and 5% risk for infection with **intracranial pressure** monitoring, this procedure is not appropriate for all patients with head injury (especially those with coagulopathy or thrombocytopenia). ICP monitoring is appropriate in patients with a **Glasgow Coma Scale** score of 3 to 8 and abnormal findings on head CT or for selected patients with normal findings on CT and risk factors for elevated ICP, such as age older than 40 years, systolic blood pressure lower than 90 mm Hg, decerebrate or decorticate posturing on motor examination, or a suspicious mechanism of injury. CT may not show overt hemorrhage or lesions, but edema may still develop quickly and lead to high ICP. Common signs of brain swelling with high ICP on CT are slit ventricles, flattening or loss of normal cortical sulci patterns, blurring of normal gray-white junctions, and effacement of the basal cisterns. Ventricular catheters are an accurate, low-cost, and reliable method to monitor ICP, thus making them preferred over parenchymal, subarachnoid, subdural, or epidural devices. They have the additional ability to be recalibrated without replacement. The risk for hemorrhage associated with different ICP monitoring devices has not been clearly defined and it is rarely of clinical consequence. The presence of actual infection versus device colonization is difficult to assess with any ICP monitoring device without associated clinical signs. Colonization rates do appear to be related to the type of device, however, with parenchymal monitors carrying the highest rates. Recently, more advanced techniques such as cerebral oxygenation, cerebral blood flow, microdialysis, and electrophysiologic monitors are being studied. Normal ICP is 0 to 15 mm Hg, but ICP is not usually treated in most centers until it rises to 20 mm Hg or higher.

**ANSWER:** C

5. Which of the following is true regarding neurogenic shock?

   A. First-line therapy consists of repetitive fluid boluses with crystalloids.

   B. Pure α-adrenergic sympathomimetics are the vasopressor drugs of choice.

C. Tachycardia and hypotension are pathognomonic signs of neurogenic shock.

D. The absence of a cervical collar can be used to rule out neurogenic snock.

E. Dopamine is the preferred vasopressor agent.

*Ref.:* 1, 5, 6

**COMMENTS: Neurogenic shock** should be suspected in any patient with cervical spinal cord trauma. It is characterized by the sudden loss of sympathetic tone and the predominance of parasympathetic tone. Sympathetic control starts in the hypothalamus and is carried down the brainstem through the spinal cord, where it exits to target organs at the thoracic and high lumbar levels. Therefore, any damage to the cervical cord may disrupt descending sympathetic neurons. Common features of neurogenic shock include hypotension, bradycardia, warm and dry extremities, peripheral vasodilation, venous pooling with decreased cardiac output, poikilothermia, and priapism. In contrast to other forms of shock, loss of sympathetic tone in patients with neurogenic shock leads to both hypotension *and* bradycardia. As smooth muscle in the vasculature relaxes and blood pressure decreases, cardiac drive is also lost and reflexive tachycardia cannot be accomplished. First-line therapy is similar to that for other forms of shock and may involve placing the patient in the Trendelenburg position, fluid resuscitation, or administration of vasopressor agents, but a few key points differ. Because of loss of vasomotor tone, massive fluid boluses with crystalloids may result in flash pulmonary edema. Pressor agents are often useful, but an agent with only α-adrenergic properties may lead to unopposed reflexive bradycardia, which may worsen cardiovascular dynamics. An agent such as dopamine with both α- and β-adrenergic properties will combat any reflexive bradycardia and is the preferred medication. In any trauma with suspected cervical injury, a cervical collar is recommended until the spine is cleared. However, the pure absence of a cervical collar should never be used to rule out either cervical trauma or neurogenic shock.

**A N S W E R :**   E

6. Which of the following is true regarding cervical trauma?

A. The mortality associated with atlanto-occipital dislocation is 100%.

B. Most mortality in cervical trauma is not the direct result of neural compression.

C. With the advent of CT, no other imaging is needed for evaluation of the cervical spine.

D. In a neurologically intact patient with neck pain, the cervical spine can be cleared immediately with normal findings on plain cervical radiographs.

E. Methylprednisolone should be started immediately in any trauma patient suspected of having cervical trauma, regardless of the findings on neurologic examination or the time of injury.

*Ref.:* 1-3, 5, 10-16

**COMMENTS:** Evaluating, treating, or possibly clearing the cervical spine in a trauma patient is a procedure that can be complex at times. In fact, the spine trauma guidelines state that there is insufficient evidence to even support treatment guidelines. Initial immobilization of a trauma victim's cervical spine is commonplace with most emergency medical service systems. The neck continues to be immobilized until the spine can be cleared by clinical assessment or radiographic imaging. The process of evaluating begins with a careful history and physical examination. In the absence of any suspicious mechanism of injury and with an asymptomatic patient (awake, alert, neurologically intact, not intoxicated, without neck pain/tenderness, and without other injuries that prevent appropriate assessment of the spine or that distract the patient), imaging is unlikely to be necessary. However, a symptomatic patient requires imaging. A three-view cervical spine series (anteroposterior, lateral, and odontoid views) is recommended, sometimes supplemented by **computed tomography** to better define suspicious or poorly visualized areas on plain cervical radiographs. The diagnostic performance of helical CT scanners has a sensitivity approaching 99% and specificity approaching 93%. Because of this, many trauma centers have proposed relying exclusively on CT to evaluate the cervical spine. However, the CT-generated artifact, especially in coronal and sagittal reconstructions, may distort the true anatomy of the cervical spine. Nonetheless, missed injuries on CT are extremely rare and the majority are ligamentous. In an awake and neurologically intact patient with neck pain, three-view plain cervical radiographs and CT are recommended to evaluate bony pathology. If pain is still present despite normal findings on radiography and CT, either **magnetic resonance imaging** or dynamic flexion/extension films are recommended. **Atlanto-occipital dislocation**, or craniocervical junction dislocation, occurs in approximately 1% of patients with cervical spine trauma and has been noted in 18% to 19% of patients with fatal cervical spine injuries at autopsy. Although the entity was previously perceived as an infrequent injury resulting in death, improved emergency management has recently provided increased survivors. Most mortality in patients with cervical spine trauma results from anoxia secondary to respiratory arrest from other injuries. The use of steroids, in particular **methylprednisolone**, after spinal cord injury is a matter of great debate. The original studies performed involved patients with known neurologic deficits seen within 8 hours of injury. A 30-mg/kg bolus, followed by a 23-hour infusion of 5.4 mg/kg/h, is the usual protocol. Even in this scenario, the degree of functional motor improvement is questionable, and side effects such as sepsis and pneumonia may occur. Therefore, no level I evidence exists to support the use of methylprednisolone for spinal cord injury, although many physicians still follow the protocol based on levels II and III data. However, in the setting of a neurologically intact patient or a patient with spinal cord injury but outside the 8-hour window, data suggest that **steroids** should not be administered.

**A N S W E R :**   B

7. Which of the following statements regarding traumatic CSF leaks is false?

A. Most are caused by basilar skull fractures and close spontaneously.

B. The risk for infection is greater with rhinorrhea than with otorrhea.

C. They often do not require immediate surgical repair to avert infection.

D. They may be observed for up to 14 days if there is no evidence of infection.

E. The presence of a traumatic CSF leak mandates the use of prophylactic broad-spectrum antibiotic coverage.

*Ref.:* 2, 3, 5, 17, 18

**COMMENTS:** The overall incidence of traumatic **cerebrospinal fluid leak** is 0.25% to 0.50%. It occurs secondary to a skull fracture that tears the dura. If a CSF leak is suspected, the fluid may be sent for determination of $\beta_2$-transferrin because this protein only exists in CSF and the vitreous of the eye. Imaging studies may then be useful in identifying the site of leakage after one is suspected. Most **traumatic cerebrospinal fluid fistulas** close spontaneously within a few days, but they may be managed in the hospital under close supervision. Placement of a lumbar drain to divert the fistula can be helpful if spontaneous resolution does not occur. The risk for persistent drainage and infection is greater with rhinorrhea than with otorrhea. If left untreated, both rhinorrhea and otorrhea may eventually lead to infection, but some patients can go for years without sequelae. Initial treatment involves bed rest, elevation of the head of the bed, and stool softeners to prevent straining. The use of prophylactic antibiotics remains a controversial issue. Proponents believe that CSF leaks are exposed to upper respiratory tract and skin pathogens and are therefore at high risk for infection. Opponents argue that despite the exposure, prophylactic antibiotics contribute to antibiotic resistance and, moreover, that prophylactic antibiotics do not decrease the risk for meningitis. The evidence available does not support the use of prophylactic antibiotics, whether a skull fracture exists in isolation or with a CSF leak. However, if meningitis is confirmed, antibiotic therapy is started based on sensitivity of the organism. Surgical exploration may be indicated for leaks refractory to observation and lumbar drainage to repair the torn dura if the site of CSF leak can be found.

**ANSWER:** E

8. Which of the following statements regarding brain injury is false?

   A. The extent of brain injury is a function of the mechanism of injury.

   B. Contusions tend to involve the anterior portions of the frontal and temporal lobes.

   C. Diffuse axonal injury (DAI) is usually an incidental and asymptomatic finding.

   D. The effects of secondary edema and hematoma enlargement may be delayed for several days.

   E. Not all brain contusions are clinically apparent on neurologic examination.

*Ref.:* 2, 3, 5, 6, 8, 9

**COMMENTS:** Localized force can damage the scalp, skull, and underlying brain tissue in the immediate area of injury. The resulting neurologic deficit is related to the area of the brain directly involved and usually produces brief or no loss of consciousness. The application of generalized force to the skull, such as that caused by impact of the head against an immovable object, allows diffuse transmission of energy and thus causes injury to the entire brain. In such a case the brain insult is generalized, with altered consciousness often being produced, and its severity is related to the mechanism of injury. For example, the injury may be the result of linear or rotational acceleration-deceleration of the brain against the cranium, such as when the head hits an immovable object. When the brain strikes the rigid skull, contusions occur in the area where the force is applied (coup injury), as well as against the opposite inner surface of the skull (contrecoup injury). The undersurface of the frontal lobes, the anterior portions of the temporal lobes, the posterior portions of the occipital lobes, and the upper portion of the midbrain are most likely to suffer contusions because

they are relatively more confined by rough bone and dural shelves. The contusion may be clinically silent initially if the involved area of brain has no demonstrable clinical function. These injuries often become most apparent days after the injury as edema accumulates and creates the effects of an intracranial mass. Occasionally, a hematoma accumulates in the area of contusion 24 to 72 hours after initial injury despite having initial normal-appearing findings on CT. This situation occurs more often in elderly persons. Rotation of the brain within the skull may cause tearing of axons and result in **diffuse axonal injury** within the white matter, a so-called shearing injury, which is often severe. Some estimate that more than 90% of patients with severe DAI remain in a persistent vegetative state. DAI most commonly affects the subcortical white matter (centrum semiovale), corpus callosum, superior cerebellar peduncle, and dorsal rostral brainstem. The severity of DAI is based on (1) the distance from the center of rotation, (2) the arc of rotation, and (3) the duration and intensity of force. Gunshot brain injuries are frequently severe because of damage caused by the bullet and the associated shock wave that travels along the path. The primary injury, bleeding, swelling, and infection result in high mortality rates.

**ANSWER:** C

9. Which of the following is true regarding brain death?

   A. Neurosurgical evaluation is required for proper determination of brain death.

   B. Once the patient demonstrates no functional neurologic findings, including loss of all cranial nerves and reflexes, brain death can be pronounced.

   C. If toxicology studies show the presence of opiates in blood or urine, brain death may still be pronounced if all other criteria are met and if the opiates were given in known low concentrations.

   D. If while performing a brain death examination the patient becomes cardiovascularly unstable, the examiner should finish quickly to pronounce brain death without delay.

   E. Confirmation with electroencephalography (EEG) is not required to pronounce brain death.

*Ref.:* 1, 6, 19

**COMMENTS: Brain death** is a confusing topic for many individuals, even within the realm of health care. Brain death is a clinical diagnosis, and the exact criteria may vary from one hospital to another. It may be legally performed by any physician, although many centers recommend either neurologic or neurosurgical consultation. The diagnostic criteria for brain death are (1) clinical or neuroimaging evidence of CNS dysfunction that is compatible with the clinical diagnosis of brain death, (2) exclusion of confounding medical conditions, (3) no drug intoxication or poisoning (the brain death examination may be performed only after laboratory-verified absence of any sedating drugs), and (4) core temperature higher than 32° C (febrile patients can be tested). Regarding the clinical criteria, findings must show (1) coma or unresponsiveness, including no cerebral motor response to pain; (2) absence of all brainstem reflexes, including absence of the pupillary response, oculocephalic reflex, cold caloric testing, corneal reflex, jaw reflex, cough reflex, or gag reflex; and (3) apnea testing. Usually, the brain death examination consists of two examinations separated in time, which is often at least 6 hours. Because the **apnea test** can destabilize an already potentially unstable patient, it is generally performed only after the second brain death examination when brain death is highly suspected. Prerequisites for the apnea test are (1) a core temperature higher than 36.5°C, (2) systolic blood pressure higher than 90 mm Hg, (3) euvolemia, (4) normal $Pco_2$, and (5) normal serum electrolyte levels. The apnea test is usually performed as follows: The patient is given 100% $O_2$ by nasal or tracheal cannula to maintain adequate oxygen saturation and prevent cardiovascular collapse. Baseline arterial blood gas studies are performed. The ventilator is disconnected, arterial blood gas studies are performed at variable intervals throughout the test, and the examiner assesses for respiratory movements. If no respiratory movements are observed *and* $Pco_2$ is greater than 60 mm Hg or has increased more than 20 mm Hg from baseline at the end of the test, the apnea test supports the clinical diagnosis of brain death. One caveat is that the patient must remain cardiovascularly stable during the examination as described in the prerequisite criteria. If at any time the blood pressure falls below the criteria, the test should be stopped and repeated. Vasopressor agents may be used during the examination. After the apnea test, confirmatory tests are optional but do not replace the three core diagnostic criteria. Some examples of confirmatory tests are **cerebral angiography** showing no intracerebral filling at the level of the circle of Willis, confirmation of no electrical activity via **electroencephalography**, **transcranial Doppler ultrasonography**, **technetium-99m hexamethylpropyleneamine oxime brain scan** showing no uptake of isotope, or **somatosensory evoke potentials** showing no activity. Each of these confirmatory tests has flaws, including EEG, and may not appear to demonstrate brain death despite the other diagnostic criteria already having been fulfilled. This is why they are purely optional. Of note, some research now recommends monitoring pH levels rather than $Pco_2$ during the apnea test.

**ANSWER: E**

10. Which statement is true regarding elevated ICP and brain herniation syndromes?

   A. The pupils are always dilated in the setting of brain herniation.

   B. After the pupils become fixed and dilated, no functional recovery is possible.

   C. Cortical sulci effacement may not be observed in the setting of increased posterior fossa pressure from a cerebellar hematoma.

   D. In a patient with a unilateral supratentorial mass and increased ICP, weakness will always be observed on the contralateral side of the body.

   E. Compression of the occulomotor nerve during brain herniation causes pupillary constriction.

   *Ref.:* 1, 5, 6, 9, 12, 17, 20

**COMMENTS:** In the setting of sustained elevated **intracranial pressure**, the brain will seek lower pressure and "herniate" across various dural attachments and bony prominences inside the cranium. **Uncal herniation** is one of the most recognized and is caused by elevated pressure in the supratentorial compartment with downward pressure on the brain. This forces the medial temporal lobe or lobes, including the uncus, through the incisura. The **occulomotor nerve** is compressed, thus impairing the parasympathetic fibers running superficially along the nerve, and dilation of either one or both pupils ensues. *Of note, some studies suggest that brainstem ischemia from raised ICP may also be responsible for at least some cases of pupillary dilation when uncal herniation was not present.* The overall mortality rate associated with **herniation**

**syndromes** leading to fixed and dilated pupils has been reported to be as high as 75%. However, if medical therapy is instituted immediately and the pupils return to normal, a small chance of survival may exist, but often with low chance for a favorable outcome. If the pupils do not respond to therapy, few patients improve to more than a vegetative state. Not all brain herniation syndromes result in dilated pupils. **Herniation of the frontal lobes** into and beneath the falx may not affect the pupils at all. Similarly, pressure from a pontine hemorrhage may disrupt the descending sympathetic fibers and result in pinpoint pupils (myosis) from unopposed parasympathetic tone. Elevated ICP in the posterior fossa is unique in that it may cause either downward pressure through the foramen magnum or upward pressure into the tentorium cerebelli. In either case, the supratentorial compartment is often "protected" from the majority of the elevated pressure by the tentorium. Therefore, despite a resultant comalike state from brainstem compression, the supratentorial compartment may appear relatively unaffected on imaging studies with normal cortical sulci patterns. "**Kernohan notch**" refers to a transtentorial brain herniation scenario in which elevated supratentorial pressure pushes the contralateral cerebral peduncle into the tentorium. This is manifested as weakness ipsilateral to the side of pressure formation because the descending corticospinal fibers have not yet decussated.

**ANSWER: C**

11. Which of the following is true regarding the management of elevated ICP?

   A. Hemicraniectomy is first-line therapy for elevated ICP.

   B. Hypertonic saline is superior to mannitol for osmotherapy.

   C. Prolonged hyperventilation is a benign method for lowering elevated ICP.

   D. Maintenance of elevated cerebral perfusion pressure (CPP) may be more important in improved neurologic outcome at the expense of high ICP.

   E. Persistent hyperventilation is a terrific method to sustain alkalization and combat acidosis in the brain for long periods.

   *Ref.:* 5, 6, 9, 21, 22

**COMMENTS** **Cerebral perfusion pressure** is calculated by the formula CPP = MAP − ICP, where MAP is mean arterial pressure. Therefore, as **intracranial pressure** rises to malignant levels, CPP falls. This is problematic in the treatment of elevated ICP, because attempts to continue perfusing the brain (elevating CPP) can occur only by elevating blood pressure (MAP). Increasing blood pressure with already elevated ICP leads to loss of the brain's normal autoregulatory mechanisms, which eventually results in even higher ICP. Much debate exists over whether to focus treatment on CPP or ICP. Early studies indicated that greater than a 20-mm Hg elevation in ICP for sustained intervals was associated with poor neurologic outcome. Later studies indicated that CPP less than 60 mm Hg was also associated with worse outcome. Recent preliminary studies, however, have shown that aggressive maintenance of CPP at a level higher than 60 mm Hg, even with prolonged ICP higher than 50 mm Hg for more than 48 hours, may still lead to a good neurologic outcome. Further randomized trials need to be performed before definitive recommendations can be made. Unfortunately, there are no level I studies indicating an optimal CPP threshold or ICP limit on which to base CPP-guided therapy. The initial steps in controlling elevated ICP include medical therapies such as raising the head of the bed, maintaining the patient's head straight, hyperventilation, and **hyperosmolar therapy**. Hyperventilation is a quick and easy way to lower ICP in theory, for lowering $P_{CO_2}$ will decrease cerebral blood flow and reverse brain parenchymal and CSF acidosis. However, hyperventilation is not without consequence. Disadvantages include induced vasoconstriction to a point where ischemia develops. The alkalization of **cerebrospinal fluid** is also very short-lived with hyperventilation. In a direct comparison of hyperventilation and no hyperventilation in patients with severe head injury, some studies have shown a statistically significant worse outcome in the hyperventilation group, mainly because of ischemia induced by the prolonged therapy. However, temporary hyperventilation is still a useful tool to lower ICP until other measures can be instituted. The usual **hyperosmolar** agents used in the setting of traumatic brain injury are **mannitol** and **hypertonic saline**. Mannitol has three postulated effects: (1) plasma expansion, which improves cerebral rheology; (2) antioxidant effect, which improves the cerebral reaction to ischemia; and (3) osmotic diuresis, which lowers MAP and then ICP in a slightly delayed fashion. This third mechanism, however, could be detrimental if diuresis decreases MAP to a point of reduced CPP. Regardless, a level III randomized controlled trial has shown improved outcome with mannitol therapy. Hypertonic saline, in contrast, reduces ICP while preserving or improving CPP. Although it is questioned whether the reduction in ICP by hypertonic saline is greater than that by mannitol, few studies have directly compared the two, and they are rarely compared in equimolar doses. Additionally, despite hypertonic saline's proved effect on control of ICP, no evidence of improved outcome exists. As a result, there is insufficient evidence to support the use of hypertonic saline over mannitol for **osmotherapy** in adults. **Hemicraniectomy** has an important role in the treatment of elevated ICP; however, it is rarely used as first-line therapy except in some cases of malignant stroke.

**ANSWER:** D

12. Which of the following statements regarding the evaluation and care of head-injured patients is the most accurate?

   A. Hypotension is often the direct result of intracranial trauma.

   B. Decerebrate posturing is a common response to diffuse cortical injury.

   C. A score of 5 on the GCS is associated with a poor prognosis.

   D. The syndrome of inappropriate antidiuretic hormone secretion (SIADH) should be suspected when the serum sodium level exceeds 150 mEq/L.

   E. Brain injury takes predominance over any other injury, and therefore initial evaluation and management should focus only on the neurologic examination.

*Ref.: 2, 3, 8, 9*

**COMMENTS:** Initial care of a head-injured patient must focus on maintenance of ventilation, control of hemorrhage, and maintenance of the peripheral circulation as in any trauma scenario. Continued hypotension and tachycardia are rarely the direct results of head trauma and should alert the examiner to the existence of a systemic hemorrhage. Normal intracranial volume is only 1300 cm$^3$ in adult females and 1500 cm$^3$ in adult males, which makes severe blood loss intracranially nearly impossible. Instead, severe intracranial trauma more commonly leads to the **Cushing triad** (hypertension, bradycardia, and irregular respirations). As soon as

possible, careful neurologic examination and documentation of the level of consciousness should be undertaken as a baseline for later comparison as the patient progresses. **Decerebrate posturing** (extension and internal rotation of the extremities, neck extension, and arching of the back) implies compression of or damage to the brainstem below the level of the red nucleus (midbrain). The **Glasgow Coma Scale** measures motor, verbal, and eye responses on scales of 1 to 6, 1 to 5, and 1 to 4, respectively. It is recorded as a sum of the highest score in each category, and the lowest possible total score is 3. Coma is defined by a GCS score of 8 or less. Patients with a score lower than 5 have a mortality rate higher than 50%. Scores of 3 are associated with mortality approaching 100%. The **syndrome of inappropriate antidiuretic hormone secretion** should be suspected when serum osmolality and sodium levels fall in association with an increase in urinary osmolality. Restriction of water intake or the use of solute diuretics may be necessary to control this problem. SIADH sometimes needs to be differentiated from cerebral salt wasting (CSW), in which brain trauma induces the active secretion of sodium. Although the resultant hyponatremia and low serum osmolality are similar to SIADH, treatment of CSW focuses more on serum sodium replacement with hypertonic saline as opposed to fluid restriction.

**ANSWER:** C

13. Which of the following statements regarding cerebral edema caused by head injury is the most accurate?

   A. CT should be performed to exclude the diagnosis of intracranial hemorrhage or a mass lesion before starting therapy.

   B. Cerebral edema caused by head injury is vasogenic and not cytotoxic in origin.

   C. Steroids are useful for the treatment of head trauma.

   D. Hypercapnia induces cerebral vasoconstriction and is useful for decreasing intracerebral blood volume.

   E. Within a few hours (1 to 3 hours) after injury, maximal cerebral edema has already formed, so further monitoring is unnecessary if the patient is clinically stable.

*Ref.: 2, 3, 6, 9, 23*

**COMMENTS:** According to the Monro-Kellie doctrine, the intracranial contents normally consist of brain tissue, intravascular blood, and CSF. If any of these components increase in volume, the others must reciprocally decrease to avoid increasing pressure. In the setting of injury, neuronal injury and death occur and lead to **cytotoxic edema**, which results in increased pressure and a compensatory reduction in blood flow and the production of **cerebrospinal fluid**. As the pressure is further elevated to high levels and cerebral perfusion continues to decrease, further neuronal death and edema occur. The onset of edema is usually slow and reaches its maximal level within 48 to 72 hours after injury. Therefore, these patients should be monitored closely, often in an intensive care unit, over the following few days because the true neurologic sequelae of edema may not initially be obvious early after injury. The progress of **cerebral edema** may be monitored by neurologic examination, **computed tomography**, and sometimes the use of **intracranial pressure**–monitoring devices. These devices are commonly used to monitor patients with altered consciousness following head injury or patients with **Glasgow Coma Scale** scores lower than 8. A baseline CT is initially obtained to identify intracranial hemorrhage or a mass lesion that may need to be evacuated surgically. Once these entities are ruled out, medical treatment is started to counter the progress of edema. This may be accomplished, but not necessarily in this order, by (1) elevating the head of the bed 15 to 30 degrees; (2) maintaining the patient's head in a straight position to facilitate cerebral venous drainage; (3) temporary hyperventilation to $P_{CO_2}$ levels of 30 to 35 mm Hg; (4) **hyperosmolar therapy** and sometimes fluid restriction to minimize edema; (5) intermittent drainage of CSF through a pressure-monitoring catheter placed in the ventricular system; (6) paralytic agents to minimize patient agitation or elevated blood pressure, which may further increase ICP; and (7) neuronal burst-suppressive medications to minimize cerebral metabolism and counter neuronal distress from low perfusion. Finally, and in rare circumstances, decompressive **hemicraniectomy** may be indicated if enough swelling occurs from the edema and the high ICP is refractory to the aforementioned medical therapies. Frequently, the first few therapies are performed and the later, more invasive therapies are pursued only in refractory cases. Exciting experimental animal models using neuroprotective agents have not shown the same beneficial effects in humans when translated to clinical trials. New research on induced hypothermia has demonstrated promise in small case studies, but larger randomized trials have not yet been performed. **Steroids** are believed to decrease vasogenic edema by limiting the permeability of the vasculature, but they have not been shown to impede cell death from trauma or limit cytotoxic edema. No meta-analysis has been performed, but the largest trial to date on traumatic brain injury demonstrated an increase in mortality with steroids, and therefore steroids are not recommended.

**ANSWER: A**

14. Which of the following statements regarding subarachnoid hemorrhage (SAH) is the most accurate?

   A. Normal findings on CT of the brain exclude the possibility of SAH.

   B. Aneurysms occur most frequently on the basilar artery.

   C. Surgical or endovascular treatment is recommended for patients who are neurologically intact and have an uncomplicated aneurysmal SAH.

   D. The use of hypertension, hypervolemia, hemodilution (triple-H therapy), and calcium channel blockers is contraindicated for the treatment of vasospasm.

   E. Aneurysms are the most common cause of SAH.

*Ref.: 4, 5*

**COMMENTS:** Trauma is the most common cause of **subarachnoid hemorrhage**, although aneurysms are the most common "nontraumatic" etiology. In the traumatic setting, patients commonly complain of only mild headache, and the neurologic sequelae are rarely as profound as observed in those with **aneurysmal subarachnoid hemorrhage**. Sudden severe headache followed by altered consciousness is the usual clinical pattern following aneurysmal SAH. Focal neurologic deficits may occur, but they are less common than those seen after occlusion of major intracranial arteries. The sequelae vary, depending on the size of the hemorrhage, and range from headache to death. Although CT is the diagnostic method of choice to confirm SAH, approximately 15% to 20% of patients with documented hemorrhage have normal findings on CT within 24 hours of the onset of SAH. It is therefore important to perform a lumbar puncture when SAH is suspected and CT is negative for SAH. Maintenance of a high red blood cell count (often >100,000/mm$^3$) in the first and last tube is indicative of SAH rather

than traumatic lumbar puncture. Furthermore, the presence of xanthochromia indicates hemorrhage, although xanthochromia may not be present if the hemorrhage occurred in the preceding few days. **Angiography** is helpful to confirm the presence of an **aneurysm** and is the gold standard for diagnosis. **Computed tomographic angiography** and **magnetic resonance angiography** are also helpful but may miss smaller aneurysms because of their limited resolution. Most intracranial aneurysms arise from the large intracranial arteries of the circle of Willis and at the origin of the vertebrobasilar arteries. The most common sites of aneurysm, in decreasing order of prevalence, are the anterior communicating artery and posterior communicating artery (nearly equal prevalence), middle cerebral artery, and vertebrobasilar system. Not all aneurysms rupture. Autopsy studies of the population as a whole indicate an approximately 4% to 5% prevalence of aneurysms. The risk for rupture and need for treatment of aneurysms found incidentally (no SAH) are much debated topics. Recent studies have used the size and location of incidentally found nonruptured aneurysms to stratify the risk for rupture, and the necessity for and type of treatment must be discussed with the patient based on the individual risk for rupture. Multiple aneurysms are present 20% of the time and tend to be symmetrical in distribution or arise from the same parent artery on opposite sides of the circulation. Aneurysms are congenital in nature (not caused by hypertension), but risk factors, predominately hypertension, are believed to induce rupture. The incidence of rupture is highest in patients between the ages of 40 and 60 years. Most aneurysms are "false" aneurysms, as opposed to "true" aneurysms, which contain all three layers of the vessel, or "pseudoaneurysms," which contain no layers and are simply surrounded by previous blood clot. They most commonly have a saccular or berry-like shape, hence the name berry aneurysm. The goal of treatment is to isolate the aneurysm from the force of systolic blood flow. This should be attempted as early as possible. After initial rupture the aneurysm thromboses, but if left untreated, it may rerupture at an incidence of 4% on the first day and 1.5% every subsequent day to a risk of approximately 20% at 2 weeks and about 50% at 6 months. It is commonly recommended that surgical correction be performed within 48 to 72 hours, if possible. Antifibrinolytics, such as ε-aminocaproic acid, have been found to decrease the rate of rebleeding during the time preceding treatment. Current options for definitive treatment involve either craniotomy for clipping or endovascular coiling (with or without stenting) of the aneurysm. Vasospasm, or delayed ischemic neurologic deficit, is a common entity in patients with SAH. Symptomatic vasospasm occurs in approximately 15% of patients with SAH, results in the highest morbidity in patients surviving the initial hemorrhage, and can be aggressively treated after the ruptured aneurysm is secured by either clips or coils. It often occurs in delayed fashion after the initial hemorrhage (usually after the third day) and is seen most commonly between the sixth and eighth days after hemorrhage up until 2 weeks. There is no definitive way to predict whether or when **vasospasm** will occur. A calcium channel blocker (nimodipine) and relative hypertension, hypervolemia, and hemodilution (triple-H therapy) are the medical therapies most commonly recommended for combating vasospasm.

**ANSWER: C**

15. Which of the following statements regarding subdural hematomas (SDHs) is false?

   A. Acute SDHs are generally unilateral and have a poorer prognosis than chronic SDHs do.

   B. Adequate treatment of an acute SDH usually consists of drainage through bur holes.

C. Chronic SDHs frequently recur.

D. Chronic SDHs should be suspected in elderly patients with progressive changes in mental status, even without a definite history of trauma.

E. SDHs carry a worse prognosis than do epidural hematomas (EDHs).

*Ref.:* 5-7, 12

**COMMENTS: Subdural hematomas** are caused by rupture of veins traversing the subdural space or by arterial bleeding from parenchymal lacerations. Their symptoms and treatment depend on the rapidity of hematoma formation. All types of SDH (acute, subacute, or chronic) have in common the presence of a decreased level of consciousness out of proportion to the observed focal neurologic deficit. **Acute subdural hematomas** cause progressive neurologic deficit within 48 hours of injury. They usually follow severe head trauma, are unilateral, often have both arterial and venous sources of bleeding, and can progress rapidly. The diagnosis should be considered in any patient with a severe head injury who exhibits deteriorated neurologic status or who is unresponsive with a focal neurologic deficit. The hematomas are solid and easily visualized on CT as a hyperdense collection or sometimes a hypodense collection in the hyperacute setting with active bleeding. In contrast to **epidural hematomas**, they are crescent shaped, cross suture lines, but do not cross dural reflections. They can be bilateral, and adjacent intracerebral hematomas are often present. Treatment requires formal craniotomy with removal of solid clot and control of bleeding points. **Subacute subdural hematomas** are defined as those more than 48 hours but less than 2 weeks old. Patients are usually less severely injured than those with acute SDHs, and marked fluctuation of the level of consciousness or headache should alert surgeons to the diagnosis. With large hematomas, third-nerve palsy with dilation of the pupils is a warning sign that midbrain compression secondary to temporal lobe herniation is occurring. CT may not identify the collection because the hematoma becomes isodense 10 to 12 days after its formation, and bilateral hematomas may be present. If the clot is completely liquefied, two bur holes may be placed followed by copious irrigation. Otherwise, formal craniotomy may be required if the hematoma is more solid than liquid. **Chronic subdural hematomas** most often develop in the elderly, frequently without a clear history of antecedent trauma. They can occur months after the initial injury and should be suspected in patients with decreasing or fluctuating mental status out of proportion to the focal neurologic deficit. The hematoma is commonly liquid, and drainage via bur holes is often adequate. However, chronic SDHs frequently recur when associated with subdural membranes, which may then require formal craniotomy to strip the superficial membrane. Subdural-peritoneal shunting may also eventually be necessary. Because of the tremendous mass effect on the brain from an SDH, mortality may be as high as 60% and can approach 90% in patients older than 80 years without surgical treatment. The mortality associated with untreated EDHs is approximately 50%, lower than that for SDHs because the dural attachments prevent the EDH from compressing the brain to the degree observed with SDH. Patients with EDH may sometimes initially have a "lucid interval," with temporary clinical improvement after the trauma followed by deterioration as the blood accumulates epidurally.

**ANSWER:** B

16. Which of the following statements regarding intracranial vascular malformations is the most accurate?

A. Arteriovenous malformations (AVMs) are the most common vascular malformations in the brain.

B. Venous angiomas commonly bleed and surgical removal is usually required.

C. AVM rupture and aneurysm rupture may cause spontaneous SAH at nearly equal frequency.

D. AVMs have a 2% to 4% incidence of hemorrhage per year.

E. Capillary telangiectases are the least common vascular malformations in the brain.

*Ref.:* 2, 5, 7

**COMMENTS: Vascular malformations** in the brain include **venous angiomas**, **cavernomas**, **capillary telangiectases**, and **arteriovenous malformations**. AVMs receive more attention than the other, more common lesions because of their propensity to cause seizures or life-threatening hemorrhage. AVMs are irregular connections of arteries to veins with irregular walls and a nidus in the center. Ten percent are associated with **aneurysms**, most commonly on the feeding artery. These irregularities lead to a 2% to 4% incidence of hemorrhage per year. Intracranial hemorrhage is the most common initial symptom, and it is mostly intraparenchymal, although **subarachnoid hemorrhage** may also occur. AVMs are the second most common cause of spontaneous SAH (4% to 10%), with aneurysms being the most common (75% to 80%). Most AVMs are symptomatic when found, whereas the other vascular malformations are commonly incidental findings. In fact, CT or MRI is necessary to detect **cavernomas** or **capillary telangiectases**, which are both angiographically occult lesions. However, capillary telangiectases are often missed on MRI as well. Cavernomas hemorrhage at a rate of about 0.7% per year. They are most commonly identified radiographically after a small hemorrhage that was manifested clinically as a headache or seizure. Capillary telangiectases and **venous angiomas** rarely hemorrhage but are the first and second most common vascular malformations overall, respectively. Neither require treatment.

**ANSWER:** D

17. Which of the following statements regarding peripheral nerve injuries is false?

A. Neurapraxic injury does not require surgical resection of the nerve root involved to eliminate pain.

B. Axonal regeneration progresses at a rate of 1 mm/day after a 10- to 20-day lag period.

C. Denervation atrophy of muscles becomes irreversible after 12 to 15 months.

D. Restoration of sensory loss is not possible after muscle atrophy secondary to denervation is complete.

E. Recovery is influenced by the cause of the injury, the patient's age, the type of nerve injured, and the severity of injury to nearby vessels and bone.

*Ref.:* 2, 3, 8

**COMMENTS:** There are several classifications of nerve injuries. The Seddon classification uses three terms to classify nerve injuries: **neurapraxia**, **axonotmesis**, and **neurotmesis**. With **neurapraxia**, anatomic continuity of the nerve is preserved, and there is often incomplete motor paralysis with little muscle atrophy and considerable sparing of sensory and autonomic function. Neura-praxia, in simplified terms, is a bruise. Operative repair is not indicated, and the quality of recovery is excellent. **Axonotmesis** is the loss of axonal continuity without interruption of the investing myelin tissue. There is complete motor, sensory, and autonomic paralysis and progressive muscle atrophy. Operative repair is not indicated, and recovery occurs at a rate of about 1 mm/day. **Neu-rotmesis** is a more severe injury, with significant disorganization within the nerve or actual disruption of continuity of the nerve and its investing myelin tissues. It is common with penetrating trauma and less common with compression injury, such as that seen with surgical positioning. Recovery is impossible without operative repair. After disruption, axonal sprouting begins within 10 to 20 days. After operative repair, distal growth occurs at a rate of 1 mm/day after the initial 10- to 20- day lag period. The degree of recovery is a function of the patient's age (with greater recovery in younger patients), type of nerve involved (pure motor or sensory nerves recover better than do mixed motor and sensory nerves), level of nerve injury (distal is better), and duration of denervation (shorter tends to be better). Early repair of the severed nerve has the advantage of clearer anatomy and a longer period for regeneration, but late repair also has advantages. If more than 12 to 15 months is required for regenerating axons to reach a denervated muscle, a significant degree of denervation atrophy will have occurred and is irreversible. In contrast, sensory loss may be recovered after prolonged periods of denervation, and thus a nerve repair can provide protective sensory function in the atrophied distal extremity. With **peripheral nerve injury**, the site of injury and nerve activity can be detected by **electromyography** only after 2 to 3 weeks. A rare late consequence of peripheral nerve injury is **causalgia**, a painful condition causing burning sensations, swelling, and skin changes in the distribution of a partially injured mixed peripheral nerve. It is believed to be caused by "sensitization" of the traumatized nerve with sympathetic hyperactivity. Treatment consists of medications or sympathectomy in intractable cases. The role of **corticosteroids** in the treatment of peripheral nerve injury is unclear, and level III evidence suggesting a beneficial role is lacking and mostly anecdotal.

**ANSWER:  D**

18. Which of the following is false regarding brain and spine tumors?

   A. Intracranial schwannomas most commonly arise from the eighth cranial nerve, and spinal schwannomas are most commonly found in the intradural and extramedullary space on sensory nerves.

   B. Spinal cord ependymomas are the most common primary adult spinal cord tumors and are commonly found in the cervical cord.

   C. Most intracranial tumors are benign.

   D. Meningiomas arise from the arachnoid layer of the brain, as opposed to the brain tissue itself.

   E. Glioblastoma multiforme (GBM) is the most common primary brain tumor and carries the worst prognosis.

*Ref.:* 2, 3, 7, 8, 10

**COMMENTS:** CNS tumors can be classified in many ways, such as the tissue of origin or even location. The main types include astrocytic tumors (including **pilocytic astrocytoma**, **anaplastic astrocytoma**, **glioblastoma multiforme**, **oligodendroglioma**, and ependymoma), neuroectodermal tumors (including ganglioglioma and dysembryoplastic neuroepithelial tumor), embryonal neuroepithelial tumors (including medulloblastoma, neuroblastoma, and pineoblastoma), choroid plexus tumors, pineal region tumors, peripheral nerve sheath tumors (including neurofibroma and schwannoma), **meningiomas**, parasellar tumors (including pituitary tumors, craniopharyngiomas, and Rathke cleft cysts), blood-based tumors (including lymphoma), germ cell tumors, and miscellaneous tumors (including dermoids, epidermoids, and colloid cysts). In both the brain and spinal cord, **metastases** are the most common tumors. The most common **brain metastases** are from lung, breast, skin, and kidney cancers. Approximately one fourth of patients who die of cancer have brain metastases on autopsy. One half of all patients with brain metastases will have a single metastasis. If it is a solitary lesion, the patient has an approximately 6-month expected longevity from systemic cancer. The lesion may be primarily surgically resected if accessible, followed by radiation therapy in certain circumstances. Whole-brain irradiation versus focused beam irradiation, along with possibly chemotherapy, is determined on an individual basis and tumor sensitivity. The spine is also a common target for metastases, most commonly from a large epidural venous system called the Batson plexus. Up to 40% of patients who die of cancer have **spine metastases** on autopsy. In the brain, **gliomas** are the most common primary tumor, with GBM being the most frequent. The World Health Organization (WHO) developed a grading system for CNS tumors in which grade I is the most benign and grade IV is the most malignant. GBMs are grade IV tumors. The prognosis of patients with GBM is poor, with median survival being 3 months without treatment. With surgery, radiation therapy, and chemotherapy, survival averages 14 months. Of the more common brain tumors, **meningiomas** arise from the arachnoid cap cells of the brain coverings and are most commonly located parasagittally. **Schwannomas** arise from sensory nerves, with the eighth cranial nerve being the most common. **Ependymomas** arise in the ventricles. Oligodendrogliomas arise in the cerebral hemispheres, usually in the frontal lobe. **Medulloblastoma** is one of the most common primary pediatric tumors, and it arises in the cerebellum of the posterior fossa. In the spinal cord, ependymomas and **astrocytomas** are the most common primary tumors, with ependymomas being more common in adults and astrocytomas more common in children. Although primary brain tumors tend to be malignant, primary spinal cord tumors tend to be benign. **Spine tumors** may be extradural (most commonly metastases), intradural and extramedullary (most commonly schwannomas, neurofibromas, or meningiomas), or intradural and intramedullary (most commonly ependymomas and astrocytomas). Because spinal ependymomas often have a dissectible plane and tend to not diffusely infiltrate the nervous tissue itself, they may be resected while maintaining stable neurologic function. They, like spinal cord astrocytomas, are commonly found in the cervical region.

**ANSWER:  C**

19. Which of the following myotome and dermatome distributions is correct?

   A. C1 has a myotome distribution as part of the ansa cervicalis with supply to the neck "strap muscles," but no dermatome distribution.

   B. T4 has a myotome distribution to the intercostal muscles and a dermatome distribution to the nipple area.

   C. L1 has a myotome distribution to the iliopsoas muscle and a dermatome distribution to the inguinal area.

D. L5 has a myotome distribution to the extensor hallucis longus and anterior tibialis muscles and a dermatome distribution to the lateral aspect of the calf and foot.

E. All of the above.

*Ref.: 5, 7, 10*

**COMMENTS:** Thirty-one paired spinal nerves provide afferent and efferent innervation to the body, except C1, which has only motor function. Compression of a spinal nerve can lead to pain, numbness, or weakness in the distribution of that spinal nerve. This is known as **radiculopathy**. When radiculopathy is manifested as pain only, certain ones mimic common medical conditions. A left-sided midthoracic radiculopathy can be mistaken for cardiac disease, a right-sided lower thoracic radiculopathy can mimic gallbladder disease, and an L1 or L2 radiculopathy can be mistaken for hernia symptoms. Fortunately, disk herniations at these levels are uncommon. Common levels for disk herniation are C5-6, C6-7, L4-5, and L5-S1. The disk herniation usually causes a radiculopathy in the nerve root paired with the lower vertebra (i.e., C5-6 causes a C6 radiculopathy). In the cervical spine, a nerve roots exits above its number-associated pedicle, and the intervertebral disk space is located near the inferior portion of the pedicle. Therefore, the herniated disk compresses the lower nerve as it exits because the higher nerve is protected by the pedicle. In the lumbar region, the given nerve root exits below and in close proximity to its number-associated pedicle, but the intervertebral disk space is located far below the pedicle. Therefore, a herniated lumbar disk often still spares the nerve exiting at that interspace (even though the pedicle is not protecting it as in the cervical spine) and instead compresses the lower nerve root heading toward the interspace below.

**ANSWER:** E

20. Regarding spinal cord injury, which of the following incorrectly describes the syndrome listed?

A. In anterior spinal artery syndrome, bilateral loss of motor and pain sensation occurs with preservation of position and vibratory sensation.

B. In posterior spinal artery syndrome, bilateral loss of position and vibration sensation occurs with preservation of motor and pain sensation.

C. In central cord syndrome, bilateral motor and pain sensation is lost, worse in the lower extremities than the upper extremities and worse in the proximal ends of extremities than in the distal ends of extremities.

D. In Brown-Sequard syndrome, ipsilateral motor and position sensation is lost along with contralateral pain and temperature sensation.

E. In cauda equina syndrome, unilateral or bilateral loss of motor and sensory function occurs in the distribution of multiple nerve roots, including bladder areflexia and stool incontinence.

*Ref.: 2, 10, 11*

**COMMENTS:** The syndromes of spinal cord injury are named according to the area of injury and have deficits related to the tracts running in that area of the spinal cord. The anterior two thirds of the spinal cord holds the corticospinal tracts and the spinothalamic tract. Injury to this area via compression or infarction of the anterior spinal artery leads to paralysis and loss of pain and temperature sensation below the level of the lesion, with sparing of proprioception, which runs in the dorsal columns. The posterior spinal cord holds the dorsal columns, which are involved in position and vibratory sense and are supplied by the paired posterior spinal arteries. Lesions in this area result in loss of these modalities below the level of the lesion, with sparing of motor and pain/temperature sensation. The cervical central spinal cord consists of gray matter, crossing fibers of the spinothalamic tract, and motor fibers to the upper extremities. Injury here causes **central cord syndrome**. Most common in the elderly with preexisting cervical stenosis, injury is caused by neck hyperextension in which hypertrophied perispinal ligaments compress the already stenosed cervical cord. This leads to weakness and loss of pain sensation in the arms more than in the legs and distally worse than proximally. Central cord syndrome was originally thought to occur as a result of somatotopy of the corticospinal tract and ischemia from cord impingement, but this theory has recently been questioned. Axial hemisection of the spinal cord from penetrating trauma leads to **Brown-Sequard syndrome**. Deficits associated with this syndrome are loss of ipsilateral motor, position, and vibratory sensation and contralateral pain and temperature sensation because of the crossing fibers of the spinothalamic tracts. The nerve roots of the cauda equina arise from the distal spinal cord at L1-2. Compression of nerve roots of the cauda equina leads to variable loss of all functions of the nerve roots involved, along with radicular pain.

**ANSWER:** C

21. Which of the following statements regarding brain abscesses is false?

A. The brain is resistant to infection despite its high glucose content.

B. The brain is extremely effective in walling off infections.

C. Brain abscesses are classified as acute, subacute, and chronic.

D. Prompt drainage is indicated for all types of brain abscesses.

E. Corticosteroids may be useful in treating this type of infection.

*Ref.: 2, 3, 7*

**COMMENTS:** The brain is generally resistant to infection because of the blood-brain barrier unless previously damaged by trauma, hemorrhage, or anoxia. Once infected, the brain is effective in walling off the infection and is capable of isolating the **abscess** from the uninvolved brain and systemic circulation, thus making sterilization by systemic antibiotics difficult. The three major sources of brain abscesses include (1) direct extension from middle ear, mastoid, and nasal sinus infections (commonly affecting the temporal lobe and cerebellar hemispheres); (2) hematogenous spread (as occurs with cyanotic heart defects or pulmonary AVMs with right-to-left shunts); and (3) direct trauma. The most common organisms are *Streptococcus* and *Staphylococcus*. Brain abscesses are classified as acute, in which they follow a course similar to and difficult to differentiate from subdural empyema; subacute, with a picture in between acute and chronic; and chronic, often with progressive neurologic deficit and an expanding mass with a longer history (2 weeks to 2 months). MRI is the most accurate indirect means of making the diagnosis and is helpful before performing surgical drainage. Treatment consists of medical measures (antibiotics) or surgical evacuation. Medical therapy requires 6 to 8 weeks of intravenous antibiotics and the use of **corticosteroids** if severe edema and mass effect are present. On follow-up imaging, if an increase in size occurs, surgical drainage should be considered. Surgery is also necessary if the abscess is causing enough mass effect to induce focal symptoms or if identification of the organism is needed to select appropriate antibiotics. Even with surgical drainage, antibiotics are still required for at least 6 to 8 weeks, and it may take longer than 10 weeks for significant resolution of the capsule and its enhancement to be observed on imaging. Seizures are a common sequelae of brain abscess. Brain abscess recurs in 8% to 10% of patients.

**ANSWER:** D

22. Which of the following is true regarding pediatric trauma?

   A. Spinal cord injury without radiologic abnormality (SCIWORA) is a diagnosis made after neurologic symptoms are present despite normal findings on MRI.

   B. Because of their inability to speak, the GCS cannot be used in infants.

   C. Age younger than 3 years, nonparietal skull fractures, isolated SDH in the absence of witnessed trauma, retinal hemorrhages, and long-bone fractures at varying stages of healing are all signs arguing against the diagnosis of nonaccidental trauma.

   D. Spinal cord injuries are relatively uncommon in young children.

   E. Interpretations of pediatric spinal radiographs are similar to those of adults, and pathologic fractures and subluxations are often easily identified.

*Ref.:* 5, 7, 9, 11

**COMMENTS: Spinal cord injury without radiologic abnormality** is an injury originally described in children in the 1980s before the advent of MRI. Signs of myelopathy were present in pediatric patients after known cervical spine trauma, but plain radiography and CT showed no pathology. Therefore, the current definition does not necessarily include the complete absence of imaging abnormalities because abnormal MRI findings may very well be present. The incidence has been reported to be as high as 36% in children with traumatic myelopathy. Because MRI has become a mainstay imaging modality in the evaluation of cervical trauma, children in whom SCIWORA has been diagnosed have been shown to exhibit ligamentous or disk injury, complete spinal cord transection, spinal cord hemorrhage, or occasionally, normal findings on MRI. SCIWORA most commonly results from hyperflexion or hyperextension movements. Because the adult **Glasgow Coma Scale** assessment is not appropriate for the functional level of infants, particularly in its verbal and motor aspects, a modified version known as the Pediatric Glasgow Coma Scale has been developed. It still uses the eye, verbal, and motor components, but to an age-appropriate level for infants. **Nonaccidental trauma** is most common in children younger than 3 years. Nonparietal skull fractures, isolated **subdural hematomas** without witnessed trauma, retinal hemorrhages, and long-bone fractures at various stages of healing are common inclusion signs for this diagnosis. Spinal cord injuries account for less than 5% of all childhood spinal injuries. The spinal ligaments are lax and the facet joints are oriented more horizontally in children, thus making vertebral body subluxation and ligamentous injury more common than fractures or cord injuries. Because of incomplete fusion of ossification centers in a pediatric patient's spine, radiolucencies may falsely appear to be fractures and make interpretation of pediatric spine imaging challenging. Such radiolucencies may occur in the anterior arch of C1

and the junction of the dens with the body of C2, a finding representing persistent synchondrosis that may mimic a fracture. In similar fashion, the tip may fail to fuse with the peg body of the dens, a condition called ossiculum terminale persistens (differs from os odontoideum), which can appear similar to an odontoid fracture. Laxity in ligaments may also allow normal movement in the pediatric spine that would be considered pathologic in adults. The high cervical levels may move up to 3 to 4 mm with flexion, which is considered a normal variant in the pediatric spine. The atlantodens interval may be particularly prominent with motion as well and be mistakenly diagnosed as instability.

**ANSWER:** D

23. Which of the following is true regarding brain metastases?

   A. More than 75% of patients who die of cancer have intracranial metastasis on autopsy.

   B. The most common primary malignancies from which brain metastases arise are lung, breast, and prostate cancers.

   C. Melanoma, colorectal, and renal carcinoma are extremely sensitive to whole-brain radiation therapy (WBRT).

   D. Patients with a single metastasis and good prognostic features often benefit from surgery followed by WBRT.

   E. Most brain metastases are chemosensitive.

*Ref.:* 2, 3, 5, 7, 8, 11, 24

**COMMENTS: Brain metastases** are the most common brain tumors in adults. They occur in 10% to 30% of adults with systemic disease and are found at autopsy in 25% of patients who have died of systemic disease. The most common primary sources are lung cancer (40% to 50%), breast cancer (15% to 25%), and melanoma (5% to 20%). Prostate carcinomas rarely metastasize to the brain. As with any cancer, treatment options for brain metastases are surgery, radiotherapy (**whole-brain radiotherapy** and **stereotactic radiosurgery**), and **chemotherapy**. Management is based on the extent of systemic disease and the number, size, location, and histology of the brain metastases. The patient's initial performance status is also crucial and is rated by the Karnofsky performance scale (KPS). Simplified, a good KPS score is one greater than 80, which describes a patient who is able to carry out normal daily activity and work without special assistance. WBRT has long been the most frequently used therapeutic modality for brain metastases. Currently, it is used for patients with multiple metastases (usually more than three), for metastases too large for radiosurgery (usually >2 to 3 cm), and for patients with disease progression after previous treatment. Radiosensitive tumors are lung and breast tumors, whereas melanoma, colon tumors, and renal tumors are fairly resistant. Commonly, WBRT is used in addition to surgery or radiosurgery, although it may be used alone, predominately in the scenario of active systemic disease with multiple large metastases. Cognitive decline following WBRT is of concern and factors into the overall treatment decision. Stereotactic radiosurgery may also be very useful in carefully selected patients. Surgery for brain metastases obtains tissue for diagnosis, provides therapy by resecting at least some of the tumor burden, and may be used to deliver brachytherapy. Like WBRT, surgery is commonly used in addition to other therapies such as WBRT, radiosurgery, or chemotherapy. Several studies have shown that patients with a single metastasis and good prognosis benefit from surgery followed by radiation therapy. Brain metastases are relatively resistant to chemotherapy. It is usually reserved for recurrence after standard therapy.

**ANSWER:** D

# REFERENCES

1. Kandel ER, Schwartz JH, editors: *Principles of neural sciences, Part II*, London, 1981, Edward Arnold.
2. Schwartz SI, Shires GT, Spencer FC: *Principles of surgery*, ed 7, New York, 1999, McGraw-Hill.
3. Sabiston DC Jr: *Textbook of surgery*, ed 15, Philadelphia, 1997, WB Saunders.
4. Ross JS, Masaryk TJ, Modic MT, et al: Intracranial aneurysms: evaluation of MR angiography, *AJR Am J Roentgenol* 155:159–165, 1990.
5. Greenberg MS: *Handbook of neurosurgery*, New York, 2001, Thieme Medical Publishers.
6. Narayan RK, Rosner MJ, Pitts LH, et al: *Guidelines for the management of severe head injury*, Chicago, 1995, Brain Trauma Foundation.
7. Schmidek HH, Sweet WH: *Operative neurosurgical techniques*, ed 3, Philadelphia, 1995, WB Saunders.
8. Greenfield LJ: *Surgery*, ed 3, Philadelphia, 2001, Lippincott, Williams & Wilkins.
9. Bullock MR, Povlishock JT: Guidelines for the management of severe traumatic brain injury. Editor's Commentary, *J Neurotrauma* 24(Suppl 1):2, 2007.
10. Way LW: *Current surgical diagnosis and treatment*, ed 10, Norwalk, CT, 1994, Appleton & Lange.
11. Menezes AH, Sonntag VK, Benzel EC, et al: *Principles of spinal surgery*, New York, 1991, McGraw-Hill.
12. Atlas SW: *Magnetic resonance imaging of the brain and spine*, New York, 1991, Raven Press.
13. Sciubba DM, Dorsi MJ, Kretzler R, et al: Computed tomography reconstruction artifact suggesting cervical spine subluxation, *J Neurosurg Spine* 8:84–87, 2008.
14. Doran SE, Papadopoulos SM, Ducker TB, et al: Magnetic resonance imaging documentation of coexistent traumatic locked facets of the cervical spine and disc herniation, *J Neurosurg* 79:341–345, 1993.
15. Bracken MB, Shepard MJ, Collins WF, et al: A randomized controlled trail of methylprednisolone or naloxone in the treatment of acute spinal cord injury, *N Engl J Med* 322:1405–1411, 1990.
16. Hadley MN, Walters BC, Grabb PA, et al: Guidelines for the management of acute cervical spine and spinal cord injuries, *Clin Neurosurg* 49:407–498, 2002.
17. Ritter AM, Muizelaar JP, Barnes T, et al: Brain stem blood flow, pupillary response, and outcome in patients with severe head injuries, *Neurosurgery.* 44:941–948, 1999.
18. Aston S, Seasley R, Thorne C, editors: *Grabb and Smith's plastic surgery*, ed 5, Philadelphia, 1997, Lippincott-Raven.
19. Greer DM, Varelas PN, Haque S, et al: Variability of brain death determination guidelines in leading U.S. neurologic institutions, *Neurology* 70:284–289, 2008.
20. Clusmann H, Schaller C, Schramm J: Fixed and dilated pupils after trauma, stroke, and previous intracranial surgery: management and outcome, *J Neurol Neurosurg Psychiatry* 71:175–181, 2001.
21. Young JS, Blow O, Turrentine F, et al: Is there an upper limit of intracranial pressure in patients with severe head injury if cerebral perfusion pressure is maintained? *Neurosurg Focus* 15(6):E2, 2003.
22. Muizelaar JP, Marmarou A, Ward JD, et al: Adverse effects of prolonged hyperventilation in patients with severe head injury: a randomized clinical trail, *J Neurosurg* 75:731–739, 1991.
23. Alderson P, Roberts I: Corticosteroids for acute traumatic brain injury, *Cochrane Database Syst Rev* 1:CD000196, 2005.
24. Ranjan T, Abrey, L: Current management of metastatic brain disease, *Neurotherapeutics* 6:598–603, 2009.

# C. Urology

*Michael R. Abern, M.D., and Kalyan C. Latchamsetty, M.D.*

1. Regarding the management of blunt renal trauma, which of the following is true?

   A. Contusions are best treated by observation until the gross hematuria subsides.

   B. Parenchymal lacerations secondary to blunt trauma require routine exploration because of the risk for secondary hemorrhage or infection.

   C. Nonexpanding retroperitoneal flank hematomas encountered during laparotomy should be explored.

   D. On exploring a perinephric hematoma, the fascia of Gerota is opened first to facilitate control of the vessels.

   E. Nonvisualization of the kidneys, on CT requires immediate operative exploration.

   *Ref.:* 1

**COMMENTS:** As with any visceral organ, a spectrum of **renal injuries** may occur following blunt trauma. Renal contusions are the most common renal injury and are managed conservatively with bed rest and observation. Parenchymal lacerations confined to the renal cortex may also be treated nonoperatively if the patient is stable. Deeper lacerations extending into the calyceal system may require primary surgical repair. When an expanding retroperitoneal hematoma is encountered, it should be explored. However, when a nonexpanding perinephric hematoma is encountered, high-dose intravenous urographic studies should be done if no other imaging study is available to evaluate the potentially injured kidney and to confirm the presence of a contralateral functioning kidney. Preoperative CT provides accurate staging, thereby allowing one to determine the best treatment modality and to manage the majority of patients by observation. The key surgical principle in the approach to an injured kidney is to obtain control of the vascular pedicle first. If the fascia of Gerota is incised first, the tamponade effect may be released, and a significant hemorrhage could occur and possibly lead to nephrectomy. Moreover, if nephrectomy is necessary, the presence of a functioning contralateral kidney is verified via intravenous pyelography (IVP) or CT before exploration. Penetrating renal injury usually requires exploration, but some patients may be managed nonoperatively, provided that adequate imaging staging is done and they are not undergoing laparotomy for associated injury. Traditionally, nonvisualization of the kidneys has been further evaluated with renal angiographic studies. Recently, spiral CT has provided adequate evaluation of the renal vessels. Nonvisualization of the renal artery may be caused by total avulsion of the renal artery and vein, renal artery thrombosis, absence of the kidney, or severe contusion resulting in major vascular spasm. If a kidney cannot be visualized on arteriography, exploration and revascularization are indicated if salvage of the kidney is possible.

**ANSWER:** A

2. Which of the following statements is true regarding renal vascular anatomy?

   A. Solitary renal arteries are seen in approximately 20% to 30% of patients.

   B. The right renal artery usually crosses ventral to the vena cava.

   C. The left renal vein usually crosses dorsal to the aorta.

   D. The right adrenal and gonadal veins typically empty into the right renal vein.

   E. The renal arteries are end arteries.

   *Ref.:* 2

**COMMENTS:** Approximately two thirds of normal kidneys are supplied by a single renal artery arising from the aorta, near the upper aspect of the second lumbar vertebra. Each renal artery has approximately five segmental branches that are end arteries. Occlusion of the segmental vessels therefore causes infarction. Renal arterial anomalies are more often present in abnormally located kidneys. Venous drainage of the kidneys often involves collateral vessels, particularly on the left side, via the gonadal, adrenal, and lumbar veins. The renal vein itself is usually singular on the left side but multiple on the right side approximately 10% of the time. Because the aorta in normal individuals lies to the left side of the vena cava, the right renal artery crosses behind the vena cava and the left renal vein crosses ventral to the aorta. This is consistent with the general anatomic principle that major systemic veins pass ventral to their associated arteries. The longer length of the left renal vein is advantageous when the left kidney is used as a donor organ during renal transplantation. The right adrenal and gonadal veins empty directly into the inferior vena cava.

**ANSWER:** E

3. Which of the following findings occurs in most patients with renal cell carcinoma?

   A. Hypertension

   B. Erythrocytosis

   C. Hematuria

   D. Acute varicocele

   E. Palpable flank mass

   *Ref.:* 3

**COMMENTS:** Among the many symptoms that have been associated with **renal cell carcinoma**, hematuria, pain, and an abdominal mass are the most common. Only 10% of patients have the classic triad of hematuria, pain, and an abdominal mass. Hypertension (37.5% of cases) may result from renal vascular compression but is more commonly seen with Wilms tumor. Fever (17%) is believed to result from tumor necrosis. A small percentage of patients exhibit erythrocytosis (1% to 5%), which has been related to the production of erythropoietin-like substances by the tumor. It is more common, however, for patients with renal cell carcinoma to have anemia (36%) than erythrocytosis. Renal vein thrombosis and a subsequent acute varicocele (3%) develop in a small percentage of patients with renal tumors. **Hematuria** occurs in about 60% of patients. Renal cell carcinomas occur in an approximate 2 : 1 male-to-female ratio. In most patients it is diagnosed during the sixth and seventh decades of life. More than 50% of renal cell carcinomas are now detected incidentally because of the increased use of imaging for a variety of abdominal symptoms. Thus, masses are rarely palpable on physical examination. The TNM staging system classifies a T1/T2 tumor as being confined to the kidney, with tumors larger than 7.0 cm classified at a higher stage (T2). T3 tumors involve the renal veins, inferior vena cava, or perinephric tissues that are confined by the fascia of Gerota. T4 tumors extend beyond this fascia. Nodal status is stratified by size, number of nodes, and whether metastatic disease is present or absent. Lesions that involve the inferior vena cava may still be cured with surgical therapy, and such involvement is not considered a contraindication to surgery.

**ANSWER: C**

4. Transitional cell cancers of the renal pelvis are best treated by which of the following?

   A. Nephrectomy

   B. Nephroureterectomy with excision of the ureter to the level of the bladder

   C. Nephroureterectomy with excision of the bladder cuff

   D. Nephroureterectomy and total cystectomy

   E. Radiotherapy

   *Ref.:* 4

**COMMENTS: Transitional cell cancers** of the renal pelvis and ureter are notable for their multicentricity and tendency to spread by direct extension to other parts of the urothelium. Approximately 30% of patients have a recurrence in the ureteral stump. For this reason, nephroureterectomy with excision of a cuff of bladder at the ureteral orifice is the preferred treatment. There is no specific role for radiotherapy in the primary treatment of these lesions. Long-term cystoscopic surveillance is necessary postoperatively because in approximately 25% of patients, a subsequent bladder tumor arises. In selected cases (e.g., solitary kidney or chronic renal disease), endoscopic or percutaneous resection or ablation of small, low-grade noninvasive tumors of the renal pelvis or ureters has produced long-term survival. Meticulous long-term postoperative surveillance, including cystoscopic studies, periodic IVP or CT, and urine cytologic examination, is essential in these circumstances.

**ANSWER: C**

5. Regarding treatment of renal cell carcinoma, which of the following statements is true?

   A. Induction chemotherapy followed by nephrectomy yields the best overall results.

   B. Radical nephrectomy involves removal of the kidney, adrenal gland, perinephric fat, fascia of Gerota, and regional lymph nodes.

   C. Regional lymphadenectomy for lesions extending outside the kidney improves postoperative survival.

   D. CT- or ultrasound-guided biopsy of the renal mass should be performed before nephrectomy.

   E. Percutaneous cryoablation or radiofrequency ablation may be used for large unresectable tumors.

   *Ref.:* 3

**COMMENTS:** Treatment of **renal cell carcinoma** and the subsequent prognosis are determined by the anatomic extent of the disease. Treatment of local disease focuses on tumor removal by radical nephrectomy. Solid renal masses are rarely subjected to biopsy, and they are diagnosed after pathologic examination of the kidneys. Surgery alone offers an excellent prognosis in patients with early lesions confined within the renal cortex. **Percutaneous ablation** of renal masses is indicated for small masses generally less than 3 cm. A survival advantage for those undergoing regional lymphadenectomy has not been established. Metastases frequently occur by hematogenous routes as well, which may negate any theoretical advantage of even more radical local surgery, although the presence of a limited volume of tumor thrombus in the vena cava with right-sided carcinomas may not adversely affect long-term outcome if the thrombus is removed completely. In the presence of distant metastases, nephrectomy may still be appropriate to control bleeding, pain, or infection. A randomized controlled study revealed that survival is increased (from 9 to 12 months) in patients who undergo nephrectomy in the face of metastatic disease versus chemotherapy with interleukin-2 alone. Recent studies have established tyrosine kinase inhibitors as the adjuvant treatment of choice for metastatic renal cell carcinoma after nephrectomy. Phase III trials have shown a 3-month survival advantage over placebo. **Immunotherapy** may result in remission of the cancer in a small percentage of patients. In select circumstances, patients with isolated metastases have benefited from resection of their metastatic disease.

**ANSWER: B**

6. A 64-year-old woman with symptoms typical of cholelithiasis undergoes ultrasound of the abdomen, which detects an asymptomatic, solid left renal mass. Which of the following should be the next examination?

   A. Excretory urographic studies

   B. Renal angiographic studies

   C. CT of the abdomen

   D. Radionuclide scanning of the urinary tract

   E. Renal biopsy

   *Ref.:* 3

**COMMENTS:** CT of the abdomen is the single most useful examination for the work-up of patients suspected of having renal cell carcinoma. In addition to confirming the solid nature of a renal mass, it can demonstrate local extension, venous and caval involvement, and distant metastases to the liver, adrenal gland, and visualized skeleton. Calcification is present in 8% to 18% of renal cell carcinomas, in contrast to about 1% of simple renal cysts. Small asymptomatic renal cell carcinomas are frequently discovered during abdominal ultrasonography and CT performed for other reasons (**incidentalomas**). Renal cell carcinoma, which probably arises from the proximal tubular epithelium, is the most common primary renal cancer; it accounts for approximately 86% of all primary malignant renal cancers. Of the remainder, 12% are Wilms tumor and 2% are renal sarcoma. The foregoing comments refer to primary renal tumors, but the most common asymptomatic **renal masses** are metastatic, with the lung being the most frequent primary site. A calcified renal artery aneurysm demonstrates opacification of the lumen on postinfusion scans. Calcified metastases to the kidney are extremely uncommon and have been reported only in patients with primary osteosarcoma elsewhere. A calcified simple cyst demonstrates a radiolucent center with peripheral ring calcification.

**ANSWER: C**

7. A 45-year-old man complains of severe flank pain and gross hematuria. Urinalysis reveals 200 red blood cells per high-power field, and his creatinine level is normal. What should the next test be?

   A. Imaging of the kidney, ureter, and bladder (KUB)

   B. IVP

   C. Ultrasonography

   D. CT of the abdomen and pelvis

   E. MRI

   *Ref.:* 5

**COMMENTS:** CT of the abdomen and pelvis is currently the best test for diagnosing nephrolithiasis. It is controversial whether the use of intravenous contrast material is necessary in patients with nephrolithiasis. The benefits of evaluating renal function and better assessing the degree of obstruction must be weighed against the disadvantages of using contrast material. The preferred CT protocol for the diagnosis of nephrolithiasis or other genitourinary pathology includes three phases: plain, venous phase (to visualize the renal parenchyma and vasculature), and 5- to 10-minute delay (to visualize the collecting system). The use of oral contrast material is not necessary and it may obscure the visibility of stones. IVP and ultrasound are acceptable but are not the preferred choices. To complete the work-up for **gross hematuria**, lower tract evaluation with cytologic and cystoscopic studies should be performed.

**ANSWER: D**

8. For which of the following types of renal calculi is growth not affected by manipulation of urinary pH?

   A. Cystine

   B. Uric acid

   C. Ammonium magnesium phosphate (struvite)

   D. Calcium oxalate

   E. Carbonate apatite

   *Ref.:* 6

**COMMENTS: Renal calculi** result from a variety of metabolic conditions. Determination of stone composition is important for both recognition of the underlying abnormality and institution of appropriate therapy aimed at removing the stone and preventing recurrence. Most urinary calculi (up to 75%) are calcium oxalate stones, and approximately one half of them are mixtures of calcium

oxalate and phosphate. The serum calcium level should be checked in patients with these stones, and if elevated, the parathyroid hormone level should be determined as well, Calcium phosphate and calcium oxalate stones are not generally altered by variations in urinary pH within the normal range. Ammonium magnesium phosphate (struvite) stones are next in frequency and are usually associated with infection. They form in alkaline urine, and their solubility is increased by acidic urine. Because urea-splitting organisms form ammonia and alkaline urine in the presence of infection, adequate pH manipulation cannot be obtained without control of the infection. Uric acid stones are typically radiolucent, and their solubility is increased by alkalinization. The solubility of cystine is increased in alkaline urine. However, because cystine stones are not crystalline in nature but are composed of amino acids, they are not easily pulverized by extracorporeal shock wave lithotripsy (ESWL). Stone composition is related to the ability to visualize stones on plain radiographs. Calcium-containing stones in particular are radiopaque. Ammonium magnesium phosphate (struvite) and cystine stones may also be visualized.

**ANSWER: D**

9. Which of the following is an indication for expectant management of renal calculi?

   A. Progressive renal damage

   B. Intractable pain

   C. Persistent or progressive obstruction

   D. Intractable urinary tract infection

   E. Detection of any calculi

   *Ref.:* 7

**COMMENTS:** The simple presence of a **renal or ureteral calculus** alone is not an indication for intervention by invasive techniques. Medical management, including analgesics, antibiotics, and appropriate urinary pH adjustments, often result in the spontaneous passage of stones. Smaller stones (<4 mm), in particular, can be expected to pass 90% of the time. There is no evidence that excessive hydration facilitates the passage of renal or ureteral calculi. Indeed, it may increase pain. α-Antagonist and calcium channel blocker medications have been shown to significantly decrease the time to passage of distal ureteral stones. Surgical management is indicated when calculi produce persistent obstruction, intractable pain, or a stone associated with impaired renal function. Techniques for stone removal include ureteroscopic manipulation, percutaneous nephrolithotomy, open nephrolithotomy, and ESWL.

**ANSWER: E**

10. Resection of a sigmoid cancer necessitates excision of a segment of the left pelvic ureter, with the specimen extending 3 cm distal to the bifurcation of the common iliac artery. Possible options for reconstruction include which of the following?

    A. Ileal substitution

    B. Ureteroneocystostomy

    C. Nephrectomy

    D. Psoas bladder hitch ligatures

    E. Renal autotransplantation

    *Ref.:* 1

**COMMENTS:** In this situation, simple in situ ureteroneocystostomy is not possible. An end-to-side anastomosis of the **severed ureter** to the opposite ureter (transureteroureterostomy) may be successful but may jeopardize the contralateral ureter. This approach is contraindicated in patients with a history of nephrolithiasis, transitional cell carcinoma, or recurrent pyelonephritis. A broad U-shaped flap (Boari flap) can be rotated off the bladder, fashioned in the shape of a cylinder, and anastomosed to the severed ureter. Another solution is to mobilize the bladder extensively and hitch it to the psoas muscle as high as possible, at which point ureteral implantation is performed (psoas hitch). With this technique, the bladder can often be brought as high as the common iliac artery. Mobilization of the kidney may provide 2 to 3 cm of ureteral length distally. Autotransplantation or ileal substitution of the ureter is reserved for large mid or proximal ureteral injuries. Nephrectomy may be considered for a nonfunctioning kidney with differential function consisting of less than 20% of the total glomerular filtration rate as quantified on a nuclear medicine study; however, every effort should be made to preserve the renal unit.

**ANSWER:** D

11. Which of the following is not a principle of repair of an intra-operative ureteral injury?

    A. Use of nonabsorbable suture material

    B. Spatulation of the transected ends

    C. Foley catheter drainage

    D. Drainage

    E. Intraureteral stent

*Ref.:* 1

**COMMENTS: Ureteral injuries** are usually iatrogenic and occur during the course of retroperitoneal dissection for various abdominal and pelvic conditions. In cases of transection, repair should be carried out with absorbable suture material and an indwelling intraureteral stent. Nonabsorbable sutures should be avoided because they may serve as a nidus for calculus formation. Extensive ureteral dissection should be avoided to preserve the segmental blood supply. Spatulation reduces the incidence of anastomotic stricture in the severed ureter. Drains should be placed to accommodate any anastomotic leak. When injury involves the pelvic ureteral segment, ureteroneocystostomy may be preferable. Percutaneous (or open) nephrostomy serves to divert urine from the repair site, thereby facilitating healing at the anastomotic site. Foley catheter drainage is important in the immediate postoperative period because an intraureteral stent allows reflux of bladder urine to the anastomosis.

**ANSWER:** A

12. A properly constructed cutaneous ureteroileostomy (ileal conduit) should do which of the following?

    A. Provide an adequate reservoir for storage of urine

    B. Prevent ureteral reflux

    C. Require catheterization for emptying

    D. Separate the urinary and fecal streams

    E. Allow urinary continence

*Ref.:* 8

**COMMENTS:** The use of an isolated segment of ileum to serve as a conduit between the ureters and the skin has become the most common form of urinary diversion and is the standard against which all other diversions are measured. **Ileal conduits** are used for patients after cystectomy, as well as for those with other indications for supravesical diversion. Large bowel is useful as a conduit because of the ease of creating an antireflux ureterointestinal anastomosis. Continent urinary reservoirs are fashioned from colon or small bowel (or both) and require periodic catheterization if anastomosed to skin. Continent reservoirs offer patients even greater control of urinary function and are well accepted. In selected cases, complete neobladders, fashioned from bowel, may be attached directly to the urethral remnant to eliminate the need for catheterization. The purpose of constructing an ileal conduit is to create a route (unidirectionally within the conduit) for transport of urine. It is not a reservoir for storage. Stasis in the bowel segment predisposes to infections, stone formation, and ureteral reflux. Stasis also promotes the absorption of electrolytes and may result in hyperchloremic metabolic acidosis. Some degree of ureteral reflux can normally be expected with an ileal conduit.

**ANSWER:** D

13. The preferred treatment of muscle-invasive bladder cancer involves which of the following?

    A. Radical cystectomy

    B. Preoperative irradiation and radical cystectomy

    C. Preoperative chemotherapy and radical cystectomy

    D. Radiation therapy alone

    E. Intravesical chemotherapy

*Ref.:* 9

**COMMENTS:** In the United States, radical cystectomy is the preferred treatment of **muscle-invasive bladder cancer**. Preoperative radiation therapy has not been shown to increase survival after radical cystectomy. The role of partial cystectomy with muscle invasion is limited because of a high local recurrence rate (approximately 50%). Lesions confined to the mucosa can be treated by transurethral resection, fulguration, or intravesical chemotherapy. A careful surveillance program must then be maintained. Treatment of lesions with submucosal invasion has been controversial with regard to whether intravesical chemotherapy is appropriate and the necessary extent of surgical resection. Certainly, intravesical therapy is of no value for high-grade invasive cancer. In the United States, radical cystectomy is the preferred treatment. The 5-year survival rate of patients with muscle invasion following cystectomy is only 50%, and the major cause of death is distant metastatic disease. Recent studies have shown a modest survival benefit with neoadjuvant chemotherapy for locally advanced tumors that may otherwise be unresectable. Because combination chemotherapy (with methotrexate, vinblastine, Adriamycin [doxorubicin], and cisplatin [MVAC]) in patients with advanced disease has yielded response rates of 50% to 70%, these agents now are being considered before cystectomy when muscle invasion is present. Complete response rates with MVAC alone, however, have been disappointing (10% to 15%).

**ANSWER:** A

14. In a male patient with a pelvic fracture secondary to blunt trauma, retrograde urethrographic examination demonstrates disruption of the membranous urethra. Which of the following constitutes appropriate initial treatment?

A. Passage of a transurethral catheter

B. Suprapubic cystostomy

C. Urethrostomy

D. Retropubic repair

E. Percutaneous nephrostomy tubes

*Ref.:* 10, 11

**COMMENTS: Blunt pelvic trauma** is the most common cause of urethral injury. **Urethral disruption** may cause the classic triad of blood at the meatus, a palpable bladder, and inability to urinate. Approximately 10% of pelvic fractures in males result in urethral injury. **Urethral injuries** are classified as posterior (proximal to the urogenital diaphragm) or anterior (distal to the membranous urethra). Disruption usually occurs at or above the membranous portion of the urethra because the anterior prostatic and membranous portions are relatively fixed by the puboprostatic ligaments and the urogenital diaphragm. Urethral injury should be suspected if blood is noted at the meatus or if the patient is unable to void clear urine. Passage of a catheter should not be attempted under these circumstances. Instead, a retrograde urethrogram should be obtained. In select cases, a urologist may attempt passing a catheter retrogradely in patients with minimal disruption. The risk of inserting the catheter is that partial disruption may be converted to complete disruption. In most cases, if urethral injury is confirmed, treatment should initially be accomplished with suprapubic cystotomy. A punch cystostomy can be performed if the bladder is palpable and no contraindications exist, such as extreme obesity, suprapubic surgical scars, or the presence of an abdominal hernia. Perineal urethrostomy does not divert the urine proximal to the site of injury and is of no value in such a situation. Immediate retropubic surgical realignment has a place in selected clinical situations, such as major bladder neck laceration, prostatic fragmentation, or severe dislocation of the prostate with severely displaced bone fragments. In most cases, however, current results suggest that the complications of incontinence, stricture, and impotence are minimized by performance of suprapubic cystostomy and delayed repair. Percutaneous nephrostomy tubes will not decompress the bladder and therefore leave the patient at risk for bladder rupture. Penetrating urethral injuries, in contrast, can often be treated by initial repair and urinary diversion.

**ANSWER: B**

15. Regarding bladder trauma, which of the following statements is true?

A. Rupture is usually extraperitoneal when associated with pelvic fracture.

B. A single-view retrograde cystogram in the emergency department demonstrates most significant bladder injuries.

C. Primary closure is generally indicated for extraperitoneal ruptures.

D. Intraoperative injury usually requires repair with a suprapubic cystostomy.

E. Injuries at the dome of the bladder are typically extraperitoneal.

*Ref.:* 10, 11

**COMMENTS:** Bladder injury may result from blunt or penetrating trauma or may occur during pelvic operations. When associated with pelvic fracture, the site of injury is usually extraperitoneal because it has been caused by the shearing force of the pelvic fracture. Extraperitoneal rupture without pelvic fracture is an infrequent occurrence. Isolated extraperitoneal bladder rupture is treated with 7 to 10 days of Foley catheter drainage. Blunt injury without pelvic fracture is associated with intraperitoneal rupture, particularly if the bladder is full at the time of injury, and results in perforation, typically at the dome of the bladder. **Bladder injury** should be suspected in any patient with lower abdominal trauma if there is any hematuria or the patient is unable to void. Single-view cystography may miss a significant injury. Anterior, posterior, lateral, oblique, and in particular, postvoid films are necessary. Alternatively, a CT cystogram may be performed by injecting 300 to 400 ml of contrast material through a Foley catheter followed by CT of the pelvis. The usual treatment of intraperitoneal rupture involves a two-layer, watertight closure with absorbable suture and transurethral or suprapubic bladder drainage. Iatrogenic injury recognized at the time of an operation does not generally require suprapubic cystotomy but does require repair with absorbable suture and urethral catheter drainage for 5 to 7 days. It is also necessary to be vigilant that the Foley catheter does not become obstructed, such as with blood, and cause the bladder to become distended.

**ANSWER: A**

16. Which of the following is true regarding the management of a patient with benign prostatic hyperplasia (BPH)?

A. All patients with complaints of prostatism should undergo therapy.

B. Patients with BPH have an increased risk for prostate cancer.

C. Initial therapy usually consists of nonoperative therapy.

D. Surgery is indicated only in patients who fail medical management.

E. The disease arises from the peripheral zone of the prostate.

*Ref.:* 12

**COMMENTS:** Unlike prostate cancer, which arises in the periphery of the gland, **benign prostatic hyperplasia** arises in the transitional zone of the prostate gland. The incidence of BPH is approximately 50% at 50 years of age and increases to approximately 80% in men entering their eighth decade of life. Patients are traditionally treated with medical therapy first, if the symptoms warrant it, and then undergo surgical therapy in the event of medical failure. Most patients are treated initially with medical therapy consisting of 5α-reductase inhibitors or α-adrenergic blocking agents that act on prostatic smooth muscle. 5α-Reductase inhibitors inhibit the conversion of testosterone to dihydrotestosterone, which is the active agent responsible for BPH. Indications for surgical management include recurrent urinary tract infection, recurrent gross hematuria, worsening renal function, failure of medical management, or the presence of bladder stones. The presence of a normal-sized prostate on rectal examination does not exclude obstruction by BPH. BPH occurs in most men, and the incidence increases with advancing age. It is not a risk factor for the development of prostate cancer. It should be noted, however, that the usual transurethral prostatectomy or open surgery does not remove all the prostate tissue, and prostate cancer can occur following removal of the prostate for benign disease.

**ANSWER: C**

**17.** Regarding prostate-specific antigen (PSA), which of the following statements is true?

A. PSA is a better serum marker for prostate cancer than acid phosphatase.

B. PSA is produced by both benign and malignant prostate tissue.

C. As an immunohistochemical marker, determination of the PSA level has been able to establish whether a metastatic adenocarcinoma is of prostatic origin.

D. A PSA level greater than 10 ng/dL in a patient with prostate cancer may be cured surgically.

E. All of the above.

*Ref.:* 13

**COMMENTS: Prostate-specific antigen** is the best marker for prostate cancer and the first organ-specific marker in all of cancer biology. It is produced by both benign and malignant prostate tissue. Although age-specific reference ranges have been proposed, most would consider a normal PSA level to be less than 4 ng/mL. As an immunohistochemical marker, the PSA level is much more accurate and specific than the prostatic acid phosphatase level, which can be elevated in association with nonprostatic cancers, bone disorders, and liver abnormalities. In addition, the acid phosphatase level is not generally elevated with early prostate cancer. An elevated PSA level does not necessarily imply escape beyond the capsule and surgical incurability, although high values are often associated with bulky lesions. In contradistinction, an elevated acid phosphatase level in an individual with prostate cancer usually signifies extensive local or metastatic disease.

**ANSWER:** E

**18.** One hour after a prolonged transurethral resection of the prostate (TURP), a 70-year-old man with mild coronary artery disease experiences bradycardia, hypertension, confusion, nausea, and headache. What is the most likely cause?

A. Hyperkalemia

B. Hypokalemia

C. Hypernatremia

D. Hyponatremia

E. Anemia

*Ref.:* 14, 15

**COMMENTS:** The patient is most likely suffering from transurethral resection (TUR) syndrome, which is caused by excessive absorption of irrigating solution and results in **hyponatremia**. The usual irrigation fluid is 1.5% glycine, which has an osmolarity of 200 mOsm/L, as compared with the normal serum osmolarity of 290 mOsm/L. Excessive systemic absorption of the irrigating solution can result in a dilutional hyponatremia, hypoproteinemia, and ultimately, decreased serum osmotic pressure. Extremely low sodium levels (<110 mEq/L) may result in severe cerebral edema and subsequent seizures. Treatment of **transurethral resection syndrome** traditionally consists of terminating the procedure as rapidly as possible, administration of furosemide (Lasix) intraoperatively or postoperatively, and instillation of a 0.9% NaCl (and in severe cases 3% NaCl) solution over a 3- to 6-hour period. Newer bipolar resecting equipment allows irrigation with 0.9%

normal saline, which has drastically decreased the probability of TUR syndrome occurring. However, these patients may still suffer from fluid overload as a result of absorption of isotonic fluid.

**ANSWER:** D

**19.** A 60-year-old man in good general health has an asymptomatic prostate nodule. His PSA level is 9 ng/mL, and biopsy confirms adenocarcinoma (Gleason III + III) on one side. Bone scanning does not reveal any evidence of metastatic disease. Which of the following therapies is appropriate?

A. Transurethral prostate resection

B. Radical prostatectomy

C. Orchiectomy

D. Diethylstilbestrol

E. Injection of luteinizing hormone–releasing hormone (LHRH) agonist

*Ref.:* 16

**COMMENTS:** Carcinoma of the prostate is the most common non–skin-related cancer in men older than 65 years and is the second most common cause of cancer death in the male population. Histologically, most of these lesions are adenocarcinomas. Squamous cell carcinoma and sarcomas of the prostate are rare. No definite etiologic factors have been established, but age, race, and family history are important predictors. Most prostate cancers arise in the periphery of the gland and are asymptomatic until urinary obstruction or symptoms of metastases develop. More than one half of the prostate nodules detected on examination are malignant. When a prostatic nodule is detected, a PSA level should be obtained, followed by transrectal ultrasound imaging and biopsy. If **prostate cancer** is found, a bone scan may be obtained to rule out evidence of metastatic disease. In addition, a chest radiograph and possibly a serum acid phosphatase level are obtained preoperatively. Treatment of localized prostate cancer consists of radical prostatectomy or external beam or interstitial implanted radiotherapy, depending on the physician's and patient's preference. Watchful waiting or active surveillance has been studied for men with low-grade and low-stage prostate cancer, but men undergoing definitive surgical or radiation therapy enjoy a significant improvement in overall and prostate cancer–specific survival. Many new experimental and investigational modalities are being used for the treatment of prostate cancer. **Radical prostatectomy** consists of removing the entire prostate and seminal vesicles and may be done through the retropubic or perineal route. Staging pelvic lymph node dissection is often performed before prostatectomy. If the lymph nodes are grossly enlarged, they are sent for frozen section, and the operation is usually terminated if cancer has spread to the lymph nodes. Tables have been established that predict the likelihood of positive margins and lymph node involvement based on the clinical stage, PSA level, and Gleason score. Hormonal therapy with estrogens or LHRH agonists is indicated for metastatic disease but is not appropriate primary therapy.

**ANSWER:** B

**20.** An asymptomatic 76-year-old man has a hard, irregular prostate, an elevated acid phosphatase level, a PSA level of 53 ng/mL, and multiple osteoblastic lesions in the lumbosacral spine. Biopsy of the prostate reveals a moderately differentiated adenocarcinoma. Which of the following therapies is indicated?

A. Transurethral prostate resection

B. Radical prostatectomy

C. Hormonal therapy

D. Radiation therapy

E. Cytotoxic chemotherapy

*Ref.:* 17

**COMMENTS:** The treatment of locally advanced or **metastatic prostate cancer** is palliation. The primary method of therapy is hormonal manipulation, which consists of bilateral orchiectomy or the administration of LHRH agonists (e.g., leuprolide) and possibly testosterone-blocking agents (e.g., flutamide). Exogenous estrogens, such as diethylstilbestrol, are not used often because of their associated increased incidence of thromboembolic disease. Hormonal therapy is the primary means of palliating bone pain, obstructive uropathy, and the general debility of metastatic disease. Use of early versus delayed hormonal therapy is controversial, and a survival benefit for initiating hormonal therapy before the onset of symptoms has yet to be proved but may benefit select patients with positive nodes. When hormonal treatment fails to palliate, TURP is performed to relieve obstruction or local radiotherapy is used to palliate painful or bulky metastasis. Chemotherapy is not particularly useful, although protocols are forthcoming for hormone-refractory prostate cancer. Radical prostatectomy is not indicated in men with metastatic disease.

**ANSWER: C**

21. An 11-year-old boy complains of scrotal swelling and pain. His parents note that the size of his scrotum seems to fluctuate. What is the probable diagnosis?

A. Testicular tumor

B. Spermatocele

C. Chronic epididymitis

D. Acute or subacute epididymitis

E. Hydrocele

*Ref.:* 11, 18

**COMMENTS: Hydrocele** can be idiopathic or secondary to a process such as epididymitis, trauma, mumps, or tuberculosis. Typically, it is a nontender, translucent mass. It can obscure palpation of the testes, and it is important to be aware of this in young men because as many as 20% of acute hydroceles are secondary to testicular tumors. If a mass with all the characteristics of a hydrocele empties when the patient is in the supine position, there is probably a **patent processus vaginalis**. In patients who have a fluctuating hydrocele or are younger than 12 years, an inguinal approach is necessary to perform high ligation of the hydrocele. Hydroceles in adults require treatment only when symptomatic, but in children they may require treatment if persistent. A **spermatocele** is a simple or multiloculated cyst at the head of the epididymis and usually requires no treatment unless it is symptomatic. It transilluminates and can be palpated as being discrete from the testes. **Epididymitis**, if acute, leaves the patient with an exquisitely tender scrotum whose skin may be red and edematous. There may be a mass, but this is often difficult to appreciate because the patient does not permit a deliberate examination. With chronic epididymitis, the mass is nontender and firm and can cause beading of the entire vas deferens. If a draining sinus tract is also present, the most

likely cause is tuberculosis. Testicular cancer is the most serious condition in the scrotum, and a solid mass arising from the testicle is considered cancer. The mass is usually firm, cannot be transilluminated, and is not tender. If it is tender, it may be so as a result of bleeding of a tumor into the testicle. Ultrasonic examination of the testicle, along with determination of tumor markers, has greatly facilitated making a diagnosis in such a clinical setting.

**ANSWER: E**

22. A 14-year-old boy is brought to the emergency department with a 4-hour history of acute, severe left scrotal pain. Examination reveals a high-riding left testicle with severe pain on palpation. Urinalysis does not reveal any evidence of red or white blood cells. Which of the following is the treatment of choice at this point?

A. Heat, scrotal elevation, and antibiotics

B. Manual attempt at detorsion

C. Analgesics and re-examination

D. Doppler examination to assess testicular blood flow

E. Surgical exploration

*Ref.:* 11

**COMMENTS:** When examining the acutely painful scrotum, one should attempt to differentiate epididymitis from **testicular torsion**, but it may not be possible. Doubtful cases should be treated as testicular torsion until proved otherwise. Because irreversible testicular ischemia occurs within 4 hours when there is complete torsion, prompt surgical exploration is indicated even if the diagnosis is uncertain. Doppler examination may be helpful for assessing testicular blood flow. Nuclear medicine scans also are reliable and must be used judiciously. Manual detorsion is not usually successful but can be done when the scrotum is not swollen. It may relieve pain, but exploration is still necessary because residual torsion may still exist. At the time of exploration, the involved testis should be anatomically fixated and detorsion performed. The contralateral testis should undergo a similar procedure prophylactically because the same anatomic abnormality may be found in both testes.

**ANSWER: E**

23. The anatomic abnormality found with torsion of the testicle in adolescents most commonly involves which of the following?

A. Intravaginal torsion of the spermatic cord

B. Extravaginal torsion of the spermatic cord

C. Torsion of the appendix testis

D. Torsion of the appendix epididymis

E. Torsion of the contralateral testis

*Ref.:* 11, 19

**COMMENTS:** There are two types of **torsion of the testicle**. In neonates, torsion of the spermatic cord occurs before attachment of the gubernaculum, which allows torsion of the entire testicle and tunica vaginalis. This is called **extravaginal torsion**. The second type of torsion usually occurs in adolescents and older men and is called **intravaginal torsion** of the spermatic cord. By this time, the tunica vaginalis is fixed to the dartos fascia and cannot twist. Intravaginal torsion is most commonly associated with a long mesenteric attachment between the cord and the testes and epididymis, which allows the testicle to rotate (producing the "bell clapper" deformity), and torsion can therefore occur within the tunica vaginalis. This deformity is often bilateral, and fixation of the contralateral testis should be performed at the time that the testicular torsion is corrected. Nonetheless, bilateral torsion is exceedingly rare at initial evaluation. Regarding the appendix testis and the appendix epididymis, torsion of these appendages can produce acute pain and swelling similar to torsion of the spermatic cord, but it does not result in testicular infarction. Transillumination may reveal the "blue dot" sign representing the infarcted structure. Exploration is sometimes required to exclude testicular torsion.

**ANSWER:** A

24. Which of the following is true regarding varicocele?

   A. Varicoceles occur more commonly on the right side.

   B. Varicoceles are associated with infertility.

   C. Varicoceles occur in about 40% of men.

   D. Varicoceles are often associated with testicular tumors.

   E. Varicoceles are not usually palpable on physical examination.

*Ref.:* 20

**COMMENTS: Varicoceles** are seen in approximately 15% to 20% of the male population but in up to 40% of infertile men. Varicoceles have not been found to be associated with testicular tumors. They are much more common on the left side—because the gonadal vein drains into the renal vein, it usually maintains higher pressure than the right side. They have been associated with diminished sperm count, decreased sperm motility, and abnormal sperm morphology. In infertile patients with abnormal findings on semen analysis, varicocelectomy often improves the semen analysis. Physical examination of the scrotum reveals a large group of veins palpable within the scrotum, which has been described as a "bag of worms."

**ANSWER:** B

25. A 65-year-old man is unable to void after an abdominoperineal resection. Postvoid residuals have been 600 to 800 mL. The treatment of choice is which of the following?

   A. Chronic Foley catheterization

   B. TURP

   C. Clean intermittent catheterization

   D. Transurethral sphincterotomy

   E. α-Blockers alone

*Ref.:* 21

**COMMENTS:** Bladder dysfunction has been reported in 10% to 50% of patients following abdominal perineal resection or other major pelvic surgery. The type of voiding dysfunction that occurs is dependent on the specific nerve involved and the degree of

injury. Patients with **urinary retention** are best treated by clean intermittent catheterization. Most (>80%) resolve over a period of 3 to 6 months. The use of a chronic indwelling catheter is a reasonable choice in some patients, but the risk for infection is higher with chronic catheterization than with intermittent catheterization. The use of α-blockers alone or TURP is unlikely to be successful. Transurethral sphincterotomy does not treat the underlying problem and may result in incontinence.

**ANSWER:** C

26. Which of the following are not treatments or characteristics of nonseminomatous germ cell tumors of the testis?

   A. Radiation therapy

   B. Retroperitoneal lymph node dissection

   C. Elevated α-fetoprotein (AFP)

   D. Elevated hCG

   E. Chemotherapy for advanced disease

*Ref.:* 22

**COMMENTS:** The most common solid tumor in a young male is a **seminoma**. About 95% of testicular masses are of germ cell origin. Germ cell tumors are divided into seminomatous and nonseminomatous germ cell tumors. **Nonseminomatous germ cell tumors** include tumors of the following histologic types: embryonal cell carcinoma, yolk sac tumor, choriocarcinoma, and teratoma. Clinically, stage I seminomas (confined to the testis) are treated with prophylactic radiotherapy of the retroperitoneal lymph nodes to eliminate any chance of failure in the retroperitoneum. Select patients are now treated by surveillance alone. Higher-stage seminomas (visible adenopathy in the retroperitoneum or lung metastasis) are best treated with chemotherapy. An elevated hCG level is seen in 5% to 10% of patients with seminomas, but if an elevated AFP level is found, the tumor is considered nonseminomatous. Treatment of clinical stage I nonseminomatous germ cell tumors is controversial but consists of either retroperitoneal lymph node dissection, primary chemotherapy, or surveillance. Elevated AFP and β-hCG levels may be seen in patients with nonseminomatous germ cell tumors. For patients with bulky retroperitoneal disease or visceral metastasis, treatment consists of combination chemotherapy.

**ANSWER:** A

27. Appropriate treatment of a painless solid testicular mass in a 28-year-old man includes which of the following?

   A. Preoperative CT for staging

   B. Incisional biopsy via a scrotal incision

   C. Incisional biopsy via an inguinal incision

   D. Orchiectomy via a scrotal incision

   E. Orchiectomy via an inguinal incision

*Ref.:* 22

**COMMENTS:** During the work-up of a patient with a testicular tumor, serum should be obtained for determination of AFP and β-hCG levels because these tumor markers are elevated in many patients with **testicular cancer**. CT of the abdomen and pelvis for staging is performed after the diagnosis is made and should not delay orchiectomy The primary diagnostic and therapeutic maneuver is **orchiectomy**, and it should be carried out via an inguinal incision with early clamping of the vessels. If the presence of a testicular mass is confirmed, an orchiectomy should be performed. Rarely, the testicle suspected of being involved with cancer may be affected by a benign condition. Yet even in this situation, the best treatment is often orchiectomy. A scrotal approach is contraindicated because it does not permit control of the testicular vessels before manipulation of the testicle, which may dislodge tumor cells into the venous drainage. In addition, with such an approach, cells from the biopsy specimen may spill into the scrotum and subsequently spread tumor via the scrotal lymphatic drainage to the superficial inguinal nodes, or they may seed locally.

**ANSWER:** E

28. A 32-year-old man arrives at the emergency department with an exquisitely painful and "woody"-feeling penile erection of 18 hours' duration. Which of the following is not a therapeutic option?

A. Aspiration of blood from the corpora cavernosa

B. Irrigation of the corpora cavernosa with a dilute solution of papaverine

C. Creation of a communication between the glans penis and a corporal body with a biopsy needle or scalpel blade

D. Side-to-side anastomosis between the corpus spongiosum and corpus cavernosum

E. Exchange transfusions

*Ref.:* 23

**COMMENTS: Priapism** is a prolonged pathologic penile erection in the absence of sexual stimulation, and there are two major types: ischemic (or "low flow") and nonischemic ("high flow"). Blood gas analysis of aspirated corporal blood shows acidosis and hypoxemia in ischemic priapism, and the patient experiences pain. Nonischemic priapism is not usually painful and requires only conservative management and reassurance, but ischemic priapism requires emergency treatment. Most cases of priapism are idiopathic. Some known causes are sickle cell disease, leukemic infiltration of veins draining the penis, and certain medications, such as anticoagulants and antidepressants. Frequently, simple aspiration of blood from the corpus cavernosum alone can cause lasting detumescence. If this fails, irrigation of the corpus with a dilute solution of epinephrine or norepinephrine may work. This has the dual effect of decompressing the corpus and the venous obstruction that goes with it, as well as diminishing arterial flow. Papaverine is used to treat impotence. It increases penile blood flow by directly relaxing vascular smooth muscle. The glans penis is an extension of the corpus spongiosum and is not usually affected by priapism. Shunts between it and the corpus cavernosa created with biopsy needles or scalpel blades or removal of a portion of the glandular corporal septum may provide a path of egress for blood trapped in the penis. If all else fails, formal spongiosum-to-cavernosum shunts may be created. There is a high incidence of impotence after priapism lasting 24 hours or longer. When priapism is secondary to sickle cell anemia, exchange transfusions and other medical therapies, including oxygenation, hydration, and alkalinization, may be indicated.

**ANSWER:** B

29. A 40-year-old man with a history of alcoholism comes to the emergency department with changes in mental status and scrotal pain. Physical examination reveals a temperature of 102.2°F and an ecchymotic and exquisitely tender scrotum with palpable crepitus. What are the immediate next steps in management?

A. CT of the pelvis to the midthigh

B. Incision and drainage of the scrotal skin and culture of the retrieved fluid

C. Plain radiograph of the pelvis

D. Duplex ultrasonography of the scrotum

E. Wide débridement of the affected tissues

*Ref.:* 21

**COMMENTS:** This patient has evidence of a necrotizing infection of the scrotal tissue consistent with **Fournier gangrene**. It is a necrotizing fasciitis that arises from urethral, rectal, or perineal skin flora. The etiology is usually polymicrobial, including aerobic and anaerobic bacteria. It is characterized by subcutaneous crepitus, tenderness, and foul-smelling necrotic tissue. This life-threatening infection must be widely débrided without delay, and broad-spectrum antibiotic therapy and aggressive fluid resuscitation are necessary. Imaging studies may confirm the presence of subcutaneous gas, but surgery should not be delayed because the diagnosis is clinical.

**ANSWER:** E

30. Which of the following events is necessary for normal micturition?

A. Increase in sympathetic tone to the detrusor resulting in bladder contraction

B. Increased activity of cholinergic nerves in the lower urinary tract

C. Stimulation of α-adrenergic receptors at the bladder neck

D. Cerebellar coordination of voiding reflex

E. Increase in intra-abdominal pressure

*Ref.:* 11, 24

**COMMENTS:** Normal **micturition** is a complex process requiring coordination of the autonomic and voluntary nervous systems. Voluntary relaxation of the external urinary sphincter (innervated by the sacral spinal nerve roots) initiates normal urination. When the bladder fills, autonomic afferent nerves transmit a signal to the pons that coordinates relaxation of the bladder neck and contraction of the bladder via an increase in parasympathetic tone and inhibition of sympathetic tone in the lower urinary tract. α-Adrenergic receptors mediate closure of the bladder neck and therefore facilitate urine storage. α-Blockers facilitate voiding by relaxing smooth muscle in the bladder outlet. Some patients with detrusor areflexia may void via maneuvers such as the Valsalva or Credé maneuver, which increases intraabdominal pressure.

**ANSWER:** B

31. Which of the following matches a layer of the scrotum with its corresponding fascial layer in the abdominal wall:

A. Cremasteric fascia—Internal oblique muscle

B. Tunica vaginalis—External oblique fascia

C. Dartos fascia—Transversalis fascia

D. External spermatic fascia—Scarpa fascia

E. Internal spermatic fascia—Peritoneum

*Ref.: 25, 26*

**COMMENTS:** As the testes descend, the scrotal wall is formed from layers of the abdominal wall. The Scarpa fascia is continuous with the dartos fascia. The external oblique aponeurosis corresponds to the external spermatic fascia and is attached to the external inguinal ring. The internal oblique muscle gives rise to the cremasteric muscle and fascia. The transversalis fascia is continuous with the internal spermatic fascia. The transversus abdominis muscle terminates superior to the triangle of Hesselbach and therefore does not have a scrotal counterpart. The tunica vaginalis is a bilayered scrotal structure that is continuous with the peritoneum. They are connected by the processus vaginalis, which normally closes in infancy. Persistence of the processus vaginalis may result in a hydrocele.

**ANSWER:** A

**32.** Which of the following is true regarding circumcision?

A. It is protective against penile cancer

B. It may increase HIV transmission

C. It decreases penile sensation

D. The fascia of Buck must be closed before skin closure

E. Hypospadias is a contraindication

*Ref.: 27, 28*

**COMMENTS: Circumcision** is removal of the preputial skin. The fascia of Buck is deep to the dartos fascia and should not be entered during circumcision. No reports have definitively proved any decrease or increase in penile sensation after circumcision. **Penile cancer** is most commonly squamous cell carcinoma, occurs in men with phimosis as a result of chronic irritation of the underlying skin, and is virtually nonexistent in circumcised men. At the time of circumcision the glans penis should be inspected carefully for suspicious lesions and the surgical specimen analyzed. In high-risk young adult populations in Africa, circumcision has been shown to reduce the rate of acquiring HIV by 50%. It has been shown that the inner prepuce has a high concentration of Langerhans cells that contain receptors for HIV. Hypospadias is not a contraindication to circumcision; however, because the preputial skin is often used for urethral reconstruction, circumcision should be deferred until the hypospadias is repaired.

**ANSWER:** A

**33.** Which of the following is true regarding enterovesical fistulas?

A. Barium enema is the most sensitive imaging test.

B. An oral charcoal test will localize a fistula to the small bowel.

C. Pneumaturia is the most common initial sign/symptom.

D. A definitive diagnosis can be made 90% of the time with cystoscopy.

E. Inflammatory bowel disease is the most common cause.

*Ref.: 29*

**COMMENTS: Enterovesical fistulas** are abnormal connections between the bowel and bladder. The sigmoid colon is the most common site, and sigmoid diverticulitis accounts for 70% of cases. Patients are initially seen with pneumaturia or air in the urine 50% to 80% of the time and fecaluria or symptoms of urinary tract infection 40% of the time. CT of the abdomen and pelvis with oral contrast enhancement is the most sensitive imaging modality for detecting an enterovesical fistula. The classic triad of findings on CT are a thickened bladder wall adjacent to a thickened loop of bowel, air in the bladder in the absence of instrumentation, and colonic diverticula. Barium enema has low sensitivity for the detection of fistulas; however, the first voided specimen after the test may be centrifuged and examined radiographically to increase its diagnostic yield. Oral charcoal administration and subsequent blackening of the urine will make the diagnosis of enterovesical fistula but will not provide anatomic information. Cystoscopy will reveal changes in the bladder mucosa, but a fistula tract is identified only approximately 35% of the time. Any endoscopically identified fistula tract in the setting of previous malignancy should undergo biopsy to evaluate for a malignant fistula.

**ANSWER:** C

## REFERENCES

1. McAninch JW, Santucci RA: Renal and ureteral trauma. In Wein AR, Kavoussi LR, Novick AC, et al, editors: *Campbell-Walsh urology*, ed 9, Philadelphia, 2007, WB Saunders.
2. Anderson JK, Kabalin JN, Cadeddu JA: Surgical anatomy of the retroperitoneum, adrenals, kidneys, and ureters. In Wein AR, Kavoussi LR, Novick AC, et al, editors: *Campbell-Walsh urology*, ed 9, Philadelphia, 2007, WB Saunders.
3. Campbell SC, Novick AC, Bukowski RM: Renal tumors. In Wein AR, Kavoussi LR, Novick AC, et al, editors: *Campbell-Walsh urology*, ed 9, Philadelphia, 2007, WB Saunders.
4. Sagalowsky AI, Jarrett TW: Management of urothelial tumors of the renal pelvis and ureter. In Wein AR, Kavoussi LR, Novick AC, et al, editors: *Campbell-Walsh urology*, ed 9, Philadelphia, 2007, WB Saunders.
5. Bhayani SB, Siegel CL: Urinary tract imaging: basic principles. In Wein AR, Kavoussi LR, Novick AC, et al, editors: *Campbell-Walsh urology*, ed 9, Philadelphia, 2007, WB Saunders.
6. Pearle MS, Lotan Y: Urinary lithiasis: etiology, epidemiology, and pathogenesis. In Wein AR, Kavoussi LR, Novick AC, et al, editors: *Campbell-Walsh urology*, ed 9, Philadelphia, 2007, WB Saunders.
7. Lingeman JE, Matlaga BR, Evan AP: Surgical management of upper tract calculi. In Wein AR, Kavoussi LR, Novick AC, et al, editors: *Campbell-Walsh urology*, ed 9, Philadelphia, 2007, WB Saunders.
8. Dahl DM, McDougal WS: Use of intestinal segments in urinary diversion. In Wein AR, Kavoussi LR, Novick AC, et al, editors: *Campbell-Walsh urology*, ed 9, Philadelphia, 2007, WB Saunders.
9. Schoenberg MP, Gonzalgo ML: Management of invasive and metastatic bladder cancer. In Wein AR, Kavoussi LR, Novick AC, et al, editors: *Campbell-Walsh urology*, ed 9, Philadelphia, 2007, WB Saunders.
10. Morey AF, Rozanski TA: Genital and lower urinary tract trauma. In Wein AR, Kavoussi LR, Novick AC, et al, editors: *Campbell-Walsh urology*, ed 9, Philadelphia, 2007, WB Saunders.
11. Olumi AF, Richie JP: Urologic surgery. In Townsend CM, Beauchamp RD, Evers BM, et al, editors: *Sabiston textbook of surgery: the biological basis of modern surgical practice*, ed 18, Philadelphia, 2008, Saunders.
12. Kirby R, Lepor H: Evaluation and nonsurgical management of benign prostatic hyperplasia. In Wein AR, Kavoussi LR, Novick AC, et al,

editors: *Campbell-Walsh urology*, ed 9, Philadelphia, 2007, WB Saunders.

13. Gretzer MB, Partin AW: Prostate cancer tumor markers. In Wein AR, Kavoussi LR, Novick AC, et al, editors: *Campbell-Walsh urology*, ed 9, Philadelphia, 2007, WB Saunders.

14. Fitzpatrick JM: Minimally invasive and endoscopic management of benign prostatic hyperplasia. In Wein AR, Kavoussi LR, Novick AC, et al, editors: *Campbell-Walsh urology*, ed 9, Philadelphia, 2007, WB Saunders.

15. Ho HS, Yip SK, Lim KB, et al: A prospective randomized study comparing monopolar and bipolar transurethral resection of prostate using transurethral resection in saline (TURIS) system, *Eur Urol* 52:517–524, 2007.

16. Catalona WJ, Han M: Definitive therapy for localized prostate cancer: an overview. In Wein AR, Kavoussi LR, Novick AC, et al, editors: *Campbell-Walsh urology*, ed 9, Philadelphia, 2007, WB Saunders.

17. Nelson JB: Hormone therapy for prostate cancer. In Wein AR, Kavoussi LR, Novick AC, et al, editors: *Campbell-Walsh urology*, ed 9, Philadelphia, 2007, WB Saunders.

18. Sandlow JI, Winfield HN, Goldstein M: Surgery of the scrotum and seminal vesicles. In Wein AR, Kavoussi LR, Novick AC, et al, editors: *Campbell-Walsh urology*, ed 9, Philadelphia, 2007, WB Saunders.

19. Schenck FX, Bellinger MF: Abnormalities of the testes and scrotum and their surgical management. In Wein AR, Kavoussi LR, Novick AC, et al, editors: *Campbell-Walsh urology*, ed 9, Philadelphia, 2007, WB Saunders.

20. Sigman M, Jarow JP: Male infertility. In Wein AR, Kavoussi LR, Novick AC, et al, editors: *Campbell-Walsh urology*, ed 9, Philadelphia, 2007, WB Saunders.

21. Schaeffer AJ, Schaeffer EM: Infections of the urinary tract. In Wein AR, Kavoussi LR, Novick AC, et al, editors: *Campbell-Walsh urology*, ed 9, Philadelphia, 2007, WB Saunders.

22. Richie JP, Steele GS: Neoplasms of the testis. In Wein AR, Kavoussi LR, Novick AC, et al, editors: *Campbell-Walsh urology*, ed 9, Philadelphia, 2007, WB Saunders.

23. Burnett AL: Priapism. In Wein AR, Kavoussi LR, Novick AC, et al, editors: *Campbell-Walsh urology*, ed 9, Philadelphia, 2007, WB Saunders.

24. Yoshimura N, Chancellor MB: Physiology and pharmacology of the bladder and urethra. In Wein AR, Kavoussi LR, Novick AC, et al, editors: *Campbell-Walsh urology*, ed 9, Philadelphia, 2007, WB Saunders.

25. Brooks JD: Anatomy of the lower urinary tract and male genitalia. In Wein AR, Kavoussi LR, Novick AC, et al, editors: *Campbell-Walsh urology*, ed 9, Philadelphia, 2007, WB Saunders.

26. Turnage RH, Richardson KA, Li BD, et al: Abdominal wall, umbilicus, peritoneum, mesenteries, omentum, and retroperitoneum. In Townsend CM, Beauchamp RD, Evers BM, et al, editors: *Sabiston Textbook of surgery: the biological basis of modern surgical practice*, ed 18, Philadelphia, 2008, WB Saunders.

27. Jordan GH, Schlossberg SM: Surgery of the penis and urethra. In Wein AR, Kavoussi LR, Novick AC, et al, editors: *Campbell-Walsh urology*, ed 9, Philadelphia, 2007, WB Saunders.

28. *Male circumcision and risk for HIV transmission and other health conditions: implications for the United States*. Centers for Disease Control and Prevention Fact Sheet, February 2008. Available at www.cdc.gov/hiv/resources/factsheets/circumcision.htm.

29. Rovner ES: Urinary tract fistula. In Wein AR, Kavoussi LR, Novick AC, et al, editors: *Campbell-Walsh urology*, ed 9, Philadelphia, 2007, WB Saunders.

# CHAPTER 32

# Pediatric

*Shaun Daly, M.D., and Ai-Xuan L. Holterman, M.D.*

**1.** Which of the following statements is true regarding daily fluid requirements?

  A. Premature infants weighing less than 2 kg require only up to 80 mL/kg/day of fluid.

  B. Neonates and infants weighing 2 to 10 kg require 200 mL/kg/day of fluid.

  C. Infants and children weighing 10 to 20 kg require 1000 mL/day plus 50 mL/kg/day of fluid for every kilogram over 10 kg.

  D. Children heavier than 20 kg require 1500 mL/day plus 30 mL/kg/day of fluid for every kilogram over 20 kg.

  E. All of the above.

*Ref.:* 1-3

**COMMENTS:** See Question 2.

**A N S W E R :** C

**2.** Which of the following is true in the pediatric population?

  A. The daily sodium requirement is 8 mEq/kg.

  B. The daily potassium requirement is 4 mEq/kg.

  C. The daily protein requirement is 2 to 3.5 g/kg/day in infants.

  D. The minimum daily carbohydrate requirement is 2 to 3 mg/kg/min in neonates.

  E. Fat infusions should be started at 1.5 g/kg/day and titrated up to 3.5 to 4 g/kg/day.

*Ref.:* 1

**COMMENTS: Free water maintenance** requirements include replacement of insensible losses from the skin and lungs and the free water necessary to clear metabolic solutes in the urine. It does not include treatment of preexisting deficits or ongoing fluid losses. Numerous formulas are applicable to the calculation of maintenance requirements. **Daily electrolyte requirements** include sodium at 2 to 5 mEq/kg and potassium at 2 to 3 mEq/kg. Dextrose is administered to provide a glucose substrate at a minimum rate of 4 to 6 mg/kg/min. Fat infusions are started at 0.5 g/kg/day and advanced up to 2.5 to 3 g/kg/day. Protein requirements are 2 to 3.5 g/kg/day in infants, as opposed to requirements of about 1 g/kg/day in adults.

**A N S W E R :** C

**3.** A 5-week-old boy has a 5-day history of vomiting and weight loss of 0.4 kg (from 4.0 to 3.6 kg). His anterior fontanelle is flattened and his mucous membranes are dry. Laboratory data are as follows (mEq/L): sodium, 132; potassium, 3.2; chloride, 91; and bicarbonate, 28. Which of the following statements about this infant is true?

  A. Characterization of the emesis as bilious is crucial to aid in the diagnosis.

  B. Palpation of the abdomen will not help with the diagnosis.

  C. Ultrasound imaging of the abdomen will not add to the diagnosis.

  D. The most likely diagnosis is intussusception.

  E. The condition should be corrected by emergency surgery.

*Ref.:* 1-3

**COMMENTS:** Age is important in sorting out the differential diagnosis. Duodenal atresia is seen only in newborns. **Pyloric stenosis** typically produces symptoms in infants between 3 and 12 weeks of age. **Intussusception** most commonly occurs in children between 3 and 18 months of age. Pyloric stenosis is usually manifested as nonbilious vomiting, which progressively becomes projectile as a result of the blockage occurring proximal to the ampulla of Vater. **Duodenal atresia** most commonly occurs distal to the ampulla of Vater and will be accompanied by bilious vomiting. The extent of dehydration and electrolyte imbalance depends on the duration of the symptoms. Early in the course, fluid and electrolyte levels can be normal. If the condition is diagnosed late, infants are more likely to have severe metabolic derangements and dehydration. Physical examination can reveal a palpable thickened pylorus manifested as a pathognomonic olive-sized mass in the upper part of the abdomen. Sometimes gastric waves are seen through the epigastrium. If the pyloric mass cannot be palpated by an experienced examiner, ultrasound imaging is the first choice for diagnostic study, but an upper gastrointestinal contrast-enhanced study can also be done. Correction of fluid and electrolyte abnormalities takes precedence over surgery, which can be undertaken electively.

**A N S W E R :** A

**4.** For the infant in Question 3, which of the following is the most common electrolyte abnormality?

  A. Hypokalemia

  B. Hyperkalemia

C. Hypocalcemia

D. Hyperchloremia

E. Hypercalcemia

C. Sepsis

D. Pulmonary sequestration

E. Respiratory distress syndrome

*Ref.:* 1

*Ref.:* 1

**COMMENTS:** The **electrolyte imbalances** commonly seen in infants with hypertrophic pyloric stenosis are those associated with **gastric outlet obstruction**, namely, hypokalemic, hypochloremic metabolic alkalosis and paradoxical aciduria. The electrolyte abnormalities reflect the extensive loss of gastric contents from emesis in **hypertrophic pyloric stenosis**. **Paradoxical aciduria** and hypokalemia result from the urinary loss of acid ($H^+$) and potassium at the expense of sodium and water retention to preserve fluid volume. Hypochloremia is secondary to loss of bicarbonate from emesis with resulting contraction alkalosis. Disturbances in calcium are not classically a common electrolyte imbalance seen in infants with hypertrophic pyloric stenosis. Correction of fluid and electrolyte imbalances is essential before proceeding to surgery.

**ANSWER: A**

5. Which of the following solutions is appropriate for initial intravenous therapy in the infant in Question 3?

A. Lactated Ringer's solution at 25 mL/h

B. Five percent dextrose in water ($D_5W$) + 0.1% normal hydrochloride (HCl) at 30 mL/h

C. $D_5W$ + 0.20% normal saline solution + KCl, 30 mEq/L at 25 mL/h

D. $D_5W$ + 0.45% normal saline solution + KCl, 30 mEq/L at 16 mL/h

E. $D_5W$ + 0.45% normal saline solution + KCl, 30 mEq/L at 24 mL/h

*Ref.:* 1-3

**COMMENTS:** Appropriate **fluid therapy** requires the administration of maintenance fluid in addition to replacement for the estimated deficit and ongoing fluid losses. The estimated initial replacement volume for the first 24 hours includes maintenance of 100 mL/kg (400 mL/24 h, or 16 mL/h), plus replacement of approximately one half of the estimated deficit. Because weight loss is 40 g, or 10% of body weight, one half of this deficit would be 200 mL/24 h, or 8 mL/h. The initial rate of fluid replacement should be adjusted to maintain a urine output of 1 to 2 mL/kg/h. An initial bolus of isotonic saline solution at 20 mL/kg may be appropriate for severely dehydrated patients. Sodium, potassium, and chloride must be supplied for both maintenance and replacement of gastric losses as a 5% dextrose with 0.5% normal saline solution and KCl at 30 mEq/L. Ongoing assessment of fluid and electrolyte correction should be performed and adjusted as necessary by monitoring serum electrolytes and urine output. The operation should proceed only after appropriate fluid and electrolyte correction.

**ANSWER: E**

6. Major indications for the initiation of extracorporal membrane oxygenation (ECMO) in a newborn include all of the following except:

A. Diaphragmatic hernia

B. Meconium aspiration syndrome

**COMMENTS:** Meconium aspiration syndrome, respiratory distress syndrome, persistent pulmonary hypertension, sepsis, and congenital diaphragmatic hernia are all major indications for the initiation of **extracorporal membrane oxygenation**. Meconium aspiration syndrome is the most common indication for neonatal ECMO. Selection criteria include failure of conventional therapy with an alveolar-arterial oxygen gradient of greater than 620 for 12 hours (or 6 hours in patients with extensive barotrauma and requiring high inotropic support) or an oxygen index higher than 40. Exclusion criteria include gestational age less than 34 weeks, birth weight less than 2 kg, irreversible pulmonary disease, uncorrectable cyanotic congenital heart disease, intractable coagulopathy or hemorrhage, intracranial hemorrhage, or a history of more than 10 to 14 days of high-pressure mechanical ventilation. Follow-up hematocrit, platelet count, fibrinogen, and activated clotting time values and daily cranial ultrasound are required.

**ANSWER: D**

7. Which of the following statement concerning pediatric trauma is true?

A. Trauma is the second leading cause of death in children between 1 and 15 years of age.

B. Acceptable indications for computed tomography (CT) include the presence of a painful distracting injury, significant head injury, or an unclear examination.

C. Indications for operative intervention include documentation of injury to the spleen or liver on CT.

D. Intraosseous access is the preferred means for delivering fluids or blood in a child younger than 10 years.

E. Surgical cricothyroidotomy is an acceptable means of airway control for a child younger than 12 years.

*Ref.:* 1, 2

**COMMENTS:** For children between the ages of 1 and 15 years, **trauma** is the leading cause of death. Motor vehicle accidents, falls, bicycle accidents, and child abuse are the most common causes of traumatic death. The priorities of **resuscitation** are airway, breathing, and circulation. Fluid resuscitation is given as 20-mL/kg boluses. If intravenous access cannot be obtained in a timely manner, a specially designed needle can be used to deliver fluids or blood through an intraosseous route in children younger than 6 years, most commonly via the tibia. The needle is placed 1 to 2 cm below the tibial tuberosity through the anteromedial surface of the tibia under sterile conditions. If hypovolemic shock is refractory to two crystalloid boluses, blood transfusion should be initiated. CT is commonly used to evaluate pediatric trauma patients. CT is indicated when there is an injury elsewhere causing pain, a significant head injury precluding a reliable examination, or if there is an equivocal examination in general. Even though injuries to the liver and spleen are common, the need for operative intervention is not absolute. Surgical **cricothyroidotomy** should not be attempted in a child younger than 12 years because of the risk of inadvertent airway injury.

**ANSWER: B**

8. A 6-month-old infant requires blood transfusion after injury. Which of the following regimens is the most appropriate initial replacement?

   A. 10 to 20 mL/kg of packed red blood cells (PBRCs)

   B. 30 to 40 mL/kg of PBRCs

   C. 10 to 20 mL/kg of PBRCs + 10 to 20 mL/kg of platelets

   D. 10 to 20 mL/kg of PBRCs + 10 to 20 mL/kg of fresh frozen plasma

   E. 40 to 60 mL/kg of whole blood

   *Ref.:* 1, 2

**COMMENTS:** Blood volume for infants is usually estimated at 80 mL/kg of body weight. When **blood transfusions** are required, PRBCs are typically used, and the initial volume replacement is 10 to 20 mL/kg body weight. Coagulation deficits can develop rapidly in infants requiring more blood replacement. Fresh frozen plasma at a volume of 20 mL/kg and platelets at a volume of 10 to 20 mL/kg can be given if necessary.

**ANSWER:** A

9. A 3-month-old child is admitted to the hospital for irritability and a 4-hour history of right scrotal fullness. Testicular torsion is suspected. Which of the following is false?

   A. Physical examination may reveal a horizontal testicular lie (bell clapper deformity).

   B. The chance of testicular salvage decreases after 6 hours of symptoms.

   C. Ultrasound is the test of choice to assist in the diagnosis.

   D. Contralateral orchiopexy is not indicated.

   E. Testicular scan may assist in the diagnosis.

   *Ref.:* 1

**COMMENTS: Testicular torsion** is a surgical emergency and must be diagnosed rapidly. Doppler ultrasound is the diagnostic test of choice to assess blood flow to the testicle. Rapid diagnosis is essential because longer than 6 hours of testicular ischemia significantly decreases the salvage rate. Contralateral orchiopexy is indicated to prevent future torsion of the contralateral testicle. The **bell clapper deformity** refers to the horizontal lie of a testicle as a result of the failure of normal posterior anchoring of the gubernaculum, epididymis, and testis to the tunica vaginalis, thereby predisposing the testis to torsion.

**ANSWER:** D

10. Which of the following is the indicated treatment for a non-communicating hydrocele in a 2-month-old infant?

    A. Observation

    B. Needle aspiration

    C. Hydrocelectomy through a groin incision

    D. Hydrocelectomy through a scrotal incision

    E. Repair of the hernia and hydrocelectomy

    *Ref.:* 1-3

**COMMENTS:** Most noncommunicating **hydroceles** in young children are asymptomatic and will resolve as the fluid is absorbed. If the hydrocele persists past 12 months of age, peritoneal communication is likely, and hydrocelectomy with ligation of the patent processus vaginalis is indicated. In children, these operations are performed through the groin. Aspiration of the hydrocele is not recommended. If the hydrocele is noncommunicating, it will resolve and thus make aspiration unnecessary. If the hydrocele is communicating, the fluid will reaccumulate, and an operation will be necessary.

**ANSWER:** A

11. The following are true of inguinal hernias in the pediatric population except:

    A. Inguinal hernias are more common in females than in males.

    B. The most common structure found in an incarcerated inguinal hernia in girls are the ovaries.

    C. Laparoscopic evaluation of the contralateral groin is not always needed.

    D. High ligation of the hernia sac without repair of the inguinal floor is appropriate.

    E. Routine contralateral exploration is not indicated.

    *Ref.:* 1-3

**COMMENTS:** Repair of **inguinal hernias** in infants is recommended because the patent processus vaginalis does not close after birth and the risk for incarceration is high. In girls, the ovaries are the most common incarcerated organs in an inguinal hernia. High ligation plus excision of the hernia sac is adequate treatment, and routine repair of the inguinal floor is unnecessary. Inguinal hernias are more common in males than in females by a ratio of almost 6:1. The distal part of the hernia sac should be opened widely to prevent postoperative hydrocele. Operative management of a clinically normal contralateral groin has long been controversial. Many surgeons adopt a more selective approach over routine contralateral exploration. Laparoscopic examination through the hernia sac can identify a **patent processus vaginalis** of the contralateral groin but requires general anesthesia. Not all patients with a patent processus vaginalis will progress to a clinically significant hernia, but certainly patients without a patent processus vaginalis do not require contralateral exploration.

**ANSWER:** A

12. Which of the following statements is false in regard to branchial cleft remnants?

    A. Branchial fistulas are more common than external sinuses, which are more common than branchial cysts.

    B. First branchial cleft remnants are typically located along the anterior border of the sternocleidomastoid muscle.

    C. Second branchial cleft remnants are the most common branchial cleft remnants.

    D. Third branchial cleft remnants are typically located in the suprasternal notch or clavicular region.

    E. Second branchial cleft remnants are typically located along the anterior border of the sternocleidomastoid muscle.

    *Ref.:* 1

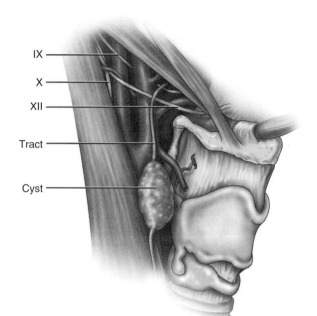

**Figure 32-1.** Second branchial cyst in relation to the cranial nerves.

**COMMENTS:** Structures of the head and neck are derived from six pairs of branchial arches with intervening external clefts and internal pouches. Failure of these structures to regress leads to **congenital branchial fistulas**, sinuses, or cysts, with fistulas, sinuses, and cysts occurring in decreasing order of frequency. First branchial remnants are typically located in the front or back of the ear or in the region of the mandible. Second branchial remnants, which are the most common, are typically located along the anterior border of the sternocleidomastoid muscle. Third branchial remnants are typically located at the sternal notch or the clavicular region. Figure 32-1 shows a second branchial cyst in relation to the cranial nerves. The tract emerges superior to cranial nerve IX and will cross anterior to cranial nerves IX and XII. The cyst itself lies anterior to cranial nerves X and XII.

**ANSWER: B**

13. Which of the following statements is most accurate regarding branchial cleft anomalies?

A. Third arch anomalies are common.

B. Type II first arch branchial anomalies are the most common overall.

C. The glossopharyngeal nerve is associated with the third branchial arch.

D. Second arch anomalies end in the piriform sinus.

E. Second arch anomalies travel deep to the internal carotid artery.

*Ref.:* 4, 5

**COMMENTS: Branchial cleft anomalies** can include cysts, fistulas, and sinus tracts, depending on the extent of development of the arch. Diagnosis depends mainly on understanding the associated anatomy of these structures. Treatment is surgical and may require a stair step incision, depending on the length of the tract.

**Branchial arch defects** travel deep to the structures derived from its arch and superficial to the structures of the following arch. **First arch anomalies** are divided into type I and type II. The trigeminal nerve is derived from the first arch. Type I anomalies are duplications of the external auditory canal. Type II anomalies many times appear at the angle of the mandible and pass up through parotid gland. Both types can be intimately associated with the facial nerve, a second arch derivative. **Second branchial arch anomalies** are by far the most common and are characterized by a tract along the anterior border of the sternocleidomastoid muscle. They pass deep to the external carotid artery and superficial to the internal carotid artery and end at the tonsillar fossa. **Third arch anomalies** are rare and appear lower in the neck. They travel and enter the pharynx at the piriform sinus. They pass deep to third arch structures such as the internal carotid artery and glossopharyngeal nerve but superficial to the vagus nerve, a fourth arch analogue. Fourth arch anomalies are extremely rare.

**ANSWER: C**

14. A 12-month-old infant is admitted to the hospital for lower gastrointestinal bleeding. Which of the following is false regarding the probable admitting diagnosis for this infant?

A. Most of the lesions are detected incidentally at autopsy or laparotomy.

B. It is typically found on the mesenteric side of the bowel.

C. It results from incomplete closure of the omphalomesenteric (vitelline) duct.

D. Typically, gastric mucosa is indirectly responsible for the gastrointestinal hemorrhage.

E. It occurs in 2% of the population.

*Ref.:* 1

**COMMENTS:** A **Meckel diverticulum** is the most common congenital anomaly of the small intestine and occurs in 2% of the population. It is most commonly diagnosed at autopsy or found incidentally during exploratory laparotomy. It arises from incomplete closure of the omphalomesenteric (vitelline) duct. A Meckel diverticulum occurs on the antimesenteric border of the ileum, most commonly between 4 and 60 cm from the ileocecal valve. Gastric mucosa is commonly found in the diverticulum (in about 50% of cases) and can lead to ulcer formation and cause painless lower gastrointestinal bleeding as the most common initial symptom. Approximately 5% of Meckel diverticula contain ectopic pancreatic tissue.

**ANSWER: B**

15. Which of the following is the most common malignancy found in children?

A. Lymphoma

B. Leukemia

C. Neuroblastoma

D. Nephroblastoma

E. Rhabdomyosarcoma

*Ref.:* 1-3

**COMMENTS: Malignancy** is second only to trauma as the leading cause of childhood death. In infants, it is the third most frequent cause of death after prematurity and congenital anomalies. Approximately 40% of childhood malignancies are leukemia. The most common solid tumor in children younger than 2 years is neuroblastoma, which accounts for 6% to 10% of all childhood cancers. In children older than 2 years, the most common solid tumor is Wilms tumor.

**ANSWER:** B

16. Which of the following statements concerning biliary atresia is true?

   A. Without treatment, the average survival is 5 years.

   B. The hallmark pathologic findings in biliary atresia are giant cell transformation and hepatocellular necrosis.

   C. The Kasai procedure typically includes a choledochojejunostomy anastomosis.

   D. Ultrasound of the liver and gallbladder is an integral part of the diagnostic work-up for biliary atresia.

   E. Biliary atresia is the third most common indication for pediatric liver transplantation.

*Ref.:* 1, 2

**COMMENTS: Biliary atresia** is characterized by progressive, irreversible fibrosis of the extrahepatic and intrahepatic bile ducts. There is no proved effective medical therapy. If surgical correction is not performed, the obliterative process progresses, and biliary cirrhosis and portal hypertension develop, followed by death by 2 years of age. Severe cholestasis, bile duct proliferation, and inflammatory cell infiltration are pathologic findings seen with biliary atresia. These findings are distinct from the hepatocellular necrosis and giant cell transformation seen with neonatal hepatitis. Biliary atresia is the most common indication for pediatric liver transplantation. The work-up for suspected biliary atresia includes ultrasound imaging of the liver and gallbladder, hepatobiliary iminodiacetic acid (HIDA) scanning, and percutaneous liver biopsy. In biliary atresia, the extrahepatic bile ducts cannot be seen on ultrasound imaging, and the gallbladder is diminutive or absent. Surgical diagnosis is made with an intraoperative cholangiogram demonstrating lack of opacification of the intrahepatic biliary tree. The goals of the **Kasai procedure** are to restore biliary flow by performing a Roux-en-Y portojejunostomy after resection of the gallbladder, extrahepatic bile ducts, and the fibrotic portal plate. A long-term successful outcome is generally low if the procedure is performed after 90 days of life. Cholangitis is the most common postoperative complication with the Kasai procedure.

**ANSWER:** D

17. With regard to the Kasai procedure for the treatment of biliary atresia, which of the following statements is true?

   A. It is most successfully performed after 3 months of age.

   B. Cholangitis rarely complicates a successful procedure.

   C. Portal hypertension remains problematic despite a successful operation.

   D. If hepatic transplantation is needed, an initial Kasai enterostomy is not indicated.

   E. Cholangitis is an infrequent late complication.

*Ref.:* 1-3

**COMMENTS: Biliary atresia** occurs as part of a spectrum of anomalies of infantile obstructive cholangiopathy. In utero viral infection has been implicated as the cause, although the evidence for such has not been proven. A HIDA scan and ultrasound imaging of the bile ducts are the mainstays among imaging tests to support the diagnosis. Variable patterns of ductal involvement of the intrahepatic and extrahepatic biliary tree are seen, with 10% of patients initially having extrahepatic disease only. The goals of treatment are to establish biliary flow and prevent the late complications of biliary cirrhosis and hepatic failure. **Hepatoportoenterostomy** is most successful in establishing bile drainage when performed during the patient's first 2 months of life. The success rate falls dramatically after 3 months of age. Cholangitis, biliary cirrhosis, hepatic failure, and portal hypertension remain late problems despite the fact that bile drainage is achieved. Attempts to reduce later cholangitic complications include prolonged use of antibiotics and steroids to minimize inflammation and infection. Hepatic transplantation has been successful in the treatment of this problem but has not replaced biliary enteric anastomosis as the initial procedure. An unsuccessful hepatoportoenterostomy does not preclude later hepatic transplantation.

**ANSWER:** C

18. Which of the following always requires surgical correction during infancy?

   A. Meconium ileus

   B. Umbilical hernia

   C. Meconium plug

   D. Hirschsprung disease

   E. All of the above

*Ref.:* 1-3

**COMMENTS: Large bowel obstruction** cannot be differentiated from small bowel obstruction in infants on plain radiographs because of the lack of haustral markings. Classic **Hirschsprung disease** is characterized by aganglionosis of the rectosigmoid segment and should be suspected whenever an infant fails to pass meconium within the first 24 hours of life. Longer intestinal segments may be involved. Rarely, total colonic aganglionosis may be present. Infants with Hirschsprung disease have intestinal obstruction that requires surgical intervention. A meconium plug often occurs in the distal part of the colon and is frequently seen in infants of diabetic mothers. It can be treated with hypertonic water-soluble radiographic contrast–enhanced enemas. Patients with **meconium ileus** have distal ileal obstruction and microcolon from disuse. The diagnosis of cystic fibrosis must be considered in patients with meconium ileus. In the majority of cases, a Gastrografin enema relieves the obstruction without the need for surgery. **Umbilical hernias** are rarely an indication to operate during infancy unless the hernia is incarcerated or strangulated, has a large defect, or occurs in the setting of ventriculoperitoneal shunts.

**ANSWER:** D

19. Which of the following is true concerning Hirschsprung disease?

   A. More common in females

   B. Absent ganglion cells in both the Auerbach and Meissner plexuses

C. Failure to pass meconium in the first 48 hours of life

D. Best diagnosed by lower gastrointestinal contrast-enhanced study

E. Atrophy of submucosal nerve endings seen on rectal biopsy specimens

*Ref.:* 2, 3

**COMMENTS:** The primary clinical manifestation of **Hirschsprung disease** is intestinal obstruction with failure to pass meconium in the first 24 hours of life or chronic constipation in older infants and children. Hirschsprung disease is more common in males than in females. Affected infants are prone to the development of enterocolitis, which carries a high mortality rate if not recognized and treated promptly. In newborn babies in whom dilation of the bowel proximal to the aganglionic segment may not have developed, findings on barium enema may be normal. Anal manometric measurements demonstrate failure of relaxation of the internal sphincter in response to rectal distention. Definitive diagnosis is based on the rectal biopsy specimen demonstrating submucosal hypertrophied nerve endings, absent **ganglion cells** in the Auerbach and Meissner plexuses, and acetylcholinesterase staining. Full-term infants with Hirschsprung disease but without enterocolitis may be treated by single-stage pull-through. The remaining patients are managed mostly by serial intestinal biopsy to determine the level of normal ganglionated intestine and leveling colostomy followed by pull-through 3 to 6 months later. Anastomosis of the normally innervated colon to the anus is the basis of all three **pull-through procedures** (Swanson, Duhamel, and Soave).

**ANSWER:** B

20. A previously well 3-week-old infant exhibits a sudden onset of bilious vomiting. Which of the following is the most likely diagnosis?

A. Pyloric stenosis

B. Duodenal atresia

C. Malrotation of the midgut

D. Intussusception

E. Tracheoesophageal fistula, H type

*Ref.:* 1-3

**COMMENTS:** See Question 21.

**ANSWER:** C

21. For the scenario described in Question 20, which would be the most appropriate initial diagnostic test?

A. Upper gastrointestinal contrast-enhanced study

B. Abdominal ultrasound

C. Barium enema

D. Abdominal radiograph

E. CT

*Ref.:* 1-3

**COMMENTS:** Infants with **intestinal obstruction** exhibit bilious emesis. Fifty percent of children with **malrotation** have bilious emesis during the first few weeks of life. Infants with malrotation

are at risk for **midgut volvulus**. Infants with a previous history of normal feedings in whom a sudden onset of bilious vomiting develops should be immediately evaluated for midgut volvulus. Midgut volvulus is demonstrated by upper gastrointestinal series showing an abrupt cutoff from failure of contrast material to pass beyond the distal duodenum or a corkscrew pattern of partial obstruction from the torsed intestines (or both), whereas malrotation is demonstrated by an aberrant course of the duodenum and duodenal-jejunal junction. A barium enema can be misleading in the diagnosis of malrotation because the position of the cecum cannot be relied on to rule in or rule out malrotation. As soon as a diagnosis is made, the infant should be taken immediately to surgery. Pyloric stenosis or tracheoesophageal fistula is not accompanied by bilious vomiting. The symptoms of infants with **H-type tracheoesophageal fistula** are usually feeding difficulties and recurrent pneumonia. The main symptoms associated with intussusception are colicky abdominal pain and bloody stools. **Duodenal atresia** may mimic malrotation in the first 24 to 48 hours of life, but at 3 weeks of age, duodenal atresia should already have been diagnosed and treated. Importantly, malrotation of the midgut is frequently associated with duodenal atresia and should be searched for at the time of repair of duodenal atresia.

**ANSWER:** A

22. All of the following are true of the Ladd procedure for midgut volvulus except:

A. Midgut volvulus twists in a counterclockwise direction and needs to be untwisted in a clockwise manner.

B. Ladd bands refer to congenital bands extending across the duodenum from the ascending colon to the retroperitoneum in the right upper quadrant.

C. There is no proved benefit with pexis of the cecum, duodenum, or both.

D. An incidental appendectomy is often performed to prevent confusing future signs and symptoms of appendicitis.

E. Midgut volvulus twists in a clockwise direction and needs to be untwisted in a counterclockwise manner.

*Ref.:* 1

**COMMENTS:** Operative management of **malrotation** involves counterclockwise reduction of the midgut volvulus when present. Nonviable bowel is resected. If viability is in question, second-look laparotomy should be performed in 24 hours to reassess and treat the intestine appropriately. The peritoneal bands (**Ladd bands**) between the ascending colon and the posterior abdominal wall in the right upper quadrant are divided, and the duodenum is mobilized so that the small bowel can be positioned in the right side of the abdomen and the colon in the left side of the abdomen. Pexis of the cecum or duodenum has not been proved to be of benefit in preventing midgut volvulus. Because of the abnormal position of the appendix, appendectomy is routinely performed to avoid future difficulty in the clinical diagnosis of appendicitis.

**ANSWER:** A

23. Which of the following is the most common anatomic type of tracheoesophageal malformations?

A. Proximal atresia and distal tracheoesophageal fistula

B. Complete esophageal atresia without fistula

C. H-type esophageal fistula

D. Proximal fistula and distal esophageal atresia

E. Proximal and distal tracheoesophageal fistulas

*Ref.:* 1

**COMMENTS:** There are five readily identified anatomic variants of **esophageal atresia** and **tracheoesophageal fistula**. Type A, with an incidence of 6%, is true esophageal atresia and no tracheoesophageal fistula. Type B, with an incidence of 2%, is distal esophageal atresia with a proximal tracheoesophageal fistula. Type C, the most common variant with an incidence of 85%, refers to proximal esophageal atresia with a distal tracheoesophageal fistula. Type D, with an incidence of 1%, is a proximal and distal tracheoesophageal fistula. Type H, with an incidence of 2%, refers to an intact esophagus with a single tracheoesophageal fistula. Other anatomic variants may be present, and *t*racheoesophageal fistula can occur in association with *v*ertebral, *a*norectal, and *r*enal and or *r*adial anomalies, which together are components of the VATER syndrome.

**ANSWER:** A

24. A 1-month-old neonate has an umbilical hernia in which the defect is estimated to be 1 cm in diameter. Which of the following statements is true?

A. The likelihood of spontaneous closure in this neonate is low, and the hernia should be repaired.

B. Indications for early repair of an umbilical hernia include a history of incarceration, a large skin proboscis, and the presence of a ventriculoperitoneal shunt.

C. Repair of the hernia defect should include the placement of mesh.

D. Complete closure of the umbilical ring may be expected in only 30% of children by the age of 4 to 6 years.

E. All of the above

*Ref.:* 1

**COMMENTS:** **Umbilical hernias** occur as a result of persistence of the umbilical ring. By the age of 4 to 6 years, closure of this ring can be expected in 80% of children. In patients with umbilical hernias with greater than a 2-cm defect, spontaneous closure is less likely. Umbilical hernias are usually repaired early if the defect is greater than 2 cm, there is a history of incarceration, or a large skin proboscis or a ventriculoperitoneal shunt is present. Repair of an umbilical hernia involves an infraumbilical semicircular incision, separation of the hernia sac from the overlying skin, repair of the fascial defect, pexis of the base of the umbilicus to the fascia, and closure of the skin. The fascial closure is rarely under tension and does not require prosthetic mesh.

**ANSWER:** B

25. The most common cause of duodenal obstruction at birth is:

A. Malrotation

B. Duodenal atresia

C. Annular pancreas

D. Choledochal cyst

E. Midgut volvulus

*Ref.:* 1-3

**COMMENTS:** **Vomiting** within the first 24 hours of life in the absence of abdominal distention suggests duodenal atresia in a neonate. **Malrotation** with **midgut volvulus** is the most common and the most devastating cause of duodenal obstruction beyond the neonatal period. The duodenal obstruction can be caused by extrinsic compression by the peritoneal Ladd bands that extend from the abdominal wall to the anomalously located cecum in the right upper quadrant. Alternatively, the catastrophic complication of malrotation is midgut volvulus and intestinal infarction from torsion of the superior mesenteric vessels about the narrow mesenteric pedicle by which the midgut is suspended. An **annular pancreas** may cause duodenal obstruction as a result of duodenal stenosis. Choledochal cysts are rare and manifested as jaundice and an abdominal mass.

**ANSWER:** B

26. Regarding jejunal atresia, which of the following statements is false?

A. It is caused by failure of embryologic recanalization of the gut.

B. Associated anomalies are more common with duodenal atresia than with jejunal atresia.

C. Cystic fibrosis may be present in roughly 10% of patients with jejunal atresia.

D. The most common significant associated morbidity is short gut syndrome.

E. It is not usually associated with trisomy 21.

*Ref.:* 1-3

**COMMENTS:** **Intestinal atresia** is believed to arise from an in utero vascular accident. Multiple atresia occurs in approximately 10% of patients. Many forms exist, from a simple web or stenosis to long segments of atretic intestines or complete intestinal disruption with varying degrees of mesenteric defect. Intestinal atresia is usually accompanied by bilious vomiting and abdominal distention. Passage of **meconium** does not exclude the diagnosis. Cystic fibrosis may be present in approximately 10% of patients with jejunoileal atresia. **Duodenal atresia** is frequently associated with trisomy 21 (Down syndrome). The most common and significant morbidity associated with jejunoileal atresia is short gut syndrome.

**ANSWER:** A

27. An 8-hour-old newborn has mild respiratory distress and excessive drooling. An abdominal radiograph shows complete lack of air in the gastrointestinal tract. What is the most likely diagnosis?

A. Bilateral choanal atresia

B. Pyloric atresia

C. Duodenal atresia

D. Esophageal atresia with a distal tracheoesophageal fistula

E. Esophageal atresia without a tracheoesophageal fistula

*Ref.:* 1-3

**COMMENTS:** See Question 28.

**ANSWER:** E

**28.** The VACTERL association most commonly includes which of the following?

    A. Ankylosis

    B. Imperforate anus

    C. Eye deformities

    D. Congenital cystic lung malformation

    E. Choanal atresia

*Ref.:* 1

**COMMENTS:** Neonates have a gasless gastrointestinal tract at birth. As they start to swallow soon after birth, air reaches the colon within 6 to 12 hours. In pure **esophageal atresia** without an associated fistula, swallowed or inspired air does not reach the distal end of the gastrointestinal tract and abdominal films demonstrate no air in the gastrointestinal tract. Esophageal atresia is suggested when an infant drools excessively because of esophageal obstruction or spits up during attempted feedings. When an orogastric tube is passed in an infant with esophageal atresia, a chest radiograph showing the tube coiled in a blind pouch helps in making the diagnosis. About 85% to 90% of patients with a **tracheoesophageal malformation** have a blind proximal pouch with a distal tracheoesophageal fistula, also known as esophageal type C. Respiratory symptoms are secondary to aspiration from the esophageal pouch or retrograde reflux of gastric contents from the fistula into the lung. In esophageal atresia with a tracheoesophageal fistula, inspired air reaches the stomach and small bowel through the tracheoesophageal fistula. Contrast-enhanced studies and bronchoscopy may be useful in select cases to confirm the diagnosis and demonstrate the location of the fistula. Recognition of the anatomy of the anomaly is important for establishing appropriate initial treatment and definitive repair. Air fails to pass from the stomach into the duodenum and small bowel in neonates with pyloric atresia, a rare congenital anomaly. Radiographic studies show extreme distention of the stomach with air-fluid levels. Neonates, being obligatory nasal breathers, have major respiratory problems when born with bilateral choanal atresia but do not have difficulty swallowing air. The **VACTERL association** refers to *v*ertebral anomalies, imperforate *a*nus, *c*ardiac defects, *t*racheo*e*sophageal fistula, *r*adial and *r*enal malformation, and *l*imb defects.

**ANSWER:** B

**29.** A 3000-g infant is born with esophageal atresia and a distal tracheoesophageal fistula. If the infant does not exhibit respiratory distress and associated anomalies are not present, which of the following is the preferred treatment?

    A. Gastrostomy, cervical esophagostomy, and delayed repair

    B. Gastrostomy, sump tube drainage of the proximal pouch, and delayed repair

    C. Fistula ligation and delayed esophageal repair

    D. Division of the fistula with primary esophageal anastomosis

    E. Primary repair with colonic interposition

*Ref.:* 1-3

**COMMENTS:** The timing and type of surgical intervention for **esophageal atresia** and **tracheoesophageal fistula** depend on the maturity of the infant and associated cardiorespiratory problems or other congenital anomalies that have an impact on the mortality associated with primary repair. Medically stable infants weighing more than 2500 g are treated by primary repair with fistula division, closure of its tracheal end, and end-to-end anastomosis of the esophageal segments. Unstable infants with respiratory problems can be treated by gastrostomy and sump drainage of the blind proximal pouch. Because loss of ventilatory pressure can occur through the open tracheoesophageal fistula or retrograde aspiration of gastric contents into the lungs can exacerbate the pulmonary symptoms, some infants may benefit from primary fistula ligation without esophageal repair, with or without gastrostomy placement. The final esophageal repair is accomplished after the complicating cardiorespiratory problems have been addressed.

**ANSWER:** D

**30.** Common complications following repair of esophageal atresia and tracheoesophageal fistula include all of the following except:

    A. Esophageal strictures

    B. Anastomotic leak

    C. Tracheomalacia

    D. Recurrent fistula

    E. Gastroesophageal reflux

*Ref.:* 1-3

**COMMENTS: Gastroesophageal reflux** and **tracheomalacia** are commonly associated with esophageal atresia and tracheoesophageal fistula in infants. Gastroesophageal reflux is believed to be related to the underlying esophageal dysmotility and perhaps to dysfunction of the lower esophageal sphincter, which frequently requires fundoplication. Anastomotic leakage, stricture, and recurrent fistula formation are known operative complications.

**ANSWER:** C

**31.** Which of the following statements concerning necrotizing enterocolitis (NEC) is true?

    A. The initial insult in NEC is to the intestinal mucosa.

    B. The jejunum is the most frequently involved site.

    C. Operative intervention is indicated after resuscitation.

    D. Progression of NEC is halted after surgical therapy.

    E. The cecum is frequently not involved.

*Ref.:* 1, 2

**COMMENTS: Necrotizing enterocolitis** is a disease that affects the intestinal tract of neonates. Clinical and experimental data have shown that the cause of NEC is multifactorial, with risk factors including perinatal stress, maternal cocaine use, and prematurity. The initial injury with NEC is observed in the intestinal mucosa. The spectrum of severity ranges from isolated mucosal injury to transmural bowel necrosis. Although the terminal ileum and right colon are the most commonly affected sites, the disease can be segmental or affect the entire gastrointestinal tract. The initial treatment of infants with NEC is nonsurgical and consists of nasogastric decompression, bowel rest, broad-spectrum antibiotics, optimal fluid management, and parental nutrition. Operative intervention, such as bowel resection with proximal enterostomy, is indicated to treat the acute complications of NEC, which include intestinal perforation, necrosis, persistent bleeding, or obstruction. Operative intervention, however, does not prevent progression of the disease, which can continue after resection and may require additional surgical therapy.

**ANSWER:** A

32. A premature infant with a history of neonatal respiratory distress requiring ventilatory support is being fed oral formula. Abdominal distention develops, and blood-streaked stool is passed. Appropriate management includes which of the following?

A. Anoscopy for a probable neonatal fissure

B. Barium enema to rule out intussusception

C. Restriction of oral intake to clear liquid to prevent mucosal injury

D. Antibiotic-directed treatment of specific pathogens cultured from the stool

E. Cessation of oral feeding, institution of nasogastric drainage, intravenous antibiotics, total parenteral nutrition, and serial abdominal examinations and radiographic studies

*Ref.:* 1-3

**COMMENTS:** See Question 33.

**ANSWER:** E

33. Which of the following are indications for surgery in an infant with NEC?

A. Pneumatosis intestinalis

B. Portal venous gas

C. Pneumoperitoneum

D. Bloody stools

E. All of the above

*Ref.:* 1-3

**COMMENTS: Necrotizing enterocolitis** affects premature infants with a history of neonatal stress who received oral feedings. The pathophysiologic processes involve mucosal ischemia, bowel necrosis, perforation, peritonitis, and sepsis. Clinical manifestations are initial intolerance of formula, abdominal distention, blood-streaked stool with progression to systemic sepsis, metabolic acidosis, and thrombocytopenia. The initial treatment is directed at prevention of further mucosal injury and septic complications. Oral feedings are stopped, nasogastric tube decompression is instituted, broad-spectrum antibiotics are administered, and fluid and electrolyte support is provided. Close monitoring with physical examination, serial radiographs, and biochemical assessment for signs of deterioration is mandatory. **Pneumatosis intestinalis** is a pathognomonic radiographic finding of NEC that is caused by invasion of the bowel wall by gas-forming organisms. Portal venous gas indicates the presence of gas-forming organisms translocated to the portal circulation. Neither of these radiographic findings is an absolute indication for surgery, however. Indications for surgical intervention are perforation, persistent necrosis as evidenced by

progressive clinical deterioration such as worsening metabolic acidosis, thrombocytopenia, and hemodynamic instability. During surgery, the necrotic bowel is resected, and the ends of the retained bowel are brought out as enterostomies. Bowel preservation is a high priority during surgery to avoid complications associated with short bowel syndrome. A second-look operation in 24 hours can be performed if bowel viability is questionable at the first operation.

**ANSWER:** C

34. Which of the following statement concerning the physiology of the newborn is true?

A. Perfusion is best monitored clinically by distal pulses.

B. Newborns preferentially breathe through their mouths rather than their noses.

C. Cardiac output in the newborn period is primarily rate dependent.

D. Newborns have normal levels but are functionally deficient in immunoglobulins and C3b complement.

E. Adequate capillary refill is less than 5 seconds.

*Ref.:* 1

**COMMENTS:** Capillary refill is the best way to clinically monitor cardiac perfusion in a newborn. Adequate **capillary refill** is less than 1 second. Unlike adults and older children, cardiac output in the newborn is directly related to the child's heart rate, and the child's ability to increase cardiac output depends on the increase in heart rate and not stroke volume. Newborns are obligate nose breeders. Respiratory distress in the newborn is heralded by nasal flaring, grunting, and intercostal and substernal retractions. Newborns are immunodeficient from low immunoglobin and C3b levels.

**ANSWER:** C

35. A newborn is evaluated for respiratory distress because of severe hypoxia several hours after birth. The patient appears dyspneic, tachypneic, and cyanotic. The abdomen is noted to be scaphoid. Which of the following is true of this newborn?

A. This condition can be diagnosed prenatally with fetal ultrasound.

B. An upper gastrointestinal contrast-enhanced study is required to diagnose this condition.

C. The survival rate is extremely low.

D. Emergency surgical intervention is required within hours of birth.

E. Emergency placement of a chest tube is required.

*Ref.:* 1

**COMMENTS:** This patient most likely has congenital diaphragmatic hernia. The incidence of **congenital diaphragmatic hernia** is reported to be the range of 1 in 2000 to 5000 live births. The most common diaphragmatic defect is in a posterolateral location and is known as a Bochdalek hernia. A less common site for the defect is anteromedial (retrosternal), in which case it is known as a **Morgagni hernia**. Congenital diaphragmatic hernias can be diagnosed on prenatal ultrasound. A plain chest radiograph demonstrating an intrathoracic location of the gastric air bubbles, nasogastric tube, or intestines is diagnostic. Rarely is an upper gastrointestinal study needed. Before it was understood that **pulmonary hypoplasia** and pulmonary hypertension are the causes of morbidity and mortality in infants with congenital diaphragmatic hernia, emergency repair was recommended. However, because emergency repair does not improve the outcome, pediatric surgeons will wait between 24 and 72 hours for cardiorespiratory stabilization before proceeding to surgical repair. The survival rate of infants with congenital diaphragmatic hernia is in the range of 70% to 90%. A chest tube may be needed in situations in which a tension pneumothorax could occur following the institution of high-pressure ventilation.

**ANSWER:** A

36. During treatment of an infant with congenital diaphragmatic hernia, all of the following may be required except:

    A. Chest tube insertion

    B. ECMO

    C. High-frequency oscillatory ventilation

    D. Immediate surgery

    E. Nitric oxide

    *Ref.:* 1

**COMMENTS:** The primary physiologic disturbance in infants with **respiratory distress** caused by **congenital posterolateral diaphragmatic hernia** is related to pulmonary hypoplasia and high pulmonary vasculature resistance (pulmonary hypertension) because of pulmonary arteriolar vasoconstriction. The initial resuscitation must include prompt correction of hypoxia, metabolic acidosis, and hypothermia to relieve the pulmonary vasoconstriction. High pulmonary vascular resistance produces right-to-left shunting via the patent ductus arteriosus, thus further compromising the infant's cardiopulmonary status. Initial treatment involves endotracheal intubation for respiratory distress, placement of an orogastric tube, and maintenance of adequate vascular volume. Infants intubated with high-pressure ventilation are prone to the development of pneumothorax, and tube thoracostomy may be required. Treatment consists of gentle ventilation to recruit alveoli and avoid barotrauma with the use of high-frequency oscillatory ventilation or the addition of a pulmonary vascular dilator such as inhaled nitric oxide. **Extracorporeal membrane oxygenation** may salvage infants who remained critically ill despite conventional support. Surgical repair is performed after resuscitation and stabilization of the infant's cardiopulmonary status. Definitive surgical repair is usually carried out via an abdominal approach. Biomesh or synthetic material may be used if primary approximation of the diaphragmatic defect is not possible.

**ANSWER:** D

37. All of the following are true of bronchopulmonary malformations except:

    A. Associated anomalies are extremely rare in patients with pulmonary sequestration.

    B. CT, magnetic resonance imaging (MRI), or both are indicated before surgical intervention in those with pulmonary sequestration.

    C. Congenital lobar emphysema occurs in a histologically normal lung and is caused by air trapping secondary to abnormal cartilaginous support of the feeding bronchus.

    D. A congenital cystic adenomatoid malformation typically has a bronchial communication and receives its blood supply from the normal pulmonary circulation.

    E. Pulmonary sequestrations are associated with congenital cardiac defects.

    *Ref.:* 1

**COMMENTS: Pulmonary sequestrations** are either intralobar or extralobar and are associated with congenital cardiac defects. The vascular supply and drainage of pulmonary sequestrations frequently include anomalous systemic and pulmonary vessels, such as the aorta and azygous veins, which can complicate surgical excision. CT angiography, magnetic resonance imaging, or both are therefore important for mapping the blood supply before removal of the pulmonary sequestrations. Both types may be complicated by a large intravascular shunt leading to cardiac insufficiency, and intralobar sequestrations are commonly complicated by infections and bleeding. Congenital lobar emphysema is caused by overdistention of histologically normal lung because of air trapping as a result of abnormal cartilaginous support of the feeding bronchus. **Congenital cystic adenomatoid malformations**, unlike pulmonary sequestrations, typically have bronchial communications and normal blood supply. Because of the high risk for infection and the potential for malignant degeneration, resection is recommended for all these lesions.

**ANSWER:** A

38. With regard to defects of the abdominal wall, which statement is correct?

    A. In gastroschisis, the herniated bowel contents are covered by a membrane.

    B. Gastroschisis is frequently associated with cardiac malformations.

    C. Chromosomal abnormalities are often present with omphalocele.

    D. Treatment of abdominal wall defects is immediate surgical closure of the fascial defect.

    E. In omphalocele, a silo bag is placed to cover the exposed intestine.

    *Ref.:* 1

**COMMENTS:** Both **omphalocele** and **gastroschisis** are neonatal abdominal wall defects. In omphalocele, the umbilical cord arises from the layers of peritoneum and amnion covering the abdominal wall contents. In contrast, in gastroschisis, the abdominal wall defect is to the right of the umbilical ring and is complete with herniation of the intestines. Approximately 50% of infants born with omphalocele have other malformations, including cardiac and chromosomal abnormalities. Anomalies associated with gastroschisis are rare, with the major exception being intestinal atresia. The initial management of abdominal wall defects consists of nasogastric decompression, intravenous fluids, broad-spectrum antibiotics, and protection of the abdominal wall contents. In omphalocele, the sac is covered with a sterile occlusive dressing, and a work-up for associated anomalies should be initiated. In gastroschisis, a silo bag is placed to cover the exposed intestines. Complete medical evaluation and resuscitation of the infant with protection of the abdominal contents take precedence over surgical closure.

**ANSWER:** C

39. An asymptomatic 3-year-old boy is found to have a palpable abdominal mass on routine examination. Which of the following is true regarding the most likely diagnosis in this child?

   A. The current overall survival rate of these patients is about 50%.

   B. The hereditary form of this tumor is more aggressive and more common.

   C. Common metastatic foci are in the lungs and liver.

   D. There is no role for preoperative chemotherapy in the treatment of this childhood tumor.

   E. Measurement of serotonin metabolites in the urine aids in the diagnosis and in monitoring the course of the disease.

*Ref.:* 1

**COMMENTS:** The differential diagnosis for this mass is **Wilms tumor** and **neuroblastoma**. This patient has a Wilms tumor. Neuroblastoma is the third most common pediatric malignancy. More than 80% of cases are seen before the age of 4 years. They arise from neural crest cells, and the tumor originates most frequently in the adrenal glands. Two thirds of these tumors are first noticed as an asymptomatic mass. The use of preoperative chemotherapy is based on the stage of the tumor. Determination of **serum catecholamines** or their metabolites (or both) is used to aid in diagnosis and monitoring of the disease. The patient should be evaluated with abdominal CT, which usually shows displacement of an intact kidney. Bone metastasis, proptosis, and periorbital ecchymosis may develop. Spontaneous regression of neuroblastoma in infants has been well described, especially in tumors with a nearly triploid number of chromosomes that also lack N-myc amplification and loss of chromosome 1p. Wilms tumor is an embryonal tumor of renal origin and the most common primary malignant kidney tumor in childhood. It is commonly manifested as an asymptomatic abdominal mass. Abdominal and thoracic CT, MRI, or both are used preoperatively to distinguish Wilms tumor from neuroblastoma and assess for bilateral Wilms tumor, liver or lung metastasis, and vascular invasion such as tumor thrombus within the inferior vena cava. Urine examination for **vanillylmandelic acid** (VMA) also helps distinguish Wilms tumor from neuroblastoma. VMA will be produced and levels elevated in children with neuroblastoma, whereas it will not be produced and levels will be normal in those with Wilms tumor. The most common germline mutation is the Wilms tumor gene-1. Hereditary Wilms tumor is uncommon. Wilms tumor is associated with Denys-Drash syndrome, WAGR syndrome (*W*ilms tumor, *a*niridia, *g*enitourinary abnormalities, and mental *r*etardation), and Beckwith-Wiedemann syndrome; thus, patients with these syndromes need to be screened for Wilms tumor. Preoperative chemotherapy is indicated for the treatment of invasive Wilms tumor. The current overall survival rate after surgical resection exceeds 85%.

**ANSWER:** C

40. A 6-month-old infant has a history of an acute onset of crampy abdominal pain and leg withdrawal of 12 hours' duration. Rectal examination shows guaiac-positive stool. Which of the following is the most likely diagnosis?

   A. Bleeding Meckel diverticulum

   B. Acute appendicitis

   C. Kidney stone

   D. Infected urachal cyst

   E. Intussusception

*Ref.:* 2, 3

**COMMENTS: Ileocolic intussusception** should be strongly suspected in a child between the ages of 3 and 18 months with colicky abdominal pain and guaiac-positive stools. Acute appendicitis, infected urachal cyst, and nephrolithiasis can occur in this age group but are not accompanied by bloody stools. A bleeding Meckel diverticulum is usually painless, and frank bloody stool is seen.

**ANSWER:** E

41. Cystic hygromas are most commonly complicated by which of the following?

   A. Infection

   B. Hemorrhage

   C. Respiratory distress

   D. Malignancy

   E. All of the above

*Ref.:* 1-3

**COMMENTS: Cystic hygroma** is a congenital lymphangiomatous malformation that commonly occurs in the posterior region of the neck, the axilla, the groin, or the mediastinum. These lesions can attain a large size, and all of the complications mentioned have been described. Malignant degeneration is rare. Infection, however, is the most common complication.

**ANSWER:** A

42. Progressive abdominal distention and bilious vomiting develop in a newborn. Radiographic studies reveal distended bowel loops of various size with air-fluid levels and a "soap suds" appearance in the right lower quadrant. Which of the following procedures should be performed next?

   A. Laparotomy

   B. Paracentesis

   C. Gastrografin lower gastrointestinal radiographic studies

   D. Gastrografin upper intestinal radiographic studies

   E. Sweat chloride test

*Ref.:* 1-3

**COMMENTS:** Postnatal distal intestinal obstruction with the classic radiographic findings of "soap bubbles" suggests the diagnosis of **meconium ileus**. Nearly all affected infants have cystic fibrosis. Abnormalities in salt and water exchange across the intestinal lumen lead to a thick inspissated meconium plug causing distal ileal obstruction. With uncomplicated meconium ileus, a **Gastrografin enema** may be both diagnostic and therapeutic. The detergent and hyperosmolar effects of the contrast material may loosen the thick meconium and relieve the obstruction. Surgery is indicated if the obstruction does not respond to the Gastrografin enema or if complications such as peritonitis or perforation are present. The usual operative treatment includes exteriorization of the intestines to allow postoperative irrigation of the inspissated meconium with a water-soluble agent or *N*-acetylcysteine. A positive sweat chloride test is diagnostic of cystic fibrosis and can be performed electively. Paracentesis and lavage have no role in the work-up or treatment of meconium ileus.

**ANSWER:** C

43. Select the true statement regarding the operative management of intussusception.

   A. Resection should be performed without an attempt at intra-operative manual reduction.

   B. Primary ileocolic anastomosis may be performed if bowel resection is necessary.

   C. After successful reduction by barium enema in a 1-year-old child, delayed surgery should be performed because of the risk for recurrence.

   D. After successful reduction by barium enema, exploration is indicated to rule out associated pathologic processes.

   E. Appendectomy should never be performed after successful operative manual reduction.

*Ref.:* 1

**COMMENTS:** See Question 43.

**ANSWER:** B

44. Contraindications to attempted reduction of an intussusception via air/barium enema in a child include which of the following?

   A. Pneumoperitoneum

   B. Initial evaluation after 48 hours of symptoms

   C. Recurrence after hydrostatic reduction

   D. Age older than 5 years

   E. Recurrent symptoms in the immediate postoperative period

*Ref.:* 1

**COMMENTS: Ileocolic intussusception** should be strongly suspected in a child between the ages of 3 and 18 months with colicky abdominal pain and guaiac-positive stools. A barium or preferably an air enema should be performed promptly for diagnosis and reduction of the intussusception via hydrostatic or pneumatic pressure. In approximately 80% of children, successful radiologic reduction is the only therapy needed. An attempt at nonoperative reduction is contraindicated in children with perforation or peritonitis. In such cases, prompt surgery is required. When nonviable bowel is encountered at the time of exploration, resection is carried out without an attempt at reduction. Otherwise, reduction by gentle digital pressure on the intussusceptum is attempted. Resection is performed if the intussusception is not manually reducible. Primary anastomosis can be performed. After successful operative manual reduction, an appendectomy is usually performed. Recurrence is

not considered to be an absolute indication for surgery, and a second and third attempt may be successful. A 1-year-old child most likely has "idiopathic" intussusception with no anatomic leading point. Children older than 5 years are more likely to have surgical lead points such as an intestinal polyp, **Meckel diverticulum**, or tumor (**lymphoma**). Further work-up and appropriate surgery to prevent recurrences are needed. Intussusception recurs in 5% to 10% of patients regardless of whether the intussusception has been reduced radiographically or operatively. Treatment involves repeated air enema, which is successful in most cases.

**ANSWER:** A

45. The "double-bubble" sign seen on abdominal radiographs of neonates is suggestive of all of the following conditions except:

   A. Duodenal atresia

   B. Normal newborn radiographic finding at delivery

   C. Malrotation of the midgut

   D. Meconium ileus

   E. Duodenal stenosis

*Ref.:* 1-3

**COMMENTS:** The radiographic **double-bubble sign** usually signifies duodenal obstruction (Figure 32-2). It has been believed

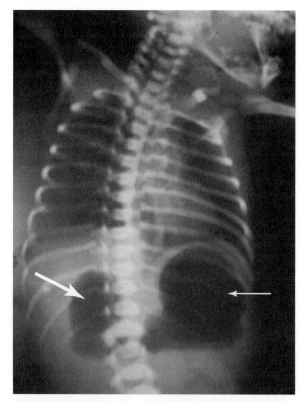

**Figure 32-2.** The classic double-bubble sign (*arrows*) seen on a radiograph. *(Reprinted with permission from Kimura K, Loening-Baucke V: Radiologic decision making: bilious vomiting in the newborn: rapid diagnosis of intestinal obstruction,* Am Fam Physician *61:2791, 2000. Copyright © 2000 American Academy of Family Physicians. All Rights Reserved.)*

to be pathognomonic of duodenal atresia. Infants are born with a gasless abdomen. After taking the first few breaths, they start swallowing air. This column of air usually takes 6 to 12 hours to reach the distal end of the colon. Therefore, an abdominal film taken a few minutes after delivery might show a double bubble and yet be normal in the absence of other clinical signs of intestinal obstruction such as bilious emesis. The double-bubble sign can also be seen in infants with malrotation and midgut volvulus, but air is present in the distal intestines. This is an operative emergency to avoid progression to vascular necrosis of the entire midgut. Immediate diagnostic upper gastrointestinal study and operative treatment are essential. Both **ileal atresia** and **meconium ileus** are manifested as distal small bowel obstruction. The radiographic findings of ileal atresia and meconium ileus are multiple dilated loops of intestine with air-fluid levels, along with the presence of "soap suds" for meconium ileus.

**ANSWER: D**

46. The treatment of choice for duodenal atresia is which of the following?

    A. Duodenojejunostomy

    B. Duodenoduodenostomy

    C. Duodenostomy with delayed repair

    D. Gastrojejunostomy

    E. Roux-en-Y enterostomy

*Ref.:* 1

**COMMENTS:** Once the diagnosis is made, surgery can be deferred until after medical stabilization and work-up for associated anomalies. **Duodenoduodenostomy** is the preferred operation because it provides physiologic continuity to the gastrointestinal tract. An intraluminal duodenal windsock diaphragm or partial webs should be sought intraoperatively by passing a Foley catheter into the distal part of the duodenum. If no resistance is encountered on withdrawal of the Foley catheter from the duodenum, continuity is ensured; otherwise, the obstruction is untreated.

**ANSWER: B**

47. Which of the following is the most reliable test for establishing the diagnosis of gastroesophageal reflux in pediatric patients?

    A. Esophagography

    B. Esophagoscopy with biopsy

    C. Upper gastrointestinal contrast-enhanced study

    D. Monitoring of the pH of the esophagus for 12 to 24 hours

    E. Nuclear scanning after the ingestion of radioactive milk

*Ref.:* 1-3

**COMMENTS:** All of the studies listed are useful in documenting the presence of **gastroesophageal reflux**, but an abnormal finding on a 12- to 24-hour esophageal pH study is most sensitive and specific for gastroesophageal reflux as the cause of the symptoms.

**ANSWER: D**

48. Which of the following is false regarding teratomas in the pediatric population?

    A. Sacrococcygeal teratomas are treated by excision of the tumor alone and by addition of coccygectomy as needed.

    B. The sacrococcygeal site is the most common location for the tumor in neonates.

    C. Most neonatal sacrococcygeal teratomas are benign.

    D. Elevations in the α-fetoprotein level confirm the diagnosis.

    E. Evidence of hydrops and a large teratoma carries a poor prognosis.

*Ref.:* 1

**COMMENTS: Teratomas** are tumors arising from more than one of the three embryonic germ layers and contain tissue that is foreign to the anatomic site in which they are found. The sacrococcygeal region is the most common site for neonatal teratomas. In adolescents, the gonads are a more common site for teratomas. Most neonatal **sacrococcygeal teratomas** are benign. Without coccygectomy, complete tumor extirpation is associated with a higher rate of recurrence. Patients must be monitored carefully after surgical intervention because recurrence can be seen even with benign tumor. Levels of α-fetoprotein markers are always elevated at birth because of components of maternal origin. Levels are expected to continue to decrease and normalize after excision with subsequent follow-up and should be monitored to detect incomplete resection or tumor recurrence. Prenatal intervention is advocated for fetuses with evidence of hydrops and a large sacrococcygeal teratoma because the prognosis is poor in these cases.

**ANSWER: D**

49. Hepatoblastomas in children are characterized by all of the following except:

    A. Usually occur in children younger than 3 years

    B. Associated with Beckwith-Wiedemann syndrome

    C. Often extensively invasive and multifocal

    D. Better response to preoperative chemotherapy

    E. Elevated α-fetoprotein levels

*Ref.:* 1

**COMMENTS: Hepatoblastomas** usually occur before 3 years of age, whereas hepatocellular carcinoma may be found in children and adults. Hepatoblastoma is most often unifocal, whereas hepatocellular carcinoma is often invasive and multicentric. Hepatoblastoma is associated with hemihypertrophy, very low birth weight, familial adenomatous polyposis, and Beckwith-Wiedemann syndrome, whereas hepatocellular carcinoma is associated with underlying chronic liver injury such as occurs with perinatally acquired infection with hepatitis B and C viruses, mutations in c-met, tyrosinemia, biliary cirrhosis, and $\alpha_1$-antitrypsin deficiency. α-Fetoprotein levels parallel disease activity in both hepatoblastoma and **hepatocellular carcinoma**. The overall survival rate is 70% for hepatoblastoma and 25% for hepatocellular carcinoma. Chemotherapy is more effective for hepatoblastoma than for hepatocellular carcinoma.

**ANSWER: C**

**50.** A 2-year-old boy is seen in your office with a midline neck mass that has been present for 2 months. On examination, the mass is 2 cm in size, is not tender or pulsatile, and moves with protrusion of his tongue. Ultrasound of the neck demonstrates a midline cystic lesion sitting deep to the strap muscles with no surrounding lymphadenopathy or other pathology. The thyroid gland is noted in the normal location. Findings on thyroid function studies are normal. Which of the following statements is true regarding this mass?

A. Simple excision of the mass is sufficient.

B. This mass most likely represents ectopic thyroid tissue.

C. The rate of recurrence is very high after appropriate therapy.

D. These lesions can be found along the base of tongue and hyoid bone.

E. Most lesions are associated with a draining cutaneous fistula tract.

*Ref.:* 4-6

**COMMENTS:** The most likely diagnosis is a **thyroglossal duct cyst**. The differential diagnosis for a midline neck mass in a child would also include a dermoid cyst, lymphadenopathy, ectopic thyroid, thymic cyst, or a ranula. Thyroglossal duct cysts arise from remnants of the thyroid gland that descended from the foramen cecum at the tongue base down to its anatomic position in the neck. The hyoid bone is a common location to find the cyst. Most do not have a draining fistula tract, as with branchial cleft remnants. Ultrasound and thyroid function tests should be performed to be certain that there is thyroid tissue in the normal anatomic location so that the patient is not rendered hypothyroid in the postoperative period. Surgical treatment involves removal of the cyst tract along with the central hyoid bone—the **Sistrunk procedure**. Simple cyst excision alone results in high rates of recurrence, whereas a Sistrunk procedure has reported recurrence rates of less than 5%.

**ANSWER:** D

**REFERENCES**

1. Warner BW: Pediatric surgery. In Townsend CM, Beauchamp RD, Evers BM, et al, editors: *Sabiston textbook of surgery: the biological basis of modern surgical practice,* ed 18, Philadelphia, 2008, WB Saunders.
2. Hackman D, Grikscheit TC, Wang KS, et al: Pediatric surgery. In Brunicardi FC, Andersen DK, Billiar TR, et al, editors: *Schwartz's principles of surgery,* ed 9, New York, 2010, McGraw-Hill.
3. Rowe MI, O'Neill IA, Grosfied IL, et al, editors: *Essentials of pediatric surgery,* St. Louis, 1995, CV Mosby.
4. Lorenz RR, Netterville JL, Burkey BB: Head and neck. In Townsend CM, Beauchamp RD, Evers BM, et al, editors: *Sabiston textbook of surgery: the biological basis of modern surgical practice,* ed 18, Philadelphia, 2008, WB Saunders.
5. Bailey BJ, Johnson JT, Newlands SD: *Head and neck surgery— otolaryngology,* ed 4, Philadelphia, 2006, Lippincott Williams & Wilkins.
6. Cummings CW, Haughey BH, Thomas JR, et al: *Cummings otolaryngology: head and neck surgery,* ed 4, Philadelphia, 2005, CV Mosby.

# CHAPTER 33

# Plastic and Reconstructive Surgery, Including Hand Surgery

*Gordon H. Derman, M.D.; Samuel M. Maurice, M.D.;*
*Niki A. Christopoulos, M.D.; and Steven D. Bines, M.D.*

1. Which of the following statements regarding the blood supply of a skin graft is true?

   A. Active uptake of nutrients and serum by the skin graft is a process called imbibition.

   B. Before imbibition, inosculation, or capillary alignment, is essential for graft survival.

   C. At 48 hours, efferent and afferent blood flow to and from the graft is established.

   D. Capillary buds from the recipient bed have been shown to form anastomoses with graft vessels and to invade the graft directly.

   E. The return of venous circulation precedes that of arterial circulation.

   *Ref.:* 1-4

**COMMENTS:** A skin graft survives initially by **plasmatic imbibition**, or **passive diffusion** of nutrients from the recipient bed to the graft. This phase lasts 24 to 48 hours, depending on the abundance of blood supply in the recipient bed. During this phase, the graft is ischemic and undergoes significant weight gain because the plasmatic circulation occurs essentially from the recipient bed to the graft only. At the end of 48 hours, the process of inosculation occurs. During this phase, which lasts 2 to 4 days, capillaries from the recipient bed align with capillaries from the graft. This circulation is initially immature and prone to blood pooling and pendulum-like flow. The final stage of revascularization, which occurs on average 5 to 7 days after grafting, is marked by the formation of a mature circulation with afferent and efferent blood flow established. Revascularization occurs both by the formation of anastomoses between recipient vessels and graft vessels and by neovascularization. Return of the arterial circulation precedes return of the venous circulation. This delay in return of venous circulation to the skin graft supports the practice of elevating a newly skin-grafted extremity. The delay in establishment of a venous circulation also explains the initial pink appearance of the graft, which later changes to blue or purple because of venous insufficiency.

**ANSWER:** D

2. Which of the following statements regarding the use of split-thickness and full-thickness skin grafts is true?

   A. A split-thickness skin graft undergoes approximately 10% shrinkage of its surface area immediately after harvesting.

   B. A full-thickness skin graft undergoes approximately 10% shrinkage of its surface area immediately after harvesting.

   C. Secondary contraction is more likely to occur after adequate healing of a full-thickness skin graft than a split-thickness skin graft.

   D. Sensation does not return to areas that have undergone skin grafting.

   E. Skin grafts may be exposed to moderate amounts of sunlight without changing pigmentation.

   *Ref.:* 1-5

**COMMENTS:** Skin grafts are considered to be **full thickness** when they are harvested at the dermal-subcutaneous junction. **Split-thickness** skin grafts are those that contain epidermis and variable partial thicknesses of underlying dermis (split thickness). Epithelial cells from epidermal appendages deep to the plane of graft harvest resurface the donor site of a split-thickness skin graft in approximately 1 to 3 weeks, depending on the depth. When a skin graft is harvested, there is immediate shrinkage of the surface area of the graft. This process is known as primary contraction and is caused by recoil of the elastic fibers of the dermis. The thicker the skin graft, the greater this immediate shrinkage, with full-thickness grafts shrinking by approximately 40% of their initial surface area and split-thickness grafts shrinking by about 10%. **Secondary contraction** is caused by contractile myofibroblasts in the bed of a granulating wound interacting with collagen fibers. Secondary contraction is greater in wounds covered with split-thickness grafts than in those covered with full-thickness grafts. The amount of secondary contracture is inversely proportional to the amount of dermis included in the graft, not the absolute thickness of the graft. Sensation may return to areas that have been grafted as long as the bed is proper and not significantly scarred. Although sensation is not completely normal, it is usually adequate for protection. This process begins at about 10 weeks and is maximal at 2 years. Early exposure of skin grafts to sunlight after grafting may lead to permanently increased pigmentation of the graft and should be avoided. Dermabrasion or application of chemical peels may be of benefit for reducing this pigmentation.

**ANSWER:** A

**3.** All of the following represent random-pattern flaps (as opposed to axial-pattern flaps) except:

A. Z-plasty

B. V-Y flap

C. Rhomboid flap

D. Omental flap

E. Interpolation flap

*Ref.:* 1, 2, 4, 6

**COMMENTS:** Flaps are defined according to the nature of their blood supply. A **random flap** derives its blood supply from the dermal-subdermal plexus, in contrast to an **axial flap**, which derives its blood supply from a direct, usually named cutaneous artery. The area supplied by a specific named vessel is called as an angiosome. **Random flaps** are generally used to reorient a wound in a different direction or to close a small defect. Examples of random flaps include the Z-plasty, simple rotation flap, advancement flap, and transposition flap. A **simple rotation flap** is usually semicircular and is "slid" over the recipient site for closure. An **advancement flap** is moved directly forward to cover a defect without rotation around a pivot point. A **V-Y flap**, a commonly used advancement flap, is frequently used to close small defects in the finger or eyelid areas. **Transposition flaps** involve rotation around a pivot point to a defect that is adjacent to the donor site. A **rhomboid flap** is a type of transposition flap in which a rhomboid-shaped flap is transposed to cover an adjacent defect with primary closure of the donor site. An **interpolation flap** is another type of transposition flap. It involves rotation around a pivot point but is used to cover a defect that is nearby but not directly adjacent to the donor site. **Axial flaps** are generally used to cover larger defects more distant from the donor site. A flap that crosses two angiosomes will undergo necrosis of the "watershed" area. Examples of axial flaps are the midline forehead flap (supratrochlear artery), deltopectoral flap (perforating branches of the internal mammary artery), and omental flap (gastroepiploic arteries). An **island flap** is a type of axial flap in which a segment of tissue is carried on a vascular pedicle that has been skeletonized and is without overlying skin at the base to allow greater flap mobility.

**ANSWER:** D

**4.** Which of the following statements regarding wound healing is true?

A. The inflammatory response to an acute wound is transient vasodilation.

B. Lymphocytes are the cells most critical to wound healing.

C. Platelets are the first cells to populate the wound, followed by lymphocytes, macrophages, and then neutrophils.

D. A granulating wound is considered to be in the proliferative stage of wound healing.

E. Rising transforming growth factor-α (TGF-α) levels indicate that the wound is in the proliferative stage.

*Ref.:* 7

**COMMENTS:** The process of **wound healing** undergoes three phases: **inflammatory**, **proliferative**, and **maturation**. The inflammatory phase begins with a period of **transient vasoconstriction**, initiation of the coagulation cascade, and subsequent aggregation and degranulation of platelets. Platelets are the initial cells present in wounded tissue, followed by neutrophils (24 to 48 hours), macrophages (48 to 96 hours), and lymphocytes (5 to 7 days). Neutrophils produce inflammatory products and phagocytose microbes and foreign bodies in the wound bed. Macrophages become the predominant cell population after about 48 hours until the influx of fibroblasts during the proliferative period. Macrophages are the cells most critical to wound healing because they secrete many cytokines and growth factors (such as TGF-β) that orchestrate many of the subsequent processes of wound healing. The role of lymphocytes is poorly defined, but they are not believed to be critical to wound healing. Once the levels of TGF-β rise, the wound moves into the proliferative phase of angiogenesis, fibroplasia, and epithelialization. A granulating wound is considered to be in the proliferative phase. Maturation is characterized by cross-linking and remodeling of collagen, which results in a more organized wound matrix.

**ANSWER:** D

**5.** Regarding free flaps and their vascular supply, all of the following are true except:

A. The predominant blood supply to a free transverse rectus abdominis myocutaneous (TRAM) flap is the superior epigastric artery.

B. The predominant blood supply to a free latissimus dorsi myocutaneous flap is the thoracodorsal artery.

C. The predominant blood supply to a free fibular osteocutaneous flap is the peroneal artery.

D. The predominant blood supply to a free dorsalis pedis fasciocutaneous flap is the anterior tibial artery.

E. Preoperative angiograms are avoided because of risk for capillary runoff.

*Ref.:* 1, 8

**COMMENTS:** The aforementioned free flaps are widely used for free tissue transfer. Their use should follow three principles: (1) the flap should be of adequate size, with a constant pedicle; (2) use of the flap should result in a mild secondary defect; and (3) the flap should provide functionality, as well as adequate cosmesis. The pedicle of the **free latissimus dorsi flap** comes from the thoracodorsal artery, which gives one branch to the latissimus dorsi and another to the serratus anterior muscles. The latissimus dorsi can be transferred on the thoracodorsal artery itself, or it can be harvested at the level of the subscapular artery to provide a longer, larger pedicle. The **free transverse rectus abdominis flap** is classically based on the deep inferior epigastric artery. When used as a pedicle flap (e.g., pedicled TRAM flap for breast reconstruction), it is generally based on the superior epigastric artery, which is a branch of the external iliac artery. The **free fibular osteocutaneous flap** is based on the peroneal artery. The **dorsalis pedis flap** (dorsum of the foot) is based on the anterior tibial artery. Documenting the blood flow present in the three leg vessels is critical before harvesting these flaps, and it is also extremely helpful when the leg is the recipient site as well. Arteriograms are often used to assist in planning and helping avoid tissue necrosis or loss of the foot.

**ANSWER:** A

**6.** A 35-year-old woman who underwent augmentation mammoplasty with silicone breast implants notices a flattening on the left side and is worried about rupture of her implant. The most sensitive and specific modality for diagnosing implant rupture would be:

A. Physical examination

B. Ultrasound

C. Computed tomography (CT)

D. Mammography

E. Magnetic resonance imaging (MRI)

*Ref.:* 9-11

**COMMENTS:** Many implant ruptures are silent and diagnosed only at the time of implant exchange or at the time of routine imaging. MRI has a sensitivity and specificity of greater than 90% for detecting rupture of silicone implants. Mammography, ultrasound, and CT have all been used to detect implant rupture, but they are less sensitive and specific than MRI. Intracapsular rupture on MRI is demonstrated by the so-called linguine sign, or multiple low-density lines representing the implant shell folding on itself. Extracapsular rupture is diagnosed by a high-intensity focal area (representing free silicone) in the surrounding tissues outside the capsule. The U.S. Food and Drug Administration currently recommends serial MRI evaluation for patients with silicone breast implants. The first MRI study is performed 3 years after implant surgery and then every 2 years for the life of the implant. If rupture is noted, removal of the implant with or without replacement is recommended.

**ANSWER:** E

7. Which of the following is true regarding pressure sores?

A. Stage II ulcers are characterized by nonblanching erythema with the skin grossly intact.

B. The effect of pressure-related ischemia is most pronounced at the epidermal layer of the skin, with the underlying muscle being least susceptible to pressure-related ischemia.

C. A pressure sore with exposed bone is classified as stage IV.

D. A pressure sore with an overlying blister is classified as stage III.

E. Only fasciocutaneous flaps can be used to reconstruct full-thickness pressure sores.

*Ref.:* 1, 12, 13

**COMMENTS:** Continuous pressure on tissues, if severe enough and for a long enough time, results in ischemic necrosis of the tissue, which leads to a pressure sore. Ischemic injury occurs when external pressure exceeds capillary pressure, usually between 12 and 32 mm Hg. An inverse relationship exists between pressure and time until ulceration. A pressure of 40 to 80 mm Hg applied continuously to tissue over a 4-hour period results in temporary microvascular changes and edema. If the pressure continues for an 8-hour period, it may lead to permanent microvascular changes and the development of a pressure ulcer. Underlying soft tissue, especially muscle, is more vulnerable to pressure-related ischemia than the overlying skin is. This results in the "tip of the iceberg phenomenon" whereby the underlying soft tissue damage is often more severe than the visible wound would indicate. Pressure sores are most common over dependent bony pressure points, such as the buttocks, sacrum, and heels (in a supine patient), and over the ischial tuberosities (in a sitting patient). Pressure sores are

classified according to a four-stage system developed by the National Pressure Ulcer Advisory Panel.

**Stage I** pressure sores appear as nonblanching erythema with some edema and tenderness, and the skin is intact. Treatment consists of removal of pressure from these areas with frequent turning and the use of specially designed beds to distribute the pressure evenly (e.g., Clinitron or KinAir bed). Meticulous skin care and protective dressings are often used to avoid maceration, friction, and shear forces. **Stage II** ulcers represent a partial-thickness loss of skin involving the epidermis and dermis. The ulcer is superficial and manifested as a blister, abrasion, or shallow crater. It can be treated with the conservative means listed for stage I plus moist dressings, wound cleansing, and possibly the placement of topical antibiotics (e.g., silver sulfadiazine [Silvadene] or bacitracin ointment). Superficial ulcers usually heal spontaneously as long as there is no devitalized tissue and subsequent pressure is avoided. **Stage III** ulcers have areas of full-thickness skin loss with subcutaneous destruction that may extend down to, but not through the underlying fascia. Mechanical, enzymatic, or sharp débridement of devitalized tissue and conservative treatment with moist dressings, absorbable dressings, or vacuum-assisted wound closure (VAC) devices may allow closure by secondary contracture, scarring, and epithelialization. **Stage IV** pressure sores represent full-thickness loss of skin and underlying soft tissue, along with involvement of muscle, bone, or joint. These sores often contain necrotic debris and may therefore require débridement and control of cellulitis or osteomyelitis (or both) before definitive treatment. Stage IV ulcers usually require excision of bone prominences and flap closure. Myocutaneous or fasciocutaneous flaps are generally used for coverage.

**ANSWER:** C

8. Which of the following statements regarding the differentiation of keloid scars from hypertrophic scars is true?

A. A hypertrophic scar grows beyond the boundaries of the initial scar or injury.

B. Differentiation between the two is by histologic diagnosis and cannot be determined clinically.

C. Keloids are most often seen in dark-skinned individuals.

D. They are both characterized by increased lysis of collagen at the cellular level.

E. Keloid scars respond better to treatment than hypertrophic scars.

*Ref.:* 14, 15

**COMMENTS:** Differentiation between **hypertrophic scarring** and **keloid scarring** is based mainly on clinical examination. Both keloids and hypertrophic scars are raised and may be tender, pruritic, or associated with a burning sensation. A keloid scar overgrows the boundaries of the initial injury, whereas a hypertrophic scar lies within the boundaries of the initial injury. Light microscopic examination alone shows the same basic architecture for both lesions: increased collagen production and decreased lysis of the collagen with perivascular sclerosis. Keloid scars occur more commonly in persons with dark skin, but this fact in itself does not help differentiate between the two, and they are certainly seen in all groups. Treatment of hypertrophic scars and keloids is usually multimodal and includes intralesional steroid injections, excision, compression therapy, silicone gel sheeting, and radiation treatment. Treatment outcomes for hypertrophic scars are usually better than those for keloid scars.

**ANSWER:** C

**9.** A 10-year-old girl is brought to a surgeon's office because of hypoplasia of her right breast. On closer examination she is also found to have asymmetry of the chest wall itself. Which of the following is true regarding this syndrome?

A. The syndrome affects 1 in every 1000 live births.

B. Deformity of the thoracoacromial joint is a characteristic of this syndrome.

C. Absence of the sternum is a characteristic of this syndrome.

D. Absence of the sternal head of the pectoralis muscle is a characteristic of this syndrome.

E. Pectus excavatum is part of this syndrome.

*Ref.:* 16, 17

**COMMENTS: Poland syndrome** is a congenital defect with an incidence of about 1 in every 30,000 births. The precise mechanism causing Poland syndrome has not been elucidated, but some data suggest an early insult to the subclavian and vertebral arterial systems in the developing embryo. The chest wall anomaly, a hallmark of the syndrome, includes partial absence of the sternal head of the pectoralis major muscle, hypoplasia or aplasia of the breast and subcutaneous tissue, and possibly complete absence of the pectoralis minor muscle. Other muscles around the chest wall may be affected, including the serratus anterior, supraspinatus, external oblique, and latissimus dorsi muscles. Although the sternum may be normal, the ribs and costal cartilages may be hypoplastic or absent. The upper extremities and the hand may be affected in the form of hypoplasia, possibly with syndactyly. Definitive breast reconstruction is usually addressed after puberty following full development of the contralateral breast. Intervention in the preadolescent years may be considered if the psychosocial impact of the deformity is significant.

**ANSWER: D**

**10.** A 35-year-old man with no drug allergies is evaluated for a dog bite injury to his left forearm sustained 24 hours earlier. The wound is a complex, stellate laceration, approximately 2 cm deep with devitalized tissue. It is contaminated with dirt and saliva. His last tetanus booster was 7 years ago. Appropriate treatment would include:

A. Tetanus toxoid and broad-spectrum antibiotic coverage, including coverage for *Eikenella corrodens*

B. No tetanus toxoid but broad-spectrum antibiotic coverage, including coverage for *Staphylococcus epidermidis*

C. Tetanus toxoid and broad-spectrum antibiotic coverage, including coverage for *Pasteurella multocida*

D. Tetanus toxoid, tetanus immune globulin, and broad-spectrum antibiotic coverage, including coverage for *E. corrodens* and *P. multocida*

E. Tetanus immunoglobin followed by débridement only

*Ref.:* 18, 19

**COMMENTS:** When considering prophylaxis against **tetanus** in patients with acute wounds, the wounds must first be classified as tetanus prone or non–tetanus prone based on characteristics of the wound. **Tetanus-prone wounds** include wounds older than 6 hours, wounds with stellate or avulsive configurations, and wounds

resulting from crush, missile, burn, or frostbite injuries. Other characteristics of a tetanus-prone wound include a depth greater than 1 cm, evidence of contamination or infection, and the presence of devitalized, denervated, or ischemic tissue. Non–tetanus-prone wounds are less than 6 hours old. They are usually linear (often resulting from injury by a sharp object, such as a knife or piece of glass) and are less than 1 cm deep. They show no evidence of infection or contamination. The underlying tissue is generally healthy appearing, without areas of devitalized, denervated, or ischemic tissue. For tetanus-prone wounds, tetanus toxoid and tetanus immune globulin are administered if the patient has not received three previous doses of toxoid or if the patient's immunization status is unknown. If the patient has received three or more previous doses of tetanus toxoid, a repeat booster is administered only if it has been longer than 5 years since the patient's last tetanus toxoid booster.

For non–tetanus-prone wounds, tetanus immune globulin is not administered. **Tetanus toxoid** is administered if the patient has not received three previous doses of toxoid, if the patient's immunization status is unknown, or if it has been 10 years since the patient's last tetanus toxoid booster. Antibiotic prophylaxis is usually administered for animal and human bite wounds, especially if medical attention is delayed (>12 hours), the injury involves an anatomically sensitive area (e.g., face, scalp, hand, or foot), or the patient is diabetic or immunosuppressed. Infections that occur after a bite are generally polymicrobial in nature and involve a mixture of aerobes and anaerobes. *P. multocida* is the major pathogen in dog and cat bites. *E. corrodens, Staphylococcus aureus, S. epidermidis,* α- and β-hemolytic streptococci, and *Corynebacterium* species are common pathogens isolated from human bite wounds. Amoxicillin-clavulanate is the drug of choice for **bite wounds** because it provides broad-spectrum aerobic and anaerobic coverage, including coverage for both *P. multocida* and *E. corrodens*.

**ANSWER: C**

**11.** A 60 year-old diabetic woman currently being treated for right lower extremity cellulitis is brought to the emergency room from her nursing home with an exquisitely tender erythematous rash on her right leg associated with bullae formation. On arrival, her temperature is 38.9° C, her blood pressure is 82/43 mm Hg, and her heart rate is 128 beats/min. The next step in management should be:

A. Admission to the intensive care unit, blood cultures, broad-spectrum antibiotics, and close serial examinations for at least the next 2 hours

B. Complete blood count, basic metabolic profile, and MRI of the right lower extremity

C. Admission to the intensive care unit, fluid resuscitation, débridement of the bullae, and Gram stain and culture of the blister fluid before initiating antibiotic coverage for *S. aureus*

D. Stabilization of the patient and immediate transfer to the operating room for wide débridement of all involved tissue

E. Immediate dosing with 100 mg of hydrocortisone intravenously followed by repeated doses every 8 hours and antibiotic coverage for *S. aureus*

*Ref.:* 20-22

**COMMENTS:** This clinical scenario is suggestive of a **necrotizing soft tissue infection**. Necrotizing soft tissue infections are characterized by erythema and severe pain that is classically out of proportion to the findings on physical examination. Tenderness is often present beyond the areas of erythema. Other signs that may be present include crepitus, bullae, blebs, and skin necrosis, which are late signs indicative of extensive tissue destruction and vascular thrombosis. Patients often demonstrate signs of sepsis, including fever, hypotension, tachycardia, changes in mental status, and oliguria/anuria. In equivocal cases, diagnostic studies may prove helpful, but they should not delay operative treatment. CT, MRI, or plain radiography may reveal subcutaneous air, subcutaneous edema, or fat stranding. The presence of soft tissue gas warrants immediate operative treatment, but its absence does not exclude the diagnosis. Aggressive resuscitation, administration of broad-spectrum antibiotics, and immediate operative exploration provide immediate diagnosis and treatment. In the operating room, all necrotic and infected tissue should be aggressively débrided back to viable tissue. Gram stain and aerobic and anaerobic cultures should be obtained. Steroids are not indicated in the presence of a necrotizing soft tissue infection. **Impetigo** is a non-necrotizing soft tissue infection. It is an often pruritic, erythematous bacterial infection of the epidermis typically attributed to *S. aureus*. It is characterized by blisters, bullae, or vesicles that subsequently rupture to form honey-crusted plaques and erosions. Patients do not typically exhibit toxicity and are not exquisitely tender. The diagnosis is made by Gram stain and culture of the blister fluid. Treatment usually consists of the application of mupirocin ointment, administration of antistaphylococcal antibiotics, or both.

**ANSWER: D**

12. Treatment with a negative-pressure wound dressing (VAC dressing) is best avoided in the following situations except:

    A. Wound dehiscence following ilioinguinal lymph node dissection with exposure of the femoral vessels

    B. Mediastinitis following cardiac surgery

    C. A stage 4 sacral decubitus ulcer with untreated sacral osteomyelitis

    D. A lower extremity wound with underlying necrotic muscle

    E. A necrotic wound with exposed prosthetic graft material

*Ref.:* 23-25

**COMMENTS: Vacuum-assisted wound closure** involves applying a porous sponge and occlusive dressing to the wound, followed by the application of negative pressure over the entire wound surface. Although the exact mechanism by which VAC therapy promotes wound healing is unknown, it is believed to provide more robust and faster wound granulation than possible with conventional means by increasing wound perfusion and blood flow, removing wound exudate, and providing a mechanical force drawing the wound edges together. VAC dressings have been used for both acute and chronic wounds. Unlike wet-to-wet dressings, VAC dressings provide no wound débridement and therefore should be used only after the wounds have been properly débrided. VAC dressings applied over exposed vessels or grafts have been associated with massive hemorrhage and should be used only after coverage of vital structures (e.g., by a sartorius or rectus muscle flap in the case of exposed femoral vessels). VAC therapy is contraindicated in patients with osteomyelitis, and appropriate débridement of involved bone and appropriate antibiotic treatment are necessary before VAC placement. VAC therapy has been used successfully in patients with mediastinitis after cardiac surgery following débridement as both primary treatment and as a bridge to definitive therapy with flap coverage.

**ANSWER: B**

13. Which of the following statements regarding skin incisions and excisions is false?

    A. Skin incisions should usually be oriented parallel to the long axis of the underlying muscle.

    B. Lines of minimal tension parallel skin lines.

    C. The long axis of underlying muscles is usually perpendicular to skin lines.

    D. During an elliptical excision, the long axis should be four times the length of the short axis.

    E. The dog-ear deformity is a result of infection after incision.

*Ref.:* 1, 2, 4

**COMMENTS:** In most anatomic areas, skin lines represent lines of minimal tension (**Langer lines**), or relaxed skin tension lines. Incisions in these areas should be made parallel to these lines to result in the narrowest possible scar. These lines of minimal tension generally run perpendicular to the long axis of underlying muscles. When excising lesions involving the skin, the long axis should be four times the length of the short axis. This approach will minimize the formation of mounds of excess skin at the peripheries of the incision (dog-ear deformity).

**ANSWER: A**

14. All of the following recipient beds are unlikely to support a split-thickness skin graft except:

    A. Muscle without overlying fascia

    B. Tendon without paratenon

    C. Nerve without perineurium

    D. Bone without periosteum

    E. Subcutaneous tissue with organized clot

*Ref.:* 1-4

**COMMENTS:** The condition of the recipient bed is one of the most important predictors of **graft success**. Proper "take" of a split-thickness skin graft depends on adequate vascularization of the recipient bed. Muscle with or without its fascia intact is an excellent, well-vascularized recipient site for split-thickness skin grafts. Although less well vascularized, tendon with its paratenon intact, nerve with its perineurium intact, and bone with its periosteum intact can also support a split-thickness skin graft. However, tendon devoid of paratenon, nerve lacking perineurium, and exposed bone without periosteum are unlikely to support a skin graft. Other keys to maximizing take of a skin graft include maximizing patient nutrition and taking steps to prevent the common causes of graft failure, such as hematoma or seroma (most common), infection, and shear force on the graft. Thicker grafts have a higher rate of failure when a wound is more likely to be compromised by vascular insufficiency, hematoma, or infection. For this reason, thinner split-thickness skin grafts are generally preferred when the recipient site for a graft is suboptimal, such as in irradiated wounds. For wounds in which the most normal final appearance and the least contraction is desired, as on the face or hands, full-thickness skin grafts are preferred. Donor sites are typically from the upper eyelid or the postauricular region. Full-thickness grafts are also used when hair production is required. The skin graft may also be meshed, or "pie-crusted," to facilitate drainage of fluid at the expense of cosmesis. Wound infection as determined by clinical examination or a quantitative wound culture (showing >10$^5$ bacteria per gram of tissue) mandates treatment of the wound with débridement, frequent dressing changes, and in some cases, culture-directed antibiotics before skin grafting.

**ANSWER:** A

15. Which of the following statements regarding techniques of breast reconstruction is true?

  A. Frequent problems associated with silicone implants for single-stage breast reconstruction include an inadequate skin envelope leading to excess tension with possible skin necrosis or wound dehiscence.

  B. Breast reconstruction with a tissue expander involves placement of the expander in a submuscular pocket, closure of the wound, and immediate full expansion to match the size of the opposite breast.

  C. When a latissimus dorsi myocutaneous flap is used for breast reconstruction, placement of an implant is not usually necessary.

  D. A TRAM flap survives on vessels that run longitudinally in a plane superficial to the anterior rectus sheath.

  E. A free TRAM flap is anastomosed to the subclavian artery.

*Ref.:* 1, 26, 27

**COMMENTS: Breast reconstruction** following mastectomy is an important aspect of breast cancer therapy for cosmetic and psychological reasons that does not adversely affect cancer recurrence rates or patient survival. Options for breast reconstruction include the use of (1) tissue expanders or implants, (2) pedicled myocutaneous flaps, or (3) free tissue transfer. A **tissue expander** reconstruction is the least complex and involves placing a tissue expander in a submuscular pocket beneath the pectoralis major and serratus anterior muscles and serially expanding the device during weekly outpatient visits. After full expansion, the tissue expander is exchanged for a permanent implant in the operating room. A permanent implant in most instances cannot be placed at the time of mastectomy because of an inadequate skin envelope. Drawbacks include the need for weekly office visits and a second operation, difficulty creating natural-looking breast ptosis, and capsular contracture. **Myocutaneous flap** reconstruction is particularly well suited to patients who have an inadequate amount of local skin remaining after mastectomy, a poor-quality skin envelope, skin that has been damaged from previous radiation therapy, or loss of the pectoralis major muscle, such as following radical mastectomy. The **latissimus dorsi** myocutaneous flap is considered a hybrid procedure in which autogenous tissue is used, but an implant is also required. The flap pedicled on the thoracodorsal vessels is particularly useful for replacing the pectoralis major muscle in a radical mastectomy defect. The **transverse rectus abdominis myocutaneous flap** may be performed both in a pedicled fashion and as a free flap. TRAM flaps allow a completely autogenous reconstruction. A pedicled TRAM flap is based on the superior epigastric vessels. This technique results in the presence of an often bothersome epigastric bulge. Problems with fat necrosis, especially in smokers, are not uncommon. To combat this problem, the free TRAM flap involves transferring the flap based on the more robust deep inferior epigastric artery, which is anastomosed to the recipient vessels in the chest (either the thoracodorsal vessels or internal mammary vessels). The superior and inferior epigastric arteries lie within the rectus sheath.

**ANSWER:** A

16. Which of the following statements regarding vascular anomalies is true?

  A. Newborns with capillary malformations (port-wine stains) involving the ophthalmic trigeminal dermatome should undergo MRI of the head.

  B. A 2-month-old with a stable hemangioma on the left upper extremity that has failed to regress should be treated with a pulsed dye laser.

  C. Arteriovenous malformations respond well to a course of systemic steroids in the majority of cases.

  D. Most venous malformations (70%) regress by 7 years of age; therefore, observation is the treatment of choice.

  E. Injection sclerotherapy is effective in the treatment of arteriovenous malformations.

*Ref.:* 2, 28

**COMMENTS:** The International Society for the Study of Vascular Anomalies divides the classification of **vascular anomalies** into two categories: **vascular tumors**, including hemangiomas, hemangioendotheliomas, and angiosarcomas, and **vascular malformations**. Vascular malformations are further subdivided into slow-flow malformations (e.g., capillary, lymphatic, and venous malformations) and high-flow malformations (e.g., arterial and arteriovenous malformations). For example, the still commonly used term "cavernous hemangioma" may denote either a deep infantile hemangioma or a mislabeled venous malformation. The vernacular "strawberry angioma" is sometimes used to describe a superficial infantile hemangioma, whereas the term "port-wine stain" refers to a capillary malformation. A **hemangioma** is a vascular tumor of infancy that usually appears within the first 2 weeks of life and slowly regresses during childhood. Fifty percent regress by 5 years of age and 70% by 7 years of age. The appearance depends on the depth of the hemangioma. A hemangioma of the superficial dermis appears as a raised erythematous or violaceous lobulated lesion; a hemangioma of the deep dermis may exhibit only a slightly raised skin surface and is characterized by a bluish hue. Observation of hemangiomas is appropriate because most of these lesions involute spontaneously. Corticosteroids, interferon, and even surgery may be required for large lesions obstructing the rapidly maturing eyes, airways, or small lumens. **Vascular malformations** are congenital lesions of abnormally formed vascular channels. They never regress and often expand. A **capillary malformation** (port-wine stain) is a vascular malformation that results in a flat, uniformly dark red cutaneous lesion that is present at birth and does not involute. Capillary malformations are treated by pulsed dye laser. Therapy yields the best outcome if initiated in infancy or early childhood. When a port-wine stain of the face occupies the ophthalmic trigeminal nerve distribution (V1), MRI of the head should be considered to evaluate for Sturge-Weber syndrome, which is associated with ipsilateral leptomeningeal and ocular vascular anomalies. **Lymphatic malformations** (also known as lymphangiomas or cystic hygromas) are composed of abnormally formed lymphatic channels. They are often present in the head and lateral neck region. These lesions expand and contract, depending on the flow of lymphatic fluid. They often enlarge and become tender during periods of upper respiratory infection. Although sclerotherapy has assumed a role in managing these lesions, surgical excision is the only potential curative treatment. **Venous malformations** are blue, soft, compressible lesions that are present at birth and swell with dependency. They seldom involute. They may be associated with gigantism of the involved part of the body. Sclerotherapy is generally the first-line treatment, but great care must be taken to avoid systemic passage of the sclerosant. Excision may be hazardous because of the risk for hemorrhage and should be reserved for patients with significant associated functional or cosmetic disability. **Arteriovenous malformations** are high-flow lesions. Usually, they are treated when dangerous signs and symptoms arise, such as bleeding or manifestations of high-output congestive heart failure. Treatment consists of arterial embolization 24 to 72 hours before surgical resection.

**ANSWER:** A

17. Which of the following statements regarding nasal trauma is true?

   A. A septal hematoma should not be disturbed but should be left to absorb on its own.

   B. Diagnosis of nasal fractures requires dedicated maxillofacial CT.

   C. Naso-orbitoethmoid fractures should be managed by closed reduction and splinting.

   D. Patients with telecanthus usually require reattachment of their medial canthal tendons.

   E. Nasolacrimal duct stenting is avoided because of the risk for stricture.

*Ref.:* 1, 29

**COMMENTS:** When evaluating a patient who has suffered **nasal trauma**, a careful physical examination is mandatory. Nasal projection, contour, deviation, and any lacerations should be noted. The nasal septum should be examined for signs of a **septal hematoma**. If undiagnosed, a septal hematoma can lead to necrosis and erosion of the nasal septum and result in a "saddle nose" deformity. When identified, a septal hematoma should be incised and drained, and either quilting sutures or a nasal stent should be placed to prevent reaccumulation. Fractures of the nasal bones are diagnosed clinically, and dedicated radiographs are rarely necessary. Nasal fractures are usually treated by closed reduction, splinting, and intranasal packing. If nasal packing is used, antibiotics should be prescribed because cases of toxic shock syndrome have been reported with intranasal packing. **Naso-orbitoethmoid fractures** are generally the result of a high-energy impact. This injury is associated with fracture of the nasal bones, ethmoid complex, medial orbital walls, nasofrontal junction, and septum. The nasolacrimal duct may also be injured. Closed reduction is not sufficient to repair these injuries. These patients typically require bone grafting, repositioning and reattachment of the medial canthal tendons, and frequently, repair of the nasolacrimal duct over a stent.

**ANSWER:** D

18. Which of the following regarding reconstruction of lip defects is false?

   A. Proper alignment of the vermilion border is one of the most important cosmetic aspects of primary closure of lip defects.

   B. Upper lip defects involving less than one third of the upper lip can be repaired by primary closure.

   C. Lower lip defects involving less than one half of the lower lip can be repaired by primary closure.

   D. Lip defects involving the commissure can be reconstructed with an Abbe flap.

   E. Cheek advancement flaps are used to avoid microstomia.

*Ref.:* 30

**COMMENTS: Defects of the lip** can usually be closed primarily unless they involve more than one third of the length of the upper lip or up to 30% to 50% of the length of the lower lip or are in close approximation to the commissure. The most important cosmetic aspects of primary closure of a lip defect are proper apposition of the vermilion border and multilayered closure. Even a slight "step-off" of vermilion apposition is noticeable. For larger lip defects, the best cosmetic results are achieved by replacing a lip defect with lip tissue (i.e., replacing "like with like"). This is often accomplished by using lip tissue from the opposite lip. The Abbe, or lip switch, flap uses a full-thickness wedge of up to a third of either the upper or lower lip. Based on the labial artery, this flap is rotated to cover the defect, with the pedicle divided 10 to 14 days later. This technique is best for reconstruction of the central philtral area of the upper lip. The **Abbe flap** cannot be used for defects involving the commissures. Lip defects involving the commissure require rotation flaps from the opposite lip (e.g., Estlander or Karapandzic flaps). The **Estlander and Karapandzic** flaps involve sliding upper lip elements around the commissure to fill lower lip defects. These flaps reposition the commissure medially. Some defects are too large to allow repair of "like with like" without resulting in microstomia. In these cases, replacement of lip tissue through local advancement of cheek tissue (e.g., Webster-Bernard flap) or by free flap reconstruction (e.g., radial forearm flap) is required.

**ANSWER:** D

19. Which of the following statements regarding the facial nerve is true?

   A. The three major branches of the facial nerve are the ophthalmic, maxillary/buccal, and mandibular.

   B. Injury to a buccal branch of the facial nerve medial to the lateral canthus should be tagged or reapproximated within 72 hours.

   C. A sural nerve graft may be used when a gap between the cut ends of the facial nerve precludes primary repair.

   D. Injury to the marginal mandibular branch of the facial nerve results in no significant functional sequelae.

   E. Gold upper eyelid implants are used sometimes in early reconstruction.

*Ref.:* 1, 2, 31

**COMMENTS:** The **facial nerve**, cranial nerve VII, has five major branches—the frontal/temporal, zygomatic, buccal, marginal mandibular, and cervical. The frontal branch runs just deep to the superficial temporal fascia. The zygomatic, buccal, and marginal mandibular branches run deep to the superficial musculoaponeurotic system after traversing the substance of the parotid gland. Repair or identification plus tagging of facial nerve injuries is generally undertaken within the first 72 hours following transection because after transection, the facial muscles will contract for up to 72 to 96 hours after the injury. Generally, injuries to the zygomatic and buccal branches medial to the lateral canthus are not repaired because of difficulty identifying these small branches and because of multiple interconnections, which makes sacrifice of a peripheral branch insignificant most of the time. However, injury to peripheral branches of the frontal and marginal mandibular branches should be repaired whenever possible because injury results in significant functional loss. Bell palsy is the most common cause of facial paralysis, followed by facial trauma. Reconstruction for facial paralysis can be divided into early and late reconstruction. Early reconstruction involves approximation of the cut nerve ends or reconstruction with a nerve graft (usually the sural nerve) to span a defect that cannot be approximated in a tension-free manner. For proximal facial nerve injuries, a cross-face nerve graft to the contralateral facial nerve may be undertaken. After about 18 months, the facial muscles will atrophy and lose function. Once this happens, reconstruction with muscle transfers is usually undertaken (e.g., gracilis muscle transfer with or without a cross-face nerve graft). Static reconstructions with gold upper eyelid implants, browlifts, and blepharoplasty are also options for delayed reconstruction.

**ANSWER:  C**

20. Which of the following statements regarding frontal sinus fractures is true?

    A. Frontal sinus fractures usually occur in isolation as a result of blast injuries.

    B. Nondisplaced fractures of the anterior wall of the frontal sinus require operative exploration, mucosal stripping of the sinus, and rigid fixation.

    C. Treatment of frontal sinus fractures with significant disruption of the posterior wall and associated cerebrospinal fluid (CSF) leak involves cranialization of the sinus.

    D. Anterior wall fractures involving the nasofrontal duct require stenting the nasofrontal duct with a Silastic stent for 2 weeks.

    E. Cranialization involves decompressing the sinus into the pericavernous lymphatics.

*Ref.:* 1, 29

**COMMENTS: Frontal sinus fractures** are usually the result of a high-energy impact. The majority of frontal sinus fractures are associated with other maxillofacial and intracranial injuries. Frontal sinus fractures are generally diagnosed by CT. All patients suspected of having a frontal sinus injury should be evaluated for signs of CSF rhinorrhea, which indicates a dural tear. Treatment of a frontal sinus fracture depends on the number of walls involved, the status of the nasofrontal duct, and the degree of displacement. Isolated fractures of the anterior wall are treated only if there is considerable displacement. If the nasofrontal duct is involved in the fracture, the frontal sinus is demucosalized, the nasofrontal duct is plugged with a bone graft, and the sinus is obliterated with cancellous bone or fat. Fractures of the posterior wall raise suspicion for a dural laceration. Observation of isolated, nondisplaced posterior wall fractures without evidence of CSF leak is advocated by some, whereas others advocate exploration of all posterior wall fractures. For displaced fractures of the posterior wall, a team approach with a neurosurgeon is preferred. If there is significant loss of the posterior wall, the sinus is cranialized. **Cranialization** involves removing the posterior wall, plugging the nasofrontal duct with bone graft, demucosalizing the sinus, and replacing the sinus with a pericranial flap.

**ANSWER:  C**

21. Which of the following is true regarding the repair of orbital floor fractures?

    A. Cosmetically unacceptable enophthalmos is not an indication for surgical repair.

    B. Diplopia is an indication for surgical exploration.

    C. Exposure of the orbital floor via a subciliary incision is associated with less risk for lower lid retraction than is exposure via a transconjunctival incision.

    D. Marked periorbital swelling is an indication for urgent surgical exploration.

    E. Treatment of complex bone fractures take precedence over that of globe injuries.

*Ref.:* 1, 29

**COMMENTS:** The diagnosis of an **orbital floor fracture** is suspected when periorbital ecchymosis and subconjunctival hematoma are present. Patients may also exhibit anesthesia in the sensory distribution of the infraorbital nerve, which lies beneath the orbital floor. Orbital floor fractures may also be manifested as diplopia and enophthalmos. Diplopia may result from restriction of extraocular movement because of contusion or entrapment of the inferior rectus or inferior oblique muscles in the fracture segment. Enophthalmos, or posterior displacement of the globe, results from increased orbital volume (as the floor is displaced inferiorly) or is caused by disruption of the ligamentous support of the globe. Initial evaluation of a patient with a suspected orbital fracture includes testing for visual acuity, extraocular muscle movement, and pupillary reflexes. A forced duction test whereby the insertion of the inferior rectus is grasped with forceps and manually rotated (after topical anesthetic is instilled) helps identify extraocular muscle entrapment. If visual acuity is affected or globe rupture is suspected, ophthalmologic consultation is mandatory. Globe injury always takes precedence over bone repair. Fine-cut maxillofacial CT is performed with both axial images and coronal reconstructions to better characterize the nature of the fracture and aid in identification of an entrapped extraocular muscle. The indications for surgical repair of orbital floor fractures include diplopia, entrapment of extraocular muscles, and enophthalmos. Surgery may be performed immediately or delayed until the edema has resolved, usually within a 2- to 3-week period from the time of injury. Exposure is usually achieved with either a transconjunctival incision or subciliary or subtarsal incisions. Subciliary and subtarsal incisions carry a greater risk for lower lid retraction. Many materials have been used to reconstruct the orbital floor, including titanium mesh, polyethylene sheets, and bioresorbable mesh.

**ANSWER:  B**

22. Which of the following wounds would most likely require free flap reconstruction?

    A. Open wound of the knee with an exposed total knee prosthesis

    B. Open wound with exposed sternum following coronary artery bypass surgery

    C. Full-thickness resection of the chest wall for tumor with exposed lung

    D. Fracture of the distal third of the tibia with an open wound and exposed bone without hardware in the wound

    E. Pen fractures of the midhumerus

*Ref.:* 1, 32, 33

**COMMENTS:** Open tibial fractures have a high incidence of infection and nonunion, and they necessitate extended hospital stays. The zone of injury is always larger than is clinically apparent. Replacement of the tissue deficit is a critical part of the treatment, and myocutaneous flaps have led to a significant decrease in the incidence of infection and nonunion. Local muscle flaps are not dependable for defects involving the distal third of the leg because they are usually involved in the zone of injury and may not be available that far distally. For this reason, free flap transfer of muscle or skin (or both) from a distant site is the treatment of choice for lower third defects. When considering free flap coverage for traumatic wounds, it should be noted that the recipient vessels are frequently traumatized within the zone of injury and require extensive débridement. These defects are often repaired in less than 1 week, or repair is delayed until 3 months for successful reconstruction. The other wounds mentioned require muscle coverage but can be treated with a local muscle flap unless the flap has been used previously and failed. In such instances, a free flap can be used in a salvage procedure.

**ANSWER:** D

23. A 65-year-old woman with insulin-dependent diabetes mellitus underwent coronary artery bypass grafting using the left inferior mammary artery, and a sternal wound infection developed. All of the following flaps are appropriate for repair except:

    A. Bilateral pectoralis flaps

    B. Omental flap based on the left gastroepiploic vessel.

    C. Bilateral rectus abdominis flaps

    D. Latissimus flap

    E. Omental flap based on the right gastroepiploic vessel

    *Ref.:* 1, 9

**COMMENTS: Sternal wound infections** are a potential complication of heart surgery. Use of the internal mammary artery interrupts blood flow to the superior epigastric artery, which provides the blood supply to the pedicled rectus abdominis flap. In this patient, a bilateral rectus abdominis flap is a poor choice because the left rectus muscle's superior vascular pedicle (i.e., the superior epigastric artery) has been interrupted. Bilateral pectoralis muscle flaps are an excellent choice for sternal wound repair. Each pectoralis muscle is fully dissected and advanced to the midline. The thoracoacromial artery supplies the pectoralis muscle. An omental flap is also a viable choice. It may be based on the right or left gastroepiploic vessel. The latissimus flap, though not ideal, can be mobilized to repair a sternal wound. It is based on the thoracodorsal vessels.

**ANSWER:** C

24. The most common cause of free flap necrosis is:

    A. Arterial thrombosis

    B. Venous thrombosis

    C. Arterial spasm

    D. Venous spasm

    E. Trauma from manipulation of a compromised flap

    *Ref.:* 2, 34-37

**COMMENTS:** The nature of a tissue defect may require the transfer of distant tissue to fill the defect. **Free flaps** involve severing the nutrient vessels of the flap to be transferred and reanastomosing

these vessels to vessels in the vicinity of the recipient site. This nearly always requires thoughtful planning and precise microvascular surgical technique with the aid of an operating microscope. In experienced hands, free flap success rates approach 95%. A well-controlled postoperative environment, along with maintenance of a warm patient room and avoidance of tobacco, caffeine, and vasoconstrictive medications, is essential. Success depends on careful postoperative monitoring, which involves clinical assessment of flap color, temperature, and capillary refill and Doppler assessment of blood flow. All flaps must be observed closely during the immediate postoperative period following transfer to avoid possible circulatory compromise. A purple-blue or dusky coloration, flap swelling or congestion, and rapid capillary refill are often early signs of venous insufficiency. Increased dark-colored bleeding and hematoma formation may also be seen. Unchecked, this will progress to loss of capillary refill and arterial inflow because of high venous pressure. Arterial insufficiency is manifested as pale flap color, reduction in flap temperature, and loss of capillary refill. Venous thrombosis is the most common cause of flap necrosis. Arterial insufficiency is not usually responsible for **flap failure**. Complications such as excessive tension, vessel kinking, or hematoma can eventually lead to venous thrombosis. A seriously compromised flap requires immediate attention, and treatment may involve taking down a dressing, removing tight sutures, changing the position of an extremity or the head and neck, or exploring the flap in the operating room. There should be a low threshold for returning to the operating room because prompt exploration of a failing flap improves salvage rates. The patient must also be examined for systemic causes such as hypovolemia, hypotension, or hypoxia. Heparin, aspirin, low-molecular-weight dextran, and leech therapy may serve as useful adjuncts.

**ANSWER:** B

25. Which of the following statements is true?

    A. Women with breast augmentation implants have a significantly increased risk for the development of breast carcinoma in comparison with those with nonaugmented breasts.

    B. When breast cancer is diagnosed in a patient with silicone breast augmentation implants, it is more likely to be at an advanced stage than when diagnosed in nonaugmented breasts.

    C. Patients with silicone breast implants require a modification of conventional mammographic techniques to obtain optimal visualization of the breast parenchyma.

    D. The concentration of silicone in the breast milk of women with silicone implants is slightly greater than that in the breast milk of women without implants.

    E. Epidemiologic studies have clearly demonstrated a cause-and-effect relationship between breast implants and the development of collagen vascular disease.

    *Ref.:* 1, 10, 27, 38

**COMMENTS:** Much confusion exists about the potential hazards and risks associated with **silicone breast implants**. Patients with breast implants do not have an increased risk for the development of breast carcinoma. In fact, epidemiologic studies have actually shown a lower risk for breast cancer in women who have had breast augmentation with silicone implants than is expected in the general population. When breast carcinoma is diagnosed in a patient with breast implants, it is not at a more advanced stage than when it develops in a patient without breast implants. Conventional mammographic techniques need to be modified when performing imaging studies on patients with breast implants. The Eklund modification involves compression of the implant and displacement of the breast parenchyma away from the implant. The silicone concentration of breast milk in patients with augmented breasts is not significantly different from that of nonaugmented women. At present, there is no clear-cut documentation of an increased incidence of collagen vascular disease in patients with silicone breast implants, nor is there any proved cause-and-effect relationship between the two.

**ANSWER: C**

26. Which of the following statements regarding cleft lip and cleft palate is true?

A. Cleft lip is an uncommon abnormality that occurs in approximately 1 in every 50,000 live births.

B. Repair of a cleft lip is generally delayed until the patient is at least 6 months old.

C. Structures anterior to the uvula are part of the primary palate.

D. With a soft palate cleft, the palatal musculature is abnormally inserted onto the posterior margin of the hard palate.

E. Later closure has the most detrimental effect on maxillary growth.

*Ref.:* 1, 2, 39

**COMMENTS:** The most common congenital craniofacial abnormality treated by plastic surgeons is **cleft lip and palate**. It is secondary only to clubfoot as the most frequent congenital deformity. The incidence of cleft lip with or without cleft palate has a variable racial distribution, with an incidence of 2.1 per 1000 in Asians, 1 per 1000 in white individuals, and 0.4 per 1000 in African Americans. Isolated cleft palate does not exhibit racial heterogeneity, with an incidence of 0.5 per 1000. Cleft lip may occur as an isolated abnormality or may be associated with clefts of the alveolar ridge, hard palate, and soft palate. Typically, the "rule of 10's" determines the timing of lip repair: when the hemoglobin level is greater than 10 g/100 mL, the patient is older than 10 weeks, and the patient weighs more than 10 lb. At some centers, clefts of the lip are repaired at even earlier ages. The incisive foramen marks the dividing line between the primary and secondary palate. The **primary palate** (the lip and hard palate anterior to the incisive foramen) and the **secondary palate** (the hard palate posterior to the incisive foramen, soft palate, and uvula) develop from different embryologic structures, which results in different degrees of susceptibility to genetic and environmental influences. Hence, it is possible to have isolated clefts of either the primary or secondary palate, as well as complete clefts of the entire palate. When the soft palate is cleft, the levator palatini muscle, which normally forms a muscular sling across the palate, is abnormally inserted on the posterior border of the hard palate. Restoration of the normal muscular anatomy is believed to play an important role in normal speech development. Contraction of normal palatal musculature produces velopharyngeal closure, which is critical to most sounds in the English language. Patients who lack this closure mechanism have a characteristic speech marked by hypernasality; nasal air emissions; weak pressure consonants, or plosives (p, t, and d); and compensatory articulation consisting of consonant omissions ("og" for "dog"), substitutions, or distortions. The development of normal speech in patients with cleft palate may be optimized if the palate is closed before the age of 12 months; however, later closure may

have less detrimental effects on future maxillary growth. Patients with cleft palate have an increased incidence of middle ear infections and resultant hearing loss.

**ANSWER: D**

27. Which of the following statements regarding examination of an acutely injured hand is true?

A. All fingers (except the thumb) when flexed at the metacarpophalangeal (MCP) and proximal interphalangeal (PIP) joints point to the scaphoid tubercle.

B. Normal two-point discrimination in the palm and volar side of digits is 2 mm or less.

C. A laceration over the distal phalanx of a finger raises suspicion for a zone II flexor tendon injury.

D. A severed finger should be soaked in a cool, dilute antiseptic solution (e.g., 1 : 100,000 povidone-iodine [Betadine]/ normal saline solution) until replantation is possible.

E. Pain on palpation in the area of the anatomic "snuffbox" should raise suspicion of fracture of the lunate bone.

*Ref.:* 40-43

**COMMENTS:** Examination of an **acutely injured hand** should be a systematic process that includes thorough evaluation of both bone and soft tissue structures. A complete history and physical examination are mandatory. The time, place, and method of injury, as well as the hand dominance of the patient, are essential components of any hand examination. Neurovascular status is then checked. The Allen test is used to assess the vascular supply to the hand, whereas neurologic function can be assessed accurately via light touch and two-point discrimination. If the patient can discriminate between one point and two, this is normal. However, two-point discrimination greater than 8 mm should raise suspicion for a nerve injury. Certain autonomous zones are useful for evaluating individual nerve function: the median nerve, on the flexor aspect of the index finger beyond the distal interphalangeal (DIP) joint; the ulnar nerve, on the flexor aspect of the little finger beyond the DIP joint; and the radial nerve, on the dorsal web space along the thumb.

The bony architecture of the hand is evaluated by both x-ray and physical examination. If they are not open, many types of fractures (e.g., boxer's fractures) can be reduced and splinted in an emergency department situation with the aid of a hematoma block or a wrist block. Metacarpal fractures need special attention because even though radiographic evidence may suggest a stable, nondisplaced fracture, a rotational deformity may exist, which if not treated, will cause functional disability. The best way of assessing a rotational deformity is by observing the hand as it is flexed at the MCP and PIP joints. Normal fingers point to the scaphoid tubercle. Flexor tendon injuries are categorized according to five anatomic zones. **Zone II** begins proximally at the distal palmar creases and ends distally over the middle portion of the middle phalanx. Bunnell called this area "no-man's land" because even though injuries may be relatively easy to repair, both flexor tendons run through the area inside the sheath and significant scarring can subsequently occur, with difficulty restoring long-term function. An amputated finger part should be wrapped in gauze soaked in sterile saline solution only and placed in a plastic bag or sterile urine cup, if available, which is then placed in ice water until replantation is possible. Soaking the finger in antiseptics such as Betadine may injure tissue and adversely affect the ability to replant it. Distal amputations properly cooled immediately after injury may be viable for up to 24 hours. The scaphoid is the most commonly injured wrist bone (accounting for almost two thirds of all carpal bone fractures), and a history of a fall onto outstretched hands should prompt an examiner to look for a scaphoid fracture. Tenderness in the anatomic snuffbox, formed by the abductor pollicis longus and the extensor pollicis longus on the dorsum of the hand, should raise suspicion of a scaphoid fracture, which can be seen on radiographs. However, sometimes standard radiography is not diagnostic, and further studies are necessary (i.e., MRI, CT, or a bone scan) to rule out the diagnosis. A missed scaphoid fracture can lead to serious complications such as avascular necrosis of the bone, chronic arthritis, and chronic wrist pain.

**ANSWER:** A

28. Which of the following statements regarding the placement of hand incisions is true?

   A. Palm incisions should be placed in the skin creases.

   B. It is better to err on the volar aspect than the dorsal aspect when placing incisions on the side of the digit.

   C. Incisions on the volar side of the digit must cross the interphalangeal (IP) flexion creases transversely.

   D. Dorsal skin incisions should cross skin creases transversely or obliquely.

   E. The key principle in planning hand incisions is to maximize motion to avoid contractures.

*Ref.:* 40, 43

**COMMENTS:** There are several key principles in planning **hand incisions**. Whenever possible, the incision should be designed along lines that undergo no change in length with motion. Those on the palm should run parallel to the skin creases or across them obliquely because the blood supply in this region comes straight upward into the skin. Digital incisions should be placed dorsal to the midlateral line through the midaxial line, which is exactly neutral between flexion and extension. This line is determined by connecting the most dorsal points of the IP joint creases when the finger is in a flexed position. Oblique incisions connecting these points (Bruner), or volar zigzag incisions, are also an excellent approach that provides full exposure to the entire palmar side of the digit. A line marking the change in character between the dorsal and volar skin of the digit is also a useful landmark. Given a choice, it is far better to err in placing an incision dorsally than on the volar aspect of the side of the digit because the volar incisions may form a bridging scar. Skin incisions on the dorsum of the hand and digits should cross skin creases transversely, obliquely, or over the middorsum when between joints. In a rheumatoid hand, incisions that cross the skin of the dorsal surface of the wrist should be longitudinal or minimally curved to avoid slough of a distally based flap.

**ANSWER:** D

29. A surgeon is called to examine a 30-year-old painter who cut the palm of his right hand with a dirty razor blade. Examination reveals a 2-cm clean laceration at the base of the long finger. MCP joint flexion is intact, but the patient cannot flex either IP joint in that finger. The injury is 1 hour old. What is the diagnosis?

   A. Lacerated flexor digitorum superficialis tendon

   B. Lacerated flexor digitorum profundus tendon

   C. Combined flexor digitorum superficialis and profundus laceration

   D. Laceration of the intrinsic muscles to the long finger

   E. Median nerve transection

*Ref.:* 40, 44, 45

**COMMENTS:** See Question 30.

**ANSWER:** C

30. The immediate treatment plan for the patient described in Question 29 should include which of the following?

   A. Plans for immediate tendon repair (within 6 hours) to avoid the hazards of delayed tendon anastomosis

   B. Wrist block anesthesia, extension of the skin wound along proper incision lines, and exploration to confirm the diagnosis

   C. Careful cleansing and irrigation of the wound, placement of an appropriate dressing or simple sutures, and hand immobilization before definitive primary surgical repair some time within 2 weeks

   D. Cleansing of the wound, primary skin closure, hand immobilization, and outpatient follow-up visits because this injury will require free tendon graft reconstruction 6 weeks after injury

   E. Cleansing of the wound, closure, and then physical therapy starting 2 weeks after the injury

*Ref.:* 40, 44, 45

**COMMENTS:** Flexion of the MCP joint is a function of the intrinsic muscles and can persist in the face of extrinsic flexor muscle and tendon injury. The goal of **flexor tendon repair** is restoration of IP joint flexion. Flexor tendon repair demands meticulous attention to detail and, whenever possible, should be performed by a hand surgeon. The character of the wound, the nature of the injury, the degree of contamination, and the time between injury and definitive treatment determine whether primary or delayed repair is performed. Proper wound cleansing, dressing, immobilization, and prophylactic antibiotics allow delay of primary repair if a hand surgeon is not immediately available. If there is a question about the degree of contamination or if the initial wound treatment has been delayed beyond several hours, thus making primary closure hazardous, delayed repair after 2 to 14 days may be performed. This allows the presence or absence of infection to be clearly established. Many experts believe that this type of delay does not significantly alter the ultimate outcome of the repair. Tendon injuries with grossly contaminated wounds, those with significant tendon loss, or wounds with significant associated injuries to the soft tissue, bone, nerve, or blood vessels should be treated by secondary repair in 3 to 6 weeks—after the wounds have stabilized, the infection has cleared, and edema formation has subsided.

**ANSWER:** C

31. Which of the following statements regarding the most common metacarpal fractures is true?

   A. They are commonly known as Bennett fractures.

   B. They are commonly known as boxer's fractures.

C. They most often involve the distal metacarpal of the index and long fingers.

D. Physical examination is the most effective means of assessing the degree of angulation.

E. They usually require open reduction and internal fixation.

*Ref.:* 40, 42, 46, 47

**COMMENTS: Metacarpal fractures** commonly result from hitting an object with a clenched fist. They usually involve the distal metacarpal of the fifth and occasionally the fourth fingers and are known as "boxer's fractures." The metacarpal head is displaced palmward, and pain, swelling, and some loss of knuckle prominence are the usual physical findings. Associated lacerations should be treated as human bites until proved otherwise, and early exploration, with the administration of intravenous antibiotics, is recommended. Because swelling usually masks the degree of angulation, a lateral radiograph is needed for accurate evaluation. Each finger should be individually flexed to the palm to assess the degree of rotational deformity. During flexion, the fingers normally point to the scaphoid tubercle. Deviation from this alignment allows estimation of the rotational deformity. The usual treatment is closed reduction followed by immobilization of the involved and adjacent digits, with the MCP joint placed in 65 to 90 degrees of flexion and the IP joints placed in full extension. Unstable or multiple metacarpal fractures often require open reduction and internal fixation. Metacarpal shaft fractures require reduction and immobilization. Percutaneous Kirschner wires or a plate and screws for internal fixation are frequently required if the fracture is unstable, particularly if the fracture is oblique or comminuted. A Bennett fracture is a fracture at the base of the thumb metacarpal.

**ANSWER: B**

32. An 8-year-child is taken to the emergency department after slamming his right index finger in a door. There is a laceration on the pulp of the finger and a subungual hematoma. A radiograph shows a tuft fracture. Your treatment plan should include which of the following:

A. Leave the laceration open, dress the finger with antibiotic ointment, and place it in a finger splint.

B. Perform a finger block, remove the nail plate, repair any nail bed laceration, and repair the pulp laceration.

C. Use Kirschner wire fixation of the fracture, remove the nail plate, and repair the nail bed.

D. Perform operative exploration with internal fixation of the tuft fracture and repair the nail bed and pulp lacerations.

E. Place the epichondrial fold over the nail plate.

*Ref.:* 40, 47

**COMMENTS: Distal phalangeal fractures** are among the most common fractures seen in the hand, and of these, tuft fractures are the most common. These fractures are often comminuted and are frequently associated with a nail bed injury. Treatment involves removal of the nail plate, irrigation, repair of the nail bed with absorbable suture, replacement of the nail plate under the eponychial fold to prevent scarring of the fold to the nail plate, and use of a hand or finger splint. Such management allows a new nail to grow out from under the eponychial fold. Most of these fractures can be reduced at time of nail bed repair and protected with a splint for 3

to 4 weeks. Kirschner wire fixation and operative repair are rarely indicated.

**ANSWER: B**

33. Which of the following statements regarding hand infections is false?

A. The relatively avascular environment of the synovial sheaths makes them resistant to infection.

B. One third of hand infections have mixed flora.

C. Treatment of human bite wounds includes aggressive cleansing and antibiotic therapy, and they should be left open to heal secondarily.

D. A common organism isolated in a human bite injury to the hand is *E. corrodens*.

E. The organisms most commonly isolated from hand infections are penicillinase-producing staphylococci.

*Ref.:* 40, 48-50

**COMMENTS: Hand infections** are potentially serious because of the superficial locations of the hand's bones and joints; the high density of relatively avascular tendons, fat, and synovium; and the ease of spread through the synovial sheaths because of constant flexion and extension. Staphylococci are present in nearly 80% of hand infections and are often resistant to penicillin. One third of hand infections contain mixed flora and frequently include β-hemolytic streptococci, *Escherichia coli*, *Proteus* spp., and *Pseudomonas* spp. In human bites, a high percentage of anaerobic organisms may also be present, with *E. corrodens* known to be a significant contributor. Drainage procedures are reserved to decompress loculations of pus. Cellulitis without fluctuance is treated by immobilization, elevation, antibiotics, and frequent reexamination. The empirical use of antibiotics is indicated for severe infections, with appropriate changes in therapy being made when culture and sensitivity results are available. All complex infections should be drained in the operating room with proximal tourniquet control. Distal-to-proximal wrapping to obtain a bloodless field, as used during elective hand surgery, is contraindicated to avoid spreading the infection. **Human bites** should be cleansed vigorously, treated with antibiotics (including anaerobic coverage), and left open to close secondarily. Because of the superficial locations of the tendons and MCP joints, human bites (usually from a punch) should be treated vigorously. Motion of the skin, tendons, and joints in various planes helps spread infection and cover drainage paths, thereby trapping bacteria. Extension of the wound, with formal joint exploration in an operating room, is often required.

**ANSWER: A**

34. Which of the following statements is true?

A. Paronychia occurs in the digital pulp of the finger.

B. A felon is an infection around the margin of the nail bed.

C. Finger felon, or paronychia, has the potential to cause tenosynovitis.

D. The deep structures of the hand are protected from subcutaneous abscesses of the palm by the superficial palmar fascia.

E. The versatile "fish mouth" incision is used for draining both pulp and paronychial infections.

*Ref.:* 40, 49, 50

**COMMENTS:** Subcutaneous abscesses of the volar surface of the hand often follow small puncture wounds or infection of superficial blisters. Pain and swelling are confined to the area of inflammation and are not increased with minor tendon motion. Loculations should be drained because they have the potential of tracking to the dorsum of the hand. A **felon** is an infection of the pulp of the fingertip that can lead to deep ischemic necrosis, osteomyelitis, or both because of the presence of compartmentalizing septa that prevent expansion as the pressure increases. Sharp pain and tenderness out of proportion to the amount of swelling are characteristic. The pulp space must be drained by dividing the septa before tissue necrosis occurs. As a result of the proximity of the pulp and paronychial space to the tendon sheath, extension of this infection can lead to tenosynovitis. The once popular fish mouth incision is now discouraged because of the potential for painful scarring and neuroma formation. **Paronychial infections** involve the margins of the nail plate and are often caused by hangnails, manicure trauma, or small foreign bodies. *Staphylococcus* is the usual offending organism. Early cases can be treated with warm soaks and antibiotics, but abscesses must be drained, with resection of a portion of the overlying proximal nail plate often being required. Unattended superficial infections may spread to deeper compartments, such as the tendon sheaths. Likewise, deep compartment infections frequently spread to neighboring bursa and web spaces.

**ANSWER:** C

35. Which of the following statements regarding tenosynovitis is true?

A. Infections of the flexor sheath of the little finger more often extend to the thumb than to the adjacent ring finger.

B. A flexor tendon sheath infection causes the involved finger to assume a position of mild extension at all joints.

C. The involved digit is rarely swollen and often exhibits little pain.

D. By definition, deep palmar space infections involve the flexor tendons.

E. Because of potential for contracture, conservative management without drainage is contraindicated.

*Ref.:* 40, 48, 50, 51

**COMMENTS:** Infection of the synovial sheaths of the flexor tendons is a serious problem that requires prompt appropriate treatment. The tendons are relatively avascular and are characterized by poor natural resistance to infection. This may be compounded in patients with diabetes mellitus or those who are immunosuppressed. Although anatomy varies, the sheath of the little finger is often continuous with the ulnar bursa, which in turn is directly adjacent to the radial bursa, which extends to the flexor sheath of the thumb. A. Kanavel (from Cook County Hospital in Illinois) described four cardinal findings of **pyogenic tenosynovitis**: (1) the infected digit becomes uniformly swollen along the length of the flexor tendon sheath, (2) the involved digit assumes a slightly flexed position, (3) there is tenderness over the entire flexor tendon sheath, and (4) passive extension causes disproportionate pain. If there is no frank purulence, conservative measures may be successful and surgery may be avoided. Such measures include elevation of the extremity, splint immobilization, intravenous antibiotics, and close observation. If no response is seen within 24 to 48 hours, surgical drainage with copious irrigation is indicated. Immediate surgical drainage should be considered at any time if the disease process progresses despite treatment. Surgical drainage is accomplished with a longitudinal incision on the side of the digit along the axis of joint motion. The incision is placed on the ulnar side of the digit if palmar spread is suspected. Placement of irrigating catheters within the sheath and systemic antibiotics may be used as adjuncts to surgical therapy, but they are not always needed if thorough irrigation is performed. The deep palmar space is located between the flexor tendons and the metacarpals in the palm. It is divided into the thenar space and the midpalmar space at the level of the third metacarpal, where a vertical septum extends between the metacarpal and sheath of the long finger flexor tendons. Infection here is manifested as localized, tender swelling and must be drained with an appropriate incision.

**ANSWER:** A

36. Which of the following statements regarding replantation of the hand is false?

A. Single digits (other than the thumb) are uncommonly replanted except in children.

B. The amputated part may tolerate cool ischemia for up to 24 hours if there is no significant avascular muscle mass.

C. Bleeding from the proximal part is ideally treated with pressure rather than clamping.

D. A history of heavy smoking, diabetes mellitus, hypertension, and Raynaud phenomenon are relative contraindications to replantation.

E. Replantation above the elbow is contraindicated.

*Ref.:* 40, 52, 53

**COMMENTS: Replantation** is a highly specialized procedure that is best performed by a team of replantation surgeons. Single digits are less frequently replanted, except in children or if there is a sharp noncrushing cut at the level of the middle phalanx distal to the splitting of the superficialis tendon. The hand and thumb are always considered for replantation unless definite contraindications exist or the extremity was not properly preserved. The thumb is the most important digit, and as much of its length as possible should be preserved. An index finger amputated proximal to the PIP joint loses its ability to pinch, and the brain naturally switches the pinching to the long finger. Attempts to preserve length distal to the PIP joint should be made, but if the digit is painful, is insensate, or "gets in the way," the patient may best be served by transection through the metacarpal (ray amputation) because the long finger can assume the role of primary pinch. Loss of little finger length proximal to the PIP joint may also best be treated by ray amputation. Distal amputations properly cooled immediately after injury may be viable for up to 24 hours. Central finger amputations (long and ring fingers) near the MCP joint can cause bothersome spaces in the clenched fist that can be treated by transfer of the adjacent peripheral finger with its metacarpal to fill the space. Amputations above the elbow are considered for replantation (particularly in children) because even partial success can convert an above-elbow to a below-elbow stump for future rehabilitation. Guillotine amputations are the injuries that are most favorable for replantation.

**ANSWER:** E

**37.** Which of the following statements regarding peripheral nerve injury is false?

    A. Nerve repair is progressively less effective if delayed beyond 2 months after surgery.

    B. Nerve repair is best performed under 4 to 15 times magnification.

    C. Nerve repair is best performed in a fashion that minimizes tension across the repair.

    D. Regeneration may be followed clinically by observing distal progression of the Tinel sign.

    E. The use of conduits can assist in nerve regeneration.

*Ref.:* 40, 54, 55

**COMMENTS: Nerve injuries** result from stretching or compression (neurapraxia) or from transection. Neurapraxic injuries carry a better prognosis than do transection injuries. Nerve injuries do not need to be repaired at the time of injury, but it is believed that the results are progressively worse if repair is delayed beyond 6 months, when the distal nerve tubules have contracted and the new axons can no longer grow distally. Occasionally, repair delayed for up to 2 years has been successful, particularly in children. Most surgeons perform a careful epineural repair, but repair of the individual fascicular bundle is also required in large, mixed peripheral nerves. Recovery after repair begins with return of function starting proximally. Regenerating axons grow down the distal nerve sheath at a rate of approximately 1 mm/day. Distal progression of the Tinel sign (tingling felt after percussion over the growing nerve) usually follows the start of regeneration. Recently, successful nerve regeneration with healing has been achieved with vein grafts, synthetic tubes, and cadaver allograft, which act as conduits for nerve growth across the repair.

**ANSWER:** A

**38.** A 35-year-old mechanic is seen 1 hour after high-pressure injection of an oil solvent into his right index finger while cleaning his spray apparatus. The finger is slightly swollen and erythematous. Sensation is intact. He is able to flex and extend all joints with mild discomfort. What is the most appropriate treatment at this point?

    A. Ice, elevation, and re-examination in 24 hours

    B. Ice, elevation, oral antibiotics, and re-examination in 24 hours

    C. Elevation, intravenous antibiotics, and hospital admission for close observation with frequent assessment of vital signs, sensibility, and circulation

    D. Urgent wide surgical drainage and débridement of the digit and palm to remove all tissue containing the solvent

    E. Urgent drainage of the digit only to avoid contamination of the palmar space.

*Ref.:* 40, 49, 56

**COMMENTS: High-pressure solvent injection** injuries often initially appear deceptively benign. The entrance site is small, the digit is not necessarily painful, and the patient tends to minimize the degree of injury. Despite this appearance, urgent wide surgical drainage, irrigation, and débridement of the digit and hand are required to prevent rapid progression of a severe inflammatory response, compartment syndrome, and digital loss. Similar problems can be seen with paint, paint thinners, and grease injected under pressure. Extensive injuries have been known to have fluid forced all the way up to the wrist. Application of ice, elevation, and antibiotics are all important aspects of management to reduce the inflammatory response and prevent digital compartment syndrome and infection, but they are only temporizing measures. The intense inflammatory response to the solvent will lead to digital compartment syndrome and tissue necrosis unless wide surgical drainage of the digit and hand is performed urgently (even before the inflammatory response is obvious). As with tendon sheath infections, the solvent quickly tracks proximally along the flexor tendon sheath into the palm, and aggressive, wide opening and débridement into the palm are required. Subcutaneous tissue containing the solvent should be débrided while preserving vital structures whenever possible. Repeated débridement is often required. Standard radiographs often reveal radiopaque material and help define the extent of extravasation. Stiffness is a common long-term complication—if the digit can be salvaged at all. Even with appropriate management, the results are often not optimal.

**ANSWER:** D

**39.** A 36-year-old man is involved in a common industrial mishap in which he sustains a phenol burn. Which of the following antidotes can most effectively minimize skin destruction?

    A. Alcohol

    B. Sodium bicarbonate

    C. Propylethylene glycol

    D. Calcium gluconate

    E. Balanced salt solution

*Ref.:* 57, 58

**COMMENTS:** Propylethylene glycol applied directly to the burned areas is the treatment of choice. If it is not available, glycerol is the best second choice. **Phenol burns** not only affect the skin locally but, if absorbed systemically, can also cause toxic effects. For this reason, using soap and water is not recommended because it would dilute the concentration in the phenol burns and prevent the formation of a thick eschar, which acts as a barrier preventing further absorption of phenol. Calcium gluconate is used for the immediate treatment of hydrofluoric acid exposure. Patients exposed to hydrofluoric acid (most commonly when etching glass or cleaning aluminum) are usually seen several hours after exposure with pain about the nails and fingertips. Injection of a 10% solution of calcium gluconate is required without delay to prevent further symptoms and tissue destruction.

**ANSWER:** C

**40.** A 70-year-old mechanic sustains a "pinching" amputation when his dominant long finger is caught between a garage door pulley and the belt. There is loss of the volar two thirds of the pulp skin, along with exposed subcutaneous tissue. Select the most appropriate reconstruction:

    A. Sterile dressing changes with topical antibiotics and closure by contracture and epithelialization

    B. Full-thickness hypothenar skin graft

    C. Split-thickness skin graft

    D. V-Y advancement flap

    E. Replantation

*Ref.:* 40, 59-61

**COMMENTS:** **Fingertip amputation** is one of the most common hand injuries. The mechanism of injury, the orientation and location of the amputation, and the age, gender, general condition, and hand dominance of the patient are integral to decision making and planning of the reconstruction. Reconstructions that require prolonged immobilization in "unsafe" positions, such as a thenar flap or a cross-finger flap, are not recommended in older individuals. If properly cared for and free of crush-avulsion injury, the amputated part can be defatted, meticulously sutured back, and used for a salvage procedure. Microvascular replantations have been successful even as far distal as the midnail but are not generally performed for fingertip injuries. In this particular case, a hypothenar skin graft is best. It provides glabrous skin (the unique non–hair-bearing skin found on the volar aspect of the digits and palms, as well as the soles), which matches the other digits and resists contracture and hypersensitivity. Sensibility, an important factor with all hand grafts, is similar to that achieved with flaps. The V-Y advancement flap is best used with straight transverse amputations. A split-thickness skin graft would be too thin, and allowing the wound to heal by contracture and epithelialization is a good option when there is only soft tissue loss, but the orientation should be such that the tissues can contract to cover the defect. The broad surface area described here would not be satisfactory for this method of healing.

**ANSWER:** B

41. Which of the following statements is false?

    A. Jersey finger refers to an intra-articular fracture of the DIP joint.

    B. Mallet finger results from traumatic avulsion of the extensor tendon insertion into the distal phalanx.

    C. Skier's (ski pole injury) thumb results from disruption of the ulnar collateral ligament at the thumb MCP joint.

    D. Kienböck disease refers to idiopathic lunatomalacia.

    E. Rolando and Bennett fractures are fractures of the base of the thumb metacarpal.

    *Ref.:* 40, 47, 62

**COMMENTS:** There are numerous common names for disorders of the hand. Understanding the cause of the disorder sheds light on the common name. For instance, **jersey finger** is traumatic avulsion of the flexor digitorum profundus at the DIP level. It is an injury sustained most commonly by rugby and football players as the tendon avulses from the bone with forceful gripping, such as when grabbing a jersey. **Mallet finger** is the extensor counterpart of jersey finger and is a traumatic disruption of the extensor mechanism at its insertion into the distal phalanx that is usually caused by forced flexion at the joint, such as occurs when "jamming" one's long finger while catching a softball. Injuries to the extensor insertion into the dorsum of the distal phalanx result in the **mallet deformity**. Frequently, no fracture can be seen. If such an injury is associated with no fracture or is associated with a fracture and the fragment is small, dorsal splinting with the joint in 0 to 10 degrees of hyperextension for 6 to 8 weeks provides good results. If more than one third of the articular surface is displaced with the avulsed tendon and volar subluxation of the distal phalanx occurs, open reduction plus internal fixation is advised. A **boutonnière deformity** results from disruption of the central extensor tendon at its insertion into the dorsum of the base of the middle phalanx. Immobilization of the PIP joint at zero degrees of extension with dynamic extension splinting for 6 to 8 weeks is recommended whenever possible. The name **gamekeeper's thumb** is derived from Scottish gamekeepers'

practice of breaking the necks of rabbits by twisting their necks. Repetitive trauma of this type tended to weaken the ulnar collateral ligament of the thumb and cause both pain and laxity of the thumb at the MCP joint in this area. **Skier's (ski pole injury) thumb** is specifically an acute traumatic avulsion of the ulnar collateral ligament, although gamekeeper's thumb is sometimes used incorrectly to describe this situation.

Robert Kienböck, an Austrian professor of radiology, was the first to describe a syndrome of idiopathic lunatomalacia in 1910—**Kienböck disease**. It is most commonly manifested as a stiff, painful, and weak wrist in a young adult male. A Bennett fracture is a fracture at the base of the thumb metacarpal. It is inherently unstable, but its management tends to be less complicated and its prognosis much better than that of a Rolando fracture. The latter is a comminuted, intra-articular fracture at the base of the thumb metacarpal that exhibits a T or Y fracture pattern in which the articular surface is split at the base of the first metacarpal.

**ANSWER:** A

42. Which of the following statements regarding burns of the hands is false?

    A. Full-thickness dorsal burns cause scarring, which prevents flexion contractures.

    B. Loss of the extensor tendons is often treated by joint fusion to prevent contractures from unopposed flexion forces.

    C. Partial superficial-thickness burns are best treated by sterile débridement, splinting, and occupational therapy.

    D. Deep partial-thickness burns require early débridement and grafting with sheet grafts.

    E. Splinting in a safe position should be performed whenever possible.

    *Ref.:* 40, 57, 58, 63

**COMMENTS:** Treatment of **hand burns** must begin as soon as possible. Although the injury to the hand may be complex, certain principles must be followed. Proper dressing should be applied and the hand splinted in a "safe" position whenever possible. Destruction of extensor tendons results in flexion contractures unless the tendons and skin are reconstructed or the joints are fused in the appropriate position. Superficial partial-thickness burns should be débrided of superficial necrotic tissue. Deep partial-thickness and full-thickness burns are best treated by early full-thickness or tangential excision and skin grafting. This allows early initiation of occupational hand therapy to prevent stiffness and contractures.

**ANSWER:** A

43. A surgeon is called to the emergency department to evaluate a 42-year-old man who after 14 hours in subfreezing temperatures has frostbite on his left index, middle, and ring fingers down to the level of the PIP joint. Which of the following treatment plans should be undertaken?

    A. Plan to amputate the involved areas within the next 6 hours.

    B. Begin gradual rewarming of the involved area by immersion in a water bath (35° C to 39° C).

    C. Splint the hand and administer tetanus immunoglobulin, provide elevation, begin oral antibiotics, and discharge for follow-up in 48 hours.

D. Begin rapid rewarming of the involved area by immersion in a water bath at 40° C to 44° C.

E. Administer tetanus toxoid and gradually rewarm the involved area.

*Ref.:* 40, 56, 58

**COMMENTS:** Tissue destruction secondary to **frostbite** is the result of direct cellular injury through the formation of extracellular ice crystals and through vascular impairment as a result of intense invasive constriction, shunting, stasis, and endothelial damage. The frozen extremity should be rewarmed rapidly in a warm bath carefully maintained at 40° C to 44° C until flushing of the digital pads is observed (usually about 30 minutes). Gradual warming allows continued tissue injury and is not indicated. Parenteral analgesics may be required during the rewarming period. Because it takes at least 2 weeks for demarcation to occur, amputation should be delayed until after this acute period. Splinting and elevation do not address the issue of tissue damage. The intense care just listed requires hospitalization, especially for observation during the first 48 hours. The patient should not be discharged until the wounds are under control, although the patient need not remain in the hospital until demarcation and surgery, if the latter should become necessary. Tetanus immunization status must always be checked and supplemented as necessary for frostbite and burn injuries.

**ANSWER:** D

## REFERENCES

1. Burns JL, Blackwell SJ: Plastic surgery. In Townsend CM Jr, Beauchamp RD, Evers BM, et al, editors: *Sabiston textbook of surgery: the biological basis of modern surgical practice,* ed 18, Philadelphia, 2008, WB Saunders.

2. Losee JE, Gimbel M, Rubin JP, et al. Plastic and reconstructive surgery. In Brunicardi FC, Andersen DK, Billiar TR, et al, editors: *Schwartz's principles of surgery,* ed 9, New York, 2010, McGraw-Hill.

3. Senchenkov A, Valerio IL, Manders EK: Grafts. In Guyuron B, Eriksson E, Persing JA, et al, editors: *Plastic surgery: indications and practice,* Philadelphia, 2009, WB Saunders.

4. Thorne CH: Techniques and principles in plastic surgery. In Thorne CH, Beasley RW, Aston SJ, et al, editors: *Grabb and Smith's plastic surgery,* ed 6, Philadelphia, 2007, Lippincott Williams & Wilkins.

5. Paletta CE, Pokorny JJ, Rumbolo PM: Skin grafts, Volume 1. In Mathes SJ, editor: *Plastic surgery,* ed 2, Philadelphia, 2006, WB Saunders.

6. The reconstructive triangle: a paradigm for surgical decision making, Volume 1. In Mathes SJ, Nahai F, editors: *Reconstructive surgery: principles, anatomy, & technique,* New York, 1997, Churchill Livingstone.

7. Ethridge RT, Leong M, Phillips LG: Wound healing. In Townsend CM Jr, Beauchamp RD, Evers BM, et al, editors: *Sabiston textbook of surgery: the biological basis of modern surgical practice,* ed 18, Philadelphia, 2008, WB Saunders.

8. Strauch B, Yu HL, editors: *Atlas of microvascular surgery: anatomy and operative approaches,* ed 2, New York, 2006, Thieme.

9. Agnese DM, Povoski SP, Souba WW: Benign breast disease. In Ashley SW, Barie PS, Cance WG, et al, editors: *ACS surgery: principles & practice,* New York, 2007, WebMD.

10. Khosla RK: Augmentation mammaplasty, Volume 10, Number 21. In Kenkel JM, editor: *Selected readings in plastic surgery,* Texas, 2008.

11. U.S. Food and Drug Administration. Breast Implant Questions & Answers. Online at: http://www.fda.gov/MedicalDevices/Products andMedicalProcedures/ImplantsandProsthetics/BreastImplants/UCM 063719.

12. Myers WT, Phillips LG: Pressure sores. In Guyuron B, Eriksson E, Persing JA, et al, editors: *Plastic surgery: indications and practice,* Philadelphia, 2009, WB Saunders.

13. Bauer J, Phillips LG: Pressure sores, *Plast Reconstr Surg* 121:1–10, 2008.

14. Gosain AK, Nacamuli R: Embryology of the head and neck. In Thorne CH, Beasley RW, Aston SJ, et al, editors: *Grabb and Smith's plastic surgery,* ed 6, Philadelphia, 2007, Lippincott Williams & Wilkins.

15. Barbul A, Efron DT: Wound healing. In Brunicardi FC, Andersen DK, Billiar TR, et al, editors: *Schwartz's principles of surgery,* ed 9, New York, 2010, McGraw-Hill.

16. Sugarbaker DJ, Lukanich JM: Chest wall and pleura. In Townsend CM Jr, Beauchamp RD, Evers BM, et al, editors: *Sabiston textbook of surgery: the biological basis of modern surgical practice,* ed 18, Philadelphia, 2008, WB Saunders.

17. Mathes SJ, Seyfer AE, Miranda EP: Congenital anomalies of the chest wall, Volume 6. In Mathes SJ, editor: *Plastic surgery,* ed 2, Philadelphia, 2006, WB Saunders.

18. Norris RL, Auerbach PS, Nelson EE: Bites and stings. In Townsend CM Jr, Beauchamp RD, Evers BM, et al, editors: *Sabiston textbook of surgery: the biological basis of modern surgical practice,* ed 18, Philadelphia, 2008, WB Saunders.

19. Sullivan SR, Engrav LH, Klein MB: Acute wound care. In Ashley SW, Barie PS, Cance WG, et al, editors: *ACS Surgery: principles & practice,* New York, 2007, WebMD.

20. Anaya DA, Dellinger EP: Surgical infections and choice of antibiotics. In Townsend CM Jr, Beauchamp RD, Evers BM, et al, editors: *Sabiston textbook of surgery: the biological basis of modern surgical practice,* ed 18, Philadelphia, 2008, WB Saunders.

21. Manahan MA, Milner SM, Freeswick P, et al: Necrotizing skin and soft tissue infections. In Cameron JL, editor: *Current surgical therapy,* ed 9, Philadelphia, 2008, CV Mosby.

22. Malangoni MA, McHenry CR: Soft tissue infection. In Ashley SW, Barie PS, Cance WG, et al, editors: *ACS Surgery: principles & practice,* New York, 2007, WebMD.

23. Disa JJ, Halvorson EG, Hidalgo DA: Open wound requiring reconstruction. In Ashley SW, Barie PS, Cance WG, et al, editors: *ACS Surgery: principles & practice,* New York, 2006, WebMD.

24. Argenta LC, Morykwas MJ, Mark MW, et al: Vacuum-assisted closure: state of clinic art, *Plast Reconstr Surg* 117(7 Suppl):127S–142S, 2006.

25. V.A.C. Therapy Clinical Guidelines: A reference source for clinicians (July 2007), available at www.kci1.com/Clinical_Guidelines_VAC.pdf.

26. Wilhelmi BJ, Phillips LG. Breast reconstruction. In Townsend CM Jr, Beauchamp RD, Evers BM, et al, editors: *Sabiston textbook of surgery: the biological basis of modern surgical practice,* ed 18, Philadelphia, 2008, WB Saunders.

27. Granzow JW, Levine JL, Chiu ES, et al: Breast reconstruction with perforator flaps, *Plast Reconstr Surg* 120:1–12, 2007.

28. Mulliken JB: Vascular anomalies. In Thorne CH, Beasley RW, Aston SJ, et al, editors: *Grabb and Smith's plastic surgery,* ed 6, Philadelphia, 2007, Lippincott Williams & Wilkins.

29. Manson PN: Facial injuries. In Cameron JL, editor: *Current surgical therapy,* ed 9, Philadelphia, 2008, CV Mosby.

30. Boutros S: Reconstruction of the lips. In Thorne CH, Beasley RW, Aston SJ, et al, editors: *Grabb and Smith's plastic surgery,* ed 6, Philadelphia, 2007, Lippincott Williams & Wilkins.

31. Manktelow RT, Zuker RM, Neligan PC: Facial paralysis reconstruction. In Thorne CH, Beasley RW, Aston SJ, et al, editors: *Grabb and Smith's plastic surgery,* ed 6, Philadelphia, 2007, Lippincott Williams & Wilkins.

32. Shaw WW, Hidalgo DA, editors: *Microsurgery in trauma,* Mount Kisco, NY, 1987, Futura.

33. Klein AW: Filler materials. In Thorne CH, Beasley RW, Aston SJ, et al, editors: *Grabb and Smith's plastic surgery,* ed 6, Philadelphia, 2007, Lippincott Williams & Wilkins.

34. Kane MAC: Botulinum toxin. In Thorne CH, Beasley RW, Aston SJ, et al, editors: *Grabb and Smith's plastic surgery,* ed 6, Philadelphia, 2007, Lippincott Williams & Wilkins.

35. Kwei SL, Weiss DD, Pribaz JJ: Microsurgery and free flaps. In Guyuron B, Eriksson E, Persing JA, et al, editors: *Plastic surgery: indications and practice,* Philadelphia, 2009, WB Saunders.

36. Bui DT, Cordeiro PG, Hu QY, et al: Free flap reexploration: indications, treatment, and outcomes in 1193 free flaps, *Plast Reconstr Surg* 119: 2092–2100, 2007.

37. Trussler AP, Rohrich RJ: Blepharoplasty, *Plast Reconstr Surg* 121:1–10, 2008.

38. Lemmon JA: Reduction mammaplasty & mastopexy, Volume 10, Number 19. In Kenkel JM, editor: *Selected readings in plastic surgery,* Texas, 2008.

39. Hopper RA, Cutting C, Grayson B: Cleft lip and palate. In Thorne CH, Beasley RW, Aston SJ, et al, editors: *Grabb and Smith's plastic surgery*, ed 6, Philadelphia, 2007, Lippincott Williams & Wilkins.
40. Sunil TM, Kleinert HE, Miller JH, et al: Hand surgery. In Townsend CM Jr, Beauchamp RD, Evers BM, et al, editors: *Sabiston textbook of surgery: the biological basis of modern surgical practice*, ed 17, Philadelphia, 2004, WB Saunders.
41. Green DP: General principles. In Green DP, Hotchkiss RN, Pederson WC, et al, editors: *Green's operative hand surgery*, ed 5, Philadelphia, 2005, Churchill-Livingstone.
42. Stern PJ: Fractures of the metacarpals and phalanges. In Green DP, Hotchkiss RN, Pederson WC, et al, editors: *Green's operative hand surgery*, ed 5, Philadelphia, 2005, Churchill-Livingstone.
43. Chang B: Principles of upper limb surgery. In Thorne CH, Beasley RW, Aston SJ, et al, editors: *Grabb and Smith's plastic surgery*, ed 6, Philadelphia, 2007, Lippincott Williams & Wilkins.
44. Boyer MI, Taras JS, Kaufmann, RA: Flexor tendon injury. In Green DP, Hotchkiss RN, Pederson WC, et al, editors: *Green's operative hand surgery*, ed 5, Philadelphia, 2005, Churchill-Livingstone.
45. Zidel P: Tendon healing and flexor tendon surgery. In Thorne CH, Beasley RW, Aston SJ, et al, editors: *Grabb and Smith's plastic surgery*, ed 6, Philadelphia, 2007, Lippincott Williams & Wilkins.
46. Jobe MT, Calandruccio JH: Fractures, dislocations, and ligamentous injuries. In Canale ST, editor: *Campbell's operative orthopaedics*, ed 10, St. Louis, 2003, CV Mosby.
47. Friedman DW, Kells A, Aviles A: Fractures, dislocations, and ligamentous injuries of the hand. In Thorne CH, Beasley RW, Aston SJ, et al, editors: *Grabb and Smith's plastic surgery*, ed 6, Philadelphia, 2007, Lippincott Williams & Wilkins.
48. Wright PE: Hand infections. In Canale ST, editor: *Campbell's operative orthopaedics*, ed 10, St. Louis, 2003, CV Mosby.
49. Stevanovic MV, Sharpe F: Acute infections in the hand. In Green DP, Hotchkiss RN, Pederson WC, et al, editors: *Green's operative hand surgery*, ed 5, Philadelphia, 2005, Churchill-Livingstone.
50. Chao JJ, Morrison BA: Infections of the upper limb. In Thorne CH, Beasley RW, Aston SJ, et al, editors: *Grabb and Smith's plastic surgery*, ed 6, Philadelphia, 2007, Lippincott Williams & Wilkins.
51. Wolfe SW: Tenosynovitis. In Green DP, Hotchkiss RN, Pederson WC, et al, editors: *Green's operative hand surgery*, ed 5, Philadelphia, 2005, Churchill-Livingstone.
52. Goldner RD, Urbaniak JR: Replantation. In Green DP, Hotchkiss RN, Pederson WC, et al, editors: *Green's operative hand surgery*, ed 5. Philadelphia, 2005, Churchill-Livingstone.
53. Jones NF: Replantation in the upper extremity. In Thorne CH, Beasley RW, Aston SJ, et al, editors: *Grabb and Smith's plastic surgery*, ed 6, Philadelphia, 2007, Lippincott Williams & Wilkins.
54. Jobe MT: Nerve injuries. In Canale ST, editor: *Campbell's operative orthopaedics*, ed 10, St. Louis, 2003, CV Mosby.
55. Birch R: Nerve repair. In Green DP, Hotchkiss RN, Pederson WC, et al, editors: *Green's operative hand surgery*, ed 5, Philadelphia, 2005, Churchill-Livingstone.
56. Wright PE: Special hand disorders. In Canale ST, editor: *Campbell's operative orthopaedics*, ed 10, St. Louis, 2003, CV Mosby.
57. Germann G, Philipp K: The burned hand. In Green DP, Hotchkiss RN, Pederson WC, et al, editors: *Green's operative hand surgery*, ed 5, Philadelphia, 2005, Churchill-Livingstone.
58. Klein MB: Thermal, chemical, and electrical injuries. In Thorne CH, Beasley RW, Aston SJ, et al, editors: *Grabb and Smith's plastic surgery*, ed 6, Philadelphia, 2007, Lippincott Williams & Wilkins.
59. Browne EZ, Pederson WC, Lister GD, et al: Skin grafts and skin flaps. In Green DP, Hotchkiss RN, Pederson WC, et al, editors: *Green's operative hand surgery*, ed 5, Philadelphia, 2005, Churchill-Livingstone.
60. Tymchak J: Soft-tissue reconstruction of the hand. In Thorne CH, Beasley RW, Aston SJ, et al, editors: *Grabb and Smith's plastic surgery*, ed 6, Philadelphia, 2007, Lippincott Williams & Wilkins.
61. Eaton CJ: Thumb reconstruction. In Thorne CH, Beasley RW, Aston SJ, et al, editors: *Grabb and Smith's plastic surgery*, ed 6, Philadelphia, 2007, Lippincott Williams & Wilkins.
62. Golimbu CN: Radiologic imaging of the hand and wrist. In Thorne CH, Beasley RW, Aston SJ, et al, editors: *Grabb and Smith's plastic surgery*, ed 6, Philadelphia, 2007, Lippincott Williams & Wilkins.
63. Donelan MB: Principles of burn reconstruction. In Thorne CH, Beasley RW, Aston SJ, et al, editors: *Grabb and Smith's plastic surgery*, ed 6, Philadelphia, 2007, Lippincott Williams & Wilkins.

# Fundamentals of Surgical Technology

# CHAPTER 34

# Principles of Ultrasound and Ablative Therapy

*Joseph R. Durham, M.D., F.A.C.S., R.P.V.I.; José M. Velasco, M.D.;
Vikram D. Krishnamurthy, M.D.; and Tina J. Hieken, M.D.*

1. Which of the following most accurately represents the average speed at which ultrasound waves move through the human body?

   A. 350 m/s

   B. 2000 m/s

   C. 500 cm/s

   D. 1540 m/s

   E. 800 m/s

   *Ref.: 1*

**COMMENT:** Sound moves through biologic tissue at a speed that is dependent on tissue density. Sound moves more slowly through less dense matter, such as air (330 m/s), and more quickly through high-density material, such as bone (4050 m/s). The average **speed of sound** through human tissue is 1540 m/s. Specific examples of propagation speeds through tissue are 1459 m/s for fat, 1520 m/s for brain, 1550 m/s for liver, 1560 m/s for kidneys, and 1580 m/s for muscle. Because most soft tissues have similar density and therefore sound passes through them at a similar speed, ultrasound machines are designed on the assumption that the speed of sound through soft tissues is 1540 m/s.

**ANSWER: D**

2. Concerning acoustic impedance, which of the following statements is true?

   A. It can be amplified by increasing the gain on the ultrasound equipment.

   B. It is influenced by the density of the tissue and the velocity of the sound wave.

   C. It permits the operator to distinguish between two structures even if their densities are the same.

   D. It is calculated by multiplying the amplitude of the waves by the density of the tissue.

   E. The greater the difference in impedance between two tissues, the less energy is reflected to the transducer.

   *Ref.: 1*

**COMMENT:** Diagnostic ultrasonography is centered on the analysis of sound waves that have been reflected back to the ultrasound transducer. Impedance is the acoustic resistance to sound traveling in a medium. **Acoustic impedance** is dependent on the speed of sound in the tissue and the density of the tissue and can be calculated as acoustic impedance = density × velocity. Sound wave properties are not the only parameters that shape ultrasound physics. The medium (tissue) carrying the sound is a major contributor to events. The compressibility of a material determines, in part, the way that sound is carried along within that material. Because sound forms compressions and rarefactions, the ability of the tissue to be compressed and stretched determines just how well sound can be propagated through the tissue. Hard tissues (e.g., bone) are difficult to compress and thus *impede* the formation of compressions and rarefactions when they carry sound waves. As a result, hard materials have high acoustic impedance when compared with softer tissues (e.g., muscle), which have low acoustic impedance. Therefore, the ease with which sound is transmitted through a substance is termed *impedance*. The interface between two adjacent tissues serves as a major source for reflecting sound waves back to the transducer. When two adjacent tissues have different impedance values, the sound wave reflects back to the transducer. The greater the difference in impedance between the two tissues, the less energy is transferred to the next tissue and more energy is reflected back. Fortunately, differences in impedance between most soft tissues are small. These small differences are enough to cause a reflection of the sound waves to provide the information for generating an image; at the same time, the differences are small enough to allow enough amplitude for passage of some sound waves past the tissue interface into deeper tissues. These small differences in impedance are sufficient to make ultrasound a workable diagnostic modality. Increasing the gain on the machine does not affect any of these parameters.

**ANSWER: B**

3. Which of the following statements regarding transducers is false?

   A. Higher-frequency transducers have poor penetration and good resolution

   B. The higher the frequency, the shorter the wavelength.

   C. Longer wave lengths result in deeper penetration.

D. Axial resolution is independent of frequency.

E. The piezoelectric effect is defined as the "conversion of electrical to mechanical energy."

*Ref.: 1*

**COMMENT: Ultrasound transducers** contain crystals. When a sound wave mechanically deforms one of the crystals, voltage is produced. The corollary is also true: when a crystal has voltage applied to it, it deforms and a sound wave is generated. This is described as the piezoelectric effect and has practical applications to the field of ultrasonography. The crystals used in ultrasound machines initially act as speakers that send out and receive sound waves. The returning sound that is reflected back causes the crystals to vibrate and generate voltage.

High-frequency transducers provide high-resolution images at the expense of tissue penetration. In ultrasonography, three types of resolution exist: axial resolution, lateral resolution, and temporal resolution. **Axial resolution** is the ability to distinguish one object from another object below it. It is dependent on frequency. By definition, a higher frequency means a shorter wavelength. Because the depth of penetration is dependent on the wavelength, a higher frequency results in less tissue penetration. **Lateral resolution** is the ability to differentiate between two objects that are next to each other. It is independent of frequency and is dependent on the width of the beam. **Temporal resolution** is the perception of real-time movement and is dependent on the frame rate.

**ANSWER:  D**

4. Which of the following descriptors regarding echogenicity is not true?

A. Hyperechoic tissues are brighter than the surrounding tissue.

B. Hypoechoic tissues are less dark than the surrounding tissue.

C. Isoechoic tissues are similar in appearance to surrounding tissue.

D. Anechoic tissues appear as black sonographic images.

E. Simple cysts are hyperechoic.

*Ref.: 1*

**COMMENT: Echogenicity** refers to the appearance of a specific tissue or structure on the ultrasound image relative to its ability to reflect the ultrasound wave. A region in a sonographic picture in which echoes are brighter than those in nearby structures is referred to as hyperechoic. In contrast, hypoechoic areas appear darker than surrounding areas. Isoechoic areas appear similar to surrounding structures, and anechoic areas appear dark or black, without echoes, on a sonographic image. Simple cysts appear as anechoic images with posterior enhancement.

**ANSWER:  E**

5. Which of the following artifacts is often associated with visualization of the diaphragm?

A. Reverberation

B. Posterior enhancement

C. Mirror image

D. Comet tail

E. Black boundary

*Ref.: 1*

**COMMENTS:** See Question 8.

**ANSWER:  C**

6. Which of the following artifacts is often associated with visualization of a simple cyst?

A. Reverberation

B. Posterior enhancement

C. Mirror image

D. Comet tail

E. Black boundary

*Ref.: 1*

**COMMENTS:** See Question 8.

**ANSWER:  B**

7. Which of the following artifacts is often associated with visualization of a bullet?

A. Reverberation

B. Posterior enhancement

C. Mirror image

D. Comet tail

E. Black boundary

*Ref.: 1*

**COMMENTS:** See Question 8.

**ANSWER:  D**

8. Which of the following artifacts is often associated with visualization of bone?

A. Reverberation

B. Posterior enhancement

C. Mirror image

D. Comet tail

E. Black boundary

*Ref.: 1*

**COMMENTS:** Although the utility of ultrasound is unquestionable, certain problems do exist with it. **Artifacts** are errors in ultrasound images that occur because the machine design is based on assumptions that are not always true. Reverberation takes place when sound waves are trapped between two areas and the waves are forced to bounce back and forth. Some of this trapped energy eventually returns to the transducer. However, the temporal delay leads to an artifact in the image. A reverberation artifact often resembles a ladder, with hyperechoic areas representing the rungs. Reverberation artifact usually occurs with strong specular reflectors such as bone. Ultrasound images of fluid-filled structures, such as cysts, sometimes display an artifact known as posterior enhancement. This artifact occurs because the ultrasound machine makes the assumption that sound waves are uniformly attenuated by tissue. Fluids are efficient at transmitting sound waves. As the sound travels through a cyst and reaches the tissue below it, the attenuation changes. The ultrasound machine interprets this change incorrectly, and posterior enhancement is the result. Posterior enhancement appears as a hyperechoic (bright) area below the fluid-filled structure. When sound waves are reflected by a curved surface, such as the diaphragm or bladder, instead of by a flat surface, a mirror-image artifact may appear. When the transducer sound waves strike a piece of metal, the metal can act as a bell and continue "ringing" for a longer time than the actual contact between the ultrasound wave and the metal object. As this additional sound energy returns to the transducer, it is incorrectly interpreted as having come from a deeper location. The result is a hyperechoic line extending from the metallic object that resembles a comet tail. The black boundary artifact is an artificially created black line located at fat-water interfaces such as muscle-fat interfaces. It results in a sharp delineation of the muscle-fat boundary that is sometimes visually appealing but not an anatomic structure. This is an artifact seen on magnetic resonance imaging (MRI), not on ultrasound.

**ANSWER:** A

9. Which of the following is not a sonographic characteristic of an inflamed gallbladder?

   A. Gallbladder distention

   B. Pericholecystic fluid

   C. Wall thickness of 2 mm

   D. Sonographic Murphy sign

   E. Gallstones

*Ref.:* 1

**COMMENTS:** The sonographic diagnosis of **cholelithiasis** is generally indicated by the presence of a mobile, hyperechoic, intraluminal object with posterior shadowing. If these three criteria are not met, the diagnosis is less certain. Gallbladder distention, pericholecystic fluid, a sonographic Murphy sign, and gallstones can all be seen on a sonogram in the presence of cholecystitis. Gallbladder wall thickness is considered abnormal if it is greater than 3 mm.

**ANSWER:** C

10. Which of the following are not characteristic of the sonographic appearance of a malignant thyroid nodule?

    A. Hypoechoic in comparison with surrounding tissue

    B. Peripheral calcifications

    C. Irregular margins

    D. Absence of cystic areas

    E. Heterogeneity

*Ref.:* 1

**COMMENTS:** Ultrasound has proved useful in the evaluation of **thyroid carcinoma**. Thyroid cancers are often seen as heterogeneous hypoechoic lesions with irregular borders. When microcalcifications are present (psammoma bodies), they are located in the interior of the lesion, not at the periphery. Cystic thyroid masses are usually benign.

**ANSWER:** B

11. Which of the following statements regarding focused abdominal sonography for trauma (FAST) is true?

    A. It can reliably evaluate the retroperitoneum.

    B. It can quickly detect the presence of pericardial fluid or a pleural effusion.

    C. It is useful in detecting a cardiac contusion.

    D. It is considered a replacement for computed tomography (CT).

    E. It can reliably detect diaphragmatic injuries.

*Ref.:* 1

**COMMENTS: Focused abdominal sonography for trauma** has become a vital component in the initial evaluation of trauma patients. Currently, the primary focus of the FAST examination is to detect fluid presumed to be blood, but as time progresses, more advanced applications will undoubtedly arise. The examination is completed quickly during a primary survey (of an unstable patient) or a secondary survey (of a stable patient) and focuses on detecting fluid in the pericardial space and dependent portions of the abdomen. The examination is divided into three parts: cardiac, abdominal, and thoracic. The cardiac examination consists of a sagittal view in the subxiphoid region. The abdominal examination focuses on longitudinal views of the left and right upper quadrants and a transverse view of the pelvis. The thoracic portion is an upward scan from the upper abdominal quadrants and can detect pleural effusions or pneumothorax. Despite the usefulness of the FAST examination, it does have limitations. The FAST examination can quickly evaluate for the presence of both pericardial fluid and pleural effusion. However, it does not evaluate the retroperitoneum and does not detect a cardiac contusion. CT still has many practical applications in trauma patients and has not been fully replaced by the FAST examination. Transabdominal ultrasound has several advantages over CT, including cost, portability, safety, and speed of the examination. However, ultrasound examinations are operator dependent. The quality of the images, or lack thereof, depends on the technical expertise of the person operating the ultrasound machine.

**ANSWER:** B

12. Regarding vascular arterial ultrasound imaging, which of the following statements is true?

    A. In Doppler ultrasound of blood flow, the reflected wave returning to the transducer has the same frequency as the transmitted wave.

    B. For Doppler ultrasound, the transducer should be held at a 90-degree angle to the body.

    C. Arterial stenosis leads to decreased flow velocity.

D. Carotid artery duplex ultrasound scanning allows assessment of arterial plaque morphology, as well as estimation of the degree of carotid artery stenosis caused by the plaque.

E. In dialysis access patients, duplex ultrasonography does not generally assess arterial inflow for arteriovenous (AV) fistulas or grafts accurately.

*Ref.:* 1

**COMMENTS: Doppler ultrasound** relies on the fact that the sound wave that has been reflected back to the transducer from a moving object has a different frequency than does the transmitted wave. The change in frequency is known as the Doppler shift, named after the Austrian physicist Christian Doppler who described it in 1842. If the transducer is held at a 90-degree angle while performing Doppler ultrasonography, regardless of the actual velocity in a blood vessel, the ultrasound machine will read zero velocity. This is because the theoretical velocity is calculated by the equation $V = \Delta f \ c/2f \cos \theta$ (where V is velocity, c is the speed of sound in soft tissue, $\Delta f$ is the change in frequency of reflected versus transmitted sound waves, f is the frequency of transmitted sound, and $\cos \theta$ is the angle between the ultrasound wave and the direction of motion of the target). Because the cosine of 90 degrees is zero, the theoretical velocity would be zero if the transducer is held at a 90-degree angle to the target. The ideal angle of insonation is 60 degrees. Analysis of the Doppler shift is used to determine the speed and direction of blood flow. Unless the arterial stenosis is so severe that blood flow is slowed almost to zero, the velocity increases in arterial stenosis. As its name implies, duplex ultrasonography uses two diagnostic modalities: (1) high-resolution gray-scale B-mode imaging (anatomic information) and (2) Doppler spectral analysis of blood flow patterns (physiologic information). B-mode imaging allows visualization of plaque location, composition, and morphology. Soft plaques and plaques with an irregular intimal surface (ulceration) may be relatively unstable and pose more risk for cerebral thromboembolic events and stroke than might dense fibrous plaques with a smooth intimal lining. Doppler spectral measurement of flow velocities allows accurate assessment of the degree of carotid artery stenosis. As with other ultrasound diagnostic modalities, the accuracy and reliability of vascular ultrasound imaging are dependent on the skill and experience of the operator. Ultrasound imaging is very useful in patients requiring hemodialysis access. Vein mapping can be performed preoperatively to determine the best vessels to support an AV fistula and postoperatively to assess fistula maturation. It can also be used to assess the arterial inflow for a fistula or graft. Ultrasound of new AV grafts may be limited by air entrained in the wall of the prosthetic graft.

**ANSWER:** D

13. Which of the following statements best describes the use of breast ultrasound imaging?

A. It should be used instead of breast biopsy.

B. It can be used to distinguish between cystic and solid masses.

C. It is considered an initial screening test to evaluate the entire breast.

D. It can be used to define microcalcifications.

E. It should not be used in lieu of stereotactically guided biopsies even if the lesion is detected ultrasonographically.

*Ref.:* 1

**COMMENTS:** As the technology of breast ultrasonography has continued to improve, the uses for which it is being applied have increased. Although breast ultrasound can aid in the performance of breast biopsy and other interventional modalities, ultrasound images cannot replace the information that biopsy provides. **Breast ultrasound** is used in the work-up of a palpable breast mass to aid in the differentiation of a cystic from a solid mass. A simple cyst in the breast appears anechoic in comparison to the surrounding breast tissue. Breast ultrasound is performed early in the work-up of breast lesions but is not generally used as a screening tool. It is difficult to adequately characterize (and often to even visualize) microcalcifications with breast ultrasound. If suspicious calcifications are seen on mammography, stereotactic biopsy should be performed for a thorough evaluation. Ultrasound-guided biopsy should be used preferentially whenever the lesion has been defined sonographically.

**ANSWER:** B

14. Regarding intraoperative ultrasound, which of the following statements is true?

A. It is very accurate in determining vessel encasement by tumor.

B. It necessitates the presence of a board-certified radiologist in the operating room.

C. It generally doubles the operative time.

D. It is less sensitive than CT in locating small pancreatic tumors.

E. Open intraoperative ultrasound is confounded by more artifacts than laparoscopic ultrasound is.

*Ref.:* 1

**COMMENTS: Intraoperative ultrasound** imaging has become an important part of the evaluation of many conditions. It may be performed both by open means and laparoscopically. In addition to being a valuable tool for determining vascular encasement by tumor, intraoperative ultrasound has also proved useful for delineating small pancreatic tumors not well seen on CT. For intraoperative ultrasound, a board-certified radiologist does not have to be present. However, the surgeon performing this test should have sufficient training and experience to be technically proficient in ultrasound imaging. Laparoscopy is being used in a growing number of situations, as is laparoscopic ultrasound imaging. **Laparoscopic ultrasound** has been used to help assess the extent of tumor invasion and to guide treatment. It can also detect small, intraparenchymal tumors in organs such as the pancreas or liver. In experienced hands, laparoscopic ultrasound can provide much of the same diagnostic information as intraoperative cholangiography and conventional intraoperative ultrasound. Newer probes with biopsy-guiding devices have made the application of laparoscopic ultrasound much more user friendly.

**ANSWER:** A

15. Endoscopic ultrasound (EUS) imaging has proved useful for all of the following except:

A. Staging esophageal tumors

B. Diagnosis of common bile duct stones

C. Detecting portal vein invasion by pancreatic cancer

D. Identifying small pancreatic tumors not seen with CT

E. Assessing metastatic disease to the liver

*Ref.:* 1, 2

**COMMENTS: Endoscopic ultrasound** imaging is useful for all of the applications described in this question except for the assessment of metastatic disease to the liver. EUS is a minimally invasive technique in which a high-frequency transducer is placed into the gastrointestinal tract. Frequency, EUS techniques allow the identification of small lesions (<2 cm), detection of lymphadenopathy, detection of vascular involvement, and the ability to perform guided fine-needle aspiration (FNA). Staging of esophageal tumors by EUS identifies patients with advanced tumors who may benefit from preoperative therapy. Pancreatic tumors as small as 3 mm may be seen on EUS. The accuracy of EUS without FNA averages 85% for determining T stage and 70% for determining N stage disease. Percutaneous biopsy of pancreatic tumors has been used primarily in patients with unresectable pancreatic cancers or in those with cancer for whom neoadjuvant protocols are being considered. Nevertheless, EUS has become the preferred technique, when possible, in either situation. EUS has a complication rate lower than that of endoscopic retrograde cholangiopancreatography (ERCP) and is as accurate as ERCP in detecting common bile duct stones.

**ANSWER:** E

16. Which of the following statements regarding the safety of diagnostic ultrasound and possible adverse effects on scanned tissues is false?

A. As sound propagates, energy is converted to heat.

B. Bone absorbs sound; therefore, an elevation in temperature is more likely at a bone-tissue interface.

C. Significant tissue damage can occur with an increase of 2.5° C (4.5° F).

D. Fetal tissue is less tolerant than adult tissue.

E. None of the above.

*Ref.:* 3

**COMMENTS:** Attention to the acronym "ALARA" (as low as reasonably achievable) will help minimize any possible bioeffects: decrease the power and decrease the time of exposure as much as possible. "…There are no confirmed biological effects on patients or instrument operators by exposures from present diagnostic ultrasound instruments. Although the possibility exists that such biological effects may be identified in the future, current data indicate that the benefits to patients of the prudent use of diagnostic ultrasound outweigh the risks, if any, that may be present." Ultrasound does generate heat and therefore warms tissue, but the degree is so slight that it is clinically undetectable in most routine applications and the physiologic effect appears to be negligible. Fetal tissue appears to be more susceptible than adult tissue.

**ANSWER:** E

17. Which of the following is not true regarding radiofrequency ablation (RFA)?

A. It may be used for benign conditions such as neuralgia and cardiac arrhythmias.

B. It cannot be applied topically for the treatment of metastatic cutaneous tumors.

C. It may be used endoscopically to treat gastroesophageal reflux disease.

D. It results in coagulation necrosis, protein denaturation, and tissue desiccation from thermal injury.

E. It is synonymous with microwave ablation.

*Ref.:* 4

**COMMENTS:** Radiofrequency ablative therapy or **radiofrequency ablation** involves the transmission of a high-frequency alternating current via electrode application into the tissue of interest. The main application of RFA is for the ablation of malignant tumors, including liver, lung, kidney, adrenal, breast, thyroid, and pancreatic tumors. Probes applied to the skin or too close to the surface of the skin can cause a thermal burn. Microwave ablation involves the transmission of microwave energy via a probe to create a rapidly alternating electrical field that induces motion of polar molecules within the lesion; generates kinetic energy, which in turn is dissipated as heat; and causes coagulation necrosis of the target. Microwave ablation may be used for liver lesions and to treat cardiac arrhythmias, prostatic hyperplasia, and endometrial bleeding, but it is limited by the very small volume of tissue treated with current equipment.

**ANSWER:** E

18. Regarding cryotherapy, which of the following is true?

A. It is not associated with significant risk for coagulopathy.

B. It is a relatively inexpensive modality.

C. It is usually performed with the patient under local anesthesia.

D. It is used for interstitial applications only.

E. It is less efficacious for lesions adjacent to major blood vessels.

*Ref.:* 4-6

**COMMENTS:** Cryotherapy is the freezing and thawing of tissue either topically or interstitially with liquid nitrogen or argon circulating through a probe. Ice crystals form in the target tissue during freezing and the tissue degrades during thawing, thereby resulting in cell death from tissue ischemia, fluid and electrolyte shifts, and protein denaturation. Freezing of all areas of the target to at least −40° C, with an additional surrounding 1-cm margin, and repeated treatment cycles are advisable to ensure that no viable tumor cells remain. Its major application has been for the treatment of unresectable primary or secondary liver tumors, as well as kidney tumors.

A major disadvantage is that cryotherapy equipment is quite expensive, and major complications of treatment include "cryoshock," coagulopathy, myoglobinuria, and hypothermia. Frequently, significant bilateral pleural effusions develop, and a severe systemic inflammatory response syndrome can even occur. Additionally, the procedure is time-consuming, patients usually require general anesthesia, and its efficacy is limited for lesions near large vessels secondary to the heat-sink effect of circulating blood.

**ANSWER:** A

**19.** With regard to ablative therapy for malignant tumors, which of the following is true?

   A. RFA is best suited for the treatment of smaller hepatocellular carcinomas (HCCs), whereas percutaneous ethanol injection (PEI) is better suited for treating larger lesions.

   B. PEI is more efficacious for the treatment of septated HCC than is percutaneous injection of acetic acid.

   C. Real-time ultrasound is the only imaging modality suitable for guiding percutaneous ablation.

   D. During treatment with cryotherapy, the formed frozen area (ice ball) denoting the treated area is visualized easily with real-time ultrasound.

   E. During treatment with RFA, the ablation zone denoting the treated area is visualized accurately with real-time ultrasound.

*Ref.:* 4, 5, 7, 8

**COMMENTS:** Initially, **radiofrequency ablation** was limited to the treatment of smaller lesions (or required multiple overlapping probe placements). Currently available larger probes (configured with retractable multiple electrode tips that extend in a radiating pattern) can now treat areas as large as 7 cm with a single ablation. **Percutaneous ethanol injection** is usually reserved for the treatment of smaller HCCs in patients not candidates for resection. Recent data suggest that RFA is superior to PEI for limited HCC in terms of local tumor control but not in terms of overall survival. Similarly, surgical resection appears to be superior to laparoscopic RFA in terms of local control of HCC, but it does not appear to improve overall survival. Because of its strong necrotizing properties, acetic acid injection has been demonstrated to be more effective than PEI for the treatment of septated lesions. Percutaneous ablations can be done with CT, MRI, or ultrasound guidance. A drawback of RFA is that treatment cannot be monitored precisely by ultrasound because gas microbubbles form in the tissue during treatment and create markedly hyperechoic areas that only roughly correspond to the treatment area. The ice ball (or cryolesion) created with cryotherapy can be monitored with real-time ultrasound. The cryolesion appears as a hypoechoic area during and after treatment, whereas edema in the surrounding tissue creates a distinctive hyperechoic halo.

**ANSWER:** D

**20.** A 59-year-old man is found to have an elevated carcinoembryonic antigen (CEA) level 3 years after resection of a T3N0 carcinoma of the sigmoid colon. CT of the abdomen reveals bilobar metastatic liver disease. The largest lesion is 4 cm. Preoperative positron emission tomography (PET) demonstrates four fluorodeoxyglucose (FDG)-avid lesions corresponding to the findings on CT and no evidence of extrahepatic disease. The patient previously underwent partial hepatectomy for trauma. The consensus opinion from your multidisciplinary tumor conference is that this patient would best be treated by RFA, followed by systemic therapy. Which of the following is true regarding the care of this patient?

   A. Laparoscopy before RFA may diagnose unsuspected extrahepatic disease in up to 30% of patients.

   B. Chemotherapy converts unresectable disease to resectable in more than 50% of patients.

   C. Systemic therapy may cause hepatic toxicity, bleeding, and hypercoagulability.

   D. The efficacy of RFA depends on the size but not the location of the metastatic lesions.

   E. Randomized controlled clinical trial data support the use of RFA over other treatment modalities for unresectable colorectal liver metastases.

*Ref.:* 6, 9, 10

**COMMENTS: Liver metastasis** will already be present at initial evaluation or will develop in approximately one half of patients with colorectal cancer. Although these patients are all considered to have stage IV disease, they are a heterogeneous group. Treatment recommendations depend on both tumor and patient characteristics. Factors reported to be of significant prognostic and predictive value, either singly or within a scoring system, include patient age, CEA level, primary tumor grade, T and N stages, size of the largest metastasis, number of metastases, presence of bilobar metastases, and the presence of extrahepatic disease. Although patients initially seen with metastatic disease should be evaluated for resection, the majority of patients are not candidates because of tumor features, performance status, or limited hepatic reserve. Increasingly over the past decade, RFA has been used to treat these patients. Percutaneous, laparoscopic, and open approaches have all been used. Because laparoscopy or celiotomy may disclose extrahepatic disease in approximately 10% of patients and because laparoscopic or open intraoperative ultrasound may identify more disease than diagnosed by preoperative imaging, as well as for technical reasons, either of these operative approaches is considered superior to percutaneous ablation of hepatic metastases from colorectal cancer. Aggressive systemic therapy is variably reported to convert 10% to 30% of patients from unresectable disease to potentially resectable disease. However, the commonly used agents oxaliplatin and camptothecin-11 (CPT-11; irinotecan) frequently cause hepatic steatosis, which may decrease functional hepatic reserve. Moreover, bevacizumab can cause both coagulopathy and thrombosis, and thus surgical treatment should be delayed until at least 6 weeks after the cessation of therapy. Both tumor size and location affect the success of RFA; complete ablation of tumors near large blood vessels may be limited by the inability to achieve target temperatures in the tumor. A recent systematic review of evidence about the efficacy and utility of RFA for hepatic metastases from colorectal cancer by an American Society of Clinical Oncology panel noted that the data were insufficient to form a practice guideline and that the large body of literature is composed of single-arm, retrospective, and prospective trials; no randomized control trial data exist. Their review concluded that overall survival of patients without extrahepatic disease was improved by hepatic resection. Contemporary series of appropriately selected patients report a 5-year survival rate of 25% to 58% for these patients. With RFA, reported 5-year survival rates vary widely from 14% to 55%, as do reported local recurrence rates of 4% to 60%.

**ANSWER:** C

**21.** After successful treatment by RFA, which of the following is the most appropriate recommendation for follow-up?

   A. Ultrasound examination 1 week postoperatively and then at 3-month intervals

   B. MRI 2 weeks after surgery and then at 6-month intervals

   C. MRI every 3 months after surgery

   D. CT 1 week postoperatively and then at 3-month intervals

   E. PET-CT every 3 months after surgery.

*Ref.:* 6

**COMMENTS:** Although intraoperative ultrasound is used to facilitate proper placement of the **radiofrequency ablation** probe and for intraoperative monitoring, it is not sensitive for distinguishing the difference between treated tissue and tumor recurrence. CT or MRI best visualizes the adequacy of ablation following treatment. The appropriate follow-up imaging schedule is either CT or MRI 1 week postoperatively, followed by repeated studies at 3-month intervals thereafter. Tumor marker studies are usually done at 3-month intervals as well. After RFA, peritumoral hyperemia is seen on cross-sectional imaging as rim enhancement around the ablation zone, which is indistinguishable from tumor enhancement. Persistent rim enhancement, months after treatment, is diagnostic of recurrent (or residual) disease. PET may also help diagnose recurrence, but findings in the treated area or areas in the perioperative period are usually nonspecific.

**ANSWER:** D

22. Which of the following ablative modalities is approved by the Food and Drug Administration (FDA) for the treatment of biopsy-proved breast fibroadenomas?

   A. RFA

   B. High-frequency ultrasound ablation

   C. Cryoablation

   D. Laser ablation

   E. Microwave ablation

*Ref.:* 11

**COMMENTS: Cryoablation** is currently approved by the FDA for the treatment of core needle biopsy–proved fibroadenomas. The use of ablative technology for or as an adjunct to the treatment of small invasive breast cancers is an area of active investigation.

**ANSWER:** C

23. With regard to ablative therapy for breast cancer, which of the following is true?

   A. RFA, cryotherapy, and laser ablation can all be performed with ultrasound guidance.

   B. Laser ablation and RFA create similar-size zones of ablation.

   C. Similar information regarding margin status and tumor size and histology can be obtained after treatment with ablation alone or surgical excision.

   D. The ablation zone created by RFA cannot be distinguished from residual carcinoma on postablation MRI.

   E. In the majority of cases, no viable tumor cells are found after complete RFA.

*Ref.:* 11

**COMMENTS: Laser ablation** requires that the lesion be targeted with MRI or stereotaxis, whereas cryoablation and RFA can be done with real-time ultrasound guidance. With current technology, laser ablation creates a smaller coagulation zone than RFA does, 2.5 to 3 cm versus 3 to 7 cm, respectively. Histopathologic information on tumor size, grade, and histology is not obtained when the tumor is ablated, although some of this information may be obtained from the preprocedure diagnostic core needle biopsy. On MRI, the zone of ablation differs in signal intensity from residual carcinoma. Thus, MRI can be used as a follow-up imaging modality. Pilot safety and efficacy studies of **radiofrequency ablation** followed by excision for small breast cancers report residual viable tumor cells detected in 5% to 35% of cases and complication rates (predominantly skin or muscle burns) of less than 10%. Intraoperative RFA of the lumpectomy cavity has been proposed as a one-step technique to avoid reexcision of positive or close margins, improve cosmesis, decrease treatment cost, and possibly substitute for postoperative adjuvant brachytherapy (partial breast irradiation).

**ANSWER:** E

**REFERENCES**

1. Machi J, Staren ED: *Ultrasound for surgeons*, ed 2, Philadelphia, 2005, Lippincott Williams & Wilkins.
2. Prasad P, Wittmann J, Pereira SP: Endoscopic ultrasound of the upper gastrointestinal tract and mediastinum: diagnosis and therapy, *Cardiovasc Intervent Radiol* 29:947–957, 2006.
3. American Institute of Ultrasound in Medicine, Official statements on Heat and Mammalian In Vivo Ultrasonic Biological Effects. http://www.aium.org/publications/statements.aspx (accessed 1/23/2010).
4. Neumayer L, Vargo D: Preoperative and operative surgery. In Townsend CM, Beauchamp RD, Evers M, et al, editors: *Sabiston textbook of surgery: the biological basis of modern surgical practice*, ed 18, Philadelphia, 2008, WB Saunders.
5. Velasco JM, Hieken TJ, Yamin N, et al: Colorectal hepatic metastasis. In Saclarides TJ, Millikan KW, Godellas CV, editors: *Surgical oncology: an algorithmic approach*, New York, 2003, Springer-Verlag.
6. Bilchik AJ: Colorectal cancer metastatic to the liver: radiofrequency ablation. In Cameron JL, editor: *Current surgical therapy*, ed 9, St. Louis, 2007, CV Mosby.
7. D'Angelica M, Fong Y: The liver. In Townsend CM, Beauchamp RD, Evers M, et al, editors: *Sabiston textbook of surgery: the biological basis of modern surgical practice*, ed 18, Philadelphia, 2008, WB Saunders.
8. Santambrogio R, Opocher E, Zuin M, et al: Surgical resection versus laparoscopic radiofrequency ablation in patients with hepatocellular carcinoma and Child-Pugh class A liver cirrhosis, *Ann Surg Oncol* 16:3289–3298, 2009.
9. Reissfelder C, Rahbari NN, Koch M, et al: Validation of prognostic scoring systems for patients undergoing resection of colorectal cancer liver metastases, *Ann Surg Oncol* 16:3279–3288, 2009.
10. Wong S, Mangu PB, Choti MA, et al. American Society of Clinical Oncology, 2009 clinical evidence review on radiofrequency ablation of hepatic metastases from colorectal cancer, *J Clin Oncol* 28:493–508, 2010.
11. Klimberg VS: Ablative techniques in the treatment of benign and malignant breast disease. In Cameron JL, editor: *Current surgical therapy*, ed 9, St. Louis, 2007, CV Mosby.

# CHAPTER 35

# Principles of Minimally Invasive Surgery

*Kyle A. Perry, M.D., and Jonathan A. Myers, M.D.*

1. Which of the following is not a characteristic of carbon dioxide ($CO_2$) as an insufflation gas?

    A. Rapid absorption

    B. Relatively inexpensive

    C. Minimal physiologic consequences

    D. Low risk for air embolism

    E. Readily available

    ***Ref.:*** 1

**COMMENTS:** $CO_2$ is the insufflation gas most commonly used in laparoscopic surgery because it is relatively inexpensive, does not support combustion, and is rapidly eliminated from the body. However, $CO_2$ pneumoperitoneum is associated with physiologic changes in most body systems, including cardiopulmonary and renal effects and changes in intracranial pressure and mesenteric blood flow.

**ANSWER:** C

2. Which of the following insufflation gases should not be used with electrocautery?

    A. $CO_2$

    B. Nitrous oxide

    C. Argon

    D. Helium

    E. None of the above

    ***Ref.:*** 2

**COMMENTS:** $CO_2$ is the most commonly used gas for peritoneal insufflation, but alternative gases are available. Nitrous oxide has been used for procedures performed with the patient under local anesthesia because it does not cause the acid-base disturbances associated with $CO_2$ pneumoperitoneum and may cause less post-operative pain. However, it will support combustion and cannot be used in procedures that require electrocautery. Use of the inert gases helium and argon also avoids acid-base problems; however, these agents are rarely used because they are expensive and have

low solubility, which may increase the risk for gas embolism. In addition, argon may cause significant cardiac depression.

**ANSWER:** B

3. Which body compartment is the largest reservoir for $CO_2$?

    A. Bone

    B. Skeletal muscle

    C. Lungs

    D. Peritoneum

    E. Adipose tissue

    ***Ref.:*** 3

**COMMENTS:** $CO_2$ is rapidly absorbed during laparoscopic procedures, but not all of it is eliminated rapidly. Thus, body stores of $CO_2$ increase during the course of an operation, with bone serving as the largest reservoir. Stored $CO_2$ may take several hours to eliminate, so premature extubation after a long laparoscopic operation should be avoided, particularly in patients with underlying respiratory disease.

**ANSWER:** A

4. Which of the following hemodynamic parameters decreases during laparoscopy with $CO_2$ pneumoperitoneum?

    A. Mean arterial pressure

    B. Pulmonary vascular resistance

    C. Systemic vascular resistance

    D. Heart rate

    E. Peripheral blood flow

    ***Ref.:*** 1

**COMMENTS:** $CO_2$ pneumoperitoneum produces consistent cardiopulmonary effects, but their magnitude depends on several factors, including the anesthetic agent, patient cardiopulmonary status, and metabolic factors. Cardiac effects include decreased venous return, which produces decreased preload, stroke volume, and cardiac output. Direct myocardial depression from $CO_2$ pneumoperitoneum also reduces stroke volume and cardiac output. These changes produce a compensatory increase in heart rate and systemic and pulmonary vascular resistance. Increased intra-abdominal pressure on the aorta, vena cava, and splanchnic vasculature along with the compensatory release of renin and vasopressin produces increased systemic vascular resistance and decreased peripheral blood flow.

**ANSWER:** E

5. Which of the following does not routinely increase during laparoscopic surgery?

   A. Airway pressure

   B. Pulmonary capillary wedge pressure

   C. Vital capacity

   D. Diaphragmatic excursion

   E. Intrathoracic pressure

*Ref.:* 1

**COMMENTS:** Unlike the indirect cardiac effects, almost all respiratory changes during laparoscopic surgery are directly attributable to the mechanical effects of increased intra-abdominal pressure. This produces increased diaphragmatic excursion, which in turn causes increased airway pressure and decreased vital capacity, functional reserve capacity, and thoracic compliance. The combination of these factors typically requires a 15% increase in minute ventilation for compensation, even in healthy subjects.

**ANSWER:** C

6. Which of the following characteristics regarding infection and tumor growth are related to laparoscopic surgery?

   A. Immunosuppression is increased in comparison with open surgery.

   B. The acute phase proteins interleukin-6 (IL-6) and C-reactive protein are elevated after laparotomy.

   C. The catecholamine response after laparoscopy is reduced in comparison to laparotomy.

   D. Current studies demonstrate increased port site metastasis after laparoscopic colectomy.

   E. Survival is improved after laparoscopic colon resection.

*Ref.:* 3, 4

**COMMENTS:** Reversible immunosuppression occurs after both open and laparoscopic procedures. Several acute phase proteins, such as IL-6 and C-reactive protein, which correlate with the physiologic stress response, are reduced after laparotomy. However, the magnitude of immunosuppression is considerably lower after laparoscopy. This is supported in studies that demonstrate significantly more depressed cell-mediated immunity in patients undergoing laparotomy than in those undergoing laparoscopy. A decreased stress response to laparoscopic surgery is also supported by a reduced catecholamine response to laparoscopic versus open cholecystectomy.

   Regarding tumor growth and spread of neoplasms, early studies demonstrated the existence of port site metastasis after

laparoscopic colon surgery. Theories for this include aerosolization of neoplastic cells in the peritoneum, direct implantation of cells during removal of specimens, and local trauma from the procedure resulting in hematogenous spread. However, the Clinical Outcomes of Surgical Therapy (COST) study, published in 2003, demonstrated that "in experienced hands, laparoscopic and open colectomy were equivalent techniques with no oncologic disadvantage to patients."

**ANSWER:** C

7. Which of the following patients would not be an appropriate candidate for diagnostic esophagogastroduodenoscopy (EGD)?

   A. A 30-year-old man with a 6-year history of heartburn and regurgitation poorly controlled with antacids

   B. An 80-year-old man with a history of peptic ulcer disease who has an acute onset of severe epigastric pain and tenderness, leukocytosis, and tachycardia

   C. A 45-year-old woman with hematemesis following a bout of violent emesis

   D. A 57-year-old man with worsening dysphagia and odynophagia

   E. A 45-year-old woman with a 2-year history of Barrett's esophagus without evidence of dysplasia

*Ref.:* 5

**COMMENTS:** EGD is generally indicated when its results will cause a change in management. Common indications include, but are not limited to the evaluation of gastroesophageal reflux disease, dysphagia/odynophagia, and upper gastrointestinal bleeding, as well as surveillance of premalignant conditions such as Barrett's esophagus. EGD is not generally recommended for the evaluation of symptoms that are considered functional and is specifically contraindicated in patients with a known or suspected visceral perforation.

**ANSWER:** B

8. Which of the following conditions represents a contraindication to advanced laparoscopic operations?

   A. Pregnancy

   B. Morbid obesity

   C. Contraindication to general anesthesia

   D. Previous laparotomy

   E. Cirrhosis

*Ref.:* 1

**COMMENTS:** The indications for laparoscopic surgery are generally the same as those for open surgery, but several factors may complicate or increase the difficulty associated with laparoscopic surgery. High-risk (American Society of Anesthesiologists [ASA] class IV) patients are not ideal candidates for laparoscopic surgery because of the prerequisite for establishing pneumoperitoneum. Gasless laparoscopy with regional anesthesia has been used in the past to avoid the use of gas insufflation. Yet high-risk patients may not tolerate the increased intraabdominal pressure required for adequate visualization. Morbid obesity, previous abdominal surgery, and pregnancy are no longer considered contraindications to laparoscopy; however, these patients are at high risk for the development of complications of surgery and anesthesia, so adequate preoperative preparation is essential. Morbidly obese patients may be difficult to intubate and might require large doses of muscle relaxants. Proper positioning is paramount to prevent nerve injuries. Selecting an appropriate access point for establishing pneumoperitoneum is important in those who have previously undergone laparotomy. Ultrasound imaging of the abdominal wall (visceral sliding technique) and selection of the left upper quadrant as a point of entry (Palmer's point) are useful techniques. These considerations are important in pregnant patients to maintain adequate fetal blood flow and prevent uterine injury. Although it increases the likelihood of complications, early cirrhosis with preserved hepatic synthetic function is no longer considered an absolute contraindication to laparoscopy.

**ANSWER: C**

9. Which of the following are appropriate techniques for endoscope insertion during EGD?

   A. Direct vision

   B. Blind tip manipulation and patient swallowing

   C. Digital manipulation of the endoscope in the posterior pharynx

   D. All of the above

   E. None of the above

*Ref.: 5*

**COMMENTS:** Advancement of the endoscope beyond the cricopharyngeus muscle and into the esophagus is a challenging part of the EGD examination. Several techniques exist to accomplish this, and it is important for endoscopists to be familiar with all of them. The safest method is to pass the scope into the esophagus under direct vision. In responsive patients capable of swallowing, the shaft of the endoscope can be held over the tongue and advanced slowly as the patient swallows. Finally, in an unconscious patient, the fingers may be placed in the mouth posterior to the tongue and used to keep the endoscope in the midline and guide the tip into the esophagus.

**ANSWER: D**

10. Which of the following is not an appropriate technique for initial trocar placement during laparoscopic surgery?

    A. Veress needle insufflation followed by blind trocar placement

    B. Open placement of a Hasson cannula without pneumoperitoneum

    C. Optical trocar placement

    D. Blind trocar placement without pneumoperitoneum

    E. All of the above are acceptable

*Ref.: 2*

**COMMENTS:** Initial intraperitoneal access for laparoscopic surgery may be obtained with a number of open or closed approaches. One standard closed method involves inserting a Veress needle to achieve insufflation, most commonly at the umbilicus or in the left upper quadrant, followed by blind trocar placement. Another closed technique involves using an optical trocar to visualize the abdominal wall layers during insertion. Open access techniques use a cutdown and open the fascia and peritoneum under direct vision. A blunt Hasson trocar is then placed and secured with a conical sleeve before peritoneal insufflation. Blind trocar placement alone is not a recommended technique for abdominal access. Aside from this, with appropriate training and good surgical judgment, all of the remaining methods listed can be used safely.

**ANSWER: D**

11. Following insertion of a Veress needle, what is the initial maneuver to confirm intraperitoneal placement?

    A. Saline drop test

    B. Aspiration of the needle

    C. Flushing the needle

    D. Measuring insufflation pressure

    E. Starting high-flow insufflation

*Ref.: 6*

**COMMENTS:** When using the Veress needle technique, free entry of the needle into the peritoneal cavity must be confirmed before beginning insufflation. Usually, two audible clicks are heard as the needle traverses the fascia and peritoneum. Following suspected entry, the needle is aspirated to ensure that no blood, urine, or intestinal contents are returned. Subsequently, a saline drop test is confirmatory of intraperitoneal needle placement when saline in the needle hub flows freely through the needle. Insufflation should be initiated only after confirmation of needle position. Low insufflation pressure should also be confirmed at this time.

**ANSWER: B**

12. Select the most appropriate site for initial trocar placement in a patient undergoing laparoscopic Nissen fundoplication with a previous midline scar from the xiphoid to the pubis:

    A. Umbilical

    B. Suprapubic

    C. Left upper quadrant

    D. Left lower quadrant

    E. Right upper quadrant

*Ref.: 2*

**COMMENTS:** The most appropriate site for placement of the initial trocar for a laparoscopic operation depends on several factors, including the procedure to be performed, the size and shape of the patient, the location of previous incisions, and the presence of organomegaly, hernias, or masses. Frequently, the umbilicus will be the site of choice, but alternative, nonmidline sites may be used in patients with previous abdominal surgery. The area of previous incisions should be avoided, and the chosen site should be lateral to the rectus muscle to avoid the major abdominal wall vessels.

The peritoneum is tented up along the costal margins to provide a good alternative access point. Performance of laparoscopic Nissen fundoplication requires a trocar in the left subcostal position, thus making this the best choice for this patient.

**ANSWER:** C

---

13. Thirty minutes into a laparoscopic procedure, visualization becomes inadequate to proceed. The insufflation monitor shows an intra-abdominal pressure of 20 mm Hg and no flow of $CO_2$. What is the most likely explanation?

   A. An empty $CO_2$ canister

   B. $CO_2$ leak from the abdominal wall

   C. Inadequate muscle relaxation

   D. Improper insufflator settings

   E. Dislodged insufflation tubing

   *Ref.:* 2

**COMMENTS:** When visualization inexplicably deteriorates during a laparoscopic procedure, the cause is most often inadvertent loss of the pneumoperitoneum that has been maintaining the operative exposure. This may occur for several reasons, but in this case, intra-abdominal pressure is high with no gas flow in the presence of decreased pneumoperitoneum. This scenario is most commonly caused by abdominal muscle contraction because of inadequate paralysis, but occlusion of the insufflation tubing could produce similar findings. Peritoneal gas leaks via trocar sites or through a trocar may produce impaired visualization, but this will be manifested as low pressure and a high gas flow rate.

**ANSWER:** C

---

14. Shortly following $CO_2$ insufflation, the heart rate of an otherwise healthy 50-year-old woman undergoing laparoscopic cholecystectomy decreases to 40 beats/min. What is the most likely cause of her bradycardia?

   A. Gas embolism

   B. Unrecognized hemorrhage

   C. $CO_2$ pneumoperitoneum

   D. Anesthetic drugs

   E. Capnothorax

   *Ref.:* 2

**COMMENTS:** Cardiac arrhythmias are not uncommon during laparoscopic surgery and occur in up to 25% of patients. The most frequent insufflation-associated arrhythmia is sinus bradycardia, although tachycardia and premature ventricular contractions may also occur. Bradycardia has been attributed to the vasovagal effect of stretching the peritoneum during insufflation; therefore, gradual insufflation at a low flow rate is advisable to avoid this complication.

**ANSWER:** C

---

15. During laparoscopic paraesophageal hernia repair, the patient's end-tidal $CO_2$ increases to 48 mm Hg and airway pressure rises. The patient's blood pressure and heart rate are stable. What is the most appropriate treatment at this time?

   A. Place a chest tube for capnothorax.

   B. Increase minute ventilation.

   C. Convert to an open operation.

   D. Immediately desufflate the abdomen.

   E. Proceed with the intervention.

   *Ref.:* 2

**COMMENTS:** $CO_2$ diffuses across the peritoneum into the venous circulation, where it is carried to the lungs for alveolar elimination. Hypercapnia may result, and an increase in expired $CO_2$ is typical. The mechanical effects of pneumoperitoneum increase diaphragmatic excursion and airway pressure and can be anticipated in any laparoscopic procedure. A 15% increase in minute ventilation is usually required to compensate for these effects, even in healthy patients. Some patients with severe cardiopulmonary impairment may present with severe hypercapnia that cannot be controlled in this manner and may require conversion to an open procedure. Immediate release of the pneumoperitoneum should be the surgeon's first maneuver when acute hemodynamic instability develops during the course of a laparoscopic procedure.

**ANSWER:** B

---

16. Which of the following is not a potential advantage of robotic systems versus standard laparoscopy?

   A. Improved ergonomics

   B. Reduced operative times

   C. Increased manual dexterity

   D. Reduced fatigue of assistants

   E. Elimination of tremor

   *Ref.:* 7

**COMMENTS:** Although laparoscopy has revolutionized the performance of many operations, technical problems have limited the dissemination of this technology to all areas of surgery. Such problems include the rigidity and finite movement of laparoscopic instruments, amplification of natural tremor, the need for surgeons to stand in ergonomically awkward positions for prolonged periods during complex procedures, and fatigue in camera holders and assistants during lengthy operations. Surgical robots have been developed to address some of these limitations. Robotic systems allow automated camera holding and retraction and limit the demands on assistants while allowing the surgeon to maintain a comfortable sitting position throughout the procedure. In addition, the robotic arms provide seven degrees of freedom, thus mimicking the mobility of the human wrist. However, most robotic procedures have been shown to take longer than their laparoscopic or open counterparts, mostly because of the time required to set the robot up. Moreover, the robotic arms are not attached to the operating table, and any change in patient position requires removal of the robotic arms from the patient and replacement after positioning. Currently, these systems are also limited by their large size and high cost.

**ANSWER:** B

**17.** In the United States, performance of human natural-orifice transluminal endoscopic surgery (NOTES) procedures requires which of the following according to the Natural Orifice Surgery Consortium for Assessment and Research (NOSCAR)?

A.  Informed consent

B.  Institutional Review Board (IRB)-approved research protocol

C.  Use of laparoscopy to confirm hemostasis and security of luminal closure

D.  Inclusion of cases in a national NOTES registry

E.  All of the above

*Ref.:* 8

**COMMENTS:** Since 2005, rapid development of NOTES has occurred primarily in acute animal survival models, but diagnostic transgastric peritoneoscopy and transgastric and transvaginal cholecystectomy have been successfully performed in human patients. NOSCAR was developed to guide the research, development, and clinical application of these technologies. Because these procedures all remain experimental at present, NOTES must be performed in the United States under an IRB-approved protocol with laparoscopic confirmation of hemostasis and secure luminal closure. NOSCAR has also requested that all cases be recorded in a national registry to facilitate data collection regarding their safety and efficacy.

**ANSWER:** E

## REFERENCES

1. Jamal MK, Scott-Connor CH: Patient selection and practical considerations in laparoscopic surgery. In Soper NJ, Swanstrom LL, Eubanks WS, editors: *Mastery of endoscopic and laparoscopic surgery*, ed 3, Philadelphia, 2009, Lippincott Williams & Wilkins.
2. Fingerhut A, Millat B, Borie F: Prevention of complications in laparoscopic surgery. In Soper NJ, Swanstrom LL, Eubanks WS, editors: *Mastery of endoscopic and laparoscopic surgery*, ed 2, Philadelphia, 2005, Lippincott Williams & Wilkins.
3. Are C, Raman S, Talamini M: Physiologic consequences of laparoscopic surgery. In Soper NJ, Swanstrom LL, Eubanks WS, editors: *Mastery of endoscopic and laparoscopic surgery*, ed 2, Philadelphia, 2005, Lippincott Williams & Wilkins.
4. Nagle D: Laparoscopic Colon surgery. In Cameron JL, editor: *Current surgical therapy*, ed 9, Philadelphia, 2008, CV Mosby.
5. Gupta N, MacFayden BV: Diagnostic upper gastrointestinal endoscopy. In Soper NJ, Swanstrom LL, Eubanks WS, editors: *Mastery of endoscopic and laparoscopic surgery*, ed 2, Philadelphia, 2005, Lippincott Williams & Wilkins.
6. Kaban GK, Czerniach DR, Novitsky YW, et al: Special access techniques in laparoscopic surgery. In Soper NJ, Swanstrom LL, Eubanks WS, editors: *Mastery of endoscopic and laparoscopic surgery*, ed 2, Philadelphia, 2005, Lippincott Williams & Wilkins.
7. Gould JC, Melvin WS: Surgical robotics. In Soper NJ, Swanstrom LL, Eubanks WS, editors: *Mastery of endoscopic and laparoscopic surgery*, ed 3, Philadelphia, 2009, Lippincott Williams & Wilkins.
8. Swanstrom LL, Soper NJ: New developments in surgical endoscopy: natural orifice transluminal endoscopic surgery. In Soper NJ, Swanstrom LL, Eubanks WS, editors: *Mastery of endoscopic and laparoscopic surgery*, ed 3, Philadelphia, 2009, Lippincott Williams & Wilkins.

# Practice of Surgery

# CHAPTER 36

# Special Considerations in Surgery: Pregnant, Geriatric, and Immunocompromised Patients

*Michelle A. Kominiarek, M.D., and Edward F. Hollinger M.D., Ph.D.*

1. A 22-year-old woman who is 8 weeks pregnant arrives at the emergency department with persistent nausea and vomiting. She has not been able to tolerate any liquids for the past 3 days. On physical examination, she is afebrile, her pulse is 110 beats/min, and her blood pressure is 120/70 mm Hg. Her abdomen is soft, nontender, and nondistended. Moderate ketones are found on urinalysis. The next step in her evaluation includes:

A. Intravenous hydration

B. Liver function tests

C. Right upper quadrant ultrasound

D. Parenteral nutrition

E. Abdominal computed tomography (CT)

*Ref.: 1-3*

**COMMENTS:** See Question 3.

**ANSWER:** A

2. The differential diagnosis of nausea and vomiting in pregnancy includes all of the following except:

A. Appendicitis

B. Pyelonephritis

C. Diabetic ketoacidosis

D. Drug toxicity

E. Renal insufficiency

*Ref.: 1-3*

**COMMENTS:** See Question 3.

**ANSWER:** E

3. Treatment regimens for nausea and vomiting in pregnancy include:

A. Vitamin $B_6$

B. Acupuncture

C. Ginger root

D. Dopamine antagonists

E. All of the above

*Ref.: 2, 3*

**COMMENTS:** Approximately 70% to 85% of pregnant women experience nausea and vomiting of varying intensity and for various lengths of time in pregnancy. Symptoms usually start 5 to 6 weeks after the last menstrual period. The severity and frequency of symptoms generally peak at approximately 9 weeks and then begin to subside. The diagnosis of **nausea and vomiting of pregnancy** (NVP) can be difficult to make in early pregnancy because many other conditions can cause nausea and vomiting. An important distinguishing feature of NVP is that it usually begins before 10 weeks' gestation. Nausea and vomiting that begin after 10 weeks are most likely caused by a different etiology. The differential diagnosis includes gastroenteritis, gastroparesis, achalasia, biliary tract disease, hepatitis, intestinal obstruction, peptic ulcer disease, pancreatitis, and appendicitis. Mildly elevated liver enzymes (usually <300 U/L) and serum bilirubin (<4 mg/dL) are encountered in 20% to 30% of pregnant women. Similarly, serum concentrations of amylase and lipase (up to five times higher than normal levels) are seen in 10% to 15%.

The first-line treatment of NVP consists of conservative measures (dietary modifications and vitamin supplementation) along with patient reassurance. Medications effective in reducing nausea and vomiting without an increased risk for teratogenicity include antihistamines, hydroxyzine, meclizine, dopamine antagonists (chlorpromazine, metoclopramide, perphenazine, prochlorperazine, promethazine, trifluoperazine, trimethobenzamide), and pyridoxine. Patients with severe dehydration should be admitted to the hospital and treated with isotonic crystalloid solutions that contain glucose and supplemental potassium chloride.

**ANSWER:** E

4. A surgical consultation is requested on a patient who had undergone a cesarean delivery 5 days earlier. At the bedside, the Pfannenstiel incision shows separated skin and subcutaneous tissue with an intact fascia. There are no signs of infection and the probable diagnosis is a seroma. The next step in management is:

A. Open the fascia.

B. Close the wound with interrupted sutures immediately.

C. Arrange for vacuum-assisted closure.

D. Instruct the patient on wet-to-dry dressing changes with iodine solution.

E. Débride the fascia and subcutaneous tissues.

*Ref.:* 4

COMMENT: In the United States, more than 30% of all deliveries are by cesarean section. Disruption of the skin incision is a major source of postoperative morbidity after cesarean delivery and occurs after 2.5% to 16% of procedures. **Pfannenstiel incisions** are the most common transverse incisions used in obstetrics and gynecology. **Hematomas** and **seromas**, common problems after cesarean delivery, require manual opening of the wounds to allow drainage and proper healing. An open wound can be managed in three ways: secondary closure, secondary intention with serial dressing changes, and secondary intention using negative pressure wound therapy. **Secondary closure** can be performed once a wound is free of infection or necrotic tissue and has started to granulate. This procedure, which may be performed at the bedside with the patient under local anesthesia or sedation (or both), is done within 1 to 4 days after the wound separates or the hematoma or seroma is evacuated. **Negative pressure wound therapy**, also known as vacuum-assisted closure, received U.S. Food and Drug Administration approval in 1995. In this system, controlled levels of negative pressure help accelerate wound healing by evacuating localized edema. Negative pressure treatment results in faster healing times with fewer associated complications and can be used for noninfected wounds. If **a wet-to-dry approach** is used, the solution should be nontoxic inasmuch as studies have shown that povidone-iodine, iodophor gauze, and hydrogen peroxide are cytotoxic to white blood cells (WBCs) and other vital wound-healing components. Use of these products can delay wound healing.

ANSWER: C

5. Risk factors for impaired wound healing after cesarean delivery include all of the following except:

A. Obesity

B. Diabetes

C. Chorioamnionitis

D. Prolonged rupture of membranes

E. Preterm labor

*Ref.:* 4-6

COMMENT: Risk factors for **wound breakdown** after cesarean section include prolonged duration of surgery, obesity, diabetes, patient age, coincident infection, and poor nutrition. **Obesity** increases risk, probably as a result of the poor vascularity of subcutaneous fat and the propensity for serous fluid collections and hematoma formation. Suture closure of subcutaneous fat during cesarean delivery results in a 34% decrease in the risk for wound disruption in women with fat thickness greater than 2 cm. Other methods (antibiotic solutions, subcutaneous drains) have not been shown to be effective in preventing wound complications. The explanation for the difference in **diabetic wound healing** is complex but is probably related to alterations in the inflammatory response and differences in enzyme secretion and growth factor production. Recommendations to improve wound healing in diabetics are to avoid hyperglycemia and regulate insulin doses. **Corticosteroids** increase the risk for infection by suppressing inflammation, inhibiting leukocyte function, slowing wound contraction, decreasing collagen matrix deposition, and delaying epithelialization. **Chorioamnionitis** is an infection of the membranes (chorion, amnion) surrounding the fetus. The presence of chorioamnionitis increases the risk for wound infection tenfold. Preterm labor is not a risk factor for impaired wound healing.

ANSWER: E

6. A 32-year-old gravida 4 who is 29 weeks pregnant reports left leg pain and swelling for 3 days. A diagnosis of deep venous thrombosis (DVT) is suspected. The most appropriate test to diagnose DVT during pregnancy is:

A. D dimer

B. Contrast-enhanced venography

C. Impedance plethysmography

D. Compression duplex ultrasound

E. Spiral CT of the chest

*Ref.:* 7

COMMENT: There is a predisposition for **deep venous thrombosis** to occur in the left leg (approximately 70% to 90% of cases). This is probably attributed to an exacerbation of the compressive effects of the uterus on the left iliac vein because of it being crossed by the right iliac artery. Clinical suspicion is critical for the diagnosis of DVT. However, many of the classic signs and symptoms of DVT and pulmonary embolism, such as leg swelling, tachycardia, tachypnea, and dyspnea, may be associated with a normal pregnancy. In nonpregnant patients, **D-dimer levels** have high negative predictive value and can reliably exclude the diagnosis of DVT. However, in pregnancy, the D-dimer level gradually increases, and therefore its value is not reliable in the evaluation of DVT. **Contrast-enhanced venography** should not be used in pregnant patients because it is invasive and involves a high radiation dose. Although **impedance plethysmography** has been evaluated in pregnancy and has proven accuracy in excluding DVT, it has been replaced by **duplex ultrasound** because of its higher sensitivity and specificity and wider availability.

ANSWER: D

7. Venous thromboembolism occurs four times more often in pregnant patients than in the general population. Physiologic changes that occur during pregnancy include:

A. Decreased fibrin generation

B. Increased fibrinolytic activity

C. Increased levels of coagulation factors II, VII, VIII, and X

D. Increased free protein S levels

E. Improved venous flow velocity

*Ref.:* 8

**COMMENT:** Pregnancy is classically believed to be a **hypercoagulable state**. Fibrin production is increased; fibrinolytic activity is decreased; levels of coagulation factors II, VII, VIII, and X are all increased; free protein S levels are decreased; and acquired resistance to activated protein C is common. These physiologic changes, including increased markers of coagulation activation such as prothrombin fragment and D dimer, occur in all pregnancies. In addition, a 50% reduction in venous flow velocity occurs in the legs by 25 to 29 weeks of gestation and lasts until approximately 6 weeks after delivery.

**ANSWER:** C

8. The best treatment of acute venous thromboembolism in pregnancy is:

    A. Warfarin

    B. Low-molecular-weight heparin

    C. Unfractionated heparin bridge to a therapeutic international normalized ratio with warfarin

    D. Aspirin

    E. Vena cava filter

*Ref.:* 8

**COMMENT:** Treatment and prophylaxis of **DVT** in pregnancy center on the use of unfractionated heparin or low-molecular-weight heparin because of the teratogenicity associated with **warfarin**, which is known to cross the placenta. **Warfarin-induced embryopathy** is characterized by fetal midface hypoplasia, stippled chondral calcifications, scoliosis, short proximal limbs, and short phalanges. It occurs in 5% of fetuses exposed to the drug between 6 and 9 weeks of gestation. Because neither **unfractionated heparin** nor **low-molecular-weight heparin** crosses the placenta in a significant amount, there is no possibility of teratogenesis or fetal hemorrhage with these medications. The use of retrievable **vena cava filters** should be considered only for patients in whom anticoagulation is contraindicated or in whom extensive DVT develops 2 weeks before delivery.

**ANSWER:** B

9. Appendiceal perforation is more common in pregnant patients. What percentage of pregnant patients with appendicitis are initially seen with perforation?

    A. 5%

    B. 15%

    C. 25%

    D. 35%

    E. 55%

*Ref.:* 9

**COMMENT:** **Appendicitis** is the most common nonobstetric cause of acute abdominal pain leading to exploratory laparotomy. It occurs in 1 in 1500 deliveries. **Urinary tract problems** are often the initial diagnosis because up to 20% of pregnant patients with appendicitis have pyuria, hematuria, or both. If a perforation or peritonitis occurs, the **fetal loss rate** is 10% to 35% because of preterm labor and fetal demise. Preterm labor usually occurs within

5 days of the perforation. **Delayed diagnosis** is more likely to occur in the second (18%) and third (75%) trimesters. **Perforation rates** as high as 55% in pregnant patients have been reported, as opposed to 4% to 19% in the general population.

**ANSWER:** E

10. The imaging modality of choice for pregnant patients suspected to have appendicitis is:

    A. Obstructive series

    B. Right lower quadrant ultrasound

    C. Abdominal and pelvic CT with oral and intravenous contrast enhancement

    D. Magnetic resonance imaging (MRI)

    E. Lower gastrointestinal series (barium enema)

*Ref.:* 9-12

**COMMENT:** **Ultrasonography** with a graded compression technique is the imaging modality of choice in pregnant patients with right lower quadrant pain because of its availability and lack of ionizing radiation. This approach has some limitations. **Graded compression ultrasound** may not be feasible because of the size of the enlarged gravid uterus, particularly in the third trimester. Furthermore, a normal appendix is visualized in only 13% to 50% of patients who are not pregnant. The negative predictive value of a nonvisualized appendix is, at best, 90%. Consequently, if the appendix is not visualized and no other cause of the pain can be found, further evaluation is warranted. **Computed tomography**, which is often the modality of choice in the evaluation of acute appendicitis in patients who are not pregnant, delivers an estimated radiation dose as high as 30 mGy (3 rad) to the uterus with conventional protocols. A **barium enema** is also associated with significant radiation exposure and has generally been supplanted by other imaging tests for the evaluation of acute appendicitis. MRI has not been found to be safe during pregnancy.

**ANSWER:** B

11. Which of the following is true with respect to the management of appendicitis in pregnancy?

    A. An appendectomy during pregnancy increases the risk for congenital malformations and stillbirth.

    B. Fetal mortality can approach 35% for a ruptured appendix.

    C. Negative laparotomy rates of 50% are considered acceptable in the pregnant population.

    D. To decrease the risk for congenital malformations, antibiotics should not be given.

    E. Laparoscopic appendectomy is contraindicated during pregnancy.

*Ref.:* 1, 9, 10

**COMMENT:** In pregnancy, an elevated leukocyte count is normal (9 to $15 \times 10^3$ cells/mm$^3$). In most cases, there is a gradual upward displacement of the appendix as the pregnancy progresses; however, some more recent studies suggest that there is no change in the location of the appendix during pregnancy. Hemoglobin levels decrease during a pregnancy, and hematuria is not a normal finding in a pregnant patient. An appendectomy does not increase the risk for stillbirth or congenital malformations. A higher negative laparotomy rate (up to 35%) is acceptable in the pregnant population (15% for the nonpregnant population) because of the serious consequences of delayed diagnosis. Perioperative antibiotics are appropriate in the pregnant population but should be tailored to the use of antibiotics with minimal risk for birth defects. A laparoscopic approach during pregnancy is appropriate in most gestations of less than 24 weeks.

**ANSWER: B**

12. A 39-year-old gravida 3 para 2 at 32 weeks' gestation is evaluated for a 3-day history of nausea, vomiting, and anorexia. She also reports abdominal pain, primarily located in the right upper quadrant and epigastric areas. Her blood pressure is 120/60 mm Hg with a pulse of 110 beats/min and a temperature of 98.6° F. After completing the physical examination, the diagnosis of cholelithiasis is entertained. Which of the following conditions must also be considered in the differential diagnosis?

A. Acute fatty liver of pregnancy (AFLP)

B. Syndrome of hemolysis, elevated liver enzymes, and low platelets (HELLP)

C. Appendicitis

D. Pyelonephritis

E. All of the above

*Ref.:* 1, 9, 13

**COMMENTS:** See Question 14.

**ANSWER: E**

13. The patient's pain improves with nonoperative management, including intravenous hydration, bowel rest, and analgesics. Her liver function tests, amylase, and lipase are normal. A right upper quadrant ultrasound confirms cholelithiasis without evidence of cholecystitis or obstruction. Select the safest plan for her management:

A. Immediate laparoscopic cholecystectomy

B. Endoscopic retrograde cholangiopancreatography (ERCP)

C. Plan for postpartum cholecystectomy

D. Induction of labor

E. Continuation of antibiotic prophylaxis until delivery

*Ref.:* 1, 9, 13

**COMMENTS:** See Question 14.

**ANSWER: C**

14. During pregnancy, when is the optimal time to perform abdominal operations?

A. 5 to 9 weeks

B. 10 to 13 weeks

C. 15 to 18 weeks

D. 26 to 28 weeks

E. After 32 weeks

*Ref.:* 1, 9, 13

**COMMENT: Biliary tract diseases** are the second most common gastrointestinal disorders that require surgery during pregnancy. Pregnancy predisposes to gallstone formation because of increased bile lithogenicity and decreased gallbladder contractility caused by the effects of progesterone. Gallstones occur in approximately 3% to 12% of pregnant women, but most patients are asymptomatic. The incidence of **acute cholecystitis** is 1 to 8 per 10,000 pregnancies. Early surgery is recommended to avoid biliary complications because recurrent symptoms are common during pregnancy. **Cholecystectomy** should be deferred until the second trimester whenever possible. The rationale behind this recommendation is an increased rate of fetal loss with surgery in the first trimester and a greater risk for preterm labor during the third trimester. When symptoms are mild or the patient is in the third trimester, cholecystectomy can often be delayed until after delivery. An operation may need to be performed early for patients with gallstone pancreatitis, choledocholithiasis, or unresolving acute cholecystitis, regardless of gestational age.

**ANSWER: C**

15. When performing laparoscopic operations in a pregnant patient, which of the following is recommended?

A. Antibiotic prophylaxis with a fluoroquinolone (e.g., levofloxacin)

B. Right lateral decubitus positioning

C. Limiting carbon dioxide pneumoperitoneum to 12 mm Hg for laparoscopy

D. Using an umbilical entry site for laparoscopy for gestational ages beyond 24 weeks

E. Performing open rather than laparoscopic procedures after 24 weeks' gestation

*Ref.:* 1, 9, 13

**COMMENT:** The major general consideration when performing abdominal surgery on a pregnant woman is to maintain adequate perfusion to the uterus and fetus and decreasing maternal risks. To improve venous return, the patient should always be placed in a slight left lateral position. One should also use caution with a Veress needle because the gravid uterus is located closer and closer to the umbilical site with increasing gestational age. Accordingly, one may consider a **left upper quadrant entry** (**Palmer point**) at the midclavicular line 1 to 2 cm below the costal margin, open (Hassan) entry techniques, or placing the trocars under direct visualization. Carbon dioxide pneumoperitoneum should be **limited to 12 mm Hg**. During laparotomy, retractors should not come in contact with the uterus because this could lead to uterine irritability and preterm labor.

**ANSWER: C**

16. A 17-year-old gravida 1 at 25 weeks' gestation is brought to the emergency department after a motor vehicle accident with direct abdominal trauma. She complains of abdominal pain. Initial management should include all of the following except:

A. Establishment of the airway

B. Maintenance of oxygenation

C. Fluid resuscitation

D. Administration of corticosteroids for fetal lung maturity

E. Left lateral displacement of the uterus

*Ref.:* 1

**COMMENT:** Management of a **pregnant trauma patient** parallels that of a nonpregnant patient—the initial evaluation includes establishment of the airway, maintenance of oxygenation, and fluid resuscitation. Because the gravid uterus can compress the inferior vena cava in the supine position in the late second and third trimesters, turning the patient to the left side can displace the uterus and increase cardiac output up to 30%. Although this maneuver contradicts the principle of maintaining the patient in a supine position, spinal stabilization precautions can still be taken. For example, the patient may be transported in the left lateral decubitus position or the backboard rotated to the right. Early and rapid fluid resuscitation is important even in a pregnant patient who is normotensive. Corticosteroids are important for fetal lung maturation in the event of preterm delivery; however, they can be administered after the patient is stabilized.

**ANSWER:** D

17. What is typically the earliest sign of intravascular volume depletion (hypovolemia) in a young pregnant woman?

A. Decreased systolic blood pressure

B. Increased respiratory rate

C. Increased heart rate

D. Decreased heart rate

E. Decreased capillary refill

*Ref.:* 1

**COMMENT: Trauma** complicates approximately 6% to 7% of all pregnancies. Regardless of the injury, resuscitation of the mother with treatment of **hypovolemia and hypoxia** is emphasized during the initial evaluation. Because blood volume expands during pregnancy, a third of the blood volume may be lost without a noticeable change in blood pressure or heart rate. Clinically significant blood loss of up to 2 L, or 30% of the total blood volume, may not be readily apparent. The clinician must be aware of a falsely reassuring hemodynamic state masking ongoing hemorrhage.

**ANSWER:** C

18. Which of the following radiologic examinations poses the greatest radiation exposure to a fetus?

A. Chest radiograph (two views)

B. Abdominal film (single view)

C. CT of the head

D. CT of the abdomen/pelvis

E. CT pelvimetry

*Ref.:* 14, 15

**TABLE 36-1 Estimated Fetal Exposure from Some Common Radiologic Procedures**

| Procedure | Exposure |
|---|---|
| Abdominal film (single view) | 100 mrad |
| Chest radiography (2 views) | 0.02-0.07 mrad |
| Intravenous pyelography | ≥1 rad* |
| Hip film (single view) | 200 mrad |
| Mammography | 7-20 mrad |
| Barium enema or small bowel series | 2-4 rad |
| CT of head or chest | <1 rad |
| CT of abdomen and lumbar spine | 3.5 rad |
| CT pelvimetry | 250 mrad |

*The exposure also depends on the number of films.

**COMMENT:** In pregnancy, the **cumulative radiation dose** should be less than 5 rad; this dose has not been associated with an increase in fetal anomalies or loss of pregnancy (Table 36-1).

**ANSWER:** D

19. A 25-year-old gravida 1 at 37 weeks' gestation is being evaluated for right upper quadrant abdominal pain. On examination, she is found to be afebrile with a blood pressure of 130/70 mm Hg, pulse of 110 beats/min, and respiratory rate of 18 breaths/min. She has scleral icterus. Her laboratory results are as follows:

| Test | Value | Normal Range for Pregnancy |
|---|---|---|
| Hemoglobin | 12 | 10.5-12 g/dL |
| White blood cells | 20,000 | 3200-15,000/mL |
| Platelets | 111,000 | 150,000-350,000/mm³ |
| Prothrombin time | 40 | 12.5 s |
| Blood urea nitrogen | 29 | 7-18 mg/dL |
| Creatinine | 2.8 | 0.6-0.9 mg/dL |
| Aspartate transaminase | 317 | 7-27 |
| Alanine transaminase | 297 | 1-21 |
| Total and direct bilirubin | 7.8/4.6 | <1.0 mg/dL, <0.4 mg/dL |
| Glucose | 48 | 70-110 mg/dL |

The most likely diagnosis in this patient is:

A. AFLP

B. Viral hepatitis

C. Thrombotic thrombocytopenic purpura

D. Hemolytic-uremic syndrome

E. HELLP syndrome

*Ref.:* 16

**COMMENT: Acute fatty liver of pregnancy** is rare (1 in 7000 to 16,000 deliveries). It occurs more commonly in male fetuses and twins. It is related to an autosomally inherited mutation that causes a deficiency of long-chain 3-hydroxyacyl coenzyme A dehydrogenase, a fatty acid β-oxidation enzyme. AFLP is usually manifested in the third trimester as nausea and vomiting, followed by right upper quadrant pain. A 7- to 10-day prodrome of a viral illness is common as well. Hepatomegaly is rare, but other findings include progressive jaundice, malaise, somnolence, and coma. Laboratory abnormalities include liver and renal dysfunction, coagulopathy, increased ammonia, leukocytosis (20,000 to 50,000), hypoglycemia, and pancreatitis. Although the laboratory results may also be consistent with HELLP syndrome, hypoglycemia is one of the distinguishing factors in AFLP. Treatment consists of supportive measures to correct the coagulopathy, electrolyte abnormalities, and hypoglycemia, as well as prompt delivery. Maternal mortality is very low with early diagnosis, appropriate supportive therapy, and early delivery. The fetal mortality rate associated with AFLP is less than 15%.

**A N S W E R :**  A

20. Many unplanned pregnancies occur after bariatric surgery, in part because of improved fertility rates in patients who were infertile before the procedure. Most experts recommend waiting between bariatric surgery procedures and pregnancy. Select the most appropriate time frame:

   A.  2 to 3 months

   B.  6 to 8 months

   C.  12 to 14 months

   D.  18 to 24 months

   E.  >2 years

*Ref.:* 17

**COMMENT:** Most clinicians recommend waiting at least 18 months between **bariatric surgery** and conception. In this case, the fetus is not exposed to a rapid maternal weight loss environment, and the patient can achieve full weight loss goals.

**A N S W E R :**  D

21. The leading cause of maternal morbidity and mortality in the developed world is:

   A.  Postpartum hemorrhage

   B.  Thromboembolism

   C.  Preeclampsia

   D.  Uterine rupture

   E.  Pneumonia

*Ref.:* 18, 19

**COMMENT:**  In 2006, the national **maternal mortality rate** was 13.3 deaths per 100,000 live births. Maternal mortality is defined as the number of maternal deaths (direct and indirect) per 100,000 live births. "Maternal deaths" are defined by the World Health Organization as "the death of a woman while pregnant or within 42 days of termination of pregnancy, irrespective of the duration and the site of the pregnancy, from any cause related to or aggravated by the pregnancy or its management, but not from accidental or incidental causes." Direct obstetric deaths result primarily from thromboembolic events (19.9%), hemorrhage (18.2%), hypertensive disorders of pregnancy (15.9%), and **infectious complications** (13.2%). Indirect obstetric deaths arise from preexisting medical conditions, including diabetes, systemic lupus erythematosus, pulmonary disease, and cardiac disease aggravated by the physiologic changes of pregnancy.

**A N S W E R :**  B

22. A 32-year-old woman in the first trimester of her second pregnancy comes to the emergency department because of epigastric pain, anorexia, vomiting, and low-grade fever. Which of the following findings would be considered normal in a pregnant patient?

   A.  WBC count of 20,500 cells/mm$^3$

   B.  Respiratory rate of 40 breaths/min

   C.  $P_{CO_2}$ of 32 mm Hg on arterial blood gas analysis

   D.  Amylase concentration of 500 U/L

   E.  Serum creatinine level of 1.6 mg/dL.

*Ref.:* 1, 9

**COMMENTS:** During pregnancy, a number of **physiologic changes** occur, such as increases in plasma volume and red blood cell mass. The platelet count is generally normal or slightly decreased, whereas the WBC counts increase from 3000 to 15,000 cells/mm$^3$ in the first trimester to 6000 to 16,000 cells/mm$^3$ during the second and third trimesters. Progesterone and increased $CO_2$ production contribute to the hyperpnea of pregnancy. There is a reduction in arterial $P_{CO_2}$ from the usual 40 mm Hg to 28 to 35 mm Hg and an increase in arterial oxygen tension ($P_{O_2}$) from 60 mm Hg to 100 mm Hg. This facilitates efficient exchange of gases between the mother and fetus. A respiratory alkalosis with compensatory metabolic acidosis is normal in pregnancy. The glomerular filtration rate increases, with a concomitant decrease in normal serum creatinine levels. Serum osmolality is also decreased. Serum amylase values remain normal to slightly elevated during pregnancy. A significant elevation in amylase along with abdominal pain suggests pancreatitis; in pregnancy, the most common causes of pancreatitis are gallstones and hypertriglyceridemia.

**A N S W E R :**  C

23. A 37-year-old gravida 1 at 31 weeks is taken to the emergency department with complaints of midepigastric pain, nausea, and vomiting that began 30 minutes after eating a fatty meal. Her surgical history is significant for a Roux-en-Y gastric bypass 2 years earlier. Her body mass index is currently 32 kg/m$^2$. On examination, the patient's temperature is 39° C and her abdomen is diffusely tender with rebound and guarding. The fetal heart rate was slightly tachycardic (170 beats/min), and the cervix was not dilated. The differential diagnosis should include all of the following except:

   A.  Cholelithiasis

   B.  Chorioamnionitis

   C.  Internal hernia

   D.  Pancreatitis

   E.  Preterm labor

*Ref.:* 1, 9, 17

**COMMENTS:** See Question 24.

**A N S W E R :**  E

24. The patient's amylase and lipase levels are normal. Right upper quadrant ultrasonography shows a normal gallbladder and liver. Her abdominal pain worsens, and she is tachycardic to 130 beats/min. The fetal heart rate also continues to be tachycardic (170 beats/min). What is the next step in management?

A. Laparotomy

B. Cesarean delivery

C. Intravenous methylprednisolone to induce fetal lung maturity

D. Tocolysis to prevent preterm delivery

E. ERCP

*Ref.:* 1, 9

**COMMENTS:** The number of bariatric surgery procedures performed annually has dramatically increased—from 12,480 in 1998 to 113,500 in 2005. More than 80% of these patients are female, and one half of the bariatric procedures in 2004 were performed in women of reproductive age with a mean age of 40 years. Evaluation of abdominal pain in pregnancy is complicated by difficulty in differentiating symptoms of pathology from normal, pregnancy-associated symptoms. The evaluation becomes even more difficult in a pregnant patient who has undergone bariatric surgery. Confusion regarding the cause of symptoms can lead to a critical delay in the diagnosis of **bariatric surgery complications**, including anastomotic leaks, bowel obstruction, internal hernias, ventral hernias, band erosion, and band migration. All gastrointestinal complaints such as nausea, vomiting, and abdominal pain, which occur commonly during pregnancy, should be thoroughly evaluated in a bariatric surgery patient. This patient has an acute abdomen, which is concerning for bowel obstruction or an internal hernia. Although her pregnancy may have an impact on anesthesia and postoperative care, immediate treatment should focus on her abdominal complaints. **Cesarean delivery** is not indicated. Corticosteroids (betamethasone or dexamethasone) are administered to patients between 24 and 34 weeks' gestation if delivery is anticipated within 7 days. They promote fetal lung maturity and decrease the risk for interventricular hemorrhage. Other steroids, such as prednisone or methylprednisolone, do not cross the placenta. The patient is not in labor (the cervix is not dilated), so **tocolytic agents** will not be helpful. **ERCP** can be performed during pregnancy; fluoroscopy should be limited and the fetus should be shielded, but some radiation exposure will occur. ERCP is unlikely to be helpful in this patient.

**ANSWER:** A

25. A 32-year-old woman who is 23 weeks pregnant finds a 1.5-cm firm mass during a breast self-examination. An ultrasound-guided core needle biopsy shows infiltrating ductal carcinoma. Which of the following would be the most appropriate treatment option?

A. Lumpectomy, axillary dissection, and immediate radiation therapy and chemotherapy

B. Lumpectomy, axillary dissection, immediate chemotherapy, and radiation therapy after delivery

C. Lumpectomy, axillary dissection, immediate radiation therapy, and chemotherapy after delivery

D. Immediate radiation therapy and chemotherapy followed by surgery after delivery

E. Termination of the pregnancy followed immediately by treatment of breast cancer

*Ref.:* 1

**COMMENTS:** Breast cancer that is diagnosed during pregnancy or within 1 year after delivery is termed **pregnancy-associated breast cancer**. Breast cancer represents the most common nongynecologic malignancy associated with pregnancy, and it occurs in 0.01% to 0.03% of pregnancies. It has been associated with delayed diagnosis (mean delay of 1 to 2 months). When compared with matched, nonpregnant patients, women with pregnancy-associated breast cancer have a similar stage-related prognosis but overall worse prognosis because on average they have larger primary tumors and a higher risk for lymph node involvement. **Mammography** can be performed with the fetus appropriately shielded; however, the increased density of the fibroglandular breast tissue limits its specificity. **Ultrasound imaging** is useful both for assessing the tumor and for guiding biopsy. Although **MRI** can be used during pregnancy, gadolinium crosses the placenta and may be associated with a risk for fetal abnormalities. As with breast masses in a nonpregnant patient, a tissue diagnosis is imperative. Either core-needle or fine-needle aspiration biopsy may be used. Surgical resection represents the most important component of treatment. Classically, **modified radical mastectomy** was considered the standard therapy. More recent data suggest that patients in whom breast cancer is diagnosed later in pregnancy can be treated with immediate **breast-conserving lumpectomy** and **axillary dissection**, followed by **radiation therapy** after delivery. Axillary dissection rather than sentinel lymph node biopsy has been recommended because of the more aggressive nature of pregnancy-associated breast cancer and because no radioisotope is required. Most **chemotherapeutic regimens** can be administered safely after the first trimester, although changes in plasma volume, protein content, and the volume of distribution associated with chemotherapeutic agents crossing the placenta may complicate dosing. Radiation therapy should be avoided until after delivery because of the risk to the fetus. **Pregnancy termination** to allow the full gamut of therapeutic options for breast cancer is not recommended because it has not been shown to increase patient survival.

**ANSWER:** B

26. A 43-year-old woman is profoundly neutropenic because of intensive chemotherapy for acute myeloid leukemia. She has a temperature of 103.4° F with right lower quadrant pain, guarding, and rebound tenderness, although she remains hemodynamically stable. A kidney, ureter, and bladder film shows an enlarged, fluid-filled cecum with adjacent dilated loops of small bowel. The radiologist suspects that there is some localized pneumatosis in the cecum. What is the most appropriate next step in the management of this patient?

A. Barium enema

B. Colonoscopy

C. Exploratory laparoscopy

D. CT scan of the abdomen

E. Capsule endoscopy

*Ref.:* 20, 21

**COMMENTS:** See Question 27.

**ANSWER:** D

27. Abdominal CT scan in the patient in Question 26 demonstrated marked thickening and edema of the cecum with localized pneumatosis. The appendix is not inflamed. The adjacent small bowel is thickened and mildly dilated. Which of the following would be least appropriate?

A. Rectal tube decompression of the colon

B. Broad-spectrum intravenous antibiotics

C. Administration of granulocyte colony-stimulating factor (G-CSF)

D. Stool evaluation for *Clostridium difficile* toxin

E. Nasogastric decompression of the stomach

*Ref.:* 20, 21

**COMMENTS: Neutropenic enterocolitis** (or **Typhilitis**) is a necrotizing colitis seen in patients with profound neutropenia that often occurs after myelosuppressive chemotherapy. It can also occur in patients with aplastic anemia, human immunodeficiency virus (HIV) infection, and acute leukemia or after immunosuppressive therapy for solid tumors or organ transplants. The pathogenesis appears to include mucosal injury, bacterial translocation, intramural infection, and bowel wall ischemia with eventual necrosis. **Typhilitis** is typically characterized by thickening and edema of the cecum, although the distal ileum and ascending colon may also be involved. Typical symptoms include fever and abdominal pain, usually in the right lower quadrant. Other symptoms may include nausea, vomiting, distention, and watery or bloody diarrhea. Abdominal CT is useful in differentiating typhlitis from other causes of abdominal pain, such as appendicitis, abscess, Ogilvie syndrome, or pseudomembranous colitis. Operative findings include cecal wall thickening with edema or air, a soft tissue mass, hemorrhage, or perforation. Ultrasound imaging can also be used, although it is less specific. Barium enema or colonoscopy should be avoided because of the risk for perforation or additional bacterial translocation.

Prompt surgical intervention is required for patients with peritonitis, free perforation, or persistent gastrointestinal bleeding. If surgery is required, a right hemicolectomy and diversion should be performed, with reanastomosis reserved for a later procedure when the patient has stabilized and the neutropenia has resolved. Treatment of patients who do not meet the criteria for surgery includes bowel rest, nasogastric decompression, intravenous hydration, nutritional support, and broad-spectrum antibiotics. G-CSF can be used to accelerate normalization of the leukocyte count. Anticholinergic, antidiarrheal, and opioid analgesics should be avoided because of their propensity to worsen the ileus. Blood and stool cultures and *C. difficile* toxin assays should be obtained. In patients who do not improve after a short course of antibiotics, antifungal therapy should be added. Rectal tube decompression should be avoided in neutropenic patients because of the risk for mucosal compromise and bacterial translocation.

**ANSWER: A**

28. A 62-year-old woman with long-standing end-stage renal disease who is being maintained on **peritoneal dialysis** (PD) has had several months of intermittent abdominal pain and difficulty obtaining normal dwell volumes for her peritoneal catheter. She goes to the emergency department because she was unable to adequately drain her peritoneal fluid. Review of her medical records reveals that her creatinine level has slowly been increasing for the last several months without any change in her dialysis regimen. Abdominal CT shows ascites; shortened, thickened small bowel mesentery; and diffusely thickened small bowel with areas of luminal narrowing. There are punctuate calcifications throughout the peritoneum. Which of the following is least appropriate?

A. Trial of tamoxifen therapy

B. Oral steroid pulse

C. Replacement of the PD catheter

D. Immunosuppressive therapy with azathioprine

E. Exploratory laparoscopy and enterolysis

*Ref.:* 22, 23

**COMMENTS: Encapsulating peritoneal sclerosis** (**EPS, sclerosing peritonitis**) is one of the most feared complications of **peritoneal dialysis**. EPS is characterized by a decrease in the efficacy of PD and the development of extensive intraperitoneal fibrosis, mesenteric shortening, and encasement of the bowel. It can progress to bowel obstruction. Radiologic features include mesenteric, bowel, and peritoneal thickening, often with calcifications. Loculated ascites, adherent bowel loops, and luminal narrowing of the bowel may also be visualized. The etiology of EPS is not well understood. Risk factors include the duration of PD therapy, episodes of peritonitis, and acetate dialysis. Treatment is often unsuccessful. Most patients with EPS are switched to hemodialysis (although such a switch can sometimes precipitate EPS). Steroid therapy, tamoxifen, and immunosuppressive regimens, including azathioprine or cyclosporine, have all been used to treat EPS. When bowel obstruction is present, total parenteral nutrition may be required. The role of surgical therapy for EPS remains controversial. Early results with enterectomy and anastomosis have shown high mortality, but more recent studies suggest a role for early enterolysis.

**ANSWER: C**

29. A 54-year-old woman with end-stage renal disease treated by PD complains of abdominal pain and fever. When performing her exchanges she has noted turbid fluid for the last several days. She has been undergoing PD for 3 years and has never had any complications. Which of the following statements is correct?

A. She should undergo immediate peritoneal exploration with removal of the dialysis catheter.

B. Fungal peritonitis requires long-term antifungal therapy through the PD catheter.

C. PD-associated peritonitis from coagulase-negative staphylococci can be cured with antibiotics alone in more than 80% of cases.

D. She will need to resume hemodialysis while the infection is treated.

E. Broad-spectrum empirical antibiotic therapy is required because peritoneal fluid cultures have little value.

*Ref.:* 24

**COMMENTS: Peritonitis** is a common complication of **peritoneal dialysis** and occurs about 1.4 times per patient-year of PD. It is one of the most important reasons for failure of PD and accounts for nearly one half of all technical failures. Typically, patients have abdominal pain and tenderness (75%), fever (33%), and cloudy dialysate. The diagnosis is confirmed by a fluid leukocyte count of greater than 100/mL with more than one half of the cells being neutrophils. Most infections are caused by gram-positive organisms, but gram-negative bacilli and fungi can also be responsible. Initial treatment should consist of intraperitoneal antibiotics, most commonly vancomycin or a first-generation cephalosporin. About 75% of infections are cured with culture-directed antibiotic therapy without discontinuation of PD. Persistent or recurrent infection may require removal of the PD catheter and a switch to hemodialysis. Cure rates with antibiotics alone are best for coagulase-negative staphylococci (90%) and less for *Staphylococcus aureus* (66%) or gram-negative bacilli (56%). **Fungal infections** require prompt removal of the catheter. Prompt treatment of peritoneal infections is important to reduce the formation of adhesions and the loss of peritoneal area, which can limit the patient's ability to continue with PD.

**ANSWER: C**

30. A 76-year-old man with cardiac, liver, and renal disease is admitted to the intensive care unit with fever, hypotension, and abdominal distention. An abdominal ultrasound reveals ascites. His serum albumin level is 3.2 g/dL, and the albumin concentration in the ascites fluid is 2.8 g/dL. This serum-ascites albumin gradient (SAAG) is most supportive of which of the following diagnoses?

    A. Cardiac ascites

    B. Cirrhosis

    C. Myxedema

    D. Nephrotic syndrome

    E. Alcoholic hepatitis

    *Ref.:* 24

**COMMENTS:** The most useful tests for characterizing **ascites** are cell counts, differential count, and the total protein and albumin concentrations of the fluid. If the fluid has a high neutrophil concentration, an acute inflammatory process is suggested. The **serum-ascites albumin gradient** provides one of the most useful tools for characterizing the cause of ascites (Box 36-1). SAAG is calculated by subtracting the albumin concentration of the ascites fluid from that of serum. **High-SAAG ascites** (SAAG ≥1.1 g/dL) is associated with portal hypertension. Causes include cirrhosis, alcoholic

---

**BOX 36-1   Classification of Ascites by Serum-Ascites Albumin Gradient**

**High Gradient (≥1.1 g/dL)**

Cirrhosis
Alcoholic hepatitis
Cardiac ascites
Massive liver metastases
Fulminant hepatic failure
Budd-Chiari syndrome
Portal vein thrombosis
Myxedema

**Low Gradient (<1.1 g/dL)**

Peritoneal carcinomatosis
Tuberculous peritonitis
Pancreatic ascites
Biliary ascites
Nephrotic syndrome
Postoperative lymphatic leak
Serositis in connective tissue disease

From Runyon B: Ascites: spontaneous bacterial peritonitis. In Sleisenger MH, Feldman M, Friedman LS, editors: *Sleisenger and Fordtran's gastrointestinal and liver disease: pathophysiology, diagnosis, management,* ed 7, Philadelphia, 2002, WB Saunders, p 1523.

---

or cardiac ascites, liver metastases, fulminant hepatic failure, Budd-Chiari syndrome, myxedema, and portal vein thrombosis. **Low-SAAG ascites** (SAAG <1.1 g/dL) is associated with tuberculous peritonitis, pancreatic or biliary ascites, nephritic syndrome, and lymphatic leaks.

**ANSWER: D**

31. A 64-year-old man with end-stage renal disease is visiting from Mexico. He is evaluated in the emergency department for worsening vague abdominal pain, occasional vomiting, and abdominal swelling. The pain has been present intermittently for several months but has worsened over the last few weeks. He has lost about 30 lb and has no appetite or energy. A purified protein derivative (PPD) skin test is positive, and the patient gives a history of being successfully treated for tuberculosis (TB) several years ago. Ultrasound shows moderate ascites with echogenic material within the fluid. Which of the following tests would be most appropriate to confirm a diagnosis of tuberculous peritonitis?

    A. CT of the abdomen and pelvis

    B. Percutaneous peritoneal biopsy

    C. Microscopic examination of peritoneal fluid

    D. Mycobacterial cultures of peritoneal fluid

    E. Diagnostic laparoscopy and peritoneal biopsy

    *Ref.:* 24, 25

**COMMENTS:** **Tuberculous peritonitis** is most commonly associated with individuals with **acquired immunodeficiency syndrome**; however, it can also occur in the setting of cirrhosis (especially alcoholic) and chronic renal failure. Most cases result from reactivation of latent peritoneal disease in patients with previous pulmonary TB. Typical complaints include abdominal distention from ascites and generalized abdominal discomfort. Constitutional symptoms, including fever, night sweats, anorexia, and malaise, may also be present. Most patients have a positive PPD skin test. In the absence of cirrhosis, the ascites has a **low serum-ascites albumin gradient**, high glucose, high protein, and high fluid WBCs, mainly lymphocytes. Abdominal ultrasound may show echogenic material within the ascites, whereas CT shows a thickened, nodular mesentery, lymphadenopathy, and omental thickening. **Laparoscopic peritoneal biopsy** is diagnostic. Most commonly the peritoneum is studded with multiple small whitish nodules, which on biopsy contain caseating granulomas. Blind peritoneal biopsy has much lower sensitivity than directed biopsy. Microscopic examination of the ascites for acid-fast bacteria is rarely positive, and cultures are relatively insensitive (20%) and require several weeks of incubation. Tuberculous peritonitis can be manifested as a pelvic mass with elevated CA 125, which can lead to an incorrect diagnosis of metastatic ovarian cancer. Treatment consists of 6 to 9 months of antituberculous drugs; regimens typically include rifampin, isoniazid, and pyrazinamide.

**ANSWER: E**

32. A 39-year-old HIV-positive man who is noncompliant with his antiretroviral medications wishes a second opinion because of a worsening condition that started a month earlier with abdominal pain, diarrhea, low-grade fever, and malaise. He has a history of *Pneumocystis carinii* pneumonia. Abdominal CT had shown thickening of the terminal ileum with a small

amount of surrounding fluid. Colonoscopy showed circumferential ulcers and inflamed mucosa; biopsy of the cecum and terminal ileum showed granulomas. Therefore, a diagnosis of Crohn disease was made and the patient was treated with steroids. However, 1 month later his symptoms are worse, and repeated CT shows increased cecal and peritoneal thickening, ascites, and large mesenteric lymph nodes with hypodense centers. Suspecting that the initial diagnosis may have been in error, which of the following conditions is the most likely diagnosis?

A. Crohn disease

B. Cecal carcinoma

C. Tuberculous enteritis

D. Intestinal amebiasis

E. Small bowel lymphoma

*Ref.:* 26, 27

**COMMENTS:** The differential diagnosis for ileocecal thickening or a mass includes **neoplasms** such as lymphoma, sarcoma, and adenocarcinoma; **Crohn disease**; and **infectious causes** such as amebiasis, histoplasmosis, actinomycosis, *Yersinia*, or intestinal TB. Because the symptoms of many of these conditions overlap, a careful diagnostic approach is needed. Commonly, evaluation includes imaging and colonoscopy with biopsy. Many of these conditions may result in ulcers. However, the finding of granulomas on biopsy led to the diagnosis of Crohn disease. Carcinoma or lymphoma biopsy specimens should show malignant cells. A biopsy specimen revealing **intestinal amebiasis** should show trophozoites, and stool studies and serologic evaluation should confirm the diagnosis. **Tuberculous enteritis** can be confused with Crohn disease because both have granulomas, although the granulomas in Crohn disease are infrequent, small, nonconfluent, and noncaseating. Tuberculous granulomas are larger and confluent, often with caseating necrosis. Imaging of TB may show large lymph nodes with characteristic central caseous liquefaction. Many patients will have pulmonary manifestations of previous TB infection, although active disease is often not present. Culture results may take several weeks to become positive, and it is being supplanted by polymerase chain reaction (PCR) testing of biopsy specimens. **Treatment** of intestinal TB consists of antituberculosis drugs, with surgery being reserved for patients with an abscess or fistula, uncontrolled bleeding, perforation, or complete obstruction. Misdiagnosis of TB as Crohn disease is particularly unfortunate because immunosuppressive therapy can result in miliary dissemination.

**ANSWER:** C

33. A 48-year-old man underwent HLA-matched allogeneic bone marrow transplantation for myelofibrosis with myeloid metaplasia. One month after discharge, he returned to the clinic with a 2-week history of anorexia, malaise, low-grade fevers, and difficulty swallowing. His tongue was chalky white. Esophagogastroduodenoscopy revealed white plaques throughout the esophagus, and colonoscopy showed linear, well-demarcated ulcers in the terminal ileum and cecum. He was prescribed oral nystatin and treated for his neutropenia. Two days later severe abdominal pain develops, and CT shows a perforation at the distal ileum. Which of the following is the most likely cause of the ileal perforation?

A. Epstein-Barr virus (EBV)

B. Cytomegalovirus (CMV)

C. Parvovirus

D. *Candida albicans*

E. Herpes simplex virus

*Ref.:* 28, 29

**COMMENTS: Cytomegalovirus** infection can result in serious complications in patients who are immunosuppressed, including patients with HIV infection, organ transplants, or cancer or those receiving immunosuppressive therapy. The most common site of CMV disease is the eye, and **CMV retinitis** can result in blindness. Gastrointestinal involvement can occur anywhere from the mouth to the anus, although the colon is most commonly involved. Clinical symptoms include fever, malaise, anorexia, nausea, diarrhea, abdominal pain, ileus, and bleeding. Endoscopic evaluation shows well-defined, "punched-out" ulcers. Lesions are usually limited to a segment of the gastrointestinal tract, with diffuse involvement being less common. Biopsies usually show mucosal inflammation, tissue necrosis, and vascular endothelial involvement. Visualization of **viral inclusions** by light microscopy remains the standard of diagnosis. CMV typically causes gastritis, enteritis, or colitis, but in rare cares it can result in perforation and significant gastrointestinal bleeding. Viral serology and quantitative PCR may be helpful in diagnosing CMV enteritis, but endoscopy with biopsy remains the gold standard. EBV can be associated with viral syndromes and lymphomas but rarely causes perforation. Parvovirus causes anemia. Invasive *Candida* infections very rarely cause perforation, although this patient did have findings of superficial esophageal candidiasis. **Herpes simplex virus** has cutaneous manifestations and may result in proctitis, but perforation does not usually occur.

**ANSWER:** B

34. Which of the following should not be included in the initial approach to a profoundly neutropenic patient with fever?

A. Skin, mucous membrane, and ophthalmoscopic examination

B. Inspection and cultures from central venous access

C. Digital rectal examination

D. Chest radiograph

E. Initiation of empirical antibiotic therapy

*Ref.:* 30

**COMMENTS:** Determining the cause of a fever in a **neutropenic** patient requires careful attention to detail because signs of infection or inflammation are often subtle or absent in patients with profound neutropenia. The skin, mucous membranes, and ocular fundi should be carefully examined for an infectious source. All access sites, including intravenous and central lines, should be checked for soft tissue infection or thrombophlebitis. Mucous membranes should be examined for signs of viral or fungal infection. All indwelling catheters should be cultured. Laboratory studies should include urine and blood cultures from peripheral sites and all indwelling lines. Stool should be sent for study if there are any changes in bowel habits. Lumbar puncture should be performed in patients who have altered mental status or localizing symptoms. A chest radiograph should be performed; however, the findings may be subtle or absent even with pneumonia. Chest CT may demonstrate evidence of infection not revealed on radiography. Empiric antibiotic therapy should be initiated promptly and modified on the basis of the results of examination, imaging, and culture. Anorectal infection can be very subtle in immunosuppressed patients. Routine digital rectal examination should be avoided because of the risk of provoking bacteremia. However, if prostatitis or a perirectal abscess is suspected, gentle digital rectal examination can be performed after antibiotic therapy is initiated.

**ANSWER:** C

35. Which of the following strategies is least useful for improving surgical outcomes in geriatric patients?

A. Preoperative evaluation of medical physiologic status

B. Optimization of physical and cognitive function

C. Minimization of perioperative nutritional deficiency

D. Postoperative assessment for rehabilitation options

E. Surgical risk assessment based on a specific diagnosis

*Ref.: 31-34*

**COMMENTS:** There are several important factors in achieving positive surgical outcomes in geriatric patients. Assessment of a patient's preoperative physical and cognitive function, along with optimization of these variables, is critical in elderly patients. Ignorance of these variables may result in more aggressive surgical procedures and poor outcomes. As the risks associated with surgical therapy increase, elderly patients may opt for palliative procedures, which allow resumption of preoperative independence and activities of daily life, as opposed to more radical procedures, which entail a prolonged convalescence and questionable quality of life. Elderly patients may be at risk for **malnutrition** because of physical and cognitive disabilities, poverty, and lack of awareness of the importance of a balanced diet. Patients with more than 10% weight loss and serum albumin level less than 2.5 g/dL should be considered to have **protein-energy malnutrition** and may benefit from a minimum of 7 to 10 days of nutritional repletion before surgery. Proper **preoperative rehabilitation planning** has been shown in patients with hip fractures to result in quicker resumption of independent living. Surgical risk assessment is **multifactorial** and **not based on a specific diagnosis**. Physical fitness, cognitive fitness, and social factors (e.g., family and financial support), in addition to a specific diagnosis and surgical plan, are part of a thorough preoperative risk assessment.

**ANSWER:** E

36. Regarding the following several scenarios, which one of the operations can proceed as scheduled?

A. An 80-year-old scheduled for cataract surgery who has a pulse of 60 beats/min and a blood pressure of 180/110 mm Hg and is completely asymptomatic

B. A 67-year-old scheduled for left total hip arthroplasty who has a pulse of 80 beats/min and blood pressure of 180/110 mm Hg, is asymptomatic, and takes β-blockers

C. A 65-year-old hypertensive scheduled for bilateral total knee arthroplasty who has a pulse of 90 beats/min and a blood pressure of 130/70 mm Hg and who takes angiotensin-converting enzyme (ACE) inhibitors

D. An 80-year-old scheduled for bilateral laparoscopic hernia repair who has a pulse of 42 beats/min and a blood pressure of 100/60 mm Hg and who has a pacemaker and takes β-blockers

E. None of the above operations should proceed

*Ref.: 33-35*

**COMMENTS:** Management of **hypertension** in the perioperative period remains controversial. However, several studies have consistently shown that a preoperative diastolic blood pressure higher than 110 mm Hg confers increased risk for major morbidity. Aggressive perioperative normalization may not reduce the risk. However, the patient in scenario A is scheduled for a low-risk operation, unlike the patient in scenario B. Therefore, the operation in scenario A can be performed safely as long as the patient has adequate follow-up. **Angitensin-converting enzyme inhibitors** have been associated with severe perioperative hypotension during major surgery, especially in patients who receive an epidural catheter as part of their management. The patient in scenario D may have a pacemaker malfunction that needs to be evaluated. **β-Blockers** have been shown to decrease intraoperative ischemia and should be continued. **Calcium channel blockers** and **diuretics** may be continued.

**ANSWER:** A

37. Following small bowel resection, a 75-year-old patient is agitated and calling out for his deceased wife. He requires restraints. Which of the following statements is incorrect regarding his condition?

A. Postoperative delirium may occur in up to 15% of patients 70 years or older.

B. Postoperative delirium increases the risk for other complications.

C. Preoperative assessment of cognitive function should be routine in patients older than 75 years for major elective surgery.

D. Postoperative delirium may indicate the onset of another disease process.

E. In geriatric patients, regional anesthesia is associated with a lower incidence of postoperative delirium than general anesthesia is.

*Ref.: 35-37*

**COMMENTS:** **Postoperative delirium** is a common and serious problem in the geriatric population. Delirium occurs in 15% of patients 70 years and older. The risk is greater following **orthopedic procedures**, with rates as high as 60%. Marcantonio identified seven factors to stratify risk for the development of delirium that are useful in deciding who will benefit from perioperative delirium prevention. New-onset postoperative delirium may be caused by multiple factors, including drugs, disease, and depression. Pain and nausea control is essential, as is the avoidance of anticholinergics, antihistamines, and benzodiazepines, according to the Beers criteria. Controversy exists regarding whether the anesthetic technique has an effect on postoperative delirium. However, recent studies indicate no relationship between the severity of postoperative delirium and anesthetic technique.

**ANSWER:** E

**38.** Which of the following is not true when comparing geriatric patients with younger patients?

A. Elderly patients have lower creatinine values.

B. The risk for hypothermia is greater in elderly patients.

C. Fever is a less reliable sign of infection in elderly patients.

D. Colonic pathology is the most common indication for surgery in elderly patients.

E. Cardiac complications are the leading cause of perioperative complications in the elderly.

*Ref.:* 35

**COMMENTS:** When obstetric procedures are excluded, more than 40% of operations are performed in patients older than 65 years. Elderly surgical patients represent a heterogenous group, and **physiologic age** is generally of greater importance than chronologic age. To optimize the care of older patients, it is critical to understand age-related changes in physiology. Because decreased muscle mass occurs with aging, baseline serum **creatinine** levels may decrease in the elderly despite progressive loss of renal function. Geriatric patients are at increased risk for **hypothermia** because of impaired mechanisms of heat conservation, especially during operative procedures. Decreased muscle mass and metabolic heat production, malnutrition, and increased heat loss as a result of thinning skin all contribute to this phenomenon. **Fever** is not a reliable indicator of infection in elderly patients and may be absent in up to one third of patients with serious infections. It is important to evaluate the patient's baseline temperature, with fever being suspected with an elevation in temperature of greater than 2° above baseline. Malnourished geriatric patients or the extremely old are especially unlikely to mount a febrile response to infection. **Biliary tract disease**, including acute cholecystitis, is the most common indication for surgical intervention in elderly patients. This may be related to the increased lithogenicity of bile and increased prevalence of cholelithiasis. **Cardiac complications** are the leading cause of perioperative problems and death in all age groups but are of particular importance in elderly patients because of the prevalence of preexisting cardiac dysfunction and poor functional reserve.

**ANSWER:** D

**39.** Following cholecystectomy, an 82-year-old patient has an oxygen saturation of 88% on 2 L of oxygen by nasal cannula. Which of the following is not a probable explanation for this phenomenon?

A. Maximal breathing capacity is 50% of what the patient had at age 30.

B. The cough mechanism is less effective in elderly patients.

C. The pulse oximetry reading is spurious.

D. The patient was recently repositioned from supine to a sitting position.

E. The patient required conversion from laparoscopic to open cholecystectomy.

*Ref.:* 31, 32, 35

**COMMENTS:** **Pulmonary complications** represent some of the most common adverse events in elderly surgical patients; they account for up to 50% of postoperative complications and 20% of preventable deaths. Decreased strength and endurance of respiratory muscles, decreased lung volumes, and decreased compensatory responses to hypoxia or hypercapnia make tachypnea a less reliable sign of impending respiratory failure. Furthermore, changes in the respiratory system limit the maximal breathing capacity at age 70 to about one half that present at age 30. Decreased airway sensitivity, dysfunctional mucociliary clearance, and decreased muscle strength all contribute to a decreased cough mechanism. **Shivering**, a common postoperative phenomenon, dramatically increases oxygen consumption, which could cause hypoxia. In addition, movement of the patient could result in a spurious pulse oximetry reading. The patient's positioning has a direct effect on ventilation-perfusion mismatch and the alveolar-arterial oxygen gradient. In contrast to sitting, a supine position results in closure of small airways in the dependent portion of the lung. This leads to ventilation-perfusion mismatch and may contribute to hypoxemia. Therefore, placing a patient in a sitting position should improve oxygenation. Unlike laparoscopic cholecystectomy, open cholecystectomy entails an upper abdominal incision, which results in decreased tidal volume, impaired diaphragmatic excursion with resultant hypoxemia, and an increased risk for atelectasis and pneumonia.

**ANSWER:** D

**40.** Which of the following statements regarding age-related changes in the cardiovascular system is not correct?

A. Ventricular contractility decreases.

B. Sympathetic nervous system activity decreases.

C. Mean arterial pressure increases.

D. Left ventricular afterload increases.

E. Myocardial contraction is prolonged.

*Ref.:* 31, 32, 35

**COMMENTS:** Aging is associated with **functional and structural changes** in the heart and blood vessels, as well as alterations in autonomic regulatory mechanisms. The myocardium becomes thicker and stiffer, with reduced conduction fiber density and a decrease in the number of cells within the sinus node. These changes lead to decreased contractility and increased filling pressures. The elastic arteries become larger and stiffer, which results in increased mean arterial pressure and pulse pressure. The larger, stiffer arteries lead to increased pulse wave velocity, which allows earlier reflection of the pulse waves from the peripheral circulation. The reflected waves may reach the heart during end-systole, thereby increasing **cardiac afterload**. Decreased ventricular compliance and increased afterload cause a compensatory prolongation of **myocardial contraction** and decreased early ventricular filling time. Because the ventricle has less time to fill, the contribution of the atrium becomes more significant. Thus, elderly patients are less tolerant of arrhythmias such as atrial fibrillation. The activity of the sympathetic nervous system increases, although decreased receptor affinity and alterations in signal transduction lead to decreased β-receptor responsiveness. This impairs an elderly patient's ability to increase the heart rate and ejection fraction in response to physiologic stress and may contribute to intraoperative hemodynamic lability.

**ANSWER:** B

**41.** A 74-year-old man is admitted for cardiac surgery. His preoperative creatinine level is 1.6 mg/dL. Which of the following statements about renal function in elderly patients is correct?

A. Renal blood flow decreases by 10% to 20% by the age of 80.

B. Loss of renal mass is most pronounced in the renal medulla.

C. Renal capacity to retain sodium is decreased.

D. Urinary tract infections are almost always symptomatic.

E. Bladder distention is common in elderly patients because the bladder becomes more elastic.

*Ref.:* 31-33, 35

**COMMENTS:** Nearly one fourth of all Americans 70 years or older have moderate or severely decreased renal function. With age, there is progressive loss of **renal mass** (up to 30% at 80 years), especially in the renal cortex. **Nephrosclerosis** increases, afferent and efferent arterioles atrophy, and the number of renal tubular cells decreases. **Renal blood flow** decreases by 5% to 10% per decade, with a 50% decrease being common in elderly patients. On average, the **glomerular filtration rate** decreases by 45% by age 80. However, the progressive decline in lean body (muscle) mass may result in **serum creatinine** concentrations remaining constant or even decreasing. Because of a decline in renin-angiotensin axis activity, the kidneys' capacity to conserve **sodium** decreases, thereby leading to a propensity for sodium loss when salt intake is inadequate. There is also a marked decline in the subjective feeling of **thirst** in response to increases in serum osmolarity. The kidneys become less responsive to **antidiuretic hormone**. These changes lead to an increased risk for **dehydration**. Asymptomatic **urinary tract infections** are more common in elderly patients. Urinary tract infections are responsible for 30% to 50% of all cases of bacteremia in older individuals. Increased collagen content causes the bladder to become less distensible. **Prostate hypertrophy** can impair bladder emptying in males, and decreased serum **estrogen** levels and impaired tissue responsiveness to estrogen in females predispose to **incontinence**.

**ANSWER:** C

42. A 77-year-old man is admitted after a radical prostatectomy. On postoperative day 3, a productive cough and fever develop. A chest radiograph shows a right lower lobe infiltrate. Which of the following is correct regarding immune function in older patients?

A. WBC counts increase significantly even with mild infections.

B. The T-cell response to new antigens is impaired.

C. Normal neutrophil counts decline with age.

D. Normal acute phase protein levels are decreased.

E. Normocytic anemia is uncommon in older patients.

*Ref.:* 35

**COMMENTS:** The ability to mount an **immune response** becomes blunted with age, which leads to increased susceptibility to infections and increased **tumorigenesis**. These changes are particularly apparent under physiologic stress. Elderly patients with infections often have normal WBC counts, but the differential will show a profound left shift with many immature cells. Although baseline neutrophil counts remain relatively constant, the ability of the bone marrow to increase neutrophil production when indicated is diminished. Decreased T-cell production by the bone marrow, as well as thymic involution, impairs the production and differentiation of naïve T cells and therefore leads to a weakened response

to new antigens. Chronic infection with viruses such as CMV may also alter T-cell function. **Inflammatory cytokine** levels are persistently elevated, as are levels of **acute phase proteins**. Chronic inflammation is believed to contribute to frailty, including loss of muscle mass, impaired nutrition, and decreased mobility. It may also contribute to the **normocytic anemia** commonly seen in elderly patients.

**ANSWER:** B

**REFERENCES**

1. Mikami DJ, Beery PR, Ellison EC: Surgery in the pregnant patient. In Townsend CM, Beauchamp RD, Evers BM, et al, editors: *Sabiston textbook of surgery: the biological basis of modern surgical practice*, ed 18, Philadelphia, 2008, WB Saunders.
2. Goodwin TM: Hyperemesis gravidarum, *Obstet Gynecol Clin* 35:401–417, 2008.
3. Herbert WNP, Goodwin TM, Koren G, et al: Nausea and vomiting in pregnancy. Association of Professors of Gynecology and Obstetrics Educational Series on Women's Health Issues. 2001.
4. Sarsam SE, Elliott JP, Lam GK: Management of wound complications from cesarean delivery, *Obstet Gynecol Surv* 60:462–473, 2005.
5. Chelmow D, Rodriguez EJ, Sabatini MM: Suture closure of subcutaneous fat and wound disruption after cesarean delivery: a meta-analysis, *Obstet Gynecol* 103:974–980, 2004.
6. Hellums EK, Lin MG, Ramsey PS: Prophylactic subcutaneous drainage for prevention of wound complications after cesarean delivery: a metaanalysis, *Am J Obstet Gynecol* 197:229–235, 2007.
7. Scarsbrook AF, Evans AL, Owen AR, et al: Diagnosis of suspected venous thromboembolic disease in pregnancy, *Clin Radiol* 61:1–12, 2006.
8. Marik PE: Venous thromboembolic disease and pregnancy, *N Engl J Med* 359:2025–2033, 2008.
9. Brooks DC, Oxford C: The pregnant surgical patient. In Ashley SW, editor: *ACS surgery: principles and practice*, Philadelphia, 2010, American College of Surgeons.
10. Pastore PA, Loomis DM, Sauret J: Appendicitis in pregnancy, *J Am Board Fam Med* 19:621–626, 2006.
11. Hodjati H: Location of the appendix in the gravid patient: a re-evaluation of the established concept, *Int J Gynecol Obstet* 81:245–247, 2003.
12. Pedrosa I, Levine D, Eyvazzadeh AD, et al: MR imaging evaluation of acute appendicitis in pregnancy, *Radiology* 238:891–899, 2006.
13. Malangoni MA: Gastrointestinal surgery and pregnancy, *Gastroenterol Clin North Am* 32:181–200, 2003.
14. Cunningham FG, Leveno KJ, Bloom S, et al: General considerations and maternal evaluation. In *Williams Obstetrics*, ed 23, New York, 2010, McGraw-Hill.
15. American College of Obstetrics and Gynecology. Committee Opinion #299, 2004. Guidelines for Diagnostic Imaging During Pregnancy.
16. Cappell MS: Hepatic and gastrointestinal diseases. In Gabbe SM, editor: *Obstetrics: Normal and problem pregnancies*, ed 5, Philadelphis, 2007, Churchill Livingstone.
17. American College Obstetricians and Gynecologists. Practice Bulletin #105, 2009. Bariatric Surgery and Pregnancy.
18. Heron M, Hoyert DL, Murphy SL, et al: Deaths: final data for 2006, *Natl Vital Stat Rep* 57(14):1–134, 2009.
19. Berg CJ, Chang J, Callaghan WM, et al: Pregnancy-Related Mortality in the United States, 1991-1997, *Obstet Gynecol* 101:289–296, 2003.
20. Davila ML: Neutropenic enterocolitis, *Curr Opin Gastroenterol.* 22:44–47, 2006.
21. Madoff LC, Sifri CI: Diverticulitis and typhlitis. In Mandell GL, Bennett JE, Dolin R, editors: *Mandell, Douglas, and Bennett's principles and practice of infectious diseases*, ed 7, Philadelphia, 2010, Churchill Livingstone.
22. Blake PG, Sharma A: Peritoneal dialysis. In Brenner BM, editor: *Brenner & Rector's the kidney*, ed 8, Philadelphia, 2008, WB Saunders.
23. Kawaguchi Y, Tranaeus A: A historical review of encapsulating peritoneal sclerosis, *Perit Dial Int* 25(S4):S7–13, 2005.
24. Li BD, McDonald JC, Richardson KA, et al: Abdominal wall, umbilicus, peritoneum, mesenteries, omentum, and retroperitoneum. In Townsend CM, Beauchamp RD, Evers BM, et al, editor: *Sabiston*

*textbook of surgery: the biological basis of modern surgical practice*, ed 18, Philadelphia, 2008, WB Saunders.

25. Fisher DR, Matthews JB: Surgical peritonitis and other diseases of the peritoneum, mesentery, omentum, and diaphragm. In Feldman M, Friedman LS, Brandt LJ, editors: *Sleisenger & Fordtran's gastrointestinal and liver disease*, ed 8, Philadelphia, 2006, WB Saunders.

26. Hassan I, Brilakis ES, Thompson RL, et al: Surgical management of abdominal tuberculosis, *J Gastrointest Surg* 6:862–867, 2002.

27. Hovarth KD, Whelan RL: Intestinal tuberculosis: return of an old disease, *Am J Gastroenterol* 93:692–696, 1998.

28. Kram HB, Shoemaker WC: Intestinal perforation due to cytomegalovirus infection in patients with AIDS, *Dis Colon Rectum* 33:1037–1040, 1990.

29. Keates J, Lagahee S, Crilley P, et al: CMV enteritis causing segmental ischemia and massive hemorrhage, *Gastrointest Endosc* 53:355–359, 2001.

30. Castagnola E, Viscoli C: Prophylaxis and empirical therapy of infection in cancer patients. In Mandell GL, Bennett JE, Dolin R, editors: *Mandell, Douglas, and Bennett's principles and practice of infectious diseases*, ed 7, Philadelphia, 2010, Churchill Livingstone.

31. Berger DH, Dardik A, Rosenthal RA: Surgery in the elderly. In Townsend CM, Beauchamp RD, Evers BM, et al, editors: *Sabiston textbook of surgery: the biological basis of modern surgical practice*, ed 18, Philadelphia, 2008, WB Saunders.

32. Hardin RE, Zenilman ME: Surgical considerations in the elderly. In Brunicardi FC, Andersen DK, Billiar TR, et al, editors: *Schwartz's principles of surgery*, ed 9, New York, 2010, McGraw-Hill.

33. Pavlin DJ, Pavlin EG, Fitzgibbon DR, et al: Management of bladder function after outpatient surgery, *Anesthesiology* 91:42–50, 1999.

34. ACC/AHA Guideline Update for Perioperative Cardiovascular Evaluation for Noncardiac Surgery: A Report of the American College of Cardiology/American Heart Association Task Force on Practice Guidelines (Committee to Update the 1996 Guidelines on Perioperative Cardiovascular Evaluation for Noncardiac Surgery), *Anesth Analg* 94:1052–1064, 2002.

35. Geriatric Anesthesia. In Miller RD, Eriksson LI, Fleisher LA, et al, editors: *Miller's anesthesia*, ed 7, London, 2009, Churchill Livingstone.

36. Leung JM, Liu LL: Current controversies in the perioperative management of geriatric patients, *ASA Refresher Course Anesthesiol* 29:175–187, 2001.

37. Marcantonio ER, Flacker JM, Wright RJ: Reducing delirium after hip fractures: a randomized trial, *J Am Geriatric Soc* 49:516–522, 2001.

# Ethical Principles and Palliative Care

*Martha L. Twaddle, M.D., F.A.C.P., F.A.A.H.P.M.; Tina J. Hieken, M.D.; and Mona Tareen, M.D.*

**1.** A 93-year-old woman is seen after a fall at home with complaints of right leg and wrist pain. She also gives a history of anorexia and 40-lb weight loss. On physical examination she is cachectic and has a large necrotic tumor in her left breast with significant drainage and odor. She admits to its presence but prefers to deflect questions about the history of the breast lesion. You assess her Karnofsky performance status (KPS) score to be 40% and palliative performance status (PPS) score to be 40%. Radiographs reveal a right wrist fracture and metastases to her pelvis and femur with a nondisplaced hip fracture. As you discuss goals with the patient and her daughter, the patient states that she does not want "you to make a fuss" and her goals are "to be comfortable" and "to not be a burden." She denies any depression and feels "blessed for having such a wonderful life." Which one of the following is the best course of action?

A. You tell the patient and her daughter that the median survival with stage IV breast cancer is about 2 years and recommend preoperative chemotherapy followed by a mastectomy and radiation therapy.

B. You speak privately with the daughter, who desires that her mother undergo surgery and chemotherapy. You declare the patient incompetent because you think that she is depressed and look to her daughter to serve as a designated power of attorney for health care (DPAHC).

C. You recommend radiation therapy because this may help decrease the pain of the bone metastases and recommend a single fraction as opposed to a 2-week course.

D. You recommend no surgical intervention given her goals to not pursue other treatment.

E. You recommend that the patient undergo whole-body computed tomography (CT), positron emission tomography, and magnetic resonance imaging (MRI) of the brain to formulate a treatment plan.

*Ref.:* 1-7

**COMMENTS:** This patient's goals of care are most consistent with a palliative approach to management. Given the extent of disease and her age, this approach is reasonable. The **Karnofsky performance scale** was developed in 1949 by Dr. Karnofsky as a means to measure and reflect a cancer patient's quality of life as reflected by functionality. A KPS score of 100% reflects no complaints and no evidence of disease, 50% requires help often and

frequent medical care, and 0% is death. The **palliative performance status** provides a functional assessment of ambulation, activity, cognition, self-care, and oral intake and is used as a tool in prognosis with a scale similar to the KPS (100% is normal, 0% death). Evaluation for depression and decision-making capacity is of key importance to ascertain that the patient clearly understands the consequences of her decisions, is consistent in her decision making, and is not depressed. Even patients with mild cognitive impairment may have decision-making capacity. Physicians do not determine whether a patient is "competent" because that is a legal decision. If the patient is decisional, the DPAHC is not active. The patient's goals suggest care focused primarily on comfort. Thus, chemotherapy, nonpalliative surgery, and radiotherapy, as well as an extensive radiologic work-up in this patient in whom metastatic disease is already apparent, are not indicated. Wound care for the breast lesion, pain management for the bone metastases, and a palliative care evaluation to facilitate a complex symptom management and discharge plan are recommended. A toilette mastectomy or partial mastectomy may be considered for local control of bleeding, odor, and infection, even in the presence of metastatic disease. Reduced-fraction radiation therapy will facilitate symptom management and minimize the duration of treatment.

**A N S W E R :**  C

**2.** A 48-year-old man has a recent increase in abdominal girth, 20-lb weight loss, jaundice, and confusion. He has no other significant past medical history and was working until 1 week earlier. His wife provides the history and states that the patient has had persistent complaints of abdominal and back pain unrelieved by acetaminophen or ibuprofen. His current KPS score is 40% and his PPS score is 30%. After further testing, pancreatic cancer with gastric outlet obstruction is diagnosed. Because he is symptomatic with pain and encephalopathy, you speak to his wife. She is very anxious and tells you that they have two children 6 and 8 years of age who are unaware of their father's diagnosis and the extent of his disease. All of the following are true except:

A. At the time of diagnosis, only 20% of patients with pancreatic cancer will have resectable disease.

B. Laparoscopic gastrojejunostomy can provide effective palliation of symptoms.

C. Celiac neurolysis has been demonstrated to help in pain management.

D. Acute thromboembolic disease, a common complication of advanced pancreatic cancer, is best managed with a heparin bridge to oral anticoagulation.

E. Specialized support services for children and the spouse may be of great psychological benefit earlier in the course of diagnosis and treatment.

*Ref.:* 8-12

**COMMENTS:** Although the majority of patients with **cancer of the pancreas** have advanced disease not amenable to surgical resection when initially seen, much can be done to improve the symptoms and thus quality of life. For patients with good performance status and a life expectancy of several months, laparoscopic gastrojejunostomy can provide effective **palliation** of the obstruction and allow the patient to eat. Metoclopramide may also improve any associated dysmotility. Pain is a common problem with cancer of the pancreas and can be difficult to manage, particularly if there are concomitant dysmotility issues. Endoscopic ultrasound-guided celiac plexus block is greater than 70% effective in managing the pain related to pancreatic cancer and is a reasonable option for pain management. For patients with acute thromboembolic disease, a common complication of pancreatic cancer secondary to a hypercoagulable state, studies demonstrate a significant decrease in recurrent thromboembolic events in patients treated with low-molecular-weight heparin as opposed to oral anticoagulation. In addition, management of oral anticoagulation is complicated by the malnutrition and liver dysfunction that typically accompany pancreatic cancer. Supportive care services introduced early in the care of patients (and their families) helps address the psychosocial and spiritual stresses of the illness and their ramifications on all family members.

**ANSWER:** D

3. A patient scheduled for surgery on her left lower extremity awakens from surgery to find her right leg bandaged and her left leg untouched. Which of the following is true regarding wrong-site surgery?

A. The rate of wrong-site surgeries has decreased substantially since the 2004 Institute of Medicine (IOM) initiatives.

B. The patient should receive prompt, full disclosure of the error and an apology from the surgeon.

C. A sufficient apology typically consists of saying "I'm sorry that this happened."

D. Exposure of the error successfully mitigates against the risk of a patient suing.

E. The Joint Commission's National Patient Safety Goals apply only to hospital settings.

*Ref.:* 13-18

**COMMENTS: Adverse events** are defined by the IOM as "harm that is the result of the process of health care rather than the patient's underlying disease." A **medical error** is an adverse event that could have been prevented, and thus its risk or occurrence warrants changes in procedures, systems, practice, or products. The IOM defines a medical error as "failure of a planned action to be completed as intended, or the use of a wrong plan to achieve an aim." The Joint Commission Board of Commissioners approved the Universal Protocol for Preventing Wrong Site, Wrong Procedure and Wrong Person Surgery in July 2003, and it became effective July 1, 2004, for all accredited hospitals, ambulatory surgery suites, and office-based surgical facilities. The protocol seeks to prevent these errors through active and robust strategies involving the surgical team and the patient (or representative). The three components include preoperative verification of the patient's and team's expectations of the procedure to be performed, operative site marking that is visible when the patient is draped for all right and left or multiple-site procedures, and a final **time-out** before the procedure begins to facilitate reverification. The occurrence of **wrong-site surgery** is exceeding rare (1 per 112,994 non–spine-related operations in one series) but, interestingly, has not declined since the Joint Commission's protocol was put into effect in 2004. The occurrence of a wrong-site surgery would constitute a "**sentinel event**" to be voluntarily reported to the Joint Commission with a **root cause analysis** and action plan accompanying the report. The Joint Commission maintains a database on sentinel events.

The medical profession's historical response to errors and adverse outcomes has been to deny and defend. Currently, the widespread consensus is that patients should receive a prompt, thorough **disclosure of the error** and a sincere apology. Apology in this context indicates that one should admit responsibility, show remorse, offer explanation, and make reparations. Historically, surgeons have been less apt to disclose error than have physicians in other disciplines. Research indicates that the absence of disclosure motivates many medical malpractice lawsuits and that disclosure and full apology may actually decrease liability and maintain support of true patient-centered care. However, this mitigation is not 100%. Many states have adopted laws that such disclosure is inadmissible as evidence of liability.

**ANSWER:** B

4. An 85-year-old man with a history of hypertension, peripheral vascular disease, and hyperlipidemia who was living independently at home was taken to the emergency department after being found unresponsive on the kitchen floor by his sister. On examination, his right pupil is fixed at 7 mm and his left pupil at 5 mm; both are unresponsive. The oculocephalic maneuver (doll's eyes) is negative. There is a positive but weak corneal reflex on the left; it is absent on the right. The patient gags with insertion of an endotracheal tube and demonstrates extensor posturing in both upper extremities when intubated for airway protection. CT demonstrates a large right temporal-parietal intracerebral hemorrhage, a right frontal subdural hematoma, intraventricular hemorrhage, and a 2-cm midline shift. The patient is unmarried, has no children, but does have five siblings. There is no advance directive available. You decide:

A. That urgent neurosurgical intervention is warranted because the patient may regain function even though he has only lower brainstem reflexes.

B. To obtain a neurology consultation and let the neurologist deal with decision making.

C. To hold a family meeting as soon as possible to explain the patient's poor prognosis with the goal of determining what treatment the patient would have wanted via substituted judgment.

D. To admit the patient to the intensive care unit (ICU) and treat the aspiration pneumonia and urinary tract infection with the intention of performing a tracheostomy and placing a percutaneous endoscopic gastrostomy tube after a family meeting to obtain consent.

E. To initiate a morphine drip.

*Ref.:* 19-23

**COMMENTS:** "Breaking the bad news" regarding a **poor prognosis** is the responsibility of every physician, and the ability to provide this intervention is an acquired skill that requires knowledge and practice. The most commonly followed procedure is Buckman's SPIKES method. Early communication facilitates earlier recognition of the prognosis by the family and is more likely to establish a cooperative, patient-centered plan of care. Although certainty about outcomes may be unclear early in an ICU stay, families find information helpful in anticipating outcomes and making decisions. **Family meetings** facilitate communication and improve family satisfaction, clinical decision making, and the psychological well-being of the family. In families who perceive communication to be inadequate, symptoms of post-traumatic stress disorder are more likely to develop. Ideally, patients choose their surrogate decision makers. However, the presence of a health care proxy via an **advance directive** is not always present despite all 50 states having legislation authorizing the appointment of such. The next of kin customarily serves in this role with the expectation that the decisions will be based on **substituted judgment**, that being what the patient would want if able to provide directives.

**ANSWER:** C

5. A 67-year-old woman with a history of severe chronic obstructive pulmonary disease is admitted on an emergency basis to the hospital from home. She has been admitted for pneumonia and respiratory failure four times in the last 6 months; her last hospitalization was complicated by a protracted time in the ICU in which she required biphasic positive airway pressure. She also has chronic renal insufficiency with anemia that is exacerbating her primary lung disease and controlled non–insulin-dependent diabetes mellitus. On this admission, in addition to her severe dyspnea and fever, acute emphysematous cholecystitis develops. The patient has given a "do not resuscitate" (DNR) order as part of her advance directive. She is currently considered decisional despite her serious condition; she understands that she is seriously ill, that she may soon require intubation given her progressive respiratory failure, and that she will need surgery in the very near future, depending on her response to antibiotics and supportive therapies. The patient states that she does not wish to be intubated now or resuscitated if she should die now or later in surgery. You decide:

A. To intubate her because this is a potentially reversible condition from which she can fully recover.

B. To call her husband because he is her surrogate and ask him for permission to move ahead with intubation as well as rescinding the DNR order.

C. To respect her wishes and elect to not intubate her given her advance directives, yet continue to provide antibiotics and supportive care to facilitate possible recovery.

D. To call her primary physician and ask him to reverse her DNR order so that you can move ahead with what is best for her.

E. To proceed with surgery.

*Ref.:* 3, 24-29

**COMMENTS:** Patients have the right to refuse treatments, even those that are likely to be beneficial and have a reasonable chance to remediate or resolve a serious condition. This patient has an **advance directive** and has had time to reflect on her values, draw conclusions based on her past experiences, and make decisions

regarding future care. Despite her current condition, she maintains **decision-making capacity** (she is consistent in her directives, she understands her illness and her prognosis without specific treatments, and she is able to draw to a conclusion). Her care would include providing support to her husband regarding her decisions, adding small doses of hydromorphone for dyspnea given her impaired creatinine clearance, and planning a family meeting to discuss surgery. Involving her husband and primary care physician is appropriate, but not to change or overrule the patient's advance directive. Reversal of a DNR order preoperatively remains a tremendous challenge for institutions. Position papers of the American College of Surgeons, the Association of Operating Room Nurses, and the American Society of Anesthesiologists speak strongly against policies requiring automatic cancellation of existing DNR orders for patients undergoing anesthesia based on the principle of patient **autonomy**. Careful attention to the decision-making process and identification of the health care proxy are very important when this is done. The goals of care may need to be further negotiated as the patient receives supportive interventions. The outcome may not what the physician believes is "best" yet may be consistent with what the patient desires. The patient may indicate that she wishes to pursue surgery with some parameters regarding the extent of perioperative interventions. Supportive care interventions include treatment of the infection and relief of the abdominal pain with intravenous analgesics. Morphine should be avoided given the patient's renal failure to circumvent the accumulation of morphine-6-glucoronide and its side effects. Preferred analgesics for patients with advanced renal disease and renal failure include hydromorphone, fentanyl, and methadone. Given her multiple comorbid conditions, she is at high risk for delirium and should be reassessed frequently for the onset of global confusion, progressive sleep abnormalities, and agitation.

**ANSWER:** C

6. A 58-year-old African-American woman with stage IV colon cancer has been admitted multiple times for pneumonia and recurrent partial bowel obstruction over the past month. She is now in the ICU with peritonitis, gram-negative sepsis, acute renal failure, and a suspected bowel perforation. When the patient was decisional, she had expressed to her family that she wanted "everything done" and that "God will cure me." Her mother and sister are frequently at the bedside and express a range of emotions, including anger. Her sister cannot understand why "you aren't doing anything to help her!" In particular, the sister, acting as the patient's surrogate decision maker, is insistent that you move forward with surgery to repair the bowel and states this is necessary for religious reasons. The next best step in your approach to this patient is to:

A. Consult the palliative care service to hold a family meeting to discuss the goals and prognosis before instituting hemodialysis or operating on the patient.

B. Operate because of the patient's and family's goals and their religious beliefs after the sister signs fully informed consent.

C. Tell the patient and the family that surgery in her case is futile care and sign off the case.

D. Call the hospital risk management department.

E. Delay surgical intervention and avoid confrontation with the family until full discussion of the case with the patient's clergy can take place.

*Ref.:* 9, 20, 23, 24, 28, 30-33

**COMMENTS:** Surgeons are faced with patient and family member requests for what may be called **"futile" care**, although this term is best avoided in family discussions because it implies a value judgment. Clearly, this family does not think that treatment is futile, and discussion may be eclipsed by the meaning of a word as opposed to focusing on the issues. The surgeon is confronted with a request for care that is unlikely to benefit the patient, who appears to be dying, and complicated by the family's expressions of anger and their stated religious beliefs. A palliative care team or ethics consultation is beneficial in this situation; these services have been shown to improve symptom control, enhance patient and family satisfaction, lower costs, and even increase organ donations. Ideally, the surgeon provides primary palliative care and does not abdicate resolution of the issue but actively collaborates with the consultants. The surgeon has a responsibility to explain the clinical situation, the options for care, and the probable outcomes of each option. A second opinion may be offered. **Religious traditions** may affect decisions about treatment and withholding and withdrawing of life-prolonging care. The medical team should make "reasonable accommodation" for such beliefs. In this case, the family is asking for treatment of no benefit and probable harm, thereby potentially accelerating death. Involving chaplaincy or a member of the patient's religious community can be of value but is not a substitute for direct discussion with the family. Studies show that African Americans tend to prefer life-prolonging measures. They may see death as a struggle to overcome or to deny and suffering as something spiritual to be endured; this may be at odds with a palliative care approach. Honest open communication, compassion, and respect can align the surgeon with the family so that the surgeon is seen as an advocate seeking to do what is best for the patient. Alerting risk management services is often advisable but is not the most pressing priority.

**ANSWER:** A

7. A 52-year-old woman is now at postoperative day 5 after debulking surgery for stage IIIC ovarian cancer. She is passing some flatus, but her recovery is complicated by protracted nausea and vomiting. She has received odansetron, chlorpromazine, and droperidol without improvement in her symptoms, and she continues to complain of nausea, to vomit intermittently, and to require intravenous fluids for hydration. The patient tells you that when her food is brought in and she sits up to eat, her nausea increases significantly and she vomits. Her protracted symptoms are most likely related to:

A. Centrally mediated nausea from the smell of the food.

B. Bowel dysmotility and edema.

C. Stimulation of the vestibular apparatus.

D. Manipulation of the uterus and ovaries in surgery.

E. Anesthesia.

*Ref.:* 34-38

**COMMENTS:** **Nausea**, like pain, is a complex symptom that requires a thorough history to elucidate the cause and best treatment. **Vomiting** is controlled by the vomiting center in the brain, which is located in the medulla and serves to process all the stimuli that elicit nausea. The chemoreceptor trigger zone in the floor of the fourth ventricle is outside the blood-brain barrier and can be directly stimulated by changes in blood chemistry, toxins, or pharmaceuticals. Centrally mediated nausea from the cortex is not as well understood but can trigger nausea via smells and learned triggers. Dysmotility from postoperative ileus, bowel edema, decreased peristalsis from

opioids, or inflammatory changes in the viscera may also affect the vomiting center via gastrointestinal neurologic mechanisms. There is also a strong correlation between postoperative pain and nausea; improved pain control may concomitantly decrease nausea without direct treatment of the symptoms. An often overlooked type of nausea is **vestibular nausea**, caused by activation of the vestibular apparatus, which may be triggered by drugs such as opioids, dehydration, and postural changes. Vestibular nausea is more common in women, and those with a previous history of motion sickness may be at increased risk. This patient's history is significant for nausea after a change in posture. Ondansetron, chlorpromazine, and droperidol address centrally mediated nausea; none will alleviate vestibular nausea, which is best treated by scopolamine applied as a transdermal patch or diphenhydramine.

**ANSWER:** C

8. A 66-year-old man is seen 4 months after right thoracotomy and upper lobectomy for stage I adenocarcinoma of his right lung. He appears anxious and depressed, has suffered a 12-lb weight loss, and complains of pain along the area of the healed incision. He describes the pain as a deep pressure with shooting, electrical qualities. He experiences severe pain when his undershirt rubs against the area and says that if the area is rubbed or touched repeatedly, the resultant surge of pain will last for several days. On examination, the thoracotomy incision is well healed, numb, yet markedly dysesthetic to touch. Given his deteriorating condition, the patient is convinced that the cancer has returned and seeks your help. As you counsel the patient, you explain that:

A. He would probably benefit from radiation therapy directed to the intercostal area.

B. The pain is suggestive of locally recurrent disease secondary to implantation of tumor cells in the incision, and you order CT of the chest.

C. His pain is consistent with a post-thoracotomy neuropathic pain syndrome and it should resolve over time without intervention.

D. His pain is consistent with a post-thoracotomy neuropathic pain syndrome and prompt treatment with a combination of medications may reduce or remit his pain.

E. His pain is suggestive of a centrally mediated phenomenon, and you order an MRI of the brain to evaluate for brain metastases.

*Ref.:* 39-44

**COMMENTS:** **Neuropathic pain** is defined by the International Association for the Study of Pain as "pain initiated or caused by a primary lesion or dysfunction in the nervous system." It may follow injury to the nervi nervorum or nerve axons in peripheral pain syndromes or be centrally mediated from lesions of the spinal cord or brain. The diagnosis is made principally by eliciting a history of the characteristic **dysesthesias**, which may be manifested as a searing sensation of heat, electrical shocks, or stabbing pain coupled with abnormal evoked pain. The latter, known as **allodynia**, is pain caused by nonnoxious stimuli, such as the brush of clothing or a light touch. Hyperalgesia may be present, in which a painful stimulus is greatly exaggerated, or hyperpathia, in which repeated nonpainful stimuli seemingly accumulate and cause an intensified pain response. Neuropathic pain persists after the primary cause has resolved. In this case, healing of the thoracotomy is complete, but the pain persists. In some individuals the pain will not begin until several weeks after surgery. There may be physical findings that accompany the neuropathic pain, such as changes in the color of the skin (pallor or redness), abnormal sweating or coldness, loss of hair, or atrophy. Frequently, however, other than the abnormal neurologic findings, the area of concern appears normal. The pain may mistakenly be dismissed as a psychological problem given the paucity of physical findings. Neuropathic pain presents a particular challenge to treat in that it tends to be less responsive to traditional analgesics, such as opioids, because the pain is not a result of activation of the pain receptors (nociceptors) but a dysfunction or lesion of the nerve itself. Treatment often involves polypharmacy with tricyclic antidepressants or anticonvulsants (or both) coupled with opioids. Topical local anesthetics may also be of benefit, in some cases combined with the anesthetic and *N*-methylaspartate receptor antagonist ketamine. Despite treatment, neuropathic pain may never fully resolve and can result in a chronic pain syndrome. There is a suggestion that the more rapidly the pain is controlled, the less likely it will persist. It is not uncommon that serious illness or new pain stimuli may worsen previous symptoms.

**ANSWER:** D

9. A 47-year-old woman is evaluated 2 years after the diagnosis of serous epithelial ovarian carcinoma because of a 3-month history of unpredictable bowel function, intermittent nausea and vomiting, abdominal pain, expanding abdominal girth, and weight loss. She is admitted 3 weeks after chemotherapy with protracted vomiting and no bowel movement for 7 days. Her physical examination is notable for temporal wasting, oral thrush, a protuberant tender abdomen with shifting dullness, and a palpable firm mass in the left lower quadrant. Imaging reveals multiple sites of partial small bowel obstruction, ascites, and enlarging pelvic tumors despite treatment. The initial approach most likely to alleviate this patient's symptoms is:

A. Endoscopic stenting of the obstructions.

B. Placement of a venting percutaneous gastrostomy tube.

C. Palliative surgery to relieve the obstruction.

D. Medical management with corticosteroids, octreotide, and opioid analgesics.

E. Palliative surgery to bypass the obstruction followed by pelvic radiation therapy.

*Ref.:* 45-48

**COMMENTS: Bowel obstruction** is a common complication of ovarian cancer and may be part of the manifestation of the disease. Likewise, after debulking surgery, some patients are at risk for small bowel obstruction secondary to adhesions. These patients may benefit significantly from surgery to relieve the obstruction. However, a frequent complication of advanced ovarian cancer is malignant bowel obstruction that is not amenable to a surgical intervention, even one aimed purely at control of symptoms. This patient has several markers for a poor prognosis, including a palpable tumor, compromised nutritional status with weight loss, ascites, multiple sites of obstruction, and tumor progression while undergoing chemotherapy. In this scenario, the nonsurgical interventions must be considered carefully. Given the disease progression while undergoing chemotherapy, the patient is not likely to respond to further chemotherapy. Radiation therapy for the bulky pelvic disease is associates with a low response rate and significant morbidity. The administration of dexamethasone, 8 mg/day, to address bowel inflammation and edema and octreotide to diminish

intestinal secretions, along with intravenous fluids and analgesics such as morphine, are very effective in relieving malignant bowel obstructions from ovarian, gastric, and colon cancers. These medications are available as a compounded suppository, which may facilitate outpatient therapy. Placement of a venting gastrostomy tube may alleviate vomiting but renders the patient unable to take oral alimentation; in the presence of palpable abdominal disease and ascites, this is controversial. Most recommend against the use of total parenteral nutrition (TPN) for patients with progressive malignant bowel obstruction unless their performance status is high. If TPN is considered, a clear and thorough discussion of the goals of the therapy, the desired outcomes, and the signs and symptoms of negative outcomes such as infection, worsening ascites, jaundice, or edema should take place before TPN is initiated.

**ANSWER:** D

10. An 82-year-old Taiwanese Chinese widow who speaks little English is evaluated for anemia, melena, and hematemesis. Endoscopy reveals a friable gastric carcinoma; biopsy confirms adenocarcinoma. You are asked to evaluate the patient for a surgical consultation. The family intercepts you in the hallway and asks that you not tell the patient her diagnosis. Her son, a 62-year-old businessman, states that he and his siblings will discuss the surgery with you and that he will sign all the necessary consents. The best course of action is:

A. To insist on obtaining informed consent from the patient and ask the family to provide interpretation.

B. To state that you must fully disclose the findings to the patient and will then ask her permission to have her son act on her behalf.

C. Through a hospital interpreter, to explore with the patient how she prefers to make decisions about her medical care and how much information about diagnoses and test results that she prefers to know.

D. After discussion with the family (without the patient), to allow the son to sign consents for the patient's surgery while acknowledging and respecting their cultural preferences.

E. To ask the patient's primary care physician, who speaks Chinese, to talk to the son and obtain consent for surgery.

*Ref.:* 20, 21, 30, 33, 49-52

**COMMENTS:** The approach to medical decision making will vary across cultures and ethnicities. In general, **Asian cultures** that are influenced by Confucianism ascribe to the family playing the central role in medical decision making. In many situations such as this, when the husband is deceased, the first-born male child or the oldest child will step forward as the decision maker. This scenario can cause significant moral distress for a physician who ascribes to the Western ethical construct of **autonomy** and self-determination. The United States is a culturally and religiously diverse nation. The current system of health care decision making based on patient **autonomy** does not appeal to all patients, and imposition of this approach may cause tremendous suffering. Family members of immigrants who were born in the United States may not be as observant of traditions, so ethnicity alone may not be helpful in understanding how patients make decisions. As physicians, we must be sensitive to the unique ways in which families make health care decisions and seek to clarify these issues before making any assumptions or moving ahead with any discussions. In this case, asking the patient through an interpreter how she prefers to make decisions and how much information she would like about her condition will allow her to direct decision making to her son and family should she so desire. Alternatively, she may make it clear that she would like to make her own decisions and that the family's desire to "protect" her does not reflect her preferences. Ideally, conversations with patients are conducted via a nonbiased interpreter and not a family member. In this situation, a family member acting as interpreter may not convey to the patient what the physician is truly saying.

**ANSWER:** C

11. A resident making rounds with an eminent professor of surgery presents a case to him. In the patient's room the professor calls the resident "stupid" and berates his decision making and evaluation of the patient, which is indeed incorrect. The patient is visibly upset. Which of the following is not true regarding disruptive physicians?

   A. The majority of cases of disruptive physician behavior are reported only when the offense is severe.

   B. Disruptive behavior may include inappropriate language, disrespectful behavior, refusal to complete tasks, and physical abuse, such as throwing objects.

   C. Disruptive physician behavior is most often directed at nurses and other allied health workers.

   D. Disruptive physician behavior is the most frequently reported type of complaint to disciplinary boards.

   E. Fear of reprisal is an uncommon reason for the underreporting of disruptive physician behavior.

*Ref.:* 49, 53, 54

**COMMENTS:** The American Medical Association's Code of Medical Ethics defines **disruptive physician behavior** as any "personal conduct, whether verbal or physical, that negatively affects or that potentially may affects patient care." It is incumbent on surgeons to model their professional behavior toward other physicians, nurses, allied health care workers, and their students and residents in a circumspect manner. There is strong evidence that trainees learn abusive behavior from their mentors and emulate it in their own practices. When care by colleagues needs remediation, such discussion should be done promptly, but privately and away from patient care areas. It is always appropriate to maintain a sober decorum in patient care areas. Although disruptive physician behavior is not often reported, it is the most frequently reported issue to disciplinary boards, more than one half of the cases are directed against nonphysician health care workers, and the most frequently cited reason for hesitancy in reporting is fear of reprisal.

**ANSWER:** E

12. A 14-year-old Jehovah's Witness who was in a motor vehicle accident undergoes emergency splenectomy and packing of a liver laceration. In the recovery room he is hypotensive and tachycardic and his hemoglobin is 6 g/dL. His parents refuse to give permission for transfusion of any blood products. The most appropriate next step in the care of this young patient is to:

   A. Repeat the hemoglobin test.

   B. Transfuse 2 units of packed red blood cells.

   C. Administer erythropoietin.

   D. Obtain a court order and then transfuse 2 units of packed red blood cells.

   E. Withhold transfusion.

*Ref.:* 55, 56

**COMMENTS:** Since their 1945 ban on all blood products, **Jehovah's Witnesses** are best known to health care workers for their refusal of transfusion for themselves and their minor family members, regardless of the possibility of significant morbidity or death in the absence of transfusion. However, the courts have recognized, and the Supreme Court has upheld, that parents are expected to act in their child's best interests at all times and that although parents have the right to freely practice and exercise their own religious beliefs, this does not include the right to expose their children to illness or death. This principle applies regardless of whether the life of the child is in imminent danger. Repeating the hemoglobin determination in the clinical scenario just described is unlikely to alter the need for transfusion. Erythropoietin first acts by increasing the reticulocyte count with a noticeable increase in hemoglobin and hematocrit at 2 to 6 weeks after administration, too slow to be of benefit in this acutely ill child.

**ANSWER:** D

13. A surgeon wishes to perform a new procedure on a patient. Which of the following does the surgeon need to do beforehand?

   A. Obtain informed consent from the patient, including disclosure that the procedure in question is new; the physician's experience, training, and qualifications for performing the procedure; the rationale for recommending this procedure; and its attendant risks, benefits, and possible outcomes.

   B. Obtain an institutional review board (IRB) waiver to treat the patient in this manner, followed by a standard preoperative informed consent.

   C. Obtain IRB approval for the proposed treatment after submitting a formal IRB application describing the experimental surgery and then obtain a special informed consent for experimental procedures.

   D. Obtain approval from hospital administration and the department chair and then obtain a special informed consent for experimental procedures.

   E. Obtain approval from hospital administration and the department chair and then obtain a standard preoperative informed consent.

*Ref.:* 57, 58

**COMMENTS:** Surgical innovation is a constant feature of the practice of surgery, and the introduction of a new procedure may be necessary to provide optimum care for an individual patient, as well as to improve surgical patient care in general. Rare disorders and unusual clinical scenarios demand that surgeons "think outside the box." The basis of **informed consent** is that the patient is provided with sufficient relevant information in a noncoercive setting to arrive at a prudent decision. In the setting of new surgical procedures, it is especially important to stress the completeness of this consent as outlined in choice A. Informed consent requires discussion of the nature of the intervention and the expected benefits, risks, and consequences. Patients also need to know, especially in this case, alternatives to the proposed treatment and their risks, benefits, and consequences. Physicians are not required to inform a patient of alternatives for care that they do not believe are medically indicated but rather alternatives that other reasonable physicians would recommend.

The **institutional review board** does not have any role in the care of individual patients outside the research setting. The National Commission for the Protection of Human Subjects of Biomedical and Behavioral Research serves to identify the basic ethical principles that underlie biomedical and behavioral research involving human subjects. In this scenario, there is no plan to conduct any formal research study. Hospital administration has no role in policing surgical conduct; individual institutional policies regarding departmental approval for novel procedures vary, as does the specificity of the surgical privileges that surgeons are granted. As surgeons wish to perform newly developed procedures after the completion of their formal training, departments may require evidence of additional training such as via a seminar with a hands-on laboratory component, proctoring by colleagues or national experts, and outcomes reporting for a defined number of cases.

**ANSWER:** A

14. A 65-year-old man with a very recent diagnosis of cholangiocarcinoma is brought to the emergency room by his exhausted wife. She reports that he is "in severe pain" and that neither of them have slept in days because of his symptoms. She says that he has been seeing people who are not present, such as the patient's father, who is deceased. On examination, he is disoriented, grimacing and groaning, and persistently trying to pull off his clothing and the bedsheet to get out of the gurney. He is repetitively saying "let's go" and becomes combative when examined. He has been taking a long-acting morphine, 60 mg every 12 hours by mouth, and his wife has been giving him several doses of a short-acting morphine concentrate through the night without any improvement. He has taken another 10 mg six times over the past 8 hours. He is not hypoxemic. After correcting the metabolic derangements, he remains confused and agitated. You decide:

A. To admit the patient and start intravenous morphine, as well as a benzodiazepine, for his anxiety. You recommend wrist restraints to keep him from pulling out his intravenous line.

B. The problem is related to too much medication, so you stop the long-acting morphine and change the analgesic to a hydrocodone-acetaminophen combination.

C. To double the long-acting morphine given how much short-acting medication that he has required and initiate treatment with a benzodiazepine for anxiety.

D. The clinical scenario is most consistent with delirium, which is probably multifactorial in etiology. You admit the patient and initiate intravenous morphine, haloperidol, and lactulose.

E. To obtain psychiatric consultation regarding this acute psychotic episode.

*Ref.:* 26, 59-63

**COMMENTS: Delirium** is one of the most common neuropsychiatric symptoms of advanced cancer; it occurs in up to 83% of patients near the end of life. The diagnosis is based on the clinical picture and connotes an elevated risk for mortality. The findings may be subtle—an acute onset of global confusion or changing cognition, a waxing and waning of attention and organized

thinking, altered levels of consciousness, and psychomotor symptoms of agitation (hyperactive or agitated delirium) or lethargy (hypoactive delirium). Delirium may be the sole manifestation of a serious illness, but there are often many contributing causes. Such causes include medications such as opioids (the worst being meperidine), dopaminergic and anticholinergic drugs, sedatives such as benzodiazepines, and corticosteroids; electrolyte disturbances from volume depletion, renal failure, or hepatic encephalopathy; sepsis; and accumulated physiologic stress from uncontrolled pain, disrupted sleep patterns, or chronic activation of the sympathetic nervous system. Delirium can be reversed in more than 50% of cases; however, in a patient at the end of life, its onset may reflect a transition toward death.

In this case, the causes of delirium may be poorly controlled pain, medication side effects from morphine and its metabolites, volume depletion secondary to insufficient oral intake, hepatic changes related to obstruction and advanced disease, and sleep deprivation. Treatment of delirium is multifactorial and starts with controlling the environment to limit overstimulation. Treatment of the agitation or the abnormal lethargy of apathetic delirium with antipsychotic medications such as haloperidol is indicated. Antipsychotics, including the newer alternative medications such as olanzapine and risperidone, are preferred over benzodiazepines, although the latter may be added for improved efficacy. Long-acting opioids require a functional gastrointestinal tract to be effective, so in this case, changing the morphine to a continuous infusion may be beneficial. Combination medications that includes acetaminophen are not recommended in patients with hepatic dysfunction because they are at greater risk for hepatotoxicity and overdosing. The ceiling dose of an opioid is not related to its analgesic potential but is determined by dose-related side effects such as intractable nausea, sedation, or myoclonus. In this case it may be beneficial to rotate to another opioid such as hydromorphone with the use of equianalgesic conversion tables while keeping in mind that if the side effects are related to the accumulation of morphine-6-glucoronide, they may take several days to clear even after the change. Lactulose diminishes the absorption of ammonia, which contributes to hepatic encephalopathy. Severe or **refractory delirium** sometimes requires therapeutic sedation to control the symptoms. Sedation is often considered a last option to relieve the distress of intractable symptoms or refractory suffering. Medications prescribed for the controlled sedation of intractable symptoms and suffering are usually provided via an intravenous infusion. The intended outcome is to control the symptoms and relieve the suffering through an altered level of consciousness. In fact, it is sometimes observed that an individual may awaken and be free of symptoms and suffering for intervals even while sedating infusions are being administered.

The ethical **principle of double effect** does apply in this setting of therapeutic sedation—the good intent (relief of suffering) is pursued while an unintended bad effect (such as death) will also foreseeably occur. However, the *sole intent* of the intervention of therapeutic sedation is to relieve refractory symptoms and uncontrolled suffering, not to hasten death. If death occurs during this intervention, it reflects the terminal state of the patients receiving the intervention, and the intervention is not a form of euthanasia, nor does it constitute physician-assisted suicide. **Therapeutic sedation** differs from palliative or **terminal sedation** in that the sedation is routinely decreased at predetermined intervals to continually reassess its necessity.

**ANSWER:** D

15. An 84-year-old woman is admitted for the third time to the ICU from a local nursing home with aspiration pneumonia. She has a 10-year history of Alzheimer dementia, is now fully

bedbound and incontinent, can speak no more than six words, and can no longer smile. During her last admission a feeding tube was placed. Now her kidneys are failing and her son requests that she receive dialysis. You are asked to see her for placement of a dialysis catheter and for further assessment regarding the placement of an arteriovenous shunt. You assess that the son's understanding of his mother's condition is very limited; he is focused on correcting medical problems when they arise and indicates to you that resolution of the problems will lead to improvement in his mother's cognition. You decide that the son's requests are based on denial and:

A. You refuse to place the catheter and the shunt according to the ethic of nonmaleficence.

B. You refuse to place the catheter according to the ethical imperative of justice.

C. You go ahead with the surgery according to the ethic of patient autonomy as expressed through her DPAHC (her son) and her living will.

D. You request an ethics consultation.

E. You request and attend a family meeting with the son, the social worker, the patient's primary care physician, and the intensive care physician to better elucidate the goals of care.

*Ref.: 24, 49, 64, 65*

**COMMENTS:** The moral duty or principled approach is often cited in the discussion of **medical ethics**. Table 37-1 lists the principles and definitions and how they specifically apply to physicians.

The process of applying the principles is not intended to be rigid or programmatic but rather to give guidance to those making complex decisions. In every decision, weighing the principles is often the discussed intellectual process, and no individual principle is intended to be supreme over the others. Overreliance on any one principle can lead to a dogmatic approach to decision making, which then risks truncating candid discussion, understanding, and joint decision making. As discussed in the article by Pawlik and Curley, our character gives us orientation and direction and

provides the foundation on which we approach our ethical struggles. When we approach patients and families as human beings, are professionally trained with expertise in our medical discipline, and are overarchingly committed to doing what is best for the patient, we are more likely to effectively communicate with patients and their families and reach a plan of care that is based on aligned values. Requesting an ethics consultation can always be of value to review the principles that are active, but it does not serve as a substitute for an effective family meeting. Such meetings allow medical professionals to hear what the patient, family, or both understand regarding the medical issues (as opposed to what they have been told) and to thoughtfully discuss the patient's condition and prognosis and what value or impact that treatments and procedures may have on the underlying condition (treating the pneumonia or correcting the renal failure does not reverse the Alzheimer dementia). Time-limited trials of interventions may be beneficial for patients and families confronting end-stage diagnoses and further strengthen the sense of collaboration and commitment between the surgeon, patient, and family.

**ANSWER:** E

## REFERENCES

1. Alvarado M, Ewing CA, Elyassnia D, et al: Surgery for palliation and treatment of advanced breast cancer, *Surg Oncol* 16:249–257, 2007.
2. Emanuel EJ, Emanuel LL: Proxy decision making for incompetent patients: an ethical and empirical analysis, *JAMA* 267:2067–2071, 1992.
3. Ganzini L, Volicer L, Nelson W, et al: Ten myths about decision making capacity, *J Am Med Dir Assoc* 6:S100–S104, 2005.
4. Karnofsky DA, Burchenal JH: The clinical evaluation of chemotherapeutic agents in cancer. In MacLeod CM, editor: *Evaluation of chemotherapeutic agents*, Columbia, 1949, Univ Press, pp 196.
5. Lau F, Downing M, Lesperance M, et al: Using the palliative performance scale to provide meaningful survival estimates, *J Pain Symptom Manage* 38:134–144, 2009.
6. Lau F, Maida V, Downing M, et al: Use of palliative performance scale in end-of-life prognostication in a palliative medicine consultation service, *J Pain Symptom Manage* 37:965–972, 2009.
7. Lee KF, Ennis WJ, Dunn GP: Surgical palliative care of advanced wounds, *Am J Hosp Palliat Med* 24:154–160, 2007.
8. Nakura EK, Warren RS. Palliative care for patients with advanced pancreatic and biliary cancers, *Surg Oncol* 16:293–297, 2007.
9. Ross EL, Abrahm J: Preparation of the patient for palliative procedures, *Surg Clin North Am* 85:191–207, 2005.
10. Kaufman M, Singh G, Das S, et al: Efficacy of endoscopic ultrasound-guided celiac plexus block and celiac plexus neurolysis for managing abdominal pain associated with chronic pancreatitis and pancreatic cancer, *J Clin Gastroenterol* 44:127–134, 2010.
11. Khorana AA, Fine RL: Pancreatic cancer and thromboembolic disease, *Lancet Oncol* 5:655–663, 2004.
12. Lee AY, Levine MN, Baker RI, et al: Low-molecular-weight heparin versus a coumarin for the prevention of recurrent venous thromboembolism in patient with cancer, *N Engl J Med* 349:146–153, 2003.
13. Universal protocol for preventing wrong site, wrong procedure, and wrong person surgery: The Joint Commission on Accreditation of Healthcare Organizations. National Patient Safety Goals 2009; http://www.jointcommission.org/NR/rdonlyres/868C9E07-037F-433D-8858-0D5FAA4322F2/0/RevisedChapter_HAP_NPSG_20090924.pdf (accessed November 22, 2009)
14. Fein SP, Hilborne LH, Spiritus BM, et al: The many faces of error disclosure: a common set of elements and a definition, *J Gen Intern Med* 22:755–761, 2007.
15. Institute of Medicine Committee on Quality of Health Care in America. *To err is human: building a safer health system.* Washington, D.C., 2000, National Academies Press.
16. Kwaan MR, Studdert DM, Zinner MJ, et al: Incidence, patterns, and prevention of wrong-site surgery, *Arch Surg* 141:353–357, 2006. discussion 357-358.
17. Gallagher TH: A 62 yo woman with cancer who experienced wrong site surgery, *JAMA* 302:669–677, 2009.

### TABLE 37-1 Principles and Definitions of Medical Ethics

| Autonomy | Self-rule, self-determination | Physicians must respect patients' rights to make decisions regarding their medical care |
|---|---|---|
| Beneficence | An action done for the benefit of others | Physicians seek to promote the welfare of their patients |
| Nonmaleficence | To do no harm | Physicians refrain from providing ineffective treatments or harming patients |
| Confidentiality | The information shared is private and will not be disclosed | Physicians respect the confidentiality of their patients and will not disclose this information except under certain mandates |
| Justice | Fairness and equality | The process for making medical decisions is fair and just and like-situated patients will be treated in a similar manner. Resources will be allocated justly |

18. Gallagher TH, Studdert D, Levinson W: Disclosing harmful medical errors to patients, *N Engl J Med* 356:2713–2719, 2007.
19. Azoulay E, Pochard F, Kentish-Barnes N, et al: Risk of post-traumatic stress symptoms in family members of intensive care unit patients, *Am J Respir Crit Care Med* 171:987–994, 2005.
20. Bradley CT, Brasel KJ: Core competencies in palliative care for surgeons: interpersonal and communication skills, *Am J Hosp Palliat Med* 24:499–507, 2008.
21. Buckman RA: Breaking bad news: the S-P-I-K-E-S strategy, *Commun Oncol* 2:138-142, 2005.
22. Emanuel EJ, Emanuel LL: Proxy decision making for incompetent patients. An ethical and empirical analysis, *JAMA* 267:2067–2071, 1992.
23. Kirchhoff KT, Song MK, Kehl K: Caring for the family of the critically ill patient, *Crit Care Clin* 20:453–466, ix–x, 2004.
24. Pawlik TM, Curley SA: Ethical issues in surgical palliative care: am I killing the patient by "letting him go"? *Surg Clin North Amer* 85:273–286, 2005.
25. Caruso LJ, Gabrielli A, Layon AJ: Perioperative do not resuscitate orders: caring for the dying in the operating room and intensive care unit, *J Clin Anesth* 14:401–404, 2002.
26. Casarett DJ, Inouye SK: Diagnosis and management of delirium near the end of life, *Ann Intern Med* 135:32–40, 2001.
27. Dean M: Opioids in renal failure and dialysis patients, *J Pain Symptom Manag* 28:497–504, 2004.
28. Dunn GP: Surgical critical care: surgical palliative care. In Cameron JL, editor: *Current surgical therapy*, ed 9, Philadelphia CV, 2008, Mosby, p 1179.
29. Sjogren, P: Clinical implications of morphine metabolites. In Portenoy RK, Bruera EB, editors: *Topics in palliative care*, Vol 1, New York, 1997, Oxford University Press, pp 163.
30. Crawley LM, Marshall PA, Lo B, et al: Strategies for culturally effective end-of-life care, *Ann Intern Med* 136:673–679, 2002.
31. Crawley L, Payne R, Bolden J, et al: Palliative and end-of-life care in the African American community, *JAMA* 284:2518–2520, 2000.
32. Olick RS, Braun EA, Potash J: Accommodating religious and moral objections to neurological death, *J Clin Ethics.* 2:183–191, 2009.
33. Weiner JS, Roth J: Avoiding iatrogenic harm to patient and family while discussing goals of care near the end of life, *J Palliat Med* 9:451–463, 2006.
34. Gan TJ, Meyer T, Apfel CC, et al: Consensus guidelines for managing postoperative nausea and vomiting, *Anesth Analg* 97:62–71, 2003.
35. Herndon CM, Jackson KC, Hallin PA: Management of opioid-induced gastrointestinal effects on patients receiving palliative care, *Pharmacotherapy* 22:240–250, 2002.
36. Mannix KA: Gastrointestinal symptoms: palliation of nausea and vomiting. In Doyle D, Hanks G, Cherny NI, et al, editors: *Oxford textbook of palliative medicine*, ed 3, Oxford, 2004, Oxford University Press, pp 459–468.
37. Philip BK: Etiologies of postoperative nausea and vomiting, *Pharm Ther Supp July* 18s–24s, 1997.
38. Faranak KK, Henzi I, Tramèr MR: Treatment of established postoperative nausea and vomiting: a quantitative systematic review, *BMC Anesthesiol* 1:2, 2001.
39. Chong MS, Bajwa ZH: Diagnosis and treatment of neuropathic pain, *J Pain Symptom Manage* 25:S4–S11, 2003.
40. Gilron I, Watson PN, Cahill CM, et al: Neuropathic pain: a practical guide for the clinician, *Can Med Assoc J* 175:265–275, 2006.
41. Kingery WA: A critical review of controlled clinical trials for peripheral neuropathic pain and complex regional pain syndromes, *Pain* 73:123–139, 1997.
42. Lynch M, Clark A, Sawynok J, et al: Topical amitriptyline and ketamine in neuropathic pain syndromes: an open-label study, *J Pain* 6:644–649, 2005.
43. Milch RA: Neuropathic pain: implications for the surgeon, *Surg Clin North Am* 85:225–236, 2005.
44. Pappagallo M: Optimizing pharmacologic treatments for patients with neuropathic pain, *Am J Cont Med Educ* 8–11, 2007.
45. Bozzetti F, Cozzaglio L, Iganzoli EB, et al: Quality of life and length of survival in advanced cancer patients on home parenteral nutrition, *J Clin Nutr* 21:281–288, 2002.
46. Jatoi A, Podratz KC, Gill P, et al: Pathophysiology and palliation of inoperable bowel obstruction in patients with ovarian cancer, *Supportive Oncol* 2:323–327, 2004.
47. Philip J, Depczynski B: The role of total parenteral nutrition for patients with irreversible bowel obstruction secondary to gynecological malignancy, *J Pain Symptom Manage* 13:104–111, 1997.
48. Ripamonti C, Twycross R, Baines M, et al: Clinical-practice recommendations for the management of bowel obstruction in patients with end-stage cancer. Working Group of the European Association for Palliative Care, *Support Care Cancer* 9:223–233, 2001.
49. Carson RA: Ethics in surgery. In Townsend CM, Beauchamp RD, Evers BM, et al, editors: *Sabiston textbook of surgery: the biological basis of modern surgical practice*, ed 18, Philadelphia, 2008, WB Saunders.
50. Haffner L: Translation is not enough: Interpreting in a medical setting. 2, *West J Med* 157:255–259, 1992.
51. McLaughlin LA, Braun KL: Asian and Pacific Islander cultural values: considerations for health care decision making, *Health Social Work* 23:116–126, 1998.
52. Parker SM, Clayton JM, Hancock K, et al: A systematic review of prognostic/end-of-life communication with adults in the advanced stages of a life-limiting illness: patient/caregiver preferences for the content, style, and timing of information, *J Pain Symptom Manage* 34:81–93, 2007.
53. American Medical Association: *E.9.045 Code of Medical Ethics: Current opinions with Annotations: 2006-2007.* Chicago, 2006, American Medical Association.
54. Mueller PS, Snyder L: Dealing with the "disruptive" physician colleague. In Medscape CME Activities: *http://cme.medscape.com/viewarticle/590319*; accessed 4/20/09.
55. Rutherford EJ, Brecher ME, Fakhry SM: Hematologic principles in surgery. In Townsend CM, Beauchamp RD, Evers M, et al, editors: *Sabiston textbook of surgery: the biological basis of modern surgical practice*, ed 18, Philadelphia, 2008, WB Saunders.
56. Woolley S: Children of Jehovah's Witnesses and adolescent Jehovah's Witnesses: what are their rights? *Arch Dis Child* 90:715–719, 2005.
57. Lieberman I, Herndon J, Hahn J, et al: Surgical innovation and ethical dilemmas: a panel discussion, *Cleve Clin J Med* 75:S6:S13–S21, 2008.
58. The Belmont Report: Ethical Principles and Guidelines for the protection of human subjects of research. The National Commission for the Protection of Human Subjects of Biomedical and Behavioral Research April 18, 1979. *http://ohsr.od.nih.gov/guidelines/belmont.html*, accessed 11/28/09
59. Brietbart W, Rosenfeld B, Roth A: The memorial delirium assessment scale, *J Pain Symptom Manage* 13:128–137, 1997.
60. Lawlor PG, Gagnon B, Mancini IL, et al: Occurrence, causes, and outcome of delirium in patients with advanced cancer, *Arch Intern Med* 160:786–794, 2000.
61. Inouye SK: Delirium in older persons, *N Engl J Med* 354:1157–1165, 2006.
62. Roth-Roemer S, Fann J, Syrjala K: The importance of recognizing and measuring delirium, *J Pain Symptom Manage* 13:125–127, 1997.
63. Twaddle ML: Therapeutic sedation protocol, *Midwest Palliative & Hospice Care Center*, 2001.
64. Lo G: Patient or surrogate insistence on life-sustaining interventions. In *Resolving ethical dilemmas: a guide for clinicians*, ed 2, Philadelphia, 2000, Lippincott Williams & Wilkins, pp 128.
65. Roy DJ: Euthanasia and withholding treatment. In Doyle D, Hanks G, Cherny N, Calman K, editors: *Oxford textbook of palliative medicine*, ed 3, Oxford, 2004, Oxford University Press, p 84–97.

# CHAPTER 38

# Evidence-Based Surgery and Applications of Biostatistics

*Edward F. Hollinger, M.D., Ph.D.*

1. As part of an effort to reduce length of hospital stay, kidney transplant patients were placed on a clinical pathway. All of the first seven patients placed on the pathway did well except the last patient, in whom pancreatitis developed and necessitated a month in the intensive care unit. The lengths of stay for these patients were 3, 4, 4, 5, 6, 7, and 41 days. What are the mean, median, and mode of the length-of-stay data?

   A. Mean = 10, median = 5, mode = 4

   B. Mean = 5, median = 10, mode = 5

   C. Mean = 10, median = 4, mode = 1

   D. Mean = 10, median = 5, mode = 41

   E. Mean = 5, median = 5, mode = 1

   *Ref.: 1-3*

**COMMENTS:** The mean, median, and mode are all measures of the **central tendency** of a data set. Both mean and median summarize the center of the data set. The **mean** is calculated by summing all of the observations and dividing by the number of observations. The **median** is the data value in which one half of the data points fall above it and one half below it. The median can be determined by listing the data points in rank order (as in the example). The median is the middle point of the ranked data. For odd sample sizes, one half of the remaining observations fall to the left of this value and the other one half fall to the right of this value. For even sample sizes, the median is the mean of the two middle values. As in this example, the mean is sensitive to outliers (the patient with a length of stay of 41 days); for these data sets the median may more correctly represent the data. The **mode** is the most frequently occurring value in the data set. For a normal distribution, the mean, median, and mode are approximately the same value.

**ANSWER:** A

2. Which of the following data types (i.e., nominal, ordinal, interval, ratio) correctly describe the variables (i.e., gender, respiratory rate, Apgar scores, date of month)?

|   | Gender (M/F) | Respiratory Rate | Apgar Scores (1-10) | Date of Month |
|---|---|---|---|---|
| A. | Nominal | Ordinal | Interval | Ratio |
| B. | Nominal | Ratio | Ordinal | Interval |
| C. | Interval | Ratio | Ordinal | Nominal |
| D. | Ordinal | Interval | Ratio | Nominal |
| E. | Nominal | Interval | Ordinal | Ratio |

   *Ref.: 2, 4*

**COMMENTS:** Experimental data can be classified as **categorical** or **quantitative**. Categorical data can be further divided into nominal and ordinal variables. **Nominal data** are classified into groups or named categories in which the order is arbitrary, for example, a "race" variable that can take on the values of black, white, Hispanic, or other. Means and medians are not meaningful for nominal data, although the mode represents the value most commonly measured. **Ordinal data** are nonquantitative variables that are ordered by some meaningful criteria, such as cancer staging (I to IV) or Likert scales (1 = strongly agree, 2 = agree, etc.). Modes and medians most appropriately represent ordinal data; although means can be calculated (and mean ranks form the basis for many nonparametric statistical tests), they must be used with caution. Quantitative data are represented by an ordered scale with equal distances between values. Calculations of arithmetic means and standard deviations (SDs) can be performed for quantitative data. **Interval data** have equal distance between values but with an arbitrary zero point, such as temperature scales or dates. **Ratio data** also have an ordered scale with equal intervals between values but with a meaningful zero point, for example, patient weight or blood pressure. Ratios are meaningful for ratio data but not for interval data because the ratio depends on the scale chosen. For instance, a central venous pressure (CVP) of 20 cm $H_2O$ is twice as great as a CVP of 10 cm $H_2O$ (ratio data), but a 60° F (15° C) day is not twice as warm as a 30° F (−1° C) day (interval data).

**ANSWER:** B

3. Which of the following is true about descriptive statistics?

   A. A histogram graphically depicts the means of experimental observations from a population.

   B. A skewed distribution will be highly symmetrical.

   C. For a normal distribution, 95% of data points will fall within 1 SD of the mean.

D. Mean, median, and mode are all approximately the same for a normal (gaussian) distribution.

E. The 50th percentile of any data set is equivalent to the mean.

*Ref.:* 1, 2, 5

**COMMENTS:** A **frequency distribution** is obtained by dividing the range of observed values into intervals and then counting the number of observations that fall into each interval. Frequency data can be depicted graphically in bar charts, histograms, and frequency polygons. These graphs allow quick evaluation of the distribution of the data. A distribution is **symmetrical** if the two halves are mirror images. If more observations are clumped to one end of the distribution, it is **skewed**. The flat or peaked shape of a distribution is called **kurtosis**. A **normal (gaussian) distribution** is symmetrical (skew = 0) and graphically appears bell shaped. For normal distributions, the mean, median, and mode all have approximately the same value. Approximately 68% and 95% of data points fall within 1 and 2 SD of the mean, respectively. **Percentile ranks** are used to describe the location of a data point within a data set. A percentile is a value on a scale of 0 to 100 that specifies the percentage of a distribution that is equal to or below it. For example, an individual who scores in the 80th percentile on an examination has performed as well as or better than 80% of all examinees. The 50th percentile of any data set is equivalent to the median.

**ANSWER:** D

4. Which of the following is true?

A. Variance is the sum of the absolute differences between each sample point and the mean.

B. The sample SD will be small if the sample size is large.

C. The standard error of the mean (SEM) is independent of sample size.

D. SEM can be obtained by dividing the sample SD by the square of the sample size ($N^2$).

E. SD is better than SEM for describing scatter in the data.

*Ref:* 1, 3, 5

**COMMENTS:** The **distribution** of a random variable is a representation that gives the probability that the variable takes different values or ranges of values. Experimental data sets typically represent a **sample** of observations from a distribution. The characteristics of a distribution, such as population mean, population SD, and population variance, are called **parameters**. The corresponding characteristics of the sample, such as sample mean, sample SD, and sample variance, are called **statistics**. The **variance** is the sum of the squares of the difference between each sample point and the mean. The **standard deviation** is the square root of the variance. Both variance and SD quantify how much individual data values vary from the mean. The sample SD is an estimate of the population SD calculated by using deviations from the sample mean. The sample SD is not proportional to the sample size; it will be large if the data are highly scattered, even if the sample size is large. The **standard error of the mean** is a measure of the variability in the distribution of sample means from the population mean. Because larger samples allow the sample mean to better approximate the population mean, SEM decreases as sample size increases. SEM is calculated by dividing the sample SD by the square root of the sample size (SEM = SD/$\sqrt{N}$). If the SD is small and the sample

size is large (yielding a small SEM), the sample mean is an accurate estimate of the population mean. The SD better represents the scatter of the data, whereas SEM estimates the variability of an estimate of the sample mean.

**ANSWER:** E

5. Which of the following is correct about descriptions and estimations of populations?

A. The 95% reference range will contain all of the data 95% of the time.

B. To calculate a 95% confidence interval (CI), the sample must contain 95% of the population.

C. Nonparametric statistics are most useful if the population distribution is normal and the sample size is large.

D. The 95% CI of the mean becomes smaller as the dispersion of the data decreases or the sample size increases.

E. The number of degrees of freedom is inversely proportional to the sample size.

*Ref.:* 3, 5

**COMMENTS:** For data that are approximately normally distributed, the sample mean and SD can be used to calculate a **reference range**. The 95% reference range, or (mean − 1.96 SD) to (mean + 1.96 SD), will contain approximately 95% of the data. A **confidence interval** reflects the accuracy of the sample parameter (often the mean) in estimating the value of the corresponding population parameter. In calculating CIs, two criteria must be met: the distribution of the sample parameter of interest must be approximately normal (generally valid if the sample size is large enough), and the population SD must be well approximated by the sample SD. In this case, the 95% CI of the mean can be calculated from the **normal distribution** as sample mean ± (1.96 × SEM). For small sample sizes, the assumption of a normal distribution of the sample means may not apply. If the sample size is very small and the population distribution is distinctly not normal, nonparametric statistical methods should be used. However, even if the sample size is relatively small, CIs can usually be calculated by using the *t*-distribution (to determine the multiplier for SEM in the CI equation) in place of the normal distribution. The *t*-distribution looks much like the bell-shaped normal distribution but has a flatter peak and more drawn-out tails. The size of the tails relative to the peak is inversely proportional to the **degrees of freedom** of the *t*-distribution, which is determined by the sample size − 1. As the number of degrees of freedom increases (with increasing sample size), the tails become smaller, and the *t*-distribution more closely approximates a normal distribution. The reference range is most useful in describing the population, whereas the CI is more useful in estimating the precision of a population value from a single sample of measurements.

**ANSWER:** D

6. Seventy-five surgical residents are surveyed to determine whether overnight calls have an impact on their driving habits. The relative risk (RR) of having a traffic accident after calls versus before calls is found to be 2.4 with a 95% CI of 0.4 to 4.8. Which of the following are true?

A. The null hypothesis for this study (no difference in accident rates) is an RR of 0.

B. A *P* value of .05 represents a stronger association than does *P* = .007.

C. The *P* value for this study will probably be greater than .05.

D. CIs are not useful for hypothesis testing.

E. This study proves that overnight calls do not increase the risk of having an automobile accident.

*Ref.: 3, 5, 6*

**COMMENTS: Hypothesis testing** is the process by which conclusions are drawn in an objective, probabilistic manner. The goal of hypothesis testing is to determine whether an observed difference between two groups is caused by the controlled variable or to chance. The **null hypothesis** is typically defined to be that there is *no* difference between the groups. The **alternative hypothesis** is usually the postulate that there *is* a significant difference between two study arms. The ***P* value** (probability) measures how likely it is that any observed differences between groups are not caused by chance. Although *P* can take any value between 0 and 1, a result is termed often significant if $P < .05$; that is, the probability that the observed difference between groups was caused by chance is less than 5%. In this case the null hypothesis is rejected. If the calculation yields a nonsignificant *P* value, no conclusions about differences between the groups can be made and the null hypothesis is retained. Even though the *P* value quantifies the strength of association ($P = .0001$ suggests a stronger association than $P = .05$), it does not provide any measure of the size of the effect. Thus, a small *P* value does not necessarily imply a clinically significant effect. Providing exact *P* values is helpful in quantifying the strength of association (rather than simply stating $P < .05$). The **confidence interval** gives a range of values within which it is likely that the true population value lies. If the expected value of the null hypothesis does not lie within the 95% CI, the null hypothesis can generally be rejected. For example, when examining RR, the null hypothesis is that the two groups do not have different risks for the end point of interest (RR = 1). If the 95% CI for the RR includes the value 1, the null hypothesis cannot be rejected.

**ANSWER:** C

7. Which of the following is true about hypothesis testing?

A. A type I error is the probability of concluding that no difference exists when in fact it does.

B. A type II error is the probability of concluding that a difference exists when it does not.

C. The Bonferroni adjustment attempts to minimize the risk of incorrectly finding differences between groups when multiple comparisons are made.

D. Power increases with sample size and effect size but decreases as type I error (alpha) increases.

E. Underpowered studies often show statistically significant differences when in fact none exist.

*Ref.: 3, 6, 7*

**COMMENTS:** A **type I error (alpha)** is the probability of falsely rejecting the null hypothesis or saying that there is a difference between groups when there actually is not. The alpha level is set a priori, or before a study is conducted. Alpha is typically set at 0.01 or 0.05 for clinical, behavioral, and basic science research. Type I error increases in proportion to the number of tests performed on the same data set. When performing multiple comparisons between two or more groups, the risk that a statistically significant difference between the groups is caused by chance increases as more variables are compared. The **Bonferroni adjustment** reduces the alpha level by dividing by the number of hypotheses that are tested. This attempts to maintain the type I error for the entire study at the preselected level. A **type II error (beta)** is the probability of failing to reject the null hypothesis when it is in fact false or, in other words, failing to observe a difference when one actually exists. A type I error is **a false positive**, whereas a type II error is a **false negative**. The **power** of a statistical test is the probability that the test will reject the null hypothesis when the alternative hypothesis is true (i.e., that it will not make a type II error). Power is equal to 1 − beta. In other words, power is the probability of correctly identifying a difference between the study groups when one actually exists in the populations from which the samples were selected. It is best to perform a power calculation when designing a study. This usually entails selecting a level for alpha, determining the effect size (generally from previous data, clinical expertise, or both), and then calculating the necessary sample size. Power increases with larger sample sizes, greater true differences between populations, and higher acceptance of false-positive results (higher alpha). Many studies that appear to demonstrate no difference between groups may simply be underpowered.

**ANSWER:** C

8. A study is performed to determine the impact of enteric spillage on the rate of anastomotic leak for bowel anastomosis. The following data are obtained:

| Enteric Spillage | | Anastomotic Leak | |
| --- | --- | --- | --- |
| | | Yes | No |
| | Yes | 20 | 80 |
| | No | 10 | 190 |

What is the relative risk for an anastomotic leak?

A. 1

B. 2

C. 4

D. 5

E. 8

*Ref.: 1, 3*

**COMMENTS:** See Question 9.

**ANSWER:** C

9. Referring to the data in Question 8, for about how many patients must enteric spillage be avoided to prevent one anastomotic leak?

A. 2

B. 3

C. 5

D. 7

E. 10

*Ref: 1, 3*

**COMMENTS:** The **relative risk** (or risk ratio) is the likelihood of experiencing the outcome in the group with the risk factor divided by the likelihood of experiencing the outcome in the group without the risk factor. In this example, RR = (20/100)/(10/200) = 4. That is, patients with enteric spillage are four times more likely than those without to have a subsequent anastomotic leak. The **absolute risk reduction** (ARR) is the differences in the percentages of patients experiencing the outcome in the groups with and without the risk factor. In this example, ARR = (20/100) − (10/200) = 0.15, or 15%. The **number needed to treat** (NNT) represents the number of patients treated (or in this case the number of patients who must avoid the risk factor) to prevent one episode of the outcome. The NNT is the inverse of the ARR, or in this case 1/0.15 = 6.7. In this example, one needs to avoid seven episodes of enteric spillage to eliminate one anastomotic leak.

**ANSWER:** D

10. Which of the following is true about nonparametric statistics?

    A. They have greater power than the corresponding parametric tests.

    B. They require fewer assumptions about the form of the population from which the data are obtained.

    C. They are generally more sensitive to outliers.

    D. They are usually less robust than corresponding parametric statistics.

    E. One example is the unpaired *t*-test.

*Ref.: 3, 8, 9*

**COMMENTS:** Traditional statistical tests are called **parametric** because they require estimation of the parameters that define the distribution. They often require assumptions about the format of the distribution. One commonly required assumption is that the underlying distribution (or a suitable transformation of the data) is normal or nearly normal. In cases in which these assumptions are not valid, **nonparametric** statistical analysis may be used. Nonparametric tests require few or no assumptions about the format of the data. They can be helpful in dealing with nominal or ordinal (categorical) data that cannot be meaningfully ordered or when there is no fixed interval between categories (e.g., cancer stages, demographic data such as race, or temperature data). They are often more robust than traditional methods (because fewer assumptions are required) and may be easier to apply. They are also usually less sensitive to **outliers** in the data. However, nonparametric tests frequently lack power when compared with parametric tests, so a larger sample size is required. They are also generally geared toward hypothesis testing rather than estimation of effects.

**ANSWER:** B

11. A study is performed to assess the impact of weight loss surgery on diabetes. A total of 64 obese, diabetic patients undergo gastric bypass. Glycosylated hemoglobin ($HbA_{1c}$) is measured for each patient 2 months before and 6 months after surgery. For patients before surgery the mean and SD of $HbA_{1c}$ were 9.2 and 2.1. After surgery, the corresponding values were 6.8 and 1.9. Which test would be most appropriate for comparing the two samples?

    A. Unpaired *t*-test

    B. Paired *t*-test

    C. One-way analysis of variance (ANOVA)

    D. Mann-Whitney U test

    E. McNemar test

*Ref.: 1-3, 8*

**COMMENTS:** See Question 12.

**ANSWER:** B

12. Many of the obese diabetic patients also had gastroesophageal reflux disease (GERD). The investigators decided to assess whether gastric bypass surgery decreased the incidence of GERD. Before surgery, 46 (of 64) patients reported GERD. After surgery, only 32 of the patients reported GERD symptoms. What test would be most appropriate for determining whether the decrease in GERD was caused by chance?

    A. Unpaired *t*-test

    B. Paired *t*-test

    C. One-way ANOVA

    D. Mann-Whitney U test

    E. McNemar test

*Ref.: 1-3, 8*

**COMMENTS:** The choice of statistical test depends on multiple factors: the expected distribution of the population (normal, scattered), the types of outcomes measured (categorical, continuous, time to event), the number of groups, whether the data are paired, and the number of factors that are tested. The *t*-test is a parametric test for examining the difference between means for two independent samples. The **paired *t*-test** compares the means for a single sample before and after some intervention (e.g., systolic blood pressure for the same patients before and after the administration of atenolol) or for two samples in which the patients are paired (e.g., a study patient and a matched control). **Analysis of variance** is a parametric test for comparing the means for three or more unpaired samples. All of these tests require the typical assumptions for parametric tests (nearly normal distribution, similar sample SDs, etc.). The **Mann-Whitney U test** (also called the Wilcoxon rank sum test) is the nonparametric analog to the *t*-test. It is more robust (in large part because it is less sensitive to deviation from population normality or outliers) and can be used for ordinal data. The **McNemar test** is a nonparametric test that can be used to compare nominal data (e.g., race, true/false, gender). This test requires that the data be paired (e.g., same patient before and after treatment).

**ANSWER:** E

13. Which of the following is true about regression and correlation?

    A. The dependent variable is used to predict the independent variable.

    B. Multiple regression generally refers to more than one outcome variable.

    C. In logistic regression, the outcome variable is categorical.

    D. Two variables are uncorrelated if they have a negative correlation coefficient.

    E. Correlation usually implies causation.

*Ref.: 3, 10*

**COMMENTS: Regression methods** are statistical models used to predict the value of a dependent variable from one or more independent variables. **Multiple regression** generally refers to models with more than one independent variable. In linear regression, the outcome variable is normally distributed, whereas in logistic regression, the outcome variable is dichotomous. Frequently, instead of predicting one variable or another, we wish to determine whether there is a relationship between two variables. A **correlation coefficient** reflects the strength of the relationship between two random variables. A positive correlation coefficient means that as one variable increases, the other variable increases. A negative correlation means that as one variable increases, the other variable decreases. It is important to recognize that "correlation does not imply causation"; that is, an observed correlation may not reflect a causal relationship between two variables. For example, several epidemiologic studies have shown that women taking hormone replacement therapy (HRT) hae a lower than average incidence of coronary artery disease (CAD), which led to postulating that HRT was protective against CAD. Randomized, controlled studies, however, demonstrated that HRT was actually associated with a small but significantly increased risk for CAD. Reanalysis of the epidemiologic studies showed that women taking HRT were more likely to be from higher socioeconomic groups. Thus, the use of HRT and the observed decrease in CAD were coincident effects of a higher socioeconomic status rather than the postulated (causal) protective effect of HRT.

**ANSWER: C**

14. Researchers have developed a rapid bedside assay for detection of a new strain of influenza virus. The assay is applied to patients with respiratory symptoms (group 1) and respiratory symptoms with fever (group 2). Each patient was also tested with the "gold standard" polymerase chain reaction evaluation to determine whether influenza was present. The results are shown in Table 38-1. Which of the following statements is not correct?

   A. The prevalence of the new influenza strain in group 1 is 1%.

   B. The RR for flu (patients with a positive rapid assay versus those with a negative one) in group 1 is about 75.

   C. The odds ratio (assay positive versus assay negative) for having the influenza strain in group 2 is 81.

   D. The incidence of the influenza strain in group 2 is 10%.

   E. An RR of 1 implies that the event is equally probable in both groups.

*Ref.: 1, 3*

**TABLE 38-1  Evaluation of Rapid Assay for Influenza**

| | Influenza Present | Influenza Absent | Total |
|---|---|---|---|
| **Group 1: Symptoms Only** | | | |
| Rapid assay + | 9 | 99 | 108 |
| Rapid assay − | 1 | 891 | 892 |
| Total | 10 | 990 | 1000 |
| **Group 2: Symptoms + Fever** | | | |
| Rapid assay + | 90 | 90 | 180 |
| Rapid assay − | 10 | 810 | 820 |
| Total | 100 | 900 | 1000 |

**COMMENTS: Prevalence** is the number of patients in a sample who currently have disease divided by the total number of patients sampled. The prevalence is calculated from the column totals; for group 1 it is 10/1000 = 1%. It is important to distinguish incidence from prevalence. In epidemiologic studies, it is often desirable to determine the **incidence**, which is the number of *new* cases of a disease that occur during a specified period. However, when calculating incidence, only cases newly diagnosed during the study period are counted (rather than the total number of observed cases). The **odds** of an event are defined as the probability of the event occurring divided by the probability of it not occurring. The **odds ratio** compares the odds of something occurring in two different groups. The odds of a patient in group 2 with a positive assay having influenza is 90/90 = 1; that is, the patient is equally likely to have or to not have influenza. The odds ratio for group 2 (assay positive versus assay negative) is calculated as (90/90)/(10/810) = 81. **Relative risk** is a more intuitive concept that compares the **probabilities** of two events rather than the odds. The RR for disease is calculated as the incidence in one population divided by the incidence in the other. If the incidence cannot be determined, we can still compare risk for disease in two populations by using the odds ratio (the odds of disease in the exposed group divided by the odds of disease in the nonexposed group). For group 1, the RR of having influenza in patients with positive assays versus those with negative assays is given by (9/108)/(1/892) = 74.3. An RR of 1 implies that the event is equally probable in the two groups.

**ANSWER: D**

15. Referring to Question 14, which of the following statements is not correct?

   A. The sensitivity of the new influenza assay in group 1 is 90%.

   B. The accuracy of the new influenza assay in group 2 is 90%.

   C. The positive predictive value (PPV) of the assay in group 1 is 8%.

   D. The negative predictive value (NPV) of the assay in group 2 is 50%.

   E. Sensitivity and specificity are better intrinsic measures of a test than PPV and NPV.

*Ref.: 1, 3*

**COMMENTS:** When interpreting diagnostic tests, it is common to be able to reduce the data to a 2 × 2 grid. For each of the groups in the table, the test results can be reduced to

| | Influenza Present | Influenza Absent |
|---|---|---|
| Rapid assay + | True positive | False positive |
| Rapid assay − | False negative | True negative |

The sensitivity and specificity are characteristics of tests that are independent of the population tested. **Sensitivity** represents the proportion of actual positives that are correctly identified as such. For a diagnostic test, it is the number of patients with disease who test positive (true positive [TP]) divided by the total number of patients with the disease (TP plus false negative [FN]): **Sensitivity = TP/(TP + FN)**. **Specificity** assesses the proportion of negatives that are correctly identified. For a diagnostic test, it is defined as the number of patients without disease who test negative (true negative [TN]) divided by the total number of patients in the sample without disease (TN plus false positive [FP]): **Specificity**

= **TN/(TN + FP)**. Sensitivity is a measure of the test's ability to detect the disease, whereas specificity is a measure of the test's ability to detect the absence of disease. For this example, the prevalence of disease in these two populations is different, but the sensitivity and specificity of the test do not change across the populations tested. In this example, the sensitivity and specificity are (coincidentally) the same (90%). In general, as one improves either the sensitivity or the specificity of a test, the other is degraded. **Accuracy** measures how closely the test value represents the true value. **Accuracy = (TP + TN)/(TP + TN + FP + FN)**. PPV and NPV are characteristics of tests that depend on the prevalence of disease in the population tested. **Positive predictive value** is the number of patients who test positive and have the disease divided by the total number who test positive in the sample: **PPV = TP/(TP + FP)**. **Negative predictive value** is defined as the number of patients who test negative and do not have the disease divided by the total number who test negative in the sample: **NPV = TN/(TN + FN)**. PPV is a measure of the test's ability to predict the presence of disease, whereas NPV is a measure of the test's ability to predict the absence of disease. It is important to realize that PPV and NPV can change dramatically as the prevalence of disease in a population changes. In this example, when prevalence changes from 1% (group 1) to 10% (group 2), PPV increases from 8% to 50%. The new assay may be a good screening test for the population in group 2 but a poor one for group 1, where most positive tests are falsely positive. This is often the case when testing low-prevalence populations (even with a highly sensitive and specific test). It is critically important to understand the population for which PPV and NPV were calculated; extrapolating these parameters to a different population with a different prevalence of disease may yield misleading results.

**ANSWER:**   D

16. Which of the following is true of a screening test?

A. If the prevalence of the disease is low, the test must be highly sensitive.

B. Increasing the sensitivity of the test also usually increases its specificity.

C. Treatment before the development of clinical disease should reduce the morbidity and mortality of the disease more than treatment initiated after clinical manifestations of disease are present.

D. Length-time bias occurs when a new test diagnoses the disease earlier but there is no effect on the disease outcome.

E. The best studies for assessing whether a screening test will increase a population's health are well-designed case-control studies.

*Ref.:* 1, 11

**COMMENTS:** The PPV of a screening test improves if the test is applied to a population with a high prevalence of disease. If the prevalence of disease is low, the test must have high specificity (to avoid large numbers of false-positive results), in addition to acceptable sensitivity. Measures taken to improve specificity usually tend to reciprocally decrease sensitivity. Obviously, screening is useful only when it diminishes morbidity and mortality rates. A screening program is beneficial when early treatment (based on screening test results) improves morbidity and mortality more than does treatment initiated later, when disease is detected clinically. **Lead-time bias** occurs when a new test diagnoses the disease earlier but there is no effect on the outcome of the disease. Although survival time

from diagnosis to death is longer (when compared with the old test), the actual length of survival is the same. **Length-time bias** occurs when screening overrepresents less aggressive disease. For example, more aggressive cancers generally have a shorter clinically occult phase than do less aggressive tumors and consequently are less likely to be detected on fixed-interval screening. However, the aggressive tumors also have poorer outcomes, so although the screening test appears to improve outcomes, this improvement is in fact caused by the less aggressive cancers being overrepresented in the population in whom cancer was identified by screening. **Selection bias** occurs when the differences in outcome seen with screening reflect the willingness of different populations to be screened rather than a true alteration of the disease process. Although expensive and time-consuming, **randomized controlled trials** are the best method for avoiding bias when evaluating screening protocols.

**ANSWER:**   C

17. Which of the following is true?

A. Type I errors are associated mainly with tests with poor sensitivity.

B. Internal validity reflects the confidence that a study can be generalized to patients beyond the limited study group.

C. Bias is best addressed by increasing the size of each group in the study.

D. Selection bias occurs when the researcher spends more time supervising the care of patients in the treatment group than those in the control group.

E. None of the above.

*Ref.:* 1, 11

**COMMENTS:** Good **internal validity** is defined by a statistical association that is not caused by chance, confounding with other causal factors, or bias introduced into the study design. That is, internal validity reflects the confidence that the intervention of interest is the actual cause of a study's outcome. Internal validity is subject to **chance**, **bias**, and **confounding**. There are two types of chance-related errors. **Type I errors** occur when the researcher rejects the null hypothesis when it is in fact true (an effect is observed when there is really none). Type I errors (alpha) are associated with tests with poor **specificity**. **Type II errors** occur when the null hypothesis is not rejected despite the fact that it is not true (no effect is observed when in truth one exists). Type II errors (beta) are associated with tests with poor **sensitivity**. A **confounding variable** is an effect that independently influences the measured outcome and is unevenly distributed among the two groups of patients. Confounding is addressed during the study design by randomization, although it can also be addressed during the analysis by statistical risk adjustment (usually with multivariate regression analysis). **Bias** occurs when there is a methodologic difference in the handling of the comparison groups. Bias can occur when participants are enrolled by different criteria (selection bias), when there is participant attrition, when noncomparable information is collected from the various groups (observational bias), or when inaccuracies are introduced during data collection (classification bias). Efforts to control bias include blinding and prospective study design. The **external validity** of a clinical study is the degree to which its findings can be generalized to other patients in other settings. Good external validity is also required to postulate a cause-and-effect relationship. A study is considered to have good external validity if the association demonstrated is biologically credible (i.e., consistent with other observations and theories) and is generalizable to clinically relevant populations beyond the group selected for study. Selecting the appropriate population for study can be challenging and often requires balancing internal validity against external validity.

**A N S W E R :**   E

---

18. Which of the following is true regarding observational (case-control or cohort) studies?

   A. Patients with the disease of interest are randomized into treatment and nontreatment groups.

   B. Case-control studies should not be used when a single disease has multiple causes.

   C. Case-control studies are useful for assessing temporal relationships between causative agents and disease.

   D. Incidence and RR can be measured directly in cohort studies.

   E. Cohort studies are most useful for commonly occurring exposures and diseases.

   *Ref.:* 11

**COMMENTS:**  When properly conducted, **observational studies** can provide conclusions nearly as compelling as those drawn from **interventional studies** (randomized controlled trials). In **case-control studies**, patients with the disease of interest are selected from a population and compared with representative, nondiseased individuals from the same population. There are several advantages of case-control studies. They are generally faster and less expensive. They are useful when there is a long latent period between exposure and disease or if the disease is rare, and multiple causes of a single disease can be studied with a case-control design. However, there are several disadvantages of case-control studies. They are inefficient when the exposure is rare. The incidence of disease or RR cannot be directly calculated (the odds ratio must be used instead). Finally, temporal relationships can be difficult to measure in case-control studies, and case-control design is prone to bias. In **cohort studies**, a population is selected and monitored for the development of exposure and disease over time. Cohort studies are more useful when exposure is rare. They can examine multiple effects of an exposure and may demonstrate temporal relationships. When performed prospectively, bias is minimized, and incidence and RR can be measured directly. Disadvantages include greater expense, inefficiency for studying rare diseases, and the need for complete follow-up and detailed record keeping.

**A N S W E R :**   D

---

19. Which of the following is true about interventional studies (randomized controlled trials)?

   A. Randomization and large sample size generally reduce the effects of confounding variables.

   B. Randomization serves to eliminate observational bias.

   C. The effects of poor compliance with therapy can be eliminated with an "intention-to-treat" design.

   D. Interventional studies are usually cheaper than observational studies such as case-control studies.

   E. Randomized controlled trials are less subject to ethics concerns than observational studies.

   *Ref.:* 11

**COMMENTS:  Interventional studies** that are designed well and conducted properly can generate a level of validity greater than that of observational studies. Interventional studies include an adequate sample of a study population, and subjects are randomly assigned to treatment or control conditions. Proper randomization not only equalizes the prevalence of known confounding factors in each group but also makes the prevalence of unknown factors equal. In a **single-blind study**, the researcher knows the details of the treatment but the patient does not. In a **double-blind study**, both the investigator and the patient are unaware of the assignment to the intervention or control conditions. Double-blind studies are preferred because they help eliminate observation bias. The "**intention-to-treat**" research design requires that a patient be assigned to the treatment group for the duration of a study, regardless of whether treatment can be completed. This method can enhance the generalizability of a study. There are, however, several problems when performing controlled trials. Poor compliance of subjects with therapy can bias the study results toward the null hypothesis. The ethical considerations of randomizing a potentially effective therapy to a treatment group are significant for researchers considering an interventional study design. Feasibility issues, such as high cost and time-intensive data collection, can make interventional studies impractical. In addition, the placebo effect—the phenomenon by which the perception of receiving a therapy tends to improve an individual's assessment of well-being—can dramatically alter results if the treatment cannot be effectively blinded.

**A N S W E R :**   A

---

20. A researcher decides to perform a meta-analysis to determine the best form of induction immunosuppression for living related-donor kidney transplantation. Which of the following is true with regard to meta-analysis?

   A. Meta-analysis techniques cannot increase the power of an investigation.

   B. Meta-analysis methods can eliminate observational or selection bias.

   C. Many of the statistical techniques used in meta-analysis are unique to meta-analysis.

   D. Meta-analysis can be used to assess effect sizes and CIs.

   E. "File drawer" or publication bias refers to the overinclusion of studies supporting the null hypothesis.

   *Ref.:* 11

**COMMENTS:  Meta-analysis** is a statistical technique used to synthesize the literature on a particular topic. A meta-analysis is essentially a study of a group of studies and is conducted to increase the power of an investigation or to resolve inconsistencies among study results. Meta-analysis methods cannot control for bias in the original studies. The steps of a meta-analysis are to (1) formulate a research question, (2) search the literature, (3) establish incorporation criteria for including studies in the meta-analysis, (4) decide which dependent variables (or summary measures) are useful, and (5) select a model as a framework for the statistical analysis on the extracted data. Statistical analyses conducted as part of a meta-analysis typically include calculations of effect size and CIs, as well as homogeneity tests. Limitations of meta-analysis include a lack of control for bias in the original studies. A good meta-analysis of badly designed studies will still result in suspect (or misleading) results. Some meta-analyses add a study-level variable that quantifies the methodologic quality of each study to examine the impact of study quality on the effect size. Furthermore, meta-analysis is often limited to published studies. **Publication bias**, or the "file drawer effect," refers to studies that remain unpublished because they do not show a statistically significant result. Many meta-analyses now include a calculation of the number of studies supporting the null hypothesis that would need to be included for an effect to no longer be reliable. The **Simpson paradox** is an apparent paradox in which the successes of groups seem reversed when the groups are combined. This can occur when frequency data are given nonrigorous causal interpretation. The paradox disappears when causal relationship are derived systematically. Finally, a synthesis of research studies may provide evidence about the overall effectiveness of a test or treatment protocol, but not the specific details that would help guide implementation.

**ANSWER:** D

21. A study is initiated to determine whether preoperative administration of an antibody directed against vascular endothelial growth factor increases disease-free survival in patients with colon cancer treated by segmental colon resection. Which of the following is correct?

    A. Survival analysis can be used only if the end point is death of the patient.

    B. If a subject dies during follow-up, the case is considered "censored."

    C. The hazard function represents the probability of a subject surviving a given length of time.

    D. The Kaplan-Meier estimator can be used to compare two survival curves.

    E. The Cox proportional hazards model allows examination of covariates underlying the survival curves.

*Ref.:* 2, 12

**COMMENTS: Survival analysis** involves examination of time-to-event data, that is, the elapsed time from a defined starting point (e.g., birth, disease diagnosis, organ transplantation) until an explicit event (e.g., death, end of remission, transplant organ failure). For example, a study may examine the longevity of patients receiving chemotherapy for lymphoma. Many of the subjects included will not have died before the study ends or they are lost to follow-up. When the terminal event has not occurred at the end of the given follow-up time, the case is considered to be **censored**. Obviously, excluding these subjects from the analysis would be misleading (e.g., in a study of chemotherapy, the subjects still alive with long follow-up are the successful results). The **survival function** S(t) represents the probability of a subject surviving until time t, whereas the **hazard function** h(t) represents the conditional probability of dying at time t after having survived to that time. A graph of the survival function against time is the **survival curve**. The **Kaplan-Meier estimator** is a way to approximate the survival curve from data when some of the observations are censored. A Kaplan-Meier plot shows an estimate of the survival curve in which survival is plotted (against time) as a series of horizontal steps with decreasing magnitude. Each step represents a subject who has undergone the terminal event; survival is regarded as a constant between steps. Censored losses are represented on a Kaplan-Meier plot by vertical tic marks. As the number of observations increases, the Kaplan-Meier plot better represents the true survival curve. The **log-rank test** is a nonparametric test used to test the hypothesis that there is no difference between two survival curves. However, it does not provide any analysis of the variables underlying the

difference. The **Cox proportional hazards model** (Cox regression) allows examination of additional covariates. For example, a study of cancer patient survival with and without adjuvant chemotherapy might include patient age at diagnosis, tumor size, and stage of disease as covariates.

**ANSWER:** E

22. Which of the following represents the most effective evidence for screening or treatment modalities?

    A. Randomized controlled trial

    B. Controlled trial without randomization

    C. Multicenter case-control study

    D. Uncontrolled trial with dramatic results

    E. Expert committee recommendations

*Ref.:* 13

**COMMENTS:** Evidence-based medicine attempts to rank the different types of available clinical evidence on the basis of their rigor and how well they control limitations in internal and external validity. Multiple ranking systems have been developed. One of the simplest (and frequently quoted) is the hierarchy developed by the **U.S. Preventive Services Task Force**:

Level I:    Evidence obtained from at least one properly designed randomized controlled trial.

Level II-1: Evidence obtained from well-designed controlled trials without randomization.

Level II-2: Evidence obtained from well-designed cohort or case-control analytic studies, preferably from more than one center or research group.

Level II-3: Evidence obtained from multiple time series with or without the intervention. Dramatic results in uncontrolled trials might also be regarded as this type of evidence.

Level III:  Opinions of respected authorities, based on clinical experience, descriptive studies, or reports of expert committees.

    This system has been criticized for its limitations; for example, it does not account for study power, multiple institutions, blinding, and other criteria. Multiple additional grading criteria have been developed to further stratify the quality of available clinical evidence.

**ANSWER:** A

23. A patient with colon cancer wishes to enroll in a study of a new chemotherapeutic agent. Which of the following is not an essential element of informed consent?

    A. A description of any risks or discomfort that the subject may experience

    B. A review of alternative courses of treatment

    C. A description of the methods for keeping the subject's medical records private

    D. Disclosure of the financial support for the study

    E. A statement that participation in the study is voluntary

*Ref.:* 14

**COMMENTS: Informed consent** requires that the following information be conveyed to each subject:

1. A statement that the study involves research, an explanation of the purposes of the research and the expected duration of the subject's participation, a description of the procedures to be followed, and identification of any procedures that are experimental
2. A description of any reasonably foreseeable risks or discomfort that the subject may experience
3. A description of any benefits to the subject or to others that may reasonably be expected from the research
4. Disclosure of appropriate alternative procedures or courses of treatment, if any, that might be advantageous to the subject
5. A statement describing the extent, if any, to which confidentiality of records identifying the subject will be maintained
6. For research involving more than minimal risk, an explanation regarding whether any compensation and whether any medical treatments are available if injury occurs and, if so, what they consist of or where further information may be obtained
7. An explanation of whom to contact for answers to pertinent questions about the research and research subjects' rights and whom to contact in the event of a research-related injury to the subject
8. A statement that participation is voluntary, that refusal to participate will involve no penalty or loss of benefits to which the subject is otherwise entitled, and that the subject may discontinue participation at any time without penalty or loss of benefits to which the subject is otherwise entitled

**ANSWER:** D

# REFERENCES

1. Davis AT: Biostatistics. In O'Leary JP, editor: *The physiologic basis of surgery*, ed 4, Philadelphia, 2008, JB Lippincott.
2. Shott S: *Statistics for health professionals*, Philadelphia, 1990, WB Saunders.
3. Guller U, DeLong ER: Interpreting statistics in medical literature: a *vade mecum* for surgeons, *J Am Coll Surg* 198:441–458, 2004.
4. Whitley E, Ball J: Statistics review 1: Presenting and summarizing data, *Crit Care* 6:66–71, 2002.
5. Whitley E, Ball J: Statistics review 2: Samples and populations, *Crit Care* 6:143–148, 2002.
6. Whitley E, Ball J: Statistics review 3: Hypothesis testing and P values, *Crit Care* 6:222–225, 2002.
7. Norman G, Streiner D: *Biostatistics: the bare essentials*, Hamilton, Ontario, Canada, 1998, BC Decker.
8. Whitley E, Ball J: Statistics review 4: Sample size calculations, *Crit Care* 6:335–341, 2002.
9. Whitley E, Ball J: Statistics review 6: Nonparametric methods, *Crit Care* 6:509–513, 2002.
10. Rosner B: *Fundamentals of biostatistics*, ed 5, Belmont, Calif, 2000, Wadsworth.
11. Hennekens CH, Buring JE: *Epidemiology in medicine*, Boston, 1987, Little Brown.
12. Bewick V, Cheek L, Ball J: Statistics review 12: survival analysis, *Crit Care* 8:389–394, 2004.
13. Harris RP, Helfand M, Woolf SH, et al: Current methods of the U.S. Preventive Services Task Force: a review of the process, *Am J Prev Med* 20(Suppl 3):21–35, 2001.
14. 45 CFR 46.116(a) retrieved 10/14/09 from the U.S. Department of Health and Human Services, Office for Human Research Protections. Available at www.hhs.gov/ohrp/humansubjects/guidance/45cfr46.htm.

# Core Competencies and Quality Improvement

*Anthony W. Kim, M.D.*

1. How many core competencies emerged from the Accreditation Council for Graduate Medical Education (ACGME) Outcomes Project?

   A. 2

   B. 3

   C. 4

   D. 5

   E. 6

   *Ref.:* 1

**COMMENTS:** In 1999, the Outcomes Project of the ACGME identified six **core competencies** to create the framework for resident training. The overall purpose of establishing these competencies was to ensure that the trainee learned how to be competent and compassionate in treating patients. The six core competencies are (1) patient care, (2) medical knowledge, (3) practice-based learning, (4) interpersonal and communication skills, (5) professionalism, and (6) systems-based practice. The ACGME implemented a 10-year time line for residencies to integrate these competencies into their training paradigms.

**ANSWER:** E

2. Which of the following specific statements is part of the patient care core competency requirement?

   A. Set learning and improvement goals.

   B. Incorporate formative evaluation feedback into daily practice.

   C. Demonstrate manual dexterity appropriate for the resident's level.

   D. Participate in the education of patients and families.

   E. Communicate effectively with patients, families, and the public.

   *Ref.:* 1

**COMMENTS:** Demonstrating manual dexterity appropriate for the resident's level is the first component of the **patient care core competency**. According to ACGME, residents must be able to

provide patient care that is compassionate, appropriate, and effective for the treatment of health problems and the promotion of health. To meet the requirements of this core competency, residents should be able to complete the following: (1) demonstrate manual dexterity appropriate for the resident's level; (2) develop and execute patient care plans appropriate for the resident's level, including management of pain; and (3) participate in a program that must document a clinical curriculum that is sequential, comprehensive, and organized from basic to complex. Choices A and B are from the practice-based learning core competency. Choices D and E are from the systems-based practices core competency.

**ANSWER:** C

3. In achieving medical knowledge core competency, the ACGME states that residents will participate in an educational program that should include the fundamentals of basic science as applied to clinical surgery. This will include the elements of wound healing; homeostasis, shock, and circulatory physiology; hematologic disorders; immunobiology and transplantation; oncology; surgical endocrinology; surgical nutrition and fluid and electrolyte balance; and the metabolic response to injury, including burns. Which of the following elements is also part of the medical knowledge core competency?

   A. Bioinformatics and information systems in health care systems

   B. Wound closure techniques

   C. Principles of cardiac surgery

   D. Applied surgical anatomy and surgical pathology

   E. Technical aspects of a cholecystectomy

   *Ref.:* 1

**COMMENTS:** To achieve the **medical knowledge core competency**, residents must demonstrate knowledge of established and evolving biomedical, clinical, epidemiologic, and social-behavioral sciences and understand how this knowledge is applied to patient care. Therefore, residents should be able to perform the following: (1) critically evaluate and demonstrate knowledge of pertinent scientific information and (2) participate in an educational program that includes the fundamentals of basic science as applied to clinical surgery, including applied surgical anatomy and surgical pathology; the elements of wound healing; homeostasis, shock, and circulatory physiology; hematologic disorders; immunobiology and transplantation; oncology; surgical endocrinology; surgical nutrition and fluid and electrolyte balance; and the metabolic response to injury, including burns. Choices A, B, C, and E are not relevant to fundamental basic science knowledge.

**ANSWER: D**

4. Residents are expected to develop certain skills and habits so that they can meet all of the following goals to satisfy the criteria for the practice-based learning and improvement core competency except:

   A. Use an evidence-based approach to patient care.

   B. Participate in mortality and morbidity conferences that evaluate and analyze patient care outcomes.

   C. Use information technology to optimize learning.

   D. Locate, appraise, and assimilate evidence from scientific studies related to their patients' health problems.

   E. Promote the participation of their patients in a clinical trial.

*Ref.:* 1

**COMMENTS:** For the ACGME **practice-based learning** and **improvement core competencies**, residents must demonstrate the ability to investigate and evaluate their care of patients, to appraise and assimilate scientific evidence, and to continuously improve patient care based on constant self-evaluation and lifelong learning. Residents are expected to develop skills and habits to be able to meet the following goals:

   1. Identify strengths, deficiencies, and limits in one's knowledge and expertise.
   2. Set learning and improvement goals.
   3. Identify and perform appropriate learning activities.
   4. Systematically analyze practice by using quality improvement methods and implement changes with the goal of improvement in practice.
   5. Incorporate formative evaluation feedback into daily practice.
   6. Locate, appraise, and assimilate evidence from scientific studies related to their patients' health problems.
   7. Use information technology to optimize learning.
   8. Participate in the education of patients, families, students, residents, and other health care professions.
   9. Participate in mortality and morbidity conferences that evaluate and analyze patient care outcomes.
   10. Use an evidence-based approach to patient care.

**ANSWER: E**

5. Effectively documenting practice activities is a component of which core competency?

   A. Practice management

   B. Interpersonal and communication skills

   C. Professionalism

   D. Systems-based practice

   E. Practice-based learning

*Ref.:* 1

**COMMENTS:** The ACGME indicates that residents must demonstrate **interpersonal and communication skills** that lead to effective exchange of information and collaboration with patients, families, and other health care professionals. Residents should be able to do the following: (1) communicate effectively with patients, families, and the public appropriate to their socioeconomic and cultural backgrounds; (2) communicate effectively with physicians, other health care professionals, and health-related agencies; (3) work effectively as a member or leader of a health care team or other professional group; (4) act in a consultative role to other physicians and health care professionals; (5) maintain comprehensive, timely, and legible medical records, if applicable; (6) counsel and educate patients and families; and (7) effectively document practice activities.

**ANSWER: B**

6. Professionalism should entail which of the following to be considered meeting the criteria for this core competency?

   A. Compassion and respect for others

   B. Autonomy during caregiving

   C. Accountability to patients only

   D. Establishing and maintaining a referral base

   E. Determining standards of behavior satisfying institutional requirements

*Ref.:* 1

**COMMENTS:** Residents must demonstrate a commitment to carrying out professional responsibilities and adherence to ethical principles to satisfy the criteria outlined in the **professionalism core competency**. Residents are expected to demonstrate the following: (1) compassion, integrity, and respect for others; (2) responsiveness to patient needs that supersedes self-interest; (3) respect for patient privacy and autonomy; (4) accountability to patients, society, and the profession; (5) sensitivity and responsiveness to a diverse patient population, including but not limited to diversity in gender, age, culture, race, religion, disabilities, and sexual orientation; (6) high standards of ethical behavior; and (7) a commitment to continuity of patient care.

**ANSWER: A**

7. Residents are expected to accomplish which of the following to meet the systems-based practice core competency?

   A. Understand the nuances of all health care delivery systems.

   B. Coordinate their patient's care even outside their clinical specialty.

   C. Ensure good patient outcomes regardless of cost awareness.

   D. Participate in identifying system errors.

   E. Understand the roles of other specialists only for the purposes of patient care.

*Ref.:* 1

**COMMENTS:** Residents should develop an awareness of the larger context of the health care system and learn to call effectively on other resources in the system to provide optimal health care to achieve the ACGME **systems-based practice** core competency.

Residents are expected to function as follows: (1) work effectively in various health care delivery settings and systems relevant to their clinical specialty; (2) coordinate patient care within the health care system relevant to their clinical specialty; (3) incorporate considerations of cost awareness and risk-benefit analysis in patient- or population-based care (or both) as appropriate; (4) advocate for quality patient care and optimal patient care systems; (5) work in interprofessional teams to enhance patient safety and improve the quality of patient care; (6) participate in identifying system errors and implementing potential systems solutions; (7) practice high-quality, cost-effective patient care; (8) demonstrate knowledge of risk-benefit analysis; and (9) demonstrate an understanding of the role of different specialists and other health care professionals in overall patient management.

**ANSWER:**   D

8. With respect to a surgical skills laboratory, which statement is true?

   A. The surgical skills laboratory improves technical skills only.

   B. Currently, no standardized skills curriculum exists.

   C. Acquisition of surgical skills in the laboratory should be weighted toward the senior residency years.

   D. Team training should be taught in the operating room only after the junior- and senior-level resident surgical skills are learned in a surgical skills laboratory.

   E. The Residency Review Committee (RRC) mandates surgical skill laboratories to maintain accreditation.

*Ref.:* 2

**COMMENTS:** As of July 2008, the RRC mandated that all surgery training programs have a **surgical skills laboratory** to maintain their accreditation. A surgical skills laboratory has been shown to improve technical skills and medical knowledge. The American College of Surgeons (ACS) and the Association of Program Directors in Surgery (APDS) have developed a standardized skills curriculum consisting of three phases. Phase I has modules for junior residents, phase II has modules for senior residents, and phase III has modules for team training.

**ANSWER:**   E

9. Efforts to have residents develop and execute patient care plans appropriate for the resident's level can be reinforced by:

   A. Negative reinforcement

   B. Attendance at conferences

   C. Didactic lecture-style format of mortality and morbidity conferences

   D. Decrease in the absolute number of conferences

   E. Increase in the absolute number of conferences

*Ref.:* 2

**COMMENTS:** The development and execution of **patient care plans** appropriate for each resident's level can be reinforced during attendance at rounds and integrated into many of the conferences that are currently available, such as morbidity and mortality conferences or grand rounds. An interactive format for the morbidity and mortality conferences has been found to improve the education value of the conference for residents at all levels. Restructuring of a morbidity and mortality conference to a more competence-based learning experience (e.g., discuss ethical dilemmas, system problems, or practice-based improvement) can enhance the educational experience. Increasing or decreasing the absolute number of conferences, per se, does not have an impact on achievement of the core competency goals.

**ANSWER:**   B

10. Regarding the format of a journal club, which of the following statements is true?

    A. It is not actually helpful in teaching residents to critically review scientific information.

    B. It is a useful adjunct in surgical education, but not one of its key components.

    C. Participation in it can lead to improved reading habits.

    D. It allows the acquisition of knowledge in residency that rarely needs updating once in practice.

    E. Participation maintains medical knowledge in participants relative to their peer group.

*Ref.:* 2

**COMMENTS:** The institution of a **journal club** can help residents learn early how to critically review the literature and is viewed as a key component of resident medical education. Residents who participate in a journal club have been shown to have improved reading habits and improved medical knowledge relative to their peers who do not participate. Other innovations such as a multifaceted Internet-based journal club can further enhance the critical reviewing ability of residents.

**ANSWER:**   C

11. Identify the four steps in practice-based learning and improvement?

    A. Identify areas for improvement, engage in learning, apply the new knowledge and skills to a practice, and check for improvement.

    B. Seek knowledge, identify areas of weakness in scientific knowledge, aim to add to the knowledge, and await constructive feedback.

    C. Learn about new techniques, apply new techniques, refine new techniques, and individualize techniques.

    D. Look for improvement in current practice, observe others with a better practice model, attempt a new model in the current paradigm, and teach others the new practice model.

    E. Identify areas that are innovative, learn innovation, apply innovation, and teach innovation.

*Ref.:* 2

**COMMENTS:** The four steps involved in the cycle for **practice-based learning and improvement** include the following: (1) identify areas for improvement, (2) engage in learning, (3) apply the new knowledge and skills to a practice, and (4) check for improvement. Learning this cycle should begin early in training so that this behavior becomes second nature as practicing surgeons.

**ANSWER:** A

12. Surgeons need to improve their communication skills with respect to palliative care. Which of the following is not such an area?

    A. Preoperative visit

    B. Intraoperative communication with the patient's family

    C. Discussion of poor prognosis

    D. Discussion of surgical complications

    E. Discussion of death

*Ref.:* 2

**COMMENTS:** The four areas in which surgeons can improve their **communication skills** with respect to the palliative care arena and include the preoperative visit, discussion of a poor prognosis, discussion of surgical complications, and discussion regarding death. It is imperative to the growth of the trainee as a surgeon to learn the ability to communicate compassionately. Numerous techniques are available for learning this skill and have ranged from the creation of an entire curriculum to the use of standardize patients as an instrument of training.

**ANSWER:** B

13. The consequences of poor communication are associated with:

    A. Decreased medical errors

    B. Efficient use of time and resources

    C. Safe patient care sign-out during shift change

    D. Adverse events leading to significant mortality

    E. Increased patient contact time

*Ref.:* 2

**COMMENTS: Poor communication** is directly linked to delays in patient care, improper use of resources, and serious adverse events that lead to significant morbidity and mortality. Web-based systems can facilitate sign-out and lead to a better quality of sign-out, decreased time and resources in gathering objective data, improved patient contact time, and improved continuity of care.

**ANSWER:** D

14. Which of the following operations has the highest risk for preventable adverse events?

    A. Abdominal aortic aneurysm repair

    B. Coronary artery bypass graft/valve surgery

    C. Lower extremity bypass graft

    D. Hysterectomy

    E. Colon resection

*Ref.:* 2

**COMMENTS:** Eight operations carry **high risk for preventable adverse events**, including the following: (1) lower extremity bypass graft (11%), (2) abdominal aortic aneurysm repair (8%), (3) colon resection (6%), (4) coronary artery bypass graft/valve surgery (5%), transurethral resection (4%), cholecystectomy (3%), hysterectomy (3%), and appendectomy (1.5%).

**ANSWER:** C

15. Which of the following errors represents an error in prevention?

    A. Inadequate monitoring or follow-up treatment

    B. Failure to use indicated tests

    C. Use of outmoded tests or therapy

    D. Failure to act on results of monitoring or testing

    E. Avoidable delay in responding to an abnormal test result

*Ref.:* 3

**COMMENTS:** The types of errors that can occur include errors in diagnosis, errors in technique, and errors in judgment. Framed alternatively, the **types of errors** that can occur and be classified include errors in diagnosis, errors in treatment, errors in prevention, and other types of errors. Errors in diagnosis included those attributable to a delay in diagnosis, failure to use an indicated test, use of outdated tests or therapy, or failure to act on the results of monitoring or testing. Errors in treatment include errors in performance of an operation, procedure, or test; errors in administering treatment; errors in dose or method of administration of a drug used; avoidable delay in treatment or in responding to an abnormal test result; or inappropriate care. Errors in prevention include failure to provide prophylactic treatment or inadequate monitoring or follow-up of treatment. Other errors include failure to communicate, equipment failure, and other system failures.

**ANSWER:** A

16. As an educator, part of teaching professionalism to trainees includes demonstrating to residents how to do which one of the following?

    A. Develop a strong leadership style

    B. Manage conflicts

    C. Maintain a balance between surgery and life

    D. Continue academic productivity with a busy practice

    E. Understand compromises in patient welfare and financial, societal, or administrative forces

*Ref.:* 2

**COMMENTS:** Teaching residents how to navigate through difficult situations and manage conflict is a very important aspect of professionalism. Four principles for successful **conflict resolution** include the following: (1) maintaining objectivity by not focusing on the participants but on the problem, (2) relinquishing the position of power and inflexibility to concentrate on individual interests, (3) creating outcomes in which both parties will have gains, and (4) making sure that there are objective criteria for negotiating the process.

**ANSWER:** B

17. Learning how to teach and become facile in systems-based practice competency can be achieved by various methods. Which of the following is an example of a method used?

   A. Maintaining a journal of issues discussed during quality improvement meetings and reflecting on how these issues may affect their practice of medicine.

   B. Using a single format (didactic or group discussion) to deliver public health policy messages.

   C. Leading by example in developing cost-containment efforts in the hospital in the hope that others will participate.

   D. Identifying problems within a specific hospital, discovering the root cause, and not ceasing until these problematic issues are resolved.

   E. Avoiding the inclusion of residents in hospital committees because of limited tenure at the hospital, a need to fulfill service requirements, and an obligation to uphold work hour limitations.

*Ref.:* 2

**COMMENTS:** There are several methods for educating residents on **systems-based practice learning**. Such methods have included maintaining a journal of issues that are discussed during meetings and reflecting on how these issues will affect the way that the practice of medicine is carried out in the future. Other methods include incorporating a longitudinal systems-based practice into a curriculum that includes group discussion, didactic lectures, and hospital training sessions. Including residents in cost reduction efforts that entail the identification of inefficiencies, creation of improvement plans, and implementation has been shown to be educational. Standard conferences such as grand rounds, morbidity and mortality conferences, and morning reports have also been modified to teach certain principles within the systems-based practice teaching efforts.

**ANSWER:** A

18. The Institute of Medicine defined safety, specifically as which of the following?

   A. Implementation of preventive measures

   B. Freedom from accidental injury

   C. Zero tolerance for mistakes

   D. Avoidance of human errors

   E. Prevention of mistakes caused by a larger system

*Ref.:* 3

**COMMENTS:** The **Institute of Medicine** has defined **safety** as freedom from accidental injury. It defined error as failure of a planned action to be completed as intended or the use of a wrong plan to achieve an objective. Safety is believed to depend on avoiding two types of errors. The first type of error is one in which the correct action does not proceed as intended, an error of execution. The second type of error is one in which the original intended action is not correct, an error in planning. It is recognized that not all errors produce harm individually. Large systems fail because recognized or unrecognized multiple faults occur together to cause an accident. An accident damages the system and disrupts the end result.

**ANSWER:** B

19. Which site or venue is the area that is at greatest risk for surgical errors?

   A. Operating room

   B. Surgical intensive care unit

   C. Hospital wards/floors

   D. Emergency department

   E. Ambulatory care sites

*Ref.:* 3

**COMMENTS:** The operating room is the highest **risk site for surgical errors**, followed by the surgical intensive care unit, the ward, ambulatory care sites and consulting sites, and the emergency department. Therefore, considerable effort should be made to reduce processes that can facilitate errors in the operating room.

**ANSWER:** A

20. Areas with high risk for error have all but which of the following characteristics:

   A. Multiple individuals involved in care

   B. Low acuity

   C. Need for rapid decision making

   D. Instructional setting

   E. High volume

*Ref.:* 3

**COMMENTS:** Areas that are at **high risk for errors** have similar characteristics, including multiple individuals being involved in care, high acuity, multiple distractions and interruptions, the need for rapid decisions, narrow margins for safety, high volume and unpredictable patient flow, communication obstacles, and an instructional setting.

**ANSWER:** B

21. The Joint Council on Accreditation of Healthcare Organizations (JCAHO) mandates that the time-out immediately precedes a procedure must be conducted in the location where the procedure will be performed. Documentation of a checklist created by each institution must be provided and must include a minimum of all of the following except:

   A. Correct patient identity

   B. Correct site

   C. Agreement on the procedure to be performed

   D. Specific confirmation of antibiotic administration

   E. Availability of correct implants and any special equipment

*Ref.:* 3

**COMMENTS:** The JCAHO requires that correct patient identity, correct site and side, agreement on the procedure to be performed, correct patient position, and availability of correct implants and any special equipment or special requirements be confirmed before the procedure—the **time-out**. Confirmation of antibiotic administration, although useful, is not mandatory and is dependent on the institution. Each institution should have processes and systems in place for reconciling differences in staff responses during the time-out.

**ANSWER:** D

22. Which organization is responsible for maintaining a joint venture with the National Surgical Quality Improvement Program (NSQIP)?

    A. American Board of Surgery

    B. ACGME

    C. Association for Surgical Education

    D. RRC

    E. ACS

*Ref.:* 4

**COMMENTS:** Quality of care has been examined by analyzing various indicators that can be classified into three main categories: structure, process of care, and outcomes. The **National Surgical Quality Improvement Program** was initially administered solely in the Veterans Administration but has now been implemented in many private sector hospitals through an alliance with the **American College of Surgeons**. In part, the NSQIP is designed to provide a comprehensive view of surgical quality. The ACS NSQIP focuses on the systems of care at its participating sites, not the individual provider of surgical care.

**ANSWER:** E

23. The Surgical Care Improvement Project (SCIP) differs from the NSQIP in what major difference?

    A. The SCIP does not partner with the ACS, but rather the JCAHO.

    B. The NSQIP focuses on individual providers of care, whereas the SCIP does not.

    C. The NSQIP focuses primarily on process measures.

    D. The SCIP focuses primarily on surgical outcomes.

    E. The SCIP focuses primarily on process measures.

*Ref.:* 5

**COMMENTS:** The **Surgical Care Improvement Project** is a national partnership of organizations (including the ACS) committed to improving the safety of surgical care through a reduction in postoperative complications. Initiated by the Center for Medicare Service (CMS) and the Centers for Disease Control and Prevention (CDC), the SCIP partnership is a multi-year national campaign to substantially reduce surgical mortality and morbidity through collaboration efforts. Although the focus of the ACS NSQIP has been the measurement of surgical outcomes, the SCIP will focus primarily on process measures. The SCIP partnership is targeting areas where the incidence and cost of complications are high, including surgical site infections, adverse cardiac events, deep venous thrombosis, and postoperative pneumonia. The program will focus on surgical process measures such as the timing, choice, and duration of prophylactic antibiotic administration. It is anticipated that as the SCIP expands, additional relevant data will be included and will be in alignment with the ACS NSQIP dataset. Both the ACS NSQIP and SCIP have as their core mission the improvement of

care for surgical patients. As a member of the SCIP partnership, the ACS NSQIP has developed a data collection tool to capture the SCIP measures and enable participating sites to meet the CMS SCIP reporting requirements.

**ANSWER:** E

24. What is true regarding the American Board of Surgery In-Training Examination (ABSITE)? Please select only one of the following:

    A. ABSITE performance has a direct correlation with performance on the American Board of Surgery Qualifying Examination.

    B. ABSITE scores for a program do not correlate with mandatory reading programs because it is individual resident dependent.

    C. ABSITE scores for a program do not correlate with focused problem-based learning education programs.

    D. ABSITE results are not a useful tool to gauge the general medical knowledge *and* patient care knowledge of surgical trainees and therefore cannot assess competency.

    E. ABSITE performance is inferior in evaluating trainee performance in comparison with ward (clinical) evaluations.

*Ref.:* 2

**COMMENTS:** The **American Board of Surgery In-Training Examination** is one tool that has been used, in part, to try to assess the general medical knowledge and patient care knowledge of surgical trainees. It is used in conjunction with clinical (ward) evaluations and is neither worse nor better than this method of evaluation. There has been a direct linear correlation between ABSITE performance and American Board of Surgery Qualifying Examination performance (written examination). ABSITE scores have been found to be higher in programs that have established a mandatory reading program and focused problem-based learning education program.

**ANSWER:** A

## REFERENCES

1. ACGME Program Requirements for Graduate Medical Education in Surgery. Available at http://www.acgme.org/acWebsite/downloads/RRC_progReq/440_general_surgery_01022008_u08102008.pdf. Effective January 1, 2008. Accreditatioin Council on Graduate Medical Education. Accessed April 5, 2011.
2. Liz LTH, Berger DH, Awad SS, et al: Accreditation Council for Graduate Medical Education Core Competencies. In Brunicardi FC, Andersen DK, Billiar TR, et al, editors: *Schwartz's principles of surgery*, ed 9, New York, 2010, McGraw-Hill. Available at http://www.accesssurgery.com/content.aspx?aID=5012505.
3. Jones RS, Way LW: Surgical patient safety. In Townsend CM, Beauchamp RD, Evers BM, et al, editors: *Sabiston textbook of surgery: the biological basis of modern surgical practice*, ed 18, Philadelphia, 2008, WB Saunders. Available at http://www.mdconsult.com/das/book/body/163578292-2/0/1565/113.html
4. Finlayson SRG, Birkmeyer JD: Critical assessment of surgical outcomes. In Townsend CM, Beauchamp RD, Evers BM, et al, editors: *Sabiston textbook of surgery: the biological basis of modern surgical practice*, ed 18, Philadelphia, 2008, WB Saunders. Available at http://www.mdconsult.com/das/book/body/163578292-2/0/1565/113.html
5. *http://www.facs.org/cqi/scip.html.* Accessed October 5, 2009.